CARDIAC INTENSIVE CARE

CARDIAC INTENSIVE CARE

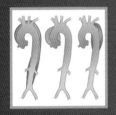 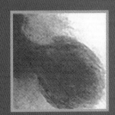 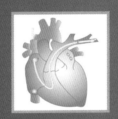 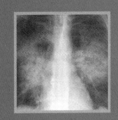 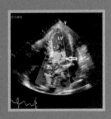

David L. Brown, MD

Professor of Medicine (Cardiovascular Disease)
Washington University School of Medicine
St. Louis, Missouri

THIRD EDITION

ELSEVIER

ELSEVIER

1600 John F. Kennedy Blvd.
Ste 1600
Philadelphia, PA 19103-2899

CARDIAC INTENSIVE CARE, THIRD EDITION ISBN: 978-0-323-52993-8

Notices

Knowledge and best practice in this field are constantly changing. As new research and experience broaden our understanding, changes in research methods, professional practices, or medical treatment may become necessary.

Practitioners and researchers must always rely on their own experience and knowledge in evaluating and using any information, methods, compounds, or experiments described herein. In using such information or methods they should be mindful of their own safety and the safety of others, including parties for whom they have a professional responsibility.

With respect to any drug or pharmaceutical products identified, readers are advised to check the most current information provided (i) on procedures featured or (ii) by the manufacturer of each product to be administered, to verify the recommended dose or formula, the method and duration of administration, and contraindications. It is the responsibility of practitioners, relying on their own experience and knowledge of their patients, to make diagnoses, to determine dosages and the best treatment for each individual patient, and to take all appropriate safety precautions.

To the fullest extent of the law, neither the Publisher nor the authors, contributors, or editors, assume any liability for any injury and/or damage to persons or property as a matter of products liability, negligence or otherwise, or from any use or operation of any methods, products, instructions, or ideas contained in the material herein.

Previous editions copyrighted 2010, 1998.

Library of Congress Control Number: 2018944851

Executive Content Strategist: Robin Carter
Senior Content Development Specialist: Jennifer Shreiner
Publishing Services Manager: Catherine Jackson
Senior Project Manager/Specialist: Carrie Stetz
Design Direction: Amy Buxton

Printed in China

Last digit is the print number: 9 8 7 6 5 4 3 2

Working together
to grow libraries in
developing countries

www.elsevier.com • www.bookaid.org

This edition of *Cardiac Intensive Care* is dedicated to the students, residents, and fellows who teach and inspire me much more than I do in return.

"If you always do what you always did, you will always get what you always got."
Albert Einstein

With the aim of improving survival from in-hospital cardiac arrest after myocardial infarction, in 1961, Desmond Julian, the legendary British cardiologist, proposed a "special intensive-care unit…staffed by suitably experienced people throughout 24 hours, since it is unreasonable to expect good results when the care of patients is entrusted to [the] inexperienced." With central tenets of regionalized specialty care, collaborative teamwork with specialized nursing, and continuous physiologic monitoring, the initial coronary care units were reported to achieve impressive reductions in mortality after myocardial infarction. Since then, the characteristics of the patients we care for, the medical problems that we encounter, and the technologies that we deploy in the cardiac intensive care unit (CICU) have all changed radically. The fast-paced progression of cardiac critical care toward increasing complexity requires that those who oversee or practice in the CICU embrace a forward-looking culture of continuous redesign and quality improvement; to do so effectively also requires the practitioner to maintain a broad fund of knowledge that keeps to the cutting edge while building on the fundamentals of cardiovascular medicine and critical care.

Now in its third edition, *Cardiac Intensive Care*, edited by David L. Brown, MD, is uniquely positioned with a focus on cardiac critical care, distilling more than a half century of advances in state-of-the-art contemporary cardiac intensive care. This textbook delivers a comprehensive and deep treatment of the pathophysiologic principles, foundational basic and clinical science, and pragmatic clinical practice essential to the diagnosis, assessment, and treatment of patients with cardiac critical illness. From the basics of recognition and management of mechanical complications of myocardial infarction and cardiogenic shock to the essential topics of medical ethics and end-of-life care in the CICU, authoritative experts present the landmark studies, latest advances, and practical pearls in the field. The liberal incorporation of figures and videos enhances the accessibility of the material to the reader.

While advances in practice have markedly improved survival and quality of life in many domains of cardiovascular medicine, the nature of the conditions and severity of illness encountered in the CICU continue to confer unacceptably high rates of morbidity and mortality. These facts challenge the field to respond with new research and insightful attention to evolving organizational models and individual processes of care. This textbook is a welcomed companion for practitioners seeking to provide state-of-the-art care in the high-stakes environment of cardiac intensive care.

David A. Morrow, MD, MPH
Professor of Medicine
Harvard Medical School;
Director, Levine Cardiac Intensive Care Unit
Brigham and Women's Hospital
Boston, Massachusetts

PREFACE

The first edition of *Cardiac Intensive Care* was published in 1998 and the second in 2010. New editions of textbooks attempt to keep pace with the rapid changes in patient demographics, new understanding of pathophysiology, and advances in treatment. Formats of textbooks evolve as technology improves and our understanding grows regarding how and where learners do the actual learning. The third edition of *Cardiac Intensive Care* is no exception. As all patient care begins with a grounding in ethics and the ability to perform an accurate history and physical exam, those topics are covered in the beginning of the book. I continue to believe that a strong grounding in the pathophysiology of cardiovascular disease is mandatory to make accurate diagnoses and appropriate treatment decisions. Thus the first chapters of the new edition focus on the scientific underpinnings of cardiac intensive care. However, as the field has evolved, chapters on specific topics such non–ST segment myocardial infarction, unstable angina, coronary spasm, complications of interventional procedures, emergency coronary bypass surgery—all common admission diagnoses to the cardiac intensive care unit (CICU) in the past—are no longer pertinent to the current CICU and have been omitted. The new edition has chapters on takotsubo cardiomyopathy, acute myocarditis, cardiorenal syndrome, electrical storm, distributive shock, and temporary mechanical circulatory support devices—all of which are commonly encountered in today's CICU. In recognition of the complexity and advanced illness of current CICU patient populations, along with the recognition of the limitations of care and our obligation to ensure quality of life as opposed to quantity of life, we have added a chapter on palliative care. We have also added audio clips of heart sounds and videos of procedures and diagnostic imaging in the online version of this book, available at Expert-Consult.com. My hope is to make this textbook more of a living document than previous editions, with online and social media discussions of topics relevant to cardiac intensive care.

At the twentieth anniversary of the publication of the first edition, the loss of contributors to earlier editions is inevitable. Giants of cardiology who contributed their time and expertise to writing chapters in earlier editions who are no longer with us include H.J.C. Swan, Kanu Chatterjee, Bill Little, Ralph Shabetai, Burt Sobel, Bob O'Rourke, and Mark Josephson. Their contributions to teaching, mentoring, research, and patient care continue to live on and inspire the next generations of physicians.

A project of this magnitude would not be possible without the contributions of many. I would be remiss if I did not acknowledge the critical contributions of Jennifer Shreiner and Carrie Stetz from Elsevier, whose tireless efforts along with constant but gentle encouragement have kept the third edition (more or less) on schedule. The artists and copyeditors at Elsevier are the best in the business. Responsibility for any mistakes or typographical errors that find their way into the finished book falls on my shoulders, not theirs. In addition, I am deeply indebted to the contributing authors. Book chapters do not return much in the way of academic currency, but I am eternally grateful to the selfless chapter authors who contributed their time and expertise without the expectation of anything in return other than a free copy of the book. Without them, this book would not have been possible. I would also like to express my heartfelt gratitude to my boss, Doug Mann (who also edits a cardiology textbook for Elsevier that you may have heard of), for hiring me to work at Washington University, for always supporting my various academic endeavors, and for being a superb role model as a person and an academic cardiologist. Finally, I thank my family for tolerating the time I spent working on this and other projects.

David L. Brown

Masood Akhtar, MD, FHRS, MACP, FACC, FAHA
Aurora Cardiovascular Services
Director of Electrophysiology Research
Aurora Sinai/Aurora St. Luke's Medical Centers;
Adjunct Clinical Professor of Medicine
University of Wisconsin School of Medicine and Public Health
Milwaukee, Wisconsin

William R. Auger, MD
Profess of Clinical Medicine
UCSD Healthcare
La Jolla, California

Richard G. Bach, MD
Professor of Medicine
Washington University School of Medicine;
Director, Cardiac Intensive Care Unit
Director, Hypertrophic Cardiomyopathy Center
Barnes-Jewish Hospital
St. Louis, Missouri

Raquel R. Bartz, MD, MMCI
Division Chief, Critical Care Medicine
Department of Anesthesiology
Duke University School of Medicine
Durham, North Carolina

Eric R. Bates, MD
Professor of Internal Medicine
Department of Internal Medicine
Division of Cardiovascular Diseases
University of Michigan
Ann Arbor, Michigan

Brigitte M. Baumann, MD, MSCE
Professor
Department of Emergency Medicine
Cooper Medical School of Rowan University
Camden, New Jersey

Richard C. Becker, MD
Professor
Department of Internal Medicine
University of Cincinnati College of Medicine
Cincinnati, Ohio

Dmitri Belov, MD
Assistant Professor of Medicine
Director, Advanced Heart Failure
Department of Cardiology
Albany Medical Center
Albany, New York

Andreia Biolo, MD, ScD
Professor of Medicine
Coordinator, Post-Graduate Program in Cardiology
Federal University of Rio Grande do Sul;
Heart Failure and Cardiac Transplant Group
Section of Cardiology
Hospital de Clinicas de Porto Alegre
Porto Alegre, Brazil

Daniel Blanchard, MD
Professor of Medicine
Director, Cardiology Fellowship Program
University of California–San Diego
La Jolla, California

David L. Brown, MD
Professor of Medicine (Cardiovascular Disease)
Washington University School of Medicine
St. Louis, Missouri

Clifton W. Callaway, MD, PhD
Professor of Emergency Medicine
Executive Vice-Chairman of Emergency Medicine
Ronald D. Stewart Endowed Chair of Emergency Medicine Research
University of Pittsburgh School of Medicine
Pittsburgh, Pennsylvania

Matthew J. Chung, MD
Interventional Cardiology Fellow
Department of Internal Medicine
Cardiovascular Division
Washington University School of Medicine
St. Louis, Missouri

Richard F. Clark, MD
Professor
Department of Emergency Medicine
University of California–San Diego School of Medicine;
Director
Division of Medical Toxicology
UCSD Medical Center;
Medical Director, San Diego Division
California Poison Control System
San Diego, California

Wilson S. Colucci, MD
Professor of Medicine and Physiology
Boston University School of Medicine;
Chief, Section of Cardiovascular Medicine
Co-Director, Cardiovascular Center
Boston Medical Center
Boston, Massachusetts

Leslie T. Cooper Jr, MD
Chair
Cardiovascular Department
Mayo Clinic
Jacksonville, Florida

Harold L. Dauerman, MD
Division of Cardiology
University of Vermont Larner College of Medicine
Burlington, Vermont

Elyse Foster, MD
Professor of Medicine
Department of Cardiology
University of California–San Francisco
San Francisco, California

Stephanie Gaydos, MD
Congenital Cardiology Fellow
Medical University of South Carolina
Charleston, South Carolina

Mark Gdowski, MD
Cardiology Fellow
Barnes-Jewish Hospital
Washington University School of Medicine
St. Louis, Missouri

Timothy Gilligan, MD, MS, FASCO
Associate Professor of Medicine
Department of Hematology and Medical Oncology
Vice-Chair for Education, Taussig Cancer Institute
Director of Coaching, Center for Excellence in Healthcare Communication
Cleveland Clinic
Cleveland, Ohio

Michael M. Givertz, MD
Medical Director, Heart Transplant and Circulatory Support Program
Brighman and Women's Hospital;
Professor of Medicine
Harvard Medical School
Boston, Massachusetts

Prospero B. Gogo Jr, MD
Division of Cardiology
University of Vermont Larner College of Medicine
Burlington, Vermont

Sarah J. Goodlin, MD
Chief of Geriatrics
VA Portland Health Care System
Associate Professor of Medicine
Oregon Health & Science University
Portland, Oregon

Barry Greenberg, MD
Distinguished Professor of Medicine
Director, Advanced Heart Failure Treatment
    Program
University of California–San Diego
La Jolla, California

David Gregg IV, MD
Associate Professor of Medicine and
    Cardiology
Medical University of South Carolina
Charleston, South Carolina

George Gubernikoff, MD
Director, Noninvasive Cardiology
Medical Director, Center for Aortic Diseases
NYU Winthrop Hospital
Mineola, New York

Colleen Harrington, MD
Assistant Professor of Medicine
Division of Cardiovascular Medicine
UMass Memorial
Worcester, Massachusetts

Nazish K. Hashmi, MD
Assistant Professor
Department of Anesthesiology
Duke University Medical Center
Durham, North Carolina

Alan C. Heffner, MD
Director of Critical Care
ECMO Medical Director
Pulmonary and Critical Care Consultants
Carolinas Medical Center
Charlotte, North Carolina

Bettina Heidecker, MD
Head, Heart Failure and Cardiomyopathies
Charité, Campus Benjamin Franklin
Berlin, Germany

Maureane Hoffman, MD, PhD
Pathology and Laboratory Medicine Service
Durham Veterans Affairs Medical Center;
Department of Pathology
Duke University Medical Center
Durham, North Carolina

Brian D. Hoit, MD
Professor of Medicine, Physiology, and
    Biophysics
Case Western Reserve University;
Director of Echocardiography
Harrington Heart & Vascular Center
University Hospital Cleveland Medical
    Center
Cleveland, Ohio

Ruth Hsiao, MD
Chief Medical Resident
Department of Internal Medicine
University of California–San Diego
La Jolla, California

Robert C. Hyzy, MD
Medical Director, Critical Care Medicine
    Unit
Professor of Medicine
Division of Pulmonary and Critical Care
    Medicine
University of Michigan Medical School
Ann Arbor, Michigan

Jacob C. Jentzer, MD
Assistant Professor of Medicine
Department of Cardiovascular Diseases
Division of Pulmonary and Critical Care
    Medicine, Department of Internal
    Medicine
Mayo Clinic
Rochester, Minnesota

Joyce Ji, MD
Resident Physician
Department of Internal Medicine
Barnes-Jewish Hospital
St. Louis, Missouri

Lauren H. Jones, MD
Anesthesiology Resident
Department of Anesthesiology
Duke University Medical Center
Durham, North Carolina

Ulrich Jorde, MD
Professor of Medicine
Section Head
Heart Failure, Cardiac Transplantation, and
    Mechanical Circulatory Support
Vice-Chief, Division of Cardiology
Montefiore Medical Center
Albert Einstein College of Medicine
New York, New York

Rochelle Judd, NP
Adult Congenital Cardiology Nurse
    Practitioner
Medical University of South Carolina
Charleston, South Carolina

Jason N. Katz, MD, MHS
Associate Professor of Medicine
Associate Professor of Surgery
Divisions of Cardiology and Pulmonary &
    Critical Care Medicine
University of North Carolina School of
    Medicine;
UNC Health Care System Director,
    Cardiovascular Critical Care, Mechanical
    Circulatory Support, and the
    Cardiogenic Shock Program
Medical Director, UNC Mechanical Heart
    Program
Medical Director, Cardiac Intensive Care
    Unit
Medical Director, Cardiovascular and
    Thoracic Surgical Intensive Care Unit
    and Critical Care Service
UNC Center for Heart and Vascular Care
Chapel Hill, North Carolina

Mohamad Kenaan, MD
Clinical Assistant Professor
Michigan State University College of
    Human Medicine
Division of Cardiovascular Medicine
Spectrum Health–Meijer Heart Center

Briana N. Ketterer, MD
Hospice and Palliative Care Fellow
University of Pittsburgh Medical Center
Pittsburgh, Pennsylvania

Holly Keyt, MD
Assistant Professor of Medicine
University of Texas Health San Antonio
San Antonio, Texas

Jon A. Kobashigawa, MD
Associate Director
Cedars-Sinai Heart Institute;
Director, Advanced Heart Disease Section
Director, Heart Transplant Program
Cedars-Sinai Medical Center
Los Angeles, California

Richard Koch, MD
Fellow
Medical Toxicology
University of California–San Diego
San Diego, California;
Staff Physician
Naval Hospital Sigonella
Sigonella, Italy

Sándor J. Kovács, PhD, MD
Professor of Medicine, Physiology,
    Biomedical Engineering, and Physics
Washington University in St. Louis
St. Louis, Missouri

Alexander Kuo, MD
Instructor
Harvard Medical School;
Physician
Department of Anesthesia, Critical Care,
    and Pain Medicine
Massachusetts General Hospital
Boston, Massachusetts

Milla J. Kviatkovsky, DO, MPH
Assistant Clinical Professor of Medicine
Department of Hospital Medicine
University of California–San Diego
La Jolla, California

A. Michael Lincoff, MD
Vice Chairman
Department of Cardiovascular Medicine
Cleveland Clinic
Cleveland, Ohio

Mark S. Link, MD
Professor of Medicine
Director, Cardiac Electrophysiology
Department of Internal Medicine
Division of Cardiology
University of Texas Southwestern Medical
    Center
Dallas, Texas

Jacob Luthman, MD
Cardiology Fellow
Department of Internal Medicine
University Hospitals Cleveland Medical
    Center
Cleveland, Ohio

Judith A. Mackall, MD
Director
Cardiac Device Clinic
Division of Cardiology
University Hospitals Cleveland Medical
    Center;
Associate Professor of Medicine
Case Western Reserve University
Cleveland, Ohio

Rohit Malhotra, MD
Associate Professor
Department of Internal Medicine
Division of Cardiology
University of Virginia
Charlottesville, Virginia

Pamela K. Mason, MD
Associate Professor
Department of Internal Medicine
Division of Cardiology
University of Virginia
Charlottesville, Virginia

Jason Matos, MD
Clinical and Research Fellow
Department of Medicine
Division of Cardiology
Beth Israel Deaconess Medical Center
Boston, Massachusetts

Sharon McCartney, MD
Assistant Professor
Department of Anesthesiology
Duke University Medical Center
Durham, North Carolina

Theo E. Meyer, MD, DPhil
Professor of Medicine
Chief, Clinical Cardiology
University of Massachusetts Medical School
UMass Memorial Medical Center
Worcester, Massachusetts

Alicia Minns, MD
Assistant Clinical Professor of Emergency
    Medicine
University of California–San Diego
La Jolla, California

Joshua D. Mitchell, MD
Cardiology Fellow
Washington University Medical Center
St. Louis, Missouri

**Narain Moorjani, MB ChB, MRCS, MD,
    FRCS(C-Th), MA**
Consultant Cardiac Surgeon and Clinical
    Lead for Cardiac Surgery
Royal Papworth Hospital;
Associate Lecturer
University of Cambridge
Cambridge, United Kingdom

Jonathan D. Moreno, MD, PhD
Cardiology Fellow
Department of Medicine
Division of Cardiology
Washington University in St. Louis
St. Louis, Missouri

Michael S. O'Connor, DO, MPH
Staff Anesthesiologist
Assistant Professor
Cleveland Clinic Lerner College of
    Medicine;
Department of Cardiothoracic
    Anesthesiology
Anesthesia Institute
Cleveland Clinic
Cleveland, Ohio

Marlies Ostermann, PhD, MD, FICM
Department of Nephrology
King's College London
Guy's & St. Thomas' Hospital & Critical
    Care
London, United Kingdom

Demosthenes G. Papamatheakis, MD
Assistant Professor
Department of Medicine
UC San Diego Health
La Jolla, California

Nimesh Patel, MD
Cardiology Fellow
Department of Internal Medicine
University of Texas Southwestern Medical
    Center
Dallas, Texas

Richard M. Pescatore II, DO
Chief Resident
Department of Emergency Medicine
Cooper Medical School of Rowan University
Camden, New Jersey

Jay I. Peters, MD
Professor and Chief
Pulmonary and Critical Care Medicine
University of Texas Health Science Center
San Antonio, Texas

**Abhiram Prasad, MD, FRCP, FESC,
    FACC**
Professor of Medicine
Department of Cardiovascular Diseases
Mayo Clinic
Rochester, Minnesota

**Susanna Price, MBBS, BSc, MRCP,
    EDICM, PhD, FFICM, FESC**
Consultant Cardiologist and Intensivist
Royal Brompton Hospital;
Honorary Senior Lecturer
Imperial College
London, United Kingdom

Thomas M. Przybysz, MD
Critical Care Physician
Carolinas Medical Center
Charlotte, North Carolina

Claudio Ronco, MD
Director
Department of Nephrology, Dialysis, and
    Transplantation
Director
International Renal Research Institute
San Bortolo Hospital
Vicenza, Italy

Michael Shehata, MD
Associate Professor of Medicine
Program Director, Cardiac
    Electrophysiology Fellowship
Heart Rhythm Center
Cedars Sinai Heart Institute
Los Angeles, California

Jeffrey A. Shih, MD
Assistant Professor
Department of Internal Medicine
Division of Cardiovascular Medicine
University of Massachusetts
Worcester, Massachusetts

Daniel M. Shivapour, MD
Interventional Cardiology Fellow
Department of Cardiovascular Medicine
Cleveland Clinic
Cleveland, Ohio

Adam Shpigel, MD
Cardiology Fellow
Washington University School of Medicine
St. Louis, Missouri

Bryan Simmons, MD
Staff Anesthesiologist and Intensivist
Aurora St. Luke's Medical Center
Milwaukee, Wisconsin

Daniel B. Sims, MD
Assistant Professor of Medicine
Director, Moses Cardiac Intensive Care Unit
Department of Cardiology
Montefiore Medical Center
Albert Einstein College of Medicine
New York, New York

Hal A. Skopicki, MD, PhD
Chief of Cardiology
Director, Heart Failure and Cardiomyopathy
    Center
Co-director, Ventricular Assist Device
    Program
Stony Brook University Heart Institute
Stony Brook University School of Medicine
Stony Brook, New York

Martin L. Smith, STD
Director of Clinical Ethics
Department of Bioethics
Cleveland Clinic
Cleveland, Ohio

Burton E. Sobel, MD†
Division of Cardiology
University of Vermont Larner College of
    Medicine
Burlington, Vermont

Nishtha Sodhi, MD
Structural Heart Disease Fellow
Cardiovascular Department
Barnes-Jewish Hospital of Washington
    University
St. Louis, Missouri

Ali A. Sovari, MD, FACC, FHRS
Cardiac Electrophysiologist
Cedars-Sinai Medical Center
Oxnard, California

Dina M. Sparano, MD
Assistant Professor of Medicine
Case Western Reserve University School of
    Medicine
Director, Lead Management Program
Associate Program Director,
    Electrophysiology Fellowship Program
University Hospitals Cleveland Medical
    Center
Harrington Heart & Vascular Institute
Cleveland, Ohio

Peter C. Spittell, MD
Consultant
Department of Cardiology
Mayo Clinic
Rochester, Minnesota

Christie Sun, MD
Toxicology Fellow
Department of Emergency Medicine
University of California–San Diego
La Jolla, California

Roderick Tung, MD, FACC, FHRS
Associate Professor of Medicine
Director, Cardiac Electrophysiology & EP
    Laboratories
University of Chicago Medicine
Center for Arrhythmia Care/Heart and
    Vascular Center
Chicago, Illinois

Peter D. Wagner, MD
Distinguished Professor of Medicine and
    Bioengineering
University of California–San Diego School
    of Medicine
La Jolla, California

Daniel E. Westerdahl, MD, FACC
Advanced Heart Failure Cardiologist
Chair, Department of Cardiology
Providence St. Vincent Medical Center
Portland, Oregon

Ryan E. Wilson, MD
Interventional Cardiology Fellow
Gill Heart Institute
University of Kentucky
Lexington, Kentucky

Jonathan D. Wolfe, MD
Cardiology Fellow
Department of Cardiology
Barnes-Jewish Hospital
Washington University in St. Louis
St. Louis, Missouri

Paria Zarghamravanbakhsh, MD
Department of Medicine
Mount Sinai-Queens Hospital
New York, New York

Shoshana Zevin, MD
Internal Medicine
Shaare Zedek Medical Center
Jerusalem, Israel

Khaled M. Ziada, MD, FACC, FSCAI
Gill Heart Institute
University of Kentucky
Lexington, Kentucky

Jodi Zilinski, MD
Aurora Cardiovascular Services
Aurora Sinai/Aurora St. Luke's Medical
    Centers;
Adjunct Assistant Clinical Professor of
    Medicine
University of Wisconsin School of Medicine
    and Public Health
Milwaukee, Wisconsin

Peter Zimetbaum, MD
Richard and Smith Professor of
    Cardiovascular Medicine
Harvard Medical School;
Associate Chief and Clinical Director of
    Cardiology
Beth Israel Deaconess Medical Center
Cambridge, Massachusetts

†Deceased.

CONTENTS

AUDIO AND VIDEO CONTENTS

CARDIAC INTENSIVE CARE

PART I

Introduction

1

Evolution of the Coronary Care Unit: Past, Present, and Future

Jason N. Katz, Richard C. Becker

Originating during a time of recognized unmet medical need and advances in medicine, the coronary care unit (CCU) emerged as one of the most important advances in the care of patients with life-threatening cardiovascular conditions. It has evolved further with technology, including mechanical circulatory support, to become a portal of entry for critically ill patients requiring a high level of support and vast resources. The emergence of contemporary cardiac intensive care units (CICUs) has introduced paradigm shifs in staffing, necessary skill sets, training, and cost for hospitals and health systems. This chapter offers a historical perspective of CCUs and their journey to the contemporary era of CICUs that provide high-acuity tertiary and quaternary care in the United States (Fig. 1.1). Also discussed are several pertinent constructs for academic medical centers with busy CICUs, including education, training of physician and nonphysician providers, and the importance of research as a vehicle to drive discovery and advanced care.

ORIGINS OF THE CORONARY CARE UNIT

Several seminal descriptions of acute myocardial infarction (MI)—a frequently fatal event at the time—underscored a clear medical unmet need.[1,2] Other than morphine and supportive measures, there were very few options to effectively manage patients with acute MI.

Early Days of Resuscitation

The first impactful therapy to attenuate the most common and life-threatening complications of MI, ventricular tachycardia and ventricular fibrillation, emerged with open-chest[3,4] and, later, closed-chest defibrillation.[5,6] Soon after these original descriptions,[7] the overall construct of a CCU designed with specific goals to detect and treat fatal ventricular arrhythmias rapidly evolved.

Desmond Julian was the first to articulate the general construct of a CCU. In his original 1961 presentation to the Royal Thoracic Society,[8] he described five cases of cardiac massage with the goal to resuscitate patients with acute MI. He came to the profound conclusion that "many cases of cardiac arrest associated with acute myocardial ischaemia could be treated successfully if all medical, nursing, and auxiliary staff were trained in closed-chest massage, and if the cardiac rhythm of patients…was monitored by an electrocardiographic link to an alarm system." His vision for the CCU was founded on the following four basic principles:

- Continuous electrocardiogram monitoring with arrhythmia alarms
- Cardiopulmonary resuscitation with external defibrillator capabilities
- Admission of patients with acute MI to a single unit of the hospital where trained personnel, cardiac medications, and specialized equipment were readily available
- The ability of trained nurses to initiate resuscitation attempts in the absence of physicians

Approximately 3 years later, the first CCU was established at the Royal Infirmary of Edinburgh. Soon thereafter, several clinicians in North America developed specialized units devoted exclusively to the treatment of patients with suspected MI. Meltzer[9] created a two-room research unit with an aperture in the wall

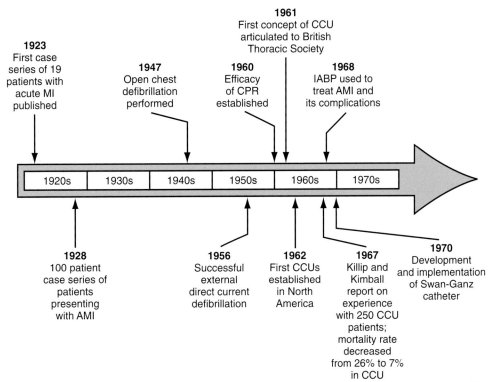

Fig. 1.1 Evolution of the coronary care unit over time. *AMI,* Acute myocardial infarction; *CCU,* coronary care unit; *CPR,* cardiopulmonary resuscitation; *IABP,* intraaortic balloon pump; *MI,* myocardial infarction.

through which defibrillator paddles could be passed from one patient to the other. Brown and associates[10] established a four-bed unit with an adjacent nursing station and arrhythmia surveillance provided using a converted electroencephalogram unit with electrocardiogram amplifiers.

Day,[11] a contemporary of Meltzer, Brown, and Julian, built mobile "crash carts" in an attempt to resuscitate patients with acute MI who were admitted to general medical wards. He recognized that delays in arrhythmia detection significantly limited the success of subsequent resuscitation attempts. As a result of his observations, an 11-bed unit was established at Bethany Hospital in New York staffed by "specially trained nurses who could provide expert bedside attention, interpret signs of impending decompensation and quickly institute CPR." Day is largely credited with introducing the term *code blue* to describe resuscitation efforts for cyanotic patients following cardiac arrest and the term *coronary care unit.*

A Paradigm Shift—Prevention of Cardiac Arrest

Julian[12] described the "second phase" of CCUs as an expansion from a sole focus on resuscitation to prevention of lethal arrhythmias and advanced care. Killip and Kimball[13] published their experience of 250 patients with acute MI treated in a four-bed CCU at New York Hospital–Cornell Medical Center and reported that aggressive medical therapy reduced in-hospital mortality from 26% to 7%. This led Killip and Kimball to conclude that "the development of the coronary care unit represents one of the most significant advances in the hospital practice of

medicine."[13] Not only did it seem that patients with acute MI had improved survival if treated in a CCU, but also all in-hospital cardiac arrest patients seemed more likely to survive if geographically located in the CCU. "Although frequently sudden, and hence often 'unexpected,' the cessation of adequate circulatory function is usually preceded by warning signals."[13] Thus began the era of CCUs throughout the world, with a categorical focus on the prevention of cardiac arrest.

Lown and colleagues[14] detailed the key components of the CCU at the Peter Bent Brigham Hospital in Boston. The foundation of their CCU centered on assembling a "vigilant group of nurses properly indoctrinated in electrocardiographic pattern recognition and qualified to intervene skillfully with a prerehearsed and well-disciplined repertoire of activities in the event of a cardiac arrest."[14] With a CCU mortality of 11.5% and an in-hospital mortality of 16.9%, these clinician-investigators hypothesized that an aggressive protocol for arrhythmia suppression after MI could virtually eradicate sudden, unexpected death. While cumulative data did not support routine preventive antiarrhythmic therapy in MI,[15] the fundamental construct of advanced care for patients at risk for post-MI complications established a foundation for contemporary CCUs.

Additional developments in the care of patients with acute MI—including the use of intraaortic balloon counterpulsation,[16] the implementation of flow-directed catheters for hemodynamic monitoring,[17] and either pharmacologic or mechanical myocardial reperfusion therapy[18]—contributed to the advance and wide-scale availability of CCUs.

VALIDATING THE BENEFIT OF THE CORONARY CARE UNIT

With the advent of CCUs and recognition that intensive care rendered on a "24-7" basis required substantial resources with resulting cost, the medical community posed fundamental questions about outcomes. Early comparisons of CCUs and general medical wards suffered from their observational nature and lack of analytic rigor. For example, the previously described study performed by Killip and Kimball[13] attributed a near 20% decline in mortality to the successful implementation of the CCU environment. Other observational studies conducted in the United States[19] and Scandinavia[20,21] drew similar conclusions, with lower mortality rates and greater resuscitation success in patients with acute MI treated in a CCU setting.

Several investigators[22] attributed the decline in mortality rates from ischemic heart disease in the United States to the presence of CCUs. From 1968 to 1976, estimates suggested a decline in mortality of approximately 21%. This, in turn, translated to saving 85,000 lives over the observation period.[23,24] The key to improved outcomes was likely the specialized care received in the CCU setting. This theme continued to play out during the era of reperfusion for acute MI.[25] Few would challenge the importance of specialized resources and care in the management of patients with complex cardiovascular disease.[26]

Economic Impact of the Cardiac Intensive Care Unit

Intensive care units (ICUs) are places of high resource use and high expenditure. Accordingly, they contribute significantly to the economic burden of health care.[27] While ICUs constitute less than 10% of hospital beds in the United States, estimates suggest that they consume more than 20% of total hospital costs and nearly 1% of the US gross domestic product.[28,29] It has been reported that ICU costs have increased by nearly 200% in the years 1985 to 2000.[30] These observations underscore the importance of patient selection and resource utilization. Contemporary data support similarities in resource use, morbidity and mortality, and in-hospital length of stay for ICUs and CICUs.[31–34]

PATIENT SELECTION IN THE CARDIAC INTENSIVE CARE UNIT

The current cost of health care in the United States dictates utilization of services that are carefully aligned with patient needs. The $3 trillion of health care expenditures suggests that this tenet is not being followed optimally. While CCUs were developed initially to manage arrhythmias among patients with acute MI, it is becoming increasingly clear that monitoring capabilities, staffing, and expertise can be provided on dedicated cardiology floors for many patients. Accordingly, each institution must establish metrics of acuity and complex care that take full advantage of CICUs and the resources therein.[35]

The appropriate organizational structure is of great importance in contemporary CICUs. We believe that whether an open- or closed-unit model is employed, the key to delivering optimal care is aligning provider skill set with specific patient needs.

This is particularly important within an ICU where changes in patient status occur suddenly and require immediate recognition and action. While medical ICUs and CICUs may seem more similar than dissimilar, it is the responsibility of all institutions to recognize specific needs and staff their units accordingly[36] (Fig. 1.2).

The CCU landscape has evolved substantially over the past several decades to a unit better described as a CICU. As a result of diagnostic platforms, advanced pharmacotherapeutics, mechanical circulatory assist devices, and novel interventional techniques, cardiologists have impacted the natural history of MI significantly. Consequently, the mortality rates for acute MI have steadily declined.[37,38] At the same time, however, the care of patients with other complex cardiovascular diseases and noncardiac critical illness is steadily increasing in the CICU. An aging US population, acute and chronic sequelae of nonfatal MI, comorbid medical conditions, and complications of implantable devices all result in increased susceptibility to critical illness in high-risk patients. Many, if not all, of these patients are likely to be admitted to the modern-day CICU. What were previously purely resuscitative and preventive units for patients with MI have now arguably transformed into critical care units for patients with cardiovascular disease. In fact, many institutions now refer, either formally or informally, to their CCU as the CICU.

In a descriptive analysis of US critical care units, Groeger and colleagues[39] highlighted mortality statistics, resource use data, and patient characteristics of modern CICUs; their results were remarkably comparable to composite data from contemporary medical ICUs.[33,34] The severity of illness, quantified by a classic measure of critical illness (the APACHE [Acute Physiology, Age, and Chronic Health Evaluation] II score), was the greatest independent predictor of in-hospital mortality in a CICU cohort of patients—suggesting that risk stratification in the CICU could be conducted in a manner similar to other ICUs, where the APACHE II score is well established.

If the contemporary CICU has become an ICU for patients with complex cardiovascular disease, reassessment of patient selection, resources, cost, and required training for faculty, nurses, and support staff must be undertaken. A growing body of evidence supports the ability of critical care specialists to improve the care of ICU patients,[40–42] and it is anticipated that patients in the CICU would derive similar benefit.[39]

DEFINING THE CONTEMPORARY CARDIAC INTENSIVE CARE UNIT

Several contemporary databases have been used to illustrate the demographic, clinical, and operational characteristics of ICUs in the United States.[39,43,44] In turn, these datasets have been used to establish practice guidelines, generate hypotheses for clinical research undertakings, and accelerate quality improvement initiatives in critical care medicine. Our longitudinal assessment of Duke University Hospital provided an early glimpse of a sea change in academic CCUs.

We created a single-center, administrative database containing 2 decades of diagnostic, procedural, demographic, and outcome-related variables from the Duke CCU and clearly demonstrated

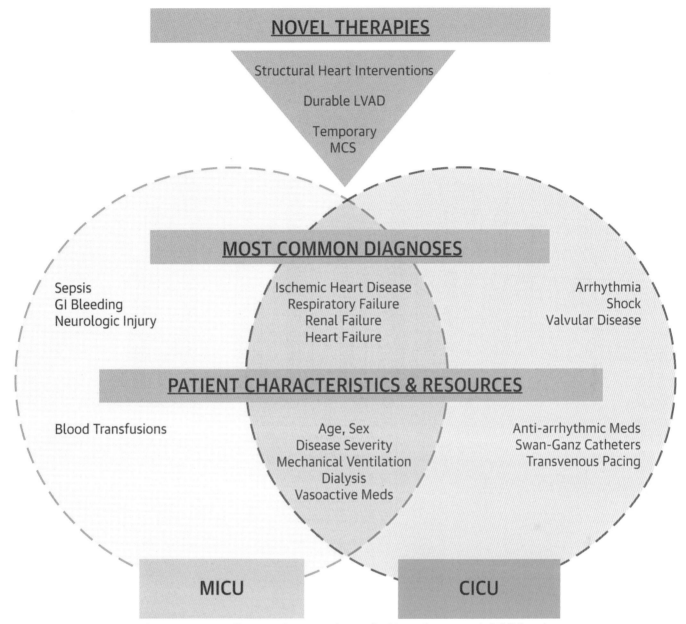

Fig. 1.2 Similarities and differences between the medical intensive care unit (MICU) and coronary intensive care unit (CICU). *LVAD,* Left ventricular assist device; *MCS,* mechanical circulatory support. (From Katz JN, Minder M, Olenchock B, et al. The genesis, maturation, and future of Critical Care Cardiology. *J Am Coll Cardiol.* 2016;68:67-79.)

a growing critical care burden and increased implementation of critical care resources over time (Figs. 1.3 and 1.4).

Ongoing Evolution of Cardiac Intensive Care Units

Multiple nonrandomized studies offer general support for the beneficial role of the CCU in the management of patients with acute MI. As a result, there has been a rapid proliferation of these specialized units in the United States and worldwide since their introduction into the medical vernacular more than 4 decades ago. At the same time, data support significant evolutionary changes within contemporary CICUs. Observational studies suggest that although the mortality for acute MI has steadily declined, there is a greater burden of noncoronary cardiovascular

disease and critical illness. For these patients, the role and impact of CICU care are uncertain. This uncertainty has numerous implications related to patient outcomes, resource use, and costs of care. As we continue to work toward better defining the changing landscape of the CICU and its place within the current health care system, several key topics need to be addressed.

Multidisciplinary Clinical Integration and the Cardiac Intensive Care Unit Model

Because of the multiplicity and complexity of critical care delivery, and the advancing critical care burden in the contemporary CICU, the development of practice models for efficient and effective patient care will be an important part of the continued

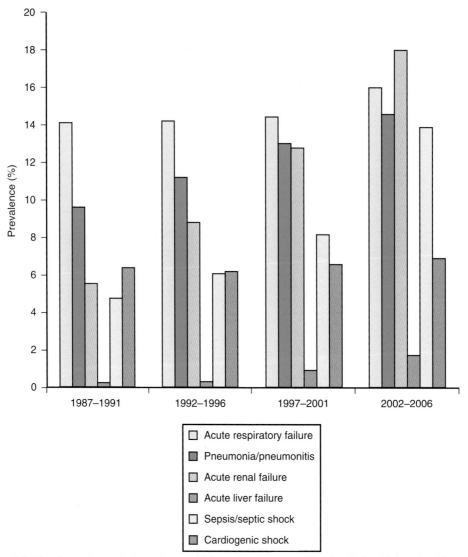

Fig. 1.3 Unadjusted trends in selected high activity illnesses in the Duke University Hospital coronary care unit (unpublished data 1987–2006).

evolution of the CCU. At the same time, landmark documents from the National Academy of Medicine (formerly the Institute of Medicine) have attacked several "dysfunctional" processes of past and current health care systems, with particular attention focused on the elimination of "isolationist decision-making and ineffective team dynamics" that may put patient care at risk.[45,46] A careful appraisal of the role of multidisciplinary care in the CICU will therefore be essential moving forward.

Currently, several models of health care delivery are employed in ICUs; they include the *open model, closed model*, and *hybrid models*. Each of these critical care platforms have distinct advantages and disadvantages from patient-care and systems-based perspectives. In a *closed ICU model*, all patients are cared for by an intensivist-led team that is primarily responsible for making clinical decisions. In a contemporary CICU, this leader might be a general cardiologist, a cardiologist with critical care expertise, or an intensivist adept in the care of patients with complex cardiovascular illness. In an *open ICU model*, the patient's primary physician determines the need for ICU admission and discharge

and makes all management decisions. A *hybrid ICU model* represents a blend of the two more traditional critical care delivery models. The available evidence increasingly supports a closed or hybrid ICU format for delivering high-quality, cost-effective care compared with the open model.[47,48]

Governing bodies for the major critical care medicine organizations universally espouse the benefits of multidisciplinary critical care.[49,50] It is believed that shared responsibility for ICU team leadership is a fundamental component for providing optimal medical care for critically ill patients. A multidisciplinary approach to CICU management seems equally reasonable in light of growing patient complexity. Potential members of CICU teams, all of whom would be intimately involved in the day-to-day care of patients, might include a cardiologist, intensivist, pharmacist, respiratory therapist, critical care nurse, and social worker or case manager. The goal of this integrated team is to provide the highest quality care, while limiting adverse events, curbing ineffective resource use and associated cost, and providing an efficient patient transition out of the intensive care setting.

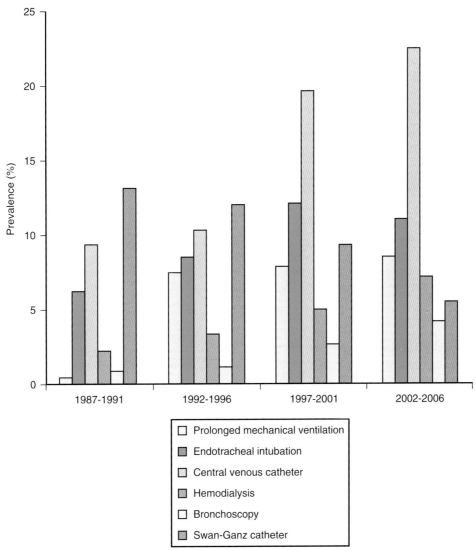

Fig. 1.4 Unadjusted trends in selected critical care procedures performed in the Duke University Hospital coronary care unit (unpublished date 1987–2006).

Management Algorithms

Best practice in patient care is achieved by following the best available evidence and standardizing processes and procedures within a working environment. We believe that standard operating procedures are particularly important in CICUs and even more so in those within an academic medical center experiencing a near constant turnover of residents, fellows, and students from nursing, pharmacy, physical therapy, respiratory therapy, and other trainees. Protocols that would have previously been attributable to MICUs are now quite relevant to CICUs.[51] Several examples are shown in Fig. 1.5.

EDUCATION AND TRAINING IN THE CARDIAC INTENSIVE CARE UNIT

Most CICUs employ nurses with critical care backgrounds. With a growing number of patients with complex cardiovascular disease admitted to the CICU, there is a significant need for training more nurses skilled in cardiovascular critical care. At the same time, an existing nursing shortage[52] raises a potential barrier to growth and, more important, achieving excellence in patient care in the CICU.

As discussed previously, the diversity of critical illness in today's CICU poses many challenges to general cardiologists who have traditionally staffed these units. To achieve optimal alignment of physician skills and patient needs, there are several fundamental options: providing cardiologists with requisite skills in critical care delivery (in the form of continuing medical education), training cardiologists with advanced specialization in critical care medicine, introducing a cardiology-critical track during fellowship training, or including an intensivist on the CICU team.[41,42,53]

The American College of Cardiology Core Cardiovascular Training (COCATS) Statement revised four requirements in 2015 to reflect the evolution and complexity of the CICU.[54] Moreover, for the first time, critical care cardiology was seen as a vital and requisite component of cardiology fellowship programs.

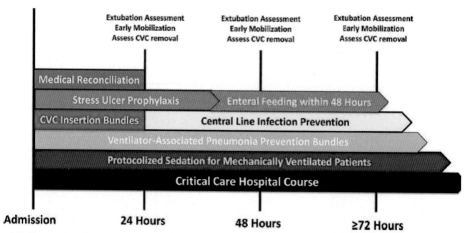

Fig. 1.5 Examples for processes, procedures, and management algorithms in a contemporary coronary care unit. *CVC,* Central venous catheter. (From van Diepen S, Sligl WI, Washam JB, et al. Prevention of critical care complications in the coronary intensive care unit: protocols, bundles, and insights from intensive care studies. *Can J Cardiol.* 2017;33:10.)

The new training guidelines outline the essentials of critical care cardiology that should be taught to all fellows. Critical care training should be integrated into the fellowship program and include the evaluation and management of patients with acute, life-threatening cardiovascular illnesses, exposure to noninvasive and invasive diagnostic modalities commonly used in the evaluation of such patients, familiarity with both temporary and long-term mechanical circulatory support devices, and understanding of the management of the critically ill patient.

The advent of critical care fellowships, including those for cardiologists,[55] specifically addresses the heightened burden of complex illness among hospitalized patients, including those within a CICU (Fig. 1.6). Hill and colleagues[56] assessed preparedness among critical care fellowship trainees in the United States. In a 19-item survey, they assessed trainee confidence in the management of cardiac critical care illnesses and the performance of cardiac-specific critical care interventions as suggested by the Accreditation Council for Graduate Medical Education. Respondents reported lower confidence in managing cardiovascular as compared with noncardiovascular diseases in the ICU setting. In addition, they reported lower competence in performing cardiovascular procedures specific to the ICU. While this survey represents a relatively modest number of trainees ($n = 134$), it should raise awareness and a thorough evaluation of curricula, training methods, and assessment tools in current cardiology critical care training programs.

Technology Needs in Contemporary Cardiac Intensive Care Units

Beyond the continuous telemetry monitoring and defibrillator capabilities that represent the foundation and origins of CCU care, contemporary needs include the ability to provide noninvasive and invasive hemodynamic monitoring, mechanical ventilation, fluoroscopic guidance for bedside procedures, continuous renal replacement therapy, methods for circulatory support (e.g., intraaortic balloon counterpulsation, percutaneous and implantable ventricular-assist devices, extracorporeal circulatory assist circuits), and portable echocardiography. Additionally, clinical information systems for standardization of care, monitoring outcomes, and tracking quality are vital. These clinical information systems often include electronic clinician order entry and real-time nursing data entry as well.

Finally, there has been a growing enthusiasm for telemedicine, especially for more rural health care facilities with limited resources for critical care. This technology has also been advocated as a way to navigate the impending crisis of insufficient critical care specialists to meet the growing demands for their skills[57] and has a potentially viable role in the operation of many CICUs in the United States and other countries.

RESEARCH IN THE CARDIAC INTENSIVE CARE UNIT

The evolution of the CICU also provides a fertile environment from which to conduct novel research. Existing platforms for CICU-based critical care investigation have included the ongoing development and implementation of mechanical circulatory support devices, the creation of models for the study of sepsis-associated myocardial dysfunction, and the execution of clinical analyses to study the impact of bleeding and transfusion on patient outcomes. The potential for future platforms in basic, translational, genomic, and clinical study is seemingly limitless. The generation of knowledge culminating from such research will inevitably lead to improvements in patient care, including more efficient CICU operational models, standardization of cardiac critical care delivery, creation of physician decision-support tools, and advanced personnel training. Key components for developing a successful, translatable, and reproducible platform of CICU-based critical care research include the creation of uniform computerized databases for efficient data abstraction, the organization of dedicated cardiac acute care research teams, and the establishment of focused multicenter and international

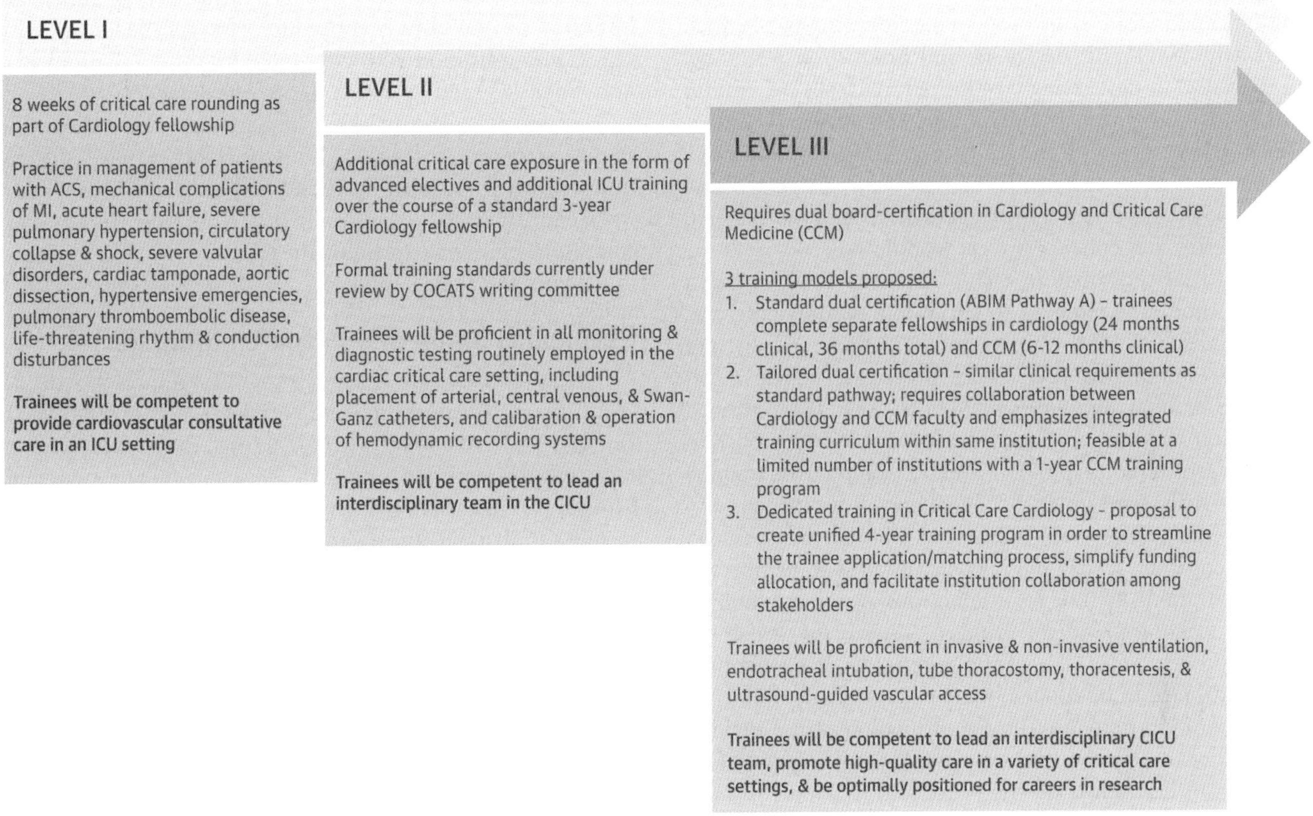

LEVEL I

8 weeks of critical care rounding as part of Cardiology fellowship

Practice in management of patients with ACS, mechanical complications of MI, acute heart failure, severe pulmonary hypertension, circulatory collapse & shock, severe valvular disorders, cardiac tamponade, aortic dissection, hypertensive emergencies, pulmonary thromboembolic disease, life-threatening rhythm & conduction disturbances

Trainees will be competent to provide cardiovascular consultative care in an ICU setting

LEVEL II

Additional critical care exposure in the form of advanced electives and additional ICU training over the course of a standard 3-year Cardiology fellowship

Formal training standards currently under review by COCATS writing committee

Trainees will be proficient in all monitoring & diagnostic testing routinely employed in the cardiac critical care setting, including placement of arterial, central venous, & Swan-Ganz catheters, and calibration & operation of hemodynamic recording systems

Trainees will be competent to lead an interdisciplinary team in the CICU

LEVEL III

Requires dual board-certification in Cardiology and Critical Care Medicine (CCM)

3 training models proposed:
1. Standard dual certification (ABIM Pathway A) – trainees complete separate fellowships in cardiology (24 months clinical, 36 months total) and CCM (6-12 months clinical)
2. Tailored dual certification – similar clinical requirements as standard pathway; requires collaboration between Cardiology and CCM faculty and emphasizes integrated training curriculum within same institution; feasible at a limited number of institutions with a 1-year CCM training program
3. Dedicated training in Critical Care Cardiology – proposal to create unified 4-year training program in order to streamline the trainee application/matching process, simplify funding allocation, and facilitate institution collaboration among stakeholders

Trainees will be proficient in invasive & non-invasive ventilation, endotracheal intubation, tube thoracostomy, thoracentesis, & ultrasound-guided vascular access

Trainees will be competent to lead an interdisciplinary CICU team, promote high-quality care in a variety of critical care settings, & be optimally positioned for careers in research

Fig. 1.6 Proposed levels of competency and training models for achieving board eligibility in critical care cardiology. (From Katz JN, Minder M, Olenchock B, et al. The genesis, maturation, and future of Critical Care Cardiology. *J Am Coll Cardiol.* 2016;68:67-79.)

research networks with the necessary tools for implementing novel research constructs. Additionally, contributions from academic organizations, government agencies, philanthropic groups, and industry to provide funding and other resources for project support and investigator career development in the field of cardiovascular critical care will be crucial. Box 1.1 lists potential research areas for future study.

Research Processes

A successful acute care research program must have an infrastructure that is dynamic and scalable to varying environments and conditions, including prehospital identification and processing of potential study subjects. Essential components for operationalizing clinical trials conducted or initiated in the prehospital setting include an experienced steering committee, an in-depth assessment of feasibility, specifically trained research coordinators either in the field or readily available employing a teleresearch platform, a tailored recruitment strategy, a facile and experienced institutional review board (IRB), and a mechanism for electronic informed consent (e-consent, see below) employing individuals or family members.

The acute care research team should develop training materials, including an operations manual, quick reference guide (pocket size) for both the on-site technicians and research personnel,

BOX 1.1 Potential Topics for Acute Care Research in the Coronary Care Unit (CCU)

Systems-of-care, operations, and organizational models
Predictive models of clinical decompensation and intervention
Circulating biomarkers of cardiovascular critical illness
Device development (e.g., smart beds and risk integration)
Escalation of care algorithms
Economic analyses of CICU-based critical care delivery
Practice patterns for pharmacotherapy in the CICU and new drug development for cardiovascular critical illness
Genomic studies of critical illness susceptibility in CICU patients
Optimal mechanical ventilation strategies for cardiac patients and optimal weaning protocols
Role of telemedicine, medical informatics, and other electronic innovations in the CICU
Development and implementation of training and learning models to improve cardiac critical care delivery
Effectiveness of multidisciplinary clinical integration in the CICU
Informed consent for research participation in a critical care setting
Application of current critical care quality metrics for CICU quality-of-care initiatives

and certification documents. All training materials should be available through an acute care research-dedicated website. A communications team consisting of the following is essential: writers, editors, graphic designers, and production personnel who specialize in developing customized materials for clinical studies—including paper and electronic data forms, e-consent platform (developed with the study team and IRB), in-service manuals, posters, pocket cards, and project websites. These trial-specific aids have been shown repeatedly to speed enrollment, reduce queries, and enhance project workflows.

Clinical trial coordinators, technicians, and other research personnel should be required to log in to a secure acute care research website to view training modules that carefully and thoroughly summarize prehospital processes, policies, and procedures. Annual retraining should be required for continued participation with notices for renewal sent at least 1 month in advance of certification expiration. Additional supportive training materials—such as streaming videos, an operations manual, and quick reference guide—should be available through the website to allow for "any time" review and reference by all staff members. A web-based training method is advantageous over the traditional in-person training paradigm primarily due to the scalability of this approach. Regardless of the number of new personnel or sites that need to be trained, there should be no additional costs, preparation time, travel, or coordination time—making training efficient, effective, and seamless. Anyone, anywhere and any time, can be trained on the process. It is critical to have processes firmly in place from the outset of conducting acute care research.

Informed Consent

The informed consent process in acute care research can be challenging. In nonacute care settings, patients and their families have time to consider whether the research best benefits the patient's interest and can voluntarily choose to participate or decline participation in the research study. Due to the nature of research in acute care settings, obtaining informed consent is time sensitive and it can be problematic when patients are physically or mentally unable to provide consent for themselves and there is a delay in identifying the legally authorized representative (LAR) or next of kin.

Some of the informed consent barriers identified in clinical research in acute care settings are improper communication with the acute care population, inability to identify LAR or next of kin in timely manner and patients' incapacity to understand informed consent (study procedure, risk and benefits, and so on). Communication with culturally diverse populations (e.g., non–English speaking) needs to be considered.

The research team working in acute care research settings should be trained professionals with the ability to make educated, time-sensitive decisions. There should be a properly distributed workload. The study team should be comfortable with properly communicating and explaining the risks and benefits of research to patients and their families.

Developing an On-site Research Program

A successful acute care research program requires a dedicated group of investigators, coordinators, and administrators. The University of Cincinnati Medical Center established an acute care research program under the auspices of our Center for Clinical and Translational Science and Training (CCTST) and includes individuals from varying backgrounds with extensive research experience. Our collaborative approach utilizes a learning development model of analysis, design, development, implementation, and evaluation (an ADDIE model). The goal is to establish a strong foundation for education, training, and design to be used specifically for acute care research.

CONCLUSION

The CCU revolutionized the care of patients with acute MI, and the CICU now offers an environment of highly skilled professionals working as teams to improve the care of patients with a broad range of complex cardiovascular conditions that are life threatening or potentially life altering. Patient selection, appropriate resource utilization, and standardized processes of care collectively represent the key to achieve optimal outcomes at a cost that is justifiable in an era of affordable care. Education, training, and research must be a priority moving forward.

Acknowledgment

We thank Tim Smith, MD, for reviewing the manuscript.

The full reference list for this chapter is available at ExpertConsult.com.

2

Ethical Issues in the Cardiac Intensive Care Unit

Michael S. O'Connor, Martin L. Smith, Timothy Gilligan

Every human being of adult years and sound mind has a right to determine what shall be done with his own body.

U.S. Supreme Court Justice Cardozo[1]

Ethical challenges abound in intensive care units (ICUs). Treatment in ICUs represents one of the costliest and most aggressive forms of Western medicine. ICU patients are the sickest and the most unstable, and they often cannot participate in health care decision making. Patients' families and loved ones are often left reeling by the sudden onset of serious illness. These factors bring to the ICU a host of difficult and troubling ethical issues. Our societal discomfort with human mortality, combined with media that exaggerate what modern medicine can accomplish, can exacerbate the discord that often arises when engaging these ethical challenges. Responding in an informed, compassionate, and ethically supportable manner is an essential part of high-quality critical care medicine.

The primary defining characteristics of cardiac ICU (CICU) patients are cardiovascular instability and life-threatening illness that require intensive monitoring, advanced life-support techniques, or both. Many such patients have poor prognoses; a substantial percentage die without leaving the hospital. Hence clinicians working in critical care must be comfortable working in the presence of death and dying and must be prepared for the attendant ethical challenges that often arise. These issues include, but are not limited to, writing do-not-resuscitate (DNR) orders, negotiating with family members or surrogates who do not want a patient to be told about a terminal diagnosis or prognosis, trying to determine what level of treatment an irreversibly ill patient without decision-making capacity would choose if able, and withholding or withdrawing life support. As medicine's ability to preserve the physiologic functioning of critically ill patients has improved, physicians, other clinicians, patients, and their families are increasingly faced with questions of when and how to terminate life-sustaining treatment.

When addressing these issues, clinicians are best served by remembering that their primary responsibility is to act in the patient's best interest by maintaining open and honest communication with patients, their surrogates, and with each other. Acting in the patient's best interest means providing the high-quality treatment and care for those who will likely survive the CICU and facilitating a peaceful and dignified death for those who will not.

Economic and resource utilization issues complicate further the work of ICU professionals. In the United States, CICU beds cost from $4000 to $10,000 per day.[2,3] In the current climate of increasing pressures to limit health care costs, the pattern of increased financial costs accrued by patients with poor prognoses in ICUs has drawn increased scrutiny, prompting the study of strategies to avoid prolonged futile ICU treatment.[4] The practice of providing tens of thousands of dollars' worth of advanced care to ICU patients who have essentially no chance of recovery is ethically problematic, given the potential to deplete patients' savings and to drive them and their families into bankruptcy. Furthermore, health care resources are limited, in terms of dollars, ICU beds, and personnel time and effort. With many CICUs routinely filled to capacity, allowing patients with no real chance of improvement to occupy CICU beds may prevent other patients with a high probability of benefiting from intensive care from being able to gain access to the CICU. Although there is general opposition to withholding potentially beneficial therapies solely for economic reasons, in the current political and economic climate, critical care physicians and other clinicians should become conversant with ICU economics and develop sound stewardship practices of CICU resources.

This chapter provides a basic overview of the ethical challenges that arise in critical care medicine. After a review of basic principles, guidelines, and methods of bioethics, as well as a discussion of the ethical challenges related to health care economics in the ICU, this chapter focuses on specific ethical issues related to withholding and withdrawal of life support. Brief discussions of euthanasia and cross-cultural conflict are also included. Some cases are presented to illuminate how the frameworks and practices described in this chapter may be applied.

WESTERN BIOETHICS

Bioethics addresses two distinct but overlapping areas: the generic issue of what it means to provide health care in a manner consistent with basic moral values and the more specific challenge of identifying principles and guidelines for proper conduct that can be widely agreed on by the health care professions. For example, although confidentiality in medicine, as in law, is a strict ethical rule, it derives less from abstract moral values and more from its necessity for the effective provision of treatment and care. For the purposes of this chapter, the term *bioethics* represents guidelines for proper and principled conduct by health care professionals.

Although Western bioethics dates to the ancient Greeks, it only started to develop into a discipline of its own in the 1950s, largely as a result of new dilemmas posed by powerful new medical therapies. As medicine developed and strengthened its ability to maintain physiologic functioning in the face of ever greater insult and injury to the human body, patients—and more often their surrogates, families, and health care professionals—found themselves struggling with a central question of when treatments are life sustaining versus death prolonging. The 1976 New Jersey Supreme Court decision in the case of Karen Ann Quinlan established that advanced life support could be withdrawn from patients who have essentially no chance to regain any reasonable quality of life.[5] Since that time, many other legal decisions, state and federal laws, and reports and consensus statements from various professional societies and regulatory commissions have helped define in what manner, under what circumstances, and by whose authority advanced or basic life support can be forgone.[6–16]

A variety of methods for "thinking ethically" have been identified and used during the decades-long evolution of the field of bioethics.[17] We have selected three methods that have been the most influential in bioethical analysis to date and that are the most helpful for addressing clinical situations in the CICU. The three methods are (1) principlism, (2) consequentialism, and (3) casuistry. Clinicians should not feel compelled to choose one of these methods over the others as their primary way for ethical analysis and reflection. Instead, using some combination of the three methods in most cases can be the most helpful.

Principlism

Principlism holds that actions must be evaluated based on their inherent qualities and the motivations or intentions underlying the actions. When applied to the clinical setting, principlism asserts that clinicians have specific obligations, moral duties, and rules that, in most circumstances, should be followed and fulfilled.[18] Beauchamp and Childress have identified four fundamental principles and duties from which all other bioethical principles and duties can be derived: patient autonomy, beneficence, nonmaleficence, and justice.[19] However, it is impossible for clinicians to perform their duties without sometimes violating one or more of these fundamental principles. Indeed, many ethical dilemmas present a clash between these principles; in such situations, health care professionals must choose which principle to uphold and which to relinquish.

Patient Autonomy. Autonomy refers to the fundamental common law right of patients to control their own bodies. As the U.S. Supreme Court ruled in 1891 in a case unrelated to health care: "No right is held more sacred or is more carefully guarded by the common law than the right of every individual to the possession and control of his own person, free from all restraints or interference by others, unless by clear and unquestionable authority of law."[20] In medical terms, patient autonomy means the right of self-determination, including the right to choose for oneself among various recommended therapies. Autonomy also implies a respect for adult patients capable of making their own decisions. The principle of autonomy stands in contrast to paternalism, which presumes that physicians and other health care professionals know best and decide for the patient or authoritatively direct patients to the "right decisions." The delineation between respect for autonomy and paternalism can be captured by affirming that in the decision-making process, clinicians have a role to inform, educate, advise, recommend, guide, and even try to persuade patients but should never engage in manipulation or coercion.

Respect for autonomy means that adult patients with decision-making capacity have the right to refuse medical treatments even if the treatments are life sustaining. It follows that, except in emergency situations, patients must consent to any treatments they receive and they must understand the risks, benefits, and reasonable alternatives of any proposed therapies or procedures for this consent to be meaningful. Withholding information from patients is a threat to their autonomy.

The acuity of CICU patients' illnesses should not be used as an excuse for failing to obtain informed consent for treatment in general or for procedures in particular. Physicians have the responsibility to ensure that the health care provided is in accord with patient wishes. For patients lacking decision-making capacity, a patient-designated surrogate or a close family member should be identified to help plan an appropriate level of treatment consistent with the best available knowledge of what the patient would have wanted. Patients do not have the right to demand specific treatments; only licensed health care providers have the authority to determine which of the therapies under their purview are indicated for a patient.

Minors do not enjoy the same decisional rights as adults and are generally not viewed as sufficiently autonomous by law to make their own health care decisions. Instead, these decisions usually fall to the minor's parents or legal guardian. However, U.S. courts have consistently been willing to overrule parents in cases in which there is evidence that the parents' decisions are not consistent with the best interests of their child. For example, although adult Jehovah's Witnesses can refuse medically indicated blood transfusions for themselves, they cannot make the same refusal on behalf of their children.

Beneficence. The principle of beneficence represents health care professionals' responsibility and ethical duty to benefit their patients. This duty encompasses the promotion of patients' health and well-being as well as reducing suffering when possible. At its most basic level, beneficence is necessary to justify the practice of medicine, because if professionals do not benefit their patients, there is no rationale for the work. One caution related to the principle of beneficence is that professionals may judge "patient benefit" primarily in physiologic categories related to medical goals and outcomes. However, from the patient's perspective, benefit may include not only medical outcomes but also psychosocial-spiritual outcomes, interests, and activities that help to define the meaningfulness and quality of a patient's life. Thus, a recommended intervention with the likelihood of a good medical outcome but which would not allow a patient to continue a significant interest or activity could be judged differently by the patient than by the health care team because of differing perceptions of "benefit."

More philosophically, beneficence as a principle in medicine supports the sanctity of human life and asserts the significance of human experience. In this regard, health care professionals practice beneficence not only by curing diseases, saving lives or alleviating pain, nausea, and other discomforts but also by expressing empathy and kindness—by contributing to patients' experiences that they are cared for and that their suffering is recognized. In the CICU, with critically ill patients near the end of life, presence, compassion, and humanity are sometimes the greatest forms of care and benefit that clinicians can offer.

Nonmaleficence. Nonmaleficence requires physicians and other clinicians to avoid harming patients. More colloquially cited as "first, do no harm," the principle of nonmaleficence warns clinicians against overzealousness in the fight against disease. Unfortunately, opportunities to do harm in medicine abound. Almost every medication and procedure can cause adverse effects and simply being in the hospital and in the ICU puts patients

at risk for blood clots and infection by a more dangerous group of microorganisms than they would likely encounter at home. Unnecessary tests may unearth harmless abnormalities, the work-up of which may result in significant complications. An unnecessary central venous line may result in a pneumothorax, bloodstream infection, or thrombus. Unnecessary antibiotics may result in anaphylactic shock, Stevens-Johnson syndrome, acute tubular necrosis, pseudomembranous colitis and toxic megacolon, or subsequent infection by resistant organisms. Many clinicians tend to feel much more comfortable with acting than with refraining from acting; hence, in the face of clinical uncertainty, many physicians are inclined to order another test or try another medication. It is essential that physicians constantly and consistently assess the potential benefits and the potential harms (including financial costs) that may result from each test and treatment they prescribe for each patient.

There are also other harms specific to the CICU. When patients languish on mechanical ventilation or invasive circulatory assistance without a reasonable possibility of recovery, physicians violate the principle of nonmaleficence. For many or most patients, the ICU can be an uncomfortable and undignified setting, filled with unfamiliar and jarring sights and sounds. Being sustained on mechanical ventilation ranges from unpleasant to miserable unless the patient is unconscious or heavily sedated. The only justification for putting patients through such experiences is an expectation that they have a likelihood of returning to some reasonable quality of life as determined by the patient's values. When physicians' care and treatments serve only to prolong the process of dying and suffering, they violate nonmaleficence.

Just as physicians can harm their patients by providing excessively aggressive treatments, they can also harm patients by withholding care from them. When patients remain in the CICU for prolonged periods of time or their disease and complications are particularly troubling, physicians may be inclined to spend less time with sicker persons or to focus on flow sheets and documentation rather than on these challenging patients. Illness, however, is often a lonely and frightening experience; abandonment by clinicians adds to patient suffering.

Justice. Justice in clinical ethics means a fair allocation of health care resources, especially when the resources are limited. In the United States, on the macro-allocation level, there has been a failure to achieve a just health care system by any standard. The quality and accessibility of medical care available remains largely a function of an individual's socioeconomic status and racial/ethnic categorization. Americans in disadvantaged economic, ethnic, or racial groups receive less care, lower-quality care, suffer greater morbidity and mortality from illness, and die younger in most disease-specific categories than do other citizens. The principle of justice demands that health care resources be allocated not according to the ability to pay but rather according to need and to the potential of treatment to benefit the individual.

On a micro-allocation level, the principle of justice plays a role in the CICU in terms of triage. With a limited number of beds, those in charge of the unit must decide which patients have the greatest need and the greatest potential to benefit.

Moreover, because intensive care represents a very expensive form of medical intervention, consuming over 13% of U.S. hospital costs and 4% of total U.S. health care expenditures,[21] there is a strong national interest in curtailing wasteful ICU use. The concepts of futility and rationing help in analyzing the challenge of triage but, as Jecker and Schneiderman have observed, the two terms have different points of reference.[22,23] Determinations of futility are related to whether identified goals of treatment are achievable.[24,25] Further, futility can have two distinct meanings, referring either to treatment that has essentially no chance of achieving its immediate physiologic purpose or outcome or that has essentially no chance of meaningfully benefiting the patient.[26] For example, treating a bacterial pneumonia in a brain-dead patient would be considered not futile with the former definition and certainly futile with the latter. The threshold for futility is a contentious subject; some have argued that the impossibility of arriving at widely accepted objective, quantitative standards renders use of the term inappropriate.[27,28]

Futility differs conceptually from rationing in that futility applies to an individual patient's likelihood of benefiting from treatment, whereas rationing refers to the distribution of limited resources within a population. Rationing is fair only when it is applied in an even-handed way for patients with similar needs, without regard to race, ethnicity, educational level, or socioeconomic status. Futility affects triage decisions because futile treatment violates the principles of beneficence and nonmaleficence. Such wasteful use of medical care also violates the principle of justice when resources are limited. Rationing comes into play when there are more patients who need ICU care than there are beds, mechanical ventilators, or other critical care resources available. As health care costs continue to climb, physicians may find increasing pressures in the CICU to limit treatment for patients with poor prognoses. The ethical test in such circumstances is whether rationing is necessary and whether it is applied in a fair manner (i.e., whether similar cases are treated similarly). To maintain a clear understanding of what physicians are doing, it is essential that assertions of futility do not become either a mask behind which rationing or hospital cost-saving decisions can hide or a means of bullying patients or their families into accepting treatment-limitation decisions.[24,29,30]

The four principles of bioethics can help untangle and clarify many complex and troubling dilemmas. In different cases, each of the individual principles may seem more or less important, but they are all usually pertinent in some way. These principles can certainly come into conflict with each other, which can then signify the presence of an ethical dilemma. Practically, the principles can help to pose a series of significant, patient-centered questions for clinicians: Am I respecting my patient's autonomy? Has the patient consented to the various treatments? Do I know my patient's resuscitation status? Is my therapeutic plan likely to benefit my patient? Am I doing all I can to improve my patient's well-being? Am I minimizing patient harm? Have I identified goals of treatment or care with my patient (or the surrogate) and are those goals achievable? Is there an appropriate balance between potential benefit and risk of harm? Is my plan of care consistent with the principle of justice?

Consequentialism

The second method for "thinking ethically" about clinical and ICU situations is consequentialism, which has its root meaning in the Western philosophical theory of teleology ("telos" in Greek means "ends"). Consequentialist reasoning judges actions as right or wrong based on their consequences or ends. This method of reasoning and analysis requires an anticipatory, projected calculation of the likely positive and negative results of different identified options prior to decisions and actions being carried out. For example, a physician may be requested by family members not to disclose a poor prognosis to their hospitalized loved one because, in their view, the disclosure will cause the patient to experience distress and to lose hope. Because the patient should be at the center of a "calculation of consequences" for this scenario, the first question should be this: How will the disclosure or nondisclosure impact the patient, both positively by way of benefits or negatively by way of harms? The patient is not the only one who will experience consequences as a result of this particular decision, however. Other stakeholders who can be affected positively and negatively include the patient's family members (will they be angry and feel betrayed if the poor prognosis is disclosed or will they ultimately feel relieved?), bedside nurses and other involved health care professionals (will they feel distress if they are expected to participate in a "conspiracy of silence" or if the patient asks them a direct question about the prognosis?), the hospital (will disclosure or nondisclosure be in accord with organizational values, such as respect for patients and compassion?), and even the wider community and society (how will other and future patients be affected if they come to know that physicians at this particular hospital disclose or do not disclose poor prognoses to patients?). When applying consequentialism, the projected and accumulated benefits and harms for all involved should be weighed against each other with the goal of maximizing benefits and minimizing harms.

One challenge of calculating consequences for the options in each medical situation is how to be sufficiently thorough in anticipating what the projected outcomes and results might be. For many situations, experienced physicians and other clinicians, using their knowledge of previous cases and building on their collective wisdom, can reasonably project medical, legal, and psychosocial-spiritual consequences for the different options. A more problematic challenge when using consequentialism is determining how much weight to assign each of the various beneficial and burdensome consequences. For example, should a potential legal risk to the physician and hospital that could result from a specific bedside decision be given more weight than doing what is clearly in a patient's best medical interests? In the end, after identifying and weighing projected burdens and benefits of reasonable options, clinicians using consequentialism would be ethically required to choose and act on the option that is likely to produce the most benefit and to avoid the option(s) likely to bring the most harm.

Casuistry

The third method of analysis that can lead to ethically supportable actions is casuistry,[31] a word that shares its linguistic roots with the word "cases." Although the term may not be familiar to many clinicians, the method itself is likely to be familiar to them. Casuistry is based on practical judgments about the similarities and differences between and among cases. Both medicine and law use this methodology when they look to previous and precedent cases to provide insight about a new case at hand. For example, when a patient presents to a physician with a specific set of symptoms and complaints and after the physician analyzes the results of various diagnostic tests, a skilled and knowledgeable physician is usually able to arrive at a specific diagnosis. The diagnosis is based on attention to the details of the patient's symptoms and test results but is also based on the physician's training and experience of having personally seen or having read in the published literature about similar or identical cases. Casuistry in ethical analysis uses a parallel kind of reasoning.

According to casuistry, attention must first be given to the specific details, features, and characteristics of the ethical dilemma at hand. Then, the goal is to identify known previous cases that are analogous to the new case and had reasonably good and ethically supportable outcomes. If such a previous or paradigm case can be identified for which a consensus exists about correct action, then this previous case can provide ethical guidance for the new case at hand. For example, a 25-year-old ICU patient with Down syndrome and an estimated cognitive ability of a 4-year-old is in need of blood transfusions. Her family members are Jehovah's Witnesses and adamantly object to the transfusions based on their religious beliefs. Using casuistry and appealing to similar cases, the ICU team notes that there is an ethical and legal consensus related to pediatric patients of Jehovah's Witness parents to override parental objections to blood transfusions and to act in the patient's best interests. Because the 25-year-old patient's cognitive ability is similar to that of pediatric patients who do not have the cognitive ability to commit themselves knowingly and voluntarily to a set of religious tenets, the ethically supportable option in the pediatric cases (i.e., overriding parental objections to blood transfusions) could be extended to this case.

An additional feature of casuistry is that as cases are compared and similarities and differences are identified, moral maxims or ethical rules of thumb can emerge that can also be helpful for current and future cases and dilemmas. Such moral maxims include adult, informed patients with decision-making capacity can refuse recommended treatment; a lesser harm to a patient can be tolerated to prevent a greater harm; and physicians are not obligated to offer or provide treatments that they judge to be medically inappropriate. One challenge of casuistry is to pay sufficient attention to the relevant facts and details of the new case to be able to identify previous cases that are similar enough to provide guidance for the case at hand.

An effective use of casuistry by physicians and health care teams can lead to the buildup of a collective wisdom and practical experience from which to draw when new ethical dilemmas arise. Parallel again to physicians building up medical experience and wisdom over time, physicians can establish an ethical storehouse of knowledge and insight based on previous cases and ethical dilemmas that they have experienced, heard about, or read about.

PRACTICAL GUIDELINES FOR ETHICAL DECISION MAKING

In addition to the three methods discussed earlier, the following four practical guidelines can facilitate the process of ethical decision making:
1. Recognize patients as partners in their own health care decisions.
2. Establish who has authority for decision making.
3. Establish effective communication with patients and their loved ones through routinely scheduled family meetings.
4. Determine patient values and preferences in an ongoing manner.

Patient Partnership

All decision making—and, indeed, all health care—must take place with the recognition that patients are partners in their own health care decisions. The American Hospital Association has supported this partnership model for decision making by addressing patient expectations, rights, and responsibilities.[32] Among these expectations and rights, the most salient are the right of patients to participate in medical decision making with their physicians and the right to make informed decisions, including both to consent to and to refuse treatment. In order to exercise these rights, patients need accurate and comprehensible information about diagnoses, treatments, and prognosis. More specifically, patients need a description of the treatment, the reasons for recommending it, the known adverse effects of the treatment and their likelihood of occurring, possible outcomes of the treatment, alternative treatments and their attendant risks and likely outcomes, the risks and benefits involved in refusing the proposed treatment, and the name and position of the person or persons who will carry out or implement the treatment plan. In cases in which someone other than the patient has legal responsibility for making health care decisions on behalf of the patient, all of the patient's expectations and rights apply to this designee as well as the patient. According to the President's Commission for the Study of Ethical Problems in Medicine and Biomedical and Behavioral Research: "Ethically valid consent is a process of shared decision-making based upon mutual respect and participation, not a ritual to be equated with reciting the contents of a form that details the risks of particular treatments."[33]

Authority or Medical Decision Making

Establishing the source of authority for making health care decisions for a patient is a common problem in critical care medicine. Although adult informed patients with decision-making capacity retain this authority for themselves, many ICU patients are unable to participate in decision making. Whatever the patient's condition, however, the patient remains the only true source of ultimate authority and the physician must assemble and review the best available evidence of what the patient would want done. If a patient lacking decision-making capacity has prepared a living will or a health care power of attorney, these documents should be obtained and reviewed. Close family members and loved ones should also be consulted; they may have spoken with the patient about what level of treatment the patient would want in the event of critical illness. In most (but not all) cases, they know the patient best and have the patient's best interest at heart. Having reviewed current clinical circumstances, treating physicians should provide interventions consistent with their best understanding of what the patient would have wanted. Physicians play the role of guides and advisors, evaluating a patient's medical problems, presenting and explaining options for diagnosis and management, and facilitating thoughtful decision making. Except in emergencies or when treatment is clearly futile, physicians should not proceed with management plans until those with true authority to consent to or refuse treatment have approved the plans.

Communication

Explaining medical problems and treatment options to patients and their loved ones, determining patient quality-of-life values and desires, and achieving consensus for a management plan all require effective communication skills.[34] Communication can be especially difficult and important in the CICU setting. Patients and their loved ones are often distressed or intimidated both by the severity of the patient's condition and by the unfamiliar environment. With many basic life functions taken over by the nursing and medical staff and their various machines and devices and with visiting hours sometimes restricted, patients and their loved ones may feel powerless and experience anxiety or anger from the loss of control. Honest, effective, and recurrent communication can help diminish these feelings and decrease the alienation that attends ICU admissions.

High-stakes communication can be conducted more effectively when there is a trusting relationship: taking a little time to get to know the patient and the family and what the patient's life was like prior to the illness is a wise investment. If clinicians start by building a relationship and establishing trust, communication becomes easier.[34,35] Key communication skills include the ability to listen attentively[36] and to express empathy and compassion. Physicians and nurses must be able to employ tact without compromising honesty and to acknowledge and respond to strong emotional expressions without withdrawing or becoming defensive or antagonistic. Clinicians often must read between the lines and recognize subtle cues about what matters most to patients and their loved ones. Effective communication prevents and defuses conflict; helps patients and families work through their anxieties, fears, and anger; and is the most important skill in negotiating the difficult ethical dilemmas arising in the CICU setting.

Establishing effective communication requires time and planning. Clinicians must remind themselves that although ICU care may become routine for them, it is rarely that way for patients or their loved ones. Discussions with a patient's family members or loved ones should take place either at the bedside, if the patient is able to participate, or in a private conference or waiting room; a hospital corridor is an inappropriate location. Because patients and their loved ones will likely feel overwhelmed by the patients' illnesses and the ICU environment, communication should be simple and to the point, with more technical details provided as requested. Encouraging the various parties to ask questions and express their feelings helps to counteract any

intimidation they may feel and communicates to them that the professional at the bedside cares about their concerns.

Finally, for communication to be effective, information should be conveyed in language and at a level of detail that the listener can understand clearly. Medical jargon, an overly sophisticated vocabulary, excessive detail, or an inappropriate emotional tone can defeat what is otherwise a sincere effort to communicate. Clinicians should always ask patients or their loved ones to summarize what they have heard; this is an easy way to assess their comprehension and to correct misunderstandings.

Several types of inadequate communication occur regularly in CICUs. The most common problems result either from focusing on trends rather than on the patient's overall condition or from drawing attention to minor favorable signs when the overall prognosis remains dismal. If a patient is not likely to survive to CICU discharge but is not deteriorating, describing the patient to family members as stable will most likely mislead them. A more truthful report might be: "Your wife is as sick as any person could be and the odds are overwhelming that she will not survive." A similar problem arises in telling a couple that their son with multiorgan failure has improved when in fact there has only been a slight reduction in his oxygen requirement and his overall prognosis remains poor. Such inappropriate "good news" may make the physician feel better, but it can be cruelly misleading by engendering false hopes and needlessly interfering with their grieving process. It is essential to tell the truth and to provide accurate prognostic information in emotionally sensitive ways.

A second common problem is for patients and their families to receive conflicting information or advice from different physicians involved in a patient's care. Alternatively, different consulting services may each address a specific aspect of the patient's treatment without helping the patient and family to integrate disparate pieces of data into a coherent overall understanding of the patient's condition, prognosis, and treatment options. Multidisciplinary care conferences that include the intensivist, relevant consulting physicians, nursing, and—when appropriate—social work and case management should be held periodically to ensure that there is a coherent, shared perspective of the patient's overall management plan. Formal, structured multidisciplinary conferences that include patient and family and that are held within 72 hours of ICU admission have been shown to reduce the burdens of intensive care for dying patients.[4]

When clinicians find that effective communication is not taking place and conflict is developing, they should recruit assistance from an ethics consultant or another facilitator such as a chaplain, social worker, or psychotherapist. Clinicians should think of facilitators as valuable resources and not view their use as a failure. CICU physicians are generally busy with a demanding set of patients and have limited time to talk to patients and their families, yet these patients often have very high communication needs. Bringing in an ethics consultant or other facilitator to supplement the CICU team's efforts can help meet these needs without overtaxing the CICU physicians.

In addition, working with critically ill and dying patients can be highly stressful and emotionally draining, both on a case-by-case basis and as an accumulating problem over time. Clinicians may feel burned out or may seek to protect themselves by creating emotional distance from their patients. Although clinicians cannot delegate all communication responsibilities, the assistance of a facilitator can reduce the stress on all parties involved. Not only can facilitators bring additional communication skills to the situation, but they often have more time for establishing rapport and, as third parties with fresh perspectives, can bring new insight to ethical dilemmas. We recommend requesting a facilitator early whenever it appears that ethical decision making will be difficult.

Determining Patients' Values and Preferences

The fourth practical guideline in ethical decision making is determining a patient's values and preferences regarding quality of life and medical care. ICU medicine can be a painful and distressing experience for the patient. Whether and for how long such an ordeal is appropriate are questions that in the end can be answered only by the patient and are also dependent on prognosis, on how the patient defines quality of life, and how sensitive the patient is to the discomforts and indignities of the illness and hospitalization. These questions become most significant for chronically or terminally ill patients who are dependent on advanced life support. Clinicians must strive to learn each patient's views regarding what constitutes a meaningful and acceptable life compared with a mere prolongation of physiologic functioning. Patients have different preferences about how aggressively they wish to be treated and when they want their physicians to forego life-sustaining treatment. Moreover, since patients' views often change over time, even during the same hospitalization, patients' perspectives should be reviewed on a regular basis. Whenever possible, discussions with patients about these matters should take place with family members and loved ones present so that all parties have the same understanding of the patient's preferences, wishes, and values. Otherwise, if the patient later loses decision-making capacity, the family may balk at following the patient's wishes.

When patients do not have decision-making capacity, physicians and clinical team members must turn to surrogate decision makers, advance directives, or both. Decisions about life support and end-of-life care are among the most personal decisions to be made. For surrogate decision makers, being asked to make such decisions on a loved one's behalf frequently elicits feelings of grief, guilt, confusion, and being overwhelmed. Physicians can perform a tremendous service for their patients' families and loved ones by discussing resuscitation status, life support, and terminal-care issues with patients before they lose decision-making capacity. Patients are not generally eager to hold such discussions; however, this does not excuse avoidance of the subject, especially with patients who have life-threatening diseases.[37]

WITHHOLDING AND WITHDRAWING OF LIFE SUPPORT

Withholding or withdrawing life support is one of the most difficult actions that a physician may have to perform. Having been trained to prolong life and overcome disease, clinicians may feel like failures when allowing a patient to die whose life could have been prolonged with life support. Clinicians, however, are not omnipotent. Death is the natural conclusion to life; although death is often viewed as an enemy in hospitals, it can also sometimes be a welcome end. For severely ill patients with irreversible conditions, the only choices available may be a prolonged and miserable dying versus a more rapid, comfortable, and dignified death. In these cases, death can represent an end to suffering, prevent a life that has been happy from ending with prolonged misery, and can allow survivors to mourn and proceed with their lives. A relatively pain-free and dignified death is sometimes the best option that physicians can offer.

Legal Precedents

Legal guidelines for withholding and withdrawing life support come predominantly from state court rulings; federal guidance has been minimal in this regard. State court rulings, however, apply only within that state's boundaries; they have no formal legal standing in other states, although they may be cited by other state courts. Hence, although the right to refuse medical treatment is protected both by common law and by the U.S. Constitution, the exact limitations of this right and the conditions under which life support can be withdrawn from patients lacking decision-making capacity vary from state to state. There exists significant variability among states regarding what the courts will accept as clear and convincing evidence that a patient without decision-making capacity would have wanted life support foregone. As in all human affairs, various court rulings can be somewhat arbitrary, reflecting the background, politics, and moral perspectives of judges who made these rulings. Physicians and hospitals must be familiar with their state's legal positions on withholding and withdrawing life support. Although malpractice and criminal actions resulting from withholding or withdrawing life support have been extremely rare, this likely stems from the extreme reluctance, bordering on refusal, of physicians and hospitals to terminate life support contrary to the wishes of the patient's family. Instead, legal action tends to result from a medical team's refusal to withdraw treatment.

Patients With Decision-Making Capacity. The right of adult informed patients with decision-making capacity to refuse both advanced life support and medically supplied nutrition and hydration is well established in the United States through case law and hospital policies.[38] For instance, the case of *Bouvia v. Superior Court*[39] concerned a young, quadriplegic woman with cerebral palsy who was suffering unrelenting pain and directing that the hospital withhold her medically supplied tube feedings so that she could die. The hospital refused. In its 1986 ruling, the California State Court of Appeals found that "to insist on continuing Bouvia's life … at the patient's sole expense and against her competent will, thus inflicting never ending physical torture on her body until the inevitable, but artificially suspended, moment of death … invades the patient's constitutional right of privacy, removes her freedom of choice and invades her right to self-determination."

Patients Lacking Decision-Making Capacity. The 1976 Karen Ann Quinlan case[5] involved a 22-year-old woman who was in a persistent vegetative state. Her father, who had been appointed her legal guardian, requested that mechanical ventilation be withdrawn, asserting that she would not have wanted to be kept alive under such circumstances. Her physicians refused to comply. The case was ultimately decided by the New Jersey Supreme Court, which evaluated "the reasonable possibility of return to cognitive and sapient life as distinguished from … biological vegetative existence."[5] The decision indicated that advanced life support provided a clear benefit to the patient only if it would result in "at very least, a remission of symptoms enabling a return toward a normal functioning, integrated existence." The court thus ruled that life support could be withdrawn from patients if they had essentially no chance of regaining any reasonable quality of life.

The New Jersey Supreme Court's ruling based Ms. Quinlan's right to have the ventilator removed on her constitutional right to privacy. In the absence of any indication from the patient herself of her preferences or values, the court found that the family and physicians were entitled to exercise substituted judgment on the patient's behalf, with the family's decision taking precedence over that of the physicians.

The major challenge in cases like Quinlan involving patients lacking decision-making capacity is deciding who is the appropriate decision maker. While state courts have consistently recognized the right of patients to refuse treatment, including medically supplied nutrition and hydration, they have been much less consistent about the question of how decisions should be made for patients who cannot decide for themselves. States that allow surrogate decisions in the absence of clear and convincing evidence about what the patient would have wanted have tended to follow a standard of either substituted judgment or best interest. The substituted judgment standard allows a surrogate to make one's best judgment about what the patient would have decided if the patient had decision-making capacity. The best interest standard applies when it remains unclear what the patient would have decided. In this eventuality, the surrogate and the medical team base the decision on the weighing of benefits and harms related to each treatment option.

The concept of proportionate treatment can help guide best-interest decision making: "Proportionate treatment is that which, in the view of the patient, has at least a reasonable chance of providing benefits to the patient, which benefits outweigh the burdens attendant to the treatment. Thus, even if a proposed course of treatment might be extremely painful or intrusive, it would still be proportionate treatment if the prognosis was for complete cure or significant improvement in the patient's condition. On the other hand, a treatment course which is only minimally painful or intrusive may nonetheless be considered disproportionate to the potential benefits if the prognosis is virtually hopeless for any significant condition."[40]

Many states have codified the substituted judgment standard, enacting laws that give families the right to make decisions on behalf of patients lacking decision-making capacity. For patients who did not identify a surrogate decision maker before they lost decision-making capacity, most states identify a hierarchy among relatives so that it is relatively clear who the decision maker should be. Most of these statutes, however, apply only to patients who are terminally ill.[41]

It is important to recognize that, from a legal and ethical perspective, no distinction is made between nutrition and hydration provided through a medical device (such as a gastrostomy or nasogastric tube or intravenous line) and other forms of life-sustaining treatment such as mechanical ventilation. As one California case ruled, "… medical procedures to provide nutrition and hydration are more similar to other medical procedures than to typical human ways of providing nutrition and hydration. Their benefits and burdens ought to be evaluated in the same manner as any other medical procedure."[40]

A different problem arises for persons who have never had decision-making capacity because they have never been in a condition in which they could meaningfully indicate what level of health care they would want if they were critically ill. Such patients include young children and persons with severe intellectual disability. Different states have dealt with this problem differently. Some have ruled that the right to refuse medical treatment must extend to incompetent patients, because human dignity has value for them just as for those who have decision-making capacity and that, therefore, legal guardians or conservators have the right to make such decisions on behalf of their wards.[42] In such cases, some courts have opined that decisions about foregoing treatment from patients who have never been competent should be based on an attempt to "ascertain the incompetent person's actual interests and preferences."[43] In other words, the decision should be that which the patient would make if the patient were competent but able to take into account one's actual incompetency. Other courts have ruled that it is unrealistic to try to determine what a patient who had never been competent would have wanted, and that, for legal purposes, such patients are like children.[44] Some courts have specifically rejected the substituted judgment standard, finding that a third party should not have the power to make quality-of-life judgments on another's behalf.

Many legal issues regarding the termination of life-sustaining treatment remain unresolved. The courts have given essentially no guidance around whether physicians have the authority to terminate life support for patients lacking decision-making capacity against the wishes of the patient's family. In general, the courts have respected physicians' rights to refuse to provide treatments that are judged to be medically inappropriate, but the applicability has yet to be established. In most cases involving attempts by hospitals or physicians to use a futility argument to justify foregoing life-sustaining treatment requested or demanded by patients or their family, the courts have ruled in favor of continuing treatment.[45]

Advance Directives

Since the *Quinlan* decision,[5] state legislatures and the federal government have passed laws designed to increase the authority of individuals to control the level of treatment they want to receive when they are incapable of participating in decision making. These laws set standards for several types of documents but primarily for living wills and medical powers of attorney (MPA). Collectively, these documents are known as written advance directives. These documents usually have legal standing only within the state where they are completed and only if they conform to the state's statutory language, although some states grant some degree of validity to other states' advance directives. These documents can assist loved ones and health care professionals in determining what an individual would have wanted, especially if the patient is an irreversible condition such as a terminal illness or a persistent vegetative state. Health care providers can play a key role in encouraging patients to engage in advance care planning that culminates in completion of written advance directives.

Living Wills and Medical Powers of Attorney. Living wills indicate what level of life support and other medical treatments patients would want under specified circumstances. The specific forms of treatment covered by living wills vary among states and are sometimes restricted to life-sustaining treatments. Some state laws specifically exclude medically supplied nutrition and hydration from the treatments that can be withheld or withdrawn. With the exception of Missouri, however, state courts have ruled that these exclusions refer only to nonmedical feedings.[46] The requirement that living wills provide for a wide range of unforeseeable eventualities forces the documents to be general in nature and hence limits their usefulness.[6,47] For example, Walker and colleagues, in their study of 102 elderly persons in Florida, found both that there was a wide range of resuscitation status preferences among patients who had completed living wills and that the language of the living wills was too vague in most cases to determine their preferences.[48]

MPAs provide more flexibility than living wills because they name a surrogate decision maker who is authorized to make health care decisions on the patient's behalf if the patient loses decision-making capacity. The advantage of an MPA lies in the authority it grants the designated agent to make decisions based on the specific details of the patient's circumstances and condition. Unfortunately, studies have found that spouses and other close family members are often inaccurate at predicting what their loved one would want.[49] In addition, both living wills and MPAs are limited by the well-documented fact that patients' desires to receive aggressive medical care can change over time.[50–52] What level of care a healthy person imagines wanting during a hypothetical illness may be very different from what that person wants when ill.[50] On the one hand, as patients grow increasingly ill, they may be willing to settle for an ever lower quality of life. On the other hand, when facing a long illness, they also may grow weary of hospitalization and invasive or otherwise burdensome medical procedures or treatments and decline treatment that they previously thought they would have wanted.

Patient Self-Determination Act. The U.S. federal government encouraged the use of advance directives when it enacted the 1990 Patient Self-Determination Act (PSDA).[53] The law requires hospitals, long-term care facilities and other health care institutions to (1) provide patients with written information regarding advance directives and their right to accept or refuse treatment; (2) document in patients' medical records whether advance directives have been completed; and (3) provide education about advance directives for patients, their families, and the facility's staff. Health care institutions failing to follow the PSDA may

have their federal Medicare and Medicaid reimbursements withheld. Despite this legislation, however, studies in the 1990s reported that only a minority of hospitalized patients had their advance directives acknowledged and that physicians were usually unaware of them when their patients with life-threatening illness preferred not to be resuscitated.[54,55] A study of hospitalized patients with life-threatening diagnoses found that fewer than 50% of physicians knew when their patients did not want to receive cardiopulmonary resuscitation (CPR). However, the proportion of elderly Americans who have completed advance directives is reported to have increased.[56]

Deciding to Withhold or Withdraw Life Support

Physicians withhold or withdraw life support in two general circumstances: (1) when the patient or the patient's surrogate refuses further treatment or (2) when the physician of record determines that further treatment is medically futile or inappropriate. Ideally, such momentous decisions by physicians will be based on individual patient preferences and objective medical information. However, studies of ICU health care professionals found that personal characteristics of physicians are significantly associated with their decision making about withholding or withdrawing life support.[57–60] These factors include age, religion, number of years since graduation, amount of time spent in clinical practice, level and type of specialization, and type of hospital and number of ICU beds where the physician works. Moreover, in the study by Cook and colleagues,[58] in which ICU health care professionals chose an appropriate level of care for 12 patient scenarios, there was extreme variability among clinicians' decisions: in only 1 of the 12 scenarios did more than half of the respondents make the same choice and opposite extremes of treatment were chosen by more than 10% of the respondents in 8 of the 12 cases. That physicians' personal characteristics influence their decision making should not be surprising; rather, it should caution against intransigence and remind physicians of their own potential biases and of the likelihood that other equally competent professionals may disagree with their decisions. Moreover, these findings reemphasize the importance of ascertaining patients' values and preferences; if life support decisions can be significantly influenced by physicians' personal characteristics, leading to physicians disagreeing on appropriate levels of treatment, then decision making should be based on the values and desires of the individual patient.

One challenge in end-of-life decisions is the uncertainty associated with predicting patient outcomes. The common use of the word *futility* implies that there exist accurate tools for identifying which patients are likely to improve or recover. However, despite the existence of multiple prognostic and severity scoring systems useful in predicting aggregated group outcomes, foreseeing the outcome of individual patients remains an inexact science.[61] Hence, in most ICU cases, *futility* remains an ephemeral and ill-defined concept requiring physicians to depend on their clinical judgments to determine when further treatment has virtually no chance to return the patient to a reasonable quality of life.

There is a broad consensus among medical societies, critical care physicians, and ethicists that withdrawing and withholding life support do not differ ethically from one another.[6,9,11,62–64] Nonetheless, physician surveys have repeatedly found that many physicians feel differently about the two actions.[65–67] Withdrawing a life-sustaining intervention, especially if the patient dies soon afterward, may feel more like causing death than withholding that same intervention. However, because the two actions of withholding and withdrawing share the same justification, motivation, and end result, there is no moral basis for differentiating them. Indeed, physicians are in a stronger position to assert that they have "tried everything" through time-limited trials to save the patient when withdrawing interventions than when declining to initiate a life-saving intervention in the first place.

Withholding and Withdrawing Basic Life Support. Denying basic life support (e.g., medically supplied nutrition and hydration, oxygen) represents a challenging step in medicine. Whereas more advanced life support may be viewed as "heroic" or "extraordinary," basic life support is simply that which everyone depends on to live; it may not appear to be part of medicine so much as part of normal human existence. Allowing a patient to die of malnutrition or dehydration may even seem like murder to some physicians. However, as noted previously, state courts have generally concluded that medically supplied nutrition and hydration are akin to other medical treatments. Ethicists[68–70] and medical societies have likewise generally denied an ethical distinction between terminating advanced and basic life support, although there has been some disagreement with this position.[71] Nonetheless, denying a patient without decision-making capacity medically supplied nutrition and hydration remains ethically and legally controversial.[72] Physicians should be familiar with their own state's laws and legal precedents; hospital attorneys can be of assistance in this regard. As always, the problem lies in identifying the patient's preferences when the patient cannot decide.

Whatever their personal views, clinicians should consider four major points. First, any medical intervention should serve what the patient considers to be in one's best interest as determined by open and forthright communication with the patient and the patient's family and loved ones. Second, close family members and loved ones should be included in the decision-making process. This not only serves to protect the best interests of the patient but to help prevent conflict regarding the course of treatment chosen. Third, physicians should anticipate the range of different medical courses that the patient is likely to follow and determine what the patient would want done for each predicted development. This anticipation makes possible a coherent medical plan that facilitates goal-centered decision making and that does not need to be reconceptualized with every change in the patient's condition. Finally, physicians often find that withdrawing a life-sustaining intervention is psychologically more troubling than withholding it. While this can never serve as justification for withholding treatment, it emphasizes the desirability of not starting interventions without a thoughtful evaluation of whether they are consonant with the patient's best interests.

If the patient or the patient's family wants everything done to prolong the patient's life and these wishes appear inappropriate, a direct, logical challenge to such expressed wishes will often fail, whereas a nonjudgmental and compassionate exploration of underlying feelings will often result in more reasonable decisions. In the rare event that a family's decisions appear clearly at odds with the patient's best interests, physicians must remember that their first responsibility is to care for the patient.

Withholding Advanced Life Support. The major difference between withholding and withdrawing advanced life support concerns the context in which the decision is made. A decision to withhold these treatments generally takes the form of a DNR order. Unlike other medical treatments, patients are presumed to have consented to CPR unless they have specifically refused it. Because CPR must be attempted immediately to increase the likelihood of being effective, physicians and patients should make resuscitation status decisions prior to the need for CPR. Thus, the patient or surrogate should be asked to make decisions about treatments that may or may not become necessary during the patient's hospital stay. Conversely, the decision to withdraw advanced life support involves treatments already in place; thus, no hypothetical reasoning is necessary.

In discussing resuscitation status with patients, physicians have a responsibility to convey an understanding of what is involved in CPR and mechanical ventilation, the probability of survival to hospital discharge if CPR is attempted, the near certainty of death if CPR is withheld and why the physician does or does not recommend a DNR order. Physicians should stress that, regardless of resuscitation status, all other treatments and care will continue as previously planned. Limits are being set, but a DNR order does not mean that the medical team is giving up on or abandoning the patient. Determining a patient's resuscitation status represents an essential part of providing responsible care to critically ill patients, yet studies continue to show that communication about this issue remains very poor and most physicians do not know their patients' preferences.[55] Research has demonstrated that physicians and family members cannot accurately predict patient preferences; thus, there is no substitute for talking with patients.[73,74]

Several major impetuses have focused increased attention on determining patients' resuscitation status preferences, including studies showing poor post-CPR survival, an increased emphasis on patient autonomy and the right to refuse treatment, and growing concern about wasteful health care expenditures. Many studies have examined post-CPR survival, with 5% to 25% of patients surviving to discharge.[75–79] Of note for the CICU, patients resuscitated from ventricular arrhythmias, including ventricular fibrillation after myocardial infarction, have fared significantly better, with up to 50% surviving to discharge. Karetzky and colleagues' study of CPR survival in ICU and non-ICU patients found that resuscitation was successful for only 3% of ICU patients receiving CPR, compared with 14% of non-ICU patients.[80]

CPR, especially in the ICU setting, is an invasive and frequently brutal intervention that can be justified only if it has a reasonable chance of benefiting patients and if it is in accord with patient wishes. Judgments of reasonableness must be informed by patient values and preferences, because this is a subjective determination: a 5% chance of survival to discharge may be acceptable to some patients but not to others. For patients to make informed decisions, they require clear and accurate information about the probability of survival.[81] Two surveys of more than 200 elderly patients found that respondents consistently overestimated the likelihood of survival to discharge following CPR; in one of the studies, the overestimation was by 300% or more.[82,83] Both studies found that patients' decisions to accept or refuse CPR was strongly influenced by the probability of surviving to discharge. In the second study, Murphy and colleagues[83] found that the percentage of elderly patients who said they would opt for CPR following cardiac arrest during an acute illness fell from 41% to 22% after they were informed of the probability of survival.

Considering the limited effectiveness of CPR and given the evidence that most elderly patients assert that they would not want CPR under many circumstances, there can be little ethical justification for not discussing CPR with this patient population. Patients should also be asked what they would want done following a successful resuscitation if, after 72 hours of aggressively sustaining their lives, physicians determine that they have little or no chance to regain a reasonable quality of life. To avoid conflict, physicians should include patients' loved ones in these discussions and should ensure that there is consensus among the various members of the medical team. For patient resuscitation status decisions to be respected, they must be documented in a readily accessible location in the medical record. Health care institutions using electronic medical records (EMR) have an opportunity for immediate access to resuscitation status documentation if DNR orders are placed in a prominent place in the EMR. Physicians who feel that they cannot participate in resuscitation status decision making probably should not provide care for critically ill patients.

Many physicians find discussions about resuscitation status with patients difficult. Time limitations, stress, and the emotional difficulty of such discussions all contribute to this problem. These conversations become particularly challenging when terminally ill patients wish to have CPR attempted despite their physician's counsel that death is imminent or that CPR will not be effective. When such conflicts arise, thoughtful and empathic communication can lead to a mutually acceptable resolution. Humans are endowed with a strong will to live; it is not surprising that even chronically and terminally ill patients find it difficult to accept death. When patients will not consent to a DNR order, they often will agree to having life support withdrawn if, after a successful resuscitation, the physician determines that the patient has virtually no chance of regaining a reasonable quality of life as defined by the patient's values.

The most contentious DNR problem centers on the question of medical futility. Can physicians write DNR orders contrary to patients' or surrogates' wishes when physicians judge that CPR would be medically futile? This is a complex dilemma in which ethical principles and duties are in conflict (e.g., patient autonomy, nonmaleficence, professional integrity). Moreover, as noted previously, futility in medicine remains a term without a widely accepted definition.[24–26] In the literature regarding DNR orders written against patient wishes, two basic points of view emerge. Some have argued that determining what range of treatments to offer a patient must remain the physician's prerogative. When a physician determines that a certain therapy should be withheld because it is futile (i.e., because it has no reasonable

likelihood of benefiting the patient), then the patient's preferences become irrelevant. This position asserts that physicians have the professional responsibility to judge whether a specific medical intervention has what the physician considers to be a reasonable chance of benefiting the patient.[84]

Opponents of this perspective argue that determinations of what is reasonable and what constitutes a benefit is a subjective judgment that reflects the decision maker's underlying values.[28,85] In this view, the value judgment of what constitutes an acceptable likelihood of offering a meaningful benefit is best made by the patient. This second perspective argues for a physiologic definition of futility by which a treatment is futile only if it cannot achieve its immediate physiologic objective. Waisel and Truog write: "CPR is futile only if it is impossible to do cardiac massage and ventilations. As long as circulation and gas exchange are occurring, CPR is not futile, even if no one expects improvement in the patient's condition."[85]

Hospitals have adopted different policies regarding futility-based DNR orders, with some requiring physiologic futility and others allowing physicians greater leeway. The states of New York and Missouri have enacted statutes that specifically require a patient's consent or the consent of the patient's surrogate (when the patient lacks decision-making capacity) before a DNR order may be written. In contrast, Texas's Advance Directives Act allows health care facilities to discontinue life-sustaining treatment if the hospital's ethics committee agrees with the patient's physicians that the treatment is medically futile.[29,86] The issue of how to respond to patients who demand futile medical treatment is drawing increased attention in the context of rapidly rising health care costs and the difficulty many Americans have accessing care.

In resolving individual cases of conflict about appropriate levels of treatment, health care professionals should use both clinical judgment and a clear consideration of patients' values and expressed goals. Assertions of medical futility must not be employed as a means of avoiding difficult discussions with patients and their loved ones. Before writing a DNR order contrary to a patient's wishes, a physician must communicate this intention to the patient and family and allow them the opportunity, if possible and safe, to transfer to a physician or institution willing to honor their wishes. It also is essential for physicians to be aware of their state's laws and their hospital's specific policy for handling such cases.

Withdrawing Advanced Life Support. The withdrawal of advanced life support is usually followed quickly by death. Therefore, it is one of the most anguishing medical decisions for patients, loved ones, nurses, and physicians. When physicians have discussed life support and critical care preferences with their patients in advance and developed an appreciation of the patient's goals and quality-of-life values, decisions about whether to withdraw life support are often much clearer and less conflictual. There are no strict guidelines for deciding how or when to withdraw advanced life support, although many position papers have been published.[7,9,64,87] In general terms, life support is withdrawn when a patient has virtually no chance of regaining a reasonable quality of life or when the burdens of continued treatment outweigh the benefits. Withdrawal is usually considered only for patients who have terminal and irreversible conditions, but there are exceptions. Each patient must be evaluated in terms of the specific clinical context and the patient's expressed values and wishes. Patients and their families have a right to know the best and most current data regarding the patient's condition and prognosis and the efficacy of available treatments. Outcome prediction studies[88] can be helpful, but physicians should not exaggerate medicine's ability to make predictions about individual patients.

Patients on mechanical ventilators should not be presumed to lack decision-making capacity. To be judged as having decision-making capacity, patients must be able to appreciate their circumstances and their condition, understand the respective consequences of accepting or rejecting recommended treatments, demonstrate rational decision making, and articulate a choice.[89] Psychiatric consultation may be useful when decision-making capacity is questionable. For a patient to give informed consent for the withdrawal of life support, all narcotics must have been discontinued long enough for the patient to be clear-headed and any treatable depression must have been clinically addressed.

Although most patients on advanced life support lack decision-making capacity, some do not. Physicians must make a rigorous effort to solicit the patient's wishes concerning the continuation or withdrawal of treatment. Patients with decision-making capacity who wish to have life support withdrawn must be carefully evaluated. They have an ethical and legal right, as noted previously, to refuse medical treatments, even if these treatments are necessary to maintain life. Conversely, some patients on advanced life support often suffer severe reactive depressions and, if they survive their critical illness, are grateful that their requests to discontinue life support were not honored. Hence, evaluating patient requests and refusals can be extremely difficult. When patients with curable illnesses request that life support be withdrawn, physicians should vigorously reevaluate the patient's decision-making capacity.

When considering the withdrawal of advanced life support, physicians should always seek unanimity among the members of the health care team and actively solicit members' opinions. Nurses spend more time with ICU patients than anyone else, and their long hours at the bedside can give them valuable information and insights, especially regarding areas such as family dynamics and the range of the patient's alertness or discomfort over the course of the day. Problems can develop when any professional feels excluded from the decision-making process.

Withdrawing life support is a stressful proposition, and decision making by patients and family members cannot be rushed. The negotiations represent delicate processes that have their own timing, integrally involved with coming to accept the inevitability of death and loss. As discussed previously, facilitators can assist in these situations. When patients lack decision-making capacity, physicians should engage family members and patient surrogates to work toward consensus on all life support decisions.

When there is conflict between the family and medical team, establishing time-limited goals based on clinical judgment and outcome studies can facilitate resolution. Families often feel overwhelmed when advised that life support should be withdrawn. They frequently experience grief, guilt, anger, and confusion—and

they may resist the physician's advice. Identification of concrete temporal milestones by which progress can be evaluated often helps facilitate the development of acceptance and coping. For example, family members might be told, "If we see no signs of improvement over the next 72 hours, then we believe you should consider withdrawing life support. We believe your loved one is suffering and has essentially no chance to regain any reasonable quality of life. To withdraw life support would allow your loved one a more peaceful and dignified death."

Time-limited goals serve the function of providing perspective. They remind the family to step back from day-to-day management concerns and consider the overall circumstances. The interlude provided by these goals also allows families and loved ones an opportunity to adjust what may have been unrealistic expectations of recovery and to express pent-up emotions. Physicians must be able to tolerate expressions of anger or hostility without becoming defensive or withdrawing. The anger usually subsides when the family understands that the physician is compassionate, supportive, and understanding.

When proposing that life support be discontinued, communication skills are centrally important. One effective approach is to say, "It is my best judgment, and that of the other doctors and nurses, that your loved one has virtually no chance to regain a reasonable quality of life. We believe that life support should be withdrawn, which means your relative will probably die." This statement contains two important components: it is qualified in a way that acknowledges uncertainty and encourages shared decision making; it also clearly states that death is the anticipated result of withdrawing treatment. Without such information, true informed consent cannot be achieved.

At times of critical illness, grief-stricken or guilty family members may press for disproportionate treatment to relieve their own distress. An open and understanding exploration of the underlying feelings usually resolves such difficulties. Sometimes an honest disagreement persists: what seems disproportionate to the physician seems reasonable to the family. Several guidelines can help in such circumstances: (1) the physician's primary responsibility is to the patient; (2) in most cases, the family has the patient's best interests at heart and knows the patient better than the medical team; (3) ethicists, chaplains, social workers, and ethics committee members can assist in facilitating an agreement on the treatment plan; and (4) care can sometimes be transferred to a physician who agrees to comply with the family's wishes.

Health care professionals should avoid direct involvement in cases that conflict with their ethical values. Clinical judgment may be compromised by the tension and resentment that can arise in such circumstances. If possible, treatment and care should be transferred to another physician in these situations. When such involvement is unavoidable, the physician's disclosure of his or her own feelings to understanding colleagues or a psychotherapist make optimal care more likely.

Patients lacking decision-making capacity who have left no indication of quality-of-life values or life support preferences can present special challenges. In such circumstances, physicians must be familiar with their hospital's policies, state's laws, and legal precedents concerning substituted medical judgments. If a thorough discussion of the patient with family and loved ones fails to yield sufficient information about the patient's values, the hospital ethics committee should engage a multidisciplinary group composed of physicians, nurses, patient advocates (e.g., a social worker, chaplain, or ombudsman) and the patient's family or loved ones. The group can then negotiate decisions based on the patient's best interests. Legal recourse rarely becomes necessary.

When implementing a decision to withdraw life support, the emphasis should be to maximize patient comfort and minimize emotional trauma to the family and loved ones. Whereas curtailing inotropic support may not result in distress, withdrawing mechanical ventilation can present the potential for extreme discomfort, especially if the patient is abruptly extubated and experiences airway obstruction. We advocate rapidly dialing down the supplemental oxygen, pressure support and intermittent mandatory ventilation (IMV) rate while maintaining a protected airway. Air hunger and anxiety should be controlled with intravenous morphine as necessary.[90]

CROSS-CULTURAL CONFLICT

To achieve maximum potential as physicians, patients' cultural values and beliefs must be understood to appreciate what their illness signifies to them and what they want from physicians.[91] Cultural patterns have great influence on how individuals and families view illness, medicine, dying and death, and on their behavioral response during periods of critical illness. People facing death tend to fall back on their traditional cultural or religious beliefs.[92] It is increasingly common that health care providers in the United States find themselves in cross-cultural situations, confronted with the cultural dimensions of ethical decision making. Cross-cultural ethical issues in medicine have received increasing attention since the mid-1980s and there has been growing acceptance within the medical community that bioethics is, at least in part, culturally determined.[93–99] This means that ethical decision making in medicine depends on the specific cultural context in which the decision is being made and that the ethical principles that Anglo-Americans hold dear may seem unimportant to people from other societies.

Anglo-American bioethics accords paramount status to the individual, underscoring the principles of individual rights, autonomy, and self-determination in decisions regarding health care. The fundamental ethical principle of patient autonomy has its basis in Western philosophy as well as in American cultural values that emphasize liberty, privacy, and individual rights. The central importance of individuals maintaining control over their body translates into the right to accept or refuse medical interventions. For individuals to be able to make medical decisions, they require an accurate understanding of their medical condition and any proposed treatments; thus, truth telling and informed consent are also stressed in Western medical ethics. Knowledge and understanding form the basis of informed consent and autonomous decision making.[100]

Many other cultures view human identity in profoundly different ways, with much less emphasis on the individual. Many cultures have more relational understandings of human identity (i.e., persons are defined by their relationships to others rather than by their characteristics as individuals) and the Western emphasis on individual rights and autonomy may not make sense to them.[101] Respecting communal or familial hierarchies is more important in some cultures than asserting individual autonomy. It is not that the interests of the family outweigh the interests of the individual; rather, the individual is conceived of primarily as a member of a family. The responsibility to show filial duty and protect the elderly may be what the family views as the most important factor in the care of terminally ill patients.

The most common source of medical conflict resulting from these relational value systems concerns the disclosure of terminal diagnoses and negative prognostic information; many cultures object to informing patients of terminal diagnoses, especially diagnoses of cancer. A 1995 study of different ethnic groups' attitudes toward patient autonomy found that Korean-Americans and Mexican-Americans generally believed that patients should not be told about terminal diagnoses and that the family, not the patient, should make life-support decisions. European-Americans and African-Americans, by comparison, were more likely to favor full disclosure and patient participation in decision making.[102,103] The objection to disclosing distressing information stems from several different beliefs. Some Asian cultures view the sick person as needing protection, like children. Telling patients upsetting diagnoses, from this perspective, only adds to their suffering, whereas healthy family members are in a stronger position to bear the bad news and make appropriate decisions. In addition, some cultures often view telling individuals that they are dying as bad luck, much like a curse.[102]

When a family does not want a patient to know about a diagnosis, physicians face a difficult ethical dilemma, because patient autonomy and the need for informed consent are central to American medical ethics and jurisprudence. From a legal standpoint, courts have ruled that physicians should not be liable for honoring a patient's specific request not to disclose information.[104,105] Regarding issues of autonomy, Gostin[101] and Pellegrino[97] both argue that patients have the right to use their autonomy to choose not to be informed.

In the end, physicians must determine for themselves how to negotiate conflicts between their own value systems and those of their patients. It is not reasonable to assert that physicians should strive to follow basic ethical principles and then claim that it is acceptable to toss these principles aside when they conflict with a patient's values. When conflict arises, open communication is essential; a willingness to accommodate can serve all parties well. For such culturally conflictual situations, Freedman has proposed a strategy of "offering truth" to the patient rather than "forcing truth."[106] Using this strategy, a physician would ascertain directly from the patient how much the patient wants to know about test results, diagnosis, and prognosis; the patient's expressed wishes would then be honored. At the very least, physicians should remain sensitive to cultural differences and maintain an open-minded and respectful attitude about other cultural beliefs and practices. Physicians should remember that a family's cultural background can be a source of tremendous strength during the crisis of critical illness; violating a patient's cultural mores should be avoided whenever possible.

In striving to understand a patient's cultural background, the pitfall of stereotyping must be avoided. Within a given culture, there can be great variation among individuals; thus, there is no substitute for talking directly to patients and their families to determine their cultural values and beliefs. Among patients who are immigrants, patients and their family frequently span more than one generation, with different levels of retention of traditional cultural practices. Hence, it is important to note the contribution of various elements in the cultural fabric, such as socioeconomics, education, and degree of acculturation. The role of culture must be seen in context with other factors that come into play in a patient's decision making or behavior, such as economic considerations and individual attributes. Culture is only one component in a complex matrix of influences.

CONCLUSION

The two major goals of CICU physicians are to save salvageable patients and to facilitate a peaceful and dignified death for those who are dying. The difficulty of achieving certainty and consensus regarding in which of these two categories an individual patient belongs leads to challenging ethical issues. These issues are best approached in an ordered and thoughtful manner. Whether the issue is a family insisting on treatment that the physician believes is futile or a ventilator-dependent patient requesting that life support be withdrawn, thinking ethically about these situations by being attentive to the four basic ethical principles (autonomy, beneficence, nonmaleficence, and distributive justice), by calculating consequences and by using casuistry can facilitate a thorough analysis and help to resolve disagreements. In addition, four guidelines provide a procedural approach to ethical problems: (1) respect the role of patients as partners, (2) determine who has authority to make health care decisions for the patient, (3) establish effective communication with the patient and family, and (4) determine in an ongoing manner the patient's quality-of-life values and desires.

From an ethical and legal perspective, patients with decision-making capacity have a clearly established right to refuse medical treatments. Although some physicians may object to withholding or withdrawing life-sustaining treatment, patients have a clear and incontestable right to refuse life support and other treatments, even when such refusal results in their death. Providing treatment against a competent patient's refusal can constitute battery. At the same time, patients do not have the right to demand specific treatments; only the physician can decide what therapies are appropriate to offer to a patient. The authority for decision making becomes less clear with legally incompetent patients; different states have different judicial precedents and laws concerning when treatment must be provided and how life-sustaining treatment may be withdrawn from incompetent patients. Some states allow family members to provide substituted judgment for incompetent patients, whereas others require clear and convincing evidence that the patient, before becoming incompetent, had indicated wanting life support to be withdrawn. Patients can protect their ability to help determine what types of medical care they receive by engaging in advance care planning and documenting their wishes in living wills or, preferably, medical powers of attorney.

Decisions about withholding or withdrawing life support occur frequently in CICUs and they are a painful and difficult process for many physicians. The essential principle in these decisions is that end-of-life decision making must reflect the individual patient's goals and quality-of-life values. At the same time, physicians are not obliged to provide futile treatments.

Good communication skills are the most powerful tool in ethical conflicts. When questions about life and death are treated in a patient, nonjudgmental and sensitive manner, ethical conflicts arise less often and tend not to become as intractable. Physicians should encourage patients, families, and other members of the health care team to express their thoughts and feelings about difficult cases. Whenever possible, decision making should take place by means of consensus. The following cases illustrate ethical dilemmas and options for handling them.

CASE 1

A 29-year-old man with a history of tricuspid valve replacement 2 years ago due to infective endocarditis (IE) secondary to intravenous drug use (IVDU) is transferred from an outside hospital. He presented with fever due to prosthetic valve endocarditis (PVE) and admits to relapse into drug use despite rehabilitative care. The outside hospital refuses to do a second valve replacement and transfers the patient to an alternative hospital willing to consider one.

The ethical conflict in this case is the appropriateness of a repeat tricuspid valve replacement for an intravenous drug user with IE and a high risk of recidivism. This case also illustrates the use of Beauchamp and Childress's four principles in evaluating difficult ethical problems.[19] The principles supporting the position of not offering a repeat valve replacement include justice and nonmaleficence. This patient has a high risk of relapse and a third PVE, supporting the opinion that a second operation is "futile" in that it will simply get infected yet again. For this reason, the outside hospital recommends treatment with long-term intravenous antibiotics as the best strategy in this complex case, given the patient's noncompliance with his rehabilitative treatment program. Health care policy analysts would also cite that we have a duty of stewardship of scarce medical resources that promote expansion of access to health care, especially when the insurance is Medicaid. The outside hospital surgical team also argues they have an obligation not to subject the patient to the higher risk of surgery, and they need to consider risks to the surgery team, such as the risk of hepatitis C associated with accidental needlestick injuries.

That said, the strongest principle in support of proceeding with surgery is beneficence: clinicians have a duty and obligation to provide the best care to our patients regardless of circumstances. Justice also argues that we treat everyone the same, whether it is an IVDU in need of a repeat valve replacement or a smoker with poor dietary habits in need of a second coronary artery bypass procedure after 2 years. It is not the clinician's place to judge patients or treat them differently for past moral failing or legal trouble, which remains in the purview of our justice system or other societal institutions. Clinicians are in no position to punish patients for their self-destructive or socially undesirable behavior by withholding treatment.

What argument or principle is most persuasive? Several excellent articles discuss the ethical dilemmas in this type of case.[107–109]

CASE 2

A 56-year-old man has an uneventful aortic valve replacement and 3-vessel coronary artery bypass graft surgery. He is extubated 4 hours after the procedure and then experiences a witnessed cardiac arrest with ventricular tachycardia followed by ventricular fibrillation. Despite 25 minutes of uninterrupted advanced cardiac life support, including chest compressions, there is no return of spontaneous circulation. The surgical team decides to open the patient's chest and initiate venous-arterial extracorporeal membrane oxygenation (VA-ECMO) emergently without informing the patient's family.

The ability of EMCO to replace the function of the heart and lungs in rapid response to cardiac or pulmonary failure allows this technology to be used as a bridge to recovery, transplant, ventricular assist devices (VAD), or decision when the event is acute and prognosis uncertain. Given the expanding applications for ECMO with only limited evidence supporting its use, ethical issues are inevitable in the initiation and management of this therapy. The data for VA-ECMO for extracorporeal CPR (ECPR), acute cardiogenic shock, and as a bridge to transplantation are limited. The use of resource-intensive technology in the absence of data that support a direct benefit to the patient raises ethical issues on the acceptable use of expensive, unproven interventions and begs for a health care policy consensus. The argument that supports the use of ECPR in this patient is the fact that he underwent an elective open-heart surgery and had an uneventful procedure but then experienced an unexpected complication (coronary artery dissection).

Resuscitation continues while the patient is emergently placed on VA-ECMO and his oxygenation and hemodynamics are stabilized. Serial echocardiography examinations over the next 72 hours show no improvement in ventricular function and continuous renal replacement therapy is started using the ECMO circuit. Neurologic examination is negative for stroke but the patient remains poorly responsive, presumably owing to metabolic encephalopathy. The surgical team approaches the conflicted family members for consent on changing ECMO to a VAD after a week of maintenance on ECMO. They also discuss the potential for listing the patient for heart transplantation given his age and few comorbidities.

This case describes the use of ECPR as a bridge to decision when the prognosis remains uncertain. ECMO extends the boundaries of what we commonly consider the limits of cardiac resuscitation and now taxes the family to consider some difficult options. Furthermore, they are asked to make decisions for a patient who is intubated and incapacitated and to do so with limited understanding of the technology (VAD) and therapy (heart transplantation) being proposed. The discussion points in this case include reviewing the standards of substituted judgment in incapacitated patients versus best interest as well the responsibility of the clinical team to assist families in decision making under duress. A discussion on the use and benefits of shared decision making as a model for reducing conflicts and improving communication can also be discussed here. Several excellent articles discuss the ethical challenges of such cases.[110–112,114]

CASE 3

A 76-year-old man was diagnosed with American Heart Association (AHA) stage C ischemic heart failure 6 years ago. His symptoms have worsened over the intervening years despite maximal medical therapy and frequent hospitalizations and intubations for shortness of breath. He is readmitted to the hospital for the third time in 6 months with severe dyspnea, fatigue, and confusion. The clinical attending requests intubation for mechanical ventilation. However, the patient confides to the bedside nurse that he does not want to be on a ventilator again and only wants treatment to relieve his shortness of breath. He tells the nurse that he has had enough. When the nurse informs the clinical team, the attending refuses to consider the patient's request or the need for palliative care and a DNR order, pointing out that the patient is too ill to make an informed decision. The nurse's distress motivates her to consult the Clinical Ethics service because she believes the patient's wishes are not being respected.

Ethical dilemmas in end-of-life (EOL) care are numerous in the setting of end-stage heart failure. The prevailing ignorance of patients and caregivers about the high risk for death is compounded by the reluctance of health care providers to discuss the terminal condition of end-stage heart failure and assist their patients in EOL planning. Best practice in EOL care should include a discussion on values, goals, and preferences as well as exercise of Advanced Directives (ADs) in the event that a patient loses capacity for decision making. Advance directives include the living will (LW), in which a patient lists preferences about future treatments; a durable power of attorney for health care (DPAHC), in which a patient designates

a surrogate for making future health care decisions; and a combined AD, which includes both an LW and a DPAHC.

One of the most prominent challenges for ethically supportable decision making at the end-of-life stage in heart failure is poor or ineffective communication between patients and clinicians. This may be related to discomfort in addressing a terminal illness, inadequate training and education in discussing EOL, and uncertainty around when to broach the subject of EOL planning. In addition, there is also a lack of understanding in the roles of palliative care and hospice at EOL. Other EOL dilemmas in this case include moral distress among the nursing staff, evaluating capacity for decision making, DNR order and caring for a terminal patient who may or may not have an AD or surrogate decision maker.

In this case, the bioethical framing of the nurse's concern is that the patient's autonomy is being violated in that he is at risk of being subjected to a treatment that he does not want. Nonmaleficence could also be invoked if there is concern that the patient could be harmed by the burdens and suffering that can ensue from intubation and mechanical ventilation. The clinical team may feel that they can help the patient with aggressive life support by prolonging his life and thus cite the principle of beneficence. In this case, however, because patients have a legally established right to refuse care, the issue would boil down to whether the patient has decision-making capacity and, if not, determining what he would have wanted if he did. The ethical challenges of decision making in advanced heart failure are discussed in several excellent articles.[115–118]

CASE 4

A 45-year-old man develops cardiogenic shock after a myocardial infarction and undergoes emergency coronary artery bypass surgery at a community hospital. However, he remains in cardiogenic shock after separation from cardiopulmonary bypass; thus, the surgical team places the patient on VA-ECMO and sends him via ambulance to an affiliated tertiary care center for further management. The patient is in profound shock upon arrival despite maximal flows on VA-ECMO; an echocardiogram reveals a clot through the heart and pulmonary vessels. The patient is not expected to survive, nor is he a transplant candidate. He has no advance directive; thus, the clinical team recommends a DNR order to the family. The family refuses, expressing their anger that the patient is not considered for transplant and insists on continued resuscitation. Given the patient's underlying disease and superimposed irreversible multiple organ failure, the clinical team debates ordering a "unilateral DNR."

DNR orders are at the heart of the futility mystery, especially since CPR is a highly invasive, low-success procedure. This case raises the following questions:

1. What is the meaning of DNR and CPR when a patient is on VA-ECMO?
2. Should a DNR discussion be avoided in this situation or is the clinical team obligated to invoke a "unilateral DNR" order?
3. What are the objections to CPR in this patient besides futility and nonmaleficence?
4. What is the process for resolving conflicts between clinicians, patients, and surrogates in medically futile situations when there are cultural differences and distrust?

In many circumstances, ECMO may be able to provide sufficient cardiopulmonary support to avoid death in the setting of cardiogenic shock. In other cases, ECMO provides only partial support and organ failure continues to decline and becomes irreversible. In the context of irreversible organ failure with clot throughout the cardiopulmonary circulation, the ICU team sees CPR as harmful and disrespectful to a dying patient. Since CPR is a default option in the care of all patients who experience sudden death in US hospitals, clinicians must request patients and family to consent to DNR or DNAR (do not attempt resuscitation) orders when death is expected.

It is accepted that clinicians are not required to perform CPR when it is medically futile. However, one legal consequence of discontinued medical treatment that ends with a patient's death is the risk of legal action, including criminal prosecution. Clinicians are wise to seek agreement with patients and surrogates before writing a "unilateral DNR" order. Attempts to resolve conflicts between physicians, patients, and surrogates regarding futile treatments should be made by a procedural approach that includes safeguards to ensure that a patient's wishes are respected and protected. Writing a unilateral DNR order over the objection of surrogates and families should be reserved for exceptionally rare circumstances after attempts to resolve differences have been tried and exhausted. As always, clinicians must be familiar with relevant state and federal laws as well as hospital policies. Several key articles discuss the challenges in these types of cases.[119–122]

The full reference list for this chapter is available at ExpertConsult.com.

3

Physical Examination in the Cardiac Intensive Care Unit

Hal A. Skopicki, George Gubernikoff, David L. Brown

The trouble with doctors is not that they don't know enough, but that they don't see enough.

Sir Dominic J. Corrigan (1802–1880)

In the cardiac intensive care unit (CICU), the ubiquitous presence of advanced technology and highly sensitive laboratory assessments/testing has resulted in an overreliance on imaging and testing at the expense of the skills required to examine critically ill patients. Yet, at the moments of initial patient contact, acute decompensation, and serially after therapeutic interventions, the ability to integrate an outstanding physical evaluation into the diagnostic assessment of the patient remains critical. Since, in the words of William Osler, "Medicine is the art of uncertainty and the science of probability," the physical examination should be used in concert with laboratory analyses and diagnostic imaging, to limit the uncertainty and increase the probability of optimal patient care.

The ideal physical examination requires time, patience, a quiet room, and the ability to think and examine simultaneously. Although these elements are rarely present in the CICU setting, it is precisely through the tangle of electrocardiogram leads and intrusive sounds of pumps, cardiac monitors, ventilators, and conversations that well-prepared physicians can optimize the management of critically ill patients by focusing their senses and performing the physical examination to the best of their abilities.

GENERAL ASSESSMENT

The general assessment should include a broad evaluation of the patient's emotional status, appearance, and nonverbal cues. Although apprehension may be part of a patient's natural temperament, abrupt-onset or escalating anxiety should elicit serious diagnostic concern until acute and life-threatening processes (e.g., escalating ventricular arrhythmias, impeding pulmonary edema, crescendo angina, extension of a myocardial infarction [MI], aortic dissection) can be ruled out. Reassuring the patient may gain time for further investigation. A patient who needs to sit up to catch his or her breath suggests the presence of pulmonary edema or a large pleural effusion, whereas a patient who finds relief of chest pain while sitting up and leaning forward may have acute pericarditis. The inability to get comfortable in any position often occurs with abdominal and genitourinary disorders, such as cholecystitis, penetrating ulcers, nephrolithiasis, ischemic bowel, and colonic obstruction. Cachexia, with decreased generalized muscle mass or temporal muscle wasting, suggests long-standing disease and is often seen with heart failure, renal or hepatic failure, cancer, or nutritional disorders.

VITAL SIGNS

When asked to examine a critically ill patient, careful consideration of the vital signs is often the difference between successful and unsuccessful outcomes. Being called on to evaluate a patient who is acutely decompensated necessitates that the physician obtain vital signs that are current and accurate. "Tachycardia" can occur when a cardiac monitor inadvertently counts the T wave. Similarly, "hypotension" may be urgently reported only to reveal an improperly situated or sized blood pressure cuff.

A critical aspect of vital sign assessment is the evaluation of trends. A patient whose heart rate has increased from a consistent baseline of 60 to 70 beats/min to 100 beats/min should be a cause for concern, similar to a patient who appears with an initial heart rate greater than 120 beats/min. Likewise, a patient with a respiratory rate that has gone from 12 to 22 breaths/min should be considered as seriously as one who initially presents with acute tachypnea.

Temperature

Because core body temperature is carefully controlled within a narrow range, the detection of hyperthermia or hypothermia offers important clinical clues. Normal oral body temperature is approximately 37°C (98.6°F) with early morning temperatures approximately 1°C lower compared with later in the afternoon. By convention, fever is defined as an oral temperature greater than 38°C (> 100°F), although it is common practice to consider temperatures greater than 38.4°C (> 101.1°F) in hospitalized patients to be clinically significant (albeit without significant data to support this assumption).

Hyperthermia associated with infection (for patients not receiving negative chronotropic agents or with intrinsic cardiac conduction disease) should be accompanied by an increase in the pulse rate of approximately 8.5 beats/min for each 1°C increase (the Liebermeister rule).[1] The presence of a factitious fever can be suspected if there isn't a similar temperature elevation in voided urine compared with the oral temperature. Although a hot drink can quickly increase oral temperature up to 2°C, 5 minutes later the increase is only 0.3°C.[2]

The pattern of the fever spikes should also be assessed. Intermittent (returning to normal each day) can occur in septicemia and with abscesses; sustained (with minor daily variation [i.e., <0.3°C] suggesting gram-negative infections or pneumonia), remittent (varying > 0.3°C each day but not returning to normal, which occurs in infective endocarditis), and relapsing (febrile and afebrile days suggesting the Pel-Ebstein fever of Hodgkin disease or episodic cholangitis caused by a mobile common bile duct stone). Once-daily spikes (quotidian fever) occur with liver abscesses or acute cholangitis; twice-daily spikes (double quotidian fever) suggest gonococcal endocarditis. Prolonged fever despite antibiotic therapy can also occur with connective tissue disorders, drug fever, neoplasm, abscess, or antibiotic-resistant organisms and superinfection.

The presence of hypothermia (oral temperature <35°C [95°F]) requires confirmation. Drinking ice water reduces the oral temperature up to 0.6°C (1°F) for 5 minutes.[2] False-negative hypothermic readings can also occur with ear temperatures taken in the presence of cerumen and oral temperatures recorded in the presence of tachypnea. Confirmed hypothermia requires the assessment of a patient's temperature with a rectal thermometer (which averages approximately 0.6°C [1°F] higher than the oral temperature). The differential diagnosis of true hypothermia includes ambient cold exposure, submersion, hypothyroidism, hypoglycemia, sepsis, and adrenal insufficiency. With hypothermia from submersion or exposure, warming to room temperature is necessary for adequate assessment of end-organ and neurologic function.

Respiration

The respiratory effort, rate, and pattern should be assessed in ventilated and nonventilated patients. Accessory muscle use is common with pulmonary edema, chronic obstructive pulmonary disease (COPD), asthmatic exacerbations, and pneumonia. It may be detected visually or by palpation over the sternocleidomastoid or intercostal muscles. With acute tachypnea (a respiratory rate greater than 25 breaths/min), an immediate assessment should be performed to distinguish peripheral cyanosis (dusky or bluish tinge to the fingers and toes without mucosal or buccal changes) from central hypoxemia (associated with a bluish tinge to the lips or mucosa under the tongue). Peripheral cyanosis may occur with or without hypoxemia, such as in the case of severe peripheral vasoconstriction. This condition is accompanied by cold extremities and compromised capillary refill.

Tachypnea, when secondary to hypoxia, should nearly always be associated with a reflex tachycardia. Although resting tachypnea may occur with cardiopulmonary disease, it may also be present in response to fever, pain, anemia, hyperthyroidism, abdominal distention, respiratory muscle paralysis, obesity, or metabolic acidosis. When tachypnea accompanies chest pain or collapse, acute pulmonary embolism should be included in the differential diagnosis. When tachypnea is present with a history of orthopnea, it suggests the presence of pulmonary edema, pleural effusion, or both. When tachypnea is present in a patient being weaned from a ventilator, tachypnea predicts weaning failure.[3]

Hypopnea is defined as less than 10 shallow or slow breaths per minute. It may be due to severe cardiopulmonary failure, sepsis, central nervous system (CNS) depressants (e.g., sedative-hypnotics, narcotics, and alcohol), or CNS disease (e.g., cerebrovascular accident, meningitis). Hypopnea may also occur secondary to factors that limit inspiration, such as pericarditis, pleuritis, or postoperative pain.

Breathing patterns can reveal underlying pathology (Video 3.1, Table 3.1). While most causes of hypoxia usually result in shallow, rapid respirations, exaggerated deep and rapid respirations were noted by Kussmaul to imply the presence of diabetic ketoacidosis. Apneic episodes with snoring suggest obstructive sleep apnea, a potentially treatable contributor to hypertension, right heart failure, and atrial fibrillation. Cheyne-Stokes breathing, in which periods of waxing and waning tachypnea and hyperpnea alternate with apnea, occurs in various cardiac, neurologic, and pulmonary disorders or from simple oversedation. When Cheyne-Stokes breathing occurs in the setting of uremia or heart failure, it portends a poor prognosis. Biot breathing is characterized by irregularly irregular breaths of equal depth that are associated with periods of apnea. It can be seen in patients with intracranial disease affecting the medulla oblongata. More severe damage to the medulla oblongata results in ataxic respiration, the complete irregularity of breathing, with irregular pauses and increasing periods of apnea. As this breathing pattern deteriorates further, it merges with agonal respiration.

Orthopnea (shortness of breath while supine) is most commonly present in patients with heart failure and pleural effusion, but also can occur with ascites, morbid obesity, and diaphragmatic paralysis. Alternatively, platypnea (shortness of breath when assuming the upright position) suggests the right-to-left shunting that occurs with an atrial septal defect or intrapulmonary shunt. Trepopnea (shortness of breath while lying on one side) occurs with a right pleural effusion or with unilateral lung or diaphragm

TABLE 3.1	Breathing Patterns	
Respiratory Pattern	**Consider**	**Eponym/Classification**
Deep and rapid	Diabetic ketoacidosis	Kussmaul respiration
Snoring with episodic apnea	Obstructive sleep apnea	
Waxing and waning tachypnea/hypopnea alternating with apnea	Oversedation	Cheyne-Stokes breathing
	Heart failure	
	Severe CNS process	
	Respiratory failure	
	Renal disease (uremia)	
Irregularly irregular (yet equal) breaths alternating with periods of apnea	Damage to the medulla oblongata (intracranial disease)	Biot breathing
Completely irregular breaths (pauses with escalating periods of apnea)	Severe damage to the medulla oblongata	Ataxic respiration
No breaths or occasional gasps	Severe cardiovascular or neurologic disease	Agonal breathing

CNS, Central nervous system.

disease when the healthy lung is down.[4,5] Bendopnea, or shortness of breath when bending over, is a sign of heart failure.

Pulse

The pulse should be assessed bilaterally for presence, rate, volume, contour, and regularity. An initial examination should always contain a description of the radial and carotid arteries, in addition to the brachial, femoral, popliteal and pedal pulses. This examination is important for patients with hypotension, claudication, arterial insufficiency, or cerebrovascular accident and after intraaortic balloon pump insertion. Assessing the pulse for 30 seconds is more accurate than counting for only 15 seconds.[6]

A discrepancy in bilateral upper extremity pulses (especially with decreases in rate or volume on the left side) raises the possibility of aortic dissection, subclavian narrowing secondary to atherosclerosis, or congenital webs. If such a discrepancy is present, the examiner should search for evidence of a subclavian steal phenomenon, detected as a decrease in pulse amplitude after raising or exercising the affected arm for approximately 45 seconds (the left side is affected 70% of the time; the reduction in systolic blood pressure is >20 mm Hg 94% of the time).[7] Aortic dissection is suggested by the presence of a pulse deficit, focal neurologic signs, and mediastinal widening on the chest radiograph.[8] Diminished lower extremity pulses are consistent with coarctation of the aorta or atherosclerotic disease of the abdominal aorta and/or the arterial supply of the lower extremities. Although the detection of low femoral pulse amplitude (or its absence) is crucial for assessing the risk-to-benefit ratio in patients who may require vascular access or device implantation, its diminution or absence after catheterization or intraaortic balloon pump implantation requires urgent investigation.

When tachycardia (heart rate >100 beats/min) is present, the regularity of the rhythm offers important diagnostic clues. Regular rhythm rates between 125 beats/min and 160 beats/min suggest sinus tachycardia, the presence of atrial flutter with 2 : 1 block, or ventricular tachycardia. The presence of intermittent cannon A waves in the neck veins is highly sensitive, whereas a changing intensity of the first heart sound (S_1) is highly specific for the detection of ventricular tachycardia.[9] Atrial flutter may be accompanied by rapid undulations in the jugular venous pulse (flutter waves or F waves). Because sinus tachycardia may be due to correctable causes, such as hypovolemia, hypoxia, infection, hyperthyroidism, anemia, or anxiety, or may be due to the pathologic adaptation occurring with chronic heart failure or myocardial ischemia, integration of these clinical suspicions with the nature of the underlying rhythm is important. The use of vagal maneuvers may help differentiate the causes of narrow-complex tachycardia.

The Valsalva maneuver, performed by asking the patient to bear down as if "having a bowel movement" or pushing up the abdomen against the examiner's hand placed on the middle of the abdomen, may be more effective than carotid sinus massage, performed by pressing on the neck at the bifurcation of the carotid artery just below the angle of the jaw, at terminating supraventricular tachycardia.[10,11] Paroxysmal supraventricular tachycardia (nodal reentry and reciprocating tachycardias) may be interrupted with enhanced vagal tone. Sinus tachycardia, atrial flutter, and atrial fibrillation may slow only transiently (to reveal the underlying rhythm), although an abrupt halving of the rate can occur with atrial flutter. Detection of an irregular tachycardia on physical examination suggests atrial fibrillation, atrial premature beats, or ventricular premature contractions. In atrial fibrillation, assessment of the apical rate (counting heartbeats via auscultation) is more accurate than counting the radial pulse, accounting for a "pulse deficit."[12]

Bradycardia (heart rate <50 beats/min) may be appropriate in trained athletes, but should be asymptomatic and associated with a gradual increase in heart rate with exercise.[13] Detection of a regular bradycardia in a patient with fatigue, mental status changes, or evidence of impaired peripheral perfusion or pulmonary congestion raises the possibility of pharmacologic toxicity (i.e., digoxin, β-blockers, or calcium channel blockers), hypothermia (owing to hypothyroidism or exposure), or an atrioventricular nodal or ventricular escape rhythm that occurs with complete heart block or sick sinus syndrome.

Appreciation of the pulse volume and contour is also informative (Table 3.2). Tachycardia with a bounding pulse is present with septic shock (owing to the acute reduction in afterload), hyperthyroidism, or—in combination with the sudden collapse of the pulse—with chronic aortic insufficiency (a "water hammer"

TABLE 3.2 Pulse Characteristics

Pulse Description	Consider
Bounding	Septic shock, hyperthyroidism, chronic AI
Weak and thready	Severe LV dysfunction, hypovolemia, severe MR, complete heart block, pericardial effusion
Slow rising and weak	Severe AS
Alternating between strong and weak	LV dysfunction, pericardial tamponade
Double tap (pulsus bisferiens)	Hypertrophic cardiomyopathy, AS with AI

AI, Aortic insufficiency; *AS,* aortic stenosis; *LV,* left ventricular; *MR,* mitral regurgitation.

pulse). Consistent with the presence of chronic aortic insufficiency is the accentuation of the radial pulse when the examiner lifts the whole arm above the patient's head (Mayne's sign). A weak and thready pulse may be present with severe LV dysfunction, hypovolemia, severe mitral regurgitation, or complete heart block. A weak and slow-rising carotid pulse (pulsus parvus et tardus) is consistent with a diagnosis of severe aortic stenosis, whereas a regular pulse that alternates between weak and strong (pulsus alternans) occurs with LV dysfunction or, when weakening of the pulse is associated with inspiration, pericardial tamponade. A "double tap" of the pulse during systole (pulsus bisferiens), a small one followed by a stronger and broader one, can occur with either hypertrophic cardiomyopathy or the combination of aortic stenosis and aortic insufficiency.[14,15] In the presence of a bisferiens pulse, two soft and rapid sounds can be auscultated with each cardiac cycle as the brachial artery is compressed by a blood pressure cuff proximally.[16]

Irregular rhythms are classified as either *regularly irregular,* in which the irregular beat can be anticipated at a fixed interval, or *irregularly irregular,* in which the irregular beat occurs without predictability. A regularly irregular pulse commonly occurs with second-degree atrioventricular block (either Mobitz I or II, depending on whether the PR interval is constant or lengthening before the dropped beat) or with interpolated ventricular premature beats. On the physical examination, the PR interval can be visualized as the distance between the a wave and c wave on the jugular venous pulse (JVP). This distance, before and after the dropped beat, can be diagnostic when the electrocardiogram (ECG) is unable to differentiate between Mobitz type I and Mobitz type II second-degree block. When an interpolated ventricular premature beat is present, it may be accompanied by a weakened pulse (owing to inadequate ventricular filling) that occurs at a fixed interval from the regular pulse.

An irregularly irregular pulse implies that the examiner cannot anticipate when the next beat will occur and may be due to ventricular premature beats, atrial premature beats, multifocal atrial tachycardia, or atrial fibrillation. Although ventricular premature beats and atrial fibrillation are associated with a pulse deficit (in which the auscultated apical rate is greater than the palpable radial pulse), the impulse that follows a ventricular premature beat should be stronger. It is clinically relevant to realize that significant numbers of ventricular premature beats can compromise cardiac output. Alternatively, if the beat following a ventricular premature beat is diminished (Brockenbrough sign), hypertrophic cardiomyopathy or severe LV dysfunction should be considered. No pulse deficit (or compensatory pause) should be present with atrial premature beats or multifocal atrial tachycardia. The physician can differentiate atrial premature beats from ventricular premature beats by tapping out the rhythm with one's finger. Atrial premature beats result in a beat that occurs while the finger is "up." Although a ventricular premature beat also occurs with the finger in the "up" position, the pulse resumes on the second down beat after the compensatory pause.

Blood Pressure

In the CICU, there is no rule defining "normal" blood pressure. *Adequate* blood pressure varies by patient and clinical status but is generally believed to consist of a mean perfusion pressure of at least 60 mm Hg and the absence of end-organ hypoperfusion. For accurate assessment, an adequately sized blood pressure cuff must be used (there are lines on all blood pressure cuffs to indicate adequate sizing) and should be correctly situated around the bicep (and not over clothing). A blood pressure obtained with a cuff that is too short or narrow, especially if the patient is obese or has an enlarged upper arm, may result in a factitiously elevated blood pressure.[17,18]

Although palpation of pulses is commonly used in emergency situations to estimate systolic blood pressure (i.e., palpation of a radial pulse suggests a minimum systolic blood pressure of 80 mm Hg; a femoral pulse, a blood pressure of at least 70 mm Hg; and a carotid pulse, a blood pressure of at least 60 mm Hg), the overall accuracy of this estimation has been questioned.[19] To obtain the palpable systolic blood pressure, the cuff should first be inflated until the radial pulse is no longer palpable (usually 150 to 200 mm Hg) and then slowly deflated (2 to 3 mm Hg per second) until the pulse returns.

For the auscultatory blood pressure, inflation should be repeated (inflate the cuff to 10 mm Hg above the palpable systolic blood pressure) and listen for the first and fifth (last audible) Korotkoff sounds during slow cuff deflation. The diastolic blood pressure may be difficult, if not impossible, to appreciate in the presence of fever, severe anemia, aortic insufficiency, thyrotoxicosis, vitamin B$_1$ deficiency, or Paget disease. For patients in atrial fibrillation or with significant ventricular arrhythmias, a relatively accurate blood pressure assessment is obtained by averaging three individual readings.

In patients with LV systolic dysfunction, multiple etiologies of hypotension require assessment during the physical examination. Although hypotension may be caused by overly aggressive diuresis, it may also occur because of volume overload. The presence of a tachycardia with orthostatic hypotension (a blood pressure decrease of >20 mm Hg systolic or >10 mm Hg diastolic when the patient is assessed first in the supine position and then again after 2 minutes with the patient standing or sitting with legs dangling) is consistent with volume depletion. The differential diagnosis of hypotension includes factors that reduce systemic vascular resistance (e.g., infection, inflammation, adrenal insufficiency, anesthetic agents, atrioventricular malformations, and vascular insufficiency), stroke volume (e.g., hypovolemia; aortic stenosis; severe mitral regurgitation; ventricular arrhythmias; and LV dysfunction owing to infarction, ischemia, or a cardiomyopathy), and heart rate (e.g., heart block or pharmacologic bradycardia).

Hypotension without a concomitant increase in the pulse rate (in the absence of medications that can blunt a heart rate response) raises the possibility of autonomic dysfunction. The presence of a pulsus paradoxus (a >10 mm Hg decrease in systolic blood pressure occurring at end expiration with the patient breathing *normally*) can occur with cardiac tamponade (very sensitive when occurring with tachycardia, jugular venous distention, and an absent y descent),[20,21] constrictive pericarditis (occurring with jugular venous distention that persistently augments with inspiration, a pericardial knock, hepatomegaly, and an exaggerated y descent),[22] severe hypertension, pulmonary embolism, COPD, and severe obesity.

With appropriate clinical scenarios, blood pressure should also be assessed in both arms and one leg. Leg blood pressure can be assessed by placing the blood pressure cuff around the calf and using the dorsalis pedis pulse for auscultation or Doppler interrogation. A systolic blood pressure difference greater than 10 mm Hg between arms suggests aortic dissection, proximal aortic aneurysm, or subclavian artery stenosis. With coarctation of the aorta, arm blood pressures are greater than blood pressures in the legs (this may also be accompanied by underdeveloped lower extremity musculature compared with upper extremity musculature). Leg blood pressure that is more than 15 mm Hg higher than arm blood pressure suggests aortic dissection, aortic insufficiency, or a proximal vasculitis (i.e., giant cell or Takayasu arteritis).

The pulse pressure (systolic blood pressure – diastolic blood pressure) may also be informative. A low pulse pressure may be present with the decreased stroke volume of hypovolemia, tachycardia, severe aortic or mitral stenosis, pericardial constriction, or cardiac tamponade. With appropriate clinical suspicion, it has a high sensitivity and specificity to predict a cardiac index less than 2.2 L/min per m^2 when the pulse pressure divided by the systolic pressure is less than 0.25. A wide pulse pressure (>60 mm Hg) can be seen with hyperthermia but may also suggest severe chronic aortic insufficiency or high output failure owing to severe anemia, thyrotoxicosis, atrioventricular malformation, sepsis, vitamin B$_1$ deficiency, or Paget disease. If the wide pulse pressure is present in just one arm, a search for an atrioventricular fistula distal to the site of the blood pressure cuff should be undertaken.

Weight

The daily weight is an important vital sign. Ideally, patients should be weighed on a scale and not in the bed to obtain the most accurate measurement. Monitoring the daily weight often proves to be especially helpful for patients in whom volume overload or hypovolemia is a clinical concern. When a weight appears inconsistent with prior weights or the clinical history, the clinician should not hesitate to have the patient reweighed. Noting an increase in weight may be crucial to discern the presence of volume overload in a patient with shortness of breath, whereas loss of weight should occur in patients being diuresed. A weight gain despite the presence of effective diuresis suggests increased fluid intake, either orally or via the intravenous route.

HEAD, EYES, EARS, NOSE, AND THROAT EXAMINATION

In the presence of an endotracheal or nasogastric tube, the physician first should ensure that the tube is not causing a pressure injury. If the patient has a central line or pulmonary artery catheter, the physician must ensure that it is secured and uninfected. The head, eyes, ears, nose, and throat examination can also suggest the presence of several syndromes.

In adults, a large skull suggests Paget disease (with associated high-output heart failure) or acromegaly (with frontal bossing and large features). A high arched palate, associated with a wide pulse pressure and pectus excavatum, is consistent with Marfan syndrome. Coarse hair texture or hair loss from the head, axilla, or pubic region suggests hypothyroidism. Temporal artery tenderness suggests temporal arteritis.

Eyelid xanthelasma or a corneal arcus may occur with either hypercholesterolemia or diabetes mellitus. Yellowed sclera are seen with hyperbilirubinemia, whereas blue sclera can be seen in Marfan and Ehlers-Danlos syndromes. Dry, puffy, and sunken (enophthalmic) eyes are consistent with hypothyroidism, whereas exophthalmic eyes (white sclera visible between the margin of the upper eyelid and the corneal limbus with the patient looking downward) associated with a lid lag (an immobility or lagging of the upper eyelid on downward rotation of the eye) and lid retraction (widening of the palpebral fissure) are associated with hyperthyroidism. Periorbital edema is seen with the hypoalbuminemia of hepatic disease, a protein-losing nephropathy, or the superior vena cava syndrome. The lack of periorbital edema with diffuse peripheral edema is a distinguishing feature of a cardiac versus hepatic or renal causes of peripheral edema. It is due to the inability of patients with heart failure and severe volume overload to elevate their upper torso to breathe more comfortably. Conjunctival pallor is a very specific sign of anemia; this diagnosis is reinforced by the presence of concomitant palmar and palmar crease pallor.[23]

When firmly palpating the patient's thyroid gland with the neck flexed (to relax the sternohyoid and sternocleidomastoid muscles), significant findings can include an enlarged thyroid (size appreciated larger than an inch) and the presence of nodules (4% prevalence; most are benign). It is important to note the size and site of these nodules for follow-up examinations.[24] During swallowing, the thyroid gland rises upward with the trachea to allow location of a neck mass either within or outside the thyroid gland.

JUGULAR VENOUS PULSE AND ABDOMINOJUGULAR REFLUX

The internal jugular venous pulse (JVP) is a useful manometer for central venous or right atrial pressure (Video 3.2). However, it is accurate only in indicating intravascular volume status and pulmonary capillary wedge pressure (PCWP) in the absence of, among other things, tricuspid stenosis, right ventricular (RV) dysfunction, pulmonary hypertension, and a restrictive or constrictive cardiomyopathy. The JVP should be sought by first asking the patient to lift the chin up and turn to the left against

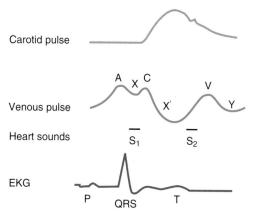

Fig. 3.1 Timing of jugular venous pressure. *ECG,* Electrocardiogram.

the resistance of the examiner's right hand. Within the triangle formed by the visible heads of the sternocleidomastoid muscle and the clavicle, the examiner should then search, with the neck muscles relaxed, for the weak impulses of the jugular vein along a line from the jaw to the clavicle. Shining a tangential light from slightly behind the neck can accentuate the visibility of the transmitted venous impulses. Simultaneous palpation of the radial pulse, assuming that the patient is in sinus rhythm, allows detection of a neck pulsation (a wave) immediately preceding the peripheral pulse (Fig. 3.1). Alternatively, one can visualize the x descent as an inward movement along the line of the jugular vein that occurs simultaneously with the peripheral pulse.

In patients with presumed volume overload, jugular venous distention may be best assessed with the patient sitting upright, a position in which the clavicle is approximately 7 to 8 cm above the right atrium (equivalent to the upper limit of normal for right atrial pressure, 5 to 7 mm Hg). The 7 to 8 cm is added to the maximal vertical distance at which any venous pulsations are seen above the clavicle to estimate the right atrial pressure. If the JVP cannot be appreciated in the upright position, an attempt can be made to visualize it sequentially with the upper body at a 45-degree angle (where only 4 to 5 cm is needed to the distance above the clavicle where the venous pulsations were seen). If venous pulsations are still difficult to discern, either of two extremes may be present: either there is no elevation of the right atrial pressure or the jugular venous pressure is so far above the angle of the jaw, even in the upright position, it is lost in the hairline. The ear lobe should always be assessed for movement in these cases.

A low right atrial pressure may be investigated further by increasing right atrial filling (i.e., with deep inspiration or passive leg elevation). The left internal jugular vein is less useful than the right internal jugular vein for estimation of right atrial pressure because of the presence of valves impeding venous return or compression of the innominate vein. When it must be used, right atrial pressure should be considered approximately 1 cm lower than the visualized left internal jugular pulse.[25,26] Likewise, the external jugular veins should be avoided in assessing jugular venous pressure because of the extreme angle with which they contact the superior vena cava and their occasional absence or diminution in the presence of elevated catecholamine levels.[27]

Although the value of sequential assessment of the JVP has been confirmed by studies of patients with LV dysfunction,[28] patients undergoing cardiac catheterization for dyspnea or chest pain,[29] and patients with suspected chronic heart failure,[30–32] it is important to confirm these findings with additional signs of volume overload in the acute setting.[33,34] When an increasing creatinine value is seen despite the presence of an elevated jugular venous pressure (with or without diuresis), the differential diagnosis includes refractory LV dysfunction requiring inotropic support, severe RV dysfunction, restrictive or constrictive cardiomyopathy or right heart failure, or underlying renal dysfunction (cardiorenal syndrome) or renovascular disease. With RV dysfunction, the assessment of JVP as a measure of PCWP becomes progressively less accurate. The JVP measured in cm of H_2O is converted to mm Hg by multiplying by 0.735.

Abdominojugular reflux is present when the height of the neck vein distention, visualized with the patient's neck at a 45-degree angle, is increased by at least 3 cm (and maintained for approximately 15 seconds) during a steady pressure of approximately 20 to 35 mm Hg applied over the right upper quadrant or mid-abdomen. (You can learn what exerting 20 to 35 mm Hg of pressure feels like by compressing an inflated blood pressure cuff against a flat surface until the sphygmomanometer reads 30 mm Hg; Video 3.2.) It is important to instruct patients not to hold their breath because the Valsalva maneuver negates the effect of abdominal pressure. The increased abdominal pressure on the mesenteric or splanchnic veins increases venous return to the RV. With RV or biventricular heart failure (and the limited ability to increase RV and LV output), distention of the internal jugular vein occurs. A positive abdominojugular reflux may also occur with tricuspid stenosis, tricuspid insufficiency, constrictive pericarditis, restrictive cardiomyopathy, pulmonary hypertension, and mitral stenosis. Although limited data are available in the CICU setting, abdominojugular reflux in patients presenting to the emergency department had a low sensitivity (33%) but a high specificity (94%; $P = .028$) for the diagnosis of heart failure. However, its sensitivity significantly increases in patients with known chronic congestive heart failure[32]; when the abdominojugular reflux is absent, it cannot be taken as evidence *against* the diagnosis of heart failure.[35]

CHEST AND LUNG EXAMINATION

The thorax should first be examined for the presence of an old sternotomy (suggesting prior coronary artery bypass grafting, valve replacement, or other heart surgery) or thoracotomy scars (suggesting prior pulmonary pathology). If the patient is intubated, the physician needs to ensure that both sides of the chest are expanding evenly (Video 3.3).

Although Laënnec's invention of the stethoscope rendered obsolete the need for the physician to place the ear directly against the chest wall to appreciate heart and lung sounds, modern technology has yet to replace the need for daily auscultation of the lungs via the stethoscope (Table 3.3). The waning ability of physicians to appreciate abnormalities in the lung examination undoubtedly limits the information available for patient management.[36] The lungs should be auscultated in an alternating and

TABLE 3.3	**Auscultation of the Lungs**
Breath Sound	**Consider**
Rhonchi	
Diffuse	COPD
Localized	Pneumonia, tumor, foreign body
Stridorous	Large airway obstruction
Wheezes	
Expiratory	Reactive small airway obstruction (asthma, allergies, β-blockers)
De novo	Nonasthmatic causes (mass, pulmonary embolism, pulmonary edema, aspiration, foreign body)
Crackles or rales	Pulmonary edema, interstitial lung disease, COPD, amiodarone toxicity

COPD, Chronic obstructive pulmonary disease.

comprehensive fashion (Videos 3.4A and 3.4B). Although the diaphragm of the stethoscope is used to detect most normal and pathologic lung sounds, the bell is more advantageous for detecting the rhonchi associated with primary tuberculosis or fungal disease in the apices.

Crackles (or rales) are discontinuous lung sounds (that sound like Velcro being pulled apart) generated when abnormally closed alveoli snap open, usually at the end of inspiration (Audio 3.1).[37] However, "clear lungs" may be present in 25% of patients presenting with heart failure.[31] The Boston Criteria for Heart Failure gives 1 point if the crackles are basilar and 2 points if they extend further.[38] Crackles have a low sensitivity but high specificity to predict the presence of LV dysfunction or an elevated PCWP.[29,30,32] Crackles may also be caused by interstitial lung disease, amiodarone toxicity, pulmonary fibrosis, or COPD (Audio 3.2).[39]

Rhonchi (coarse, dry, leathery sounds) are present in the setting of large airway (bronchial) turbulent flow caused by inflammation and congestion and are associated most commonly with pneumonia or COPD. When detected, it should be noted whether they occur during inspiration or expiration and whether they are generalized or localized. Diffuse rhonchi suggest generalized airway obstruction that occurs with COPD. Localized rhonchi suggest pneumonia or obstruction owing to tumor or a foreign body. Generally, rhonchi caused by mucous secretions subside or disappear altogether with coughing. Stridor refers to loud, audible inspiratory and, possibly, expiratory rhonchi that suggest extrathoracic large airway obstruction (Audio 3.3).

The presence of wheezes (continuous and high-pitched musical sounds) that occur during expiration often denotes reactive small airway obstruction (Audio 3.4). Because airway size is reduced in the recumbent position, wheezing should worsen when lying down. When accompanied by a prolonged expiratory phase, wheezes signify the presence of airflow through a narrowed tract that is often seen with asthma, allergies, or the toxic effects associated with β-blockade. In some patients, the presence of pulmonary edema may result in musical breath sounds similar to wheezes, called *cardiac asthma.* When wheezing is detected de novo in an older patient, a search for nonasthmatic causes, including obstructing masses, pulmonary embolism, pulmonary edema, aspiration pneumonitis, and foreign-body obstruction is

warranted.[40] Decreased or absent breath sounds in a lung field are consistent with atelectasis, pneumothorax, pleural effusions, COPD, acute respiratory distress syndrome, or pleural thickening (Audio 3.5).

Egophony (when a verbalized "e-e-e" is appreciated via auscultation as an "a-a-a") occurs in the presence of a pleural effusion but can also be heard with lung consolidation and pneumonia (Audio 3.6). Although not sensitive, egophony is specific for a parapneumonic process.[41] Lung consolidation can be confirmed further by the presence of bronchophony (when "clearer" voice sounds are heard over consolidated lung tissue). Bronchial breath sounds (breath sounds that are louder than normal; Audio 3.7) are also heard when consolidation of lung tissue is present because solid tissue transmits sound better than tissue filled with air (Audio 3.8). When bronchial breath sounds are heard and accompany a dull area to percussion at the base of the left scapula, it suggests the presence of a large pericardial effusion (the Ewart sign).

Percussion of the chest can provide important information about lung pathology (Videos 3.5 and 3.6). Expected percussion sounds are summarized here (Video 3.7). Dullness to percussion at the lung base suggests the presence of pleural effusion and, rarely, lung consolidation. If the percussive dullness responds to postural changes (i.e., diminution in the left lateral decubitus position), a pleural effusion is likely present.[42] Although left-sided pleural effusions are common after chest surgery (e.g., coronary artery bypass graft surgery after left internal mammary artery dissection) and with pancreatitis or pancreatic cancer, bilateral or right-sided effusions are more consistent with heart failure. Pleural effusions may also occur with pneumonia, hypoalbuminemia (seen with nephrotic syndrome or cirrhosis), and nearly all types of malignancy.

THORAX AND HEART EXAMINATION

The thorax should be appreciated by looking upward at the chest from the foot of the bed. This view may reveal a pectus excavatum (a congenital anterior chest wall deformity producing a concave, or caved-in, appearance that suggests Marfan or Ehlers-Danlos syndrome or right heart failure), pectus carinatum (an outward "pigeon chest," protrusion of the anterior chest wall associated with decreased lung compliance, progressive emphysema, and a predisposition to respiratory tract infections), and barrel chest deformities (with increased anteroposterior chest diameters that may be observed with obstructive forms of chronic pulmonary disease, such as COPD, cystic fibrosis, and severe asthma).

When the examiner is positioned on the right side of the patient, visible or palpable precordial pulsations may be appreciated owing to a thin body habitus or secondary to cardiac disease. Pulsations in the second intercostal space to the left of the sternal border suggest an elevated pulmonary artery pressure, whereas pulsations seen in the fourth intercostal space at the left sternal border are consistent with RV dysfunction or an acute ventricular septal defect. Apical pulsations may be secondary to systemic hypertension, LV hypertrophy, hemodynamically significant aortic stenosis, or an LV aneurysm. With the examiner standing on the right side of the patient, the LV apex or point of maximal impulse (PMI) is palpated by placing the right hand transversely across the precordium under the nipple and is perceived as an upward pulsation during systole against the examiner's hand (Video 3.8). A normal PMI is depicted here (Video 3.9). An enlarged apical impulse is variously described as an impulse detected more than 2 cm to the left of the midclavicular line in the fifth intercostal space or as greater than the size of a quarter and palpable in at least two interspaces. Recognition may be enhanced with the patient in the left lateral decubitus position or when sitting up and leaning slightly forward.

Detection of LV enlargement is a function of age: it increases steadily for men and women, occurring in 66% of men and 58% of women in the 65- to 69-year age range and 82% of men and 79% of women older than 85 years.[43] It has a sensitivity of approximately 65% and a specificity of 95%, with a negative predictive value of 94% for LV systolic dysfunction.[30] Although obesity may limit the detection of the LV apical impulse, a displaced impulse is effective in suggesting the diagnosis of heart failure, even in patients with COPD.[44] Fluid or air in the right pleural cavity, a depressed sternum, and secondary retraction of the left lung and pleura all can result in an apparent augmentation of the LV impulse, however.[45] LV enlargement is suggested further by the presence of a sustained apical impulse (persisting more than halfway between S_1 and S_2 during simultaneous auscultation and palpation). A shifted PMI as seen with LV hypertrophy is illustrated here (Video 3.10). If the LV apical impulse is detectable at end-systole, a dyskinetic ventricle is most likely. If the apical impulse seems to retract during systole, the presence of constrictive pericarditis or tricuspid regurgitation should be considered.

All auscultatory fields should be palpated with the fingertips to detect a thrill (required for the diagnosis of a grade IV/VI murmur). In addition, the presence of a palpable P_2 (an upward pulsation during diastole in the pulmonic position) suggests the presence of either secondary (acute pulmonary embolism, chronic mitral regurgitation, or stenosis) or primary pulmonary hypertension. When a pulsation is palpable in the aortic position during systole, it suggests either hypertrophic cardiomyopathy or severe aortic stenosis. Its presence over the left sternal border in the fourth intercostal space, especially in the setting of an acute MI, raises the possibility of a ventricular septal defect. A presystolic impulse (correlating with the *a* wave and equivalent to an audible S_4) suggests ventricular noncompliance and may be present with myocardial ischemia or infarction, with LV hypertrophy secondary to hypertension, aortic stenosis, acute mitral regurgitation, or hypertrophic cardiomyopathy.

Auscultation of the Heart

Cardiac auscultation in the CICU setting allows for the detection of common holosystolic (mitral regurgitation and ventricular septal defect), systolic ejection (aortic stenosis or hypertrophic cardiomyopathy), and diastolic (aortic insufficiency and mitral stenosis) murmurs that can precipitate or exacerbate a decompensation in the CICU or the presence of abnormal heart sounds (S_1, S_2, S_3, S_4) indicating underlying pathology (Table 3.4). While rapid assessment can often be lifesaving, it should not replace a more systematic investigation when acute stabilization has occurred.

TABLE 3.4 Clinical Auscultation of S_1, S_2, S_3, and S_4	
Heart Sound	**Consider**
S_1	
Accentuated	Atrial fibrillation, mitral stenosis
Soft	Immobile mitral valves, MR, or severe AI
S_2	
Accentuated	(P_2) Pulmonary hypertension; (A_2) systemic hypertension; aortic dilation
Soft	(A_2) AI, sepsis, AV fistula
A_2-P_2 Splitting	
Wide	Severe MR, RBBB, atrial septal defect (secondary), pulmonary hypertension
Paradoxical	Severe TR, WPW, LBBB, severe hypertension, or AS
Fixed	Large atrial septal defect, severe RV failure
S_3	
Present	Heart failure, HOCM, thyrotoxicosis, AV fistula, sepsis, hyperthermia
S_4	
Present	Ischemic or infarcted LV, hypertrophic, dilated, or restrictive cardiomyopathy

AI, Aortic insufficiency; *AS*, aortic stenosis; *AV*, atrioventricular; *HOCM*, hypertrophic obstructive cardiomyopathy; *LBBB*, left bundle branch block; *MR*, mitral regurgitation; *RBBB*, right bundle branch block; *TR*, tricuspid regurgitation; *WPW*, Wolff-Parkinson-White.

S_1, S_2, S_3, and S_4

An understanding of the cardiac events of systole and diastole is required before performing auscultation (Video 3.11).

S_1, best appreciated as a high-pitched and split sound at the cardiac apex, is produced at the time of mitral (M_1) and tricuspid (T_1) valve closure and occurs before the upstroke of the peripheral pulse (Audio 3.9). An accentuated S_1 is present when the mitral or tricuspid valves are widely separated in diastole (e.g., with atrial fibrillation, with a shortened PR interval, or in the presence of an obstructing myxoma) or with mitral or tricuspid valves that are difficult to open (e.g., mitral or tricuspid stenosis when the valves have become calcified). When a stenotic valve becomes nearly immobile, however, the intensity of S_1 decreases. A soft S_1 may be present when the valves are already nearly closed at the onset of systole, as occurs with moderate to severe aortic insufficiency, with advanced heart failure, with a prolonged PR interval or when the mitral valves are incompetent (from papillary muscle dysfunction, ventricular dilation, or myxomatous degeneration).

S_2, which occurs at the time of closure of the semilunar aortic (A_2) and pulmonary (P_2) valves, is probably caused by the deceleration of blood in the root of the pulmonary artery and aorta at end-systole. It is best appreciated in the second intercostal space, midclavicular line (pulmonic position) using the diaphragm of the stethoscope (Audio 3.10). Normally, the intensity of A_2 exceeds the intensity of P_2. A soft A_2 can occur in the setting of incompetent aortic valves (e.g., aortic insufficiency), a decrease in the distance that the valves have to traverse (e.g., severe aortic stenosis) or a decreased diastolic pressure closing the aortic valve (e.g., with sepsis or an atrioventricular fistula), or from physical muffling of heart sounds that occur with the air trapping of COPD. An accentuated S_2 may be caused by a loud A_2 (e.g., severe systemic hypertension or aortic dilation) or a loud P_2 (e.g., pulmonary hypertension). During auscultation, an accentuated P_2 is said to occur when the pulmonary component of S_2 is louder than S_1 in the fourth to sixth intercostal spaces (Audio 3.11). This is generally associated with a pulmonary artery systolic pressure of greater than 50 mm Hg. Associated findings may include a prominent *a* wave, an early systolic click (caused by the sudden opening of the pulmonary valve against a high pressure), and a left parasternal lift signaling the presence of RV hypertrophy.

The timing of S_2 splitting into A_2 and P_2 components should be described (Audio 3.12). Normally, A_2 precedes P_2. Wide splitting of S_2 (when P_2 is delayed relative to A_2) occurs with early aortic valve closure (e.g., severe mitral regurgitation) or delayed pulmonic valve closure (e.g., right bundle branch block, with a secundum atrial septal defect or with pulmonary hypertension). *Paradoxical splitting*, when A_2 occurs after P_2, may occur because of early pulmonary valve closure (e.g., severe tricuspid insufficiency or with preexcitation with early RV contraction); delayed activation of the LV (e.g., left bundle branch block); or the prolongation of LV contraction that occurs with hypertension, aortic stenosis, or severe systolic dysfunction. *Fixed splitting*, when the time interval between A_2 and P_2 is not increased during inspiration, may be due to a large atrial septal defect and severe RV failure. Currently, no evidence-based assessments of these findings in the critical care setting are available.

S_3, which occurs early in diastole, is best appreciated at end expiration with the bell near the apex and with the patient in the left lateral decubitus position (Audio 3.13). This low-pitched sound occurs approximately 0.16 seconds after S_2. Although often normal when detected in children and young adults, S_3 in patients older than 40 years implies an increase in the passive diastolic filling of either the RV (RVS_3) or LV (LVS_3) ventricle. An LVS_3 may be detected in patients with heart failure, hypertrophic cardiomyopathy, LV aneurysm, or with hyperdynamic states (e.g., thyrotoxicosis, arteriovenous fistula, hyperthermia, and sepsis). The presence of LVS_3 in patients with symptomatic chronic LV dysfunction has been associated with an increased risk of hospitalization for heart failure and death from pump failure.[28] The presence of S_3 in patients with advanced heart failure had 68% sensitivity and 73% specificity for detecting a PCWP greater than 18 mm Hg.[32] An RVS_3 is best appreciated with the patient in the supine position, while listening over the third intercostal space at the left sternal border. It is accentuated during inspiration because of rapid RV filling and occurs in the setting of severe tricuspid insufficiency or RV failure.

S_4 is a low-pitched sound best heard with the bell of the stethoscope at the apex in the left lateral decubitus position (Audio 3.14). It occurs just before S_1 and can be readily distinguished from a split S_1 by its ability to be extinguished by firm pressure on the bell. S_4 is believed to be due to the vigorous atrial contraction necessary to propel blood into a stiffened LV

(and is, therefore, absent in atrial fibrillation). The stiffened LV may be the result of an ischemic or infarcted LV or owing to a hypertrophic, dilated, or restrictive cardiomyopathy. Because diastolic and systolic defects can result in S_4, its presence does not contribute to their differentiation.[46] Similar to RVS_3, RVS_4 increases in intensity with inspiration. When LVS_3 and LVS_4 are appreciated, usually in the setting of tachycardia with systolic dysfunction, a summation gallop is said to be present (Audio 3.15).

Three additional diastolic sounds should be sought during routine evaluation. (1) A high-pitched early diastolic click is caused by abnormal semilunar valves (bicuspid aortic valve or pulmonic stenosis), dilation of the great vessels (aortic aneurysm or pulmonary hypertension), or augmented flow states (truncus arteriosus or hemodynamically significant pulmonic stenosis). (2) A mid-diastolic opening snap, occurring approximately 0.08 seconds after S_2 and best appreciated in the fourth intercostal space at the left sternal border or apex, is caused by the opening of a stenotic (although pliable) mitral valve. The opening snap disappears when the valve becomes severely calcified. Shortening of the interval from S_2 to the opening snap occurs as the left atrial pressure increases and indicates progressive disease severity. The opening snap of a stenotic mitral valve can be differentiated from a split S_2 by a widening of the S_2–opening snap interval that occurs when a patient with mitral stenosis stands up. (3) A dull-sounding early diastolic to mid-diastolic knock suggests the abrupt cessation of ventricular filling that occurs secondary to a noncompliant and constrictive pericardium.

Heart Murmurs: Static and Dynamic Auscultation

Heart murmurs are appreciated as systolic, diastolic, or continuous and should be further described according to their location, timing, duration, pitch, intensity, and response to dynamic maneuvers (Table 3.5). The optimal location for detecting valvular pathology must be recognized (Video 3.12). The pathophysiology of murmurs may be divided into regurgitation (Video 3.13) and stenotic (Video 3.14) defects. Although the gradations I to III are arbitrary (grade I, very faint, difficult to hear; grade II, faint, but readily identified; and grade III, moderately loud), the presence of a grade IV murmur always denotes the presence of an associated palpable thrill. Grade V is a louder murmur with a thrill; grade VI occurs when the murmur is heard with the stethoscope physically off the chest wall.

Holosystolic murmurs, with a soft or obliterated S_2, occur with tricuspid regurgitation (see Video 3.13), ventricular septal defects, and mitral regurgitation (see Video 3.13). Tricuspid regurgitation is suggested when the holosystolic murmur is best appreciated in the fourth intercostal space along the left sternal border and augments with inspiration, passive leg elevation, and isometric handgrip. The presence of pulsations in the fourth intercostal space at the left sternal border suggests either a ventricular septal defect or concomitant RV dilation or dysfunction. In the setting of an acute inferior wall or extensive anterior wall MI, the presence of a new holosystolic murmur occurring with a palpable RV lift requires that an acute ventricular septal defect be excluded. The holosystolic murmur of mitral regurgitation is best appreciated at the apex during end expiration in the

TABLE 3.5   Dynamic Cardiac Auscultation

Maneuver	Physiology	TR	PS	VSD	MR	AS	HOCM	AI
Inspiration	Increased venous return and ventricular volume	↑	↑		nc/↑			
Expiration	Brings heart closer to the chest wall	↑			nc/↑			
Leg elevation	Increased SVR; increased venous return						↓	
Mueller maneuver	Decrease CVP/BP/SNA (10 sec), then increase in BP/SNA (5 sec) and surge in BP/decrease SNA with release	↑						
Valsalva maneuver	Decreased venous return and ventricular volumes (phase 2)		↓	↓	↓	↓	↑	↓
Squatting to standing	Decreased venous return and volume	↓	↓	↓	↓	↓	↑	
Standing to squatting	Increased venous return; increased SVR			↑	↑	↑	↓	↑
Handgrip	Increased SVR; increased CO; increased LV filling pressures			↑	↑	↓	↓	↑

Inspiration also increases the murmur of tricuspid stenosis and pulmonary regurgitation.
AI, Aortic insufficiency; *AS,* aortic stenosis; *BP,* blood pressure; *CO,* cardiac output; *CVP,* central venous pressure; *HOCM,* hypertrophic obstructive cardiomyopathy; *LV,* left ventricular; *MR,* mitral regurgitation; *PS,* pulmonary stenosis; *nc,* no changes; *TR,* tricuspid regurgitation; *SNA,* sympathetic nerve activity; *SVR,* systemic vascular resistance; *VSD,* ventricular septal defect.

left lateral decubitus position and is associated with a soft S_1 (Audio 3.16). With severe mitral regurgitation, it may be associated with a slowly increasing peripheral pulse owing to partial ejection of the LV volume into the left atrium.

With acute mitral regurgitation, the murmur may be absent or may appear earlier or later in systole. When mitral regurgitation is severe, evidence of pulmonary hypertension may also be present. Posterior mitral leaflet involvement results in a murmur that radiates anteriorly whereas posterior radiation into the axilla suggests anterior mitral valve leaflet dysfunction. In more stable patients in whom positional changes are possible, prompt squatting from a standing position results in a rapid increase in venous return and peripheral resistance that causes the murmur of mitral regurgitation (and aortic insufficiency) to grow louder. A similar phenomenon occurs with isometric handgrip.

The harsh systolic ejection murmur of aortic stenosis begins shortly after S_1, peaks toward midsystole and ends before S_2 (crescendo-decrescendo; Audio 3.17). It is best appreciated in the second intercostal space to the right of the sternal border and radiates into the right neck (see Video 3.14). The absence of this radiation should bring the diagnosis into question. A systolic thrill may be palpable at the base of the heart, in the jugular notch, and along the carotid arteries. Associated findings include an ejection click (occurring with a bicuspid valve, which disappears as the stenosis becomes more severe) and, with increasing severity, a slow increase and plateau of a weak carotid pulse (pulsus parvus et tardus).[47] The severity of the obstruction is related to the duration of the murmur to its peak and not its intensity. An early-peaking murmur is usually associated with a less stenotic valve; a late-peaking murmur, suggesting a longer time for the ventricular pressure to overcome the stenosis, suggests a more severe stenosis. A nearly immobile and stenotic aortic valve can result in a muted or absent S_2. The high-pitched, diastolic blowing murmur of aortic regurgitation frequently occurs with aortic stenosis.

Hypertrophic cardiomyopathy is also associated with a crescendo-decrescendo systolic murmur. It is best appreciated *between* the apex and left sternal border, however, and although it radiates to the suprasternal notch, it does *not* radiate to the carotid arteries or neck. The murmur of hypertrophic cardiomyopathy can also be distinguished from aortic stenosis by an increase in murmur intensity (when the outflow tract gradient is increased) that occurs during the active phase of the Valsalva maneuver, when changing from sitting to standing (the LV volume abruptly decreases) and with the use of vasodilators. Hypertrophic cardiomyopathy may also be accompanied by the holosystolic murmur of mitral regurgitation owing to the anterior motion of the mitral valve during systole.

Although S_3 and S_4 are common with hypertrophic cardiomyopathy, they lack prognostic significance. Additional findings include a laterally displaced double apical impulse (resulting from the forceful contraction of the left atrium against a noncompliant LV) or a triple apical impulse (resulting from the late systolic impulse that occurs when the nearly empty LV undergoes near-isometric contraction). Similarly, a double carotid arterial pulse (pulsus bisferiens) is common because of the initial rapid increase of blood flow through the LV outflow tract into the aorta, which declines in midsystole as the gradient develops, only to manifest a secondary increase during end-systole. The jugular venous pulse reveals a prominent *a* wave owing to the diminished RV compliance associated with septal hypertrophy.

Diastolic murmurs are caused by insufficiency of the aortic or pulmonary valves (see Video 3.13) or stenosis of the mitral or tricuspid valves (see Video 3.14). Chronic aortic insufficiency is heralded by a high-frequency, early diastolic decrescendo murmur, best appreciated in the second to fourth left intercostal space with the patient sitting up and leaning forward. As aortic insufficiency becomes more severe, the murmur takes up more of diastole. When LV dysfunction results in restrictive filling, the murmur of aortic regurgitation may shorten and become softer.

Moderate to severe aortic insufficiency may also be accompanied by an Austin Flint murmur, a low-frequency, mid-diastolic to late-diastolic murmur best appreciated at the apex caused by left atrial flow into an "overexpanded" LV.[48] As Austin Flint reported, "In some cases in which free aortic regurgitation exists, the right becoming filled before the auricles contract, the mitral curtains are floated out, and the valve closed when the mitral current takes place, and, under these circumstances, this murmur may be produced by the current just named, although no mitral lesion exists." Aortic insufficiency may be accompanied by a soft S_1, prominent S_3, and a diastolic rumble. The apical impulse in chronic aortic insufficiency, which is frequently hyperdynamic and diffuse, is also often displaced inferiorly and leftward.

Severe aortic insufficiency is associated with wide pulse pressure and a multitude of eponym-rich clinical findings including a Corrigan or water-hammer pulse, the de Musset sign (a head bob with each systole), the Müller sign (systolic pulsations of the uvula; https://www.youtube.com/watch?v=CDG-Uf6cErA), the Traube sign ("pistol shot" systolic and diastolic sounds heard over the femoral artery), the Hill sign (when the popliteal cuff systolic pressure exceeds the brachial cuff pressure by more than 60 mm Hg), and the Quincke sign (capillary pulsations seen when a light is transmitted through a patient's fingernail; https://www.youtube.com/watch?v=ZzwoYTYVHSI). The Duroziez sign is elicited as an audible systolic murmur heard over the femoral artery when the artery is compressed proximally along with a diastolic murmur when the femoral artery is compressed distally.

Other diastolic murmurs include the following. (1) Pulmonary regurgitation is a diastolic decrescendo murmur that is localized over the second intercostal space (see Video 3.13). When it is due to dilation of the pulmonary valve annulus, it produces the characteristic Graham-Steele murmur. (2) Mitral stenosis is a mid-diastolic rumble that is appreciated with the bell as a low-pitched sound at the apex, immediately after an opening snap, which increases in intensity with exercise (see Video 3.14). (3) Anatomic or functional tricuspid stenosis (the latter with the delayed opening of the tricuspid valve seen with large atrial or ventricular septal defects) is associated with a mid-diastolic rumble (see Video 3.14) or with the aforementioned Austin Flint murmur of aortic insufficiency. Mitral stenosis can be differentiated from tricuspid stenosis by the localization of the latter to the left sternal border and its augmentation with inspiration.

Finally, the superficial, high-pitched, or scratchy sound of a pericardial friction rub is best heard with the patient in the sitting position while leaning forward at end expiration (Audio 3.18). This murmur may be systolic, systolic and diastolic, or triphasic and should be suspected in the postinfarction or acute pericarditis setting with pleuritic chest pain and diffuse ST segment elevations on ECG.

ABDOMINAL EXAMINATION

Examining the abdomen on admission and daily during hospitalization can unify diagnoses and potentially identify common in-hospital abdominal complications. Pancreatitis, cholecystitis, and ischemic bowel can all develop de novo in a patient days after admission to the CICU. If a wound or dressing is present, the physician should put on gloves and carefully take the dressing down (or request to be present at the time of dressing change) to examine the site. The abdomen should be inspected for obesity, cachexia, and distended or bulging flanks (the latter may be due to ascites, organomegaly, colonic dilation, ileus, or a pneumoperitoneum). A search for the stigmata of liver disease (i.e., spider angiomata and caput medusae); signs of intraabdominal hemorrhage, such as flank (Grey Turner sign) or periumbilical (Cullen sign) ecchymosis; hernias; and surgical scars should also be performed. Abdominal striae and bruises, in addition to moon facies and central obesity, may be caused by excess glucocorticoids owing to exogenous administration or endogenous overproduction (e.g., Cushing syndrome secondary to pituitary, lung, adrenal, or carcinoid tumors). Visible peristalsis and a distended abdomen argue for bowel obstruction as the cause of abdominal pain and should complement the finding of hyperactive bowel sounds.[49]

Auscultation with the diaphragm of the stethoscope should be performed over each major vascular territory in the abdomen for high-pitched systolic bruits suggesting renal artery stenosis, aortic aneurysm, hepatic or splenic vascular lesions, or the potential cause of mesenteric ischemia. An abdominal bruit may be present in 80% to 85% of patients with renal artery stenosis. Venous (continuous) hums, associated with portal venous hypertension, are best appreciated with the bell of the stethoscope, usually in the right upper quadrant.

In the CICU, it is important to assess the change in bowel sounds over time. Bowel sounds should be sought with the diaphragm of the stethoscope; although loud, high-pitched and hyperactive bowel sounds may indicate the presence of an obstructed bowel, they may also be present with gastroenteritis, inflammatory bowel disease, or gastrointestinal bleeding. Bowel sounds are considered absent only after listening for at least 3 minutes in each quadrant. Absent or decreased bowel sounds suggest the presence of a paralytic ileus (common after surgery or in the presence of hypokalemia, opiates, constipation, and hypothyroidism) or mesenteric thrombosis. Special attention should be paid to "crampy" and diffuse or periumbilical abdominal pain that progressively increases. If pain is accompanied by decreased or absent bowel sounds, distention, guarding, or rebound, the probability of ischemic or obstructive bowel disease is significantly increased. A succussion splash, defined as a palpable or audible "splash" elicited by applying a firm push to the abdomen, occurs when a hollow portion of the intestine or an organ/body cavity contains a combination of free fluid, air, or gas. A succussion splash is commonly caused by intestinal or pyloric obstruction (e.g., pyloric stenosis or gastric carcinoma) or a hydropneumothorax over a normal stomach. In critically ill patients, catastrophic intestinal rupture, bowel strangulation, or infarct must also be considered.

Palpation may reveal the presence of peritoneal signs (rebound or involuntary guarding) that are best assessed by watching the patient's facial expression during light, followed by progressively deeper, palpation. Voluntary guarding is the defensive posture patients use to avoid palpation by contracting their abdominal musculature. This is not considered a peritoneal sign and may be avoided either by distracting the patient or performing repeated examinations of the abdomen to acclimate the patient to touch. Involuntary guarding is the reflex contraction of abdominal muscles, often owing to peritoneal inflammation. Rebound tenderness occurs when the patient reports augmentation in abdominal pain after abrupt release of pressure exerted with deep palpation at the site of abdominal tenderness. Although additive to the examination, this sign is neither specific nor sensitive for peritonitis and may cause undue patient discomfort without cause. Peritoneal signs in a critically ill patient should provoke an immediate search for evidence of organ perforation, ischemic bowel, or peritonitis.

Envisioning the underlying structures is also helpful in determining potential causes of pain on palpation. Right upper quadrant tenderness is commonly associated with hepatic (e.g., hepatitis, hepatic congestion from heart failure) or gallbladder (e.g., acute cholecystitis, biliary colic) disease, a duodenal ulcer, or right lower lobe pneumonia. A positive Murphy sign (an inspiratory pause during palpation of the right upper quadrant) is a specific, but not sensitive, indicator of gallbladder disease. Right lower quadrant pain on palpation shifts the focus to the ascending colon (e.g., appendicitis or cecal diverticulitis) and tubulo-ovarian structures (e.g., ectopic pregnancy, tubo-ovarian abscess, ruptured ovarian cyst and ovarian torsion). Appendicitis is also suggested by the presence of McBurney sign, tenderness located two-thirds the distance from the anterior iliac spine to the umbilicus on the right side.

Left upper quadrant pain suggests pancreatic (e.g., acute pancreatitis or pancreatic tumor) or splenic (e.g., splenic congestion, splenomegaly, or infarction) disease or left lower lobe pneumonia. Left lower quadrant pain occurs with sigmoid and descending colonic disease (e.g., diverticulitis) or left-sided tubulo-ovarian pathology. Midline or periumbilical discomfort on palpation occurs during early appendicitis, gastroenteritis, or pancreatitis. Pancreatitis may be associated with epigastric tenderness, guarding, hypoactive bowel sounds, fever, and hypotension. Flank pain should also raise the possibility of an abdominal aortic aneurysm, pyelonephritis, and renal colic. Lower abdominal or suprapubic pain occurs with nephrolithiasis, cystitis, ectopic pregnancy, and pelvic inflammatory disease.

The discovery of an abdominal mass during palpation should include a complete description of its size, consistency (hard, soft, or nodular), and pulsatility. Not all abdominal masses indicate tumors; bowel obstruction, inflammatory bowel disease, an enlarged left lobe of the liver, and an abdominal aortic aneurysm are examples of nontumorous masses. A pancreatic mass is rarely palpable.

Percussion (Video 3.15) may reveal localized abdominal dullness, suggesting organomegaly, stool, or the presence of an abdominal mass; generalized abdominal dullness is often associated with ascites. With a suspicion of ascites, noting whether dull areas shift with changes in patient position can be informative. This shift can be detected most easily by the presence of dullness in areas of prior tympany when the patient's abdomen is percussed in the recumbent position and after the patient has been rolled approximately 30 degrees away from the examiner.

Percussion can be used to detect hepatomegaly (Video 3.16). The lower edge of the liver can be detected by placing the right hand in the right lower quadrant of the abdomen and gently moving toward the lower rib margin, approximately 2 cm with each gentle breath of the patient. If the edge is not felt, no further examination is required. If the edge is appreciated, the superior border of the liver should be determined by percussion, starting in the third intercostal space and moving down one interspace at a time until the note changes from resonant to dull. In obese patients, "scratching" with auscultation for the change from tympany to dull on superior and inferior aspects of the liver may be performed. Hepatomegaly is said to be present if the liver span is appreciated for greater than 12 cm (although the actual mean liver span along the midclavicular line is apparently 7 cm in women and 10.5 cm in men). Splenomegaly may be present if the spleen is detected while advancing the examining hand upward toward the left upper quadrant during exhalation with palpating for the spleen edge during inspiration. Percussive dullness over the spleen in the midaxillary line during inspiration also suggests splenomegaly. Finally, a rectal examination should be performed to search for potential causes of urinary tract obstruction (e.g., benign prostatic hypertrophy) or infection (e.g., prostatitis) and to evaluate the stool for gross or occult blood.

NEUROLOGIC EXAMINATION

Patients admitted to the CICU commonly have neurologic complications that may double the length of a hospital stay and increase the likelihood of death.[50] Depressed consciousness is a major contributor to prolonged ventilation. Careful attention and notation should be made on the initial examination and with changes in neurologic state.

The neurologic examination should begin with an assessment of sensorium (dementia or delirium) and the level of consciousness. Level of consciousness has been described as alert, lethargic (easily aroused with mild stimulus), somnolent (easily aroused, but requires stimulation to maintain arousal), obtunded/stuporous (arousable only with repeated and painful stimuli), and comatose (unarousable despite vigorous stimulation with no purposeful movements). If comatose, the depth of the coma can be assessed by the degree of corneal reflex loss. A continuous performance test (asking the patient to raise a hand) can be used to evaluate alertness in noncomatose patients, but a formal Glasgow Coma Scale score should be routinely monitored, along with brainstem reflex assessment, in all unresponsive or minimally responsive patients.

Frontal release signs (forced grasping) and perioral primitive reflexes (snout and pout) are found in diffuse structural and metabolic disease. Flexor and extensor postures can occur in traumatic and metabolic coma (e.g., secondary to hypoxia, ischemia, hypoglycemia, or uremia). Upper motor neuron disease (destructive, pharmacologic, infectious, or metabolic) can be implied by the coexistence of a positive Babinski response, indicated by an upward movement of the great toe (instead of a normal downward turn) in response to a forceful stroke along the lateral plantar surface of the foot from the heel toward the toes. "Fanning" of the toes is a normal phenomenon.

Delirium is an acute and reversible confusional state, occurring in 20% of all hospitalized elderly patients.[51] It can be assessed by formal screening tools that focus, at any altered level of consciousness, on an acute change in mental status from a patient's baseline that is fluctuating, with difficulty focusing attention, disorganized thinking or both.[52] Assessment of dementia is impossible in a patient who is delirious.

Pupil asymmetry, alterations in size or poor reactivity (i.e., dilated and fixed) suggest a history of cerebral anoxia, intracranial vascular events, masses, or metabolic or drug abnormalities. Although patients in a coma usually have closed eyelids, tonic lid retraction or reopening after forced closure may be present with pontine disease. The brainstem can also be examined more formally using oculocephalic maneuvers or oculovestibular testing. The presence of hand tremors can suggest thyrotoxicosis or parkinsonism (associated with a pill-rolling phenomenon); hand tremors that occur with purposeful movement suggest cerebellar pathology (e.g., alcoholism or cerebrovascular accident). In patients with evidence of diabetic neuropathy or parkinsonism, autonomic dysfunction should be suspected. Myoclonus (brief, often asymmetric, generalized body jerks lasting less than 0.25 seconds) may appear as a result of cerebral hypoxia or ischemia.

Cranial nerves (CNs) should be assessed grossly or more intently with active neurologic insults. The optic nerve (CN II) is assessed by confirming visual acuity. Pupillary reactions to light (CN III) are examined by shining a bright light obliquely into each pupil in turn, looking for papillary constriction in the ipsilateral (direct) and contralateral (consensual) eye. A decreased direct response (or dilation) indicates an afferent pathway defect (Marcus Gunn pupil) such as occurs with optic neuritis, ischemic optic neuropathy, or severe retinal disease. Fixed and dilated pupils are associated with brainstem injury but may also be due to a recent dose of atropine. A pupil that is capable of accommodation but does not respond to light (Argyll-Robertson pupil) is associated with tertiary syphilis (and should be considered if the differential diagnoses include aortic dissection or aortic insufficiency), neurosarcoidosis, and Lyme disease.[53] Anisocoria (pupil inequality >1 mm) suggests a CNS mass or bleed and may explain the precordial T wave inversions seen in a comatose patient without evidence of cardiomyopathy, myocarditis, or electrolyte abnormalities. Simple anisocoria (>0.4 mm difference between eyes) is present in nearly 40% of healthy individuals, however.[54]

Pupillary accommodation may be tested by holding a finger approximately 10 cm from the patient's nose and, while observing the pupillary response in each eye, asking the patient to alternate looking into the distance and at the finger. Narrowing should occur with focus on the near finger; dilation should occur when focusing afar. The presence of eyelid ptosis may also suggest a defect in the third cranial nerve or the presence of a posterior communicating artery aneurysm. Old age, trauma, chronic inflammation, neoplasms, and thyroid abnormalities are more commonly the cause, however.

Extraocular movements should be assessed by asking the patient to follow the examiner's finger with the eyes (without moving the head) and checking gaze in the six cardinal directions using a cross or "H" pattern (CN III, IV, and VI). The examiner should pause during upward and lateral gaze to check for nystagmus.

Trigeminal nerve (CN V) motor function can be assessed by palpating for temporal or masseter muscle strength while asking the patient first to open the mouth and then to clench the teeth. The three sensory components of the trigeminal nerve can be tested by assessing the response on both sides of the face to a sharp and blunt object lightly placed against the forehead, cheeks,

and jaw. An intact corneal reflex (eye blink when the cornea is touched by a cotton wisp) tests the sensory component of the fifth cranial nerve and the motor component of the seventh cranial nerve. Facial asymmetry, or droop, is also present with seventh cranial nerve injury (e.g., Bell palsy, cerebrovascular accident, or trauma). Bell's palsy can be differentiated from stroke by the ability of a patient with Bell palsy to close his or her eye or wrinkle the forehead. Less common causes of seventh cranial nerve injury include sarcoidosis and Lyme disease.

The eighth cranial nerve can be coarsely assessed by having the patient, with the eyes closed, detect the sound of fingers lightly rubbing together alternatively next to each ear. Sensorineural hearing loss can be associated with a genetic form of dilated cardiomyopathy.[55] A hoarse voice may be caused by tenth cranial nerve abnormalities, such as compression of the recurrent laryngeal nerve motor branch by the marked left atrial enlargement that can occur with severe mitral stenosis. The motor strength of the eleventh cranial nerve is assessed by asking the patient to shrug the shoulders against resistance. Finally, the hypoglossal nerve (CN XII) is assessed by asking the patient to protrude the tongue and move it side to side.

Assessment for sensory deficits, abnormal peripheral reflexes and muscle strength may help guide the evaluation of patients with possible systemic neurologic or myopathic disease. The sensory examination requires the attention, participation, and understanding of the patient. Light touch is tested by touching the skin with a wisp of cotton or a tissue and asking the patient to acknowledge the feeling while not looking. Pain sensation can be elicited using a sharp object; temperature sensation can be grossly ascertained using cold and warm objects. Vibration is tested with a tuning fork and needs to be compared bilaterally. Sensory deficits can offer important clues regarding the systemic, central, or peripheral location of underlying lesions. Diabetes mellitus is suggested by a "stocking-glove" distribution of sensory defects; focal hyperesthesia or anesthesia can occur with the dry beriberi of vitamin B_1 deficiency (high-output cardiac failure occurs in wet beriberi). The presence of hand tremors can suggest thyrotoxicosis or parkinsonism (associated with a pill-rolling phenomenon); hand tremors that occur only with purposeful movements suggest cerebellar pathology (e.g., alcoholism or cerebrovascular accident). Delayed ankle reflexes in a patient with cool, dry, and coarse skin with bradycardia is highly suggestive of hypothyroidism.[56,57]

Motor deficits may be difficult to evaluate in the CICU but should be initially sought in all major muscle groups by having the patient move each muscle group against resistance. Motor strength is reported as 5/5 (normal strength), 4/5 (movement against resistance, but less than normal), 3/5 (movement against gravity, but not against added resistance), 2/5 (movement at the joint, but not against gravity), 1/5 (visible muscle movement, but no movement at the joint), and 0/5 (no muscle movement). Motor deficits may be present with a cardiomyopathy in patients with Duchenne or Becker muscular dystrophy; the presence of motor and conduction defects can occur with myotonic dystrophy. Focal muscle weakness raises the possibility of a new or old upper motor neuron lesion (e.g., multiple sclerosis, intracranial mass, or cerebrovascular accident) or mononeuropathy. Symmetric proximal weakness can occur with numerous myopathies, whereas symmetric distal weakness can occur with polyneuropathy, amyotrophic lateral sclerosis and Guillain-Barré syndrome. Statins and alcohol can affect either distal or proximal muscle groups.

VASCULAR EXAMINATION

The vascular examination may begin with the auscultation of both flanks for the presence of a bruit suggestive of renal artery stenosis. Angiographically significant renal artery stenosis may be present in nearly 60% of patients with peripheral arterial disease. The aorta can often be assessed on deep palpation of the central abdomen. A pulsatile pulse immediately above the level of the umbilicus is a nonsensitive sign of an abdominal aortic aneurysm and is most readily detected in men older than 60 years. In patients complaining of exertional or positional leg pain, the absence of a pulse or the presence of arterial ulcers is often diagnostic for vascular insufficiency. In the setting of an intraaortic balloon pump or after a catheter-based coronary artery procedure, particular attention must be paid to assessing the pulses sequentially on the investigated limb.

MUSCULOSKELETAL AND INTEGUMENT EXAMINATION

The musculoskeletal examination should begin with a general assessment for global or focal muscle wasting or atrophy. During lung auscultation, one can simultaneously inspect the spine for scoliosis, lordosis, or kyphosis. Each spinous process should be inspected for focal areas of tenderness. Holt-Oram syndrome, associated with atrial and ventricular septal defects, usually manifests with upper limb skeletal deformities, including unequal arm lengths; anomalous development of the radial, carpal, and thenar bones of the hand; triphalangeal or absent thumbs; or phocomelia. Arachnodactyly (long, spidery fingers) may be found in patients with Marfan syndrome. Capillary pulsations under the fingernails may be evident with aortic regurgitation, sepsis, or thyrotoxicosis, whereas splinter hemorrhages raise the possibility of bacterial endocarditis. The presence of Osler nodes (painful reddish papules approximately 1 cm on the fingertips, palms, toes, or soles of the feet) also suggests endocarditis.

The joints should be felt for crepitus during passive motion and, in the setting of fever or focal neurologic symptoms, the neck should be assessed for evidence of nuchal rigidity. The extremities should be assessed for unilateral or bilateral edema (suggestive of heart failure, hypoproteinemia, or venous thrombosis), cellulitis, phlebitis, or ischemic extremities. While evaluating the legs, the clinician should consider if subcutaneous anticoagulation or compression boots are necessary for prevention of deep venous thrombosis.

Skin erythema and warmth suggest inflammation, as do soft tissue swelling or focal areas of tenderness. Specific skin patterns may suggest particular diseases and may prove critical to the care of patients in the CICU. A rash typically found on the palms, soles, dorsum of the hands, and extensor surfaces that begins as macules that develop into papules, vesicles, bullae, urticarial plaques, or confluent erythema is consistent with Stevens-Johnson syndrome. Other skin findings associated with disease include the malar flush (mitral facies) of mitral stenosis, brick-red coloring seen with polycythemia, bronze coloring associated with hemochromatosis, oral hyperpigmentation and brown coloring with Addison disease, "moon facies" of Cushing disease and a butterfly rash across the nose and cheeks consistent with systemic lupus erythematosus.

Approximately 4 to 5 g/dL of unoxygenated hemoglobin in the capillaries generates the blue color appreciated clinically as central cyanosis.[58] For this reason, patients who are anemic may be hypoxemic without showing any cyanosis. Central cyanosis (involving the mucous membranes of the lips, tongue, and earlobes) with warm extremities strongly suggests right-to-left shunting (usually the shunt is >25% of the total cardiac output), severe anemia (hematocrit <15%), severe hypoxia, or concomitant lung disease. Cyanosis may also occur in the presence of increased amounts of methemoglobin (e.g., with use of dapsone, nitroglycerin, or topical benzocaine) or sulfhemoglobin. Pseudocyanosis, a blue color to the skin without deoxygenated hemoglobin, may occur with the use of amiodarone, phenothiazines, and some metals (especially silver and lead). Central cyanosis often improves with supplemental oxygen. Clubbing suggests central cyanosis, right-to-left shunting with or without congenital heart disease, or bacterial endocarditis. Cyanosis in the presence of normal oximetry suggests anemia, poor cardiac output, or hypercapnia. If the lower limbs are cyanosed but the upper limbs are not, a patent ductus arteriosus should be expected. Peripheral cyanosis with cool extremities suggests the presence of low cardiac output, hypovolemia, or peripheral vasoconstriction. Warming the extremity often improves cyanosis.

Jaundice, which may be present with hepatitis, alcoholic liver disease, choledocholithiasis, pancreatic cancer, or metastatic liver disease, can be differentiated from other causes of yellow skin by the concomitant "yellowing" of mucous membranes under the tongue or in the conjunctiva of the eye. The presence of spider angiomata, palmar erythema, dilated abdominal veins and ascites increases the likelihood of a hepatocellular cause of the jaundice.[59] The finding of a palpable gallbladder (Courvoisier sign) is highly suggestive of extrahepatic obstruction.

CONCLUSION

The physical examination, if performed carefully, remains a vital and cost-effective approach to evaluating patients in the CICU. It can direct a focused and efficient diagnostic approach rather than relying on a "shotgun" approach to testing. In addition, the laying on of hands inspires confidence in the physician and forges a bond with the patient.

The full reference list for this chapter is available at ExpertConsult.com.

PART II

Scientific Foundation of Cardiac Intensive Care

4

Role of the Cardiovascular System in Coupling the External Environment to Cellular Respiration

Peter D. Wagner

The cardiovascular system exists primarily to transport oxygen and nutrients to the various body tissues and to transport carbon dioxide and other waste products from the tissues to the lungs, kidneys, or liver for disposal. It is a component of the oxygen transport pathway, linking the environment via the lungs (and chest wall) to the tissue cells by the heart and the vascular network.

The focus of this section is on cardiovascular function as it affects oxygen transport between the environment and tissue cells. Both total cardiac output and its distribution between and within organs are critical aspects of oxygen transport efficiency in health and disease. While the principles of oxygen exchange and transport in the lungs and tissues are fundamentally similar, it is worth discussing pulmonary and tissue oxygen transport separately. Normal physiologic processes are described, followed by pathophysiologic consequences of disease from the point of view of cardiac function.

CARDIOVASCULAR FUNCTION AND PULMONARY GAS EXCHANGE

Cardiac function is of importance to oxygen exchange in the lungs in a number of ways. First, total pulmonary blood flow (normally equal to cardiac output) affects partial pressure of oxygen (PO_2) of venous blood entering the lungs. Although in health this is of little significance, it is of major importance in disease. Second, the relationship between total pulmonary blood flow and the volume of blood in the pulmonary capillaries determines red cell exposure (or transit) time in the lungs. In resting normal humans, transit time is greatly in excess of what is needed. This may not be the case during exercise or in disease. Third, the distribution of pulmonary blood flow among the ~500 million alveoli[1] cannot be perfectly matched to their ventilation. This causes ventilation/perfusion ($\dot{V}A/\dot{Q}$) mismatch that interferes with arterial oxygenation. Once again, this is of little

consequence in health but is of major importance in disease of the cardiopulmonary system. Fourth, dysfunction of the left ventricle from any cause that raises diastolic filling pressure has the potential for causing pulmonary edema, especially if there has been pulmonary capillary damage from disease. Pressures are sufficiently low in health that edema does not occur at rest. On heavy exercise, mild interstitial edema can occur but the effects are subtle. Importance of left ventricular dysfunction increases dramatically when filling pressures exceed 20 to 25 mm Hg.[2] Pulmonary microvessels may even undergo a degree of physical disruption at very high vascular pressures.[3] Fifth, right ventricular hypertrophy from pulmonary diseases may impair left ventricular function, effectively decreasing left ventricular compliance through mechanical interdependence of the heart chambers.

TOTAL PULMONARY BLOOD FLOW AND OXYGEN EXCHANGE

Pulmonary oxygen exchange under steady-state conditions obeys mass balance principles. Corresponding equations can be written to describe oxygen uptake from respired air and into the pulmonary circulation.[4] These are, respectively,

$$\dot{V}O_2 = \dot{V}I \bullet FIO_2 - \dot{V}A \bullet FAO_2 \tag{1}$$

$$\dot{V}O_2 = \dot{Q}[CaO_2 - C\bar{v}O_2] \tag{2}$$

$\dot{V}O_2$ is whole body oxygen consumption; $\dot{V}I$ and $\dot{V}A$ are inspired and expired alveolar ventilation, respectively; FIO_2 and FAO_2 are inspired and expired alveolar oxygen fractional concentrations, respectively; $\dot{Q}$ is total pulmonary blood flow and CaO_2 and $C\bar{v}O_2$ are arterial and pulmonary arterial (mixed venous) oxygen concentrations, respectively. These two equations embody the principle of taking the difference between the oxygen flow rate into and out of the lungs, expressed for ventilation (Eq 1) or blood flow (Eq 2). While not completely correct, it is reasonable for clinical purposes to assume that $\dot{V}_I$ equals $\dot{V}_A$, to simplify Eq 1. Strictly, $\dot{V}_A = \dot{V}_I - \dot{V}_{O_2} + \dot{V}_{CO_2}$ (where $\dot{V}_{CO_2}$ is CO_2 output by the lungs). If the respiratory quotient (R) equals 1.0, $\dot{V}_{O_2} = \dot{V}_{CO_2}$ and $\dot{V}_A = \dot{V}_I$. Normally, $\dot{V}_{O_2}$ exceeds $\dot{V}_{CO_2}$ so that R is 0.8, on average. Under these conditions, $\dot{V}_A$ is about 1% less than $\dot{V}_I$, an unimportant difference.

In healthy lungs, alveolar P_{O_2} (proportional to $F_{A_{O_2}}$, Eq 1) is tightly related to $C_{a_{O_2}}$ (Eq 2) by the O_2-Hb dissociation curve. Thus $C_{a_{O_2}}$ can be directly computed using alveolar P_{O_2} and the O_2-Hb dissociation curve.[5] This is not true in lung disease, in which for Eq 1, $F_{A_{O_2}}$ is mean alveolar $[O_2]$ averaged over the ~500 million alveoli (weighted by the ventilation of each) and $C_{a_{O_2}}$ is arterial $[O_2]$, similarly averaged but weighted by blood flow to each of the alveoli. When ventilation and/or blood flow is distributed in a nonhomogeneous manner in lung disease, the P_{O_2} corresponding to mean alveolar gas is often much higher than that of arterial blood (corresponding to $C_{a_{O_2}}$). $C_{a_{O_2}}$ cannot then be accurately calculated from $F_{A_{O_2}}$ and the O_2-Hb dissociation curve.

Returning to the normal lung setting and Eq 1 and Eq 2, it is clear from Eq 1 that alveolar $[O_2]$, $F_{A_{O_2}}$, is a direct function of $\dot{V}_{O_2}$, $F_{I_{O_2}}$, and alveolar ventilation only. Thus so too is arterial $[O_2]$, $C_{a_{O_2}}$. The important conclusion is that changes in cardiac output, $\dot{Q}$, will have no influence on arterial $[O_2]$ or P_{O_2} in normal lungs, that is so long as $C_{a_{O_2}}$ is a direct function of $F_{A_{O_2}}$. For example, an increase in cardiac output per se with anxiety or fever would not affect arterial P_{O_2} in a normal lung (if $\dot{V}_{O_2}$, $F_{I_{O_2}}$, and ventilation remained unchanged). A fall in cardiac output from dehydration, blood loss, or myocardial infarct would also not affect arterial P_{O_2} under the same assumptions in a normal lung.

Eq 2 shows that the sole influence of cardiac output on gas exchange in a normal lung is to affect mixed venous $[O_2]$ and P_{O_2}. As cardiac output falls so too will $C_{\bar{v}_{O_2}}$ and as cardiac output rises, so too will $C_{\bar{v}_{O_2}}$. While as stated this does not affect arterial $[O_2]$ or P_{O_2} in the normal lung, this is not the case in diseases of the lungs associated with ventilation/blood flow mismatch or right to left shunting. In such diseases, it is still true that $C_{\bar{v}_{O_2}}$ must rise and fall with cardiac output just as in health (other influences staying constant). However, since arterial blood is the mixture of blood from all lung regions, a shunt (or areas of low $\dot{V}_A/\dot{Q}$ ratio) will mix blood from regions having lower $[O_2]$ than normal, reducing mixed arterial $[O_2]$ and P_{O_2}. As cardiac output falls, the $[O_2]$ and P_{O_2} of such shunts or low $\dot{V}_A/\dot{Q}$ regions will fall because such pathways essentially fail to oxygenate flowing blood above mixed venous levels. Thus the contribution of such regions to arterial blood, being tightly coupled to mixed venous $[O_2]$, is in turn closely dependent on cardiac output. The end result is more severe arterial hypoxemia as cardiac output falls and less severe hypoxemia as cardiac output rises. This is illustrated in Fig. 4.1, in which a normal lung and a lung containing as an example of disease—a 25% right-to-left shunt—are compared as cardiac output changes. Arterial oxygen saturation, a better reflection of the oxygen concentration of the blood, follows changes in P_{O_2} (Fig. 4.2). Mixed venous P_{O_2}

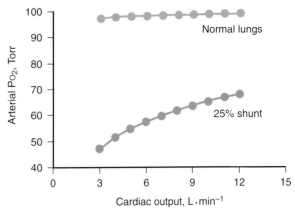

Fig. 4.1 Effect of changes in cardiac output on arterial P_{O_2} in normal and diseased lungs. In this example, the diseased lung contains a 25% right-to-left shunt. Arterial P_{O_2} is essentially independent of cardiac output in health but depends significantly on cardiac output in disease.

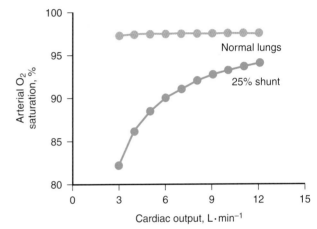

Fig. 4.2 Effect of cardiac output on arterial oxygen saturation, from the same calculations as used in Fig. 4.1. Saturation varies considerably with cardiac output in diseased but not normal lungs.

(Fig. 4.3) changes similarly in both cases (according to Eq 2) but only in the abnormal lung do arterial P_{O_2} and oxygen saturation vary with cardiac output. The clinical message is clear: the degree of arterial hypoxemia in a given patient depends not only on how much shunt (or $\dot{V}_A/\dot{Q}$ mismatch) is present but also on cardiac output. Therefore, if arterial P_{O_2} were to fall in such a patient, changes in cardiac output should be excluded if the arterial P_{O_2} change is to be interpreted as a change in health of the lung. Application of the classical shunt (or venous admixture) equation[6,7] illustrates this dramatically:

$$\dot{Q}_{VA}/\dot{Q}_T = 100 \times [C_{i_{O_2}} - C_{a_{O_2}}]/[C_{i_{O_2}} - C_{\bar{v}_{O_2}}] \quad \textbf{(3)}$$

Here $\dot{Q}_{VA}/\dot{Q}_T$ is venous admixture as a percentage of the cardiac output and $C_{i_{O_2}}$ is essentially the $[O_2]$ of normal end capillary blood in nonshunted, normal $\dot{V}_A/\dot{Q}$ regions of the lung. As $\dot{Q}_{VA}/\dot{Q}_T$ is computed over the range of cardiac output values and for the examples in Fig. 4.1, but assuming $C_{\bar{v}_{O_2}}$ staying constant ($P_{\bar{v}_{O_2}}$ constant at the normal value of 40 Torr for $\dot{Q}_T$ = 6 L $\cdot$ min^{-1} in each case, rather than the *actual* $C_{\bar{v}_{O_2}}$ associated

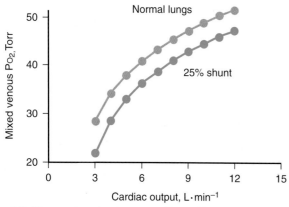

Fig. 4.3 Change in mixed venous PO_2 with cardiac output for the conditions in Figs. 4.1 and 4.2. Mixed venous PO_2 changes similarly with cardiac output both in health and disease. Absolute PO_2 is slightly higher in health at a given cardiac output.

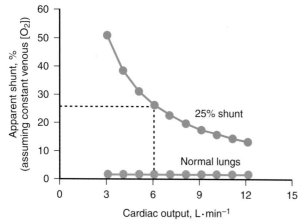

Fig. 4.4 Calculated or apparent shunt as a percentage of cardiac output when the assumption is made that oxygen concentration in mixed venous blood is constant, equaling that seen when cardiac output is 6 L · min^{-1}. This assumption leads to large errors in calculated shunt when cardiac output is reduced or increased. The dashed lines indicate conditions under which the assumption is correct so that calculated shunt is also accurate, but only at that point.

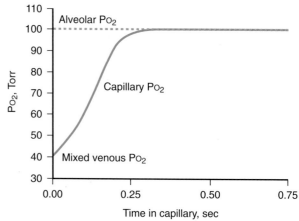

Fig. 4.5 Time course of PO_2 change along the pulmonary capillary as oxygen moves from alveolar gas into the flowing capillary blood. Starting at a mixed venous PO_2 of 40 Torr, full equilibration with alveolar gas is reached in about 0.25 seconds, leaving a large reserve in transit time under normal conditions.

with each cardiac output), it can be seen (Fig. 4.4) how badly $\dot{Q}VA/\dot{Q}T$ is overestimated when actual cardiac output is low and underestimated when cardiac output is high. Neither of the extremes of cardiac output in Fig. 4.4, that is, 3 and 12 L · min^{-1}, is beyond the range of common experience in the intensive care setting. Apparent shunt ($\dot{Q}VA/\dot{Q}T$) would be about twice the actual value when cardiac output is 50% reduced and half the real value when cardiac output is doubled if venous [O_2] is assumed to be at normal levels.

Pulmonary Transit Time

The preceding section has assumed sufficient time for oxygen to fully equilibrate across the blood gas barrier: that is, PO_2 in the capillary blood has increased from mixed venous levels all the way to alveolar PO_2 within the available red cell contact time.

Average red cell contact time normally appears to be about 0.75 seconds. This estimate is the ratio of resting capillary blood volume (75 mL, measured by the carbon monoxide technique[8]) to the corresponding cardiac output (6 L · min^{-1}). Fig. 4.5 indicates the normal PO_2 profile calculated along the pulmonary capillary and shows full equilibration in about 0.25 seconds, leaving fully 0.5 seconds in reserve.[9] While transit times in different alveoli are by no means uniform,[10] the variance in such times is still small enough that full equilibration occurs at rest even in those channels with the shortest transit and even during moderate exercise. Only during heavy exercise does failure of equilibration occur in health.[11] At altitude, however, diffusion limitation is seen even with light to moderate exercise and becomes a major factor reducing arterial [O_2] under such conditions.[12]

In cardiopulmonary diseases, diffusion limitation in the lung rarely occurs, even when patients are well enough to exercise. The exception is interstitial pulmonary fibrosis, in which diffusion limitation is usually seen during exercise and when it aggravates hypoxemia.[13] Diffusion limitation can also occur at rest in such patients.[14] However, pulmonary diffusing capacity must be below about 60% of normal before this is seen due to the above described reserve in red cell transit time.[14] Hypoxemia in cirrhosis of the liver appears to have a small component of diffusion limitation as well.

In severe cardiopulmonary diseases, such as acute pulmonary edema from left ventricular failure or acute respiratory distress syndrome (ARDS), conditions develop that reduce O_2 diffusing capacity. In particular, the normally thin (0.5 μm) blood gas barrier separating alveolar gas from capillary blood can become edematous. However, such interstitial edema is thought not to produce measurable oxygen diffusion limitation. In more advanced disease, there is alveolar filling with edema fluid and/or cellular debris. This abolishes all ventilation and affected alveoli and produces what is more commonly called *shunt* (perfusion of unventilated alveoli). One could advance the argument that such alveoli are, in fact, completely diffusion limited, since no O_2 exchange occurs at all. This becomes a semantic issue and should not detract from the more important problem of understanding the pathologic and physiologic changes with these diseases.

Distribution of Blood Flow Within the Lungs

In normal lungs, output from the right ventricle is not equally distributed among the ~500 million alveoli. Gravity affects blood flow distribution, more blood flowing through dependent than nondependent alveoli due to the weight of the blood.[15] There are nongravitational influences on blood flow distribution as well. The fractal branching nature of the vascular tree produces nonuniformity of distribution,[16] and the lack of perfect anatomic symmetry further perturbs flow patterns.[17] There may also be greater perfusion of central (proximal) than peripheral (distal) lung regions,[18] although this is presently not resolved. Given all of these independent sources of nonuniformity, a substantial degree of nonhomogeneous blood flow distribution exists and should not come as a surprise. However, it seems that the distribution of ventilation is largely matched to that of blood flow so that ventilation and blood flow are each greatest and least in the same areas.[19] This matching is not perfect, but interferes trivially with oxygen transport in the normal lung. If a perfect lung produces an arterial P_{O_2} of 100 Torr, the real lung produces in young healthy subjects an arterial P_{O_2} of 90 to 95 Torr. Given the flat O_2-Hb dissociation curve at this P_{O_2}, the effect on arterial $[O_2]$ of this 5 to 10 Torr drop is indeed negligible.

Eq 1 and Eq 2, while used earlier for considering the whole lung, can be applied at the local alveolar level, where the terms now reflect local alveolar and end-capillary oxygen levels and local $\dot{V}_{O_2}$. Still assuming equality of $\dot{V}_I$ and $\dot{V}_A$ at this level and setting Eqs 1 and 2 equal to one another yields a new relationship, Eq 4:

$$\dot{V}_A[F_{IO_2} - F_{AO_2}] = \dot{Q}[C_{c'O_2} - C\bar{v}_{O_2}]$$

$$\text{or } \dot{V}_A/\dot{Q} = [C_{c'O_2} - C\bar{v}_{O_2}]/[F_{IO_2} - F_{AO_2}] \qquad \textbf{(4)}$$

Here, $C_{c'O_2}$ is the standard term for end capillary $[O_2]$ in a local lung region, with the other terms retaining their previous definitions.

Eq 4 shows that within such a local lung region, alveolar (and end-capillary) $[O_2]$ is a unique function of the $\dot{V}_A/\dot{Q}$ ratio and the so-called boundary conditions, that is, the inspired and mixed venous oxygen levels. A third factor implicit to Eq 4 is the P_{O_2}–$[O_2]$ relationship defined by the O_2-Hb dissociation curve.

Eq 4 points out how changes in the local ratio of $\dot{V}_A$ to $\dot{Q}$ are a key factor affecting local gas exchange and thus arterial P_{O_2} and $[O_2]$.[4,6,7] Fig. 4.6 shows how local P_{O_2} depends on the $\dot{V}_A/\dot{Q}$ ratio for room air breathing and a range of three mixed venous P_{O_2} levels. At $\dot{V}_A/\dot{Q}$ ratios in the normal range (~0.3 to 3),[20] local P_{O_2} varies considerably with $\dot{V}_A/\dot{Q}$ and $P\bar{v}_{O_2}$. At lower $\dot{V}_A/\dot{Q}$ ratios typical of most cardiopulmonary diseases (i.e., below the normal range) local P_{O_2} is tied to $P\bar{v}_{O_2}$ and virtually independent of $\dot{V}_A/\dot{Q}$ ratio, as Fig. 4.6 shows. Thus as cardiac output and $P\bar{v}_{O_2}$ change, it can be seen how low $\dot{V}_A/\dot{Q}$ regions will closely reflect these changes, affecting arterial P_{O_2} as mentioned earlier.

Clearly, the quantitative manner in which blood flow is distributed within the lungs, and how this relates to the distribution

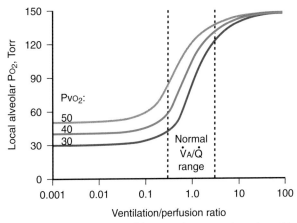

Fig. 4.6 Alveolar P_{O_2} in small lung regions as a function of local ventilation/perfusion ratio. The normal $\dot{V}_A/\dot{Q}$ range is shown. The most important observation to be made is that when ventilation/perfusion ratio is reduced below normal, alveolar P_{O_2} is tied closely to P_{O_2} in the mixed venous blood.

of ventilation and thus of $\dot{V}_A/\dot{Q}$ ratios, is a major factor in gas exchange and thus in arterial oxygenation.

In cardiopulmonary disease, areas of low or zero $\dot{V}_A/\dot{Q}$ ratio are commonly seen and are responsible for hypoxemia.[21] In the great majority of cases, areas of low or zero $\dot{V}_A/\dot{Q}$ ratio are generated by abnormalities in local ventilation, not blood flow (although, e.g., the alveolar edema underlying such effects may have its origins in primary cardiac disease). Thus, local reduction in ventilation from airways obstruction or alveolar filling (cell debris or fluid) is the usual mechanism. There are some specific situations in which hypoxemia appears to be due to primary vascular changes. The hypoxemia of chronic liver disease is due to pulmonary vascular malformations that mostly act as right-to-left shunts, the blood in them not participating in gas exchange.[22–24] Pulmonary thromboembolic disease, by obstructing some pulmonary arteries, results in exaggerated perfusion of nonembolized areas. This reduces the local $\dot{V}_A/\dot{Q}$ ratio of nonembolized alveoli and is a primary reason for hypoxemia when it occurs in such patients.[25]

Of particular relevance to the cardiovascular state in the context of pulmonary gas exchange is a curious, poorly understood, but reproducible phenomenon whereby, as total blood flow through the lung (usually cardiac output) increases or decreases, so too does fractional shunt or venous admixture.[26] Fig. 4.7 is a dramatic example of this phenomenon in a single patient with lung disease on variable right heart bypass.[27] As pulmonary blood was mechanically varied from 1 to 5 L/min per m^2, the percentage of shunt increased from 15% to over 40% of the cardiac output. To underline the magnitude of this effect, absolute shunt perfusion increased from 0.15 L/(min · m^2) to over 2 L/(min · m^2), a more than 10-fold increase. Because these changes are rapidly reversible, within minutes, it seems unlikely that the greater blood flow is actually causing more damage and therefore more shunt. There is likely some systematic change in blood flow distribution between ventilated, normal regions and the unventilated alveoli, causing the shunt to change with total blood flow.[28] This generally happens irrespective of the anatomic distribution of disease and

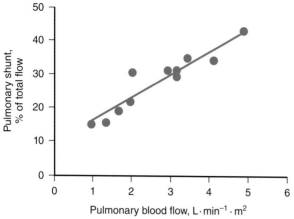

Fig. 4.7 Dependence of percentage shunt through the lungs on pulmonary blood flow in a single patient with adult respiratory distress syndrome. In this patient, on partial right heart bypass, pulmonary blood flow was varied between 1 and 5 L · min⁻¹ · m². Shunt varied between 15% and 40% in a linear manner.

therefore appears unrelated to lung structure in any systematic way. Moreover, a multitude of animal studies done under many circumstances mirror the human experience, no matter whether the cardiac output is manipulated mechanically or pharmacologically.[29] The finding that the increase in percent of shunt with cardiac output is far greater in animals breathing pure O_2 than room air and, in turn, greater than in those breathing a hypoxic gas mixture points to an interaction between hypoxic pulmonary vasoconstriction and blood flow as the basic mechanism.[30] Thus, at low blood flow rates while breathing 100% oxygen, unventilated alveoli are greatly vasoconstricted by hypoxia while ventilated units have little or no vascular tone. Any increase in total blood flow is directed mostly to the unventilated units because the higher pressure of high blood flow can overcome hypoxic vasomotor tone, while little additional blood flow can be accommodated by already relaxed, well-ventilated regions.

From the clinical standpoint, it is important to be aware of the shunt–total blood flow relationship when interpreting pulmonary gas exchange changes as cardiac output varies.

Closely related to these issues is the effect of systemic vasodilators, sometimes given to patients in left heart failure to reduce afterload. When such patients have pulmonary gas exchange abnormalities, often due to pulmonary edema from the heart failure itself, there are areas of low or zero ventilation/perfusion ratio due to edema of the alveolar wall and/or alveolar gas space.[21] Consequently, these regions are subject to hypoxic pulmonary vasoconstriction. Administration of a systemic vasodilator, such as nitroprusside, dilates not only the systemic vasculature but also the pulmonary vasculature. The latter is particularly evident in the most vasoconstricted areas having a low $\dot{V}_A/\dot{Q}$ ratio. The result is increased blood flow through these areas—that is, an increase in shunt or venous admixture.[21] Such changes accordingly act to worsen arterial hypoxemia. A reduction in arterial P_{O_2} is often not seen, however, because the simultaneous increase in cardiac output seen with vasodilators increases mixed venous P_{O_2}. From arguments given earlier in this chapter (see Figs. 4.1 and 4.6), arterial P_{O_2} would be increased by this mechanism.

The two opposing influences tend to balance, with no net change in arterial oxygenation.[21] It is important to point out, however, that despite no change in arterial $[O_2]$, if cardiac output rises, so too will total oxygen transport (the product of cardiac output and arterial $[O_2]$). This may be beneficial to cellular oxygen metabolism because it may increase oxygen availability to cells.

Left Ventricular Dysfunction and Lung Fluid Exchange

Another point of interaction between the heart, lungs, and oxygen transport occurs when left ventricular filling pressures rise for any reason (as in myocardial or valvular disease), resulting in pulmonary edema. The lungs normally allow a steady flux of both water and proteins out of the capillaries into the interstitial space. This lymph finds its way in peribronchial lymphatic channels from peripheral to central lung regions and exits the hilum of the lungs in lymph ducts that drain into the superior vena cava. Transcapillary fluid flux is described by the Starling equation:

$$J = K[(P_{MV} - P_{INT}) - \sigma(\Pi_{MV} - \Pi_{INT})] \tag{5}$$

Here, J is fluid flux across the capillary wall and K is an overall filtration coefficient proportional to permeability and surface area of the microvascular network. σ is a reflection coefficient for proteins and is 0 when the wall is freely permeable to proteins, 1 when completely impermeable; σ must be low because albumin levels in the pulmonary lymph are some 70% to 90% of those in capillary plasma.[31,32] P_{MV} and P_{INT} are intracapillary microvascular and extracapillary interstitial hydrostatic pressures, respectively. Π_{MV} and Π_{INT} are the protein osmotic pressures in the same regions. The equation therefore sums the intra- and extracapillary hydrostatic and osmotic forces. The net result is as stated positive[2] so that normally some 0.25 to 1 mL of lymph is transported across the capillary each minute. The lymphatic drainage system can easily handle this load. Its drainage efficiency is increased by one-way valves that make use of the respiratory excursions in intrathoracic pressure to pump lymph from alveoli centrally to the lymph ducts for return to the venous system.

For a structurally normal capillary, microvascular pressures have to exceed some 25 mm Hg before the rate of fluid movement out of the capillaries exceeds drainage capacity and edema develops.[2] Normal microvascular pressures are 5 to 10 mm Hg. If capillary permeability is increased by capillary damage in disease, or if plasma protein levels are very low, alveolar edema will occur at pressures much lower than 25 mm Hg, as expected.

When left ventricular dysfunction from any cause elevates pulmonary microvascular pressures sufficiently, the stage is set for clinical pulmonary edema. As explained, this causes reduced local ventilation, sometimes to the point of abolition of local gas exchange, resulting in areas of low $\dot{V}_A/\dot{Q}$ ratio and shunt. The mechanisms involved may include alveolar wall interstitial edema that reduces alveolar compliance and thus ventilation; compression of conducting airways and/or blood vessels by fluid moving centrally as lymph, increasing resistance and decreasing gas or blood flow; or alveolar flooding with edema, abolishing ventilation and gas exchange in these alveoli completely.

Ventricular Function and Lung Disease

There is increasing evidence suggesting that primary lung disease causing chronic pulmonary hypertension and resulting in right ventricular hypertrophy impedes left ventricular filling.[33,34] This is functionally equivalent to increased diastolic stiffness of the left ventricular wall. Left ventricular filling pressures are thereby increased. This increase will be transmitted back through the pulmonary microvascular bed. As pressure in that bed is raised, transcapillary fluid flux will tend to increase, raising the risk of edema (see earlier discussion). Further retrograde pressure transmission will elevate pulmonary artery pressure, worsen the load on the right ventricle, and thus set up a potential vicious circle of events impeding both cardiac and pulmonary function. While the importance of this mechanism in clinical disease states remains to be determined, there is some evidence of its pertinence to a special human disorder: high-altitude pulmonary edema (HAPE).[35] Susceptible individuals develop patchy pulmonary edema after rapid ascent and vigorous effort at altitudes of about 9000 feet and higher. While such individuals are known to have an exaggerated pulmonary vasoconstrictor response to hypoxia,[36] they also have higher left ventricular filling pressures (as estimated by pulmonary artery occlusion pressures) during exercise than HAPE-resistant subjects.[35] While this observation could reflect intrinsic variance in left ventricular stiffness per se, it is compatible with the independent ventricular effects described earlier whereby right ventricular hypertension reduces effective left ventricular compliance.

Another type of cardiac complication of lung disease comes from ventilator strategies used in patients on assisted ventilation in the intensive care setting. High respiratory inflation pressures are commonplace to overcome loss of pulmonary compliance due to fluid and cell buildup in the alveolar region. Positive end-expiratory pressure (PEEP) is also commonly maintained at end expiration to prevent alveolar collapse. When these strategies overinflate less affected alveoli, their capillaries are stretched and compressed. This raises pulmonary vascular resistance. Combined with the positive intrathoracic pressures due to PEEP, venous return and right and left ventricular function are impaired and cardiac output is reduced, often by surprisingly large amounts.[37] Balancing ventilatory strategies to maintain alveolar gas exchange while minimizing undesirable cardiovascular consequences is a classic and difficult problem in management of acutely ill patients; guidelines are continually being revised for optimal ventilatory care.[38] Until the consequences of such strategies on O_2 transport to critical organs (including the heart) can be assessed accurately, it will be difficult to rationalize a particular approach. Thus as PEEP is increased, arterial $[O_2]$ may improve due to alveolar reexpansion of previously atelectatic regions but at the cost of diminished cardiac output and thus organ blood flow.[39] Oxygen transport—the product of arterial $[O_2]$ and blood flow to each organ—may increase, not change, or fall in ways that are difficult to measure, let alone understand in terms of metabolic consequences. This remains a critical area of clinical and basic research.

CARDIOVASCULAR FUNCTION AND SYSTEMIC GAS EXCHANGE

After oxygen exchange between alveolar gas and capillary blood has taken place, oxygenated arterial blood must be transported to the various organs and tissue beds of the body. The amount of oxygen that reaches any vascular bed per unit time is given by the product of the arterial oxygen concentration and the blood flow rate through that bed, and is termed *oxygen delivery*. After reaching the microvasculature of each bed, oxygen is moved from its Hb-bound, intraerythrocytic location through a series of steps to reach intracellular mitochondria.[40] By far, the majority of oxygen taken in at the lungs is used at the mitochondrial level to produce adenosine triphosphate (ATP) for energy and thermal homeostasis of the organs. The oxygen unloading pathway in a typical tissue traverses the following sequential steps.[40] First, oxygen must chemically dissociate from the Hb molecule. In vitro studies of this reaction suggest that this is quick and not limiting to overall oxygen transport. Next, oxygen molecules in solution must diffuse out of the red cell, into the microvascular plasma and through the endothelial wall. At rest, there is sufficient time for this to proceed to completion—that is, to enable sufficient oxygen transport to meet the metabolic needs of the tissue—but during intense exercise in fit subjects, this may not be the case in the exercising muscle. The amount of microvascular surface area available within an organ is thought to be a critical variable that under some conditions (e.g., in muscle during exercise and possibly in multiple organ failure in several capillary beds) is a limiting component to the movement of oxygen from red cell to mitochondria.[41,42] The final step for oxygen is intracellular movement to reach mitochondria. All of these transport steps are reliant on passive diffusion; there are no active (energy-requiring) oxygen transport processes. However, in muscle, intracellular oxygen movement is considered to be uniquely accelerated by the binding of oxygen to myoglobin.[43,44] This reduces intracellular PO_2, maintaining a large PO_2 difference between red cell and the muscle cytoplasm that facilitates oxygen diffusion (by Fick's law of diffusion). Moreover, myoglobin molecules can move quite freely in cytoplasm, which further aids oxygen transport. Due to great metabolic need for O_2 during exercise, this mechanism is considered to be important.[45,46] Without myoglobin, maximal aerobic ATP production might be significantly reduced by the lower oxygen transport rate. Finally, both in muscle and other tissues, there may be a high concentration of mitochondria close to the cell wall, particularly near capillaries.[40] Whether this association facilitates oxygen movement directly to mitochondria or serves some other purpose, such as to facilitate metabolic clearance of waste products, is not known.

This basic process of tissue oxygen transport is common to all tissues. Quantitative features clearly will depend on individual anatomic factors that determine microvascular richness and diffusion distances. Just as in the lungs, this diffusive system is generally adequate in all organs in normal humans at rest. However, during exercise in health and possibly also in disease states, diffusive conductance may be limited to the point of constraining oxygen flux to the mitochondria and hence local metabolic rate. For example, maximal oxygen consumption is determined in part by the finite nature of the overall muscle diffusive conductance between the red cells and mitochondria.[47] The fall in maximal $\dot{V}O_2$ with hypoxia and increase in hyperoxia is further compatible with this notion. Behavior of oxygen consumption as oxygen transport to tissues is varied at rest or in disease is also compatible with a limited, finite oxygen diffusing conductance and pathway, although other factors may be responsible (see upcoming discussion).

Another important concept in oxygen transport to different organs and also within organs is that of heterogeneity. In an ideal organism, blood flow, and therefore oxygen transport to each tissue, would be precisely matched to local metabolic need. Those organs with higher $\dot{V}O_2$ would generally receive correspondingly higher blood flow. Organs with a need for high blood flow based on other functions (such as kidney and liver) disrupt this ideal. Consequently, $[O_2]$ of venous blood from various organs differs (in accord with the relationship between $\dot{V}O_2$ and blood flow $(\dot{Q})$, as Eq 2 would dictate). Even within organs, local heterogeneity may exist such that some regions are overperfused while others are underperfused. Underperfused regions may not be able to achieve their normal metabolic rate for lack of oxygen, and cellular dysfunction may result.

There is certainly blood flow heterogeneity within all organs. This has been repeatedly shown with tracer (washout or microsphere) studies.[48,49] These techniques and the related method of radioactive tracer washout, however, can measure only the distribution of blood flow per unit mass of tissue. There is no easily available, clinically accepted technology available that can measure regional blood flow in relation to oxygen consumption $(\dot{V}O_2)$. Unless local oxygen consumption and local tissue mass are tightly correlated, tracer techniques cannot give us the desired information: how uniform (or nonuniform) is the local $\dot{V}O_2$–blood flow relationship? It is by no means necessary that tissue mass and $\dot{V}O_2$ are closely related. In fact, if local $\dot{V}O_2$ depends on oxygen delivery to the region, a close relationship cannot exist; local $\dot{V}O_2$ will change with blood flow irrespective of tissue mass. We thus face a serious technological limitation on the understanding of oxygen transport/metabolism heterogeneity. This is in part why clinical application of principles of oxygen transport in the intensive care setting has been frustrating and unable to improve patient care to this point. Only when techniques are developed that assess in patients heterogeneity of $\dot{V}O_2$, blood flow, and cellular metabolism in the critical organs (brain, heart, kidney, gut), will proper use be able to be made of our theoretical understanding of oxygen transport. There has been some progress in developing methods for assessing in particular tissues how blood flow is distributed in relation to metabolic need, but these are not yet widely available in the clinical setting. One method uses MRI techniques[50] that can indicate blood flow and local metabolic use of oxygen. Another method[51] uses noninvasive near-infrared spectroscopy of the quadriceps muscles to estimate local tissue oxygenation, which is in principle determined by the local ratio of $\dot{V}O_2$ to blood flow, coupled with the same technology applied to measure local blood flow by means of indocyanine green dye as a tracer (near-infrared sensors can detect green dye). Then, multiplying the ratio of $\dot{V}O_2$ to flow by

flow itself, one derives local $\dot{V}O_2$. Preliminary results suggest that in health,[51] and even in patients with chronic obstructive pulmonary disease (COPD),[52] blood flow and $\dot{V}O_2$ may vary widely on a regional basis, but their ratio varies little. This is found at rest and across the range of exercise intensity. The methods are complex and still under development, and require significant approximations. Further development may lead to applicability in the critically ill, for whom an attractive hypothesis is that there could be general failure of vascular regulation causing impaired matching of blood flow to metabolism. This could be measured, for example, using surface optodes taped to the thigh to record muscle oxygenation indices to serve as a monitor of physiologic change.

A third physiologic phenomenon may interfere with oxygen transport within organs (in addition to finite diffusive conductance and heterogeneity). This is the so-called diffusive shunt for oxygen.[53,54] To the extent that thin-walled precapillary and postcapillary blood vessels containing arterial and venous blood, respectively, are physically juxtaposed in a tissue bed, there may be some direct diffusive escape of oxygen from the precapillary vessel into the postcapillary vessel. While the existence of this phenomenon has been demonstrated, its quantitative importance is probably small. Frozen tissue spectroscopy (measuring red cell Hb-O_2 saturation) in cross-sections of such vessel pairs fails to yield evidence of this, at least in the myocardium.[54]

A fourth factor that can also interfere with oxygen transport out of the microcirculation is anatomic nonnutritive vascular arteriovenous connections or shunts.[55] While anatomic studies clearly show the existence of such pathways, their functional significance in health, let alone in disease, remains to be firmly established. Mathematical models of oxygen transport[56] suggest that experimental data on oxygen transport are compatible with such shunts, but the key question of whether the same data can be explained without invoking such shunts has not been answered.

With this introduction, the relationship between oxygen transport and oxygen consumption can be discussed. In 1985, in a 600-page text devoted to acute respiratory failure in ARDS, less than a single paragraph was devoted to this critical topic.[57] In a more recent book on the subject, the area merited an entire chapter[58]; at recent international critical care meetings, symposia have addressed the problem and attempts have been made to tailor clinical care to maximizing O_2 transport. This issue can be laid out as follows.

In the healthy state, variations in total body oxygen transport, here referred to as $\dot{Q}O_2$, can be produced by varying cardiac output $(\dot{Q}T)$, hemoglobin concentration $([Hb])$ or arterial oxygen saturation (SaO_2). Note that $\dot{Q}O_2$ is essentially the product of these three variables:

$$\dot{Q}O_2 = k \bullet \dot{Q}T \bullet [Hb] \bullet SaO_2 \qquad \textbf{(6)}$$

Here, k is the stoichiometric binding constant for O_2 and Hb: it is the number of milliliters of O_2 that can be bound by 1 g of Hb. In theory, k is 1.39 but may be as low as 1.34 in practice due to small amounts of metHb or carboxyHb. Eq 6 ignores the normally insignificant amounts of physically dissolved oxygen in the blood (that amount to only 1.5% of total arterial $[O_2]$ in health).

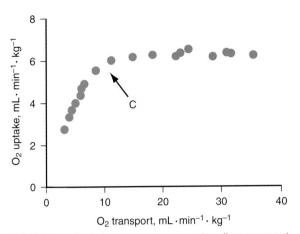

Fig. 4.8 Effect of total oxygen transport (cardiac output times arterial O_2 concentration) on total body oxygen uptake in the anesthetized dog. Above point C, at about 10 mL · min^{-1} · kg^{-1} oxygen transport, oxygen uptake is essentially independent of oxygen transport. To the left of point C, oxygen uptake falls toward the origin almost in proportion to reduced oxygen transport.

When in normal animals $\dot{Q}O_2$ is varied over a reasonable range by manipulating $\dot{Q}T$, [Hb] or SaO_2, total body O_2 consumption ($\dot{V}O_2$) is usually found to be constant—that is, independent of $\dot{Q}O_2$. However, as $\dot{Q}O_2$ is reduced further, $\dot{V}O_2$ begins to fall; when $\dot{V}O_2$ is plotted against $\dot{Q}O_2$, the falling relationship is essentially linear and heads toward the origin. Fig. 4.8 shows an example of this pattern in a normal dog.[59] The so-called biphasic $\dot{V}O_2$–$\dot{Q}O_2$ relationship shown here exemplifies the flat region of the curve where $\dot{V}O_2$ is not dependent on $\dot{Q}O_2$ and the portion at low $\dot{Q}O_2$ where as $\dot{Q}O_2$ falls so, too, does whole body $\dot{V}O_2$. Fig. 4.8 is from well-controlled studies in which—due to constant body temperature, muscle paralysis, and mechanical ventilation—overall cellular metabolic need for O_2 can reasonably be assumed to be constant. Under such conditions, the approximate (and difficult to precisely identify) junction (see Fig. 4.8, point C) of the independent and dependent portions of the curve is termed the critical point and the associated $\dot{Q}O_2$ the critical O_2 transport (or delivery) value. Note that in the literature, the term DO_2 is often used instead of $\dot{Q}O_2$. The accepted interpretation of the dependent region (below C) is that mitochondrial oxygen supply has been reduced sufficiently by the severe reduction in $\dot{Q}O_2$ that mitochondrial oxygen needs cannot be fully met. As a result, $\dot{V}O_2$ falls. A key observation is that at and below the critical point, mixed venous PO_2 has not fallen to zero. An apparent paradox therefore exists: a fall in $\dot{V}O_2$, yet failure to extract all of the O_2 out of the blood, which, had that been possible, would have at least maintained $\dot{V}O_2$ down to a lower value of $\dot{Q}O_2$. The presumption is a physical limit to O_2 transport between blood and mitochondria.

Two competing, but not mutually exclusive, hypotheses based on reduced oxygen supply have been advanced to explain $\dot{V}O_2$ dependency on $\dot{Q}O_2$.[60] The first is heterogeneity. Here, as the transport of oxygen molecules into the arterial tree is progressively reduced but above the critical point (see Fig. 4.6), sufficient oxygen flux to every organ exists. The system simply extracts the same amount of oxygen per unit time from a diminishing

arterial supply in concert with mass balance principles (see Eq 2), resulting in a mixed venous $[O_2]$ that falls progressively with $\dot{Q}O_2$. Below the critical point, oxygen extraction can no longer be maintained because, due to complex regulatory processes controlling blood flow between and within organs, some organs and/or cells within organs are deprived of flow, and thus oxygen, to ensure survival of more critical organs and cells.

The second possibility is that tissue oxygen diffusive conductance, in excess above the critical point, now is insufficient to get oxygen molecules from the tissue microvascular red cells to the mitochondria.[61] This is not because oxygen diffusive conductance suddenly falls when $\dot{Q}O_2$ is reduced below the critical value but because oxygen flux from red cells to mitochondria by diffusion depends on the product of the diffusive conductance, DO_2, and the PO_2 difference between the red cells (P_{RBC}) and the mitochondria (P_{MITO}) according to Fick's law of diffusion. Thus:

$$\dot{V}O_2 = DO_2[P_{RBC} - P_{MITO}] \tag{7}$$

Above the critical point, both P_{RBC} and P_{MITO} are well in excess of zero (or the minimal mitochondrial PO_2 necessary to sustain mitochondrial respiration), about 1 to 2 Torr according to in vitro studies.[62] At the critical point, with no change in DO_2 implied, P_{RBC} and P_{MITO} have both fallen (as $\dot{Q}O_2$ is reduced and venous PO_2 falls; see earlier discussion) and P_{MITO} has, in fact, reached the critical mitochondrial value (likely about 1–2 Torr, as mentioned) for sustaining mitochondrial $\dot{V}O_2$. As $\dot{Q}O_2$ is reduced below the critical value, P_{RBC} falls even further; P_{MITO} cannot be sustained and $\dot{V}O_2$ must fall due to mitochondrial oxygen supply limitation.

Both hypotheses could be simultaneously correct and interactive; more research is needed to clarify these and any other possibilities. In particular, a clinically applicable approach to measuring PO_2 at the mitochondrial level would be enormously beneficial, at least to our understanding of the pathophysiology. While a technique for this is under development,[63] it may never reach human clinical application due to inherent technical limitations.

A third possible factor should be mentioned: rather than $\dot{V}O_2$ passively falling due to limited oxygen supply from either heterogeneity or diffusion limitation, intracellular sensors (of O_2) could mediate a (protective) reduction in metabolic O_2 requirements. An example is the behavior of renal $\dot{V}O_2$ as renal blood flow is reduced.[64] Because most of renal oxygen consumption goes into active Na^+Cl^- reabsorption from tubular fluid and the salt load, in turn, depends on glomerular filtration and hence on blood flow, renal $\dot{V}O_2$ falls with renal blood flow (and hence with renal $\dot{Q}O_2$) because the metabolic demands on the kidney fall. This is, of course, a special case and mechanism and is not thought to reflect behavior of the other organ systems.

The preceding has not differentiated among the three possible means of reducing $\dot{Q}O_2$ mentioned at the outset: manipulating blood flow, [Hb], or SaO_2. Classical studies comparing these strategies have revealed that, for example, reducing SaO_2 or [Hb] produces the same critical point C (see Fig. 4.8) when expressed as the value of $\dot{Q}O_2$ at which $\dot{V}O_2$ begins to fall.[65] However, $\dot{V}O_2$ begins to fall at a higher venous PO_2 when oxygen transport is reduced by anemia rather than by hypoxia. This is consistent with an effect of anemia reducing the oxygen diffusional conductance (much as is the case for O_2 diffusing capacity and [Hb] in the lungs), requiring a higher driving pressure (Eq 7) to maintain $\dot{V}O_2$. Support for this idea comes from exercise studies of maximal $\dot{V}O_2$ as [Hb] is changed, demonstrating [Hb] dependence of muscle oxygen diffusional conductance.[66,67]

To this point, only whole-organism data have been described but it is important to explore the $\dot{V}O_2$–$\dot{Q}O_2$ relationship in individual organ systems. Similar biphasic $\dot{V}O_2$-$\dot{Q}O_2$ curves have been found in several organ systems: skeletal muscle,[68] liver,[69] and intestine.[70] While critical values of organ $\dot{Q}O_2$ may be different, the research conditions under which they have been measured are difficult to compare and to a rough approximation the whole body data appear to reasonably reflect these individual organ results. The implication is that, to the extent heterogeneity of oxygen transport is important to the $\dot{V}O_2$–$\dot{Q}O_2$ relationship, this is likely to be based more on intraorgan than between-organ differences in oxygen flow. However, this area needs more investigation.

As presented, it would seem that when $\dot{V}O_2$ is oxygen supply dependent (below point C of Fig. 4.8), cellular metabolism and integrity are threatened. One's natural therapeutic reaction would be to increase $\dot{Q}O_2$ by manipulating blood flow, [Hb], or arterial oxygen saturation; indeed, this has found its way into the critical care arena. This is not a trivial undertaking—of the three components of $\dot{Q}O_2$ potentially subject to manipulation, arterial oxygen saturation is of limited availability in most critically ill patients because of their lung diseases. Thus hyperoxia provides only a small improvement in oxygen saturation and moreover renders the lungs vulnerable to oxygen toxicity. Shunt reduction by ventilating the lungs with high pressures reduces cardiac output and may offset the gains in oxygen saturation. Increasing [Hb] is problematic due to risks of viral contamination of blood, limited supplies, and being confined to patients with [Hb] low enough to justify transfusion. Moreover, as [Hb] is increased, cardiac output may fall, also offsetting the gains in overall $\dot{Q}O_2$. This leaves enhancing cardiac output as the remaining major possibility. The heart in such patients is usually already under stress and pumping 2 to 3 times the usual resting volume per minute in response to the high tissue metabolic needs associated with tissue repair and fever.[71] Moreover, cardiac function may be impaired by high respiratory pressures (see earlier discussion), the myocardium may be damaged by the systemic disease processes of critically ill patients (e.g., those with ARDS), and coronary blood flow may be compromised due to prior coronary artery disease or aggressive ventilator strategies. Encouraging greater cardiac function with various inotropic or sympathomimetic agents (e.g., dopamine or dobutamine) carries significant risk under these circumstances and cannot be universally recommended until we truly understand the physicochemical basis of oxygen supply dependency of $\dot{V}O_2$ in these patients.

There are in addition two significant caveats to the entire $\dot{V}O_2$–$\dot{Q}O_2$ story. The first is delineating signal from noise. Recall that $\dot{V}O_2$ is the product of blood flow and arteriovenous $[O_2]$ difference while $\dot{Q}O_2$ is the product of blood flow and arterial $[O_2]$. Unless $\dot{V}O_2$ and $\dot{Q}O_2$ are measured by technically independent techniques, there is major covariance between $\dot{Q}O_2$ and $\dot{V}O_2$ due

to use of both blood flow and arterial $[O_2]$ in both $\dot{V}O_2$ and $\dot{Q}O_2$. Thus measurement errors in both blood flow and arterial $[O_2]$ must give an apparent correlation between $\dot{V}O_2$ and $\dot{Q}O_2$ (i.e., data compatible with O_2 supply dependency).[72] However, this would be clearly a falsely positive outcome. This problem is particularly problematic for sequential measurements in a given individual. Another manifestation of the problem is comparing patients of different size or $\dot{V}O_2$: on a plot of $\dot{V}O_2$ versus $\dot{Q}O_2$, a small patient will generally show lower values for both variables than a large patient. Normalization for body size must be performed prior to interpretation. Thus, cross-sectional surveys of single data points from many subjects may not be particularly useful in further understanding the phenomenon. In summary, before accepting data supporting a dependency of $\dot{V}O_2$ on $\dot{Q}O_2$, it is essential to be certain that appropriate methods and statistical treatment of the data have excluded false-positive correlations between $\dot{V}O_2$ and $\dot{Q}O_2$.[41,42]

The second difficulty with understanding the $\dot{V}O_2$–$\dot{Q}O_2$ relationship is a physiologic one. In all of the preceding, it has been assumed that cellular O_2 requirements are constant as $\dot{Q}O_2$ has been manipulated by the investigator. This requirement is obvious: if a patient is studied first while skeletal muscles are active and then again when paralyzed (by a muscle relaxant) on a ventilator, total body oxygen requirements will have been reduced by paralysis. Just as during normal exercise, oxygen transport (cardiac output in particular) is regulated by O_2 requirements. Thus, in this comparison, $\dot{V}O_2$ and $\dot{Q}O_2$ would have been greater prior to paralysis and a $\dot{V}O_2$–$\dot{Q}O_2$ plot would have suggested oxygen supply dependence of $\dot{V}O_2$. It is critical to understand the difference: a change in $\dot{V}O_2$ caused by a change in $\dot{Q}O_2$ constitutes true O_2 supply dependence of $\dot{V}O_2$; a change in activity of cells or tissues requiring more O_2 will generally be reflected by an increase in $\dot{Q}O_2$ to meet these needs.[64] This is an appropriate response that should not be regarded as oxygen supply dependence of $\dot{V}O_2$ in the previous context. Yet, on a diagram relating $\dot{V}O_2$ and $\dot{Q}O_2$, both scenarios will look the same.

This section may be summarized as follows: in critically ill patients, $\dot{V}O_2$ is sometimes found to vary with O_2 transport ($\dot{Q}O_2$) under conditions and at $\dot{Q}O_2$ levels that would not produce changes in $\dot{V}O_2$ in health. One must first be sure that the changes are real and not due to covariance and errors. One must then ascertain (if possible) whether the relationship is driven by a change in oxygen requirement (false O_2 supply–dependent relationship) or a change in oxygen availability (true O_2 supply dependence of $\dot{V}O_2$). Only if the latter is established can one begin to consider the pros and cons of manipulating oxygen transport variables. However, even then, options are limited as explained. In our current state of ignorance of the various intraorgan relationships between cellular metabolic normalcy and oxygen supply in critically ill patients, it will be some time before the necessary technologies are developed to allow us to make rational use of these undoubtedly important concepts.

The foregoing naturally leads into a discussion of the use of mixed venous oxygen saturation ($S\bar{v}O_2$) in assessing cardiovascular sufficiency in critically ill patients.[73] The attractiveness of continuous, accurate, real-time measurements of $S\bar{v}O_2$ using a Swan-Ganz catheter with fiberoptics allowing external spectrophotometric determination of Hb saturation has brought this issue into prominence. A rearrangement of Eq 2 and the earlier discussion provides a rational basis for interpretation of $S\overline{v}O_2$. Since

$$\dot{V}O_2 = \dot{Q}T[CaO_2 - C\overline{v}O_2], \qquad (2)$$

the right side of the equation can be reexpressed so that

$$\dot{V}O_2 = 1.34 \bullet \dot{Q} \bullet [Hb] \bullet [SaO_2 - S\overline{v}O_2] \qquad (8)$$

This transformation assumes negligible contribution of dissolved O_2 (see discussion of Eq 6). By rearrangement of Eq 8,

$$S\overline{v}O_2 = SaO_2 - \dot{V}O_2/[1.34 \bullet [Hb] \bullet \dot{Q}T] \qquad (9)$$

Provided that arterial saturation (SaO_2), $\dot{V}O_2$, and [Hb] remain constant, a fall in $S\overline{v}O_2$ indicates a fall in $\dot{Q}T$; this can be useful as a "cardiac output monitor." However, a fall in SaO_2 or [Hb] or rise in $\dot{V}O_2$ will also reduce $S\overline{v}O_2$; thus these variables have to be assessed independently to interpret $S\overline{v}O_2$. An increase in $S\overline{v}O_2$ would occur from an increase in cardiac output but would also be seen if, due to peripheral tissue heterogeneity and/or oxygen diffusion limitation, $\dot{V}O_2$ was reduced. Thus, both therapeutically beneficial and problematic phenomena can move $S\overline{v}O_2$ in the same direction, obscuring interpretation of $S\overline{v}O_2$. A further transformation of Eq 9 yields

$$S\overline{v}O_2 = SaO_2[1 - \dot{V}O_2/\dot{Q}O_2] \qquad (10)$$

Looking at Fig. 4.8, it would be expected that along the flat portion of the relationship, above the critical point C, $S\overline{v}O_2$ must fall as $\dot{V}O_2$ stays constant while $\dot{Q}O_2$ is reduced; this is clear from Eq 10. However, below the critical point C, if the $\dot{V}O_2$–$\dot{Q}O_2$ relationship is truly a straight line passing through (or near to) the origin, the ratio $\dot{V}O_2/\dot{Q}O_2$ may be essentially constant while both $\dot{V}O_2$ and $\dot{Q}O_2$ are falling. If SaO_2 is constant under such conditions, then so too will be $S\overline{v}O_2$. Thus it is quite possible that under the very conditions one wants to identify—that is, oxygen supply dependency of $\dot{V}O_2$—$S\overline{v}O_2$ could be essentially constant and thus obscure with a false sense of security the presence of the presumed cellular metabolic derangement.

It should be clear then that monitoring of $S\overline{v}O_2$ alone yields data open to many interpretations that could have either beneficial or deleterious implications.[73] Without measures of all the determinants of $S\overline{v}O_2$ (i.e., SaO_2, $\dot{V}O_2$, [Hb], and cardiac output), unique interpretation is not possible. This conclusion is further clouded by the obvious fact that $S\overline{v}O_2$ is mixed venous oxygen saturation and its relationship to oxygenation of individual critical organs is, as discussed earlier, a major unknown in critically ill patients. Moreover, it reflects PO_2 of the venous blood, not of the intracellular environment. When oxygen transport between blood and mitochondria is compromised in disease, venous PO_2 is likely to considerably exceed PO_2 at the mitochondria. This is analogous to lung disease in which alveolar PO_2 can greatly exceed arterial PO_2, a setting in which we have therefore learned not to use the alveolar value as an index of arterial—they move in opposite directions as disease worsens. The medical community has a long way to go before obtaining a clear understanding of the role of the cardiovascular system in oxygen transport in critically ill patients. Technological advances in assessing cellular metabolic function in critical organs in the context of oxygen supply and at a level that can assess functional heterogeneity within and between organs will be the key to success.

The full reference list for this chapter is available at ExpertConsult.com.

Regulation of Cardiac Output

Sándor J. Kovács

The cardiovascular system includes the four-chambered heart, arteries, veins, and lymphatics. Pulsatile arterial flow supplies tissues with oxygen and metabolic substrates, and nonpulsatile venous flow removes carbon dioxide and other metabolic products. The lymphatics ensure conservation of volume at the microvascular level. The functional integration of all these active and passive components (venous circulation, right heart, lungs and pulmonary vascular system, left heart and arterial circulation) generates the cardiac output.

The most useful conceptual framework for quantifying cardiac output (CO) is the physiologic analog of Ohm's law (V = IR; with *V* meaning voltage, *I*, current, and *R*, resistance) expressed as Pressure (mm Hg) = CO (L/min) × Resistance (mm Hg min/L). In the clinical setting, CO is usually measured using indicator dilution techniques. A common approach during right heart catheterization is to inject a bolus of cold 5% dextrose into the right atrium through the proximal port of a multilumen (Swan-Ganz) catheter and measure the resulting transient drop in blood temperature downstream, in the pulmonary artery, using a thermistor on the tip of the catheter. The recorded (temperature as a function of time) thermodilution curve obeys the Stewart-Hamilton equation and allows computation of CO.[1] Alternatively, CO can be measured using the Fick principle. Oxygen consumption rate can be measured by collecting expired gases or, less accurately, assuming a consumption value using a standard nomogram based on height, weight, and age. The difference in arterial and pulmonary venous oxygen content (A-Vo$_2$ difference, in milliliters of O$_2$/100 mL of blood) is measured. CO is calculated as:

$$CO = O_2 \text{ consumption/A-Vo}_2 \text{ difference} \quad \text{(1)}$$

Since each gram of hemoglobin (Hb) can carry 1.34 mL of O$_2$, the oxygen content of blood can be obtained as: O$_2$ content = Hb[g/dL] × 1.34 (mL of O$_2$/g of Hb) × O$_2^{\text{saturation fraction}}$ + 0.0032 × P$_{O2}$ (torr). Normally, arterial blood is 99% saturated and venous blood is 75% saturated; hence arterial blood contains about 200 mL of O$_2$/L and venous blood contains 150 mL O$_2$/L.

CO is usually normalized for body surface area and expressed as the cardiac index (CI). Normal CI at rest ranges from 2.5 to 4.2 L/min per m^2. CO can decline by almost 40% without deviating from normal limits. A low resting CI of less than 2.5 L/min per m^2 usually indicates a marked abnormality in cardiovascular performance and is almost always clinically apparent. Although resting CO or CI is an insensitive measure of cardiovascular performance in response to demand, resting values are valuable for decision making in critically ill patients.

ARTERIOVENOUS OXYGEN DIFFERENCE

Maintenance of adequate tissue oxygenation depends on the integrated function of the heart, the central and peripheral vasculature, lungs, blood, and metabolism.[2] According to the Fick principle, the oxygen extracted from the circulation and consumed by the body is equal to the product of the CO and the

A-VO$_2$ difference. Under normal circumstances at rest, oxygen delivery exceeds consumption, so that adequate tissue oxygenation is provided with an A-VO$_2$ difference of 40 ± 10 mL/L. If CO decreases, tissues extract a greater fraction of oxygen from the arterial blood, and mixed venous oxygen saturation decreases. If arterial oxygen tension and serum hemoglobin are normal, a mixed venous oxygen saturation of 70% or more is observed, indicating that oxygen delivery is sufficient to meet the physiologic need.[3]

A wide A-VO$_2$ difference and reduced mixed venous oxygen saturation may result from reduced CO, a defect in blood oxygen-carrying capacity, or pulmonary disease (impairment of gas exchange). Once tissue is no longer able to increase its extraction of oxygen, tissue hypoxia results. Under these conditions, anaerobic metabolism manifests by a precipitous increase in venous lactate levels.[4]

During exercise, oxygen consumption can increase 18-fold. This demand for increased oxygen delivery is met by a sixfold increase in CO (from 3 to 18 L/min per m^2), and a concomitant threefold increase in the A-VO$_2$ difference (from 40 to 120 mL/L), resulting in a mixed venous oxygen saturation decrease from 75% to 25%. Since CO = SV (stroke volume) × HR (heart rate), the six-fold increase in CO is *not* accompanied by a sixfold increase in HR, indicating that SV must increase as HR increases in response to increased demand.

The resting myocardium nearly maximally desaturates oxygenated (99% saturated) blood. Hence, coronary sinus oxygen saturation is low (<40%), and therefore an increase in oxygen extraction as a compensatory mechanism for inadequate coronary nutritive flow cannot be utilized by the myocardium.

REFLEX CONTROL OF CARDIAC OUTPUT

Under normal conditions, the heart has a large functional reserve; it is usually not the limiting factor in determining CO. The arterial (perfusion) pressure and CO adjust to meet the needs of the body as they vary with posture and activity. The regulatory mechanisms involve sensory and effector components. The sensory components include peripheral receptors that react to changes in blood pressure (e.g., baroreceptors in aortic arch and carotid sinuses), blood volume (e.g., stretch receptors in the atria, Bainbridge reflex), and ventilation (e.g., carotid chemoreceptors). In addition, there are loci in the cortex, hypothalamus, and diencephalon of the brain that react to emotions, anxiety, anticipation, exercise, hypoxia, and temperature. CO (as described by Ohm's law) is modulated through changes in HR, SV, and vasomotor tone (peripheral resistance) that are mediated by direct parasympathetic and sympathetic neural pathways and by circulating catecholamines. Other humoral factors—such as adrenocortical steroids, thyroid hormones, insulin, and glucagons—have been shown to have an effect on cardiac function, requiring longer time scales; the importance of these hormones for regulation of CO is unclear. It should be noted that the heart is also an endocrine organ—by virtue of the fact that the atria function as volumetric strain gauges in response to being distended (increased volume), by generating atrial natriuretic peptide (ANP), and by increasing sodium and water excretion to achieve volume control by targeting the kidney.

Direct sympathetic neural stimulation and circulating catecholamines exert a powerful stimulatory effect, increasing HR and contractile state, whereas vagal stimulation decreases HR and contractile state. The sympathetic and parasympathetic systems interact with each other in a complex fashion to influence cardiovascular performance. In general, two types of interactions exist: accentuated antagonism and reciprocal excitation.[5] Accentuated antagonism refers to the finding that the negative inotropic and chronotropic effects of vagal stimulation are more pronounced when vagal stimulation occurs in the presence of an increased adrenergic tone. Reciprocal excitation refers to the paradoxical effects of stimulation by one division on the autonomic nervous system, which results in effects normally expected from stimulation by the opposite autonomic division. The most common example of this is the production of positive inotropic effects by vagal stimulation or acetylcholine administration under experimental conditions.[5]

The factors that influence CO are summarized in Table 5.1. The CO regulatory system can become dysfunctional and result in syncope as a result of enhanced atrial and peripheral baroreceptor sensitivity, autonomic dysfunction, or complete heart block. In a critically ill cardiac patient, the normal regulatory/compensatory mechanisms are usually saturated by maximal sympathetic and catecholamine stimulation. Under these conditions, the major CO determinants are no longer the normal neurohormonal regulatory pathways but rather the interaction between pump function and load, that is, peripheral vasculature.

TABLE 5.1   Factors That Influence Cardiac Output

Factor	Effects
Sympathetic tone	↑ Contractile state, ↑ heart rate
Vagal tone	↓ Contractile state
Right vagus	↓ Sinus node activity, sinus bradycardia
Left vagus	↓ Atrioventricular conduction
Volume load	↑ Heart rate (Bainbridge reflex)
Baroreceptor stimulation (aortic arch, carotid sinus)	↓ Contractile state
Calcium administration	↑ Contractile state
Hormones (epinephrine, glucagon, thyroxine)	↑ Contractile state, ↑ heart rate
Drugs	
Positive Inotropes	
Phosphodiesterase inhibitors (milrinone, amrinone, theophylline)	↑ Contractile state, ↑ heart rate
Digitalis glycosides	↑ Contractile state, ↓ atrioventricular conduction
Adrenergic stimulants (dopamine, dobutamine)	↑ Contractile state, ↑ heart rate
Negative Inotropes	
β-adrenergic antagonists	↓ Contractile state, ↓ heart rate
Calcium channel blockers	↓ Contractile state, ↓ atrioventricular conduction

The determinants of ventricular pump function are of paramount importance.

LEFT VENTRICULAR PERFORMANCE

Pressure-Volume Loop

Although the integrity of left ventricular (LV) and right ventricular (RV) function and pulmonary and peripheral circulations is important, most cardiovascular dysfunction in adults is the result of impaired LV function. The performance of the LV can be understood by examining the relationship between LV pressure and volume during a single cardiac cycle in the pressure-volume plane (Fig. 5.1). Instantaneous intraventricular pressure is plotted on the y axis and simultaneous ventricular volume is plotted on the x axis. At end diastole (point a), ventricular pressure is relatively low and ventricular volume is relatively high. The segment ab is due to isovolumic contraction (typically <90 ms), with an increase in intraventricular pressure but no ejection. Point b represents the start of ejection, coincident with the opening of the aortic valve when ventricular pressure exceeds aortic pressure (AoP). Note that after peak AoP is reached and AoP begins to decline—the aortic valve (AoV) is still open and LV volume is decreasing. At end systole (point c), the AoV closes, and isovolumic relaxation (typically <90 ms) commences (segment cd). The mitral valve opens at point d, when ventricular pressure decreases to less than atrial pressure, and ventricular filling commences. By definition, the slope (dP/dV) of the end-diastolic pressure volume relationship (EDPVR) at a given end-diastolic volume is the chamber stiffness. Note that left ventricular pressure (LVP) continues to decrease until minimum LVP is reached after mitral valve opening, In other words, as LV volume increases, LV pressure continues to drop (dP/dV<0) until minimum LV pressure is reached.

The difference between the end-diastolic and end-systolic volumes (aortic SV) or end-systolic and end-diastolic volumes

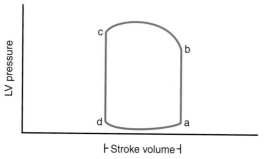

Fig. 5.1 For a single cardiac cycle, instantaneous left ventricular (LV) pressure is plotted against LV volume. Point a represents end diastole and the start of isovolumic contraction. Ventricular pressure increases without any change in volume until ejection starts at point b, which represents the opening of the aortic valve. During ejection, ventricular volume decreases. Point c represents end systole and the start of isovolumic relaxation. Aortic valve closure occurs near end systole. Ventricular pressure continues to decrease until ventricular filling starts with the opening of the mitral valve at point d. Ventricular pressure increases very slightly during diastolic filling.

(diastolic filling volume) defines the SV. The ratio of SV to end-diastolic volume (EDV) is the LV ejection fraction (LVEF). The LVEF is a clinically useful index of systolic *and* diastolic function. LVEF = SV/LVEDV is interpreted as a systolic function index. Its role as a diastolic function index is easily appreciated when rewritten as LVEF = [E-wave volume + A-wave volume]/ [LV diastatic volume + A-wave volume]. In atrial fibrillation, this reveals that LVEF = [E-wave volume]/[LV volume at diastasis], underscoring the physiologic importance of LV volume at diastasis as the **equilibrium volume** of the LV.[6] In the absence of aortic stenosis, the LV pressure at end systole is the same as the pressure in the proximal aorta and approximates systolic blood pressure (actually the pressure at the dicrotic notch in the aortic pressure-time course). The pressure-volume (PV) loop provides a useful way to analyze the effects of contractile state, preload, and afterload on CO. The area of the PV loop is the external work of the ventricle.

Effect of Alterations in Preload on the Pressure-Volume Loop

Preload (in sinus rhythm) is defined as the stretch of the myocardium by atrial systole before activation and is readily indexed by end-diastolic volume. Within physiologic ranges, the greater the stretch on the myocardium, the stronger the ensuing contraction; this is known as the Frank-Starling relationship.[7] This prestretch is absent in atrial fibrillation. From studies in isolated heart preparations in which preload, afterload, and contractile state were controlled, it has been shown that an increase in preload, produced by an increase in end-diastolic volume, results in an increase in the end-systolic pressure and SV of the ensuing beat.[8–10]

Three PV loops under three different preload conditions are shown in Fig. 5.2. For clarity, it is assumed that HR, contractile state, and afterload remain constant. Baseline conditions are represented by the shaded loop. A decrease in preload as a result of loss of blood volume, if not associated with any other change in afterload or contractile state, results in a smaller EDV and a smaller PV loop that is shifted to the left. Conversely, a volume load results in a larger PV loop that is shifted to the right. An isolated increase in preload without any change in afterload or contractile state results in increases in SV and end-systolic pressure if HR, afterload, and contractile state are unchanged. These idealized conditions do not apply precisely in vivo. Isolated changes in preload, afterload, contractile state, or HR occur rarely because these changes are usually a response to, or in themselves result in, compensatory neurohormonal reflexes, which simultaneously influence all of these variables in a complex fashion. It may be useful, however, for an understanding of cardiovascular dynamics to analyze these factors separately.

END-SYSTOLIC PRESSURE-VOLUME RELATIONSHIP

In Fig. 5.2, the end-systolic points of all three PV loops fall on a straight line. This line is termed the end-systolic PV relationship (ESPVR) and is constant for a given contractile state.[11] A similar but nonlinear relationship can be constructed for the end-diastolic points—EDPVR. Note that in atrial fibrillation diastasis defines

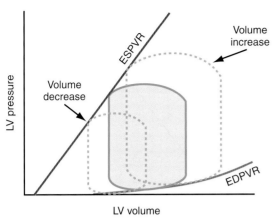

Fig. 5.2 Three different pressure-volume (PV) loops are shown representing beats at three different preloads. Control conditions are represented by the shaded PV loop. An increase in preload (e.g., a large volume load) is associated with an increase in diastolic filling and a shift in the end-systolic PV point to the left. The added stretch causes a stronger contraction and an increase in the pressure developed during systole and in stroke volume. The PV loop is larger and shifted to the right *(broken lines)*. Conversely, a decrease in preload, such as a loss of blood volume, results in a smaller PV loop that is shifted to the left *(broken lines)*. The end-systolic points of the three variably loaded beats fall on a straight line. This line represents the end-systolic PV relationship (ESPVR). A similar but curvilinear relationship is formed by the end-diastolic PV points—the end-diastolic PV relationship (EDPVR). *LV,* Left ventricular.

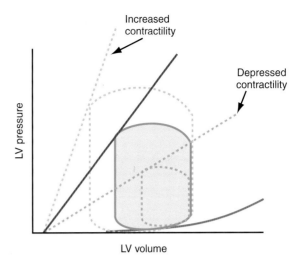

Fig. 5.3 Effect of an increase in contractile state on the pressure-volume loop and the end-systolic pressure-volume relationship. *LV,* Left ventricular.

end diastole; therefore the EDPVR and the **diastatic** pressure volume relation (DPVR) are the same. In contrast, in sinus rhythm the DPVR and the EDPVR are distinct from each other.[12] The ESPVR and EDPVR have been shown to be relatively load independent at a given contractile state[13,14]; however, the ESPVR is not absolutely load independent, probably because of the positive and negative inotropic effects of ejection.[15–17] For practical purposes, at a given contractile state, the cardiac PV loop is always bound by the ESPVR and the EDPVR. For a given contractile state, the ESPVR can conveniently be expressed as follows (see Fig. 5.2):

$$P_{es} = E_{es} (V_{es} - V_o) \qquad (2)$$

where P_{es} is end-systolic pressure, V_{es} is end-systolic volume, V_o is the volume axis intercept, and E_{es} is the slope of the ESPVR.[8,11,18] Because of its relative load independence, E_{es} has been proposed as an index of contractility.[9] V_o is interpreted as the volume at which the ventricle can no longer generate force. This "dead volume" is a function of heart size. In actuality, the linear ESPVR often crosses the P = 0 axis at negative values of volume. The explanation is that the actual ESPVR is always curvilinear, thereby avoiding negative V_o values; the linear ESPVR should be viewed as valid only in the physiologic range of SVs.

Effect of Changes in Contractile State

The contractile state of the heart refers to the intrinsic ability of the myocardium at a given load to generate contractile force. The myocardial contractile state is influenced by several endogenous and

exogenous factors (see Table 5.1). In the PV plane, an increase in contractile state results in an increase in force development—that is, higher pressure—at any given ventricular volume. Conversely, the "dead volume" of the ventricle is unchanged because heart size has not changed. These changes manifest in the PV plane as an increase in the slope of the ESPVR without a change in V_o.[11] In Fig. 5.3, preload, afterload, and HR are assumed to be constant. Under these conditions, an increase in contractile state results in an increase in SV and end-systolic pressure. Conversely, in the absence of any compensatory mechanisms, a reduction in myocardial contractility results in a reduction in systolic pressure and SV. Some common compensatory mechanisms are discussed later; first, the effect of changes in afterload must be considered.

Effect of Afterload Change

Afterload is the load that the ventricle must overcome to eject volume and, in the absence of valve disease, is determined mainly by the properties of the arterial system. An increase in afterload results in an increase in end-systolic pressure at the expense of ejection. The effect on the PV loop is shown schematically in Fig. 5.4. SV, EF, and, assuming no change in HR, CO are decreased despite a constant contractile state. This is a good illustration of the load dependence and limitations of CO and EF as clinical indices of contractile state. As shown in Fig. 5.4, an increase in afterload without a change in contractile state results in changes in the shape of the PV relationship, but the end-systolic points do not deviate significantly from the ESPVR. This is an idealized figure; as stated previously, the end-systolic points are load dependent,[15,17] but a simplified view suffices for illustration and allows the conceptual expression of the interaction between LV function and the arterial system.

To understand ventriculoarterial coupling, it is useful to view the arterial system also in terms of PV or pressure-SV relationships, as proposed by Sunagawa and colleagues.[19] In this study, the relationship between SV and arterial ESP is linear, and it is assumed that the relationship passes through the origin (Fig. 5.5). The slope of this relationship is termed the *arterial elastance*

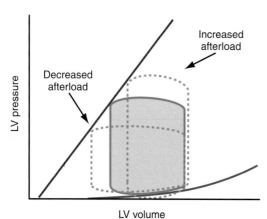

Fig. 5.4 Effect of changes in afterload is shown in three beats at different afterloads. An increase in afterload results in an increase in end-systolic pressure but a decrease in stroke volume. A decrease in afterload has opposite effects. The end-systolic pressure-volume points do not deviate significantly from the end-systolic pressure-volume relationship (ESPVR). The ESPVR is insensitive to changes in afterload.

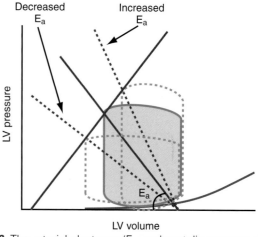

Fig. 5.6 The arterial elastance (E_a; end-systolic pressure divided by stroke volume) is superimposed on the pressure-volume loops for three variably afterload beats. An increase in afterload is represented by an increase in the slope of the arterial elastance. *LV*, Left ventricular.

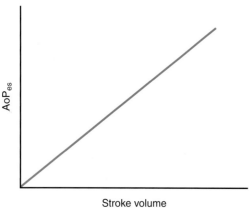

Fig. 5.5 The systolic pressure-volume relationship of the arterial system. The volume of this system at any given time is a function of the stroke volume, which determines the volume increase during systole, and of the vascular resistance to blood flow out of the arterial system and into the venous system. The change in pressure for a given change in volume is a function of the effective compliance of the arterial system. For a given cardiac cycle and assuming constant afterload, aortic end-systolic pressure (AoP_{es}) is linearly related to stroke volume. The slope of this relationship is termed the arterial elastance (E_a) and is an index of afterload.

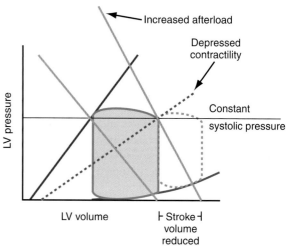

Fig. 5.7 Acute myocardial infarction results in a reduction in contractile state owing to a loss of muscle mass. This results in a decrease in the slope of the end-systolic pressure-volume relationship (ESPVR). The volume axis intercept (V_o) increases by the theoretical volume enclosed by the dead muscle, shifting the ESPVR to the right. Compensatory mechanisms result in an increase in end-diastolic volume and afterload. These changes result in a reduction in stroke volume and an increase in filling pressures.

(E_a) and is the ESP divided by the SV. E_a can be expressed in the ventricular PV plane (Fig. 5.6). E_a is represented by the slope of a line connecting the EDV on the volume axis and the upper left corner of the PV loop. This approach is simplified and not absolutely correct because the arterial PV relationship probably does not truly pass through the origin.[20] The concept of E_a and the ESPVR can be used, however, to predict analytically the effect of changes in afterload on ESP and CO.

PRESSURE-VOLUME APPROACH APPLIED TO PATHOLOGIC CONDITIONS

Acute Systolic Dysfunction

The previously described PV framework allows conceptualization of the interaction among cardiac function, preload, and afterload. Fig. 5.7 represents a hypothetical situation in a patient with an acute myocardial infarction (MI). Acute MI results in the loss of a segment of functioning myocardium, while the rest of the chamber is preserved. Assuming for simplicity that ischemia or neurohormonal stimuli do not alter the contractile state of the surviving myocardium, the ventricle can be modeled as two compartments: one with a normal ESPVR and one with an ESPVR that moves closer to the EDPVR.[21] The combined effect is to reduce the slope of the ESPVR (E_{es}), representing a reduction in overall myocardial contractility, an increase in LVEDV, a reduction in SV, and an increase in the volume intercept (V_o). The increase in V_o represents the contribution of the volume of the nonfunctioning segment of the ventricle to the dead volume.

As a result of these changes, the heart is able to maintain an adequate systemic perfusion pressure, but at the expense of an increase in EDV and EDP. The increases in EDV and EDP are mediated by neurohormonal reflexes that result in fluid retention and an increase in vascular resistance. The increase in vascular resistance is reflected in the PV plane as an increase in E_a. The clinical syndrome of heart failure as a result of acute systolic dysfunction results from the increase in end-diastolic filling pressure, which causes pulmonary congestion or peripheral edema and the reduction in SV that is the result of the decrease in E_{es} and the increase in E_a. To some extent, an increase in HR may compensate for the reduction in SV to maintain cardiac output.

Diastolic Dysfunction

Inasmuch as LV systolic function represents the role of the chamber as a simultaneous pressure and volume pump, diastolic function is best viewed as the role of the chamber as a volume (suction) pump. The chamber stores elastic strain in systole (via titin and other extracellular matrix components) that is recovered in diastole by generating mechanical recoil that aspirates atrial blood into the LV. The rate of crossbridge uncoupling (relaxation) modulates the recoil (suction) process and explains the shape of clinically observed E-waves and their relation to chamber stiffness.[22] Normal diastolic function is defined as adequate filling of the LV without exceeding a pulmonary venous pressure of 12 mm Hg.[23] From the PV approach, both the DPVR and the EDPVR are functions of diastatic and end-diastolic volume, respectively. Systolic dysfunction that increases EDV and EDP also meets this definition and clearly illustrates that systole and diastole are coupled. In this case, the abnormality is primarily in systole; however, if systole is defined as adequate ejection, given adequate filling, diastolic dysfunction manifests as an increase in LVEDP.

Isolated diastolic dysfunction commonly can result from impaired ventricular distensibility, external compression of the LV or obstruction to filling of the LV.[24–26] Impaired distensibility as a result of chronic hypertension is a common cause of diastolic dysfunction and is represented in the PV plane as a steep or left-shifted EDPVR (Fig. 5.8). With significant diastolic dysfunction, adequate filling sufficient to maintain SV is achieved only at the expense of an elevated end-diastolic filling pressure. Diastolic dysfunction, without any systolic dysfunction, can produce symptoms of pulmonary congestion and congestive heart failure.[25,27] The effect of external compression, such as pericardial tamponade or constriction, similarly results in a leftward shift of the EDPVR by reducing capacitance.

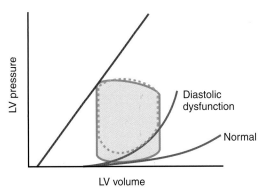

Fig. 5.8 Diastolic dysfunction resulting from impaired distensibility manifests in the pressure-volume plane as an increase in the slope or leftward shift of the end-diastolic pressure-volume relationship. The ventricle requires a higher filling pressure to distend sufficiently to receive an adequate end-diastolic volume. *LV,* Left ventricular.

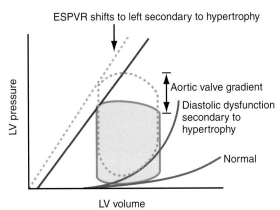

Fig. 5.9 Aortic stenosis imposes an added afterload on the left ventricle, which must generate an increased end-systolic pressure to overcome the aortic valve gradient. Concentric left ventricular hypertrophy results in a leftward shift in the end-systolic pressure-volume relationship (ESPVR) with a small increase in the slope of the ESPVR. Hypertrophy also results in diastolic dysfunction, with a steeper end-diastolic pressure-volume relationship. These changes result in a reduction in stroke volume and an increase in filling pressures. *LV,* Left ventricular.

Aortic Stenosis

Aortic stenosis is a special form of systolic dysfunction. The stenosed aortic valve imposes a resistance to ejection that must be overcome by the ventricle to maintain an adequate SV and systemic perfusion pressure. The resistance to ejection results in a pressure gradient across the valve. The effect on the ventricle is an increase in the effective E_a that, in this case, incorporates the stenotic valve and does not reflect pure arterial properties. The increase in ESP results in an increase in end-systolic ventricular wall stress. Over time, the LV compensates by concentric hypertrophy, which reduces the wall stress. The effect of this hypertrophy is to shift the ESPVR to the left. Concentric hypertrophy that ultimately remodels the chamber so that it is stiffer in diastole is also a common cause of diastolic dysfunction and manifests as an elevated EDPVR (Fig. 5.9).[28,29]

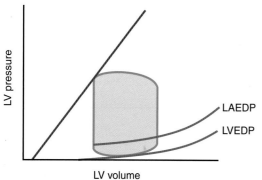

Fig. 5.10 Mitral stenosis imposes a resistance to left ventricular (LV) filling. This results in a diastolic pressure gradient between the left atrium and left ventricle. Adequate ventricular filling is maintained at the expense of an increase in left atrial end-diastolic pressure (LAEDP). *LVEDP*, Left ventricular end-diastolic pressure.

Mitral Stenosis

Mitral stenosis is a special form of diastolic dysfunction. The stenotic mitral valve imposes a resistance to left ventricular filling, which results in a pressure gradient between the left atrium and the LV. The increased atrial pressure is reflected into the pulmonary venous system and can result in symptoms of pulmonary congestion and congestive heart failure. This is best visualized in the PV plane by plotting end-diastolic left atrial pressure superimposed on the ventricular pressure (Fig. 5.10). Atrial pressure exceeds ventricular diastolic pressure throughout diastole by an amount that depends on the effective mitral valve area and the flow across the valve.[30]

Valvular Regurgitation

Mitral and aortic regurgitation result in increased ventricular filling in diastole, with an increase above normal in EDV that results in an increase in total SV. The effective SV is the difference between total SV and regurgitant volume. In acute valvular regurgitation, the increase in ventricular filling results in high filling pressures as the ventricle is forced to operate on the steep portion of its EDPVR; this can result in acute pulmonary edema. Over time, the ventricle can adapt its systolic and diastolic properties and dilate to accommodate the increase in EDV while limiting the increase in filling pressure. This shifts the ESPVR and EDPVR rightward.[28] Fig. 5.11 shows these effects for compensated, chronic valvular regurgitation. Ventricular dilation results in an increase in V_o. In the compensated phase, the contractile state is preserved and the slope of the ESPVR does not change significantly, but shifts to a higher operating volume. Chronic severe regurgitation, if uncorrected, can lead to systolic dysfunction, resulting in a dilated cardiomyopathy.

Dilated Cardiomyopathy

Chronic, severe systolic dysfunction can result from coronary ischemia, valvular regurgitation, or other causes of chronic volume overload and intrinsic myocardial pathology. The common pathophysiology is that the ventricle dilates to compensate for chronic volume overload. The ventricular dilation—imposed by regurgitation, shunts, or other abnormalities of the peripheral

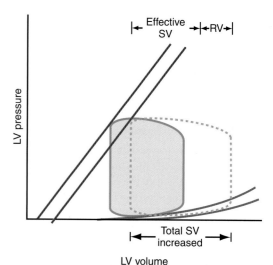

Fig. 5.11 Chronic mitral or aortic regurgitation imposes a chronic volume load on the left ventricle owing to the added burden of the regurgitant volume (RV). The increase in preload results in an increase in total stroke volume (SV), although effective stroke volume usually is unchanged. In acute regurgitation, filling pressures are markedly increased, but with chronic regurgitation, the ventricle dilates and the end-systolic pressure-volume relationship and end-diastolic pressure-volume relationship shift to the right, enabling the heart to accommodate the added volume load with smaller increases in filling pressures. *LV*, Left ventricular.

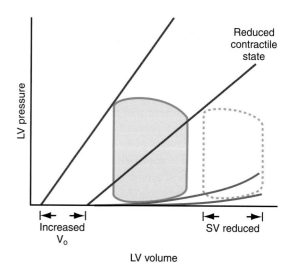

Fig. 5.12 Severe chronic systolic dysfunction results in the development of a dilated cardiomyopathy. The slope of the end-systolic pressure-volume relationship (ESPVR) is reduced, and the ESPVR and end-diastolic pressure-volume relationship are displaced to the right because of ventricular dilation. *LV*, Left ventricular; *SV*, stroke volume.

circulation or in primary myocardial disease—is the only way that the heart can maintain an adequate perfusion pressure. The changes in the PV plane are characterized by a reduction in the slope of the ESPVR as a result of a decrease in contractile state and a right shift in the ESPVR and EDPVR secondary to dilation of the LV (Fig. 5.12).[31]

LIMITATION OF THE PRESSURE-VOLUME APPROACH

For clinicians, the practical value of the PV approach lies in the conceptual framework that it provides to understand the physiologic and pathologic determinants of cardiac function and hemodynamics. Invasive and noninvasive determination of the ESPVR and EDPVR in conscious animals and humans has been described[8,31–33] but has not been implemented routinely in clinical diagnosis or therapy for several reasons. In a single heart, it is simple to interpret a change in the baseline ESPVR, but comparisons between populations or individuals are difficult because the slope and intercept of the ESPVR depend on cardiac size.

The lack of a universally acceptable correction for cardiac size makes it difficult to define a normal range for the E_{es}. This difficulty is compounded by the fact that V_o cannot be measured directly in vivo but rather is determined by extrapolation and is subject to large errors.[34] In addition, the timing of end systole is not always clear cut. End systole is defined as the upper left corner of the PV loop, but this does not always correspond with either aortic valve closure or maximal ventricular elastance, especially in mitral regurgitation.[35] Apart from difficulties in comparing PV relationships, the determination of these relationships in vivo requires alterations in loading conditions over a wide range. The changes in loading conditions themselves may directly affect the slope of the ESPVR through reflex alterations in contractile state and HR.

Last, ESPVR is depicted in this chapter as a linear relationship with a slope and an intercept that are readily determined. Several studies have suggested, however, that the ESPVR becomes nonlinear at high contractile states and with heart failure.[36–39] This nonlinearity may make a slope measurement sensitive to the range of data collection and complicate comparison. These limitations do not diminish the effectiveness of the PV relationship as a conceptual framework and an analytical tool to understand the physiologic and pathophysiologic determinants of cardiac output.

CONCLUSION

The function of the cardiovascular system is to provide adequate metabolic substrate delivery and tissue oxygenation by the circulation of oxygenated blood. Mixed venous oxygen saturation is determined by the balance between oxygen delivery and metabolism and activity-dependent oxygen consumption. Under normal conditions, the heart has a large functional reserve and cardiac output is regulated by neurohormonal mechanisms to meet the body's needs in response to posture and activity so that, at rest, mixed venous oxygen saturation is at least 70%. LV dysfunction is a common cause of cardiovascular insufficiency. In this setting, regulatory and compensatory mechanisms are characterized by maximal sympathetic autonomic stimulation; hence, CO becomes limited by LV performance. Ventricular performance and its coupling to the vasculature can be analyzed within the PV plane. This approach provides a clinically useful, mechanistic conceptual framework for understanding integrated cardiovascular function in critically ill patients.

The full reference list for this chapter is available at ExpertConsult.com.

6

Coronary Physiology and Pathophysiology

David L. Brown

A clear understanding of the physiologic control of coronary blood flow is essential to considering and treating the underlying pathophysiology in patients who are acutely ill with an acute myocardial infarction (MI) in a cardiac intensive care unit (CICU) or in patients with other severe systemic illnesses and underlying coronary artery disease (CAD).

DETERMINANTS OF MYOCARDIAL OXYGEN CONSUMPTION

The working myocardium requires a coronary blood flow of 70 to 90 mL/100 g of myocardium per minute to provide for an oxygen consumption of 8 to 15 mL/100 g of tissue per minute at rest for contraction and relaxation. This figure rapidly increases fivefold to sixfold with exercise or sympathetic arousal. At rest, the heart consumes most of the oxygen contained in its blood supply. Therefore any increase in oxygen demand must be met by an increase in coronary blood flow.

With each beat, developed muscle tension requires oxygen; total tension developed in unit time is directly proportional to the oxygen needs of the working myocardium. The frequency of developed tension (heart rate) is also quantitatively important with regard to oxygen consumption, whereas stroke volume (muscle shortening) has a smaller impact on the needs for oxygen delivery. Excitation–contraction coupling and changes in calcium flux influence contractility, which impacts the demands for oxygen delivery and myocardial blood flow.

At the level of the intact heart, myocardial oxygen demand and myocardial blood flow are determined by developed systolic wall tension, heart rate, and contractility. In the absence of coronary vascular disease or dysfunction, myocardial blood supply is determined by metabolic demands, autoregulation, blood oxygen-carrying capacity, diastolic time, neurohumoral factors, and extravascular compressive forces (Fig. 6.1). The following sections discuss the dominating controlling influences of metabolic regulation and autoregulation.

Metabolic Control

The myocardium generates aerobic energy metabolism; the prevailing tissue oxygen level provides a powerful signal for the control of blood flow through the coronary microvasculature to regulate oxygen supply and maintain physiologic tissue oxygen tension. With each beat, the myocardial tissue oxygen level exerts the most powerful effect on coronary vascular resistance within the microvasculature. Epicardial coronary occlusion causes instantaneous microvascular dilation to facilitate blood flow. Similarly, increases in myocardial work increase oxygen consumption and lead to immediate and precisely regulated dilation of microvascular vessels with increases in regional coronary blood flow to maintain the oxygen supply to tissues. Tissue oxygen tension likely signals the coronary microvasculature through local mechanisms, such as the release of adenosine, tissue levels of carbon dioxide, pH, nitric oxide, and other substances.[1-3]

Autoregulation

The heart provides pressure and blood flow to many organs (i.e., perfusion); the vascular resistance in each region of the body varies from minute to minute. As a result, alterations in pressure and flow in the ascending aorta can affect coronary circulation, which must maintain local perfusion to the myocardium (pressure × flow per unit of tissue) and meet the local needs of the heart. Aortic pressure can decrease to approximately 50 mm Hg or increase to approximately 150 mm Hg in health with the microvasculature adapting to maintain a constant and necessary level of coronary blood flow. This autoregulation is a protective mechanism and is probably mediated by the local release of nitric oxide by the

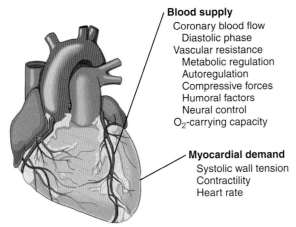

Blood supply
Coronary blood flow
  Diastolic phase
Vascular resistance
  Metabolic regulation
  Autoregulation
  Compressive forces
  Humoral factors
  Neural control
O_2-carrying capacity

Myocardial demand
Systolic wall tension
Contractility
Heart rate

Fig. 6.1 Control of myocardial blood flow and oxygen consumption and demand. (Modified from Ardehali A, Ports TA. Myocardial oxygen supply and demand. *Chest.* 1990;98:699.)

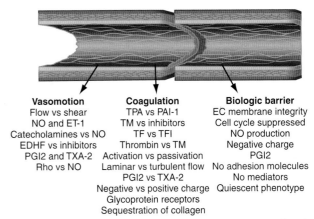

Vasomotion
Flow vs shear
NO and ET-1
Catecholamines vs NO
EDHF vs inhibitors
PGI2 and TXA-2
Rho vs NO

Coagulation
TPA vs PAI-1
TM vs inhibitors
TF vs TFI
Thrombin vs TM
Activation vs passivation
Laminar vs turbulent flow
PGI2 vs TXA-2
Negative vs positive charge
Glycoprotein receptors
Sequestration of collagen

Biologic barrier
EC membrane integrity
Cell cycle suppressed
NO production
Negative charge
PGI2
No adhesion molecules
No mediators
Quiescent phenotype

Fig. 6.2 Mechanisms present in healthy coronary arteries that control local vasomotion, maintain an anticoagulant surface, and sustain a biologic barrier that prevents infiltration and cell proliferation. *EC,* Endothelial cells; *EDHF,* endothelium-derived hyperpolarizing factor; *ET-1,* endothelin-1; *NO,* nitric oxide; *PAI-1,* plasminogen activator inhibitor-1; *PGI2,* prostacyclin; *Rho,* Rho proteins; *TF,* tissue factor; *TM,* thrombomodulin; *TXA-2,* thromboxane A_2.

endothelium and local constriction of vascular smooth muscle cells with increasing intraluminal pressure (the myogenic reflex). The preceding mechanisms are likely transduced via pressure-sensitive and flow-sensitive channels on the endothelium and vascular smooth muscle cells.[2–4] The presence of atherosclerotic narrowing in epicardial coronary arteries alone or in concert with microvascular dysfunction impairs autoregulation, narrowing the range of aortic pressure within which changing coronary resistance can maintain myocardial perfusion at different aortic pressures. Similarly, hypertension and left ventricular hypertrophy also can impair the regulation of myocardial blood flow.

VESSEL WALL AND LOCAL CONTROL OF CORONARY BLOOD FLOW

The coronary vasculature is subject to neural innervation and the effects of circulating mediators, such as serotonin, adenosine diphosphate, epinephrine, and vasopressin. These are in addition to the local mechanisms that respond to the oxygen and metabolic needs of the heart (discussed earlier). The local microvascular endothelium transduces many of these physiologic signals, including local shear force, pulse pressure, sympathetic stimulation, and blood flow itself. It responds by exerting its own local control on vascular smooth muscle cells by governing constriction and relaxation. Vascular endothelial cells possess membrane-associated channels sensitive to many circulating and local regulators, such as shear forces, flow, serotonin, and thrombin. The endothelium is also sensitive to α-adrenergic sympathetic stimulation and aggregating platelets. These signals can cause the endothelium to release vasodilators locally, such as nitric oxide, endothelium-dependent hyperpolarizing factor (EDHF), and prostacyclin or vasoconstrictors such as endothelin-1 and thromboxane. The sum total of these local mediators provides precise control of blood flow in each segment of the coronary microcirculation.

Healthy coronary arteries maintain the ability to control local vasomotion, maintain an anticoagulant surface, and present a biologic barrier that prevents infiltration and proliferation (Fig.

6.2). These key defensive mechanisms are important in maintaining health; a clear understanding of them is important to understand the effects of diseases such as atherosclerosis.

Coronary Arterial System

The coronary arterial system is composed of three compartments that have different functions (Fig. 6.3).[5] The large epicardial coronary arteries (diameter ~500 μm to ~5 mm) visualized on coronary angiography have a capacitance function and offer little resistance to blood flow. During systole, epicardial coronary arteries dilate and accumulate elastic energy as they increase their blood content by about 25%. This elastic energy is transformed into blood kinetic energy at the beginning of diastole and contributes to the prompt reopening of intramyocardial vessels that had been compressed closed by systole.[6] Prearterioles (diameter ~100 to 500 μm) represent the intermediate compartment and are characterized by a measurable pressure drop along their length. Their specific function is to maintain pressure at the origin of the next compartment within a narrow range in response to changes in coronary perfusion pressure and/or flow; proximal prearterioles are most responsive to changes in flow, whereas distal prearterioles are most responsive to changes in pressure. Finally, the distal compartment is composed of arterioles (diameter <100 μm), which are characterized by a very large pressure drop along their length. Arterioles are the site of metabolic regulation of myocardial blood flow because their tone is influenced by substances (such as hydrogen peroxide and adenosine) produced during myocardial metabolism.[7] The specific function of arterioles is the matching of myocardial blood supply and oxygen demand. Notably, each compartment is governed by distinct regulatory mechanisms. In contrast to the epicardial arteries, both prearterioles and arterioles are below the resolution of current angiographic systems and, therefore, cannot be visualized using angiography.[5] The importance of coronary microcirculation for the maintenance of appropriate

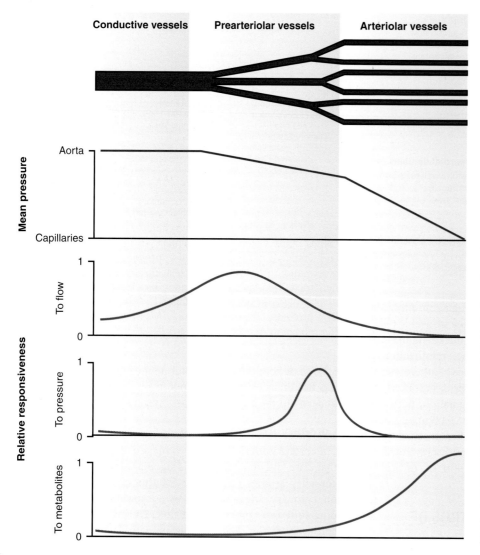

Fig. 6.3 Coronary arterial circulation. The coronary arterial system comprises large conductive vessels and the microcirculation (prearterioles and arterioles). The drop of pressure relative to that in the aorta is negligible in conductive vessels. By contrast, a considerable pressure drop occurs through prearterioles and, to a larger extent, through arterioles. Conductive vessels and (to an even greater extent) proximal prearterioles are most responsive to flow-dependent dilatation. Distal prearterioles are most responsive to changes in intravascular pressure and are mainly responsible for autoregulation of coronary blood flow, whereas arterioles are most responsive to changes in the intramyocardial concentration of metabolites and are mainly responsible for the metabolic regulation of coronary blood flow. (From Crea F, et al. Chronic ischaemic heart disease. In: Camm AJ, Lüscher TF, Serruys PW, eds. *The ESC Textbook of Cardiovascular Medicine.* 2nd ed. Oxford: Oxford University Press; 2009.)

myocardial perfusion has been recognized by physiologists since the 1950s; evidence has accrued over the past 30 years indicating that functional and structural abnormalities of this section of the circulation can be responsible for impairment of myocardial perfusion and ischemia, a condition often referred to as coronary microvascular dysfunction (CMD).[8] CMD has a high prevalence in both men (51%) and women (54%) with suspected CAD and is associated with adverse outcomes in both stable CAD and acute MI.[9]

Extravascular Compression of Coronary Blood Supply

Intracavity pressure and vascular compression achieved by contracting heart muscle act to obstruct coronary blood flow during systole, even causing reversed flow in the intramyocardial microvasculature. In health, diastolic driving pressures overcome diastolic compressive forces because the aortic diastolic pressure is higher than the pressure in the coronary sinus or right atrium. Intracavitary pressures and vascular compression are important forces influencing flow during systole and diastole. These myocardial or extravascular forces are more prominent in the inner layer of the left ventricle (i.e., the subendocardium). Flow in the

epicardium is generally 25% higher than that in the endocardium. Increases in wall stress in health and disease place greater demands for oxygen and blood flow in the subendocardial layers. This layer also exhibits the greatest susceptibility to limitations of flow (ischemia) in disease states. Increased wall tension from ventricular hypertrophy and decreased perfusion pressure from coronary stenoses and shock are more likely to jeopardize subendocardial coronary flow.[1]

Neural Control and Reflexes

α_1-Adrenergic and α_2-adrenergic innervation can produce coronary constriction. This sympathetic stimulation also produces increases in heart rate and myocardial work, increasing myocardial oxygen demand, which leads to the dominating effect of coronary vasodilation through increased metabolic demand. β_2-Adrenergic stimulation produces coronary dilation; parasympathetic stimulation dilates only the small coronary arteries. The chemoreceptors can indirectly alter sympathetic stimulation of the heart, affecting developed tension, heart rate, myocardial oxygen demand, and coronary resistance. The carotid sinus nerve mediates sympathetic stimulation and coronary dilation. The sympathetic receptors seem to cause coronary dilation and there are receptors that can also lead to coronary dilation through muscarinic pathways. Finally, continuous modulation of α-adrenergic sympathetic outflow seems to exert a tonic level of constrictor tone on the coronary circulation, which is opposed by the dilator effect of the continuous production of nitric oxide by a healthy endothelium[1–4,10]

PATHOPHYSIOLOGY

Common cardiovascular risk factors—including aging, hypertension, diabetes, insulin resistance, dyslipidemia, tobacco smoking, obesity, and chronic inflammation—impair the production of an important endothelium-derived relaxing factor, nitric oxide, by the vascular endothelium in the epicardial arteries and microvasculature. This impaired production of nitric oxide results in the failure of endothelium-dependent dilation in response to shear stress, blood flow, and the sympathetic stimulation of exercise. The lack of reflex dilation is replaced by abnormal constriction. These risk factors interfere with a wide range of endothelial functions, including nitric oxide production by uncoupling the enzymes that produce nitric oxide, oxidant stress, disabling necessary cofactors, and inhibiting the mRNA that governs the production of nitric oxide by nitric oxide synthase.

Atherosclerosis

Atherosclerosis leads to local accumulation of matrix, inflammatory cells, debris, cholesterol crystals, and smooth muscle cells within the coronary arterial wall, which ultimately can lead to the development of focal stenoses in epicardial arteries. When a stenosis is sufficiently severe, a pressure gradient develops across the lesion and, eventually, blood flow decreases as a stenosis progresses. The effect of luminal plaque and stenosis on coronary blood flow depends on the minimum cross-sectional area of narrowing; blood viscosity; vessel wall function; loss of laminar flow; development of turbulence; the severity, length, and complexity of the lesion; and the function of the microvasculature. In the presence of stenoses greater than 70%, small increases in blood flow greatly increase the pressure gradient across the stenosis. In the aforementioned circumstances, exercise increases myocardial oxygen demand, producing resistance vessel dilation, a decrease in poststenotic pressure, an increase in pressure gradient across the stenosis, and a further decrease in poststenotic perfusion pressure to the subendocardium. The minimal cross-sectional area within the stenosis is the most important measure of the lesion's rheologic effect on blood. At this point, small changes in stenosis severity produce exaggerated increases in the pressure gradient, which jeopardizes coronary blood supply. Physiologic increases in coronary blood flow are blunted when the stenosis exceeds approximately 45%, and they are abolished when the stenosis exceeds 80%. Resting coronary blood flow declines when the stenosis exceeds 90% to 95%.[11,12]

Apart from the structural disease and physical effects of stenosis on flow as described earlier, atherosclerosis is characterized by a dysfunctional endothelium that loses its ability to regulate local microvasculature vasodilation and permits abnormal and paradoxical constriction, particularly in response to the sympathetic stimulation that occurs during everyday life. This reflex constriction also has important consequences at the epicardial sites of severe stenoses. During physical exercise, exposure to cold and mental stimulation or sympathetic arousal leads to abnormal or exaggerated reflex constriction at the site of severe stenoses, leading to the development of ischemia. In atherosclerosis, the endothelium also loses other healthy functions—the maintenance of an anticoagulant surface, its antiinflammatory effect, and the local control of growth and cell proliferation. The loss of these functions permits platelet aggregation and thrombus formation locally, infiltration of inflammatory cells, local growth of smooth muscle cells, and extracellular matrix accumulation, all of which contribute to lesion progression.[1,13]

Coronary Microvascular Dysfunction

CMD can be sustained by several pathogenic mechanisms (Box 6.1).[14] Even though several of these mechanisms can be observed in the same clinical condition, their relative importance seems to vary between settings. From a pathophysiologic point of view and independently of the underlying mechanisms, CMD results in varying degrees of disruption of normal coronary physiology. CMD can be sustained by a combination of functional mechanisms that lead either to impaired dilatation or increased constriction of coronary microvessels (see Fig. 6.3 and Box 6.1). Their abnormalities eventually impair the capacity of myocardial blood flow to adapt to changes in myocardial oxygen demand.[5]

Collateral Blood Vessels

Preexisting but nonfunctioning vascular channels and collateral blood vessels connect the coronary arteries within the myocardium. If narrowing of large coronary arteries causes a decrease

---

BOX 6.1 Pathogenic Mechanisms of Coronary Microvascular Dysfunction

Type 1: In the Absence of Myocardial Diseases and Obstructive Coronary Artery Disease
- Microvascular remodeling
- Endothelial dysfunction
- Smooth muscle dysfunction

Type 2: In Myocardial Diseases Without Obstructive Coronary Artery Disease
- Microvascular remodeling
- Smooth muscle dysfunction
- Extramural compression
- Reduced diastolic perfusion time (increased intramyocardial pressure or tissue edema)
- Vascular wall infiltration
- Vascular rarefaction
- Perivascular fibrosis

Type 3: In Obstructive Coronary Artery Disease
- Endothelial dysfunction
- Smooth muscle dysfunction
- Luminal obstruction (microembolization)

Type 4: Iatrogenic
- Luminal obstruction (microembolization by plaque and thrombus debris)
- Autonomic dysfunction

in perfusion pressure, the collateral channels can open immediately and, over a period of days, can undergo passive widening to facilitate coronary blood flow between previously unconnected regions of the ventricles. Over weeks, specific cell growth leads to formation of new collateral vessels. This process is stimulated by ischemia, myocardial work, and oxygen demand with growth factors as mediators. Serotonin from platelets can cause opposite effects, such as collateral vessel constriction, and can worsen tissue perfusion. Endothelium-derived relaxing factors, such as nitric oxide, can dilate collateral vessels and facilitate regional myocardial blood flow.

Preexisting collateral vessels can partially compensate for coronary stenoses and occlusions. If the stimulus for collateral growth is persistent over months and collateral blood vessels develop, they can become capable of compensating for occlusion of large proximal epicardial arteries. Nevertheless, collateral vessels have limited ability to provide sufficient myocardial perfusion under stress and circumstances of increased demand, such as exercise or concurrent illness.

Myocardial Ischemia

Ischemia occurs when myocardial blood flow fails to deliver sufficient oxygen to meet the myocardial demand required for contraction, relaxation, and cellular metabolism. This failure is commonly caused by decreased myocardial blood flow or increased myocardial oxygen demand when blood supply is fixed by obstructive coronary artery disease and/or preexisting CMD. During ischemia, tissue oxygen tension decreases and aerobic metabolism becomes anaerobic; left ventricular relaxation and then contraction fails within seconds; and there are characteristic changes on the surface electrocardiogram (ECG) that may or may not be followed by angina pectoris.

Episodes of transient myocardial ischemia may occur in the presence of one or more atherosclerotic stenoses in the epicardial coronary arteries of 70% or greater but also occur in the absence of a severe epicardial stenosis due to spasm of the epicardial or microvascular vessels or by fixed microvascular obstruction. In addition, these atherosclerotic vessels exhibit endothelial dysfunction and, with exercise, mental arousal, or sympathetic stimulation (e.g., cold), their abnormal constriction increases the resistance at stenoses and further limits coronary blood supply, often at a time when there is an increase in myocardial oxygen demand.

While abnormal constriction occurs at atherosclerotic stenoses, myocardial oxygen demand is increased by any increase in heart rate, developed tension, and contractility, often in the presence of some degree of left ventricular hypertrophy or anemia. The mechanisms that lead to transient ischemia often include abnormalities of supply and demand, which may coexist and act in concert. During myocardial ischemia, tissue oxygen tension decreases, energy stores decline, inorganic phosphate accumulates, and intracellular calcium can no longer facilitate myocardial relaxation or contraction by myofilaments. There is temporary loss of the healthy transmembrane ion gradients while intracellular pH decreases. Myocardial relaxation fails first, and then contraction fails, followed by characteristic electrocardiogram changes with ST segment depression when there is patchy endocardial ischemia and ST elevation with severe transmural ischemia.

In acute MI, coronary blood supply is decreased further by thrombus formation superimposed on disrupted atherosclerotic plaques. If the balance between blood supply and myocardial demand is sustained and severe beyond 20 minutes (with plaque rupture, thrombosis, or sustained stimulation), the myocardial pathology described earlier is accompanied by progressive irreversible changes in myocardial membranes, enzymes, and proteins, leading to a central area of myocardial necrosis. Myocardial necrosis may result from a single episode over approximately 6 hours or may be the result of stuttering ischemic insults distributed over days. At this stage, the severity of ischemia and the development of necrosis depend almost entirely on the rapidity with which coronary blood flow can be restored.

In acute MI, restoration of coronary blood flow to the myocyte following successful reperfusion of the epicardial artery is dependent on the state of the microvasculature. In patients with ST elevation MI (STEMI), coronary microvascular dysfunction and obstruction (CMVO) occurs in up to half of patients following successful primary percutaneous coronary intervention (PCI) and is associated with a much worse outcome.[15] There are four interacting mechanisms in the pathogenesis of CMVO in STEMI: ischemia-related injury, reperfusion-related injury, distal embolization, and individual susceptibility of the microcirculation to injury[15] (Fig. 6.4).

Animal models have demonstrated that 90 minutes following a coronary occlusion, severe capillary damage occurs with endothelial protrusions and blebs that obstruct the capillary lumen.[16] Gaps in the endothelium allow erythrocytes to leave the vasculature. Interstitial edema compresses capillaries and small arterioles, further decreasing flow through these dysfunctional vessels.[17] Sodium and calcium overload result in cell swelling. The most important clinical predictors of ischemia-related injury are the duration and extent of ischemia.[15]

When ischemia lasts more than 3 hours prior to reperfusion, ischemia-associated injury is compounded by reperfusion injury.[18] CMVO is caused by further obliteration of the vessel lumen by neutrophil-platelet aggregates that release vasoconstrictor and inflammatory substances.[19] Reperfusion stimulates the production of radical oxygen species by cardiomyocytes that, along with rapid normalization of pH, leads to opening of mitochondrial membrane permeability pores, calcium overload, mitochondrial swelling, and cell disruption.[19] Neutrophils—a major source of oxidants, proteolytic enzymes, and proinflammatory mediators—may exacerbate CMVO.[19]

A third important mechanism of CMVO is distal embolization. In experimental models, myocardial perfusion starts failing when microspheres obstruct more than 50% of coronary capillaries.[20] In humans, emboli of different sizes can originate from epicardial coronary thrombus and disrupted atherosclerotic plaques during primary PCI. Spontaneous embolization prior to PCI probably occurs as well. Thrombus volume and the presence of lipid-rich plaque are associated with a greater risk of distal embolization.[21] Certain plaque features may also predispose to distal embolization. In particular, plaque erosion appears to result in more distal embolization than plaque rupture.[15]

Finally, there appears to be variation in individual susceptibility to microvascular dysfunction possibly related to the function,

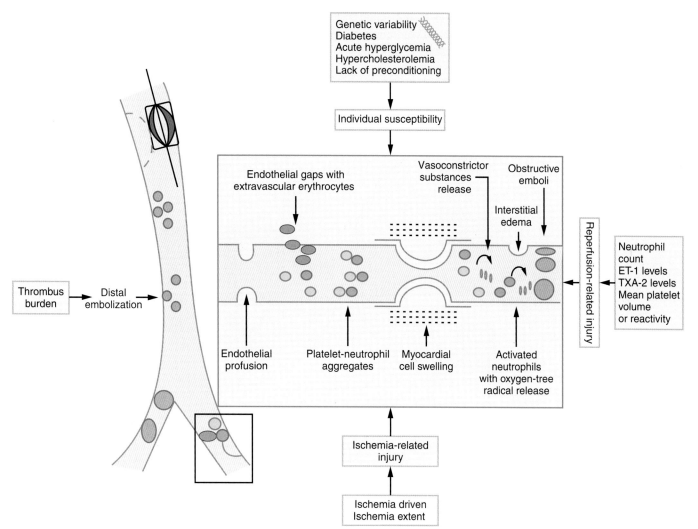

Fig. 6.4 There are four interacting mechanisms involved in the pathogenesis of coronary microvascular obstruction in humans: ischemia-related injury, reperfusion-related injury, distal embolization, and individual susceptibility (both genetic and due to preexisting coronary microvascular dysfunction) of the microcirculation to injury. Ischemic injury depends on duration and extent of ischemia and is characterized by severe capillary damage, endothelial protrusions, and blebs that block the capillary lumen, and endothelial gaps with extravascular erythrocytes *(in red)*. Interstitial myocardial edema compresses capillaries and small arterioles, further decreasing flow through these dysfunctional vessels, whereas sodium and calcium overload explains myocardial cell swelling. Reperfusion injury: The principal determinants of this phenomenon are represented by neutrophils *(in green)*, endothelin-1, thromboxane-A2, and platelets *(in yellow)*. The obliteration of vessel lumen by neutrophil–platelet aggregates is associated with release of vasoconstrictors and inflammatory mediators *(in brown)*. Furthermore, in cardiomyocytes, reperfusion stimulates the production of reactive oxygen species by mitochondria, further aggravating microvascular function. Finally, reperfusion may increase infarct size due to mitochondria swelling and cell rupture based on opening of the mitochondrial membrane permeability transition, as well as favor intramyocardial hemorrhage. Distal embolization *(in blue)* of plaque and thrombus material may mechanically obstruct the microcirculation, but it is also a source of vasoconstrictors and procoagulant substances. Both thrombus and plaque features modulate the effect of distal embolization on coronary microvascular obstruction. Individual susceptibility of the microcirculation to injury: Factors modulating individual susceptibility to coronary microvascular obstruction are presented by genetic variability, diabetes, acute hyperglycemia, hypercholesterolemia, and lack of preconditioning.

structure, and density of the microcirculation in individual patients prior to the development of acute coronary syndrome.[22]

There are a number of invasive and non-invasive techniques for diagnosing CMVO, including direct invasive measurement of coronary blood flow velocity with an intracoronary Doppler wire, Thrombolysis in Myocardial Infarction (TIMI) frame count, myocardial blush grade, TIMI perfusion grade, ST segment resolution, myocardial contrast echo, cardiac magnetic resonance, and hybrid positron emission tomography/cardiac computed tomography (PET/CT) scanning (Fig. 6.5).[15] Regardless of the

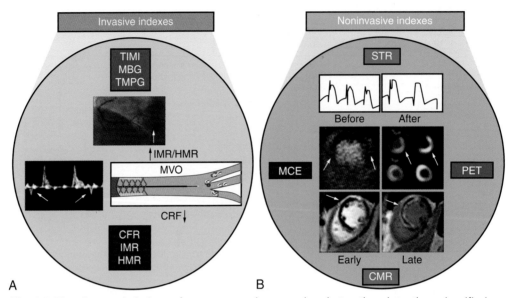

Fig. 6.5 The diagnostic indexes for coronary microvascular obstruction detection, classified as invasive *(green circle)* or noninvasive tools *(blue circle)* (B). Invasive indexes: The gold standard method for coronary microvascular dysfunction and obstruction assessment is the direct measurement of coronary flow reserve using intracoronary Doppler wire; the typical coronary microvascular dysfunction and obstruction pattern is characterized by systolic retrograde flow, diminished systolic anterograde flow, and rapid deceleration of diastolic flow. The figure at bottom left shows the systolic retrograde flow *(white arrows)* during intracoronary Doppler. The index of microvascular resistance provides a more reproducible assessment of microcirculation, independent of hemodynamic perturbations; hyperemic microvascular resistance is associated with ventricular recovery and clinical outcome after ST segment elevation myocardial infarction. The image at bottom right shows the typical pattern of coronary microvascular dysfunction and obstruction: reduced coronary flow reserve and increased index of microvascular resistance/ hyperemic microvascular resistance. Angiographic parameters of coronary microvascular dysfunction and obstruction are represented by Thrombolysis in Myocardial Infarction (TIMI) flow score, myocardial blush grade, and TIMI myocardial perfusion grade. Of note, it is becoming common practice to define angiographic coronary microvascular dysfunction and obstruction as follows: TIMI flow grade less than 3 or 3 with a myocardial blush grade or TIMI myocardial perfusion grade 0 to 1. The image at the top shows a case of angiographic coronary microvascular dysfunction and obstruction *(white arrow)* in the posterior descending branch of the right coronary artery. Noninvasive indexes: ST segment resolution represents a useful tool of coronary microvascular dysfunction and obstruction, also considering its prognostic value (see the top left image for the ST segment before opening infarct-related artery; see the top right image for the ST segment after opening infarct-related artery during coronary microvascular dysfunction and obstruction). Myocardial contrast echocardiography can be employed for coronary microvascular dysfunction and obstruction diagnosis. The typical pattern is represented by lack of intramyocardial contrast opacification *(white arrows, center left image)*. Cardiac magnetic resonance allows multislice imaging with high tissue contrast and high spatial resolution, enabling accurate quantification and localization of coronary microvascular dysfunction and obstruction and infarct size relative to the entire left ventricle. Typical signs of coronary microvascular dysfunction and obstruction are represented by lack of gadolinium enhancement during the first pass *(white arrow, bottom left image)* and lack of gadolinium enhancement within a necrotic region (late gadolinium hyper-enhancement) *(white arrow, bottom right image)*. Finally, the hybrid positron emission tomography/cardiac computed tomography allows monitoring of inflammatory reactions after reperfusion *(white arrows, center right image)*. *CFR,* coronary flow reserve; *CMR,* cardiac magnetic resonance; *HMR,* hyperemic microvascular resistance; *IMR,* index of myocardial resistance; *MBG,* myocardial blush grade; *MCE,* myocardial contrast echocardiography; *MVO,* microvascular obstruction; *PET,* positron emission tomography; *STR,* ST segment resolution; *TMPG,* TIMI myocardial perfusion grade.

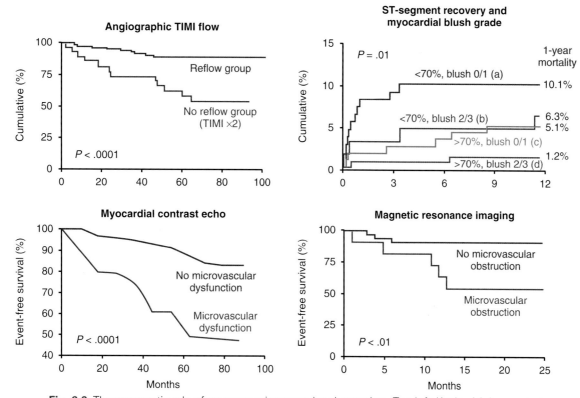

Fig. 6.6 The prognostic role of coronary microvascular obstruction. *Top left:* Kaplan-Meier survival curve showing, at long-term follow-up (100 months), that patients in the coronary microvascular obstruction group, evaluated by angiographic thrombolysis in myocardial infarction flow, had a significantly higher incidence of cardiac death (%) compared with those without coronary microvascular obstruction (log-rank *P* < .0001).[23] *Top right:* Kaplan-Meier survival curve showing cumulative adverse event rates (%), according to myocardial blush grade, among patients with and without ST segment resolution, during 1-year follow-up (log-rank, *P* = .01). In particular, among patients with ST segment resolution <70%, the cumulative adverse event rate was 10.1% for myocardial blush grade 0/1 and 6.3% for myocardial blush grade 2/3. Among patients with ST segment resolution greater than 70%, the cumulative event rate was 5.1% for myocardial blush grade 0/1 and 1.2% for myocardial blush grade 2/3.[24] *Bottom left:* Kaplan-Meier survival curve showing combined event-free survival (%) in patients with and without microvascular reperfusion, after perfused acute myocardial infarction, evaluated by myocardial contrast echocardiography. In particular, patients without microvascular reperfusion exhibit a higher cumulative 5-year combined event rate (log-rank test, *P* < .0001), than those without microvascular dysfunction.[25] *Bottom right:* Kaplan-Meier survival curve showing combined event-free survival (%) in patients with and without microvascular obstruction, after perfused acute myocardial infarction, evaluated by magnetic resonance imaging. In particular, patients with microvascular obstruction exhibit a higher cumulative 2-year combined event rate (log-rank test, *P* = .001) than those without microvascular obstruction.[26] *TIMI,* Thrombolysis in Myocardial Infarction.

modality used, the diagnosis of coronary microvascular obstruction is associated with increased mortality and reduced event-free survival (Fig. 6.6). New therapies directed at preservation and restoration of microvascular function are urgently needed to reduce morbidity and mortality from acute MI and to continue the progress achieved by revascularization of the epicardial lesion.

Acknowledgment

I acknowledge the contributions of Andrew Selwyn, MD, to this chapter in previous editions of this text.

The full reference list for this chapter is available at ExpertConsult.com.

7

Pathophysiology of Acute Coronary Syndromes: Plaque Rupture and Atherothrombosis

Nishtha Sodhi, David L. Brown

OUTLINE

The acute coronary syndromes (unstable angina, myocardial infarction [MI], sudden cardiac death) are a major cause of morbidity and mortality in developed countries. MI alone is the major cause of death in most Western countries.[1] The rapidly increasing prevalence in developing countries, specifically South Asia and Eastern Europe—coupled with an increasing incidence of tobacco abuse, obesity, and diabetes—is predicted to make cardiovascular disease the major global cause of death by 2020.[2] Although MI in patients with normal coronary arteries (MINOCA) is being increasingly recognized, atherosclerotic plaque formation within the coronary arteries with subsequent lesion disruption, platelet aggregation, and thrombus formation remains the leading cause of acute coronary syndromes in humans.

During the early 1900s, the first description of the clinical presentation of acute MI was published by Obstrastzow and Straschesko.[3] Shortly thereafter, Herrick[4] associated the clinical presentation of acute MI with thrombotic occlusion of the coronary arteries. Much has been learned since these early observations concerning the pathophysiology of coronary artery disease and the acute coronary syndromes. This chapter reviews the pathogenesis of atherosclerosis and explores the mechanisms responsible for the sudden conversion of stable atherosclerotic plaques into unstable life-threatening atherothrombotic lesions.

ATHEROGENESIS

Development

Atherogenesis, or the development of plaques within the walls of blood vessels, is the result of complex interactions involving blood elements, vessel wall abnormalities, and alterations in blood flow. Several pathologic mechanisms play an important role, including inflammation with activation of endothelial cells and monocyte recruitment,[5–9] growth with smooth muscle cell proliferation and matrix synthesis,[10,11] degeneration with lipid accumulation,[12,13] necrosis, calcification and ossification,[14,15] and thrombosis.[16] These diverse processes result in the formation of atheromatous plaques that form the substrate for future acute coronary syndromes.

Fatty Streak. Vascular injury and thrombus formation are key events in the formation and progression of atherosclerotic plaques. Fuster and colleagues[17] proposed a pathophysiologic classification of vascular injury that divides the damage into three types (Fig. 7.1). Type I injury consists of functional deviations from normal endothelial function without obvious morphologic changes. Type II injury involves a deeper form of vascular damage that includes denudation of endothelial cells and intimal damage

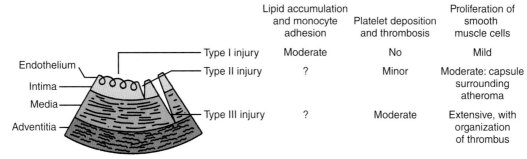

	Lipid accumulation and monocyte adhesion	Platelet deposition and thrombosis	Proliferation of smooth muscle cells
Type I injury	Moderate	No	Mild
Type II injury	?	Minor	Moderate: capsule surrounding atheroma
Type III injury	?	Moderate	Extensive, with organization of thrombus

Fig. 7.1 Classification of vascular injury and vascular response. (From Fuster V, Badimon L, Badimon J, Chesebro J. The pathogenesis of coronary artery disease and the acute coronary syndromes. *N Engl J Med.* 1992;326:242–248.)

with maintenance of an intact elastic lamina. Type III injury is represented by endothelial denudation and damage to the intima and media of the vessel wall.

The earliest finding in spontaneous atherosclerosis is an intimal lesion containing lipid-laden macrophages and a few T lymphocytes.[18] In the "response to injury hypothesis" proposed by Ross[19] and others, these "fatty streaks" are thought to result from chronic injury to the arterial endothelium induced by disturbances in coronary blood flow (type I injury) and an increased vascular permeability to lipids and monocytes (Fig. 7.2). The chronic injury is primarily a disturbance in the pattern of blood flow in certain parts of the arterial tree, such as bending, branch points, or both. Certain factors—such as hypercholesterolemia, tobacco abuse, vasoactive amines, glycosylated products, infection, and immune complexes—may potentiate the effect of type I injury on the endothelium.[20] This chronic, low-grade damage leads to the accumulation of lipids and macrophages at the site of injury, producing the characteristic fatty streak. These lipid-laden macrophages, also known as foam cells, are derived primarily from tissue macrophages. Foam cells are formed when large amounts of intracellular lipids, mainly from modified low-density lipoprotein (LDL), are taken up via a family of macrophage scavenger receptors and internalized into the macrophage.

There is growing evidence that oxidized LDL is a key active component in the generation of atheroscleroses rather than a passive substance that accumulates within macrophages. It is hypothesized that oxidized LDL has five potentially atherogenic effects: (1) monocyte chemotactic activity, (2) inhibition of macrophage migration out of the vessel wall, (3) enhanced uptake by macrophages, (4) formation of immune complexes, and (5) cytotoxicity (Fig. 7.3).

In the presence of elevated plasma LDL levels, the concentration of LDL within the intima is increased. By poorly understood mechanisms, which may involve the generation of free radicals by cellular lipoxygenases,[21,22] the LDL molecule undergoes oxidative modification (peroxidation of polysaturated fatty acids) that alters its metabolism. When the LDL contains fatty acid lipid peroxides, a rapid propagation amplifies the number of free radicals and leads to extensive fragmentation of the fatty acid chains. These fragments of oxidized fatty acids attach covalently to apoprotein B.[23,24] By means of specialized receptors, distinct from the LDL receptor, these modified apoprotein B molecules with the attached fatty acids are recognized by macrophages and

taken up by the cell (Fig. 7.4).[25] All three major cell types within the artery wall are capable of modifying LDL to a form that is recognizable by a scavenger receptor. In contrast to the LDL receptor, the scavenger LDL receptors are not down-regulated in the presence of excess ligand. Cells are able to accumulate large amounts of intracellular lipid.

Oxidized LDL within the intima may play a role in the adhesion of circulating monocytes to the arterial wall. More recent studies have shown that oxidized LDL, but not native LDL, is a powerful chemoattractant for circulating monocytes.[26] In addition, oxidized LDL is a potent inhibitor of the migration of macrophages out of the intima. By these two mechanisms, oxidized LDL may serve to attract and retain monocytes and macrophages within the vessel wall.

LDL modification by oxidation causes activation, dysfunction, apoptosis, and necrosis in human endothelial cells.[27] Activated endothelial cells express leukocyte adhesion molecules, including vascular cell adhesion molecule 1 and intercellular adhesion molecule 1, causing blood cells to adhere at the sites of activation.[27] Monocytes and lymphocytes preferentially adhere to these sites. A potent chemotactic agent, monocyte chemotactic protein 1, is produced by endothelial cells and smooth muscle cells. This same protein has been found in the intima of atherosclerotic lesions and in foam cells. Secretion of monocyte chemotactic protein 1 by endothelial or smooth muscle cells may be induced by oxidized LDL, suggesting a possible mechanism whereby lipids induce the recruitment of macrophages, leading to the formation of early atherosclerotic lesions.[28]

Within the vessel wall, monocytes undergo phenotypic modification by macrophage colony-stimulating factor, inducing them to differentiate into tissue macrophages. These macrophages are capable of expressing scavenger receptors, leading to internalization of oxidized LDL and the creation of foam cells and fatty streaks.

Plaque Formation. With time, fatty streaks progress into mature atherosclerotic plaques (Fig. 7.5). Macrophages recruited into the area may release toxic products that cause further damage, leading to denudation of the endothelium and intimal injury (type II injury). This deeper form of injury leads to platelet adhesion. Adherent platelets—along with recruited macrophages and damaged endothelium—release growth factors, such as platelet-derived growth factor (PDGF), epidermal growth

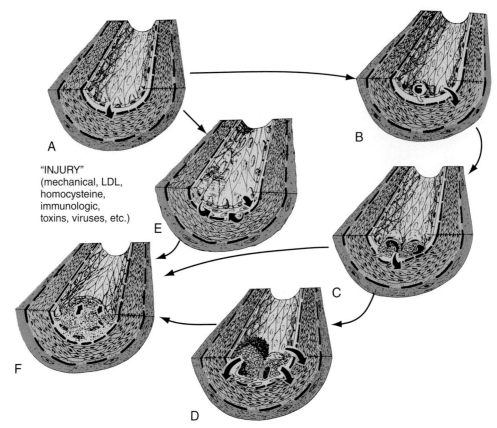

Fig. 7.2 Response-to-injury hypothesis. Advanced intimal proliferative lesions of atherosclerosis may occur by at least two pathways. The pathway shown by the *long arrows* has been observed in experimental hypercholesterolemia. Injury to the endothelium (A) may induce growth factor secretion *(short arrows)*. Monocytes attach to endothelium (B), which may continue to secrete growth factors *(short arrow)*. Subendothelial migration of monocytes (C) may lead to fatty streak formation and release of growth factors such as platelet-derived growth factor (PDGF, *short arrow*). Fatty streaks may become directly converted to fibrous plaques (*long arrow* from C to F) through release of growth factors from macrophages or endothelial cells, or both. Macrophages may also stimulate or injure the overlying endothelium. In some cases, plaques may lose their endothelial cover, and platelet attachment may occur (D), providing additional sources of growth factors *(short arrows)*. Some of the smooth muscle cells in the proliferative lesion itself (F) may synthesize and secrete growth factors such as PDGF *(short arrows)*. An alternative pathway for the development of advanced atherosclerosis lesions is shown by the *arrows* from (A) to (E) to (F). In this case, the endothelium may be injured but remain intact. (A) Increased endothelial cell turnover may result in growth factor synthesis by endothelial cells. (E) This may stimulate migration of smooth muscle cells from the media into the intima, accompanied by endogenous production of PDGF by smooth muscle cells and growth factor secretion by the "injured" endothelial cells. (F) These interactions could lead to fibrous plaque formation and further lesion progression. *LDL,* Low-density lipoprotein. (From Ross R. The pathogenesis of atherosclerosis: an update. *N Engl J Med.* 1986;314:458–500.)

factor-β, and somatomedin C. These growth factors may lead to migration and proliferation of vascular smooth muscle cells and stimulate the production of collagen, elastin, and glycoproteins. These proteins provide the connective tissue matrix of the newly formed plaque and give it structural support. Cholesterol, derived from insudated blood lipid or extruded from dying foam cells, becomes entrapped within this matrix. The lipid and connective tissue matrix are covered by a fibromuscular cap consisting of smooth muscle cells, collagen (types I and III), and a single layer of endothelial cells. This complex constitutes the mature atherosclerotic plaque (Fig. 7.6A). Vascular smooth muscle cells

synthesize and assemble the collagen fibrils and furnish the bulk of the noncollagenous portion of the extracellular matrix of the cap. The fibromuscular cap is a dynamic structure undergoing constant remodeling through the synthesis and breakdown of essential components (Fig. 7.7).

The microscopic changes that occur in spontaneous atherosclerosis have been described by Stary[18] and modified by the American Heart Association (AHA).[29] Using autopsy results from the coronary arteries and aortas of young people, Stary described five distinct lesions. A Stary I lesion, not apparent macroscopically, consists of isolated macrophages or foam cells within the intima

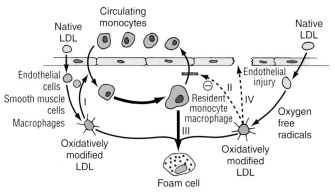

Fig. 7.3 Mechanisms by which the oxidation of low-density lipoprotein (LDL) may contribute to atherogenesis, including the recruitment of circulating monocytes by means of the chemotactic factor present in oxidized LDL, but absent in native LDL (I); inhibition by oxidized LDL of the mobility of resident macrophages and their ability to leave the intima (II); cytotoxicity of oxidized LDL, leading to loss of endothelial integrity (III); and uptake of oxidized LDL by macrophages, leading to foam cell formation (IV). Formation of immune complexes is not shown. (From Quinn MT, Parthasarathy S, Steinberg D. Endothelial cell-derived chemotactic activity for mouse peritoneal macrophages and the effects of low density lipoprotein. *Proc Natl Acad Sci U S A.* 1985;82:5949–5953.)

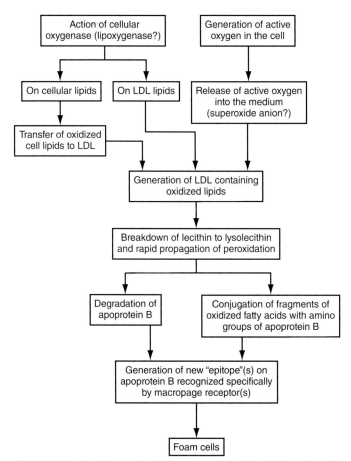

Fig. 7.4 Mechanisms of oxidative modification of low-density lipoprotein (LDL) by cells. (From Steinberg D. Metabolism of lipoproteins and their role in the pathogenesis of atherosclerosis. In Gotto AM Jr, Paoletti R, eds. Atherosclerosis Reviews, Vol 18. Stokes J III, Mancini M, eds. Hypercholesterolemia: Clinical and Therapeutic Implications. New York: Raven Press, 1988:1–23.)

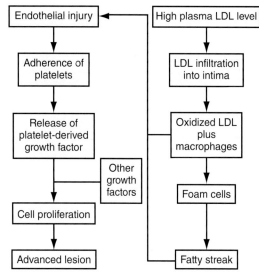

Fig. 7.5 Linkage between the lipid infiltration hypothesis and the endothelial injury hypothesis. The lipid infiltration hypothesis *(right column)* may account for fatty streaks, and the endothelial injury hypothesis *(left column)* may account for the progression of the fatty streak to more advanced lesions. *LDL,* Low-density lipoprotein. (From Steinberg D. Metabolism of lipoproteins and their role in the pathogenesis of atherosclerosis. In Gotto AM Jr, Paoletti R, eds. Atherosclerosis Reviews. Vol 18. Stokes J III, Mancini M, eds. *Hypercholesterolemia: Clinical and Therapeutic Implications.* New York: Raven Press, 1988:1–23.)

of the involved vessel. These lesions are noted in 45% of infants up to 8 months of age and eventually regress. A Stary II lesion, which is seen in adolescents, is characterized by numerous foam cells, lipid-containing smooth muscle cells, and a minimal amount of scattered extracellular lipid. Macroscopically, with Sudan IV staining, these lesions appear as a flat or raised fatty streak. In some children, more advanced lesions are noted that are characterized by an increased amount of extracellular lipid and the appearance of a raised fatty streak (Stary III) or a single confluent extracellular core (Stary IV). In adults, usually beginning in the third decade of life, two types of lesions are noted in the coronary arteries. Some plaques are mostly fibromuscular, whereas others are fibrolipid with a cap of smooth muscle cells and collagen. These latter lesions are designated as Stary V lesions.

The first three lesion types in the AHA classification are similar to those in the original Stary description. In the AHA classification, a type IV lesion has a predominance of extracellular, mostly diffuse lipid, whereas a type Va lesion has localized lipid content surrounded by a thin capsule. Additionally, type V lesions are classified further according to the amount of stenosis and fibrosis (types Vb and Vc). Type IV or Va lesions may progress slowly over time into more advanced type V lesions or undergo disruption, resulting in a type VI lesion represented by a ruptured plaque with overlying thrombus (Fig. 7.8).

The composition of nonruptured atheromatous plaques is highly variable, and the factors controlling this process are poorly understood. Mature plaques consist of two components: (1) soft, lipid-rich, atheromatous gruel; and (2) hard, collagen-rich, sclerotic tissue. The relative amounts of each component may differ with the individual plaque, but generally two populations

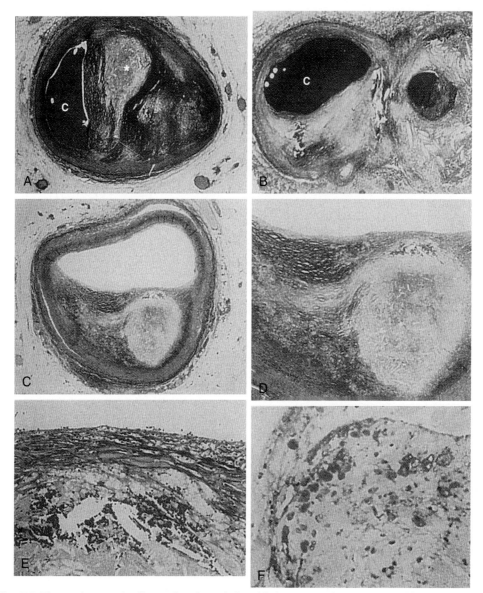

Fig. 7.6 Photomicrographs illustrating the relationship between plaque composition and vulnerability. (A) A mature atherosclerotic plaque consisting of two main components: soft lipid-rich gruel *(asterisk)* and hard collagen-rich sclerotic tissue *(blue)*. (B) Two adjacent plaques, one located in the circumflex branch *(left)* and another in the proximal side branch *(right)*. Although both plaques have been exposed to the same systemic risk factors, the plaque to the left is collagenous and stable, but the plaque to the right is atheromatous and vulnerable, with disrupted surface and superimposed nonocclusive thrombosis *(red)*. (C–E) Vulnerable plaque containing a core of soft atheromatous gruel (devoid of blue-stained collagen) separated from the vascular lumen by a thin cap of fibrous tissue infiltrated by foam cells that can be seen clearly at high magnification (E), indicating ongoing disease activity. Such a thin, macrophage-infiltrated cap is probably very weak and vulnerable, actually disrupted nearby, explaining why erythrocytes *(red)* can be seen in the gruel just beneath the macrophage-infiltrated cap. (F) Atherectomy specimen from culprit lesion in non–Q-wave myocardial infarction. At high magnification it can be seen clearly that this plaque specimen is heavily infiltrated by red-stained macrophages. (A–E) Trichrome stain. (F) Immunostaining for macrophages using monoclonal antibody PG-MI from Dako. (From Falk E, Shah PK, Fuster V: Coronary plaque disruption. *Circulation.* 1995;92:657–671.)

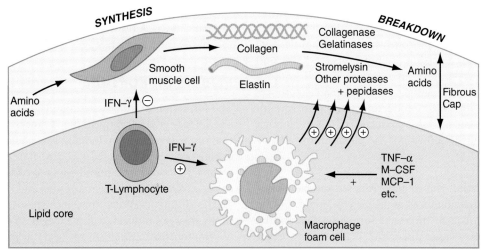

Fig. 7.7 Metabolism of collagen and elastin in the plaque's fibrous cap. The vascular smooth muscle cell synthesizes the extracellular matrix proteins, collagen, and elastin. In the unstable plaque, interferon-γ (IFN-γ) secreted by activated T cells may inhibit collagen synthesis, interfering with the maintenance and repair of the collagenous framework of the plaque's fibrous cap. The activated macrophage secretes metalloproteinases that can degrade collagen and elastin. Degradation of the extracellular matrix can weaken the fibrous cap, rendering it particularly susceptible to rupture and precipitating acute coronary syndromes. IFN-γ secreted by T lymphocytes can activate the macrophage. Plaques also contain other activators of macrophages, such as tumor necrosis factor-α (TNF-α), macrophage colony-stimulating factor (M-CSF), and macrophage chemoattractant protein-1 (MCP-1). (From Libby P. Molecular bases of the acute coronary syndromes. *Circulation.* 1995;91:2844–2850.)

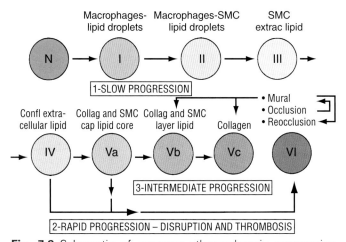

Fig. 7.8 Schematic of coronary atherosclerosis progression according to lesion morphology. See text for details. *Collag,* collagen; *Confl,* confluence; *extrac,* extracellular; *SMC,* smooth muscle cells. (From Fuster V. Mechanisms leading to myocardial infarction: insights from studies of vascular biology. *Circulation.* 1994;90:2126–2146.)

of lesions predominate (see Fig. 7.6B). One group consists of fibrointimal lesions characterized by large amounts of fibrous tissue and relatively little atheromatous gruel. The second population consists of lipid-laden lesions with a cholesterol-rich central core and a thin outer capsule.

Differences in plaque composition have important clinical implications. Plaques causing severe stenosis tend to have a higher fibrous and lower lipid content than less stenotic lesions.[30]

However, several studies have shown the less stenotic, lipid-laden plaques to be the more clinically dangerous lesions.[31] As discussed in this chapter, the soft atheromatous center may predispose the plaque to rupture, exposing the highly thrombogenic gruel and subintimal elements to blood flow and leading to the formation of thrombus and acute myocardial ischemia in many cases.

Progression of Atherosclerosis

Atherosclerosis is a dynamic process that, without intervention, is progressive. Serial angiographic studies have shown that atherosclerotic plaques tend to enlarge over time and that a significant number of lesions progress to total occlusion. The risk of progression to total occlusion seems to be related to the initial severity of the lesion, with more obstructive lesions progressing to total occlusion more frequently than less severe lesions.[32] The factors that govern plaque progression are incompletely understood, but two mechanisms have been proposed. One mechanism involves continuation of the myointimal proliferative process produced by the chronic endothelial injury responsible for the early lesions of atherosclerosis.[10] The second mechanism, which may be more important in rapidly growing plaques, involves recurrent minor fissuring of the atheromatous plaque (type Va lesion undergoing type III injury) with subsequent thrombus formation and fibrotic organization.

Chronic Endothelial Injury.   In the response-to-injury hypothesis, progression of atherosclerotic lesions occurs via the same mechanisms responsible for the initial myointimal lesion. At least two separate processes seem to be involved. One pathway involves gross endothelial cell damage and monocyte, macrophage, and platelet recruitment with growth factor secretion leading to the formation and progression of fibrous plaques. A second pathway involves direct stimulation of endothelial cells without obvious injury. This process may increase endothelial cell turnover with increased growth factor production leading to smooth muscle cell migration and increased production of PDGF. Through these interactions, further growth of the initial fibrous plaque may occur (see Fig. 7.2).[10]

Recurrent Thrombosis. The second proposed mechanism of atherosclerotic progression involves recurrent minor plaque disruption with subsequent thrombus formation followed by fibrotic organization. Plaque disruption is a common event and may be asymptomatic in many patients.[33] As discussed in greater detail later, rupture of lipid-laden plaque exposes the highly thrombogenic atheromatous core and subendothelial components of the arterial wall to the circulation. This exposure results in platelet adhesion and activation with the release of growth factors and stimulation of the coagulation cascade. This sequence of events results in the formation of thrombus, superimposed on the damaged plaque, which eventually undergoes fibrotic organization with subsequent incremental narrowing of the arterial lumen. In this model, recurrent subclinical events may lead to progressive plaque growth and, ultimately, vessel occlusion.

Several lines of evidence point to an important role of mural thrombus formation in the progression of atherosclerosis. Autopsy studies of coronary artery disease patients who died of cardiac and noncardiac causes reveal the presence of plaques with healed fissures with various stages of thrombus formation and organization and old organized coronary thrombi that are difficult to distinguish from primary atherosclerotic changes seen in the arterial wall.[33–35] In situ hybridization techniques and monoclonal antibodies directed at platelets, fibrin, fibrinogen, and their degradation products reveal increased amounts of these substances within the intima, neointima, and deeper medial layer in patients with coronary artery disease.[36,37] These observations suggest that products of organized thrombus are important in the growth of atherosclerotic plaques.

Platelets and mural thrombi may contribute to the progression of atherosclerosis by mechanisms other than the addition of organized fibrous layers to the plaque. As noted previously, adherent platelets are capable of secreting various mitogenic factors, including PDGF, transforming growth factor-β, and others. These factors may be involved in the proliferation, hypertrophy, and migration of smooth muscle cells, which are important steps in intimal thickening and plaque growth.[17] Studies from animals with thrombocytopenia or lacking von Willebrand factor (a protein required for platelet adhesion) have shown a reduced amount of atherosclerotic plaque formation and growth. Thrombin produced after vascular injury may become incorporated into the thrombus and extracellular matrix, and may be released slowly over time during periods of spontaneous fibrinolysis or remodeling of the thrombus. Thrombin may bind to platelet receptors and cause platelet activation or bind to

smooth muscle cells, resulting in proliferation. Through these mechanisms, it is possible that platelets and thrombin play a role in the early and late stages of atherosclerotic progression.

PLAQUE DISRUPTION

The formation of atherosclerotic plaques within the coronary arteries may gradually impede blood flow by progressive obstruction of the vessel lumen. Initially, these lesions are silent except during periods of increased myocardial oxygen demand. When coronary blood flow cannot be increased to meet the demand of the myocardium, ischemia results and causes characteristic exertional angina. With time, the atherosclerotic plaque may slowly enlarge, producing a greater degree of occlusion that results in symptoms with progressively lesser degrees of exertion.

The pathophysiology of acute coronary syndromes—including unstable angina, MI, and sudden cardiac death—is significantly different. These clinical entities represent a continuum of disease characterized by an *abrupt* reduction in coronary blood flow. Current concepts hold that this abruptly reduced coronary blood flow is caused by atherosclerotic plaque erosion, fissuring or rupturing that leads to the formation of thrombus that, superimposed on a preexistent lesion, severely limits flow (see Fig. 7.6B).[38–41]

The risk of plaque fissuring or rupturing is related to the intrinsic properties of individual plaques (vulnerability) and extrinsic factors acting on the plaque itself (rupture triggers). The former predisposes plaques to rupture, whereas the latter may precipitate disruption if vulnerable plaques are present.

Vulnerability

Pathoanatomic examination of intact and disrupted plaques and in vitro mechanical testing of isolated fibrous caps indicate that the vulnerability of a given plaque to rupture depends on several factors: size and consistency of the atheromatous core, thickness and collagen content of the fibrous cap covering the core, the degree of inflammation within the cap, and cap fatigue (see Figs. 7.6C–D).

Core Size and Content. The size and consistency of individual plaques vary greatly from lesion to lesion. As previously described, atherosclerotic plaques are composed of two main components whose ratio may vary within a given plaque. The typical plaque, especially in the most highly stenotic lesions, contains more hard fibrous tissue than soft atheromatous gruel. Plaques containing a larger amount of gruel tend to be identified more often beneath thrombi in acute coronary syndromes, however.[31] Several investigators have shown that the culprit lesions responsible for acute coronary syndromes tend to have a lipid-laden core occupying greater than 40% of the plaque.[42]

The composition and size of the atheromatous core are important in determining vulnerability. The core is rich in extracellular lipids, especially cholesterol and its esters.[43] Plaques are softened and made more prone to rupture by an increased amount of extracellular lipids in the form of cholesterol esters. Conversely, lipids in the form of cholesterol crystals have the opposite effect on plaque stability. However, it has been suggested, but not proven, that cholesterol crystals can perforate the intimal surface of the plaque shoulder.

Cap Thickness and Content. Fibrous caps covering the lipid cores of atherosclerotic lesions vary in thickness, cellularity, matrix composition, and collagen content, all of which are important determinants of plaque stability.[44] Disrupted caps tend to contain fewer cells that synthesize collagen than intact caps.[42,45] This lack of collagen may weaken the fibrous cap, leaving the plaque prone to rupturing, which tends to occur in areas where the cap is the thinnest and often most heavily infiltrated by foam cells. In eccentric plaques, rupturing usually occurs in the shoulder region, defined as the junction between plaque and the adjacent, less diseased vessel wall. The cap in these shoulder regions is often thin and heavily infiltrated with macrophages.[44] Superficial erosion and fissuring of plaque can also lead to thrombosis.

Inflammation. The concept that the inflammatory response may play a role in atherosclerosis dates back to Rudolph Virchow in the late 1800s, who postulated that atherosclerosis results from the local reaction of the vessel wall to the insudation of blood products. More recently, a growing body of evidence supports the concept that inflammation is involved in plaque disruption leading to acute coronary syndromes.

Several studies have shown that disrupted fibrous caps are heavily infiltrated by lipid-laden macrophages or foam cells (see Figs. 7.6E–F).[31] Postmortem examination of thrombosed coronary arteries has shown foam cell infiltration in most plaque rupture sites. Atherectomy specimens from culprit lesions responsible for acute coronary syndromes show significantly increased amounts of macrophages compared with specimens from patients with stable angina. Although the morphology of the plaque itself may vary, the cellular composition at the site of rupture is remarkably consistent with macrophages being the dominant cell.

Experimental evidence from in vitro[46] and in vivo systems[44] suggests that the macrophages present in atherosclerotic plaques are involved in active inflammation. Other components of the inflammatory response, including T lymphocytes, mast cells, and neutrophils, have been found in atherosclerotic plaques.[47] Interferon-γ, a cytokine produced within atheromas by activated T cells,[48] may play a crucial role in this process. Interferon-γ decreases interstitial collagen synthesis within the fibrous cap, inhibits smooth muscle cell proliferation, activates the apoptosis pathway in smooth muscle cells, and activates macrophages.[49] Active inflammation in areas of high stress may weaken the fibrous cap further and contribute to plaque rupture.

T-cell cytokines also induce the production of large amounts of molecules downstream in the cytokine cascade, resulting in elevated levels of interleukin-6 and C-reactive protein in the peripheral circulation, which amplifies local and systemic inflammation. Elevated levels of C-reactive protein and interleukin-6 in patients with acute coronary syndromes are associated with a worse prognosis.

When activated, macrophages are capable of causing weakening of plaque structure by several mechanisms. These cells may degrade the extracellular matrix by secreting various proteolytic enzymes. One such group of enzymes is the matrix metalloproteinases (MMPs). The MMPs are a family of zinc-dependent and calcium-dependent enzymes that are important in the resorption of the extracellular matrix in normal and pathologic conditions. These enzymes may be divided into subgroups based broadly on substrate preference.[50] The MMP subgroups include collagenases, gelatinases, stromelysin, and membrane-type MMPs that act on various substrates, including collagen, elastin, proteoglycan, lamin, fibronectin, and basement membrane components. Taken together, these MMPs are capable of completely degrading all extracellular components, and may play a role in atherogenesis and plaque disruption. In addition, MMPs can be proinflammatory by facilitating inflammatory cells.

MMPs are secreted by macrophages, smooth muscle cells, and lymphocytes found within atherosclerotic plaques. Production and secretion of MMPs is a balance between several different factors. Numerous cytokines and growth factors—including interleukin-1, PDGF, and tumor necrosis factor-α—have been shown to induce the synthesis of MMPs. Conversely, several unrelated substances have been shown to inhibit MMP production, including heparin, corticosteroids, and tumor necrosis factor-β. MMPs are secreted as proenzymes or zymogens and require an activation step to become capable of degrading the extracellular matrix. When activated, the effects of the MMPs are controlled by a family of naturally occurring specific inhibitors, the tissue inhibitors of metalloproteinases. Several lines of investigation point to a possible role for MMPs in plaque rupture. Messenger RNA transcripts of one MMP family member, stromelysin, have been identified in macrophages and smooth muscle cells in fibrous and lipid-laden plaques.[51] Other MMPs have been found in atherosclerotic, but not normal, arteries.[52] Atherectomy specimens from patients with unstable angina have shown increased intracellular gelatinase B production compared with specimens from patients with stable angina.[53]

Chronic immune stimulation within the atheroma may lead to the elaboration of several factors, including cytokines and metalloproteinases that alter the structural integrity of the fibrous cap by inhibiting collagen synthesis and increasing matrix degradation. Taken together, these factors reduce the structural integrity of the plaque, rendering the fibrous cap weak and prone to rupture in a susceptible region of the plaque. More recent studies using in situ zymographic techniques have revealed a net excess of metalloproteinase activity and matrix degradation within fibrous caps, especially at the vulnerable shoulder region of plaques.[54]

Rupture Triggers

Atherosclerotic plaques are constantly exposed to various mechanical and hemodynamic forces that may precipitate disruption of a vulnerable lesion. The importance of several external forces has been shown, including cap tension, cap and plaque compression, intraplaque hemorrhage, circumferential bending, longitudinal flexion, and hemodynamic forces.

Cap Tension. The blood pressure inside the artery exerts radial and circumferential forces across the arterial wall, which must be counteracted by tension within the wall to maintain vessel integrity. The circumferential tension is described by the law of

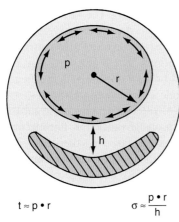

$$t \approx p \bullet r \qquad\qquad \sigma \approx \dfrac{p \bullet r}{h}$$

Fig. 7.9 Circumferential tension on the fibrous cap of an atherosclerotic plaque containing a lipid pool *(hatched area)* is determined by the law of Laplace, which relates tension *(t)* to the intralumen pressure *(p)* and the lumen radius *(r)*. The mean circumferential stress on the fibrous cap is related to circumferential tension and cap thickness *(h)*. (From MacIsaac A, Thomas JD, Topol EJ. Toward the quiescent coronary plaque. *J Am Coll Cardiol.* 1993;22:1228–1241.)

Laplace, which relates intracavity pressure (blood pressure) and lumen radius (vessel diameter; Fig. 7.9). The higher the blood pressure or the larger the luminal diameter, the greater the tension is within the wall.[55] If components within the wall are unable to bear the tension, the stress may be redistributed to the adjacent structures. In coronary artery disease, the soft atheromatous core is unable to bear the imposed load, resulting in a shift of these forces to the fibrous cap. Studies using simulated and real plaques have shown that soft eccentric pools of atheromatous gruel lead to the concentration of stress on the adjacent cap, especially near the shoulder region.[30] These areas of increased stress correlate with the actual area of plaque rupture in most specimens.[56]

The consistency of the atheromatous gruel and the thickness of the fibrous cap are important determinants of plaque rupture. Atheromatous gruel with increased amounts of extracellular lipid in the form of cholesterol esters tends to be softer. Softer plaques are less able to handle increased wall stress, and redistribute these forces to the fibrous cap, predisposing the lesion to rupture. The thickness of the fibrous cap is also an important factor in determining the ability of a given lesion to handle circumferential stress, with the thinner caps developing a greater amount of stress. Mildly to moderately stenotic lesions are associated with greater circumferential wall tension rather than more severe lesions. Active newer plaques are also noted to have positive remodeling of their vessel size as postulated by Glagov[57] and confirmed by intravascular ultrasound. This increase in vessel diameter can also contribute to increased wall stress promoting plaque rupture. These observations, along with several other factors, may help to explain why the less occlusive lesions tend to be the most clinically volatile.

Cap and Plaque Compression. In addition to rupture from the lumen into the plaque, the reverse process of disruption from the interior of the plaque into the vessel lumen may occur. This process is likely to be secondary to an increase in intraplaque pressure caused by vasospasm, intraplaque hemorrhage, plaque edema, and collapse of compliant stenosis.

Vasospasm may rupture plaques by compressing the atheromatous core and displacing the fibrous cap into the lumen.[58] Intraplaque hemorrhage is an important contributor to the transformation of stable plaques into unstable lesions.[59] Microvascular incompetence is a likely source of intraplaque hemorrhage, although the exact mechanism is unknown. The rapid accumulation of erythrocyte-derived cholesterol contributes to the expansion of the volume of the necrotic core. In addition, it serves as a potent inflammatory stimulus, resulting in greater macrophage density. These factors may increase plaque vulnerability to rerupture. Collapse of a severe but compliant stenosis because of negative transmural pressure may cause buckling of the vessel wall, which may disrupt the plaque.

Circumferential Bending. The propagating pulse wave generated by the systolic contraction of the heart produces changes in the lumen size and shape. The normal cyclic diastolic-systolic change in lumen diameter is 10%, although this number may be altered with advancing age or coronary disease.[55] The change in lumen configuration may produce deformation and bending of the atherosclerotic plaque, especially in the shoulder region.[60] Over time, these cyclic changes may weaken the plaque and lead to disruption. Sudden changes in vascular tone may also produce a bending of plaques that may cause rupture.

Longitudinal Flexion. With the beating of the heart, the coronary arteries tethered to the surface of the myocardium are subjected to longitudinal deformation. Similar to circumferential bending, this stretching of the arterial wall may weaken plaques or, with acute changes in the contractility of the heart, lead to plaque rupture.[31]

Hemodynamic Factors. Hemodynamic stress tends to be less than the mechanical forces produced by blood and pulse pressure. Hemodynamic factors, such as shear stress, can cause endothelial cell injury, however. Increased shear stress through stenotic lesions can theoretically lead to plaque disruption, although this concept has not been shown in angiographic studies.[61]

THROMBOSIS

Thrombus formation is central to the development of acute coronary syndromes. Intrinsic and extrinsic factors may combine to cause rupture of the fibrous cap with exposure of the plaque's central components to the circulating blood and subsequent thrombosis.

Platelet Biology

Aggregation and activation of platelets play an essential role in normal hemostasis and acute coronary syndromes. After injury to the vessel wall, such as in plaque rupture, platelets are involved in the body's initial response (primary hemostasis). Effective primary hemostasis requires three critical events to occur: (1)

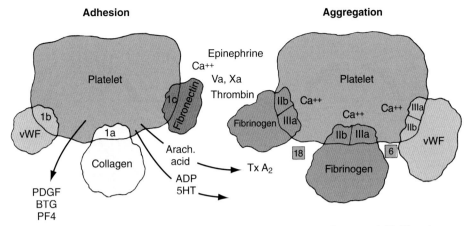

Fig. 7.10 Schematic of platelet activation and receptor sites. *1a, 1b, 1c,* and *IIb/IIIa,* glycoprotein receptor sites; *5HT,* serotonin; *ADP,* adenosine diphosphate; *Arach. acid,* arachidonic acid; *BTG,* β-thromboglobulin; *PDGF,* platelet-derived growth factor; *PF4,* platelet factor 4; *TxA₂,* thromboxane A₂; *Va,* activated factor V; *vWF,* von Willebrand factor; *Xa,* activated factor X. (From Myler RK, Frink RJ, Shaw RE, et al. The unstable plaque: pathophysiology and therapeutic implications. *J Invasive Cardiol.* 1990;2:117–128.)

platelet adherence, (2) platelet activation with granule release, and (3) platelet aggregation.

Platelet Adherence. Damage to the vessel wall exposes the highly thrombogenic subendothelial substrate and atheromatous core (specifically collagen and tissue factor) to circulating blood. Platelet adherence to the subendothelial collagen occurs almost immediately through interaction with platelet glycoprotein VI. Adhesion of platelets depends on many platelet receptors and adhesive membrane glycoproteins (Fig. 7.10).[62] Glycoprotein Ib in the platelet membrane is important in the initial contact of platelets with von Willebrand factor in the subendothelium. von Willebrand factor forms a link between receptors on platelets and subendothelial collagen fibrils, allowing platelets to remain attached to the vessel wall despite high shear forces. The membrane receptor complex, glycoprotein IIb/IIIa, binds many relevant proteins, including von Willebrand factor, fibrinogen, and fibronectin.[63] This complex plays a crucial role in initial platelet adhesion and platelet aggregation. Through this series of complex receptor-substrate interactions, the platelets form a firmly adherent monolayer and provide a foundation for further clot formation. This collagen-initiated pathway for platelet activation is independent of thrombin.

Platelet Activation and Aggregation. Platelet adhesion leads to the release of certain intracellular products that result in further platelet activity. Platelet activation and secretion are regulated by several factors, including a change in the level of cyclic nucleotides, the influx of calcium, the hydrolysis of membrane phospholipids, and the phosphorylation of crucial intracellular proteins. Binding of agonists such as epinephrine, collagen, and thrombin to platelet receptors activates phospholipase C and phospholipase A₂, membrane enzymes that catalyze the release of arachidonic acid. Through a series of complex reactions (Fig. 7.11), the released arachidonic acid is eventually converted to thromboxane A₂ and prostacyclin. These two products have

opposite effects on platelet activation and vessel wall tone. Thromboxane A₂ is a powerful stimulus for platelet activation and aggregation and produces vasoconstriction, whereas prostacyclin acts to inhibit platelet activation and is a vasodilator. By selective production (or inhibition) of these two substances, changes in the level of platelet activation and vessel wall tone may be achieved.[64]

Other active products secreted by platelets include endoglycosidases and heparin-cleaving enzymes from lysosomes, calcium, serotonin, adenosine diphosphate (ADP) from dense granules, von Willebrand factor, fibronectin, thrombospondin, and PDGF from α granules. These products have many important roles, including modification of coronary vascular tone, cellular proliferation and migration, and interaction with the coagulation system. It has been shown that PDGF is important in the proliferation and migration of smooth muscle cells after vessel damage.[10] Released ADP binds to specific receptors that change the conformation of the glycoprotein IIb/IIIa complex so that it binds von Willebrand factor, fibrinogen, and fibronectin, linking adjacent platelets into a hemostatic plug.

Coagulation Cascade

The coagulation cascade system also plays a key role in normal hemostasis (secondary hemostasis) and acute coronary syndromes. The coagulation system comprises several plasma proteins involved in a series of reactions that culminate in the production of thrombin, which converts fibrinogen to fibrin. The fibrin produced via this system is important in strengthening the primary hemostatic plug formed by platelets.

The coagulation cascade can be divided into the intrinsic and extrinsic pathways (Fig. 7.12). Both involve a series of reactions that require the formation of surface-bound complexes and the conversion of inactive precursor proteins into active proteases. The intrinsic pathway (factors XII, XIIa, XI, and XIa) is activated by exposure of blood components to the negatively charged, damaged subendothelium and medial surfaces of the vessel. The

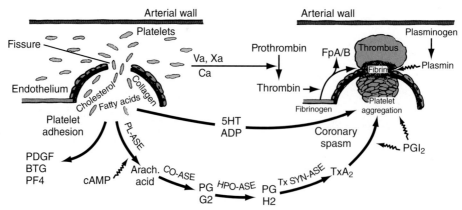

Fig. 7.11 Schematic of unstable plaque. *5HT,* Serotonin; *ADP,* adenosine diphosphate; *BTG,* β-thromboglobulin; *cAMP,* cyclic adenosine monophosphate; *CO-ASE,* cyclooxygenase; *FpA/B,* fibrinopeptide A and B; *HPO-ASE,* hydroperoxidase; *PDGF,* platelet-derived growth factor; *PF4,* platelet factor 4; *PG,* prostaglandin; *PL-ASE,* phospholipase A$_2$; *TxA$_2$,* thromboxane A$_2$; *Tx SYN-ASE,* thromboxane synthetase. (From Myler RK, Frink RJ, Shaw RE, et al. The unstable plaque: pathophysiology and therapeutic implications. *J Invasive Cardiol.* 1990;2:117–128.)

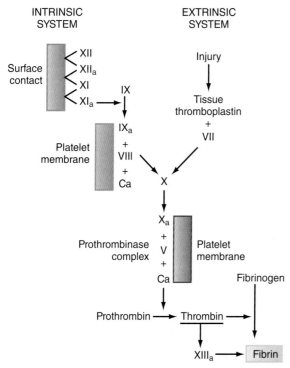

Fig. 7.12 Intrinsic and extrinsic systems of the coagulation cascade. Note interaction between clotting factors (XII, XIIa, XI, XIa, IX, IXa, VII, VIII, X, Xa, and XIIIa) and the platelet membrane. (Modified from Fuster V, Stein B, Ambrose JA, et al. Atherosclerotic plaque rupture and thrombosis: evolving concepts. *Circulation.* 1990;82[Suppl II]:II-47–II-59.)

extrinsic pathway is activated by interaction of tissue factor released from the damaged vessel wall and factor VII. Ultimately, these two pathways produce complexes that activate factor X. Activated factor X interacts with factor V, calcium, and phospholipid to form a complex that catalyzes the conversion of prothrombin to thrombin. This reaction is accelerated 1000-fold on the surface of activated platelets.

Thrombin has multiple functions in hemostasis, of which the primary function is the conversion of plasma fibrinogen to fibrin. After conversion to fibrin, the modified molecule polymerizes into an insoluble gel. The fibrin polymer is stabilized by cross-linking with other fibrin strands through the action of factor XIIIa, which results in an adherent thrombus. In addition, thrombin activates factors V, VIII, and XIII, and stimulates platelet secretion and aggregation.

Fibrinolysis

Balancing the prothrombotic events after vessel wall injury are several hemostatic mechanisms that favor fibrinolysis, decrease platelet aggregation, and cause vasodilation. Tissue plasminogen activator is the main physiologic activator of the fibrinolytic system, with Hageman factor fragments and urokinase playing a minor role. Tissue plasminogen activator converts plasminogen adsorbed to the fibrin clot to plasmin. The plasmin acts to degrade the fibrin polymer into fragments, resulting in clot lysis. Circulating thrombin stimulates several mechanisms designed to limit clot formation. The thrombin itself is inactivated by plasma protease inhibitors,[65] especially antithrombin III, which also inhibits activated factors VII, IX, and X. The thrombin also stimulates endothelial cells to release tissue plasminogen activator and produce prostacyclin and nitrous oxide, which act in concert to inhibit platelet aggregation and cause vasodilation.

Intact endothelial cells have several other important functions after vessel wall injury. These cells produce protein C, protein S, and heparin-like glycosaminoglycans that act to neutralize thrombin and activated factors V and VIII. In addition, stimulation of adenyl cyclase and accumulation of cyclic adenosine monophosphate within these cells lead to inhibition of phospholipase A$_2$ and decreased production of thromboxane A$_2$, which causes increased vasodilation.

The diverse actions of the intrinsic fibrinolytic system act to offset the thrombogenic stimulus of vessel wall injury. In the usual situation, a delicate balance is maintained that results in the formation of enough thrombus to provide hemostasis at the site of vascular injury without producing significant flow disturbance within the vessel. After a significantly strong thrombogenic stimulus (i.e., deep vessel injury), however, massive platelet activation with subsequent fibrin deposition may overwhelm the intrinsic fibrinolytic system and cause thrombus formation, thrombus growth, and vessel vasospasm that leads to a significant reduction in blood flow.

Factors That Influence Thrombus Formation

Several local and systemic factors present at the time of plaque rupture may influence the degree and duration of thrombus deposition after vessel wall injury. Interaction of these factors may account for the different pathologic and clinical manifestations of acute coronary syndromes.

Local Factors

Degree of vessel wall injury. The degree of vessel wall injury plays an important role in the biochemical response to plaque rupture. With mild amounts of vascular injury (superficial type III vascular damage), platelet adherence reaches a maximum within 5 to 10 minutes and results in a thrombus that can be dislodged by flowing blood. In contrast, deep vessel injury (deep type III injury) with exposure of fibrillar collagen results in markedly enhanced platelet deposition and thrombus formation that cannot be dislodged even at increased shear rates.[66] Tissue factor exposed by deeper injury likely contributes to the increased thrombogenicity by activating the extrinsic coagulation system.

Degree of stenosis. The amount of platelet adherence is also determined by their transport into the injured area.[63] Transport of platelets is determined by the shear rate, which is the difference in blood velocity between the center of the vessel and along the vessel wall. Shear rates increase with decreasing vessel diameter (i.e., increased stenosis) and with increasing flow. In vitro studies mimicking mild vascular injury with exposure of de-endothelialized vessels to low shear rates show the adherence of only a single layer of platelets. With the same amount of injury, but at higher shear rates, the initial platelet deposition rate and maximal extent of deposition are significantly increased.[67]

The degree of stenosis may influence the severity of thrombus formation by other mechanisms. That platelet deposition is greater with increasing amounts of stenosis suggests that platelet activation may be induced by shear forces generated by the sudden change in vessel geometry.[68] In addition, the flow characteristics of blood through the atherosclerotic lesion are partly determined by the extent of diameter stenosis. Flow is accelerated as blood passes through a stenosis and decelerates distal to the lesion. The sudden deceleration induces flow separation and recirculation vortices. The high shear rate area (the stenosis) favors platelet deposition, whereas the low shear rate area (the poststenotic recirculation zone) favors the deposition of fibrin. The combination of higher shear rates with large changes in flow dynamics seen in the more severely stenotic vessels results in a thrombus that is richer in platelets at the apex and contains larger amounts of fibrin distally.[63] These platelet-rich regions may be less amenable to fibrinolysis.[69]

Residual thrombosis. The presence of residual thrombus predisposes to recurrent thrombotic vessel occlusion by two mechanisms. The residual thrombus may encroach into the vessel lumen and cause a more stenotic lesion with increased shear rates, which may lead to further platelet activation and deposition.[66] Residual thrombus is a powerful thrombogenic stimulus. The degree of platelet deposition is increased twofold to fourfold on the surface of residual thrombi compared with on the surface of deeply injured arterial walls,[70] and the thrombi continue to grow despite heparin treatment.[71] Residual thrombi may offset the effects of the natural fibrinolytic system and add to the extent of thrombosis after plaque rupture.

Systemic Factors. Experimental and clinical studies suggest that primary hypercoagulability can enhance thrombus formation. In this model, after plaque disruption, individuals with one or two "thrombogenic risk factors" may form a small amount of thrombus that is clinically silent. In other individuals with more prothrombotic risk factors, a larger thrombus may be formed after the same degree of vessel injury, resulting in a more occlusive lesion that may produce unstable angina or acute MI.[72]

The level of circulating catecholamines at the time of plaque disruption may have important consequences. Platelet aggregation and thrombin generation can be promoted by catecholamines.[68] Such diverse factors as cigarette smoking, emotional state, and time of day have a direct effect on catecholamine levels and may provide a link between these clinically recognized risk factors and acute coronary syndromes.

Metabolic abnormalities—such as the metabolic syndrome or any of its components, including diabetes, hypertension, and obesity—may increase thrombogenicity mediated through the inflammation that they induce. Patients with hypercholesterolemia show increased platelet reactivity at sites of vascular damage[73] and hypercoagulability.[74] There is evidence that platelet reactivity and coagulation are increased in diabetics, suggesting a direct mechanism for a prothrombotic state that may be responsible for the increased incidence of MI in these patients.[68]

Finally, defective naturally occurring fibrinolysis may contribute to enhanced thrombus formation. High levels of naturally occurring inhibitors, such as plasminogen-activator inhibitor,[75] may predispose to an increased risk of acute coronary syndromes. High levels of lipoprotein(a) may also be important in ischemic heart disease. Apolipoprotein(a) is a glycoprotein present in lipoprotein(a) that has close structural homology with plasminogen.[76] This close homology may enable apolipoprotein(a) to act as a competitive inhibitor of plasminogen and cause a prothrombotic state. In addition, increased levels of other hemostatic proteins, such as fibrinogen and factor VII, have been identified in patients with ischemic heart disease.[68] Fibrinogen and factor VII activity increase with advancing age, obesity, hyperlipidemia, diabetes, smoking, and emotional stress, all factors associated with an increased risk of MI.

INTEGRATED PATHOGENESIS OF ACUTE CORONARY SYNDROMES

The acute coronary syndromes—unstable angina, non–ST elevation MI, ST elevation MI, and sudden cardiac death—all result from acute reductions in coronary blood flow. In these disease processes, atherosclerotic plaque disruption occurs and initiates a cascade of events that culminates in the formation of a thrombus overlying the damaged area. After plaque disruption and thrombus formation, there are different clinical outcomes influenced by location of the plaque (proximal vs. distal), existence of collaterals, the extent of the vessel injury, the degree of stenosis, and the thrombotic-thrombolytic equilibrium at the time of rupture (Fig. 7.13).

CONCLUSION

Coronary atherosclerosis is the most common cause of ischemic heart disease. Atherosclerosis without thrombosis is generally a benign disease, however. Disrupted atheromatous plaques are commonly associated with the formation of mural or occlusive thrombi, usually adherent to the area of damage. Certain types of plaques—those rich in lipids and surrounded by a thin fibrous cap—are the most prone to rupture. Numerous factors, intrinsic and extrinsic to the plaque itself, interact to cause the formation of a vulnerable lesion and, ultimately, plaque disruption. Erosion, fissuring, or rupturing of plaques play a fundamental role in the onset of acute coronary syndromes. In addition, repetitive damage to the plaque with thrombosis and fibrotic organization is important in the insidious progression of coronary artery disease.

Since the original clinical description of Herrick, much has been learned concerning the specific mechanisms involved in the pathophysiology of acute coronary syndromes. As discussed in subsequent chapters, this improved understanding has led to the development of treatments directed at specific steps in the pathogenesis of unstable angina, MI, and sudden cardiac death. Through these and future advances, physicians and scientists may hope to make a significant impact on the number one cause of death worldwide.

The full reference list for this chapter is available at ExpertConsult.com.

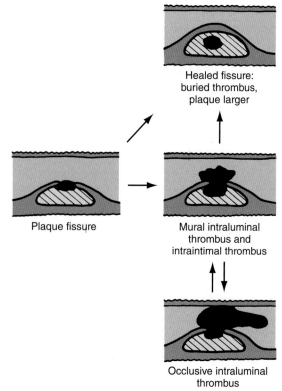

Fig. 7.13 Proposed outcome of atherosclerotic plaque fissuring. *Left panel:* Initial plaque fissure. *Upper right panel:* Fissure is sealed, and the incorporated thrombus undergoes fibrotic organization, contributing to the progression of coronary artery disease. *Middle right panel:* Fissure leads to intraintimal and intraluminal thrombosis, resulting in partial or transient reduction of coronary flow as seen in unstable angina. *Lower right panel:* Fissure results in occlusive thrombosis, which, if persistent, can lead to myocardial infarction or sudden ischemic death, particularly in the absence of collateral flow. (From Davies M, Thomas A. Plaque fissuring—the cause of acute myocardial infarction, sudden death, and crescendo angina. *Br Heart J.* 1985;53:363–373.)

8

Regulation of Hemostasis and Thrombosis

Maureane Hoffman

OVERVIEW AND DEFINITIONS

Coagulation is the clotting of blood or plasma. Hemostasis is the process by which bleeding is stopped and is the first component of the host response to injury. Its product is a hemostatic plug or hemostatic clot. Thrombosis is inappropriate clot formation within an intact vascular structure. Its product is a thrombus. Thus blood coagulation can occur at a site of injury (hemostasis), within an intact vessel (thrombosis), or in a test tube, but hemostasis is a physiologic process that can occur only in a living, bleeding organism.

Hemostasis consists of *primary hemostasis*, in which platelets adhere and are activated at a site of injury, and *secondary hemostasis*, in which the initial platelet plug is consolidated in a meshwork of fibrin. The hemostatic process represents a delicate and tightly regulated balance between effective activation of local hemostatic mechanisms in response to injury and control by regulatory mechanisms that prevent inappropriate activation or extension of coagulation reactions. The interactions of the protein components of coagulation can be studied in cell-free plasma and have been described as a "cascade" of proteolytic reactions. By contrast, the process of hemostasis occurs on cell surfaces in a tissue environment and is subject to regulation by a variety of biochemical and cellular mechanisms. The adequacy of procoagulant levels can be assessed in the routine plasma clotting assays: the prothrombin time (PT) and activated partial thromboplastin time (aPTT). Platelet number and function can be assessed in the clinical laboratory. Levels of individual plasma coagulation inhibitors and other regulatory proteins can also be assayed. However, **there is no laboratory test that can provide a global assessment of the adequacy of hemostasis or the risk of thrombosis.** Thus each laboratory test gives only a part of the picture, and the assessment of hemostatic function always requires that laboratory results be interpreted in the context of the clinical picture.

HEMOSTASIS

Because hemostasis involves more than simply getting blood to clot—it must clot at the right time and place and only to the extent needed to stop bleeding—our understanding of hemostasis must include a consideration not only of the proteins but also the cellular and tissue components that are needed to regulate the coagulation process in vivo.

Necessary Components

Vascular Bed. It is very important that blood not clot within the vascular system. In the baseline state, vascular endothelial cells provide a nonthrombogenic interface with the circulating blood. Endothelial cells do not normally express molecules that support platelet adhesion or promote activation and activity of the coagulation proteins. In addition, the antithrombotic features of the endothelial surface go beyond simply being "inert" with respect to coagulation. The endothelium also expresses molecules that actively downregulate the coagulation reactions on its surface: principally thrombomodulin to localize activated protein C (APC) to the endothelial surface and heparan sulfates to localize antithrombin (AT) to the endothelial surface. A further discussion of these mechanisms is presented in the section on thrombosis. These properties are critical to preventing coagulation from being initiated at inappropriate sites within the vasculature and preventing appropriately initiated hemostatic reactions from spreading within the vascular tree.

Extravascular Tissues. When an injury disrupts a blood vessel, it allows blood to contact extravascular cells and matrix. Extracellular matrix proteins—such as collagen, fibronectin, thrombospondin, and laminin—interact with adhesive receptors on blood platelets and support formation of the initial platelet plug at the site of injury, referred to as *primary hemostasis*. Perivascular tissues also express significant levels of tissue factor (TF).[1,2] Exposure of TF to blood initiates the process of thrombin generation on the surfaces of adherent platelets and ultimately leads to stabilization of the initial platelet plug in a fibrin clot, referred to as *secondary hemostasis*. Different tissues express different complements of matrix components and procoagulants. Thus, the local tissue environment plays a role in determining the intensity of the procoagulant response to an injury.

Platelets. Membrane receptors for collagen (glycoprotein [GP] VI) and other subendothelial and extravascular matrix proteins are present on the platelet membrane and mediate binding of unactivated platelets at sites of injury.[3–5] Platelet binding is also mediated by von Willebrand factor (vWF) bridging between collagen and the platelet receptor GP Ib. These receptor-binding events also transmit an activation signal to the platelets. Full platelet activation also requires stimulation by thrombin that is produced as the coagulation reactions are initiated. The platelet surface receptor for fibrinogen, GPIIb/IIIa, rapidly changes conformation from an inactive to an active form on platelet activation.[6] This conformational change allows platelet aggregates to be stabilized by binding to fibrinogen even before conversion to fibrin begins.

Platelet activation also initiates the synthesis of prostaglandins and thromboxanes—compounds that modulate platelet activation and promote vasoconstriction.[7] Platelet adhesion and activation at a site of injury, in concert with local vasoconstriction, provides initial hemostasis for small-caliber vessels. Once hemostasis is achieved by these mechanisms, the subsequent stabilization of the platelet plug in a fibrin meshwork can proceed more effectively than if bleeding continues. Initial hemostasis may be established even if a deficiency of plasma coagulation proteins is present. The platelet plug is insufficient, however, to provide long-term hemostasis and delayed rebleeding occurs if it is not reinforced by a stable fibrin clot during secondary hemostasis. Even after overt bleeding (loss of red blood cells) is stopped by the stable fibrin clot, leakage of plasma proteins from the microvasculature continues. A hemostatic clot structure with a densely packed core of platelets is required to form a tight vascular seal that minimizes the leakage of plasma proteins at a site of injury.[8]

It is becoming clear that, in addition to providing primary hemostasis following an overt injury, platelets also play more complex and subtle roles in maintaining vascular integrity. It has long been known that platelets maintain endothelial integrity in the microvasculature.[9] A failure of this function is responsible for petechiae resulting from thrombocytopenia. However, platelets also directly prevent microvascular bleeding at sites of inflammation[10] and angiogenesis[11] by mechanisms that are independent of fibrin generation.[12]

Coagulation Proteins. Adequate levels and function of each of a series of procoagulant proteins are required for hemostasis. The coagulation proteins can be organized into several groups based on their structural features.

The vitamin K–dependent factors include factors II (prothrombin), VII, IX, and X. These each have a structural domain in which several glutamic acid residues are posttranslationally modified to gamma carboxy-glutamic acid (Gla) residues by a vitamin K–dependent carboxylase.[13] The vitamin K cofactor is oxidized from a quinone to an epoxide in the process. A vitamin K epoxide reductase then cycles the vitamin K back to the quinone form to allow carboxylation of additional glutamic acid residues. The negatively charged Gla residues bind calcium ions. These binding interactions hold the Gla-containing proteins in their active conformation. The calcium-bound form of the Gla domain is responsible for mediating binding of the coagulation factors to phospholipid membranes. Lipids with negatively charged head groups, particularly phosphatidylserine, are required for binding and activity of the Gla-containing factors.

The carboxylation process is inhibited by the anticoagulant warfarin, which competes with vitamin K for binding to the reductase.[14] This results in the production of undercarboxylated forms of the vitamin K–dependent proteins, which are nonfunctional. The vitamin K–dependent procoagulants are zymogens (inactive precursors) of serine proteases. Each is activated by cleavage of at least one peptide bond. The activated form is indicated by the letter "a." Factors VIIa, IXa, and Xa each require calcium ions, a suitable cell (phospholipid) membrane surface, and a protein cofactor for their activity in hemostasis.

Factor IIa (thrombin) is a little different from the activated forms of the other vitamin K–dependent factors. Its Gla domain is released from the protease domain during activation. Thus, it no longer binds directly to phospholipid membranes. It also does not require a cofactor to cleave fibrinogen and initiate fibrin assembly or to activate platelet receptors. IIa that escapes the vicinity of a hemostatic plug can bind to a cofactor on endothelial cell surfaces, that is, thrombomodulin.[15] After binding to thrombomodulin, IIa can no longer activate platelets or cleave fibrinogen. Instead, it triggers an antithrombotic pathway by activating protein C (PC) on the endothelial surface.

PC and protein S (PS) are also vitamin K–dependent factors. They do not act as procoagulants but rather as antithrombotics on endothelial surfaces.[16] PC is the zymogen of a protease, while PS has no enzymatic activity but serves as a cofactor for APC.

The APC/PS complex cleaves and inactivates FVa and FVIIIa, thus preventing propagation of thrombin generation on normal healthy endothelium.

Factors V and VIII are large structurally related glycoproteins that act as cofactors. They have no enzymatic activity of their own, but when activated by proteolytic cleavage dramatically enhance the proteolytic activity of factors Xa and IXa, respectively.

Factor VIII circulates in a noncovalent complex with vWF, which prolongs its half life in the circulation. The vWF-FVIII complex binds to the platelet surface primarily via GPIb as vWF mediates adhesion of platelets to collagen under high shear conditions. Cleavage and activation of FVIII releases it from vWF so that it can assemble into a complex with FIXa on the platelet surface, where it activates FX.

FV circulates in the plasma and is packaged in the alpha granules of platelets during their development from megakaryocytes.[17] It is released upon platelet activation in a partially activated form. Both plasma and platelet-derived FV can be fully activated by cleavage by FXa or IIa. The FVa then assembles into a complex with FXa on the platelet surface, where it activates prothrombin to IIa.

TF is also a cofactor but is structurally unrelated to any of the other coagulation factors. Instead, it is related to one class of cytokine receptors.[18] This lineage emphasizes the close evolutionary and physiologic links between the coagulation system and the other components of the host response to injury. Rather than circulating in the plasma, as do the other coagulation factors, TF is a transmembrane protein.[19] TF serves as the cellular receptor and cofactor for FVIIa. It is primarily expressed on cells outside the vascular space under normal conditions, though monocytes and endothelial cells can express TF in response to inflammatory cytokines. The FVIIa/TF complex can activate both FIX and FX and is the major initiator of hemostatic coagulation.[19]

Another group of related proteins are the *contact factors*: factors XI and XII and prekallekrein (PK) and high molecular weight kininogen (HMK). These proteins share the feature of binding to charged surfaces. The only one of this group that is needed for normal hemostasis is factor XI.[20] However, the other contact factors may play a role in thrombosis in some settings. FXI is a zymogen that can be activated to a protease by FXIIa but is likely activated primarily by thrombin during the hemostatic process.[21,22] FXIa, in turn, activates FIX.

Fibrinogen provides the key structural component of the hemostatic clot. Two small peptides, fibrinopeptides A and B, are cleaved from fibrinogen by thrombin; the resulting fibrin monomer polymerizes into a network of fibers. The fibrin polymer is then stabilized further when it is crosslinked by activated factor XIII. FXIIIa is a transglutaminase present in plasma and platelets that is activated by thrombin coincident with fibrin formation.[23]

Thrombin plays a key role in activating procoagulant and anticoagulant factors; it also has a key role in triggering formation of fibrin. In addition, thrombin has cytokine-like activities that bridge the transition between hemostasis, inflammatory/immune responses, and wound healing. Thrombin is truly a multifunctional molecule that impacts the host response to injury at many levels.

Even before the structure and function of the various factors were defined, their interactions had been studied during plasma clotting. In the 1960s, two groups proposed a "waterfall" or "cascade" model of the interactions of the coagulation factors leading to thrombin generation. These schemes were composed of a sequential series of steps in which activation of one clotting factor led to the activation of another, finally leading to a burst of thrombin generation.[24,25] At that time, each clotting factor was thought to exist as a proenzyme that was activated by proteolysis. The existence of cofactors without enzymatic activity was not recognized until later. The original models were subsequently modified as information about the coagulation factors accumulated and eventually evolved into the "Y-shaped" scheme shown in Fig. 8.1.

The cascade model shows distinct "intrinsic" and "extrinsic" pathways that are initiated by FXIIa and FVIIa/TF, respectively. The pathways converge on a common pathway at the level of the FXa/FVa (prothrombinase) complex.

This scheme was not proposed as a literal model of the hemostatic process in vivo; rather, it was derived from studies of plasma clotting in a test tube and was intended to represent the biochemical interactions of the procoagulant factors. In fact, the coagulation cascade reflects very well the process of plasma clotting, as in the PT and aPTT tests. However, the lack of any other clear and predictive concept of hemostasis has meant that, until recently, most physicians have also viewed the cascade as

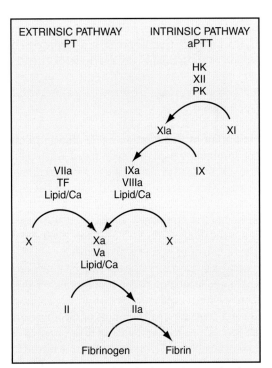

Fig. 8.1 The extrinsic and intrinsic pathways in the modern cascade model of coagulation. These two pathways are conceived as each leading to formation of the factor Xa/Va complex, which generates thrombin (IIa). *Lipid/Ca* indicates that the reaction requires a phospholipid surface and calcium ions. These pathways are assayed clinically using the prothrombin time (PT) and activated partial thromboplastin time (aPTT), respectively. *HK,* High-molecular-weight kininogen; *PK,* prekallikrein.

a model of physiology and the PT and aPTT as reflecting the risk of clinical bleeding.

The limitations of the coagulation cascade as a model of the hemostatic process in vivo are highlighted by certain clinical observations. Patients deficient in the initial components of the intrinsic pathway—FXII, high molecular weight kininogen, or PK—have a greatly prolonged aPTT but no bleeding tendency. Patients deficient in FXI also have a prolonged aPTT but usually have a mild to moderate bleeding tendency. Other components of the intrinsic pathway clearly have a critical role in hemostasis since patients deficient in factor VIII or IX have a serious bleeding tendency even though the extrinsic pathway is intact. Similarly, patients deficient in FVII also have a serious bleeding tendency even though the intrinsic pathway is intact. Thus, although the cascade model accurately reflects the protein interactions that lead to plasma clotting and is an essential guide to interpretation of PT and aPTT results, it is not an adequate model of hemostasis in vivo.

Process of Hemostasis

Having all the right ingredients is not enough to ensure an effective hemostatic process. Cellular interactions are crucial to directing and controlling hemostasis. Of course, normal hemostasis is not possible in the absence of platelets. In addition, TF is an integral membrane protein; thus, its activity is normally associated with cells, but platelets generally have little TF activity. Therefore interactions between at least these two types of cells are necessary. Because different cells express different levels of procoagulants and anticoagulants as well as have different complements of receptors, it is logical that simply representing the cells involved in coagulation as phospholipid vesicles overlooks the active role of cells in directing hemostasis. Hemostasis in vivo can be conceptualized as occurring in a stepwise process, regulated by cellular components.[26]

Step 1: Initiation of Coagulation on TF-Bearing Cells. The process of thrombin generation is initiated when TF-bearing cells are exposed to blood at a site of injury. TF is a transmembrane protein that acts as a receptor and cofactor for FVII. Once bound to TF, zymogen FVII is rapidly converted to FVIIa through mechanisms not yet completely understood but may involve FXa or noncoagulation proteases. The resulting FVIIa/TF complex catalyzes activation of FX and FIX. The factors Xa and IXa formed on TF-bearing cells have very distinct and separate functions in initiating blood coagulation.[27] The FXa formed on TF-bearing cells interacts with its cofactor, FVa, to form prothrombinase complexes and generate small amounts of thrombin on the TF cells (Fig. 8.2). The small amounts of FVa required for pro-thrombinase assembly on TF-bearing cells are activated by FXa,[28] by noncoagulation proteases produced by the cells,[29] or are released from platelets that adhere nearby. The activity of the FXa formed by the FVIIa/TF complex is largely restricted to the TF-bearing cell, because FXa that dissociates from the cell surface is rapidly inhibited by tissue factor pathway inhibitor (TFPI) or AT in the fluid phase.

In contrast to FXa, the FIXa activated by FVIIa/TF does not act on the TF-bearing cell and does not play a significant role

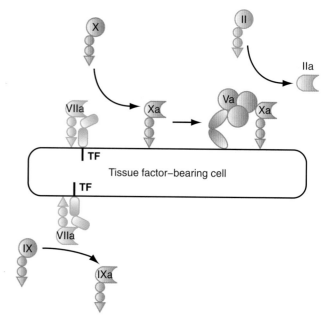

Fig. 8.2 The initiation step in a cell-based model of hemostasis. Initiation occurs on the tissue factor (TF)-bearing cell as activated FX combines with its cofactor, FVa, to activate small amounts of thrombin.

in the initiation phase of coagulation. FIXa can diffuse to adjacent platelet surfaces because it is not inhibited by TFPI and is inhibited much more slowly by AT than is FXa. FIXa can then bind to a specific platelet surface receptor,[30] interact with its cofactor, FVIIIa, and begin to activate FX directly on the platelet surface.

The small amount of thrombin produced on the TF-bearing cells is not sufficient to clot fibrinogen, but it is sufficient to initiate events that amplify the initial procoagulant signal and "prime" the clotting system for a subsequent burst of platelet surface thrombin generation. This thrombin is responsible for (1) activating platelets, (2) activating FV, (3) activating FVIII and dissociating FVIII from vWF, and (4) activating FXI.[31,32]

It is likely that most (extravascular) TF is bound to FVIIa even in the absence of an injury and that low levels of FIXa, FXa, and thrombin are produced on TF-bearing cells at all times. However, this process is kept separated from key components of hemostasis by an intact vessel wall. The very large components of the coagulation process are platelets and FVIII bound to multimeric vWF. These components normally only come in contact with the extravascular compartment when an injury disrupts the vessel wall. Platelets and FVIII-vWF then leave the vascular space and adhere to collagen and other matrix components at the site of injury.

Step 2: Amplification of the Procoagulant Signal by Thrombin Generated on the TF-Bearing Cell. Binding of platelets to collagen or via vWF during primary hemostasis leads to partial platelet activation. However, the coagulation process is most effectively initiated when enough thrombin is generated on or near the TF-bearing cells to trigger full activation of platelets. Thrombin diffuses through the fluid phase, binds to its receptor GPIb,[33] and cleaves its proteolytically activated receptors.[34] These

AMPLIFICATION

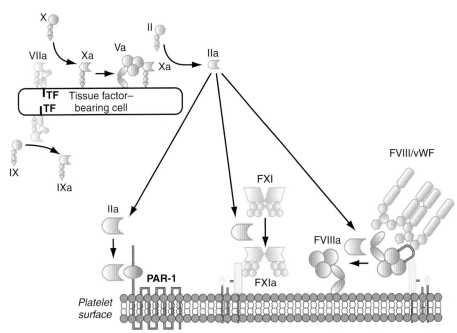

Fig. 8.3 The amplification step in a cell-based model of hemostasis. The small amount of thrombin generated on tissue factor (TF)-bearing cells amplifies the procoagulant response by diffusing to the platelet surface, where it activates platelets via the protease activated receptor-1 (PAR-1), activates FXI, and activates FVIII and releases it from its carrier molecule von Willbrand factor (vWF).

two receptor types synergize in mediating platelet activation. The small amounts of thrombin generated during the initiation step are also responsible for activation of coagulation factors XI and VIII on the platelet surface in the amplification step, as illustrated in Fig. 8.3.

Platelets not only plug the vascular defect at a site of injury but also provide the specialized membrane surface on which activation of many of the coagulation proteins takes place. Unactivated platelets express a very low level of phosphatidyl-serine, the primary procoagulant phospholipid, on their surfaces. Upon activation, phosphatidylserine is rapidly translocated from the inner to the outer leaflet of the platelet plasma membrane. It is then available to support binding and activity of the coagulation complexes.[35]

Platelet secretion of granule contents occurs somewhat more slowly after activation than does membrane surface changes. Dense and alpha-granules within the platelet cytoplasm contain numerous components that play a role in the coagulation process, such as partially activated FV, FVIII/vWF, FXIII, fibrinogen, protease inhibitors, and platelet agonists (adenosine diphosphate [ADP], epinephrine, and serotonin). Secretion of these platelet agonists further enhances platelet activation. Once platelets are activated, the cofactors Va and VIIIa are rapidly localized on the platelet surface.[36] FIXa formed by the FVIIa/TF complex can diffuse through the fluid phase, bind to the surface of activated platelets, and assemble into a complex with FVIIIa. FXI activated by thrombin on the platelet surface[32,37] can activate more FIX from the plasma to IXa. At the end of the amplification phase, the platelets accumulated at the injury site are

activated and have bound activated coagulation factors on their surfaces.

Step 3: Propagation of Thrombin Generation on the Platelet Surface. The multiple positive feedback mechanisms of the amplification phase rapidly lead to a burst of thrombin generation in the propagation phase, as illustrated in Fig. 8.4. The *tenase* (FIXa/FVIIIa) complexes progressively activate FX from the plasma to FXa on the platelet surface. FXa then associates with FVa to support a burst of thrombin generation of sufficient magnitude to produce a stable fibrin clot.

The large amount of thrombin generated on the platelet surface is responsible for stabilizing the hemostatic clot in more ways than just promoting fibrin polymerization. In fact, most of the thrombin generated during the hemostatic process is produced after the initial fibrin clot is formed. The platelet-produced thrombin also stabilizes the clot by (1) activating FXIII,[38] (2) activating the thrombin-activated fibrinolysis inhibitor (TAFI),[39] (3) cleaving the platelet PAR-4 receptor,[40] and (4) being incorporated into the structure of the clot. Activated FXIII covalently crosslinks the fibrin strands and increases resistance to plasmin degradation. TAFI also increases resistance to fibrinolysis by cleaving off lysines from the fibrin strands that serve as sites for fibrinolytic enzyme binding. Activation of platelet PAR-4 receptors promotes clot contraction. The force generated by platelets is considerable. Red blood cells trapped within the crosslinked fibrin network are compressed into a tightly packed array that contributes to the impermeable barrier needed for effective hemostasis.[41] Clot contraction also pulls together the edges of

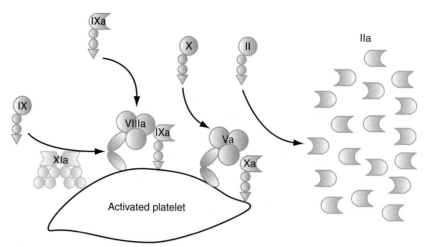

Fig. 8.4 The propagation step in a cell-based model of hemostasis. The activated coagulation factors bound to the platelet surface during the amplification phase progressively activate FX and II from the plasma, resulting in a large burst of thrombin production.

a wound and facilitates tissue repair. Excess thrombin produced during the hemostatic process can remain bound within the fibrin polymer and retains its proteolytic activity. Thus, it can rapidly activate more platelets and clot more fibrinogen if the hemostatic plug is disrupted and bleeding recommences.

The role of FXI in hemostasis has been a point of some controversy since even severe FXI deficiency does not result in a hemorrhagic tendency as severe as that in severe FVIII or IX deficiency. This can be explained if FXI is viewed as a booster of thrombin generation. FXI is not essential for platelet-surface thrombin generation, as are FIX and FVIII. Rather, FXIa activates additional FIXa on the platelet surface to supplement FIXa/FVIIIa complex formation and enhance platelet surface FXa and thrombin generation. Thus, its deficiency does not compromise hemostasis to as great an extent as FIX or FVIII deficiency.

Our knowledge of the platelet contribution to thrombin generation continues to evolve. There is evidence that there are multiple types of activated platelets. Platelets with the highest procoagulant activity are produced when they are stimulated with both thrombin and collagen; these have been referred to as COAT (*co*llagen *a*nd *t*hrombin stimulated) platelets.[42] These platelets have enhanced thrombin-generating ability due to enhanced binding of both tenase and prothrombinase components.[43,44] The in vivo relevance of the COAT platelet phenomenon is unclear, but it may be that the greatest procoagulant activity is generated on platelets that have bound to collagen matrix and also have been exposed to thrombin. When exposed collagen is covered by a platelet/fibrin layer, additional platelets that accumulate are not activated to the COAT state—tending to damp down the procoagulant signal once the area of the wound has been walled off by a hemostatic clot.[45]

Even though each phase of the cell-based model of hemostasis has been depicted as a discrete step, these phases should be viewed as an overlapping continuum of events. For example, thrombin produced on the platelet surface early in the propagation phase may initially cleave substrates on the platelet surface and continue to amplify the procoagulant response in addition to leaving the platelet and promoting fibrin assembly.

The cell-based model of hemostasis shows us that the extrinsic and intrinsic pathways are not redundant. We can consider the extrinsic pathway to consist of the FVIIa/TF complex, working with the FXa/Va complex and the intrinsic pathway to consist of FXIa working with the complexes of factors VIIIa/IXa and factors Xa/Va. The extrinsic pathway operates on the TF-bearing cell to produce small amounts of thrombin that initiate the coagulation process and amplify the initial procoagulant signal. By contrast, the intrinsic pathway operates on activated platelet surfaces to produce the large burst of thrombin that leads to formation and stabilization of the fibrin clot.

REGULATORY MECHANISMS TO CONTROL COAGULATION

Although the inability to provide effective hemostasis is a serious problem, the inability to limit coagulation to sites of hemostasis is at least as great a problem. Therefore, multiple biochemical and cellular regulatory mechanisms have evolved to limit and localize coagulation reactions. Coagulation reactions do not cascade unimpeded into a torrent of thrombin production but must instead overcome a series of regulatory barriers.

Plasma Protease Inhibitors

Several circulating protease inhibitors can inactivate one or more of the coagulation proteases. The coagulation proteases are relatively protected from inhibition while bound to a membrane surface. Proteases that escape into the fluid phase are subject to inhibition, however. Thus, the presence of inhibitors does not prevent activation and activity of coagulation but tends to confine the coagulation proteases to act on the cell surfaces on which they were activated.

AT plays a particularly important role in regulating hemostasis. AT is a serine protease inhibitor (serpin) that can inhibit most of the procoagulant factors, including IIa, VIIa, IXa, Xa, and XIa. The effectiveness of AT is increased by binding to heparinoids on the endothelial surfaces as well as by exogenous heparins.

Both hereditary and acquired deficiencies of AT lead to a significant thrombotic tendency.[46]

TFPI is also an important control mechanism. This molecule is a multifunctional Kunitz-type inhibitor.[47] One of its Kunitz domains inhibits FXa. Once it has bound FXa, another Kunitz domain can bind FVIIa in the FVIIa/TF complex. Thus, TFPI can assist in localizing FXa to the cell surface on which it was activated as well as limiting the activity of the TF pathway. Recently, it was determined that PS (see following section of endothelial antithrombotic mechanisms) serves as an important cofactor for TFPI, enhancing its affinity for FXa dramatically.[48]

Not only are the plasma protease inhibitors key players in confining a clot to the proper location but they also impose a threshold effect on activation of coagulation.[49] Thus in the presence of inhibitors, coagulation does not proceed unless procoagulant factors are generated in sufficient amounts to overcome the effects of inhibitors. If the triggering event is not sufficiently strong, the system returns to baseline rather than continuing through the coagulation process. Under pathologic conditions, the trigger for clotting may be strong enough to overwhelm the control mechanisms and lead to disseminated intravascular coagulation or thrombosis.

Endothelial Antithrombotic Mechanisms

Once a fibrin/platelet clot is formed over an area of injury, the clotting process must be terminated to avoid thrombotic occlusion in adjacent normal areas of the vasculature. If the coagulation mechanism is not controlled, clotting could extend throughout the vascular tree after even a modest procoagulant stimulus.

Endothelial cells play a major role in confining the coagulation reactions to a site of injury. Conversely, endothelial damage or dysfunction can play a major role in promoting thrombosis. Endothelial cells have several types of anticoagulant/antithrombotic activities (Fig. 8.5). The PC/PS/thrombomodulin (TM) system is activated in response to thrombin generation.[50] Some of the

thrombin formed during hemostasis can diffuse away or be swept downstream from a site of injury. When thrombin reaches an intact endothelial cell, it binds to TM on its surface. The thrombin/TM complex then activates PC, which is localized to the endothelial surface by binding to the endothelial PC receptor (EPCR). The APC can then move into a complex with its cofactor, PS, and inactivate any FVa or FVIIIa that has found its way to the endothelial cell membrane. This prevents the generation of additional thrombin in the intact vasculature. Endothelial cells also localize anticoagulant protease inhibitors to their surfaces. The protease inhibitor AT is bound to heparan sulfates expressed on the endothelial surface where it can inactivate proteases near the endothelium.[51] TFPI can also be bound to heparan sulfate or linked to the endothelial surface via a GPI anchor. Endothelial cells also inhibit platelet activation by releasing the inhibitors prostacyclin (PGI_2) and nitric oxide (NO), as well as degrading ADP by their membrane ecto-ADPase, CD39.[52]

Fibrinolysis

Even as the fibrin clot is being formed in the body, the fibrinolytic system is being initiated to disrupt it. The final effector of the fibrinolytic system is plasmin, which cleaves fibrin into soluble degradation products. Plasmin is produced from the inactive precursor plasminogen by the action of two plasminogen activators: urokinase-type plasminogen activator (uPA) and tissue-type plasminogen activator (tPA). The PAs, in turn, are regulated by plasminogen activator inhibitors (PAIs). Plasminogen is found at a much higher plasma concentration than the PAs. Therefore, the availability of the two PAs in the plasma generally determines the extent of plasmin formation. tPA release from endothelial cells is provoked by thrombin and venous occlusion.[53] tPA and plasminogen both bind to the evolving fibrin polymer. Once plasminogen is activated to plasmin, it cleaves fibrin at specific lysine and arginine residues, resulting in dissolution of the fibrin clot. The fibrinolytic system is crucial to removing an appropriate hemostatic clot as wound healing occurs. It is also essential to removing intravascular thrombi before significant tissue injury can occur. For example, the pulmonary vasculature can release large amounts of fibrinolytic enzymes to remove small thromboemboli that become lodged there.

Intravascular deposition of fibrin is also associated with the development of atherosclerosis. Therefore, an effective fibrinolytic system tends to protect against the chronic process of atherosclerotic vascular disease and the acute process of thrombosis. Conversely, defects of fibrinolysis increase the risk of atherothrombotic disease. For example, elevated levels of PAI-1, an inhibitor of fibrinolysis, are associated with an increased risk of atherosclerosis and thrombosis,[54] as are decreased levels of plasminogen.[55] The effectiveness of hemostasis in vivo depends not only on the procoagulant reactions but also on the fibrinolytic process.

CLINICAL LABORATORY TESTING

The commonly used clinical coagulation tests do not reflect the complexity of hemostasis in vivo. This does not mean that the PT and aPTT are useless. Clinicians simply need to understand

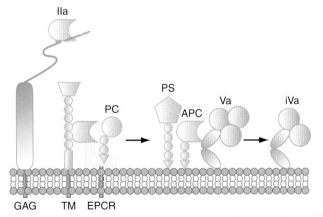

Fig. 8.5 Some antithrombotic mechanisms of the endothelial cell surface. Endothelial cells express glycosaminoglycan (GAG) molecules containing heparan sulfate to which thrombin and antithrombin can bind. They also express TM and the endothelial protein C receptor (EPCR) that localize components of the protein C (PC)/protein S (PS) system to the endothelial surface. *APC,* Activated protein C; *TM,* thrombomodulin.

what these tests can and cannot tell us. These screening coagulation tests are abnormal when there is a deficiency of one or more of the soluble coagulation factors. They do not predict the risk of clinical bleeding. Two patients with identical aPTT values can have drastically different risks of hemorrhage. All of the common coagulation tests—including the PT, aPTT, thrombin clotting time, fibrinogen levels, and coagulation factor levels—tell us something about the plasma level of soluble factors required for hemostasis. Their clinical implications must be evaluated by the ordering physician. Just because the PT and aPTT are within the normal range, it does not follow that the patient is at no risk for bleeding. Conversely, a mild elevation in these clotting times does not mean that the patient is at risk for bleeding after an invasive procedure.

The assessment of platelet function has become an issue of increasing importance in cardiac care. There is no doubt that platelets contribute substantially to acute and chronic vascular disorders. Individuals demonstrate substantial variability in platelet responses to agonists. A number of pharmacologic agents are now available to inhibit platelet function, and low platelet reactivity is associated with a reduction in atherothrombotic events in certain clinical settings. Conversely, low platelet responsiveness is associated with an increased risk of bleeding following cardiac surgery. Ideally, a test of platelet reactivity could be used to determine when a patient had achieved an adequate degree of platelet inhibition to optimally prevent future events, and to determine when platelet inhibition had been reversed sufficiently to minimize bleeding complications of an invasive procedure. At present, none of the commercially available platelet function testing systems has demonstrated sufficiently good predictive accuracy to recommend their routine use for assessment of platelet inhibition.

Many whole-blood coagulation tests are being presented as a means of evaluating overall hemostatic status in selected clinical settings. Although whole-blood tests have the advantage that they can reflect the contributions of platelets to the hemostatic process, they still do not reflect the contributions of TF-bearing cells and local tissue conditions. In addition, they suffer from the limitation that the reagents used to trigger initiation of coagulation are often not physiologic (such as kaolin). These tests of global hemostasis can be useful, especially when a rapid turnaround time is essential. They can be helpful is assessing whether a currently bleeding patient has a coagulopathy or an anatomic cause of bleeding. In summary, any laboratory test requires skilled interpretation and clinical correlation in evaluating the true risk of bleeding or thrombosis.

WHAT CAN GO WRONG WITH HEMOSTASIS?

Hemorrhage

Many patients who develop hemorrhage do not have a preexisting bleeding tendency. Bleeding following surgical or accidental trauma, or during a medical illness, is often associated with the development of an acquired coagulopathy. The hallmark of coagulopathy is microvascular bleeding: oozing from cut surfaces and minor sites of trauma, such as needle sticks. Microvascular bleeding can lead to massive blood loss. Causes of coagulopathic

bleeding include consumption of coagulation factors and platelets, excessive fibrinolysis, hypothermia, and acidosis.

Consumption of Coagulation Components. Disseminated intravascular coagulation (DIC) is the excessive consumption of coagulation factors, platelets, and inhibitors that occurs when the coagulation process is not properly localized to a site of injury. However, clotting factors and platelets can also be consumed during appropriate physiologic attempts at hemostasis. In this case, it is appropriate to replace the depleted factors with transfusion therapy.

DIC can be much more complicated to manage.[56] The mainstay of treatment is to treat the underlying disorder, such as sepsis. In early or mild/compensated DIC, administration of low-dose heparin may be considered to control the procoagulant response to inflammation, infection, or malignancy. In more severe or advanced DIC, replacement therapy may be necessary to attempt to manage the bleeding tendency associated with depletion of coagulation factors and platelets.

Excessive Fibrinolysis. The process of fibrinolysis is initiated as the fibrin clot assembles. Fibrin serves as the framework to which plasminogen binds and is activated to plasmin by tPA and uPA. Even when formation of a fibrin clot does not succeed at establishing hemostasis, a significant amount of fibrinolytic activity may still be generated and thwart subsequent efforts at hemostasis. Fibrinolytic inhibitors have proven to be useful in some circumstances.

Hypothermia. Many patients become hypothermic during medical illness or following surgical or accidental trauma.[57] Hypothermia can directly interfere with the hemostatic process by slowing the activity of the coagulation enzymes. Less well recognized is the finding that platelet adhesion and aggregation is impaired even in mild hypothermia.[58] Thus, in hypothermic coagulopathic patients, raising the core temperature can have a beneficial effect on bleeding by improving both platelet function and coagulation enzyme activity.

Acidosis. Acidosis can have an even more profound effect on the coagulation process than does hypothermia, though the two metabolic abnormalities often coexist. A drop in the pH from 7.4 to 7.2 reduces the activity of each of the coagulation proteases by more than half.[59] Thus acidosis should be considered as a possible contributor to coagulopathic bleeding in both medical and surgical patients.

Thrombosis

Disruption of the normal regulatory functions of any of the components of hemostasis can result in thrombosis. Generally, thrombosis is a multifactorial problem: congenital and acquired abnormalities in the antithrombotic activities of the vascular endothelium can synergize with enhanced platelet reactivity and alterations in procoagulant or anticoagulant levels to ultimately produce thrombosis. The risk of thrombosis in any given individual and any given time is a product of the individual's accumulated genetic, environmental, and lifestyle risk factors. Inflammation can trigger a number of responses that further predispose to thrombosis.[60] Coagulation and inflammatory responses interface at the levels of the tissue factor pathway, the PC/PS system, and the fibrinolytic system. Proinflammatory cytokines can affect all of these coagulation mechanisms. Coagulation proteases, anticoagulants, and fibrinolytic enzymes, in turn, can modulate inflammation by specific cell receptors. For example, inflammatory cytokines can promote an increase in tissue factor and a decrease in thrombomodulin by the endothelium.[61] Furthermore, activation of coagulation is closely linked with the progression of atherosclerotic vascular lesions. Progressively impaired vascular function then further predisposes to thrombosis. Ultimately, rupture of an unstable atherosclerotic plaque can expose procoagulant activity and provoke an acute thrombotic event.[62] Thus, management of cardiovascular disease often involves preventing and managing thrombosis and its consequences. Venous and arterial thrombosis tend to have different mechanisms and risk factors; thus, they are best managed by somewhat different strategies.

Venous Thrombosis. The major mechanism of venous thrombosis is related to inappropriate activation of the coagulation reactions, often on inflamed endothelium. Stasis can play an exacerbating role when activated factors are not rapidly diluted in flowing blood. Abnormalities of coagulation factors and increased levels of coagulation factors that potentially increase thrombin generation are linked to venous thrombosis.[63,64] The inherited hemostatic abnormalities most often associated with venous thromboembolism are factor V Leiden and factor II G20210A mutations, as well as deficiencies in AT, PC, and PS. Acquired abnormalities also play a major role. Major clinical risk factors for venous thromboembolism include malignancy, myeloproliferative disorders, trauma, surgery (especially orthopedic surgery), immobilization or paralysis, and prior venous thromboembolism. Minor risk factors include advanced age, obesity, bed rest, the use of hormone-replacement therapy or oral contraceptives, pregnancy and postpartum period, and inflammatory bowel disease.

Venous thrombosis is extremely common among hospitalized patients. While it is often asymptomatic, it is a significant cause of morbidity and of mortality from pulmonary embolism. The incidence of venous thrombosis can be reduced dramatically by the appropriate use of thromboprophylaxis with anticoagulants such as heparin and low-molecular-weight heparins.[65–67]

Arterial Thrombosis. Arterial thrombosis is primarily related to formation of platelet aggregates at sites of high shear and turbulent flow. As atherosclerotic plaques develop, they not only alter the nonthrombogenic nature of the endothelium but also disrupt normal laminar blood flow and produce increased turbulence. Although increased platelet reactivity can contribute to arterial thrombosis, vascular alterations play a key role in promoting platelet adhesion and activation.[68] There is also considerable evidence that TF-mediated activation of the coagulation system and thrombin generation can be important contributors to arterial thrombosis.[69] Thrombin generation at a site of plaque rupture can be the trigger for platelet activation and adhesion.[70]

The risk factors most closely linked to arterial thrombosis are smoking, hypertension, dyslipidemia, and diabetes. Inherited thrombophilia plays much less of a role in arterial than venous thrombosis.[71] Lifestyle changes can have a significant impact on the risk of arterial thrombosis. However, the most effective management is by therapies targeting platelet activation and adhesion. The results of recent studies indicate that, in addition to the efficacy of aspirin in reducing cardiac events in patients suffering from acute coronary syndromes, more potent antiplatelet and anticoagulant therapies are also valuable in high-risk patients.

What Happens After the Bleeding Stops?

Once hemostasis is completed, the process of wound healing can begin. Many of the activities involved in wound healing are influenced by thrombin. Thrombin plays a major role in platelet activation and degranulation. Several key cytokines modulating wound healing are released from activated platelets, including transforming growth factor beta (TGF-β), and platelet-derived growth factor (PDGF). Of course, the amount and rate of thrombin generated during hemostasis influences the initial structure of the fibrin clot, the framework on which cell migration takes place. In addition, thrombin has chemotactic and mitogenic activities for macrophages, fibroblasts, smooth muscle cells, and endothelial cells. Thus, generation of the appropriate amount of thrombin during the coagulation process may not only be essential for effective hemostasis but may set the stage for effective wound healing. Conversely, thrombin generation at sites of vascular injury plays a role in the development of local inflammatory changes and progression of atherosclerotic lesions.

The full reference list for this chapter is available at ExpertConsult.com.

PART III

Coronary Artery Disease

9

Diagnosis of Acute Myocardial Infarction

Matthew J. Chung, David L. Brown

Myocardial infarction (MI) describes the process of myocardial cell death caused by ischemia or the imbalance between myocardial oxygen supply via the coronary arteries and demand. In the United States each year, an estimated 1.1 million people experience an acute MI or die from coronary heart disease.[1] In 2016, it was estimated that approximately every 34 seconds one American would have a coronary event and about every 1 minute 24 seconds an individual would die from a coronary event.[1] According to the most recent World Health Organization report in 2015, coronary heart disease remains the leading cause of death worldwide. Hence the early recognition and diagnosis of acute MI is vital for the institution of therapy to limit myocardial damage, preserve cardiac function, and reduce mortality.

Acute coronary syndrome (ACS) refers to the constellation of clinical signs and symptoms caused by worsening myocardial ischemia. In the absence of myocardial damage, assessed by measuring cardiac biomarker levels, patients can be classified as having unstable angina. When myocardial damage is present, patients with ACS can be grouped into two major categories of acute MI: (1) patients with new ST segment elevation on the electrocardiogram (ECG) that is diagnostic of acute ST segment elevation myocardial infarction (STEMI), and (2) patients with non–ST segment elevation myocardial infarction (NSTEMI) who

have elevated cardiac biomarkers in an appropriate clinical setting, with or without ischemic ECG changes.[2]

Clinical trials have established the benefit of early reperfusion therapy in patients with STEMI and an early invasive strategy in patients with high-risk NSTEMI; thus a rapid and accurate assessment of patients with suspected acute MI is essential for optimal management.[2,3] This chapter describes the diagnostic modalities for the evaluation of patients with suspected acute MI.

HISTORY

There have been considerable advances in the detection of myocardial injury and necrosis in the last several decades; as a result, the definition of MI has evolved over time. Beginning in the 1950s, the World Health Organization used epidemiologic data to define acute MI as the presence of at least two of the following three criteria: (1) clinical symptoms suggestive of myocardial ischemia, (2) ECG abnormalities, or (3) elevation in serum markers indicative of myocardial necrosis.[4] Subsequently, the development of more sensitive and specific biomarkers and precise imaging techniques to detect subtle myocardial necrosis has led to further refinement of the diagnosis of MI. In 1999, a consensus conference convened by the European Society of Cardiology and the American College of Cardiology Foundation published the first universal definition of MI. With ongoing advances in the diagnosis and management of MI, this definition was updated in 2007 by a Global Task Force assembled from the European Society of Cardiology, the American College of Cardiology Foundation, the American Heart Association, and the World Heart Federation. Most recently, in 2012, the same groups assembled and published the third universal definition of MI with the goals of standardizing cardiac biomarker detection, the use of cardiac imaging in the evaluation of a patient with MI, and the classification of different types of MIs.[5]

DEFINITION OF MYOCARDIAL INFARCTION

MI is defined as myocardial necrosis caused by prolonged myocardial ischemia. The diagnosis of acute MI requires the rise and/or fall of cardiac biomarkers (preferably troponin) with at least one value exceeding the 99th percentile of a normal reference population (the upper reference limit) and at least one of the following: symptoms of ischemia, ECG changes indicative of active ischemia (new ST segment–T wave changes or new left bundle branch block [LBBB]) or infarction (new pathologic Q waves), identification of an intracoronary thrombus by angiography or autopsy, imaging evidence of a new regional wall motion abnormality, or new loss of viable myocardium.[5] The type of acute MI can be classified further depending on the etiology of the infarct (Table 9.1). Prior MI is defined as pathologic Q waves, regardless of symptoms, in the absence of nonischemic causes, pathologic findings of a healed or healing MI, or imaging evidence of a region of nonviable myocardium.

BIOCHEMICAL MARKERS OF ACUTE MYOCARDIAL INFARCTION

The ideal biochemical marker to detect an acute MI should be present in high concentration in the myocardium, absent in noncardiac tissue, released rapidly in a linear fashion after myocardial necrosis, and should remain present in the serum long enough to be easily detectable by an inexpensive and widely available assay. Table 9.2 summarizes serum cardiac markers. Cardiac biomarkers are an essential component of the criteria used to establish the diagnosis of acute MI. Cardiac troponins (I or T) have become the preferred biomarkers for the detection

of myocardial necrosis; their use is a class I indication in the diagnosis of MI.[5-7] The improved sensitivity and tissue specificity of cardiac troponins compared with creatine kinase MB (CK-MB) and other conventional cardiac biochemical markers of acute MI has been well established.[7,8] Troponins are not only useful for diagnostic implications but they also impart prognostic information and can assist in the risk stratification of patients presenting with suspected ACS.

In addition to the established biomarkers of myocardial necrosis, B-type natriuretic peptide (BNP) and C-reactive protein (CRP) are pathologically diverse biomarkers that could potentially enhance risk stratification in ACS. Additionally, several novel markers of myocardial ischemia and their usefulness during acute MI are currently being evaluated in clinical studies. However, to date, measurement of more than one specific biomarker of myocardial necrosis is unnecessary and not recommended for establishing the diagnosis of MI.[9] Furthermore, certain biomarkers should no longer be used in the evaluation of acute MI because of poor specificity secondary to their wide tissue distribution, including aspartate aminotransferase, total lactate dehydrogenase, and lactate dehydrogenase isoenzymes.[10]

TABLE 9.1 Universal Classification of Myocardial Infarction (MI)

Type	Description
1	Spontaneous MI resulting from an atherosclerotic plaque rupture, ulceration, fissuring, erosion, or dissection with resulting intraluminal thrombus
2	MI associated with ischemia due to an imbalance in myocardial oxygen supply and demand, such as in coronary endothelial dysfunction, coronary artery spasm, coronary embolism, anemia, arrhythmias, hypertension, or hypotension
3	MI resulting in cardiac death, with symptoms suggestive of myocardial ischemia, accompanied by new ischemic electrocardiogram changes, but death occurring before blood samples could be obtained, or at a time before the appearance of cardiac biomarkers in the blood
4a	MI associated with percutaneous coronary intervention
4b	MI associated with stent thrombosis as documented by angiography or autopsy
5	MI associated with coronary artery bypass graft surgery

Modified and adapted from Thygesen K, Alpert JS, Jaffe AS, et al. Third universal definition of myocardial infarction. *J Am Coll Cardiol.* 2012;60:1581–1598.

TABLE 9.2 Biochemical Markers of Myocardial Necrosis

Marker	Initial Appearance (h)	Mean Time to Peak	Return to Basal	Sampling Schedule
Myoglobin	1–4	6–7 h	12–24 h	Initially, then every 1–2 h
CK MB (tissue isoform)	2 6	18 h	48–72 h	Initially, then every 3–6 h
Cardiac troponin I	3–6	24 h	7–10 days	Initially, then every 3–6 h
Cardiac troponin T	3–6	12–48 h	10–14 days	Initially, then every 3–6 h
CK	3–12	24 h	72–96 h	Initially, then every 8 h
Lactate dehydrogenase (LDH)	10	48–72 h	10–14 days	Once at least 24 h after chest pain

Modified from Adams J, Abendschein DR, Jaffe AS. Biochemical markers of myocardial injury: is MB creatine kinase the choice for the 1990's? *Circulation.* 1993;88:750–763.

CK-MB, MB isoenzyme of creatine kinase (CK).

Detectable increases in cardiac biomarkers are indicative of myocardial injury. However, cardiac biomarker elevations are not synonymous with acute MI. Many disease states, such as sepsis, congestive heart failure, pulmonary embolism, myocarditis, intracranial hemorrhage, stroke, and renal failure can be associated with an increase in cardiac biomarkers. These elevations arise from mechanisms other than thrombotic coronary artery occlusion and require treatment of the underlying cause rather than the administration of antithrombotic and antiplatelet agents.[11,12] Acute MI should be diagnosed when cardiac biomarkers are abnormal and the clinical setting is consistent with myocardial ischemia.

Troponin

Cardiac troponins are regulatory proteins that control the calcium-mediated interaction of actin and myosin, which results in contraction and relaxation in striated muscle. The troponin complex comprises three subunits: troponin C, which binds calcium; troponin I, which inhibits actin-myosin interactions; and troponin T, which attaches the troponin complex by binding to tropomyosin and facilitates contraction. Troponin C is expressed by cells in cardiac and skeletal muscle; in contrast, the amino acid sequences of troponins I and T are unique to cardiac muscle. This difference has allowed for the development of rapid, quantitative assays to detect elevations of cardiac troponins in the serum. Troponin is the preferred biomarker for use in the diagnosis of acute MI because of superior tissue specificity and sensitivity for MI and its usefulness as a prognostic indicator.

Diagnosis. Troponin is released early in the course of acute MI. An increased concentration of cardiac troponin is defined as exceeding the 99th percentile of a normal reference population. Troponin exceeding this limit on at least one occasion in the setting of clinical myocardial ischemia is indicative of an acute MI.[5] Elevated troponin can be detected within 3 to 4 hours after the onset of myocardial injury.[12] Serum levels can remain increased for 7 to 10 days for troponin I and 10 to 14 days for troponin T (Fig. 9.1).[13]

The initial release of troponin is from the cellular cytosol, whereas the persistent elevation is a result of the slower dispersion of troponin from degrading cardiac myofilaments.[14] As a result of these kinetics, the sensitivity of troponin increases with time. At 60 minutes after the onset of acute MI, the sensitivity is approximately 90%, but maximal sensitivity of troponin (≈99%) is not achieved until 6 or more hours after the initiation of myocardial necrosis.[12] Blood samples for the measurement of troponin levels are recommended to be drawn at presentation and 6 to 9 hours later to optimize the clinical sensitivity for ruling in acute MI and the specificity for ruling out acute MI.[7]

The sensitivity and specificity of cardiac troponins is approximately 95% and 90%, respectively, with serial testing up to 12 hours after arrival at the hospital.[15] As a result of its high tissue specificity, cardiac troponin is associated with fewer false-positive results in the setting of concomitant skeletal muscle injury compared with CK-MB. This inherent characteristic of troponin is useful in the assessment of myocardial injury in patients with chronic muscle diseases, perioperative MIs, and after electrical

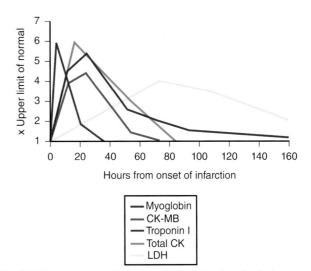

Fig. 9.1 Time course of biochemical marker levels during acute myocardial infarction. The relative timing and extent of the increase above normal values of the commonly used serum markers during acute myocardial infarction are shown. *CK,* Creatine kinase; *CK-MB,* creatine kinase MB isoenzyme; *LDH,* lactate dehydrogenase.

cardioversion or blunt cardiac trauma.[16–19] It is important to note that although cardiac troponin is highly tissue specific, its elevation does not indicate the mechanism of myocardial injury; if elevated troponins are found in the absence of myocardial ischemia, an evaluation for alternative etiologies of myocardial injury should be pursued.

More recently, there has been the ongoing development of high-sensitivity cardiac troponin assays, which are able to detect very low concentrations of cardiac troponins due to changes in how the assays are performed. High-sensitivity troponins are often abnormal earlier than conventional troponins in patients with acute MI. Because of this characteristic, high-sensitivity troponins can be used to safely and accurately rule out patients with suspected ACS more quickly than when using conventional troponins.[20] However, uncertainties about appropriate cut-off values for high-sensitivity troponins, difficulty in distinguishing between acute and chronic causes of high-sensitivity troponin elevations, and lack of clarity regarding the optimal duration of the rule-out period for acute MI have prevented the mainstream use of this assay in current practice.[21]

Thus, with the use of conventional troponin assays that do not reliably permit the very early (initial 1 to 2 hours) detection of myocardial necrosis, the diagnosis of acute MI in patients presenting within 6 hours of symptom onset must be based on the clinical scenario, ECG findings, and adjunctive imaging techniques. In the case of STEMI, reperfusion therapy should not be delayed by waiting for biomarkers confirmatory of myocardial injury.

Elevated troponins are not only vital to the diagnosis of NSTEMI but also serve to direct treatment by identifying patients who would benefit from an early invasive management strategy.[22] In the Treat Angina with Aggrastat and Determine Cost of Therapy with an Invasive or Conservative Strategy–Thrombolysis in Myocardial Infarction 18 (TACTICS–TIMI 18) study, patients with any increase in troponin who underwent early angiography (within 4 to 48 hours) and revascularization (if appropriate) achieved an approximately 55% reduction in the odds of death or MI compared with patients undergoing conservative management.[23]

Prognosis. In addition to the diagnostic value of troponin, cardiac troponins yield prognostic information. Prognosis is related partly to the extent of the increase in troponin in patients with an ischemic mechanism for myocardial injury.[24–26] Increased concentrations of troponin are associated with angiographic findings of greater lesion complexity, impaired blood flow in the culprit artery, and decreased coronary microvascular perfusion.[23]

Cardiac troponin has also been proven to be a potent independent predictor of recurrent ischemic events and the risk of death among patients presenting with ACS.[27] The Thrombolysis in Myocardial Ischemia Phase IIIB (TIMI IIIB) trial showed that in patients presenting with ACS, mortality was consistently higher among patients with elevated troponin I (>0.4 ng/mL) at the time of admission. Additionally, there were statistically significant increases in mortality with increasing levels of troponin I. Even after adjustment for baseline variables known to be significantly associated with an increased risk of cardiac events, elevated troponin I was independently associated with increased risk of mortality.[28] Additionally, the Global Use of Strategies to Open Occluded Coronary Arteries in Acute Coronary Syndromes (GUSTO-IIa) trial found that elevated troponin T (>0.1 ng/mL) was significantly predictive of 30-day mortality in patients with acute myocardial ischemia even after adjusting for ECG changes and CK-MB level.[29]

Risk Stratification. Measuring cardiac troponin is a class I recommendation for risk stratification in patients with ACS.[8] Patients presenting with clinical evidence of myocardial ischemia and elevated troponin, even at low levels, have worse outcomes than patients without evidence of abnormal troponin.[30] Peak troponin T levels after primary percutaneous coronary intervention (PCI) for STEMI are a good indicator of infarct size and an independent predictor of left ventricular function at 3 months and major adverse cardiac events at 1 year.[25]

Creatine Kinase MB

Creatine kinase (CK) is a cytosolic carrier protein for high-energy phosphates.[12] CK-MB is an isoenzyme of CK that is most abundant in the heart. However, CK-MB also constitutes 1% to 3% of the CK in skeletal muscle and is present in a small fraction in other organs, such as the small bowel, uterus, prostate, and diaphragm.[31] The specificity of CK-MB may be impaired in the setting of major injury to these organs, especially skeletal muscle.

Although cardiac troponin is the preferred marker of myocardial necrosis, CK-MB by mass assay is an acceptable alternative when cardiac troponin is unavailable.[7] The diagnostic limit for CK-MB is defined as the 99th percentile in a sex-specific reference control group.[5] All assays for CK-MB show a significant two-fold to three-fold higher 99th percentile limit for men compared with women. In addition, CK-MB can have two-fold to three-fold

higher concentrations in African Americans than whites. These discrepancies have been attributed to physiologic differences in muscle mass.[10] It is recommended that two consecutive measurements of CK-MB above the diagnostic limit in a rise-and-fall pattern be required for sufficient evidence of myocardial necrosis because of the inherent lower tissue specificity of CK-MB compared with troponin.[7]

The temporal increase of CK-MB is similar to that of troponin in that it occurs within 3 to 4 hours after the onset of myocardial injury, but in contrast to troponin, CK-MB decreases to the normal range by 48 to 72 hours (see Fig. 9.1). The rapid decline of CK-MB to the reference interval by 48 to 72 hours allows for the discrimination of early reinfarction when ischemic symptoms recur between 72 hours and 2 weeks after the index acute MI; during this time, troponin may still be elevated from the original event.[7] More recent data suggest, however, that serial troponin I levels can diagnose reinfarction if a second sample obtained 3 to 6 hours after a first sample when reinfarction is suspected increases by at least 20%.[5,32] Similar to troponin, the amount of CK-MB released is useful for estimation of infarct size, which correlates with left ventricular function, incidence of ventricular arrhythmias, and prognosis.[13]

Myoglobin

Myoglobin is a ubiquitous, heme-related, low-molecular-weight protein present in cardiac and skeletal muscle. In the setting of myocardial necrosis, myoglobin levels increase rapidly and are detectable within the first 1 to 4 hours. Elevations persist for 12 to 24 hours before being excreted by the kidneys. Myoglobin has a high sensitivity and a high negative predictive value for myocardial cell death, making it an attractive tool for the early exclusion of acute MI.[7] Myoglobin is not specific for myocardial necrosis, however, especially in the presence of skeletal muscle injury and renal insufficiency.[13]

A prospective study assessing the use of myoglobin in the early evaluation of acute chest pain revealed that an elevated myoglobin level was 100% sensitive for diagnosis of acute MI at 2 hours; the negative predictive value was also 100% with serial testing but the specificity was low, limiting the clinical usefulness of myoglobin in the evaluation of acute MI.[33] When myoglobin was directly compared with troponin in the early detection of coronary ischemia, using the 99th percentile of troponin I as a cutoff (0.07 µg/L), the cumulative sensitivity of troponin was higher.[34] A multimarker strategy including troponin and myoglobin has not been shown to yield a superior overall diagnostic performance compared with troponin alone; hence, routine measurement of myoglobin is not recommended.[34]

Adjunctive Biomarkers

Two emerging biomarkers that may be useful adjuncts in the diagnosis and prognosis of acute MI are the natriuretic peptides and inflammatory markers. BNP, a counter-regulatory peptide, and its propeptide, NT-proBNP, are released from cardiac myocytes in response to cardiac stretch. After transmural infarction, the plasma concentrations of BNP increase rapidly and peak at approximately 24 hours.[7] The peak value of BNP has been found to be proportional to the size of the infarction.[35] In patients presenting with acute MI, elevated BNP and NT-proBNP levels have been shown to predict a higher risk of death and heart failure independent of other prognostic variables.[12]

Increased concentrations of inflammatory biomarkers are detectable in a substantial proportion of patients presenting with acute MI; however, the precise basis for this relationship has not been conclusively established. Studies have implicated inflammation as a contributor to plaque disruption in ACS.[36] CRP, an acute-phase reactant protein made in the liver, has been the focus of much clinical investigation. In a cohort study of patients with STEMI, patients with increased CRP were more likely to have complications of acute MI.[37] Similarly, several studies have revealed high-sensitivity CRP to be an independent predictor of short-term and long-term outcomes in patients with ACS.[7] At this time, there are no therapeutic strategies specific to CRP or BNP and NT-proBNP; however, these biomarkers, in conjunction with troponin, may be useful for risk assessment in patients with acute MI.

Novel Cardiac Markers

Several novel markers of myocardial ischemia, such as ischemia-modified albumin, heart-type fatty acid-binding protein (H-FABP), choline, copeptin, and cystatin C, are currently being investigated in the setting of acute MI.[12] Copeptin, part of the prohormone that is cleaved to produce arginine vasopressin, is among the most thoroughly investigated of these markers. Current understanding suggests that endogenous stress, such as myocardial ischemia, leads to arginine vasopressin and copeptin release, thus allowing detection of acute ischemia and MI early after symptom onset, when conventional troponin assays are still normal. Studies have shown that when used in conjunction with conventional troponin assays, copeptin significantly improves the diagnostic accuracy for MI and enables a more expedient rule-out for MI.[38,39] The pursuit of new markers is ongoing; which markers will become clinically useful depends on several factors, including clinical efficacy, assay availability, and cost-effectiveness.

CLINICAL EVALUATION

The evaluation of a patient presenting with acute MI should begin with a targeted history that ascertains the following: (1) characterization and duration of chest discomfort and any associated symptoms; (2) prior episodes of myocardial ischemia, MI, PCI, or coronary artery bypass surgery; (3) history of hypertension, hyperlipidemia, diabetes mellitus, tobacco use, cerebrovascular disease, and other cardiovascular risk factors; and (4) assessment of bleeding risk and contraindications to anticoagulation and reperfusion therapies.[40]

The classic description of acute MI consists of crushing, substernal chest pain or vice-like tightness with or without radiation to the left arm, neck, jaw, interscapular area or epigastrium. This presentation is associated with an estimated 24% probability of acute MI; the probability decreases to about 1% if the pain is positional or pleuritic in a patient without a prior history of coronary artery disease.[41] Alternatively, the chest pain may be described as burning like indigestion, or sharp and

stabbing, which are associated with a 23% and 5% probability of acute MI, respectively.[41] Patients may commonly deny pain but describe a sensation of chest discomfort.[40] The duration of the discomfort is usually prolonged, lasting more than 30 minutes, but may wax and wane or even remit completely. There may be associated vagal symptoms of nausea, vomiting, lightheadedness, and diaphoresis. The severity of chest pain, commonly graded on a scale of 1 to 10, is not useful in discriminating ischemia or infarction from other causes of pain and should be abandoned. The performance of different chest pain characteristics in diagnosing ACS is shown in Table 9.3.[42]

Elderly patients and women more commonly have atypical presentations that mimic abdominal pathology or a neurologic event (Table 9.4).[43] One-third of all MIs are unrecognized, especially in patients without prior history of MI, and about half of these unrecognized MIs are associated with atypical presentations.[44,45] Silent myocardial ischemia is defined as objective

TABLE 9.3 Performance of Chest Pain Characteristics in Diagnosing Acute Coronary Syndrome

Symptom	Sensitivity, % (95% CI)	Specificity, % (95% CI)	Positive Likelihood Ratio (95% CI)
Radiation to both arms	11 (8.3–15)	96 (95–96)	2.6 (1.8–3.7)
Pain similar to prior ischemia	47 (42–53)	79 (77–80)	2.2 (2.0–2.6)
Change in pattern over prior 24 hours	27 (23–32)	86 (85–88)	2.0 (1.6–2.5)
"Typical" chest pain	66 (58–74)	66 (49–83)	1.9 (0.94–2.9)
Worse with exertion	38–53	73–77	1.5–1.8
Radiation to neck or jaw	24 (15–36)	84 (76–90)	1.5 (1.3–1.8)
Recent episode of similar pain	55 (50–60)	56 (54–59)	1.3 (1.1–1.4)
Radiation to left arm	40 (28–54)	69 (61–76)	1.3 (1.2–1.4)
Radiation to right arm	5.4 (3.4–8.3)	96 (95–97)	1.3 (0.78–2.1)
Associated diaphoresis	24–28	79–82	1.3–1.4
Associated dyspnea	45 (42–49)	61 (59–63)	1.2 (1.1–1.3)
Abrupt onset	76 (71–80)	32 (30–34)	1.1 (1.0–1.2)
Any improvement with nitroglycerin	71 (23–95)	35 (44–86)	(0.93–1.3)
"Typical" radiation	25–32	69–96	1.0–5.7
Burning pain	12–16	84–92	1.0–1.4
Associated nausea/vomiting	21–22	77–80	0.92–1.1
Associated palpitations	6.0 (3.5–10)	91 (88–94)	0.71 (0.37–1.3)
Associated syncope	9.0 (6.4–12)	84 (82–85)	0.55 (0.39–0.76)
Pleuritic pain	18–36	78–93	0.35–0.61

Modified from Fanaroff AC, Rymer JA, Goldstein SA, et al. Does this patient with chest pain have acute coronary syndrome? The rational clinical examination systematic review. *JAMA.* 2015;314:1955-1965. *CI,* Confidence interval.

TABLE 9.4   Atypical Symptoms of Myocardial Infarction in Elderly Patients

Symptom	PERCENTAGE OF PATIENTS WITH SYMPTOMS		
	Age 65–74 y	Age 75–84 y	Age ≥85 y
Chest pain	77	60	37
Shortness of breath	40	43	43
Sweating	34	23	14
Syncope	3	18	18
Acute confusion	3	8	19
Stroke	2	7	7

Modified from Bayer AJ, Chadha JS, Farag RR, et al. Changing presentation of myocardial infarction with increasing old age. *J Am Geriatr Soc.* 1986;34:263–266.

documentation of myocardial ischemia in the absence of angina or anginal equivalents.[46] Diabetes and hypertension are known to be associated with silent ischemia and infarction. The prognosis of acute MI patients, whether symptomatic or asymptomatic, is similar.[44]

Response of chest pain to antacids, nitroglycerin, or analgesics can be misleading and should not be relied on. Nitroglycerin can reduce pain from esophageal spasm or pericarditis (by reducing heart size) and, conversely, pain from acute MI may not always respond well to nitroglycerin because the pain is due to infarction rather than ischemia. Studies suggest that esophageal stimulation can cause angina and reduce coronary blood flow in patients with coronary artery disease. However, this response is absent in patients with heart transplant, supporting the notion of a cardioesophageal reflex, which can complicate further the use of response to treatment as a diagnostic tool.[47]

Physical Examination

Although an uncomplicated acute MI has no pathognomonic physical signs, the physical examination is crucial in the early assessment of the complications of acute MI and in establishing a differential diagnosis for the chest pain. The general assessment may reveal a restless and distressed patient with or without confusion owing to poor cerebral perfusion. A clenched fist across the chest, known as Levine sign, may be observed. The patient may appear ashen, pale, or diaphoretic and may be cool and clammy to the touch. Tachycardia and hypertension indicate high sympathetic tone and are usually consistent with anterior MI. Bradycardia and hypotension signify high vagal tone and may be seen with inferior-posterior MI with or without right ventricular involvement. Hypotension could also be secondary to the development of cardiogenic shock or a result of medications, especially nitroglycerin, morphine sulfate, or beta-blockers. Visualization of elevated jugular venous pressure may indicate significant left or right ventricular dysfunction.

Auscultation for additional heart sounds, cardiac murmurs, and friction rubs is mandatory. A soft S_1 is heard with decreased left ventricular contractility and an S_4 gallop indicates decreased left ventricular compliance.[40] Killip and Kimball proposed a prognostic classification in 1967 that is still useful today for the

evaluation of patients with acute MI.[48] The classification scheme is based on the presence of a third heart sound (S_3) and rales on physical examination. Class I patients are without S_3 or rales, class II patients have rales over less than 50% of the lung fields with or without S_3, class III patients have pulmonary edema with rales covering greater than 50% of the lung fields, and class IV patients are in cardiogenic shock. Evidence of heart failure on physical examination correlates with greater than 25% of the myocardium being ischemic.[40] A systolic murmur should prompt an evaluation for complications of MI, such as mitral regurgitation from papillary muscle rupture or the formation of a ventricular septal defect, which may also be accompanied by a palpable precordial thrill in half of cases. The chest wall should be palpated to assess for its effect on chest pain. Significant worsening of chest pain with palpation using moderate pressure is a clue that supports a musculoskeletal etiology. All peripheral pulses should be evaluated and documented. The finding of asymmetric or absent pulses, especially in the presence of tearing chest pain with radiation to the back, may indicate the presence of aortic dissection as an alternative diagnosis.

Other causes of cardiac and noncardiac chest pain that may be differentiated by physical examination include pericarditis, pulmonary embolism, pneumothorax, peptic ulcer disease, and acute cholecystitis. The initial clinical evaluation and physical examination should be directed toward expeditiously identifying the most likely etiology of each patient's presentation. The rapid triage of patients with ACS is crucial for the institution of the most appropriate early reperfusion therapy.

Electrocardiogram

The ECG is paramount in the initial assessment of patients with ACS. On arrival to the emergency department, the recommended door-to-evaluation time, which includes performing and interpreting the ECG, is 10 minutes.[40] The 12-lead ECG in the emergency department is the lynchpin of the decision pathway. The ECG aids in the diagnosis of acute MI, suggests the distribution of the infarct-related artery, and estimates the amount of myocardium at risk.[5] The presence of ST segment elevation in two contiguous leads or a new LBBB identifies patients who benefit from early reperfusion therapy, either fibrinolytic therapy or primary PCI. In the absence of a bundle branch block, the more abnormal the ECG leads, the greater the amount of ischemic myocardium.

Initial performance measures for reperfusion therapy in patients with STEMI were based on time elapsed since initial arrival at a hospital. However, newer benchmarks use first medical contact (FMC), such as arrival of emergency medical services (EMS), as time zero, emphasizing the importance of early reperfusion, which is strongly associated with outcomes.[49–51] Guidelines recommend EMS transport directly to a PCI-capable hospital for primary PCI in patients with STEMI with an ideal FMC-to-device time of 90 minutes or less. For patients with STEMI that arrive at a non-PCI-capable hospital, immediate transfer to a PCI-capable hospital for primary PCI is recommended with a goal FMC-to-device time of 120 minutes or less. In the absence of contraindications, fibrinolytic therapy should be given to patients with STEMI at non-PCI-capable hospitals

TABLE 9.5 Performance of the Electrocardiogram in Diagnosing Acute Coronary Syndrome

Electrocardiogram Finding	Sensitivity, % (95% CI)	Specificity, % (95% CI)	Positive Likelihood Ratio (95% CI)
ST segment depression	25 (16–34)	95 (92–99)	5.3 (2.1–8.6)
Any T-wave inversion, ST segment depression or Q waves	32 (24–40)	91 (85–97)	3.6 (1.6–5.7)
T-wave inversion	24 (15–38)	87 (69–95)	1.8 (1.3–2.7)

CI, Confidence interval.

Modified from Fanaroff AC, Rymer JA, Goldstein SA, et al. Does this patient with chest pain have acute coronary syndrome? The rational clinical examination systematic review. *JAMA.* 2015;314:1955–1965.

when the anticipated FMC-to-device time with transfer to a PCI-capable hospital exceeds 120 minutes. Once the decision is made to give fibrinolytic therapy, this should be accomplished within 30 minutes of hospital arrival.[50]

New LBBB or anterior infarction are important predictors of mortality.[40] In patients being evaluated for ACS, ST segment depression has a specificity of 95% and a sensitivity of 25% for diagnosing ACS (Table 9.5).[42] Conversely, the probability of acute MI in patients with chest pain and an initially normal or nonspecific ECG is low, approximately 3%.[52] Comparison with a previous ECG (if available) is indispensable and may help to avoid unnecessary treatment in patients with an abnormal baseline ECG.[53] If the initial ECG is not diagnostic of STEMI, but the patient remains symptomatic, serial ECGs at 15- to 30-minute intervals should be performed to detect acute or evolving changes.[5]

The classic evolution of acute MI on ECG begins with an abnormal T wave that is often prolonged, peaked, or depressed. Most commonly, increased, hyperacute, symmetric T waves are seen in at least two contiguous leads during the early stages of ischemia.[5] This is followed by ST segment elevation in the leads facing the area of injury with ST segment depression in the reciprocal leads. Increased R wave amplitude and width in conjunction with S wave diminution are often seen in leads exhibiting ST segment elevation.[5] This evolution may conclude with the formation of Q waves. The time course of development of these changes varies but usually occurs in minutes to several hours. A more recent study revealed that among patients presenting within 6 hours of symptom onset of STEMI, the patients who exhibited Q waves on their baseline ECG had more advanced disease with worse clinical outcomes.[54] This study underscores the need for early recognition of symptoms compatible with acute MI not only by medical personnel but also in the community.

In patients with inferior STEMI, right-sided ECG leads should be obtained to screen for ST segment elevation suggestive of right ventricle infarction (class I indication).[40] Infarction of the right ventricle associated with inferior acute MI has important therapeutic and prognostic implications.[55] Right ventricle infarction is likely when the ST segment is elevated 1 mm or more in the right precordial leads from rV_4 to rV_6. This finding has a sensitivity of about 90% and a specificity of 100% for proximal right coronary artery occlusion.[56] Other changes reported to be associated with right ventricle infarction are (1) ST segment elevation isolated to lead V_1, (2) elevated ST segments in leads

V_1 to V_4, and (3) T wave inversion isolated to lead V_2.[56] The ECG changes of right ventricle infarction are usually transient, persist for hours, and then resolve within a day.

A normal ECG can be seen in 10% of cases of acute MI.[57] One explanation for this apparent discrepancy is that the infarction may occur in an electrocardiographically silent area, such as the posterior or lateral wall in the distribution of the left circumflex artery.[58] Acute posterior injury is suggested by marked ST segment depression in leads V_1 to V_3 in combination with dominant R waves (R/S ratio >1) and upright T waves. These ECG findings are neither sensitive nor specific for posterior infarction, however, and frequently are not evident on the initial ECG.[59] In the case of patients who present with clinical evidence of acute MI but have a nondiagnostic ECG, the latest American College of Cardiology/American Heart Association guidelines state that it is reasonable to obtain supplemental posterior ECG leads, V_7 through V_9, to assess for left circumflex occlusion (class IIa indication).[2] Several studies have shown that ST segment elevation in leads V_7 through V_9 assists in the early identification and treatment of patients who are having ischemic chest pain due to acute posterior wall infarction but do not display ST segment elevation on the standard 12-lead ECG.[55,58,59]

Several conditions can potentially confound the ECG diagnosis of acute MI or cause a pseudoinfarct pattern with Q waves or QS complexes in the absence of MI. These include preexcitation, obstructive or dilated cardiomyopathy, bundle branch block, left and right ventricular hypertrophy, myocarditis, cor pulmonale, and hyperkalemia.[5]

Bundle Branch Block Patterns and Acute Myocardial Infarction. The presence of LBBB or ventricular pacing can mask the ECG changes of acute MI. In the Global Utilization of Streptokinase and Tissue Plasminogen Activator for Occluded Coronary Arteries (GUSTO)-1 trial, LBBB was seen in about 0.5% and ventricular pacing in about 0.1% of patients with acute MIs.[60] Based on this finding, Sgarbossa[61] developed criteria to evaluate for MI in the presence of left ventricular conduction abnormalities (Table 9.6). These changes in the ST segment or T waves, although very specific, are not seen in a significant proportion of patients: other modalities, such as biomarkers and adjunctive imaging, may be required for diagnosis of acute MI.

The same criteria used to assess for acute MI in the presence of LBBB are also applicable to patients with endocardial ventricular pacemakers except for the T wave criteria. The most indicative finding of acute MI in the presence of ventricular

TABLE 9.6 **Sensitivity and Specificity of Electrocardiogram (ECG) Changes in Left Bundle Branch Block for Diagnosis of Acute Myocardial Infarction**

ECG Changes	Sensitivity (%)	Specificity (%)
ST segment elevation ≥1 mm concordant with QRS polarity	73	92
ST segment depression ≥1 mm in leads V₁, V₂, V₃	25	96
ST segment elevation ≥5 mm discordant with QRS polarity	31	92
Positive T waves in leads V₅ and V₆	26	92

Modified from Sgarbossa EB. Recent advances in the electrocardiographic diagnosis of myocardial infarction: left bundle branch block and pacing. *Pacing Clin Electrophysiol.* 1996;19:1370–1379.

pacing was ST segment elevation 5 mm or greater in the leads with predominantly negative QRS complexes.[61] In right bundle branch block, the initial pattern of ventricular activation is normal; hence, the classic pattern of acute MI on ECG is usually not altered.

Imaging Techniques

Noninvasive imaging can assist in the diagnosis and characterization of acute MI but should never delay reperfusion therapy in the acute setting. Commonly used imaging techniques in acute and chronic MI are echocardiography, radionuclide ventriculography, myocardial perfusion scintigraphy using single photon emission computed tomography (SPECT), and magnetic resonance imaging (MRI).[5] Imaging techniques are useful in the diagnosis of MI by virtue of their ability to detect myocardial viability and perfusion, either directly with radionuclide techniques or indirectly with echocardiography or MRI. In the appropriate clinical setting and in the absence of nonischemic causes, demonstration of a new loss of myocardial viability meets the criteria for MI.[5]

REINFARCTION

Reinfarction may be suspected when there are recurrent clinical signs or symptoms of myocardial ischemia lasting 20 minutes or longer within the first 28 days following an initial MI. The incidence of reinfarction is reported to be less than 20%.[32] In patients who show evidence of reinfarction, an immediate measurement of cardiac troponin is recommended, followed by a second sample 3 to 6 hours later. When the first sample is elevated, reinfarction is diagnosed if there is an increase of at least 20% in the second sample; if the first sample is normal, then the criteria for a new acute MI apply.[5] Traditionally, CK-MB has been used to assess for reinfarction. However, there is increasing evidence that troponin values yield similar information; hence, it remains the preferred cardiac biomarker for diagnosing reinfarction.[32] The ECG diagnosis of reinfarction should be considered when ST segment elevation greater than 0.1 mV recurs in a patient previously having a lesser degree of ST segment elevation or with the development of new Q waves in at least two contiguous leads.[5] The reelevation of the ST segments can also be seen in threatened myocardial rupture and acute pericarditis. Their presence should prompt an expeditious evaluation for the complications of acute MI.

CONCLUSION

The rapid recognition and diagnosis of acute MI is crucial for the early institution of therapy to restore perfusion, minimize myocardial damage, and preserve cardiac function. Abnormal cardiac biomarkers, particularly troponin, have become the hallmark of acute MI but must always be interpreted in the context of the clinical scenario and ECG.

Acknowledgment

We acknowledge the contributions of Drs. Melissa Daubert and Allen Jeremias, who were coauthors of this chapter in the previous edition.

The full reference list for this chapter is available at ExpertConsult.com.

10

Use of the Electrocardiogram in Acute Myocardial Infarction

Jason Matos, Roderick Tung, Peter Zimetbaum

INTRODUCTION

The term *electrocardiogram* was first coined by Einthoven at the Dutch Medical Meeting of 1893. In 1901, he successfully developed a new string galvanometer with very high sensitivity, which he used in his electrocardiograph. His device weighed 600 pounds (Fig. 10.1). Sir Edward Schafer of the University of Edinburgh was the first to buy a string galvanometer electrograph for clinical use in 1908. The first electrocardiogram (ECG) machine was introduced to the United States in 1909 by Dr. Alfred Cohn at Mt. Sinai Hospital, New York. In 1924, Einthoven was awarded the Nobel Prize in physiology and medicine for the invention of the electrocardiograph. By 1930, the importance of the ECG in differentiating cardiac from noncardiac chest pain was well recognized; in fact, some patterns were considered so characteristic that the ECG alone could be used to confirm the diagnosis of myocardial infarction (MI).[1] This chapter reviews the contemporary use of the ECG in the diagnosis of acute MI.

INFERIOR MYOCARDIAL INFARCTION

In 80% of cases, the culprit vessel in inferior MI is the right coronary artery. The left circumflex artery is the culprit vessel in all other cases, with the rare exception of a distally extending inferoapical "wraparound" left anterior descending artery, which is suggested when there is concomitant ST segment elevation in the precordial leads.[1] ST segment elevation in lead III that exceeds the magnitude of elevation in lead II with reciprocating ST segment depressions in I and aVL of greater than 1 mm strongly suggests the right coronary artery as the culprit over the circumflex artery. The ST segment vector is directed toward the right when the right coronary artery is involved, which accounts for the elevation in lead III greater than lead II (Fig. 10.2). The added findings of ECG evidence of right ventricle (RV) MI increases the specificity for the right coronary artery and localizes the occlusion to a proximal location.[2]

Conversely, the left circumflex artery is suggested when ST segment elevation in lead III is not greater than lead II and by the absence of ST segment depression in leads I and aV$_L$.[3–5] An isoelectric or depressed ST segment with a negative T wave in lead V$_{4R}$ is very specific but insensitive for proximal left circumflex artery occlusion.[6,7] ST segment depression in leads V$_1$ and V$_2$ has been reported to be specific for the left circumflex artery, although a dominant right coronary artery can produce similar findings. The presence of ST depression in leads V$_1$ and V$_2$ with a prominent R wave in lead V$_2$ can be nonspecific and can suggest involvement of the left ventricular posterior wall or concomitant disease in the left anterior descending artery. Performing an ECG with posterior leads (V$_7$–V$_9$) can show a primary posterior wall injury pattern with ST segment elevation. A localization schema for inferior MI is summarized in Table 10.1.

RIGHT VENTRICLE MYOCARDIAL INFARCTION

In the setting of inferior MI, right-sided precordial lead recordings are strongly indicated. The presence of RV involvement portends a worse prognosis and enables the clinician to identify a subgroup of inferior MI patients with a propensity toward hemodynamic instability and shock, leading to increased in-hospital mortality.[8] RV MI is always associated with a proximal occlusion of the right coronary artery before the takeoff of the right ventricular marginal branches. The most sensitive sign is 1 mm of ST segment elevation in lead V$_{4R}$.[9] This sign is not fully specific for RV MI, however, because ST segment elevation in lead V$_{4R}$ can be seen in acute pulmonary embolus, anteroseptal MI, and pericarditis. ST segment elevation in lead V$_1$ in association with elevation in leads II, III, and aV$_F$ is highly correlated with the presence of RV infarction.[2,10] Isolated RV infarction, although rare, can be easily confused with anterior wall infarction owing to the anterior location of the RV, with ST segment elevation manifest only in the early precordial leads (V$_1$–V$_3$).[11]

ANTERIOR MYOCARDIAL INFARCTION

In acute anterior MI, ST segment elevation is present in the precordial leads. The challenge in anterior wall MI lies in identifying the site of occlusion within the vessel in relation to the septal and diagonal branches. In very proximal left anterior descending artery occlusion, before the first septal and diagonal branches, the ST segment is elevated in leads V_1 to V_3 and aV_L, with ST segment depression in aV_F.[12,13] The ST segment deviation vector points toward the base of the heart and ST segment elevation can be seen in aV_R and aV_L. ST segment elevation exceeding 2.5 mm in V_1 is also highly correlated with occlusion proximal to the first septal perforator branch.[14] Acquired right bundle branch block with a Q wave is an insensitive, but extremely specific, marker of proximal occlusion of the left anterior descending artery because the septal perforators supply blood to the right bundle (Fig. 10.3). ST segment elevation in leads V_1 to V_3 with elevation in the inferior leads suggests occlusion distal to the origin of the first diagonal branch.[13] In addition, if the ST segment in aV_L is elevated, it suggests an occlusion distal to the septal branch but proximal to the diagonal branch. If the ST segment in aV_L is depressed, it suggests an occlusion distal to the diagonal branch but proximal to the septal branch.[15] In distal left anterior descending artery occlusions, ST segment elevation is seen in leads V_3 to V_6 and in the inferior leads. A localization schema for anterior MI is summarized in Table 10.2.

LEFT MAIN OCCLUSION

When the left main coronary artery is occluded, ischemia occurs in the left anterior descending artery and circumflex artery territories. This ischemia results in an ST segment deviation vector that points toward aV_R. ST segment elevation in aV_R and V_1 is frequently present and there is higher specificity for left

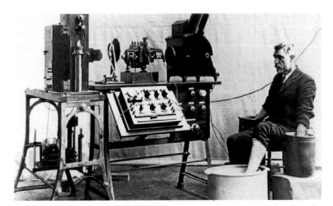

Fig. 10.1 Old string galvanometer electrocardiograph showing the big machine with the patient rinsing his extremities in the cylindrical electrodes filled with electrolyte solution.

TABLE 10.1	Inferior Myocardial Infarction: ST Segment Elevation II, III, aVF	
Right Coronary Artery	**Left Circumflex Coronary Artery**
ST segment elevation III > II	ST segment elevation II ≥ III
ST segment depression > 1 mm I, avL	ST segment elevation I, avL, V_5–V_6
ST segment elevation V_{4R} or V_1	ST segment depression V_{4R}

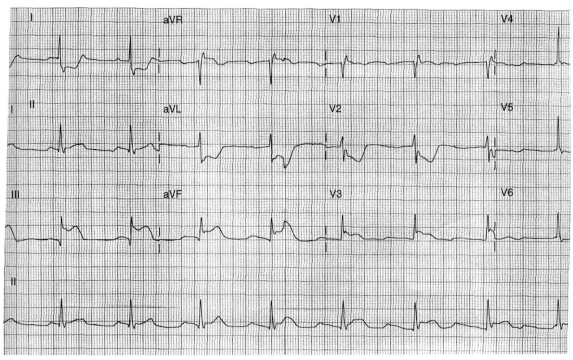

Fig. 10.2 Inferior ST elevation myocardial infarction. Elevation in lead III is greater than II and ST depressions in leads I and aVL indicate the right coronary artery as the culprit vessel. Note the posterior injury current and the presence of complete heart block. Elevation in aVR suggests concomitant right ventricular infarction due to occlusion proximal to the RV marginal branches.

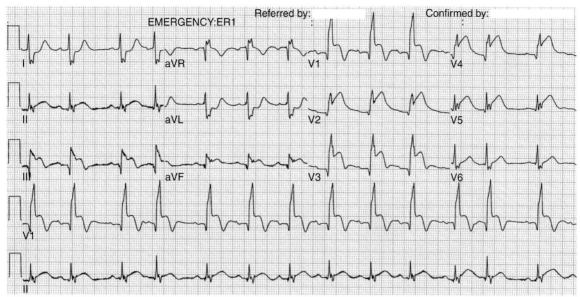

Fig. 10.3 Anterior ST elevation myocardial infarction. Occlusion of the proximal left anterior descending artery is indicated by the presence of diffuse precordial ST elevations and right bundle branch block pattern. There is elevation in the II, III, and aVF because the distal portion of the vessel wraps around the apex to supply the inferior wall.

TABLE 10.2 **Anterior Myocardial Infarction: ST Segment Elevation V_1–V_3**		
Left Main Artery	**Proximal Left Anterior Descending Artery**	**Distal Left Anterior Descending Artery**
ST segment elevation aVR > V_1	ST segment elevation V_1 (> 2.5 mm)	ST segment elevation II, III, avF
Global ST segment depressions	New right bundle branch block	
ST segment depression II, III, avF		

main occlusion when aV_R elevation is greater than V_1.[16] With the exception of aV_R and V_1, there is marked precordial and inferior ST segment depression, reflecting posterior and basal wall ischemia (Fig. 10.4).

DIAGNOSIS IN BUNDLE BRANCH BLOCK

Bundle branch block is present on the initial ECG in approximately 7% of patients presenting with acute MI.[17] Ischemia can be difficult to interpret in right and left bundle branch block because of the delayed depolarization and abnormal repolarization of the corresponding ventricle and its attendant secondary ST segment changes. In the setting of ST elevation MI, primary ST segment elevations in the precordium and new Q waves are fairly specific in the presence of right bundle branch block.

More challenging is the interpretation of acute MI in the setting of left bundle branch block, which also causes secondary ST segment repolarization changes. Because there is delay in the

left ventricular depolarization in native left bundle branch block or iatrogenic right ventricular pacing, Q waves cannot be used to diagnose infarction. Prominent notching greater than 50 ms in the QRS can indicate prior infarction, however. Two signs are extremely insensitive but have specificity approaching 85% for prior MI in the setting of left bundle branch block. The Cabrera sign refers to prominent notching in the ascending limb of the S wave in leads V_3 to V_5. A similar finding with prominent notching of the ascending limb of the R wave in lead I, aV_L, or V_6 is called the *Chapman sign*.[18,19]

Based on the Global Utilization of t-PA and Streptokinase for Occluded Coronary Arteries (GUSTO-I) trial, the Sgarbossa criteria[20] were proposed to improve specificity for diagnosis of acute MI in the setting of left bundle branch block. Primary ST segment elevation, 1 mm concordant with the major QRS vector, was given a score of 5, and discordant 5-mm ST segment elevations were assigned a score of 2. ST segment depressions greater than 1 mm in leads V_1 to V_3 were given a score of 3. A score of at least 3 was 90% specific for the diagnosis of MI. Discordant 5-mm ST segment elevations were the most specific in pacemaker-induced left bundle branch block.[21]

ABSENCE OF ST ELEVATIONS

Diagnosis of MI in the absence of ST elevations (non-ST elevation MI or NSTEMI) typically cannot be made with an ECG alone. It usually requires concurrent elevation of cardiac biomarkers, such as troponin. However, there are ECG findings that can heighten suspicion for a significant NSTEMI. Prior analysis of the Framingham and Fast Revascularization During Instability in Coronary Artery Disease (FRISC) II trial demonstrated a correlation between the number of leads with ST segment depression and coronary artery disease severity and prognosis.[22]

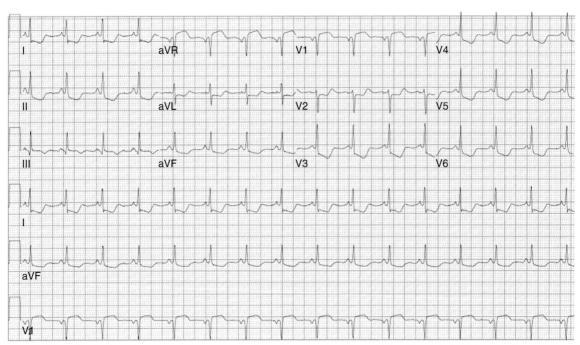

Fig. 10.4 Left main coronary artery occlusion. Elevation in aVR and VI, with global ST depressions.

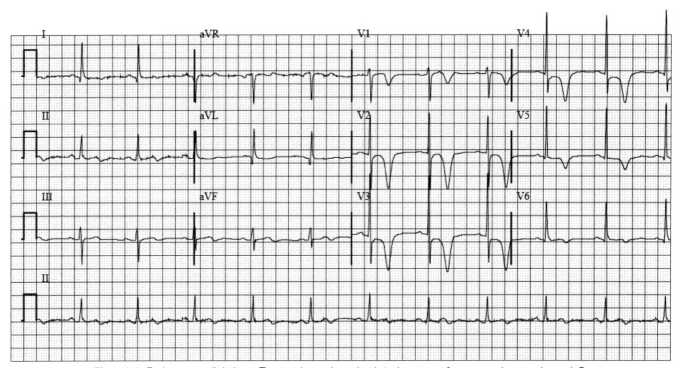

Fig. 10.5 Early precordial deep T-wave inversions in the absence of current chest pain and Q waves consistent with Wellens syndrome. This patient subsequently developed chest pain and anterior ST elevations and underwent percutaneous coronary intervention for a 95% left anterior descending artery lesion.

Aside from ST depressions, the presence of symmetric T wave inversions in early precordial leads—most commonly V_2 and V_3—can represent critical left anterior descencing (LAD) artery narrowing (Fig. 10.5). Also known as *Wellens syndrome*, this finding typically presents once chest pain has subsided and the significant LAD lesion reperfuses. Recognition of this pattern is key because early intervention could potentially limit the extent of an anterior wall MI.[15]

The full reference list for this chapter is available at ExpertConsult.com.

11

Reperfusion Therapies for Acute ST Elevation Myocardial Infarction

Harold L. Dauerman, Prospero B. Gogo Jr, Burton E. Sobel[†]

INTRODUCTION

Historical Perspective

Thrombosis was implicated as the cause of acute myocardial infarction (MI) almost a century ago. However, the pathophysiology remained obscure and, as recently as 44 years ago, many investigators believed that thrombosis was a secondary event. Chazov and Rentrop demonstrated that recanalization was achievable pharmacologically with favorable clinical consequences. Thus the concept of reperfusion therapy for acute ST elevation myocardial infarction (STEMI) was born by demonstrating that ischemic injury could be attenuated by restoration of myocardial perfusion.[1–3]

Underlying this concept was a hypothesis formulated by Dr. Eugene Braunwald: MI evolves dynamically, the magnitude of irreversible injury sustained is related to the duration of ischemia, and the clinical consequences of infarction are a reflection of the extent of irreversible injury sustained.[4] It was postulated that reduction of myocardial oxygen requirements, enhancement of myocardial perfusion, or both when implemented within the first few hours after the onset of myocardial ischemia would reduce the magnitude of irreversible injury sustained by the myocardium and improve prognosis. Thus reperfusion—first with pharmacologic agents and later with primary percutaneous coronary intervention (primary PCI)—was consistent with Braunwald's hypothesis, resulting in marked improvements in prognosis. Prior to the reperfusion era, hospital mortality from acute STEMI approached 25%[5]; with reperfusion therapy, the current STEMI mortality rates in the United States are less than 5%.[6–9]

Coronary Thrombosis and the Pathogenesis of Acute Myocardial Infarction

Although Herrick attributed fatal acute MI to a thrombotically occluded coronary artery in 1912, autopsy studies in the late 1970s did not demonstrate coronary thrombosis in patients who had died of acute MI. Thus coronary thrombosis was considered a consequence, rather than the underlying cause, of acute MI.[10,11] In 1980, DeWood and colleagues reported the results of coronary angiography performed early after the onset of acute transmural MI: within 4 hours of symptom onset, 87% of infarct-obstructed arteries were completely occluded. However, 12 to 24 hours after onset, the prevalence of coronary occlusion was only 65%. When patients with subtotal occlusion of the obstructed artery were included, the prevalence of angiographically demonstrable coronary thrombosis in the first 4 hours was 98%.[12] Over the past decade, further understanding of the pathology underlying acute

[†]Deceased.

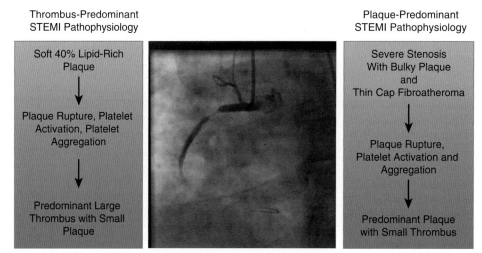

Fig. 11.1 The pathophysiology of acute ST elevation myocardial infarction requires thrombosis and occlusion of a coronary artery. Thrombosis is mediated by plaque rupture related to lipid pools, thin cap fibroatheroma, calcific nodules, and plaque erosion.

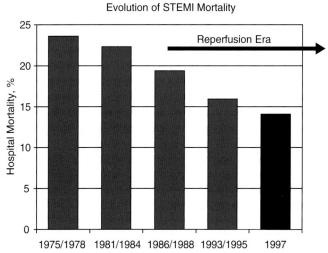

Fig. 11.2 Acute ST elevation myocardial infarction mortality occurred in 20% to 25% of patients in the hospital prior to the advent of coronary care units, arrhythmia management, and the reperfusion era. After the advent of the reperfusion era, a nearly 50% reduction in hospital mortality was observed. (Modified from Dauerman HL Lessard D, Yarzebski J, et al. Ten-year trends in the incidence, treatment, and outcome of Q-wave myocardial infarction. *Am J Cardiol.* 2000;86:730–35).

coronary occlusion has come from autopsy studies, angiography, and intracoronary imaging: underlying culprit soft lipid plaques, thin cap fibroatheromas, bulky plaques with characteristic erosion, and/or calcified nodules have all been found to predispose to plaque rupture and coronary occlusion[13–19] (Fig. 11.1). Efforts to reduce mortality have focused on both prevention of plaque rupture and rapid restoration of blood flow in thrombotically occluded coronary arteries.

This chapter addresses the developments in reperfusion therapy for STEMI responsible for a profound improvement in survival (Fig. 11.2).

THROMBOLYSIS AND REPERFUSION

Thrombolytic Agents: The First Pathway to Coronary Reperfusion

Coronary blood flow depends upon a complex balance between thrombosis, thrombolysis, and counterregulation by inhibition of both processes. From recent intravascular ultrasound and optical coherence tomography studies, we now know that underlying plaques prone to thrombosis are characterized by thin cap fibroatheromas (TCFA), lipid-rich cores, erosion of the intima, and calcified nodules[14,15,18]: the rupture of an underlying atherosclerotic plaque leads to thrombosis due to the procoagulant effects of exposed collagen, von Willebrand factor, and tissue factor in the vessel wall.[20,21] Activation of platelets accompanying the vascular injury accelerates ongoing thrombosis. Thrombin and fibrin generated by the coagulation cascade may undergo concomitant or subsequent lysis resulting from activation of the fibrinolytic system and conversion of the zymogen plasminogen to the active serine protease, plasmin, by the circulating plasminogen activators, tissue-type plasminogen activator (tPA) or urokinase plasminogen activator (uPA).[16,22] Any strategy designed to reduce myocardial damage must enhance the rapidity and extent of recanalization and promote sustained patency.

The available thrombolytic agents are plasminogen activators. These agents function as proteases that directly or indirectly hydrolyze a single peptide bond ($Arg^{561}Val^{562}$) on the inactive substrate molecule, plasminogen, to form the active serine protease enzyme, plasmin. Plasmin is responsible for the degradation of fibrin and diverse other proteins, with consequent dissolution of intravascular thrombi. First-generation agents (nonfibrin selective) include streptokinase and urokinase. Second- and subsequent-generation (fibrin-selective) agents include tPA, rPA, and molecular variants of tPA such as tenecteplase (TNK tPA). Agents that are relatively fibrin specific, such as tPA, produce less depletion of fibrinogen, less plasminemia, and less depletion of α_2-antiplasmin than that seen with nonfibrin-specific agents, such as streptokinase. The pathophysiology and development of fibrinolytic agents has been extensively reviewed by the original investigators.[3,22–29]

Streptokinase. Streptokinase (SK) is a protein present in numerous strains of hemolytic streptococci. The circulating half-life of SK is approximately 18 to 25 minutes. However, depletion of fibrinogen to less than 50% of baseline values persists for approximately 24 hours. Because of the foreign nature of the protein and the near-universal human exposure to the bacterial sources of the agent (β-hemolytic streptococci), administration of SK is complicated by inhibition of the administered drug by circulating immunoglobulin G (IgG) antibodies and problems of immunogenicity and attendant allergic reactions. Adverse reactions associated with SK (presumably attributable to plasmin-mediated activation of kininogen) limit clinical use of this agent. The overall incidence of hypotension ranges from 10% to 40%. Severe hypotension requiring pressor agents or fluids occurs in 5% to 10% of patients.[26,30–32] Other allergic reactions reported include fever, chills, urticaria, rash, flushing, and muscle pain. In the large-scale Second International Study of Infarct Survival (ISIS-2) and Global Utilization of Streptokinase and Tissue Plasminogen Activator for Occluded Coronary Arteries (GUSTO-I) trials, the incidence of minor allergic reactions was 4% to 6%.[33,34] Because of drawbacks in the use of streptokinase, it is no longer marketed in the United States. It is available internationally because of its low cost.

Tissue-Type Plasminogen Activator. tPA is an endogenous serine protease synthesized and secreted by human vascular endothelium and numerous other cells. The plasma half-life of tPA is 5 minutes, but fibrinolytic activity persists within clots for 7 hours. tPA is metabolized by the liver and inhibited in plasma by plasminogen activator inhibitor type 1 (PAI-1). An important advantage of tPA compared with SK is its affinity for fibrin-bound plasminogen. The relative fibrin specificity of tPA accounts for the more rapid clot lysis seen with tPA compared with SK. Unlike SK, tPA is not associated with immunogenicity.[28,29,35] tPA is available commercially as Alteplase. Neuhaus and coworkers introduced "front-loaded" dosing (i.e., 15 mg bolus with 50 mg given by infusion over the first 30 minutes, followed by 35 mg over the next 60 minutes). This regimen was associated with a 91% patency rate at 90 minutes, and it has now been approved by the US Food and Drug Administration (FDA).[36]

Tenectaplase and Reteplase. Third-generation agents were designed to modify the pharmacokinetics of tPA.[25] Modifications were designed to prolong the half-life, increase fibrinolytic activity, increase fibrin selectivity, or exhibit other potentially advantageous properties.[26] For example, Retavase lacks the kringle 1 domain, resulting in a prolonged half-life and thus facilitating bolus administration. However, early reocclusion necessitated a double-bolus dosing regimen. TNK tPA has three amino acid substitutions that differentiate it from wild-type tPA. They result in reduced inhibition of the plasminogen activator by PAI-1, prolongation of half-life as a result of decreased uptake by the reticuloendo-thelial system mediated by mannose receptors, and improved

efficacy following bolus injection. TNK tPA appears to induce reperfusion more rapidly than tPA in patients treated within 3 hours after onset of symptoms. The simplicity of the single-bolus dosing regimen without requiring a continuous infusion has made this the predominant fibrinolytic agent available.[23,24,37]

Magnitude and Timing

Fibrinolysis was initially evaluated using an invasive, intracoronary infusion methodology. Rentrop and colleagues, using intracoronary SK, demonstrated improved cardiac function and alleviation of chest pain accompanying recanalization compared with intracoronary nitroglycerin alone or conventional therapy.[38] The Western Washington randomized trial substantiated the efficacy of intracoronary SK in lysing coronary thrombi, with favorable effects on mortality.[6,8] However, constraints on the availability of immediate cardiac catheterization, time delays, increased costs, and risk limited enthusiasm for intracoronary administration as primary therapy for patients with acute MI.

Early patency trials employed angiographic endpoints to delineate patency 90 minutes after the administration of a thrombolytic agent. Patients with Thrombolysis in Myocardial Infarction (TIMI) 2 (slow) or TIMI 3 (normal) flow grades were considered together in delineating overall patency incidence. Even when no thrombolytic agent is given, patency rates range from 9% to 29% in the 0- to 90-minute interval.[33,39,40] Considerable "catch up" occurs (i.e., patency attributable to endogenous fibrinolysis), as judged from results of arteriography performed later. The magnitude of restoration of flow appears to be a major determinant of benefit.[41] Patients with delayed transit of contrast in the infarct-related artery (TIMI grade 2 flow) may not be exhibiting optimal or adequate recanalization. The Second Thrombolytic Trial of Eminase in Acute Myocardial Infarction (TEAM-2) study analyzed data with respect to flow in patients treated with nonfibrin-specific plasminogen activators. When TIMI flow grades were considered with respect to enzymatic and electrocardiographic markers of infarct size, no statistically significant difference was seen for TIMI flow grades 0, 1, or 2. However, better outcomes were seen with TIMI grade 3 flow. The GUSTO-I angiographic study confirmed this association between magnitude of flow restoration and outcomes.[34,37,42] Lack of patency (TIMI grade 0 or 1) was associated with the highest mortality rate (8.9%). Traditionally defined patency (TIMI grades 2 and 3) was associated with a lower mortality rate (5.7%, $P = .004$). The mortality for patients with TIMI grade 2 flow was 7.4% and numerically lower (4.4%) for those with TIMI grade 3 flow ($P = .08$). The GUSTO-I angiographic trial directly compared SK and tPA. Front-loaded tPA was associated with complete reperfusion at 90 minutes (TIMI grade 3) in 54% of patients. With SK, complete reperfusion occurred in fewer than 32% of patients. Patency trials have consistently shown more rapid and complete reperfusion with clot-selective agents.[23,28,37]

Fibrinolysis efficacy is not only related to magnitude of reperfusion but also to timing of administration.[40] Fresh clots lyse much more rapidly than older ones in which fibrin cross-linking has proceeded. Intervention within 30 to 60 minutes is likely to be particularly beneficial because more myocardium will remain viable and therefore amenable to salvage and because clot lysis will be much more rapid and complete. Accordingly, the rapidity with which patients are treated should be maximized. Current American Heart Association/American College of Cardiology (AHA/ACC) guidelines recommend the earliest possible application of therapy (within 30 minutes of emergency department arrival) with fibrinolysis for patients with STEMI (Class 1A recommendation).[1,43]

Pivotal Trials

Results of early placebo-controlled trials demonstrated consistent reduction of mortality despite differences among them with respect to entry criteria, thrombolytic agents, and adjunctive therapy. In 1986, the landmark Gruppo Italiano per lo Studio della Streptochinasi nell'Infarto Miocardico (GISSI-1) trial demonstrated a reduction in the overall 21-day mortality rate from 13% to 10.7% for 11,806 patients treated with intravenous SK rather than the usual treatment at that time. It documented a striking 47% reduction in mortality rates for patients treated with SK within 1 hour of symptom onset.[39]

The largest of all the early placebo-controlled trials was ISIS-2. It randomized 17,187 patients with acute MI to treatment with intravenous SK, oral aspirin, both, or neither. The 2×2 factorial design substantiated a reduction of mortality for patients treated with SK. Surprisingly, the effects of aspirin alone were comparable.[33] As in GISSI-1, maximal benefit was seen in patients treated early (<4 hours from symptom onset). Mortality reduction for patients treated in the interval from 12 to 24 hours after symptom onset was not significant. Time to treatment has been further evaluated in the Late Assessment of Thrombolytic Efficacy (LATE) study, in which 5711 patients presenting with acute MI that occurred 6 to 24 hours earlier were randomized to intravenous tPA or placebo. Treatment within 12 hours of symptom onset was associated with a 26% reduction of mortality for patients given tPA. In patients treated from 12 to 24 hours, no benefit was evident.[44] A meta-analysis of more than 50,000 patients has suggested that mortality can be reduced in patients treated up to, but not beyond, 12 hours.[32] The most compelling evidence indicates that the benefits of fibrinolytic induction of recanalization are minimal if it is not accomplished early, optimally within a few hours after onset of symptoms.

In 1992, the GISSI-2 trial reported no difference in the mortality rates of patients treated with intravenous SK compared with standard-dose tPA for 12,490 patients.[45] The lack of intravenous heparin and the late time to treatment appear to contribute to this phenomenon.[46] ISIS-3 compared SK with tPA and anisoylated plasminogen streptokinase activator complex (APSAC or anistreplase) in 41,299 patients. As in GISSI-2, ISIS-3 used subcutaneous heparin (in 50% of the patients) at a dose of 12,500 U begun 4 hours after enrollment. No difference in mortality could be ascribed to any of the strategies.[30,34] The need for administration of intravenous heparin with tPA has been underscored by results in the Heparin-Aspirin Reperfusion Trial (HART). A total of 205 patients with acute MI were randomized to treatment with tPA, aspirin, and intravenous heparin or tPA and aspirin alone. Even though 90-minute patency was the same (79%) with tPA with and without heparin, the patency rates between 7 and 24 hours in HART were 82% in the heparin group and only 52% in the aspirin group ($P < .0001$).[47] A high incidence of reocclusion occurred when heparin was omitted.[48] Analogous results were obtained by the European Cooperative Study Group.[46,49]

In light of these inconsistencies, the GUSTO-I trial was implemented to compare four different regimens in 41,021 patients: SK with subcutaneous heparin, SK with intravenous heparin, front-loaded tPA with intravenous heparin, and a combination of SK and tPA with intravenous heparin.[42] The 30-day mortality rate was lowest with front-loaded tPA and intravenous heparin (6.3%) and significantly less than that with combination therapy (7.0%), SK and subcutaneous heparin (7.2%), and SK and intravenous heparin (7.4%). Reduction of mortality directly depended on the rapidity and adequacy of recanalization.[41] Front-loaded tPA was associated with fewer allergic reactions, less hypotension, less overall bleeding, and a lower incidence of recurrent ischemia, reinfarction, and diverse cardiac complications than the other regimens. Overall front-loaded tPA led to more rapid and complete recanalization and an increase in the combined endpoint of survival without a stroke, equivalent to 10 lives saved per 1000 patients treated compared with either SK regimen.[34,40]

Adjunctive Therapy

The activation of circulating platelets and the blood coagulation system in patients with acute MI is a result of complex phenomena.[20] Administration of plasminogen activators paradoxically contributes to these reactions. Thrombin also activates platelets. Suppression of coagulation and platelet activation is necessary to accelerate coronary recanalization, optimize its extent, and prevent reocclusion.[21,50] One antiplatelet agent, aspirin, improved survival when used in conjunction with SK in the large ISIS-2 trial.[33] It is an established adjunctive agent that is usually given at an initial dose of 160 mg (chewable aspirin) as soon as possible when thrombolysis is planned, followed by daily doses of 81 to 325 mg.

Platelet activation is inhibited by aspirin through the blockade of cyclo-oxygenase and synthesis of thromboxane. Inhibition is incomplete, and other mechanisms can still activate platelets. In the Clopidogrel as Adjunctive Reperfusion Therapy (CLARITY)–Thrombolysis in Myocardial Infarction (TIMI) 28 trial, a 300-mg loading dose of clopidogrel was compared with placebo in patients treated with fibrinolytic drugs. Significantly more patients exhibited occlusion of the infarct-related artery at angiography or death in the placebo-treated patients (21.7%) compared with 15.0% in those treated with clopidogrel ($P = .01$). There was no difference in the incidence of mortality or the incidence of bleeding.[51] The second-generation $P2Y_{12}$ inhibitors (ticagrelor and prasugrel) have not been studied in combination with fibrinolytic therapy, but given their increased risks of bleeding in direct comparison to clopidogrel,[52,53] use of these antiplatelet therapies with fibrinolytic agents is not recommended.

In addition to preventing platelet activation, amelioration of thrombin activation is an important determinant of the success of fibrinolysis. Intravenous heparin is the most widely used agent for this purpose. The benefits of intravenous heparin (including low-molecular-weight heparin) in mechanistic trials are evident from the recanalization and patency rates delineated angiographically. In the GUSTO-I angiographic study, intravenous heparin induced greater early patency than subcutaneous heparin, even with the nonselective agent, SK.[41] Several studies have addressed the potential benefit of agents other than unfractionated heparin in combination with fibrinolytic drugs. The Assessment of the Safety and Efficacy of a New Thrombolytic Regimen (ASSENT)-3 PLUS trial studied 1639 patients after treatment with TNK plus enoxaparin compared with unfractionated heparin and demonstrated a trend toward superiority of enoxaparin ($P = .08$) but no difference in the combined endpoint of safety plus efficacy. There was a significant increase in intracranial hemorrhage (2.2% compared with 1%, $P = .047$) associated with administration of low-molecular-weight heparin, especially in elderly patients.[54,55] In the Enoxaparin and Thrombolysis Reperfusion for Acute Myocardial Infarction Treatment, TIMI Study 25, 20,479 patients were enrolled and treated with either TNK (80% of patients) or SK (20% of patients) combined with unfractionated heparin or enoxaparin. The combined endpoint of death or MI within 30 days was significantly lower with the low-molecular-weight heparin, enoxaparin (odds ratio, 0.83; 95% confidence interval [95% CI], 0.77–0.90). However, there was an increased incidence of bleeding with enoxaparin. Of note, in this study, enoxaparin dosage was reduced with respect to advanced age and other criteria, perhaps accounting, in part, for the favorable results.[56] Finally, the results of the Sixth Organization to Assess Strategies in Acute Ischemic Syndromes (OASIS-6) trial suggest that fondaparinux is a reasonable alternative as an adjunctive agent compared with unfractionated heparin for patients treated with thrombolytic drugs.[57]

Bleeding and the Elderly

Intracranial hemorrhage (ICH) is the major risk associated with the use of thrombolytic agents. With fibrinolytic drugs, stroke incidence is as high as 1.5%, with hemorrhagic stroke accounting for 0.3% to 0.7%. In the GUSTO-I trial, the risk of any stroke (including intracranial bleeding) was 1.55% for patients treated with front loaded tPA and intravenous heparin and 1.40% for patients treated with SK and intravenous heparin.[42] The difference in the total incidence of stroke seen with tPA and SK in the ISIS-3 trial was attributable largely to hemorrhagic rather than ischemic stroke (tPA, 0.7%; SK, 0.2%).[30] The imposition of stricter recruitment criteria and a lower total dose of tPA (Alteplase, 100 mg) in the TIMI trial resulted in a reduction of the hemorrhagic stroke rate to 0.6%.[32,58]

Although the relative risk reduction for death conferred by treatment with plasminogen activators is greatest in the elderly, an age greater than 65 years, weight less than 70 kg, and female gender correlate with an increased risk of ICH.[58] Elevated blood pressure is another risk factor, perhaps because prolonged, uncontrolled hypertension induces vasculopathy, rendering cerebral vessels susceptible to the adverse effects of thrombolytic agents. The risk of ICH increases with systolic blood pressures greater than 150 mm Hg and is particularly impressive in patients with systolic blood pressures exceeding 175 mm Hg. Consideration of these factors is needed to select specific treatment modalities prudently for individual patients.

BOX 11.1 Absolute and Relative Contraindications to Coronary Thrombolysis

Absolute Contraindications

Active internal bleeding
Suspected aortic dissection
Prolonged or traumatic cardiopulmonary resuscitation
Recent head trauma or known intracranial neoplasm
Diabetic hemorrhagic retinopathy or other hemorrhagic ophthalmic condition
Pregnancy
Previous allergic reaction to the thrombolytic agent (streptokinase or APSAC)
Recorded blood pressure >200/120 mm Hg
History of cerebrovascular accident known to be hemorrhagic

Relative Contraindications

Recent trauma or surgery > 2 weeks; trauma or surgery more recent than 2 weeks, which could be a source of rebleeding, is an absolute contraindication
History of chronic severe hypertension with or without drug therapy
Active peptic ulcer
History of cerebrovascular accident
Known bleeding diathesis or current use of anticoagulants
Significant liver dysfunction
Prior exposure to streptokinase or APSAC

Modified from Gunnar RM, Bourdillon PD, Dixon DW, et al. ACC/AHA guidelines for the early management of patients with acute myocardial infarction. A report of the American College of Cardiology/American Heart Association Task Force on Assessment of Diagnostic and Therapeutic Cardiovascular Procedures (subcommittee to develop guidelines for the early management of patients with acute myocardial infarction). *Circulation.* 1990;82:664–707.
APSAC, Anisoylated plasminogen streptokinase activator complex; *rtPA,* recombinant tissue-type plasminogen activator.

Selection criteria for fibrinolysis were developed by an ACC/AHA Task Force in 1990 (Box 11.1).[59] In contrast to the extensive list of absolute contraindications promulgated in GUSTO-I,[42] the only absolute criteria for exclusion were previous stroke, active bleeding, recent trauma, recent major surgery, and noncompressible vascular puncture sites. Patients with a systolic blood pressure of 180 mm Hg or higher that was unresponsive to therapy were considered to have a relative contraindication. Patients requiring cardiopulmonary resuscitation (CPR) of less than 10 minutes' duration do not appear to be at high risk for additional complications when treated with thrombolytic drugs. Clinical judgment, taking into account the extent of thoracic trauma and neurologic injury sustained, is more helpful than criteria based solely on the duration of CPR.

Treating physicians must rely on clinical acumen to best anticipate the risk/benefit ratio for an individual patient. For example, an 80-year-old woman with an acute inferior MI of 8 hours' duration and with an admitting blood pressure of 200/120 mm Hg would not likely be a good candidate for thrombolytic drugs. Conversely, a young diabetic patient with a large anterior infarction within 90 minutes of symptom onset is likely to be a good candidate.

In patients treated with thrombolytic drugs, bleeding complications need to be monitored and treated as needed. The thrombolytic, antiplatelet, and antithrombin agents should be discontinued, and reversal of heparin with protamine (1 mg per

100 U heparin) should be considered. If the patient has been treated recently with a thrombolytic agent and the concentration of fibrinogen levels is low or clotting factors depleted, administration of cryoprecipitate (10 U) or fresh frozen plasma (2 to 4 U) may be required. Aminocaproic acid (Amicar), an antifibrinolytic agent that competes with plasminogen for lysine binding sites on fibrin, should be reserved for patients with refractory bleeding unresponsive to other measures because it can precipitate thrombosis. If used, it should be given in a loading dose of 5 g intravenously, followed by 0.5 to 1.0 g/h until bleeding has stopped.[60]

PRIMARY PERCUTANEOUS CORONARY INTERVENTION

Primary Percutaneous Coronary Intervention for STEMI

Rationale and Feasability.   First-line therapy for STEMI in the late 1980s was coronary thrombolysis. Nevertheless, limitations of fibrinolysis alone were readily apparent: experience with fibrinolysis alone demonstrated that in approximately 15% of patients, recanalization fails completely and for 50% of patients, restoration of flow in the infarct-related artery is suboptimal. Last, in 10% of patients in whom recanalization is initially successful, reinfarction occurs.[61] However, in influential early TIMI trials in which strategies of PCI were performed with balloon angioplasty after thrombolysis, no clinical benefit was observed with either immediate or delayed PCI compared with conservative therapy.[62–65] In fact, immediate PCI led to a much higher incidence of bleeding and emergency coronary artery bypass graft surgery.

Given the discouraging early results of combined balloon angioplasty and fibrinolysis, several investigators explored the possibility that stand-alone balloon angioplasty would be a safe and effective alternative to stand-alone fibrinolysis for patients with STEMI. Early results by O'Neill and coworkers in comparisons of angioplasty to intracoronary streptokinase demonstrated that balloon angioplasty was superior in improving ventricular function and reducing residual stenosis in the setting of acute MI.[66] Over the next 15 years, multiple trials directly comparing stand-alone fibrinolysis to primary PCI were undertaken, eventually validating the utility of primary PCI and its superiority compared with thrombolysis in inducing more complete and more frequent recanalization of the infarct-related artery.

Key Clinical Trials.   In 1993, Primary Angioplasty in Myocardial Infarction (PAMI)—a multicenter, randomized trial that compared primary PCI with intravenous tPA in 395 patients—found no difference in the primary endpoint of posttreatment radionuclide left ventricular function, but demonstrated a trend of decreased hospital mortality with primary PCI (6.5% compared with 2.6%, $P = .06$), significantly decreased in-hospital and 6-month incidence of death and reinfarction, and a decreased incidence of ICH (0% compared with 2.0%).[67]

Despite the favorable results with PCI in this early trial, primary PCI was not widely adopted immediately as a treatment strategy

for patients with STEMI.[68] This was partly because of the substantial resources required for offering primary PCI around the clock and the relative scarcity of experienced operators able to perform emergency PCI in a high-risk setting. However, numerous studies comparing fibrinolytic therapy with primary PCI were performed throughout the later 1990s and early 2000s. The Global Use of Strategies to Open Occluded Coronary Arteries in Acute Coronary Syndromes (GUSTO-IIb) trial randomized 1138 patients to either primary PCI or fibrinolytic therapy with accelerated administration of tPA. With respect to the primary endpoint, a composite outcome of death, nonfatal MI, and disabling stroke at 30 days, primary PCI was found to be superior to fibrinolytic therapy.[69] However, the study did not demonstrate a reduction in mortality comparable to that seen in the earlier PAMI trial.

The mechanistic benefit of primary PCI as compared to fibrinolysis is clear: PCI restores TIMI grade 3 flow in more than 90% of infarct-related arteries, whereas TIMI grade 3 flow restoration is only approximately 50% to 60% after fibrinolysis. With the advent of stenting in 1993, the acute reocclusion rate fell to less than 5%, and the stent era ushered in increased use of PCI in general and potentiated the benefits of primary PCI.[70] Trials of primary PCI compared with thrombolysis were reviewed by Keeley et al. in 2003.[71] The authors evaluated 23 trials involving 7739 patients. Most patients (76%) randomized to the thrombolytic arms of these trials were treated with fibrin-specific thrombolytic agents. Primary PCI was superior with respect to short-term mortality (7% compared with 9%; $P = .0002$), reinfarction (3% compared with 7%; $P < .0001$), and stroke (1% compared with 2%; $P = .004$). With long-term follow-up, the benefits of primary PCI remained robust, with substantial reduction in mortality ($P = .0019$), nonfatal reinfarction ($P < .0001$), and recurrent ischemia ($P < .0001$). Adjunctive stenting in primary PCI was utilized in 12 of the 23 trials. The ACC/AHA guidelines in 2013 for the care of patients with STEMI list primary PCI as a class I recommendation with the highest level of supporting evidence when performed by experienced operators in a timely fashion.[1]

Adjunctive Therapy and Approach

Marked improvements in primary PCI over the past 2 decades have been a result of advancing technology (stents), pharmacology, and access approaches, as well as an emphasis on time to reperfusion (Fig. 11.3).[72] Stents, both bare metal and later drug eluting, have improved thrombus resolution and long-term outcomes after primary PCI.[73–75] Effective adjunctive medical therapy inhibits both the plasma protein-based coagulation system and the activation and aggregation of platelets. Adjunctive therapy for primary PCI has been a source of controversy for the past decade; the current ACC/AHA/European Society of Cardiology (ESC) guidelines have endorsed a broad number of effective options.[1,43] In addition, the approach to primary PCI was routinely via femoral access for the first 20 years of this reperfusion modality. Trials over the past 5 years have emphasized potential benefits of a radial artery access approach to limit bleeding and, potentially, mortality among patients undergoing primary PCI.[76–78] Changes in adjunctive therapy and approaches are summarized in the next section.

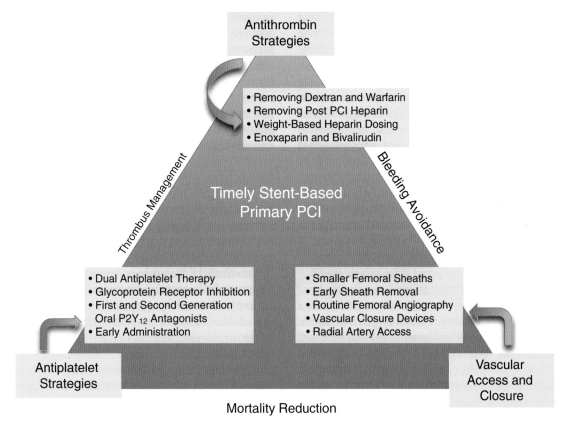

Fig. 11.3 Primary percutaneous coronary intervention has improved over the past 2 decades with active investigation in areas of stent technology, time to reperfusion, as well as adjunctive therapy and access methodology. (From Dauerman HL. Anticoagulation strategies for primary percutaneous coronary intervention: current controversies and recommendations. *Circ Cardiovasc Interv.* 2015;8.)

Oral Antiplatelet Agents: Aspirin, Clopidogrel, Prasugrel, and Ticagrelor. Aspirin is routinely utilized in primary PCI—there are no randomized trials comparing aspirin to placebo in this setting and aspirin is considered de facto therapy in all patients with STEMI unless they are known to be allergic. Results in multiple trials have established that platelet ADP receptor antagonism with $P2Y_{12}$ receptor inhibitors is beneficial in the setting of PCI; thus, a second oral antiplatelet therapy agent is uniformly prescribed at the time of primary PCI. Clopidogrel was the most commonly used $P2Y_{12}$ antagonist in primary PCI: clopidogrel is a prodrug that undergoes processing in the liver, yielding an active metabolite. Its effect on platelet inhibition may not occur for as long as 12 hours with a load of 300 mg. A 600-mg load has been shown to be more effective in rapidly inhibiting platelet aggregation. The Antiplatelet therapy for Reduction of MYocardial Damage during Angioplasty-Myocardial Infarction (ARMYDA-6 MI) trial compared standard (300 mg) versus high loading dose (600 mg) regimens of clopidogrel in the setting of primary PCI. ARMYDA-6 showed that the higher loading dose significantly reduced infarct size in a relatively small sample of 201 patients. Thus, patients who are to undergo primary PCI should probably be given a loading dose of 600 mg immediately (i.e., in the emergency department) and 75 mg daily thereafter.[79,80]

Similar to clopidogrel, prasugrel is a thienopyridine prodrug requiring conversion to an active metabolite by the hepatic cytochrome P-450 system, but prasugrel inhibits platelet activation more rapidly, more consistently, and to a greater extent. Prasugrel was compared to clopidogrel in patients presenting with acute coronary syndromes in the large multicenter Trial to Assess Improvement in Therapeutic Outcomes by Optimizing Platelet Inhibition with Prasugrel–Thrombolysis in Myocardial Infarction (TRITON-TIMI 38) trial.[52] Patients randomized to clopidogrel (300 mg oral load followed by 75 mg per day) had increased major adverse cardiovascular events, including stent thrombosis, compared to patients randomized to prasugrel, with a modest increase in the risk of bleeding. In subgroup analysis, patients who were elderly, had a prior history of cerebrovascular events, or were of low body weight did not derive a similar benefit from more aggressive platelet inhibition with prasugrel. The FDA has placed a warning urging caution regarding prasugrel treatment for elderly and low-body-weight patients and a strict contraindication for patients with prior stroke.

Unlike the other two inhibitors of the $P2Y_{12}$ platelet receptor, ticagrelor is a nonthienopyridine that does not require conversion into an active metabolite. Ticagrelor (180 mg loading dose followed by 90 mg twice per day) was compared to clopidogrel (300 mg or 600 mg loading dose followed by 75 mg per day) in the Platelet Inhibition and Patient Outcomes (PLATO) trial of patients with acute coronary syndrome.[53] The prespecified subgroup of patients ($n = 7544$) presenting for primary PCI for STEMI or new left bundle branch block had lower risks of major adverse cardiovascular events at 1 year of follow-up, with significant reductions in the risk of cardiovascular death and stent thrombosis. However, patients randomized to ticagrelor had higher risks of stroke and intracranial hemorrhage. Additionally, the benefit of ticagrelor appeared to be related to the dose of aspirin, resulting in a warning from the FDA recommending that patients taking ticagrelor receive less than 100 mg of aspirin daily. Although the ACC/AHA guidelines give all three oral P2Y$_{12}$ inhibitors equal (class 1B) recommendations for the treatment of patients with STEMI,[1] the ESC guidelines favor ticagrelor over clopidogrel due to the favorable outcomes in trials in direct comparison to clopidogrel.[43] In order to minimize decision time within the algorithm, we recommend the use of a ticagrelor loading dose for all patients being considered for primary PCI given its favorable risk profile among the oral P2Y$_{12}$ inhibitors. Whether or not prehospital loading of ticagrelor is superior to loading of the antiplatelet agent in the emergency room or catheterization laboratory is unclear based upon a single randomized clinical trial.[81,82]

Intravenous Antiplatelet Agents.

Abciximab is a chimeric antibody to the glycoprotein IIb/IIIa receptor that strongly and irreversibly binds to the receptor. In multiple trials comparing abciximab to heparin-alone strategies, patients given abciximab had higher pre-PCI infarct-related artery patency rates, better 6-month left ventricular ejection fraction, and less need for urgent target vessel revascularization. Other studies suggested broad-based benefits of abciximab in PCI, including improvements in microvascular function and selected mortality benefits, but more recent comparisons to bivalirudin/heparin/oral antiplatelet therapy show less clear benefit of routine abciximab in PCI for STEMI and a significant increase in bleeding complications.[70,83–88] Eptifibatide and tirofiban are two other commercially available intravenous glycoprotein IIb/IIIa inhibitors. Tirofiban/heparin has been recently compared to bivalirudin for primary PCI without clear evidence of benefit from tirofiban.[89] The 2013 ACC/AHA guidelines support selective use of any glycoprotein IIb/IIIa inhibitor (class IIA) in STEMI primarily in patients with inadequate loading of oral P2Y$_{12}$ inhibitors or in the setting of massive thrombus discovered during primary PCI as a bailout option.[1]

Cangrelor is an intravenously administered nonthienopyridine P2Y$_{12}$ receptor antagonist. It has a rapid onset/offset of action with a half-life in blood of 3 to 5 minutes. The Cangrelor versus Standard Therapy to Achieve Optimal Management of Platelet Inhibition (CHAMPION PHOENIX) trial randomized 10,939 patients to cangrelor versus placebo (clopidogrel 300–600 mg orally loaded 2 hours after PCI vs. cangrelor 2-hour infusion) with 1991 patients presenting with STEMI. While the overall trial results favor cangrelor across the spectrum of PCI, these results are limited by the control group: patients loaded prior to angiography with any P2Y$_{12}$ antagonists (i.e., ticagrelor or clopidogrel 600 mg) were excluded.[90] Furthermore, these results conflict with the negative results of CHAMPION PCI due to changes in protocol, definitions, or unknown factors.[91] For STEMI, the use of cangrelor may be similar to glycoprotein IIb/IIIa inhibitors in that it should be considered when there is inadequate loading of the oral P2Y$_{12}$ inhibitors at the time of PCI.

Antithrombins.

Bivalirudin, unfractionated heparin, fondaparinux, and enoxaparin are antithrombotic agents used during primary PCI. The features of these antithrombotic agents are summarized in Table 11.1 and have been examined in multiple clinical trials.[72,83,88,89,92–94] When used as adjunctive therapy in combination with glycoprotein IIb/IIIa inhibitors, unfractionated heparin should be given as a bolus in a weight-adjusted dose of 50 to 70 U/kg to target an activated clotting time of more than 200 seconds. The use of UFH alone is recommended by the ACC/AHA 2013 guidelines (class IC). Compared with unfractionated heparin, low-molecular-weight heparins are easier to administer because subcutaneous depot injections with weight-adjusted dosing is effective. The Acute STEMI Treated with Primary PCI and IV Enoxaparin or UFH to Lower Ischemic and Bleeding Events at Short- and Long-Term Follow-up (ATOLL) trial comparing unfractionated heparin and enoxaparin for primary PCI failed to demonstrate superiority of enoxaparin compared to unfractionated heparin.[92] Enoxaparin cannot be strongly recommended for primary PCI; the ESC/ACC/AHA guidelines either discourage or only cautiously recommend the use of low-molecular-weight heparins (Box 11.2).[1,43]

Bivalirudin is a bivalent direct thrombin inhibitor that is given intravenously, usually with a bolus load and continuous infusion. The Harmonizing Outcomes with RevascularIZatiON and Stents (HORIZONS) trial randomized 3602 patients with STEMI undergoing primary PCI to bivalirudin versus UFH and GP IIb/IIIa inhibitor comparators. Patients randomized to bivalirudin fared significantly better in the analysis for the primary endpoint, driven by significantly less bleeding at the expense of increased stent thrombosis.[88] These results were mostly replicated in the follow-up European Ambulance Acute Coronary Syndrome Angiography (EUROMAX) trial, except for the mortality endpoint.[83,95] On the other hand, more recent trials have failed to show any benefit of bivalirudin as compared to unfractionated heparin alone in the setting of primary PCI and again noted an increased risk of acute stent thrombosis with a bivalirudin-based regimen.[96,97]

Radial, Femoral, and Multivessel Primary PCI.

The evolution of primary PCI has involved marked changes in pharmacology, times to treatment, and, most recently, access site. These changes are summarized in Fig. 11.3. Recently, there have been multiple large clinical trials comparing radial versus femoral access in acute coronary syndromes, including primary PCI.[76,78,98] Radial access has been uniformly demonstrated to decrease access-site bleeding complications compared to the femoral approach. Agents and approaches that reduce bleeding complications have been associated with mortality reductions[99]; the radial versus femoral primary PCI trials have also suggested a reduction in death with the radial approach, presumably due to less bleeding complications.[76,78] The efficacy of radial access is linked to the volume of radial approaches performed at the institutions utilizing the approach[98]: for operators and sites that do have this expertise, though, there appears to be no harm and considerable potential benefit to routine use of radial access as a primary bleeding-avoidance strategy for primary PCI.

TABLE 11.1   Anticoagulation Options for Primary PCI

Anticoagulant	Mechanism of Action	Pharmacokinetics	Advantages	Disadvantages	Key Primary PCI Clinical Trials
Unfractionated heparin	Activation of antithrombin: indirect antithrombin	Half-life of ~60 min but depends upon bolus amount	Inexpensive and extensively studied Reversible Easily measurable anticoagulant effects	Heparin-induced thrombocytopenia (rare) Platelet activation Inactive against clot-bound thrombin Optimal dosing unclear	PAMI CADILLAC ADMIRAL HEAT ATOLL
Low-molecular-weight heparin: enoxaparin	Inhibition of Factor Xa and IIa 4:1 ratio of effect, predominantly acting on Factor Xa	Anti-Xa effects negligible after 8 hours	More reliable thrombin-inhibitory effect than heparin Partially reversible	Heparin-induced thrombocytopenia (rare) Difficult to measure anticoagulant effect	ATOLL
Fondaparinux	Indirect inhibitor of Factor Xa	Half-life of ~20 hours	Daily dosing	Heparin-induced thrombocytopenia (rare) Difficult to measure anticoagulant effect Catheter-related thrombosis	OASIS 6
Bivalirudin	Direct antithrombin	Half-life of 25 min	More reliable thrombin-inhibitory effect than heparin Does not activate platelets Short half-life No associated thrombocytopenia	Expensive Not reversible Short half-life Acute stent thrombosis risk	HORIZONS EUROMAX HEAT-PCI

Modified from Dauerman HL. Anticoagulation strategies for primary percutaneous coronary intervention: current controversies and recommendations. *Circ Cardiovasc Interv.* 2015;8.
ADMIRAL, Abciximab Before Direct Angioplasty and Stenting in Myocardial Infarction Regarding Acute and Long-Term Follow-up; *ATOLL,* Acute STEMI Treated with Primary PCI and IV Enoxaparin or UFH to Lower Ischemic and Bleeding Events at Short- and Long-Term Follow-up; *CADILLAC,* Controlled Abciximab and Device Investigation to Lower Late Angioplasty Complications; *EUROMAX,* European Ambulance Acute Coronary Syndrome Angiography; *HEAT-PCI,* How Effective Are Antithrombotic Therapies in Primary Percutaneous Coronary Intervention; *HORIZONS,* Harmonizing Outcomes with RevascularlZatiON and Stents; *OASIS-6,* Sixth Organization to Assess Strategies in Acute Ischemic Syndromes; *PAMI,* Primary Angioplasty in Myocardial Infarction.

BOX 11.2   European and US Recommendations for Anticoagulation in Primary PCI

UFH: Class I recommended, level of evidence C
- With GP IIb/IIIa receptor antagonist planned: 50–70 U/kg IV bolus to achieve therapeutic ACT
- With no GP IIb/IIIa receptor antagonist planned: 70–100 U/kg bolus to achieve therapeutic ACT

Bivalirudin: Class I recommended, level of evidence B
- 0.75 mg/kg IV bolus, then 1.75 mg/kg/h infusion with or without prior treatment with UFH. An additional bolus of 0.3 mg/kg can be given if needed
- Reduce infusion to 1 mg/kg/h with estimated CrCl <30 mL/min
- Preferred over UFH with GP IIb/IIIa receptor antagonist in patients at high risk of bleedingl class IIA, level of evidence B

Fondaparinux: not recommended as sole anticoagulant for primary PCI class III: not recommended, B

Enoxaparin: not mentioned; no recommendation level given

Bivalirudin: Class I recommended, level of evidence B
- With use of GP IIb/IIIa blocker, restricted to bailout
- Recommended over UFH and a GP IIb/IIIa blocker

- Bivalirudin 0.75 mg/kg IV bolus followed by IV infusion of 1.75 mg/kg/h for up to 4 hours after the procedure as clinically warranted. After cessation of the 1.75 mg/kg/h infusion, a reduced infusion dose of 0.25 mg/kg/h may be continued for 4–12 hours as clinically necessary

Enoxaparin: Class IIB, level of evidence B
- With or without routine GP IIb/IIIa blocker
- May be preferred over UFH
- Enoxaparin 0.5 mg/kg IV bolus

UFH: Class I recommended, level of evidence C
- With or without routine GP IIb/IIIa blocker
- Must be used in patients not receiving bivalirudin or enoxaparin
- UFH 70–100 U/kg IV bolus when no GP IIb/IIIa inhibitor is planned
- 50–60 U/kg IV bolus with GP IIb/IIIa inhibitors

Fondaparinux is not recommended for primary PCI; class III, level of evidence B.
ACT, Activated clotting time; *CrCl,* creatinine clearance; *GP,* glycoprotein; *IV,* intravenous; *PCI,* percutaneous coronary intervention; *UFH,* unfractionated heparin.

While early STEMI reperfusion strategies focused upon rapidity and completeness of culprit artery patency, many patients with STEMI have multivessel coronary artery disease: the role of nonculprit artery PCI is controversial and evolving. While the guidelines initially expressed caution and/or concern about risk of nonculprit artery PCI during STEMI,[1] more recent clinical trials suggest that complete revascularization may be attempted safely at the time of primary PCI.[100,101] Defining the efficacy and safety—along with the timing and method of nonculprit artery PCI—requires further investigation; larger randomized clinical trials are ongoing in this controversial area.[102,103]

Thrombectomy and Route of Drug Administration. The need to provide more complete coronary and microvascular reperfusion[104] spurred developments of newer fibrinolytic agents, primary PCI methodologies, and adjunctive antiplatelet/antithrombin agents. In addition, two other avenues have been pursued to improve primary PCI-based reperfusion—thrombectomy and intracoronary administration of glycoprotein IIb/IIIa inhibitors. The purpose of these two methods has not been to improve TIMI grade 3 coronary reperfusion but to decrease infarct size via decreased microvascular obstruction that occurs even in the setting of normal epicardial coronary flow. Six trials have addressed thrombectomy and intracoronary drug administration—smaller trials[105,106] have suggested beneficial effects for these methodologies. But, as shown in Fig. 11.4, these trials have since been superceded by much larger randomized clinical trials that have failed to show any clear benefit for these approaches.[107–110] Current guidelines do not support the routine use of either intracoronary drug administration or thrombectomy to aid reperfusion during primary PCI.[1,43]

PHARMACOINVASIVE THERAPY FOR STEMI

Current ACC/AHA guidelines recommend that primary PCI be performed when patients present with a goal of first medical contact to device time of 90 minutes and with the availability of skilled operators who perform more than 75 PCI procedures per year in a hospital that performs more than 36 PCI procedures for STEMI annually.[1] Fulfilling these requirements is not feasible in many US and worldwide hospitals: cost of PCI, transfer distance, transfer times, and lack of 24/7 PCI capability are among the issues that may limit universal adoption of primary PCI for STEMI in both the United States and globally.[111–115] Two options are available for patients presenting to non-PCI hospitals: rapid transfer systems and pharmacoinvasive therapy.

The available approaches for urgent treatment of STEMI—fibrinolytics and primary PCI—have often been described as competing strategies. Although numerous trials directly comparing the two have been performed over the last two decades, the two approaches are not mutually exclusive. In 2003, Dauerman and Sobel first outlined an approach called "pharmacoinvasive therapy" to describe a strategy that might combine the universal availability of fibrinolysis and the efficacy of PCI for patients that are not candidates for rapid performance of primary PCI.[116,117] As noted earlier, the two most significant factors determining infarct size and risk of mortality in patients with STEMI are the time to induction of patency of the infarct-related artery and the completeness of reperfusion.[6,41] Pharmacoinvasive therapy is designed to provide universal early reperfusion (fibrinolysis) as an initial step before routine postlytic PCI performed 3 to 24 hours after fibrinolysis.[118]

This strategy differs from two other terms: facilitated PCI and rescue PCI. Rescue is a strategy of emergent PCI after fibrinolysis if reperfusion fails (as defined by refractory chest pain and/or persistent ST elevations); evidence supporting the strategy of rescue PCI for patients after failed fibrinolytic reperfusion came from the Middlesbrough Early Revascularization to Limit Infarction (MERLIN) trial.[119] It included 307 patients randomized to conservative therapy, including repeat fibrinolysis, compared with immediate angiography with or without PCI. Although there was only a numerical trend favoring rescue PCI for the primary endpoint of 30-day mortality (9.8% compared with 11%; P = .70), rescue PCI was superior to conservative

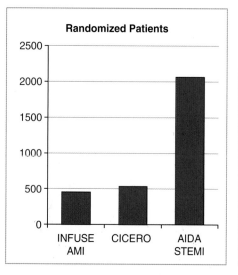

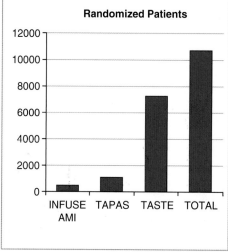

Fig. 11.4 Attempts to improve microvascular reperfusion in acute ST elevation myocardial infarction primary percutaneous coronary intervention have focused on intracoronary administration of glycoprotein IIb/IIIa inhibitors and thrombectomy devices. Initial trials suggested benefit, but much larger trials with greater than 5-fold enrollment have not shown these to be beneficial treatment strategies.[105–107,109]

treatment with respect to the combined secondary endpoint of death, reinfarction, stroke, heart failure, and urgent revascularization. These results were corroborated by those in the larger Rescue Angioplasty versus Conservative Treatment or Repeat Thrombolysis (REACT) trial, which demonstrated lower mortality in patients undergoing rescue PCI compared with the combined medical therapy or repeat thrombolysis treatment groups (hazard ratio, 0.48; 95% CI, 0.23–0.99).[120]

On the other hand, facilitated PCI is PCI for STEMI performed early and routinely after reperfusion has been facilitated by fibrinolysis: comparison of facilitated PCI with primary PCI shows no benefit of facilitating early flow with fibrinolysis (compared to primary PCI alone). Thus this strategy is not recommended. The Assessment of the Safety and Efficacy of a New Treatment Strategy for Acute Myocardial Infarction (ASSENT-4 PCI) Trial randomized patients to either primary PCI or PCI facilitated by fibrinolytic therapy given immediately before transfer of patients to the catheterization laboratory. After only 1600 of the planned 4000 patients had been enrolled, the study was stopped prematurely by the data safety monitoring board because of increased in-hospital mortality in the facilitated PCI arm (6% compared with 3%; P = .01). The incidences of stroke, reinfarction, and urgent target vessel revascularization were also unexpectedly higher in the treatment arm.[121] Based on ASSENT IV and similar negative trials, routine use of full- or half-dose fibrinolytic therapy to facilitate primary PCI for STEMI cannot be recommended.[122]

Guidelines from the 1990s recommended that only patients who have symptomatic, inducible ischemia after thrombolysis undergo angiography and possible PCI.[123] However, PCI early after thrombolysis can establish recanalization when lysis has failed and can consolidate benefit when it has succeeded. Thus, a radical change is suggested by the pharmacoinvasive approach: after fibrinolysis is given to a patient at a non-PCI center, patients are routinely transferred to a PCI center for emergent PCI if there are ongoing symptoms (rescue PCI) or urgent PCI (3 to 24 hours after fibrinolysis) as opposed to the conservative approach of fibrinolysis alone and watchful waiting at the non-PCI center. This comparison—stand-alone fibrinolysis versus a pharmacoinvasive approach for patients requiring transfer to a PCI center—has been tested in multiple large randomized clinical trials and demonstrated a clear benefit for reinfarction and recurrent ischemia with pharmacoinvasive therapy. For example, the Trial of Routine Angioplasty and Stenting after Fibrinolysis to Enhance Reperfusion in Acute Myocardial Infarction (TRANSFER-AMI) demonstrated a nearly 50% reduction in reinfarction (6.0% vs. 3.3%; P = .04) for patients treated with pharmacoinvasive therapy as compared to fibrinolysis alone (Table 11.2).[124,125]

Most important, the early concerns about PCI after fibrinolysis being linked to high rates of general bleeding and abrupt closure are not seen in the era of routine stenting and oral antiplatelet therapy.[65,66,74,125–127] On the other hand, the risk of any fibrinolytic strategy for intracranial bleeding is real and should be considered before undertaking the pharmacoinvasive approach. Recently, the Strategic Reperfusion Early after Myocardial Infarction (STREAM) trial compared primary PCI to pharmacoinvasive therapy and demonstrated similar outcomes for the primary ischemic endpoint with the two approaches. An increased risk of

TABLE 11.2 TRANSFER-AMI: Fibrinolysis Alone Versus Pharmacoinvasive Therapy

Endpoint	Standard (%)	Pharmacoinvasive (%)	P Value
Primary endpoint	16.6	10.6	.0013
Death	3.6	3.7	.94
Reinfarction	6.0	3.3	.044
Recurrent ischemia	2.2	0.2	.019
Death/MI/ischemia	11.7	6.5	.004
New/worsening CHF	5.2	2.9	.069
Cardiogenic shock	2.6	4.5	.11

Pharmacoinvasive therapy (fibrinolysis with either emergent or urgent percutaneous coronary intervention 3–24 hours after thrombolytics) is superior to stand-alone fibrinolysis as shown by decreased recurrent infarction and ischemia.[124]

CHF, Congestive heart failure; *MI*, myocardial infarction.

intracranial bleeding was noted with pharmacoinvasive therapy early in the trial, however, leading to a protocol change: for patients older than 75 years, only a half dose of fibrinolytic therapy was utilized, leading to a significant reduction in risk of intracranial bleeding.[128] A recent registry performed in Ottawa, Ontario showed similar results: ischemic/mortality/reinfarction outcomes were comparable with pharmacoinvasive therapy versus primary PCI, but enhanced risk of intracranial bleeding is noted with fibrinolysis (1.3% vs. 0%; P = .004).[127] Thus, regional approaches incorporating pharmacoinvasive therapy (as opposed to primary PCI with transfer) should (1) be restricted to those patients who require a greater than 60-minute transfer time, (2) be restricted to patients not at high risk for intracranial bleeding, and (3) utilize half-dose fibrinolysis for those older than 75 years.

REGIONAL SYSTEMS IN STEMI CARE

The choice between stand-alone fibrinolysis, pharmacoinvasive therapy, and primary PCI should not be rendered on a patient-by-patient basis. A time-dependent decision tree is required for each hospital (Fig. 11.5).[1,43,112,118,129] STEMI is a time-sensitive trauma to cardiac tissue and requires the automation and systems of care needed for similar time-sensitive situations (stroke, trauma). Thus the 2013 ACC/AHA Guidelines recommend that hospitals and regions decide on a best-practice standard to provide a system of STEMI care for the vast majority of their patients: "All communities should create and maintain a regional system of STEMI care that includes assessment and continuous quality improvement of EMS and hospital based activities" (class I, level of evidence B) (Fig. 11.6).[1]

Regional programs in primary PCI were first tested in the Danish Trial in Acute Myocardial Infarction-2 (DANAMI-2) trial.[130] This Danish trial randomized patients to fibrinolysis alone; primary PCI, if they arrived at a PCI center; and primary PCI after transfer to a PCI center from a non-PCI center. The regions of Denmark involved in this trial were organized in a spoke-and-hub model in which non-PCI centers were designated a specific referring PCI program (mean distance of approximately

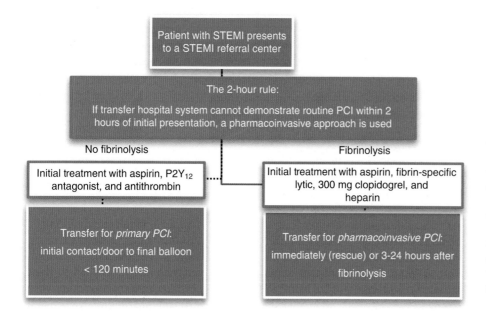

Fig. 11.5 Regional acute ST elevation myocardial infarction (STEMI) care algorithms begin with a 2-hour rule (time from presentation to percutaneous coronary intervention [PCI] <2 hours) and then triage patients to a primary percutaneous coronary intervention or pharmacoinvasive strategy accordingly. (Modified from Dauerman HL, Sobel BE. Toward a comprehensive approach to pharmacoinvasive therapy for patients with ST segment elevation acute myocardial infarction. *J Thromb Thrombolysis.* 2012;34:180–186.)

2013 ACC/AHA Guideline for the Management of ST Elevation Myocardial Infarction

All communities should create and maintain **a regional system of STEMI care** that includes assessment and continuous quality improvement of EMS and hospital-based activities.

EMS transport directly to a PCI-capable hospital for primary PCI with an ideal **FMC-to-device time system goal of 90 minutes** or less.

Immediate transfer to a PCI-capable hospital for primary PCI with an **FMC-to-device time system goal of 120 minutes** or less.

Fig. 11.6 American College of Cardiology (ACC)/American Heart Association (AHA) ST elevation myocardial infarction (STEMI) guidelines endorse regional systems of care and first medical contact goals of <90 minutes for direct presenters to percutaneous coronary intervention hospitals and <120 minutes for patients requiring transfer to a percutaneous coronary intervention hospital.[1] *EMS,* Emergency medical services; *FMC,* first medical contact; *PCI,* percutaneous coronary intervention.

30 miles from non-PCI center to PCI center). The results of stand-alone fibrinolysis versus primary PCI arms of the trial were not surprising: there was a 45% relative risk reduction in the primary endpoint of death/MI or stroke at 30 days with primary PCI. What was somewhat surprising was the similar 40% reduction in the primary endpoint with transfer-mediated primary PCI compared to fibrinolysis alone, suggesting that incorporating a defined delay (<120 minutes from initial presentation to PCI in over 90% of the DANAMI 2 transfer population) in primary PCI as part of a regional strategy could provide the best results.

These results did not immediately translate into broader incorporation of primary PCI into regional and nationwide

programs due to concerns about replicating the transfer times and coordinated spoke-and-hub models seen in the DANAMI-2 trial. Efforts to establish statewide primary PCI programs in North Carolina, Minnesota, and Vermont to replicate and expand the DANAMI-2 experience were undertaken in the mid-2000s; the results confirmed the feasibility of the DANAMI-2 approach for many hospitals and transfer patients.[131–134] These experiences helped define the need for the following key elements of successful regional primary PCI programs[129,135]:

- Simplified pharmacologic algorithms to precede primary PCI and initiated in the ambulance or non-PCI center
- Automated transfer programs (i.e., no waiting for bed availability at PCI center)
- Dedicated algorithms for care that were shared at multiple hospitals: all hospitals using a 24-hour-a-day, 7-day-a-week predictable approach to transfer for primary PCI
- Single call activation of the primary PCI team to allow for timely, automatic transfer to the catheterization laboratory
- Prehospital activation of the catheterization laboratory by emergency medical services

As the Door-to-Balloon Alliance addressed the timeliness of reperfusion among patients presenting to primary PCI centers (door-to-balloon goal <90 minutes),[9,136] Mission: Lifeline was created in the United States to address coordination of regional programs for primary PCI and timeliness of reperfusion from first medical contact to PCI among both direct presenting and transfer hospitals.[113,129,137] Similar efforts occurred in European countries demonstrating nationwide incorporation of regional transfer programs for primary PCI and improvement in STEMI outcomes.[138] Based upon DANAMI-2 and these regional programs, the ACC/AHA/ESC guidelines were revised recently to specifically include the guideline that patients presenting to non-PCI centers may be referred for primary PCI if the transfer process would allow the goal of first medical contact (or first presentation) to PCI time of less than 120 minutes (class I).[1,43] Of note, the expansion of primary PCI regional systems in the United States and some countries in Europe has not necessarily been replicated in developing countries due to cost and access issues.[112,115,139,140]

While the efforts to improve times to reperfusion for patients presenting directly to primary PCI centers have been generally successful such that over 90% of patients are achieving door-to-balloon times less than 90 minutes in the United States,[7,136] the success of regional coordination programs in achieving the guideline-mandated goal of 120 minutes has been less robust. In a recent analysis of transfer STEMI patients within 60 minutes of a PCI center, two-thirds of patients have reached the 120-minute goal (even when using first presentation as the starting point, as opposed to the more difficult first medical contact [as measured by emergency medical services' provision of a first electrocardiogram]).[141] Efforts to implement the key elements of a successful regional primary PCI program throughout 16 regions of the United States in recent years (the STEMI ACCELERATOR program) has also shown mixed success[142]: while significant improvements in surrogate metrics (i.e., use of prehospital activation, single call catheterization laboratory activation) are

clearly improved through such efforts, the percentage of transfer patients with goal-mandated reperfusion times still hovers around 50% to 60%, suggesting opportunities for further progress.

Based upon the feasibility and limitations of a regional primary PCI program, a dedicated coordinated algorithm that respects the need for timely reperfusion and availability of PCI-mediated complete reperfusion is recommended. The regional algorithm used in Vermont and upstate New York for a single PCI center and its referring community hospitals is shown in Fig. 11.7.[118,143] This algorithm mandates that each hospital in a region declares itself to be either a primary PCI or transfer to primary PCI center or pharmacoinvasive center (if greater than 60-minute transfer time to a PCI center) with dedicated pharmacologic algorithms based upon geography, distance, and transfer timing. This organizational scheme is similar to one developed in Minnesota: hospitals were designated zone 1 (primary PCI, by direct presentation or transfer) and zone 2 (pharmacoinvasive therapy with initial half-dose fibrinolysis followed by rapid transfer for PCI) with demonstration of excellent outcomes, which has led

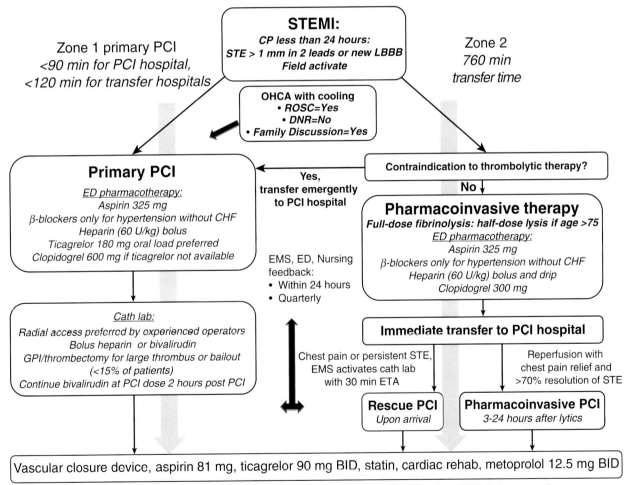

Fig. 11.7 A sample regional algorithm for ST elevation myocardial infarction (STEMI) incorporating a primary percutaneous coronary intervention (PCI) or pharmacoinvasive therapy strategy depending upon transfer time >60 minutes. Adjunctive therapy, half-dose thrombolytics in the elderly, and considerations of higher-risk groups are incorporated into this comprehensive statewide algorithm in Vermont. *BID*, Twice per day; *CHF*, congestive heart failure; *DNR*, do not resuscitate; *ED*, emergency department; *EMS*, emergency medical services; *GPI*, glycoprotein inhibitor; *OHCA*, out-of-hospital cardiac arrest; *ROSC*, return of spontaneous circulation; *STE*, ST elevation.

to wider adoption of these regionally coordinated algorithms to allow for timely and complete reperfusion across a broad spectrum of STEMI patients.[113,114,131,132]

CONCLUSIONS

Reperfusion therapy improves survival in patients with STEMI. Achieving optimal results with primary PCI depends on revascularization of the infarct-related artery within 90 minutes after presentation of the patient to the PCI hospital (or first medical contact). Primary PCI may be extended to transfer patients from community hospitals if timely transport is feasible within the goal of initial presentation to device of less than 120 minutes. Accordingly, implementation of primary PCI is appropriate for patients presenting to an interventional center or those who can be transported to one via helicopter or ambulance within 60 minutes. For patients presenting to institutions that cannot meet these primary PCI criteria and have no contraindication to thrombolysis, treatment with fibrinolysis followed by PCI (pharmacoinvasive approach) is warranted.

Appropriate adjunctive therapy should be implemented for both primary PCI and pharmacoinvasive approaches. This includes administration of aspirin and heparin for all patients with STEMI, with use of clopidogrel (300 mg) in patients undergoing fibrinolysis and potentially more potent antiplatelet therapy (ticagrelor) in patients undergoing primary PCI. With prompt and complete reperfusion as the linchpin of therapy for STEMI, 30-day mortality is routinely less than 5% in clinical trials, national registries, and clinical practice. While issues of timing and efficacy of reperfusion therapies as well as delays between symptom onset and initial presentation for treatment remain critical, the major mortality challenge facing clinicians in the STEMI population has moved to two specific populations: patients with STEMI complicated by cardiogenic shock and/or cardiac arrest. The dramatic impact of reperfusion therapy—fibrinolysis first, followed by primary PCI and pharmacoinvasive therapy—on the survival of patients with STEMI over the past 3 decades provides a model for development of future approaches and developments in this complex field.

The full reference list for this chapter is available at ExpertConsult.com.

12

Adjunctive Pharmacologic Therapies in Acute Myocardial Infarction

Richard G. Bach

OUTLINE

Acute myocardial infarction (MI) remains a major cause of death and disability worldwide. While advances in primary reperfusion therapy have resulted in significant reductions in morbidity and mortality among patients with acute MI, adjunctive pharmacologic therapies continue to play a vital role. The rapid initiation of adjunctive therapies in the cardiac intensive care unit (CICU) setting are indicated in the acute and convalescent phases of management to reduce adverse outcomes. These adjunctive treatments are directed at further reducing the short- and long-term risks of death, recurrent MI, angina, and congestive heart failure (CHF). They work by reducing ischemia and coronary reocclusion, limiting the loss of myocardium and myocardial function, preventing adverse ventricular remodeling, reducing the risk of arrhythmias, and slowing the progression of athero-sclerosis. Empiric evidence accumulated from more than three decades of clinical trial experience has demonstrated the important benefits of certain therapies while uncovering the hazards of others, such that clinicians now have evidence-based guidance on appropriate pharmacologic management following acute MI. Reinforcing the importance of a comprehensive approach to evidence-based therapies, studies have documented that more consistent application of evidence-based therapies for patients with MI significantly improves outcomes.[1,2]

Acute MI is defined as myocardial necrosis in a clinical setting consistent with acute myocardial ischemia[3] and can be divided into ST elevation MI (STEMI, including STEMI-equivalent presentations, such as left bundle branch block) and non-ST elevation MI (NSTEMI). Acute MI is commonly the consequence of an occlusive or near-occlusive coronary thrombus at the site of an eroded or ruptured atherosclerotic plaque, the pathophysiol-ogy of which is discussed elsewhere in this book. Acute MI results in loss of myocardium, acute and potentially chronic diastolic and systolic ventricular dysfunction, and increased susceptibility to potentially fatal arrhythmias. The ultimate goal of therapy for acute MI, whether primary or adjunctive, is to preserve myocardium and myocardial geometry and function and, thereby, reduce cardiovascular morbidity and mortality. Since multiple trials of reperfusion therapy for patients with STEMI have shown a consistent reduction in mortality, the primary early management of patients with acute STEMI is aimed at the occlusive coronary thrombus,[4] employing early reperfusion therapy using thrombolytic agents or mechanical devices. Early and successful reperfusion can interrupt the "march to necrosis" that progresses as a wave front from endocardium to epicardium[5] with the goal of preserving the myocardium and limiting adverse ventricular remodeling.[6] Additional evidence supports the use of adjunctive pharmacologic therapies in addition to reperfusion therapy in the management of acute MI patients.[7–10] These adjunctive therapies should also be considered as alternative therapies for STEMI patients in whom thrombolytic therapy or primary percutaneous coronary intervention (PCI) are contraindicated, for widening the time window for reperfusion when therapy cannot be instituted early, for reducing reperfusion injury in patients given late reperfusion therapy, and for achieving and maintaining complete reperfusion. Specifically, the aims of adjunctive therapy are to limit consequences of ischemia or infarction, optimize healing, and reduce adverse and recurrent events. Survivors of STEMI represent a special group of patients at greater jeopardy for increased morbidity and mortality. As a result, they stand to benefit greatly from adjunctive therapies and comprehensive secondary prevention.

This chapter focuses on evidence-based adjunctive medical therapies indicated for patients with acute MI, with a predominant focus on STEMI, which is relevant for physicians managing patients during and following the CICU phase. It also discusses and summarizes recommendations from the American College of Cardiology and American Heart Association (ACC/AHA) practice guidelines for management of STEMI and non-ST elevation acute coronary syndromes (NSTE ACS).[10,11]

ANTIPLATELET THERAPY

Platelets play a critical role in thrombus formation at sites of plaque rupture or erosion; therefore inhibiting platelets plays a central role in the treatment of STEMI and NSTE ACS. The involvement of platelets in the initiation of thrombus is a multistep process of adhesion, activation, and aggregation, each step of which involves binding and activation of certain receptors and a cascade of intracellular signaling pathways (Fig. 12.1). The importance of platelet inhibitors as therapeutic agents for acute MI was first highlighted by the Second International Studies of Infarct Survival (ISIS-2) trial,[12] in which randomization to aspirin compared with placebo among patients with STEMI reduced mortality to a similar degree compared with reperfusion by streptokinase. More recent clinical trials of inhibitors of other mediators of platelet activation and aggregation—such as the $P2Y_{12}$ receptor, thrombin receptor, and the glycoprotein IIb/IIIa receptor—have reinforced the critical importance of platelet inhibition as a therapeutic target for patients with ACS. The current standard of care for treatment of patients with ACS endorses multireceptor inhibition by routine use of aspirin in combination with a $P2Y_{12}$ antagonist, a combination commonly termed dual antiplatelet therapy (DAPT).

Aspirin

One pathway that participates in the regulation of platelet activity involves the conversion of arachidonic acid to thromboxane A_2 (TXA_2) and other prostaglandins by the platelet cyclooxygenase (COX) enzymes, COX-1 and COX-2. Constitutive COX-1 promotes platelet aggregation, thrombosis, and vasoconstriction, and protects gastrointestinal mucosa.[13] In contrast, inducible COX-2 is proinflammatory via prostaglandin E_2 (PGE_2) and antithrombotic and vasodilatory via prostaglandin I_2 (PGI_2 [prostacyclin]).[13] Aspirin (acetylsalicylic acid) exerts antiplatelet actions through acetylation of a serine residue on COX-1 to irreversibly block the production of TXA_2 which, in turn, inhibits platelet activation and aggregation. The effect of aspirin can be detected within 30 to 40 minutes of ingestion and lasts for the life of the platelet (7 to 10 days).[14,15] Low-dose aspirin appears to selectively inhibit COX-1, while higher doses inhibit both COX-1 and COX-2. Low-dose aspirin may therefore block TXA_2 production while sparing PGI_2 synthesis.[16]

The efficacy of aspirin in acute STEMI was established in the randomized ISIS-2 trial, which used a 2×2 factorial design to assess the effects of a 1-hour intravenous infusion of streptokinase (1.5 million U) or oral aspirin (160 mg) or both in patients presenting within 24 hours of the onset of symptoms.[12] At 5 weeks, aspirin reduced nonfatal reinfarction by 50%, nonfatal stroke by 46%, total cardiovascular mortality by 23% (absolute risk reduction of 2.4%) and the risk of any vascular event by 23%. Reduction of cardiovascular mortality was enhanced by the combination of antiplatelet and fibrinolytic therapy; cardiovascular mortality was decreased by 25% with streptokinase alone and by 42% with streptokinase and aspirin combined (absolute risk reduction of 5.2%), indicating that low-dose aspirin alone was as effective as streptokinase and that the combination was synergistic. Aspirin therapy also appeared to reduce the rate of reocclusion. Patients taking aspirin had fewer cardiac arrests, but slightly more minor bleeding. Aspirin did not increase the risk of cardiac rupture or bleeding requiring transfusion. A subsequent meta-analysis of MI trials using aspirin and the thrombolytic agents streptokinase and alteplase showed that aspirin reduces coronary reocclusion and recurrent ischemic events.[17]

Aspirin is generally well tolerated, but its use has been associated with an increased risk of bleeding, including serious gastrointestinal bleeding and rare intracranial (including intracerebral) hemorrhage. Adverse bleeding events appear more frequent at higher doses (>100 mg/day).[18] When aspirin is combined with other antiplatelet therapy, such as $P2Y_{12}$ antagonists, the risk of bleeding is increased. Results from the Clopidogrel in Unstable Angina to Prevent Recurrent Events (CURE) trial suggest there is an interaction between the dose of aspirin and the risk of bleeding with combined aspirin plus clopidogrel such that the risk was mitigated by use of low-dose aspirin (<100 mg).[19] For secondary prevention, the absolute benefits of aspirin are considered to far outweigh the risk of major bleeding[20]; collective evidence supports low-dose aspirin (75 to 81 mg) for long-term use.[21]

Some patients are unable to tolerate aspirin owing to hypersensitivity from one of three types of reactions: respiratory sensitivity,

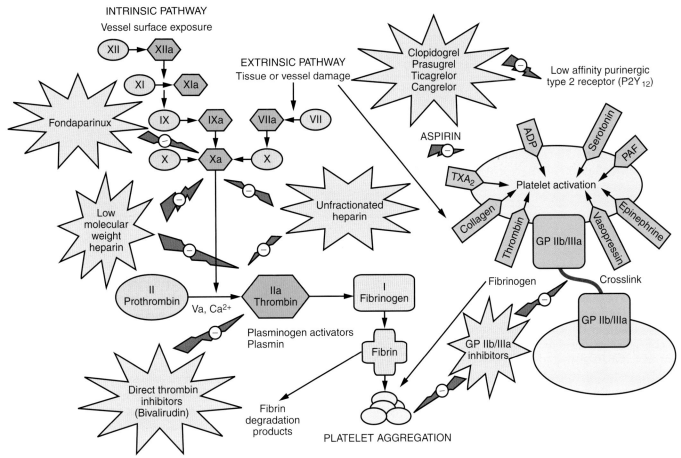

Fig. 12.1 Sites of action of antiplatelet and antithrombin agents. Low-molecular-weight heparin produces more potent inhibition of factor Xa than thrombin, whereas unfractionated heparin produces equal inhibition of factor Xa and thrombin. Direct thrombin inhibitors inhibit thrombin, but have little effect on its generation. Thrombin amplifies generation of factors VIIIa and Va, enhancing thrombus formation. Thrombin also promotes platelet activation by binding to platelet thrombin receptor. Cross-links, via ligands such as fibrinogen (factor I) to platelet glycoprotein (GP) IIb/IIIa receptors, lead to platelet aggregation. GP IIb/IIIa inhibitors act at these sites. *ADP,* Adenosine triphosphate; *PAF,* platelet-activating factor; *TXA₂,* thromboxane A₂.

cutaneous sensitivity, and systemic sensitivity.[22] Respiratory sensitivity has been designated aspirin-exacerbated respiratory disease (AERD); patients with AERD often manifest Samter's triad of asthma, aspirin sensitivity, and rhinitis/nasal polyps. Aspirin ingestion may precipitate an asthma exacerbation in patients with AERD; thus, a history of moderate or severe asthma can be considered a significant risk factor for AERD. Cutaneous reactions to aspirin consist of urticaria, which can occur alone or simultaneously with angioedema. Systemic sensitivity to aspirin results in an anaphylactoid reaction, characterized by hypotension, swelling, laryngeal edema, generalized pruritus, tachypnea, and obtundation.[22] When angioedema is accompanied by hypotension, it is generally considered an anaphylactoid reaction rather than a cutaneous reaction. Patients with respiratory or cutaneous hypersensitivity to aspirin may be candidates for aspirin desensitization[23]; patients with aspirin allergy presenting with ACS should undergo desensitization, if at all feasible. Aspirin desensitization is not feasible for individuals known to have an anaphylactoid response. For patients with irremediable

intolerance to aspirin, use of another antiplatelet agent, such as a P2Y₁₂ antagonist, is recommended.

Aspirin is also contraindicated in patients with active bleeding or with high-risk bleeding conditions (e.g., retinal hemorrhage, active peptic ulcer, other serious gastrointestinal or urogenital bleeding, hemophilia, and untreated severe hypertension). In patients with prior gastrointestinal bleeding attributed to peptic ulcer disease, addition of a proton pump inhibitor (PPI) to low-dose aspirin has been shown to reduce the risk of recurrent bleeding.[24,25] Based on these results and evidence of the large benefit of aspirin after MI,[26] aspirin combined with a PPI should be continued if possible, unless bleeding is life threatening or cannot be otherwise controlled.

Recommendations

Given the robust evidence of efficacy and safety, aspirin should be administered as soon as possible as adjunctive therapy to all ACS patients without known intolerance, including patients with STEMI, NSTEMI, and unstable angina. On presentation, STEMI

TABLE 12.1 Properties of Platelet P2Y$_{12}$ ADP Receptor Antagonists

	Clopidogrel	Prasugrel	Ticagrelor	Cangrelor
P2Y$_{12}$ receptor blockade	Irreversible	Irreversible	Reversible	Reversible
Route of administration	Oral	Oral	Oral	Intravenous
Frequency of administration	Once daily	Once daily	Twice daily	Bolus plus infusion
Prodrug	Yes	Yes	No	No
Onset of action	2–8 h	30 min–4 h	30 min–4 h	2 min
Offset of action	7–10 d	7–10 d	3–5 d	30–60 min
Interactions with CYP-metabolized drugs	CYP2C19	No	CYP3A4/5	No
Indications for use	ACS and stable CAD undergoing PCI	ACS undergoing PCI	ACS (full spectrum)	PCI not pretreated with oral P2Y$_{12}$ antagonist
Loading dose	300–600 mg	60 mg	180 mg	30 μg/kg bolus
Maintenance dose	75 mg daily	10 mg daily	90 mg twice daily	4 μg/kg/min infusion

ACS, Acute coronary syndrome; *CAD,* coronary artery disease; *PCI,* percutaneous coronary intervention.

patients should be treated with 162 to 325 mg of aspirin followed by 81 mg daily indefinitely.[10,11,26] Non–enteric-coated aspirin should be used initially and chewed to ensure rapid absorption.[27] While the dose of aspirin used for long-term maintenance therapy for secondary prevention has varied across studies,[28] evidence has accrued that low doses appear to be as effective as higher doses, yet safer. A meta-analysis that included over 190,000 patients in randomized trials reported that, compared with higher doses, doses of aspirin less than 100 mg daily provided comparable efficacy with lower bleeding rates.[18] More recently, an analysis of patient outcomes in the Treatment with ADP Receptor Inhibitors: Longitudinal Assessment of Treatment Patterns and Events After Acute Coronary Syndrome (TRANSLATE-ACS) study showed that even among MI patients treated with PCI including stent implantation, low-dose (81 mg) aspirin was associated with similar rates of adverse ischemic events but lower risk of bleeding compared with higher-dose (325 mg) aspirin.[29] Currently, recommendations endorse low-dose aspirin daily indefinitely for patients following MI, whether or not they have undergone PCI with stent implantation.[30]

Pericarditis is common in STEMI patients not treated with reperfusion, although its incidence has diminished in the era of rapid reperfusion. Its timing coincides with the subacute phase during healing. Successful early reperfusion attenuates transmural extension and explains why pericarditis is rare in the reperfusion era.[31] Although nonsteroidal antiinflammatory drugs (NSAIDs), such as ibuprofen and indomethacin, and corticosteroids have been effective for pericarditis, they can cause infarct expansion, thinning, and cardiac rupture[32-36]; thus they should be avoided or used only as a last resort. High-dose aspirin (650 mg every 4–6 hours) may be used for pain control and antiinflammatory effects.[10,37] Alternatively, colchicine[38] may be used. Short-term corticosteroids and NSAIDs may be used with extreme caution. Ibuprofen should not be used because it attenuates the antiplatelet effect of aspirin and may cause infarct thinning.[32]

P2Y$_{12}$ PLATELET ANTAGONISTS

Despite COX inhibition by aspirin, platelet activation can continue through TXA$_2$-independent pathways, leading to platelet aggregation and thrombus formation, suggesting that combining aspirin with other platelet inhibitors could provide added benefit. Additional agents that inhibit the platelet P2Y$_{12}$ adenosine diphosphate (ADP) receptor have been shown to have added efficacy in reducing ischemic events among patients with acute MI and DAPT: using a combination of aspirin and a P2Y$_{12}$ antagonist is currently recommended for secondary prevention for virtually all patients. The oral P2Y$_{12}$ antagonists include the thienopyridines, ticlopidine, clopidogrel, and prasugrel, which are prodrugs whose active metabolites irreversibly bind to and inhibit the P2Y$_{12}$ receptor and the direct acting, nonthienopyridine, reversible antagonist, ticagrelor (Table 12.1). Ticlopidine, the oldest member of this class, was shown to reduce the risk of stent thrombosis compared with prior treatments,[39] but owing to a risk of serious neutropenia, thrombotic thrombocytopenic purpura (TTP) and aplastic anemia, it was replaced by clopidogrel for the reduction of atherothrombotic events following stent implantation.[40] Ticlopidine continues to have a minor role for the uncommon patient allergic to or intolerant of clopidogrel, but the availability of newer P2Y$_{12}$ antagonists has limited its current use. A parenteral short-acting reversible P2Y$_{12}$ antagonist, cangrelor, is also available for early infusion to support PCI among patients who have not been pretreated with an oral P2Y$_{12}$ antagonist (see Table 12.1) prior to intervention.

Clopidogrel

Clopidogrel is an oral agent that blocks activation of platelets by irreversibly inhibiting the binding of ADP to the P2Y$_{12}$ receptor. Clopidogrel is a prodrug that is metabolized in the liver in a multistep process, predominantly though the cytochrome P450 isoform CYP2C19, to a short-lived active metabolite that binds to the ligand binding site of the P2Y$_{12}$ receptor (see Table 12.1). Clopidogrel has a more potent antiplatelet effect than aspirin.

In contrast to aspirin, clopidogrel produces significant platelet inhibition after 2 to 3 days, but may take 4 to 7 days to achieve its full effect,[41] reinforcing the need for a loading dose. The onset of clopidogrel antiplatelet action is reported at 2 to 6 hours after a loading dose. The platelet-inhibiting effects persist for 7 to 10 days after therapy is stopped.

Clopidogrel monotherapy has been shown to have benefits in reducing the risk of adverse ischemic events among patients with a history of or at high risk for atherosclerotic heart disease. In the Clopidogrel versus Aspirin in patients at Risk of Ischaemic Events (CAPRIE) trial,[42] which compared outcomes among patients with atherosclerotic vascular disease randomly assigned to clopidogrel versus aspirin, clopidogrel was modestly more effective in reducing the combined risk of ischemic stroke, MI, or vascular death. As a result, for long-term prevention, clopidogrel may be substituted for aspirin in patients with aspirin allergy or intolerance.[10,11]

The effect of adding clopidogrel to aspirin in the early phase of acute coronary syndromes was studied in the landmark CURE trial.[43] Patients presenting with NSTE ACS who received aspirin were randomly assigned to receive a loading dose of 300 mg of clopidogrel at the time of hospital admission, followed by 75 mg/day, versus placebo. The primary endpoint of cardiovascular death, MI, and stroke was reduced by 20% among patients randomized to clopidogrel plus aspirin. The benefit was observed early, with significant reductions in adverse ischemic events seen within 24 hours of clopidogrel administration,[44] and was consistent across the spectrum of risk and regardless of treatment strategy, with significant risk reductions evident among patients receiving medical management, PCI, or coronary artery bypass graft (CABG) surgery (although clopidogrel was associated with an increase in perioperative bleeding for patients undergoing CABG).

Despite the early hazard of increased perioperative bleeding, patients in the CURE trial who were randomly assigned to clopidogrel plus aspirin and underwent CABG surgery had improved ischemic outcomes.[45] Among patients who underwent CABG surgery, there was a 21% reduction in cardiovascular death, MI, or stroke. There was an increase in major bleeding but no significant excess of life-threatening bleeding. The investigators concluded that, overall, the benefits of starting clopidogrel on admission appeared to outweigh the risks, even among those who proceeded to CABG during the initial hospitalization.

The Clopidogrel as Adjunctive Reperfusion Therapy –Thrombolysis in Myocardial Infarction (CLARITY-TIMI) 28 study tested the effect of clopidogrel on angiographic and clinical outcome among patients younger than 75 years with STEMI who were treated with standard fibrinolytic therapy.[46] Patients were randomly assigned to receive 300 mg of clopidogrel coincident with the fibrinolytic agent followed by 75 mg/day or placebo; angiographic infarct-related artery patency and adverse events were assessed at 2 to 8 days. The results demonstrated that the addition of clopidogrel for STEMI patients receiving fibrinolytic therapy improved the patency rate of the infarct-related artery and significantly reduced adverse ischemic events with no significant increase in bleeding complications.

The effect of the addition of clopidogrel to aspirin for patients with STEMI was further studied in the Clopidogrel and Metoprolol in Myocardial Infarction Trial/Second Chinese Cardiac Study (COMMIT/CCS-2),[47] in which over 45,000 patients with suspected STEMI receiving aspirin 162 mg/day were randomly allocated to clopidogrel 75 mg daily (with no loading dose) or placebo. The results showed that adding clopidogrel to aspirin significantly reduced death, reinfarction, or stroke by 9% and mortality by 7%. The benefit was consistent among younger and older patients and among patients who did or did not receive

fibrinolytic therapy, with no significant excess risk of fatal or cerebral bleeding.

While these studies employed clopidogrel with a loading dose of 300 mg or no loading dose, subsequent studies suggested a faster onset of action and added benefit with a higher loading dose of 600 mg, particularly among higher-risk patients undergoing PCI.[48,49] In the Clopidogrel and Aspirin Optimal Dose Usage to Reduce Recurrent Events–Seventh Organization to Assess Strategies in Ischemic Syndromes (CURRENT-OASIS-7) trial,[50] patients with acute coronary syndromes were randomly assigned to double-dose clopidogrel (600 mg on day 1, 150 mg on days 2 to 7, then 75 mg daily) versus standard dose (300 mg on day 1, then 75 mg daily). Among patients undergoing PCI, compared with standard dose, double-dose clopidogrel reduced the rate of cardiovascular death, MI, or stroke, and stent thrombosis. Major bleeding was more common with double-dose than with standard-dose clopidogrel.

The cumulative data suggest that, for clopidogrel, the recommended loading dose is 600 mg with a maintenance dose of 75 mg.[10,11,30] Among patients with STEMI receiving fibrinolytic therapy, patients younger than 75 years should receive 300 mg followed by 75 mg daily. As discussed earlier, clopidogrel plus aspirin has been associated with significant increases in major bleeding with CABG surgery.[51] Clopidogrel should be withheld for 5 to 7 days before surgery, if feasible.[52]

Wide interindividual variability in the degree of inhibition of ADP-induced platelet function has been observed among patients treated with clopidogrel; so-called "high on-treatment platelet reactivity" (HPR) is reported in up to 35% of patients.[53] The mechanisms for this variability are likely multifactorial, including drug, environmental, and genetic interactions. Clopidogrel's action depends on biotransformation to its active metabolite in the liver, largely by CYP2C19, and studies have linked the presence of CYP2C19 loss-of-function alleles, such as CYP2C19*2, with an increased risk of cardiovascular events in patients with ACS or after PCI treated with clopidogrel.[54,55] As a consequence, the United States Food and Drug Administration (FDA) issued a boxed warning for clopidogrel recommending the use of other treatments for individuals known to be poor metabolizers and who have two copies of the CYP2C19 loss-of-function alleles. Studies have also suggested an increased risk of bleeding with clopidogrel among patients with CYP2C19*17 gain-of-function alleles.[56] To date, however, there has been no firm evidence from prospective studies or retrospective studies of major trials supporting the use of genetic testing (or platelet reactivity testing) to personalize the clopidogrel dose or the decision to switch to an alternate P2Y$_{12}$ antagonist.[10,11,57]

PPIs, such as omeprazole and esomeprazole, which are strong inhibitors of CYP2C19, are associated with decreased inhibition of platelet aggregation by clopidogrel. However, most clinical studies, including a prospective randomized trial, have not confirmed an adverse effect on clinical outcomes by PPI use among patients receiving clopidogrel.[58] For patients receiving DAPT who are at higher risk of upper gastrointestinal bleeding, the benefit of PPI use appears to outweigh the risk, although some have advocated for the use of a PPI with weaker inhibitory effects on CYP2C19, such as pantoprazole.

Clopidogrel therapy is generally well tolerated but may be associated with adverse effects. As discussed earlier, clopidogrel combined with aspirin increases major and minor bleeding risk, both acutely and during follow-up.[59] Clopidogrel has been associated with gastrointestinal upset and a rare incidence of thrombotic thrombocytopenic purpura.[60] Plasma exchange should be considered if thrombotic thrombocytopenic purpura develops.

Prasugrel

Prasugrel is another thienopyridine antagonist of the platelet P2Y$_{12}$ receptor. Like clopidogrel, prasugrel is a prodrug that is metabolized into an active metabolite that irreversibly binds to and blocks the ligand binding site of the P2Y$_{12}$ receptor (see Table 12.1). Prasugrel is a more potent inhibitor of ADP-induced platelet aggregation than clopidogrel and, at doses recommended, inhibits greater than 80% of in vitro ADP-induced platelet aggregation. Prasugrel also has less interpatient variability in its antiplatelet effects than clopidogrel.[61]

The efficacy of prasugrel as compared with clopidogrel on outcomes among patients with acute coronary syndromes undergoing PCI was examined in the Trial to Assess Improvement in Therapeutic Outcomes by Optimizing Platelet Inhibition with Prasugrel–Thrombolysis in Myocardial Infarction (TRITON-TIMI) 38 trial.[62] In the study, patients with STEMI or high-risk NSTE ACS who had undergone coronary angiography and were to undergo planned PCI were randomly assigned to prasugrel or clopidogrel. Treatment with prasugrel resulted in a significant reduction in cardiovascular death, MI, and stroke, and stent thrombosis, but a 32% increased risk of bleeding, including fatal bleeding. In post hoc subgroup analyses, three subgroups were identified that had less net clinical benefit or even had clinical harm in the trial. These included patients with a history of stroke or transient ischemic attack (who had an increased risk of intracranial hemorrhage), the elderly (>75 years), and those with a body weight of less than 60 kg. Among patients without any of these three risk factors, treatment with prasugrel resulted in significant net clinical benefit compared with clopidogrel. The ischemic benefit of prasugrel compared with clopidogrel was particularly evident in those with diabetes and among patients with STEMI.[63,64]

Prasugrel is administered as a 60-mg loading dose followed by a maintenance dose of 10 mg daily. A lower maintenance dose of 5 mg has been recommended in patients who weigh less than 60 kg or who are older than 75 years.[65] Due to its greater antiplatelet potency and the large increase in perioperative bleeding observed in the TRITON-TIMI 38 trial with prasugrel, it is recommended that prasugrel be discontinued 7 days prior to CABG surgery.

Ticagrelor

Ticagrelor is an oral cyclopentyltriazolopyrimidine that reversibly inhibits the platelet P2Y$_{12}$ receptor (see Table 12.1). Unlike thienopyridines, ticagrelor is not a prodrug. It does not bind to the ADP-binding site; instead, it binds to a separate site of the P2Y$_{12}$ receptor, thereby inhibiting G-protein activation and signaling. The onset of action of ticagrelor is faster than

clopidogrel, with 40% platelet inhibition in 30 minutes after dosing with a peak effect in approximately 2 hours. Ticagrelor has a plasma half-life of 8 to 12 hours. As a reversible P2Y$_{12}$ receptor inhibitor, the offset of ticagrelor action is faster than with thienopyridines.[66]

The effect of ticagrelor compared with clopidogrel for treatment of patients with ACS was examined among 18,624 aspirin-treated patients in the Platelet Inhibition and Patient Outcomes (PLATO) study.[67] At 1 year, patients randomly assigned to receive ticagrelor had a significant (16%) reduction in death from vascular causes, MI, or stroke. Of note, overall mortality was also reduced with ticagrelor. No significant difference in rate of major bleeding was observed between ticagrelor and clopidogrel, but ticagrelor was associated with a higher rate of major bleeding not related to CABG. Additional analyses from the PLATO study have shown that the efficacy of ticagrelor is preserved without excess bleeding hazard among the elderly,[68] women,[69] patients with diabetes,[70] and patients with STEMI.[71] Ticagrelor was generally well tolerated, but adverse effects included increased non-CABG-related bleeding, dyspnea, ventricular pauses (mostly asymptomatic), and increased serum creatinine.[67]

Ticagrelor also has non-P2Y$_{12}$ receptor–mediated effects that include blocking the equilibrative nucleoside transporter-1,[72] which can result in increased plasma concentrations of adenosine. The clinical significance of this observation is unknown, but adenosine has been shown to mediate in coronary vasodilation, reduction of ischemia, and reperfusion injury, along with stimulation of pulmonary vagal C fibers that cause dyspnea. An increased incidence of dyspnea was observed in the PLATO trial among patients receiving ticagrelor (14.5%) compared with clopidogrel (8.7%). Dyspnea was considered severe in only 0.4% of patients and patients with dyspnea had no related abnormalities in pulmonary function testing. A significant interaction between the aspirin maintenance dose and the benefit of ticagrelor was observed in the PLATO trial such that the greatest reduction in ischemic events was observed with ticagrelor in combination with low-dose (< 100 mg daily) aspirin.[73]

Ticagrelor is administered as a loading dose of 180 mg followed by a maintenance dose of 90 mg twice per day. When ticagrelor is prescribed for DAPT, the aspirin dose should be 81 mg daily. Although ticagrelor is a reversible P2Y$_{12}$ antagonist, due to the high level of platelet inhibition achieved, it is recommended that ticagrelor be withheld 5 days prior to CABG surgery.

Cangrelor

After oral administration of a loading dose of a P2Y$_{12}$ antagonist, the onset of antiplatelet activity is not immediate; the achievement of clinically effective platelet inhibition may be delayed by hours. This delay is more pronounced among patients with STEMI, in whom multiple factors may contribute to delayed gastrointestinal drug absorption. Among patients presenting with STEMI receiving loading doses of prasugrel or ticagrelor in the Rapid Activity of Platelet Inhibitor Drugs (RAPID) trial, effective levels of platelet inhibition were not observed until 4 hours after administration.[74] Thus many patients undergoing primary PCI within minutes of presenting with STEMI may have inadequate platelet inhibition at the time of stent implantation, which may contribute to the higher risk of stent thrombosis observed in that setting. Achievement of rapid platelet inhibition by the intravenous $P2Y_{12}$ antagonist cangrelor may have particular attractiveness for use in patients with STEMI or high-risk ACS undergoing urgent PCI who have not been adequately preloaded with an oral $P2Y_{12}$ antagonist.

Cangrelor has several unique properties as an antiplatelet agent (see Table 12.1). It is a potent, direct-acting, rapidly reversible $P2Y_{12}$ antagonist with predictable plasma levels and linear dose-dependent receptor inhibition. An effective level (>80%) of platelet inhibition with cangrelor is achieved within minutes after start of intravenous infusion. Platelet function then recovers within 60 to 90 minutes after discontinuation of the infusion.[75]

Cangrelor has been studied in a number of trials, the most important of which was the Cangrelor versus Standard Therapy to Achieve Optimal Management of Platelet Inhibition (CHAMPION) PHOENIX trial,[76] in which 10,942 clopidogrel-naive patients with coronary artery disease requiring PCI for stable angina, NSTE ACS, or STEMI received a bolus and subsequent infusion of cangrelor or placebo for at least 2 hours or the duration of the procedure, whichever was longer. Patients treated with cangrelor received a loading dose of clopidogrel at the end of infusion, while patients receiving placebo received a loading dose of clopidogrel at the time of PCI procedure. Following the procedure, patients were treated with a standard maintenance dose of oral $P2Y_{12}$ inhibitor and aspirin. The composite rate of death, MI, ischemia driven revascularization, or stent thrombosis at 48 hours was significantly lower in the cangrelor group than in the clopidogrel group and the individual rate of stent thrombosis at 48 hours was lower in the cangrelor group than in the clopidogrel group. The observed reduction of 22% in ischemic events in patients treated with cangrelor was not accompanied by a significant increase in severe bleeding or in the need for transfusions compared with patients on clopidogrel, although there was an overall increase in bleeding with cangrelor. In a notable substudy from CHAMPION PHOENIX,[77] the improved efficacy of cangrelor compared with clopidogrel was preserved among patients 75 years of age or older, and despite a 10-fold greater risk of severe bleeding complications among patients, in comparing these older patients with younger patients, cangrelor did not increase the risk of severe bleeding compared with clopidogrel.[77]

In light of these favorable results, cangrelor may be considered for use in patients with STEMI or high-risk ACS undergoing urgent PCI who have not been adequately preloaded with an oral $P2Y_{12}$ antagonist.[78] Cangrelor is administered as a 30-µg/kg intravenous bolus infused over 1 minute before PCI, followed by a 4-µg/kg per minute infusion for the duration of the procedure or at least 2 hours. During infusion, cangrelor blocks binding of the active metabolites of the thienopyridines, clopidogrel, and prasugrel to the platelet $P2Y_{12}$ receptor and those active metabolites are present in blood for a relatively short interval after administration. For this reason, a loading dose of clopidogrel should be administered *after* cangrelor is stopped. Prasugrel loading can be administered at the end of the cangrelor infusion or up to 30 minutes before cangrelor is stopped. Because ticagrelor binds to a separate site on the

$P2Y_{12}$ receptor and there is no interaction between ticagrelor and cangrelor, ticagrelor loading can be administered before or during the infusion of cangrelor.

Recommendations

Collective evidence indicates that all patients with ACS and all patients undergoing PCI with stent implantation should receive DAPT, with aspirin and a $P2Y_{12}$ antagonist, in the absence of contraindications. Aspirin should be administered immediately and the $P2Y_{12}$ antagonist should be administered as early as feasible after presentation. The selection of the $P2Y_{12}$ antagonist from among the available choices requires an assessment of multiple factors considered in the context of the available clinical trial evidence and should be individualized with attention to clinical syndrome, comorbidities, timing, and a careful assessment of ischemic risk and bleeding risk. There may also be a need to consider medication adherence and cost issues. Prasugrel is indicated for ACS patients undergoing PCI, whereas clopidogrel and ticagrelor may be considered for ACS patients with or without revascularization. Clopidogrel and ticagrelor should be withheld for 5 days and prasugrel for 7 days prior to CABG surgery. For STEMI patients undergoing primary PCI who have not been adequately pretreated with a $P2Y_{12}$ antagonist, an intravenous cangrelor infusion at the time of PCI may be considered with subsequent transition to an oral $P2Y_{12}$ antagonist. Although recent evidence suggests that the duration of DAPT may be shortened for patients whose indication for PCI is stable ischemic heart disease, a full 12 months of DAPT is recommended for patients with ACS or those undergoing PCI in the setting of ACS.[30]

GLYCOPROTEIN IIB/IIIA ANTAGONISTS

The final common pathway of platelet aggregation involves crosslinking of activated platelets via binding of the platelet glycoprotein IIb/IIIa (GP IIb/IIIa) receptor to the divalent ligand, fibrinogen (see Fig. 12.1). The GP IIb/IIIa receptor is the most abundant protein on the surface of the platelet and, with platelet activation, it undergoes a conformational change exposing the receptor binding site in a high-affinity state. The GP IIb/IIIa receptor emerged as a therapeutic target to treat cardiovascular events with the isolation of monoclonal antibodies that block the binding of the receptor to fibrinogen and were shown in animal models of coronary thrombosis to improve patency rates after fibrinolysis and reduce rethrombosis.[79]

These early studies eventually led to the clinical development of the three currently available GP IIb/IIIa antagonists, abciximab, eptifibatide, and tirofiban. These agents were studied extensively in patients with ACS and patients undergoing PCI, where they were generally shown to reduce adverse ischemic outcomes with an increase in bleeding complications. Notably, the evidence supporting the use of intravenous GP IIb/IIIa receptor antagonists in patients with ACS was established before the common use of oral DAPT.

Abciximab

The humanized chimeric monoclonal antibody, abciximab, binds to the GP IIb/IIIa receptor with high avidity after intravenous administration. The Evaluation of 7E3 for the Prevention of Ischaemic Complications (EPIC), Evaluation in PTCA to Improve Long-Term Outcome with Abciximab GP IIb/IIIa Blockade (EPILOG) and Evaluation of Platelet IIb/IIIa Inhibition for Stenting (EPISTENT) trials showed that administration of abciximab as a bolus followed by a 12-hour infusion significantly reduced the incidence of adverse ischemic events among patients undergoing PCI, a benefit that seemed enhanced among troponin-positive ACS patients. A meta-analysis of trials of abciximab use during primary PCI for STEMI reported that abciximab was associated with significant reductions in mortality and recurrent MI.[80] Nevertheless, abciximab has been associated with significantly increased rates of bleeding,[81] raising questions regarding the benefit and safety of abciximab in the contemporary era when patients are commonly pretreated with a P2Y$_{12}$ antagonist.[82] However, abciximab may be useful as adjunctive therapy to reduce acute ischemic events among select high-risk patients undergoing primary PCI with stenting or as a provisional "bail-out" agent for thrombotic complications during PCI. Of note, abciximab is not indicated for upstream use in patients with NSTE ACS.

Tirofiban

Tirofiban is a synthetic, nonpeptide, small molecule inhibitor of the GP IIb/IIIa receptor on platelets. In the Platelet Receptor Inhibition in Ischemic Syndrome Management in Patients Limited by Unstable Signs and Symptoms (PRISM-PLUS) trial,[83] upstream intravenous tirofiban reduced adverse ischemic events, both prior to and following revascularization procedures in patients with NSTE ACS. Tirofiban is indicated for reducing thrombotic complications for patients with NSTE ACS. In early PCI trials with tirofiban, outcomes were not significantly improved by tirofiban but there was concern that dosing was inadequate to achieve optimal platelet inhibition. A higher-dose regimen was developed and tested, with potentially improved outcomes[84]; the higher-dose regimen is recommended in practice guidelines for operators choosing to use tirofiban to support primary PCI.[10]

Eptifibatide

Eptifibatide is a cyclic heptapeptide inhibitor of the GP IIb/IIIa receptor. It is administered as an intravenous bolus or double bolus and continuous infusion. In the Platelet Glycoprotein IIb/IIIa in Unstable Angina: Receptor Suppression Using Integrilin Therapy (PURSUIT) trial,[85] patients with NSTE ACS were randomized to receive "upstream" eptifibatide (a bolus dose of 180 µg/kg, followed by an infusion of 2.0 µg/kg/min) versus placebo with a mean duration of infusion of 72 hours. Treatment with eptifibatide resulted in reduced rates of death or MI with an increased risk of bleeding.[85]

In the Early Glycoprotein IIb/IIIa Inhibition in Non–ST-Segment Elevation Acute Coronary Syndrome (EARLY ACS) trial,[86] in which patients with NSTE ACS being treated by an invasive strategy were routinely treated with clopidogrel and aspirin before PCI, a strategy of early administration of eptifibatide was compared with delayed, provisional administration after angiography. The results showed that ischemic outcomes were not significantly improved by upstream eptifibatide and bleeding rates were increased.[86]

As a class, the GP IIb/IIIa antagonists appear to reduce adverse ischemic events among patients with high-risk ACS but with an increase in clinically significant bleeding. The risk of serious bleeding increases with age; thus, these agents should be used with care and attention to proper dosing in the elderly.

As a monoclonal antibody, abciximab is a large protein that is cleared by the reticuloendothelial system. It has a plasma half-life of 30 minutes but remains avidly bound to platelets (it can be detected bound to platelets up to 2 weeks following administration) and recovery of platelet function may take 12 hours. The dose does not need to be adjusted for renal insufficiency. Eptifibatide and tirofiban have plasma half-lives in the 1- to 3-hour range; platelet functional recovery is seen 4 to 8 hours after discontinuation of the drug. Since they are both renally excreted, doses should be adjusted for renal insufficiency and these agents should be avoided in patients with significant renal failure. When bleeding is encountered in a patient receiving abciximab or urgent surgery is required, platelet transfusions can be administered and redistribution of the abciximab molecules can reverse the antiplatelet effect. These agents have been associated with a risk of serious thrombocytopenia, although this is uncommon and more frequent with abciximab (3% to 5%) than with the other agents.

Recommendations

Since the results of EARLY ACS and other trials in the era of more common use of P2Y$_{12}$ antagonists and DAPT pretreatment prior to PCI raised questions regarding whether there was adequate benefit of GP IIb/IIIa inhibitors to justify the increased bleeding and other safety risks, their use has become limited. More recent guidelines suggest a limited role, such that adjunctive use of a GP IIb/IIIa antagonist may be considered on an individual basis for primary PCI when heparin is used as the anticoagulant in the setting of large thrombus burden, inadequate loading with a P2Y$_{12}$ antagonist or for provisional bail-out use for thrombotic complications; use of intracoronary abciximab may be reasonable in select cases. For primary PCI patients receiving bivalirudin as the anticoagulant, routine adjunctive use of GP IIb/IIIa inhibitors is not recommended but also may be considered as adjunctive or bail-out therapy in selected cases. Upstream eptifibatide or tirofiban may be considered for patients with NSTE ACS awaiting angiography in addition to a P2Y$_{12}$ antagonist for very-high-risk patients or potentially instead of a P2Y$_{12}$ antagonist in select patients when there is reluctance to load with a P2Y$_{12}$ antagonist due to concern about the need for urgent CABG surgery.

The ACC/AHA guidelines for use of antiplatelet therapy in STEMI are summarized in the Appendix.

β-BLOCKERS

Agents that block β-adrenergic receptors (β-blockers) exert multiple actions on the cardiovascular system. β-Blockers compete with catecholamines for binding to β-adrenergic receptors; β$_1$ receptors are primarily located in the myocardium and affect sinus node rate, atrioventricular (AV) node conduction velocity and contractility; β$_2$ receptors are primarily located in bronchial and vascular smooth muscle. β-Blockers act to slow heart rate, reduce blood pressure, and reduce cardiac contractility, resulting in decreased cardiac workload, reduced myocardial oxygen consumption, and prolongation of diastolic filling time and coronary perfusion, actions that may reduce myocardial damage in the setting of MI. Given acutely, β-blockers decrease infarct size in patients who do not receive reperfusion therapy, reduce the rate of reinfarction in patients who receive reperfusion therapy, and decrease the frequency of arrhythmias.[10]

The effects of β-blockers on outcome following acute MI have been extensively tested in randomized clinical trials. These trials used different agents, different timing of initiation, and different routes of administration, yet generally demonstrated evidence of class benefit, with certain limits discussed later. Regarding later initiation and long-term use in the prefibrinolytic era, the Norwegian multicenter study[87] randomized 1884 patients to receive timolol versus placebo started at 7 to 28 days after infarction. At 33 months, the timolol-treated group showed 39% and 28% lower rates of mortality and reinfarction, respectively. In the Beta-Blocker Heart Attack Trial (BHAT),[88] the nonselective β-blocker propranolol was initiated orally 5 to 21 days following MI. At an average 25-month follow-up, there was a highly significant (26%) reduction in total mortality among patients randomized to β-blocker versus placebo. Of note, benefit of allocation to β-blocker was greatest among patients at highest risk, including those with CHF and low ejection fraction (EF), patients in whom β-blockers were felt to be relatively contraindicated and uncommonly used in clinical practice at that time.

The benefit of early administration of β-blockers for acute MI was also tested in three major trials. The International Studies of Infarct Survival-1 (ISIS-1)[89] study compared intravenous followed by oral administration of the cardioselective β-blocker atenolol to placebo in patients within 12 hours of presentation with STEMI. Randomization to atenolol was associated with a significant (15%) relative reduction in mortality at 7 days. Subsequent retrospective analysis suggested that the majority of the reduction in mortality observed in the ISIS-1 trial occurred on the day of admission or the subsequent day, potentially by reducing cardiac rupture. In the Metoprolol in Acute Myocardial Infarction (MIAMI) trial,[90] intravenous initiation of the cardioselective β-blocker metoprolol (3 × 5 mg injections at 2-minute intervals) followed by oral dosing (200 mg daily) within 24 hours of onset of symptoms was compared with placebo among patients hospitalized with acute MI. After 15 days, there was a nonsignificant (13%) lower rate of death ($P = .29$) in the metoprolol group; in subgroup analysis that stratified patients according to risk, metoprolol was associated with no difference in mortality among low-risk patients but with a 29% lower mortality among the one-third of patients considered high risk. In the later Thrombolysis In Myocardial Infarction Phase II (TIMI-II) trial,[91] patients with STEMI who were treated with alteplase were randomly assigned to receive immediate intravenous followed by oral metoprolol or deferred metoprolol (given orally after day 6). At 6 weeks, there was no overall difference in mortality between the immediate intravenous and deferred groups, but the immediate intravenous group showed a lower incidence of reinfarction and recurrent chest pain at 6 days.

Many of the early trials of β-blocker use after acute MI did not enroll patients with CHF or LV dysfunction, an important high-risk group. The Carvedilol Post-Infarct Survival Control in Left-Ventricular Dysfunction (CAPRICORN) trial[92] compared carvedilol, a nonselective β-blocker with α_1-adrenergic receptor blocking activity, initiated 3 to 21 days after MI (at 6.25 mg orally twice daily and increased to 25 mg twice daily over 4–6 weeks) with placebo in patients after acute MI with an LVEF of 40% or less. At a mean follow-up of 15 months, all-cause mortality was 23% lower in the carvedilol group than in the placebo group ($P = .03$). Of note, a later analysis[93] also observed a 59% reduction in the occurrence of atrial fibrillation or atrial flutter and a 76% reduction in the occurrence of ventricular tachycardia or ventricular fibrillation with assignment to carvedilol treatment.

More recently, the COMMIT/CCS-2 study[94] randomized 45,852 patients within 24 hours of onset of suspected MI to receive metoprolol (intravenous followed by oral) or placebo. At a mean of 15 days follow-up, no difference was observed for the co-primary endpoints, a composite of death, reinfarction, and cardiac arrest. Compared with placebo, for 1000 patients allocated to metoprolol, there were five fewer reinfarctions and five fewer ventricular fibrillation events, a benefit counterbalanced by 11 more patients developing cardiogenic shock. The excess cardiogenic shock appeared to occur early, especially during days 0 to 1 after admission, while the reductions in reinfarction and ventricular fibrillation were observed later, resulting in overall hazard during days 0 to 1 and significant later benefit. Of importance, higher rates of cardiogenic shock were observed among patients with relative hemodynamic instability or particular high-risk characteristics, including older age, increased heart rate, lower blood pressure, and signs of CHF.

Although the data from COMMIT/CCS-2 suggest that caution should be advised when considering administration of β-blockers in the early phase (within 24 hours) of acute MI, longer-term use in the convalescent phase even among patients with relative contraindications has been found to be strongly beneficial and remains recommended. A retrospective analysis of 201,752 patients in the Cooperative Cardiovascular Project concluded that after acute MI, even patients with conditions that are traditionally considered contraindications to β-blockers—such as CHF, pulmonary disease, and older age—benefited significantly from β-blocker therapy.[95] However, there are patients in whom β-blockers should be avoided. One such group is patients with STEMI precipitated by use of cocaine. Because of the theoretical risk of exacerbating coronary spasm from unopposed α-adrenergic stimulation, β-blockers should not be administered in that circumstance.

A meta-analysis of the effect of intravenous followed by oral β-blocker therapy on death, reinfarction, and cardiac arrest during the scheduled treatment periods tested in over 50,000 patients in randomized trials, including MIAMI, ISIS-1, and the low-risk subset of COMMIT demonstrated highly significant (13% to 22%) relative risk reduction for adverse events from β-blocker therapy.[94]

Cardioselective β-blockers block β_1-receptors more than β_2-receptors and thus may be preferable for patients with pulmonary and peripheral vascular disease. Some β-blockers have intrinsic sympathomimetic activity, resulting in activation of the β-receptor with less slowing of heart rate, less prolongation of AV node conduction time, and less depression of LV function. Only β-blockers without intrinsic sympathomimetic activity have been shown to reduce mortality after MI; β-blockers with intrinsic sympathomimetic activity are not indicated for secondary prevention.[96]

The overall lack of benefit observed in the COMMIT/CCS-2[94] trial may have been due to the high doses of β-blocker given to hemodynamically unstable patients. Risk factors for cardiogenic shock from this study included older age, female sex, CHF, time delay in presentation, lower blood pressure, prior history of hypertension, and elevated heart rate. One point suggested by that study is that the administration of intravenous β-blockers should be targeted for specific indications, such as patients with ongoing chest pain at rest and no contraindications, such as CHF. The ACC/AHA guidelines recommend caution with the use of intravenous β-blockade, especially in patients who are at risk for cardiogenic shock.[8,10] The short-acting intravenous β-blocker esmolol may be considered for treatment of select patients with relative contraindications and/or higher risk of adverse consequences of β-blocker use, but data in the setting of STEMI are lacking. The long-term use of oral β-blockers is recommended for secondary prevention in high-risk patients, after they have been stabilized, with gradual dose titration. There have been no adequate trials of head-to-head comparisons of different β-blockers in the setting of STEMI or ACS.

One therapeutic target is a heart rate of 50 to 60 beats/min and/or a blunting of the rise in heart rate with light activity, unless there are side effects. The dose of β-blocker can be titrated up to specified targets (Table 12.2). Regarding the length of therapy, a meta-analysis showed that β-blockers exert their effect over time and 1 year of therapy may be necessary before mortality benefits can be appreciated.[97] The Cardiovascular Cooperative Project showed a reduction of mortality with β-blockers at 2 years, even in low-risk patients.[95]

The major side effects of β-blocker therapy include hypotension, bradycardia, AV block, worsening of CHF, and exacerbation of reactive airways disease.

Relative contraindications include chronic obstructive pulmonary disease (COPD) or asthma. Patients with mild pulmonary disease not taking β-agonists benefit from β-blockers after acute MI, but patients with severe COPD or asthma taking β-agonists do not benefit.[98] After 2 years, patients with COPD receiving β-blocker therapy had a higher survival rate than patients who did not receive therapy.[95] The concern that β-blocker therapy might worsen COPD or reactive airways disease has been addressed by one meta-analysis showing that cardioselective β-blockers do not worsen pulmonary function tests in patients with mild to moderate COPD or reactive airways disease.[99] Because the benefit of β-blockers is significant, lower initial doses of cardioselective β-blockers and careful uptitration is recommended. The diagnosis of COPD or asthma should be confirmed with pulmonary function testing if there is any question of the diagnosis.

In patients with evidence of CHF, acute β-blocker therapy is contraindicated, although long-term therapy is beneficial. Older β-blocker trials were done without angiotensin-converting enzyme (ACE) inhibitors and did not assess patients with asymptomatic LV dysfunction. Data from several ACE inhibitor trials in patients with asymptomatic LV dysfunction and symptomatic LV dysfunction show that β-blockers do have additive benefit to ACE inhibitors.[100–102] Regardless of the level of LV dysfunction, β-blockers improve survival and produce benefits in post-MI patients with preserved or decreased EF.[95] In patients with peripheral artery disease, there has been concern about worsening of claudication with β-blockers; however, multiple meta-analyses and a placebo-controlled trial have shown this concern to be unfounded.[103] Long-term β-blocker therapy in STEMI survivors shows mortality benefit despite revascularization with CABG surgery or PCI.[104]

Recommendations

β-Blocker therapy is recommended for all acute MI patients without a history of intolerance or contraindications.[10] A useful regimen is oral metoprolol tartrate starting at 12.5 to 25 mg and titrated every 6 hours to a therapeutic dose during the first 24 to 48 hours, at which point the dosing interval can be changed to every 12 hours by splitting the cumulative daily dose. A lower starting dose of 6.25 mg may be considered for patients at higher risk of adverse effects. Since some data have shown greater antihypertensive effects for carvedilol compared with metoprolol, likely due to its additional α-adrenergic blocking activity, carvedilol may be considered for patients with hypertension. β-Blockers may be especially useful and should be rapidly uptitrated to therapeutic levels for patients with severe hypertension, reflex tachycardia, rapid atrial fibrillation, or postinfarction angina. If tolerated, oral β-blocker therapy should be continued for at least 2 years and, in the absence of side effects, should be continued indefinitely. Relative contraindications to β-blocker therapy

TABLE 12.2	**Target Doses for β-Blockers**			
β-Blocker	**β Selectivity**	**Partial Agonist Activity**	**Target Dose**	
Acebutolol	β₁	Yes	200–600 mg twice daily	
Atenolol	β₁	No	50–200 mg daily	
Betaxolol	β₁	No	10–20 mg daily	
Bisoprolol	β₁	No	10 mg daily	
Carvedilol[a]	None	No	6.25 mg twice daily up to 25 mg twice daily	
Esmolol (intravenous)	β₁	No	50–300 µg/kg/min	
Labetalol[a]	None	Yes	200–600 mg daily	
Metoprolol	β₁	No	50–200 mg twice daily	
Nadolol	None	No	40–80 mg daily	
Pindolol	None	Yes	2.5–7.5 mg three times daily	
Propranolol	None	No	20–80 mg twice daily	
Timolol	None	No	10 mg twice daily	

Modified from Gibbons RJ, Chatterjee K, Daley J, et al. ACC/AHA/ACP-ASIM guidelines for the management of patients with chronic stable angina. *J Am Coll Cardiol.* 1999;33:2092–2197.
[a]Labetalol and carvedilol are combined α- and β-blockers. Drugs are listed alphabetically and not in order of preference.

include heart rate less than 60 beats/min, systolic blood pressure less than 100 mm Hg, moderate to severe LV dysfunction with CHF, shock, PR interval greater than 0.24 second, second-degree or third-degree AV block, active asthma, reactive airways disease, and MI induced by cocaine use. The ACC/AHA guidelines for use of β-blockers in STEMI are summarized in the Appendix.

NITRATES

Nitrates have been used for the management of ACS for more than a century. Nitrate therapy promotes hemodynamic effects that are theoretically attractive for patients with acute MI. Administration of nitrates results in endothelium-independent release of nitric oxide, direct relaxation of vascular smooth muscle and dose-related vasodilation.[105] Nitrates may also produce vasodilation indirectly through the endothelial release of PGI_2 and may exert antiplatelet and antithrombotic effects.[106] Nitroglycerin directly dilates coronary arteries, which may relieve vasoconstriction at or adjacent to sites of thrombotic obstruction or at sites occluded owing to primary coronary vasospasm and promotes collateral flow to ischemic regions,[107] resulting in improved myocardial perfusion. Nitrates promote venodilation, resulting in a reduction in LV preload, chamber size, and wall stress.[105] Reducing preload and afterload decreases myocardial oxygen demand, which reduces myocardial ischemia and, therefore, potentially limiting myocardial infarct size. However, nitrates may also cause hypotension, resulting in decreased coronary perfusion that could be detrimental in the acute phase of acute MI.[108] Prolonged nitroglycerin infusions at high doses may produce tolerance.[109]

A pooled analysis of seven controlled randomized trials in 851 patients with acute MI conducted before the reperfusion era suggested a significant (48%) reduction in mortality by intravenous nitroglycerin.[110] The effect of nitrates on mortality was later tested in two large-scale randomized, controlled, factorial design trials, Gruppo Italiano per lo Studio della Sopravvivenza nell'Infarto Miocardico (GISSI)-3[111] and the Fourth International Study of Infarct Survival (ISIS-4).[112] In the GISSI-3 trial, 19,394 acute MI patients within 24 hours of symptom onset were randomly assigned to nitrate therapy (intravenous glyceryl trinitrate [GTN] for the first 24 hours followed by transdermal GTN 10 mg daily) or open control. At 6-week follow-up, GTN did not significantly improve outcome, resulting in a nonsignificant (6%) reduction in all-cause mortality. In ISIS-4, 58,050 patients up to 24 hours after the onset of suspected acute MI were randomized to receive 1 month of oral mononitrate (30 mg initial dose titrated up to 60 mg once daily) or placebo. At 5-week follow-up, there was no significant reduction in mortality in patients randomized to mononitrate.

A pooled analysis[112] of more than 80,000 patients treated intravenously or orally with nitrates suggested a significant (5.5%) relative reduction in short-term mortality by nitrate therapy. This effect translates into 3 to 4 fewer deaths for every 1000 treated patients.

Low-dose intravenous nitroglycerin can be administered safely to patients with evolving anterior STEMI; dose titration avoids hypotension, tachycardia, or bradycardia. Patients with inferior STEMI are more sensitive to preload reduction, especially if right ventricular infarction is present. Intravenous nitroglycerin can be recommended in the treatment of acute MI, provided that the initial systolic blood pressure is not less than 90 mm Hg. Guidelines support the use of nitroglycerin for suppressing ongoing myocardial ischemic pain and for managing acute MI complicated by CHF or pulmonary edema, along with close monitoring of blood pressure and heart rate to detect hypotension, tachycardia, or bradycardia and to avoid myocardial hypoperfusion.

The ACC/AHA guidelines[8] recognized the usefulness of low-dose intravenous nitroglycerin infusion in titrating therapy to the blood pressure response and suggested that the infusion should begin at 5 to 10 μg/min with increases of 5 to 20 μg/min until symptoms are relieved or mean blood pressure is reduced by 10% of the baseline level in normotensive patients and by up to 30% in hypertensive patients, but not below a systolic pressure of 90 mm Hg.

In contrast to acute STEMI, higher doses of nitrates have been used in unstable angina and CHF. Nitrates are available in many forms, including intravenous, sublingual sprays, rapid-acting and dissolving tablets, long-acting tablets, and slow-release patches. Use of nitrates does not preclude use of other antianginal drugs, such as β-blockers. Patients with ACS and CHF also benefit from nitrates. Nitrates should be avoided in STEMI patients with hypotension, bradycardia, tachycardia, or right ventricular infarction. They are contraindicated in patients taking phosphodiesterase inhibitors and should not be given within 24 hours of taking sildenafil, 48 hours of taking tadalafil, and probably within 24 hours of taking vardenafil.[113] Tolerance to nitrate therapy typically develops after 24 hours. If intravenous nitroglycerin is still required after tolerance develops, the dosage may need to be increased. Lower doses or nitrate-free intervals prevent the development of tolerance.

Recommendations

Based on lack of a proven long-term survival benefit in those large trials, routine nitrate therapy is not recommended in STEMI patients. However, selective use should be considered to ameliorate symptoms and signs of myocardial ischemia and may be useful to treat patients with STEMI and hypertension or CHF, as discussed earlier. The side-effect profile of nitrates includes hypotension, tachycardia, bradycardia, and headache. Rarely, methemoglobinemia can develop. Patients with inferior STEMI, especially right ventricular infarction, are more sensitive to preload reduction. Continuous long-term use of nitrates results in the development of tolerance. The ACC/AHA guidelines for nitrate use in STEMI are summarized in the Appendix.

ANGIOTENSIN-CONVERTING ENZYME INHIBITORS AND OTHER RENIN-ANGIOTENSIN-ALDOSTERONE SYSTEM INHIBITORS

Inhibition of the conversion of angiotensin I to angiotensin II by ACE inhibition, and of the binding of angiotensin to its receptor, result in vasodilation and reduction in LV afterload. These hemodynamic effects, as well as putative local tissue–level effects within the myocardium and vasculature, may result in beneficial effects on LV wall stress and remodeling, translating into clinical benefit. ACE inhibitors and angiotensin receptor blocker (ARBs) have emerged as effective adjunctive agents for preventing LV remodeling and improving survival after MI, and are recommended for the early management of acute STEMI.[10]

The renin-angiotensin-aldosterone system (RAAS) regulates blood pressure and extracellular volume. The pathway for the formation of angiotensin II (the primary effector molecule of the RAAS) begins with angiotensinogen, secreted by the liver, and its conversion to angiotensin I by renin, and conversion of angiotensin I to angiotensin II by ACE followed by subsequent degradation of angiotensin II. Angiotensin II, acting mainly via angiotensin II type 1 (AT_1) receptors,[114] exerts several important physiologic actions, including vasoconstriction as well as aldosterone and catecholamine release.

Angiotensin-Converting Enzyme Inhibitors

The beneficial physiologic effects of ACE inhibitors are related mainly to inhibition of ACE and kininase. ACE inhibition results in decreased activity of RAAS; decreased formation of angiotensin II; decreased catecholamine secretion, inotropic stimulation, heart rate, and vasoconstrictor tone; and improved collateral flow. Kininase inhibition contributes to vasodilation. The net results include increased venous capacitance and decreased preload, decreased afterload, improved perfusion, decreased infarct size, decreased chamber size and wall stress, and decreased ventricular dilation.

ACE inhibitors do not block the formation of angiotensin II that occurs via alternate pathways, and they do not prevent all aldosterone formation. ARBs selectively block the effects of angiotensin II via AT_1 receptors,[114] and aldosterone antagonists block the mineralocorticoid receptor, aldosterone. Angiotensin II degradation by ACE2 leads to formation of angiotensin-(1-7), a vasodilator that is increased during ACE inhibitor and ARB therapy and may contribute to their cardioprotective effects.[115] The rationale for using aldosterone blockade is that angiotensin II stimulates the release of aldosterone, activating the mineralocorticoid receptor. The activation of the mineralocorticoid receptor persists despite the use of ACE inhibitors, ARBs, and β-blockers.

Several clinical studies have examined the effect of very early and prolonged ACE inhibition after MI. In the Survival and Ventricular Enlargement (SAVE) trial,[116] 2231 patients with an EF of 40% or less but without overt heart failure or symptoms of myocardial ischemia were randomly assigned at 3 to 16 days after MI to receive captopril or placebo and followed for a mean of 42 months. The captopril group showed a significant (19%) reduction in all-cause mortality, a 37% reduction in the development of severe CHF, and a 25% reduction in recurrent MI. The SAVE trial showed a correlation between limitation of LV dilation and clinical benefits.[117] The collective evidence indicates that ACE inhibitor therapy after MI attenuates or delays ventricular remodeling.[118,119] This therapeutic benefit is attributed in large part to inhibition of the effects of angiotensin II and is supported by findings of increased ACE expression at the edge

of infarct scars and markedly increased LV dilation in patients with the ACE-DD genotype that is associated with increased ACE activity.[120]

Early administration of an ACE inhibitor in the acute phase of MI was tested in the second Cooperative New Scandinavian Enalapril Survival Study (CONSENSUS II),[121] in which 6090 patients presenting with acute MI were randomized within 24 hours of symptom onset to receive intravenous followed by oral enalapril or placebo. At 6 months, there was no difference in all-cause mortality by treatment assignment and, unexpectedly, the incidence of death due to progressive heart failure was increased by 26% in the enalapril group ($P = .06$). Early hypotension was significantly more frequent in the enalapril than placebo group and raised significant new concerns of hazard for ACE inhibitor administration in the early phase of AMI.

Two subsequent large-scale studies demonstrated benefit for early initiation of oral ACE inhibitor therapy among patients with AMI with or without evidence of CHF or LV dysfunction. Both the GISSI-3[111] and ISIS-4[112] trials compared an oral ACE inhibitor initiated within 24 hours of symptom onset to placebo by random assignment of very large cohorts of acute MI patients. The GISSI-3 trial randomized 19,394 patients with acute MI to lisinopril (5 mg initial dose and then 10 mg daily) or placebo, and reported a significant (12%) reduction in 6-week mortality with lisinopril treatment. The ISIS-4 trial randomized 58,050 patients with acute MI to captopril (6.25 mg initial dose titrated up to 50 mg twice daily) or placebo and reported a significant (7%) reduction in 5-week mortality with captopril treatment. These favorable results translated into approximately five lives saved per thousand treated patients by early oral administration of ACE inhibitors for patients with acute MI.

Beneficial effects of oral ACE inhibitors started early after onset of MI were also demonstrated for ramipril in the Acute Infarction Ramipril Efficacy (AIRE) trial[122] and zofenopril in the Survival of Myocardial Infarction Long-Term Evaluation (SMILE) trial.[123] Of note, with respect to long-term benefit, extended follow-up of the AIRE trial suggested that 5-year all-cause mortality was reduced 36% among patients assigned to ramipril compared to placebo. In total, 11 studies have shown improved survival conferred by ACE inhibitor use (Table 12.3),[111,112,116,122–128] and randomized clinical trials involving more than 100,000 patients have demonstrated that early ACE inhibitor use among patients with MI without contraindications significantly reduces the risk of death and major nonfatal cardiovascular events, with a benefit of 4.6 fewer deaths for every 1000 patients treated with ACE inhibitors.[129] The greatest benefits from long-term ACE inhibitor therapy are observed in high-risk patients with LV dysfunction, signs or symptoms of CHF, or both. Patients with anterior MI, age 55 to 74 years, and a heart rate greater than 80 beats/min appear to derive greater benefit.[129] Benefit occurs early, with approximately 40% of prevented deaths in the first 7 days.

Based on data showing early benefit of oral ACE inhibitor therapy in STEMI, therapy should be given early, within 24 hours, provided that there is no hypotension or other contraindications or allergy to ACE inhibitors.[10] In the ISIS-4 trial,[112] when patients were treated early with captopril, 44 deaths were prevented on

TABLE 12.3 Major Trials of Angiotensin-Converting Enzyme Inhibitors in Heart Failure and Myocardial Infarction

Trial	N	Disease	Drug	Onset	Duration	Outcome
CONSENSUS, 1987[126]	253	HF	Enalapril	—	20 mo	27% ↓ mortality; ↓ morbidity
SOLVD (symptomatic), 1991[124]	2569	HF	Enalapril	≥4 wk	41.4 mo	16% ↓ mortality; ↓ morbidity
SOLVD (asymptomatic), 1992[125]	4228	HF	Enalapril	≥4 wk	37.4 mo	8% ↓ mortality (NS); ↓ morbidity
CONSENSUS II, 1992	6090	MI	Enalapril	<24 h	6 mo	No decrease in mortality; hypotension
SAVE, 1992[116]	512	MI	Captopril	3–16 d	42 mo	19% ↓ mortality; ↓ morbidity
AIRE, 1993[122]	2006	MI	Ramipril	3–10 d	15 mo	27% ↓ mortality; ↓ morbidity
GISSI-3, 1994[111]	19,394	MI	Lisinopril	≤24 h	6 wk	11% ↓ mortality; ↓ morbidity
ISIS-4, 1995[112]	58,050	MI	Captopril	≤24 h	35 d	7% ↓ mortality; ↓ morbidity
TRACE, 1995[127]	6676	MI	Trandolapril	3–7 d	24 mo	34.7% ↓ mortality; ↓ morbidity
CCS-1, 1995[128]	13,634	MI	Captopril	≤36 h	1 mo	6% ↓ mortality; ↓ morbidity
SMILE, 1995[123]	1556	MI	Zofenopril	≤24 h	6 wk	29% ↓ mortality; ↓ morbidity
GISSI-3 (6-mo effects), 1996[201]	19,394	MI	Lisinopril	≤24 h	6 wk	6.2% ↓ mortality and LV dysfunction combined
HEART, 1997[202]	352	MI	Ramipril	≤24 h	1–14 d	↓ LV remodeling

Modified from Jugdutt BI. Valsartan in the treatment of heart attack survivors. *Vasc Health Risk Management*. 2006;2:125–138.
HF, Heart failure; *LV*, left ventricular; *MI*, myocardial infarction; *NS*, nonsignificant.

days 0 to 1, 37 deaths were prevented on days 2 to 7, and 62 deaths were prevented later. In the GISSI-3 trial,[111] patients given lisinopril within 24 hours showed early benefit, with 21 fewer deaths on days 0 to 1, 42 fewer deaths on days 2 to 7, and 12 fewer deaths later.[130]

Based on the ISIS-4 and GISSI-3 data, where the maximum dose of ACE inhibitor was achieved within 48 hours, the dose of ACE inhibitor should be rapidly titrated upward to achieve the full dose by 24 to 48 hours. Besides reperfusion and aspirin, ACE inhibitor therapy is the only other therapy shown to reduce 30-day mortality when CHF complicates STEMI. The survival benefit of ACE inhibitor therapy seems to be a class effect. The optimal duration of ACE inhibitor therapy has not been determined, especially in patients who are asymptomatic, normotensive, or non-diabetic with normal LV function. In STEMI patients, the general consensus is that ACE inhibitor therapy should be continued indefinitely.[10]

Angiotensin Receptor Blockers

Despite their proven clinical efficacy for patients with CHF and MI, not all patients tolerate ACE inhibitors. Some patients may develop intractable cough because of the effect of ACE inhibitors on kininases in the lungs. It has been recognized that ACE inhibitors are capable of blocking only part of the total production of angiotensin II in the cardiovascular system. Therefore, consideration was given to the concept that agents that directly block the angiotensin type I receptor, or ARBs, might theoretically provide equal or even superior benefit. Several trials investigated the benefits of ARBs in patients with MI and CHF, using an ACE inhibitor as comparator and on top of background therapy (Table 12.4).

In the Optimal Trial in Myocardial Infarction with Angiotensin II Antagonist Losartan (OPTIMAAL),[131] 5477 patients with CHF after acute MI were randomly assigned to losartan (50 mg once daily) or captopril (50 mg three times daily). Unexpectedly, at an average of 2.7 years, there was a nonsignificant ($P = 0.07$) relative (13%) increase in the rate of all-cause death and a

significant increase in the rate of death from cardiovascular causes seen in the losartan group, although losartan was significantly better tolerated than captopril.

In the subsequent Valsartan in Acute Myocardial Infarction Trial (VALIANT),[132] the ARB valsartan was compared with captopril and the combination of valsartan and captopril by random assignment of 14,808 patients with acute MI complicated by LV systolic dysfunction, CHF or both, with treatment initiated at 0.5 to 10 days after acute MI. At 25 months, there was no difference between valsartan and captopril observed with respect to all-cause mortality and in the rate of fatal and nonfatal cardiovascular events; combining valsartan with captopril in VALIANT increased the rate of adverse events without improving survival. Of note, valsartan met the prespecified criteria for noninferiority compared with captopril; the study concluded that valsartan started after acute MI was as effective as captopril, an agent with proven efficacy in reducing adverse events after MI. Therefore, ARBs represent an alternative approach to the inhibition of the renin–angiotensin system for patients after MI who do not tolerate ACE inhibitors.

This study established that valsartan was as effective as captopril in reducing mortality in high-risk patients after MI. The authors also performed a statistical comparison of the VALIANT results with the results of the SAVE, AIRE, and Trandolapril Cardiac Evaluation (TRACE) trials using an imputed placebo and showed that the 25% risk reduction in all-cause mortality in VALIANT was comparable to reductions in the ACE inhibitor trials. The finding that the valsartan plus captopril combination increased adverse events, including hypotension, underscores the need for careful monitoring of blood pressure when combining RAAS inhibitors after MI and supports the concern for vasodilator-induced hypotension in acute MI.

Aldosterone Antagonists

Aldosterone appears to affect multiple processes that may be deleterious to cardiovascular physiology, including plasma volume homeostasis, electrolyte balance, inflammation, collagen

TABLE 12.4 **Major Trials of Angiotensin Receptor Blockers in Heart Failure and Myocardial Infarction**

Trial	N	Disease	Angiotensin Receptor Blocker	Comparator	Outcome
ELITE, 1997[203]	722	HF	Losartan	Captopril	Unexpected 46% ↓ in mortality (secondary endpoint)
RESOLVD, 1999[204]	768	HF	Candesartan	Enalapril	Early trend in ↑ mortality and HF (secondary endpoint)
ELITE II, 2000[205]	3152	HF	Losartan	Captopril	Not superior
Val-HeFT, 2001[206]	5010	HF	Valsartan	ACE inhibitor	Not superior; ↓ composite endpoint
OPTIMAAL, 2002[131]	5477	MI	Losartan	Captopril	Not superior (noninferiority criteria not met)
CHARM—Overall, 2003[207]	7601	HF	Candesartan	ACE inhibitor	Improved primary outcome (mortality and morbidity)
CHARM—Added, 2003[208]	2548	HF	Candesartan	ACE inhibitor	Improved primary outcome (clinical, morbidity)
CHARM—Alternative, 2003[209]	2028	HF	Candesartan	ACE inhibitor	Improved primary outcome (mortality and morbidity)
CHARM—Preserved, 2003[210]	3023	HF	Candesartan	ACE inhibitor	Similar primary outcome (improved secondary outcome)
VALIANT, 2003[132]	14,703	MI	Valsartan	Captopril	Not superior, noninferior

Modified from Jugdutt BI. Valsartan in the treatment of heart attack survivors. *Vasc Health Risk Management.* 2006;2:125–138.
ACE, Angiotensin-converting enzyme; *HF,* heart failure; *MI,* myocardial infarction.

formation, myocardial fibrosis, and remodeling. The aldosterone blocker, spironolactone, was shown to reduce adverse events, including death in patients with severe CHF due to chronic LV systolic dysfunction.[133] With this as background, the Eplerenone Post–Acute Myocardial Infarction Heart Failure Efficacy and Survival Study (EPHESUS)[134] tested the use of the aldosterone antagonist eplerenone in patients with acute MI complicated by LV systolic dysfunction. In EPHESUS, 6632 patients were included, with these characteristics: 3 to 14 days after an acute MI with an LVEF of 40% or less and CHF documented by rales or an S3 on exam or chest radiograph, or at high risk by presence of diabetes. Any patient was excluded with serum creatinine greater than 2.5 mg/dL, with serum potassium greater than 5.0 mmoL/L or receiving a potassium-sparing diuretic. At a mean follow-up of 16 months, eplerenone was associated with a highly significant (15%) lower rate of all-cause mortality and 21% reduction in sudden cardiac death compared to placebo. The rate of serious hyperkalemia was increased by 1.6% in the eplerenone group. The benefit of eplerenone was observed among patients who were already treated optimally with ACE inhibitors, ARBs, diuretics, and β-blockers at the time of randomization, suggesting that the addition of eplerenone to optimal medical therapy can reduce mortality and morbidity among patients with acute MI complicated by LV dysfunction, CHF, or diabetes, with a small but significant risk of serious hyperkalemia.

Given the relatively high risk of sudden death within the first 30 days following acute MI complicated by LV dysfunction recently highlighted by data from VALIANT[135] and the lack of proven benefit of implantable cardioverter defibrillators to reduce that risk,[136] it is notable that additional analyses of the EPHESUS data suggested that within 30 days after randomization, eplerenone reduced the risk of sudden cardiac death by 37% (*P* = .051)[137] and among those at very high risk (EF ≤30%) by 58% (*P* = .008).[138]

Adverse Effects of ACE Inhibitors, ARBs, and Aldosterone Blockers

ACE inhibitors and ARBs can cause hypotension that may be symptomatic or hazardous in the setting of acute MI, acute renal failure, hyperkalemia and, rarely, angioedema. The risk of first-dose hypotension can be minimized by starting with a low dose or not beginning therapy if the patient is volume depleted and by holding or discontinuing diuretic therapy. An elevation in serum creatinine and reduction in glomerular filtration rate may be observed in some patients treated with ACE inhibitors or ARBs and is more common among patients who have bilateral renal artery stenosis, hypertensive nephrosclerosis, CHF, polycystic kidney disease, or chronic kidney disease. The rate of acute renal failure is 1% to 2%. With a glomerular filtration rate (GFR) decline of more than 30%, ACE inhibitor or ARB therapy should be stopped and the GFR allowed to return to normal.[139] ACE inhibitors and ARBs reduce aldosterone secretion, thereby impairing the efficiency of urinary potassium excretion, which can result in hyperkalemia in 3% to 4% of patients. It is more common in diabetic patients taking NSAIDs, patients taking potassium-sparing diuretics, and elderly patients.[140] The risk of acute renal failure and hyperkalemia mandate serial monitoring of serum potassium and creatinine after initiation of these agents.

Angioedema is a rare but potentially fatal complication that occurs in 0.1% to 0.7% of patients treated with ACE inhibitors.[141,142] Risk factors for angioedema include African-American race, a history of prior drug rash, age older than 65 years, and a history of seasonal allergies. Angioedema usually develops within the first week of therapy, but delayed reactions several years later have been reported. There is a high risk of recurrence if ACE inhibitor therapy is resumed after stopping owing to angioedema.[143] Angioedema has also been associated with ARB therapy despite the belief that ARBs do not affect kinin metabolism but is less common than with ACE inhibitors.[144] Patients started on ARB therapy after ACE inhibitor–induced angioedema have a higher risk of angioedema than the general population,[145] but no large trials have quantified this risk. A small retrospective review showed that 2 of 26 patients who were thought to have angioedema from ACE inhibitor therapy and switched to ARB therapy developed recurrent angioedema.[145] A careful risk–benefit assessment should be done before starting a patient who had angioedema from an ACE inhibitor on ARB therapy.[146]

A dry, hacking cough that has been described in 5% to 10% of patients treated with an ACE inhibitor may require discontinuation of the drug. The mechanism responsible for ACE inhibitor–induced cough appears to be related to increased local concentrations of kinins, substance P, prostaglandins, and thromboxane from ACE inhibitor actions on converting enzyme and kininases in the lungs.[146] Cough is much less common with ARBs, which can be substituted for patients intolerant of ACE inhibitors owing to cough. ACE inhibitors and ARBs are contraindicated during pregnancy because of the risk of renal toxicity in the fetus. The side effects of aldosterone receptor blockers include hyperkalemia and hypotension. Spironolactone can result in painful gynecomastia in men or menstrual irregularities in women. Eplerenone, being a selective mineralocorticoid blocker, does not have those side effects.

Recommendations

In view of extensive experience with ACE inhibitors in STEMI, ACE inhibitors remain the preferred RAAS inhibitor; ARBs are used in ACE inhibitor–intolerant patients.[10] Among patients with STEMI with and without LV systolic dysfunction, early initiation (within 24 hours) of oral ACE inhibitors and continued long-term treatment to reduce mortality and recurrent cardiovascular events is recommended. For STEMI patients intolerant of ACE inhibitors, ARBs also have demonstrated efficacy; valsartan is recommended as an alternative to an ACE inhibitor in ACE inhibitor–intolerant patients with a target dose of 160 mg twice daily. The aldosterone blocker eplerenone is recommended for STEMI patients with LV systolic dysfunction and an LVEF of 40% or less and either symptomatic CHF or diabetes without significant renal dysfunction or hyperkalemia who are already receiving therapeutic doses of an ACE inhibitor or ARB. Recommendations for initial and target doses of ACE inhibitors, ARBs, and aldosterone blockers are shown in Table 12.5. ACC/AHA guidelines for use of ACE inhibitors and other RAAS inhibitors in STEMI are summarized in the Appendix.

CALCIUM CHANNEL BLOCKERS

Calcium channel blockers (CCBs) have established efficacy in treating angina and hypertension. CCBs block the entry of calcium into cells or transmembrane calcium flux through voltage-dependent L-type and T-type calcium channels. The major sites of action are the vascular smooth muscle cells, cardiomyocytes, and sinoatrial and AV node cells. CCBs inhibit the slow inward calcium current, exert a negative inotropic effect on myocardium, and dilate vascular smooth muscle. As vasodilators, CCBs reduce myocardial oxygen demand and increase supply and are effective anti-ischemic and spasmolytic agents. They also reduce myocardial oxygen demand by decreasing heart rate and contractility. Despite experimental and clinical evidence of anti-ischemic, cardioprotective, and anti-remodeling effects, clinical trials and systematic reviews have raised concern about increased mortality with routine use of CCBs in acute MI.

The effect of early administration of the short-acting dihydropyridine CCB nifedipine on outcome after acute MI was

TABLE 12.5   Initial and Target Doses for Renin-Angiotensin-Aldosterone System Inhibitors

Drug	Initial Dose	Target Dose
ACE Inhibitors		
Captopril	6.25 mg three times daily	50 mg three times daily
Enalapril	2.5 mg twice daily	10–20 mg twice daily
Fosinopril	5–10 mg daily	40 mg daily
Lisinopril	2.5–5 mg daily	20–40 mg daily
Perindopril	2 mg daily	8–16 mg daily
Quinapril	5 mg twice daily	20 mg twice daily
Ramipril	1.25–2.5 mg daily	10 mg daily
Trandolapril	1 mg daily	4 mg daily
Angiotensin Receptor Blockers		
Candesartan	4–8 mg daily	32 mg daily
Losartan	25–50 mg daily	50–100 mg daily
Valsartan	20–40 mg daily	160 mg daily
Aldosterone Antagonists		
Eplerenone	25 mg daily	50 mg daily
Spironolactone	12.5–25 mg daily	25 mg daily or twice daily

Modified from Hunt SA. ACC/AHA 2005 Guideline Update for the Diagnosis and Management of Chronic Heart Failure in the Adult. *J Am Coll Cardiol* 2005;46:e1–e82.
Drugs are listed alphabetically and not in order of preference.

compared with placebo in two randomized trials involving 1177 patients.[147,148] Notably, in pooled results from these two trials, short-term mortality was significantly increased (60%) in the nifedipine-treated patients. Short-acting nifedipine should therefore not be administered to patients in the early phase of STEMI.

The effects of administration of the nondihydropyridine CCBs, verapamil and diltiazem, initiated later after acute MIs, were studied in the Danish Verapamil Infarction Trial (DAVIT II)[149] and the Multicenter Diltiazem Post-Infarction Trial (MDPIT),[150] respectively. In DAVIT II, 1775 patients 7 to 15 days were randomly assigned to verapamil or placebo. At a mean follow-up of 16 months, there was a nonsignificant (20%) lower rate of death in the verapamil group; in a subgroup analysis, among patients without heart failure in the coronary care unit, the mortality rate was reduced by 36% by verapamil ($P = .02$). In the study of acute non-Q-wave MI involving 576 patients who were randomized 24 to 72 hours after the onset of symptoms to diltiazem or placebo and followed for 14 days, assignment to diltiazem was associated with a significant (51%) reduction in the incidence of reinfarction and a 50% reduction in the frequency of refractory postinfarction angina. In MDPIT, 2466 patients were randomly assigned to receive diltiazem or placebo 3 to 15 days after acute MI and followed for a mean of 25 months. Overall mortality and adverse cardiac events were similar in the diltiazem and placebo groups, but a significant interaction was observed between diltiazem treatment and pulmonary congestion (detected radiographically) or LV systolic dysfunction (EF < 40%). Among the more than 75% of trial participants without pulmonary congestion, diltiazem conferred benefit with a significant (23%) reduction in adverse cardiac events; in the nearly 20% of patients with pulmonary congestion or LV dysfunction, diltiazem was associated with a significant (41%) increase in adverse cardiac events.[150]

A meta-analysis of the trials indicated that CCBs did not reduce mortality or morbidity in acute MI.[151] The main side effects of CCBs are hypotension, bradycardia, AV block, and worsening CHF. Potential risk to the fetus requires caution in pregnant patients.

Recommendations

In aggregate, these results suggest that, while the nondihydropyridine CCBs verapamil and diltiazem may be beneficial after acute MI for patients with no signs of CHF and preserved LV systolic function, they should be avoided for any patient with CHF or LV systolic dysfunction. Even among patients with preserved EF after AMI, the weight of evidence favors long-term use of β-blockers for all patients without contraindications, which should not be limited by prior use of CCBs. The nondihydropyridine CCBs, such as verapamil and diltiazem, may be useful for heart rate control for tachyarrhythmias when β-blocker therapy is contraindicated or ineffective. Verapamil, diltiazem, and amlodipine can be useful for treatment of angina or hypertension in select patients after STEMI when β-blockers (and/or nitrates) are ineffective, not tolerated, or contraindicated and in whom there are no serious contraindications. Routine use of CCBs in patients with STEMI, however, is not recommended (see the Appendix).

ANTIDYSRHYTHMIC THERAPY

Cardiac arrhythmias are common after STEMI both before and after reperfusion. Most episodes of ventricular fibrillation (VF) and ventricular tachycardia (VT) occur in the first 48 hours. As many as 10% of patients receiving fibrinolytic therapy in the GUSTO-I trial had sustained ventricular arrhythmias complicating their hospital course.[152] The prophylactic use of lidocaine in early MI, a routine therapy in the prefibrinolytic era, is no longer recommended and, in general, antidysrhythmic drugs should be used with great caution in patients with acute MI. In the GUSTO-I and GUSTO-IIb trials, the prophylactic use of lidocaine in STEMI patients showed no mortality benefit.[153] A meta-analysis of lidocaine use in 14 trials found a 33% reduction in the risk of primary VF, but no mortality benefit and an increased risk of bradycardia and fatal asystole.[154]

The Cardiac Arrhythmia Suppression Trial (CAST)[155] was a double-blind, randomized, controlled study designed to test the hypothesis that suppression of frequent premature ventricular complexes (PVC) with class I antidysrhythmic agents after acute MI would reduce mortality. In CAST, patients randomly assigned to receive the class I antidysrhythmic drugs (encainide, flecainide, and moricizine) showed effective suppression of the PVCs and nonsustained VT, but had worse outcomes; mortality was significantly greater among patients prescribed encainide and flecainide than patients given placebo. The results of CAST dramatically altered management of ventricular ectopy following acute MI; use of class I antidysrhythmic drugs in that setting is generally avoided.

Recommendations

A conservative approach to arrhythmia management is recommended, with close monitoring during the early post-MI period. Evidence that intravenous β-blockers decrease early VF[156] supports the routine early use of β-blockers for patients with or showing high risk for VT or VF. For significant ventricular arrhythmias, the use of intravenous amiodarone and lidocaine may be considered, in accordance with the Adult Advanced Cardiovascular Life Support 2015 American Heart Association Guidelines Update for Cardiopulmonary Resuscitation and Emergency Cardiovascular Care.[157] The ACC/AHA guidelines of ventricular arrhythmia management in STEMI are summarized in the Appendix.

MORPHINE AND OTHER ANALGESIC AGENTS

Pain relief is an important aspect of the early management of acute MI; morphine sulfate is the analgesic of choice for managing pain in these patients. Morphine binds to central nervous system receptors, preventing them from transmitting pain signals to the brain. In acute MI, morphine has analgesic, anxiolytic, and hemodynamic properties. It relieves pain that contributes to the hyperadrenergic state, decreases blood pressure via arterial dilation and venodilation, decreases heart rate via increased vagal tone and withdrawal of sympathetic tone, decreases myocardial oxygen demand, and relieves pulmonary edema. A dose of 1 to 4 mg intravenously, repeated at 5- to 15-minute intervals, is commonly used.[10]

The most common side effects of morphine are nausea and vomiting, presenting in 20% of patients. Adverse effects include hypotension, especially prominent in patients who are volume depleted, have been given vasodilator therapy, or have infarction of the right ventricle. Treatment of morphine-induced hypotension includes placing the patient in a supine or Trendelenburg position and administering intravenous saline boluses, with the addition of atropine (0.5 to 1.5 mg intravenously) for concomitant bradycardia. Rarely, the narcotic antidote naloxone (0.4 to 2 mg intravenously) or an inotropic agent may be needed. Respiratory compromise from morphine overdose can be treated with naloxone and, very rarely, may require intubation for respiratory support. Other narcotics should be considered in patients with severe side effects or allergic reactions to morphine.

It is noteworthy that an observational study reported increased mortality in NSTE ACS patients treated with morphine,[158] and has led the ACC/AHA to downgrade its recommendation from class I to class IIb.[9] More recent analyses have shown that morphine administration is associated with a significant delay in onset of effective platelet inhibition by clopidogrel,[159] ticagrelor,[160] and prasugrel[161] in patients undergoing primary PCI for STEMI, potentially by delaying gastric emptying and/or gastrointestinal absorption of the drugs.

Evidence from multiple observational studies has suggested that NSAIDs and COX-2 inhibitors (COXIBs) may be associated with an increased risk of adverse events among patients with MI receiving antiplatelet therapy, potentially due to interactions that compete with the beneficial actions of aspirin. Nonselective NSAIDs in high doses and COXIBs in all dosages have been observed to increase mortality in patients with previous MI and should be avoided.[162] Adverse effects of nonselective NSAIDs are attributed to loss of gastrointestinal protection and hemostasis via COX-1 inhibition and loss of antiinflammatory activity via COX-2 inhibition.[13] COXIB-induced reduction of PGI_2 and unchecked COX-1 activity result in continued TXA_2 production and increased risk of thrombosis that may be harmful during acute MI. COXIB-induced antiinflammatory effects may be beneficial for progression of atherosclerosis but harmful during infarct healing. Suppression of inflammation by COX inhibitors can impair infarct healing after STEMI and lead to infarct thinning, adverse LV remodeling, aneurysm formation, and cardiac rupture,[13] suggesting the need for caution.

The FDA issued a warning on the concomitant use of aspirin and the NSAID ibuprofen. Ibuprofen (but not rofecoxib, acetaminophen, or diclofenac) interferes with aspirin-induced acetylation of COX-1 and attenuates its effects. The FDA also warned that COXIBs increase cardiovascular risk; rofecoxib (Vioxx) was withdrawn from the market, although celecoxib and valdecoxib remain. Based on evidence that patients taking NSAIDs within the week before MI have an increased risk of death, hypertension, reinfarction, heart failure, myocardial rupture, or shock, NSAIDs and COXIBs are contraindicated in patients with STEMI. It is recommended that they should not be initiated in the acute phase of MI and should be discontinued in any patients using them prior to hospitalization for acute MI. A stepped-care approach to use of these agents for patients with cardiovascular disease has been recommended.[163]

Recommendations

Morphine remains recommended for the relief of continuing pain in STEMI patients.[10] Nevertheless, given recent concerns raised about the possible hazard of morphine administration, initial efforts to relieve pain by relieving ischemia with nitrates and β-blockers are reasonable with morphine use restricted to select patients in whom the need appears to outweigh the risks. NSAIDs and COXIBs are contraindicated and should be avoided in patients with STEMI. The ACC/AHA guidelines regarding use of morphine and other analgesics are summarized in the Appendix.

CHOLESTEROL-LOWERING THERAPY

In the hospital phase of acute MI treatment, determination of a patient's lipid profile and initiation of interventions to manage dyslipidemia and promote secondary prevention have been part of routine management, although recent guidelines suggest that all such patients should be treated without attention to lipid levels or targets. Hydroxymethylglutaryl–coenzyme A (HMG-CoA) reductase inhibitors (statins) have been extensively investigated and are established as an important drug class for both lowering atherogenic lipids and reducing future adverse cardiovascular events.

Statins are competitive inhibitors of the rate-limiting step in cholesterol synthesis. All statins reduce low-density lipoprotein (LDL) cholesterol; some also increase high-density lipoprotein (HDL; e.g., simvastatin, rosuvastatin) and reduce triglycerides (e.g., atorvastatin, rosuvastatin). Aggressive lipid lowering has been shown to decrease atheroma burden and is beneficial in all patients with coronary artery disease. The Reversal of Atherosclerosis with Aggressive Lipid Lowering (REVERSAL) trial showed that aggressive lipid lowering prevented progression of atheroma in patients with known coronary artery disease.[164] In A Study to Evaluate the Effect of Rosuvastatin on Intravascular Ultrasound-Derived Coronary Atheroma Burden (ASTEROID), very-high-intensity statin therapy induced regression of coronary atherosclerosis.[165] Although the mechanism of benefit is not completely understood, abundant evidence shows reduction in mortality with lowering of cholesterol in patients with hypercholesterolemia after MI[166]; even patients with mild cholesterol elevation[167,168] or normal LDL levels[169] derive benefit.

The benefit of statin therapy for secondary prevention has been well established by 25 years of clinical investigation. Several trials have specifically studied the effect of statins on outcome in patients following ACS or acute MI. In the Cholesterol and Recurrent Events (CARE) trial,[168] 4159 patients with total cholesterol levels less than 240 mg/dL were randomized to pravastatin 40 mg/day or placebo 3 to 20 months after acute MI. After a median follow-up of 5 years, the rate of fatal coronary events or nonfatal MI was reduced by 24%, the frequency of stroke by 31%, the rate of coronary bypass surgery by 26%, and the rate of coronary angioplasty by 23%.

In the Myocardial Ischemia Reduction with Aggressive Cholesterol Lowering (MIRACL) trial,[170] 3086 patients with unstable angina or non-Q-wave MI were randomly assigned to treatment with high-dose atorvastatin (80 mg/day) or placebo between 24 and 96 hours after admission. At 16-week follow-up, atorvastatin reduced LDL cholesterol by an average of 52%. The primary composite endpoint of death, nonfatal MI, cardiac arrest with resuscitation, or recurrent symptomatic myocardial ischemia was reduced 16% by atorvastatin.

The question of the benefit of early initiation of statins after acute MI was addressed in a prospective, nonrandomized cohort study using the Swedish Register of Cardiac Intensive Care (RIKS-HIA).[171] The study population consisted of nearly 20,000 patients with a first MI, of whom 5528 received statins at or before discharge and 14,071 did not. Early statin treatment started before hospital discharge was associated with a 25% reduction in 1-year mortality. Similarly, in an observational study[172] of patients with ACS from the GUSTO IIb and PURSUIT trials, the mortality rate at 6 months was 33% lower among the 3653 patients discharged on lipid-lowering agents compared with the 17,156 patients who were not.

The question of whether intensive (vs. moderate) lipid lowering would have greater benefit for high-risk patients with ACS was tested in the Pravastatin or Atorvastatin Evaluation and Infection Therapy–Thrombolysis in Myocardial Infarction 22 (PROVE IT-TIMI 22) trial.[169] In that study, 4162 patients were randomly assigned to 40 mg of pravastatin or 80 mg of atorvastatin within 10 days of hospitalization for an ACS. During the trial, the median cholesterol levels of the pravastatin and atorvastatin groups were 95 mg/dL and 62 mg/dL, respectively. By 2 years, there was a significant (16%) reduction in the composite of death from any cause, MI, unstable angina requiring rehospitalization, revascularization, and stroke among patients assigned to atorvastatin treatment. The study demonstrated that among patients with recent ACS, compared with standard treatment to moderate goals, intensive lipid-lowering treatment provides significantly greater protection against death and major cardiovascular events.

These data suggested that, after STEMI, patients should be started on high-intensity statins and continued after discharge to reduce short- and long-term adverse cardiovascular events. Starting therapy while the patient is in the hospital improves adherence with no noted adverse effects[173] and adherence improves survival.[2] The modified Adult Treatment Panel (ATP) III guidelines in 2004[174] suggested that, for high-risk patients, the recommended LDL-C treatment goal is less than 100 mg/dL. However, a target of less than 70 mg/dL represents a reasonable therapeutic option for persons considered to be at very high risk, such as patients after AMI.

Of note, however, the most recent ACC/AHA guideline for treatment of blood cholesterol[175] did not support titrating cholesterol-lowering drug therapy to achieve optimal LDL-C or non-HDL-C levels. Instead, they strongly recommended that all individuals 75 years of age or younger who have clinical atherosclerotic cardiovascular disease (ASCVD), including all patients following acute MI, should be treated with high-intensity statin therapy unless contraindicated. High-intensity therapy was defined as treatment that lowers LDL-C by more than 50%; moderate-intensity statin therapy lowers LDL-C by 30% to 50%, and low-intensity statin therapy lowers LDL-C by less than 30%. High-intensity statins include atorvastatin at 80 mg daily and rosuvastatin at 20 mg daily. The guidelines also stated that for such patients, when high-intensity statin therapy is contraindicated or when characteristics predisposing to statin-associated adverse effects are present, moderate-intensity statins should be used as the second option, if tolerated.

There is recent evidence that lowering LDL cholesterol to levels below previous targets provides additional benefit. The Improved Reduction of Outcomes: Vytorin Efficacy International Trial (IMPROVE-IT)[176] randomly assigned 18,144 patients who had been hospitalized for an ACS within the preceding 10 days to simvastatin at 40 mg or a combination of simvastatin (40 mg) and ezetimibe (10 mg; simvastatin–ezetimibe). Over a follow-up of 7 years, the average LDL cholesterol for the simvastatin monotherapy group was 69.5 mg/dL compared with 53.7 mg/dL in the simvastatin–ezetimibe group. At 7 years, the addition of ezetimibe to simvastatin resulted in a significant reduction in the composite endpoint of cardiovascular death, MI, unstable angina requiring rehospitalization, coronary revascularization, or stroke with no increase in side effects. The investigators concluded that, when added to statin therapy, ezetimibe resulted in incremental lowering of LDL cholesterol levels and improved cardiovascular outcomes.

The effect of more powerful lipid lowering by a new class of agents, the proprotein convertase subtilisin–kexin type 9 (PCSK9) inhibitors, has recently been investigated. Evolocumab is a monoclonal antibody PCSK9 inhibitor that has been shown to lower LDL cholesterol levels by approximately 60%. The effect of evolocumab on outcomes for patients with ASCVD was assessed in the Further Cardiovascular Outcomes Research With PCSK9 Inhibition in Subjects With Elevated Risk (FOURIER) trial,[177] in which 27,564 patients with ASCVD and LDL cholesterol levels of 70 mg/dL or higher who were receiving statin therapy were randomly assigned to receive evolocumab or placebo. At 48 weeks, the median LDL cholesterol level in the evolocumab group was 30 mg/dL and, in 42% of patients, evolocumab lowered LDL cholesterol to 25 mg/dL or lower. Over 2.2 years of follow-up, evolocumab treatment significantly reduced the risk of cardiovascular death, MI, stroke, hospitalization for unstable angina, or coronary revascularization without an increase in adverse events other than infrequent minor injection site reactions. Currently, the PCSK9 inhibitors are costly, with restricted indications for use that state it can be prescribed as an adjunct to diet and maximally tolerated statin therapy for the treatment of select adults with heterozygous familial hypercholesterolemia or ASCVD who require additional lowering of LDL-C.

Recommendations

STEMI patients represent a high-risk ASCVD group in need of aggressive secondary prevention; high-intensity statin treatment (e.g., atorvastatin 80 mg daily or rosuvastatin 20 mg daily) is recommended for all patients without contraindications or a history of intolerance. Additional cholesterol-lowering interventions have been shown to be beneficial, as discussed earlier, and may be considered on an individual basis for select patients for whom statin therapy is not feasible or does not achieve the desired lowering of LDL. The ACC/AHA guidelines for lipid management in STEMI are summarized in the Appendix.

ANTICOAGULANTS

The use of anticoagulants in the acute and convalescent phases of STEMI has evolved with dramatic changes in management strategy. Current parenteral anticoagulants potentially useful during the acute phase of STEMI include unfractionated heparin (UFH), low-molecular-weight heparin (LMWH), fondaparinux, and bivalirudin (Table 12.6). The selection of one of these agents for early management may vary based on reperfusion strategy, as discussed later, and assessment of the patient's risk of bleeding. Oral anticoagulants include the vitamin K–dependent antagonist, warfarin, and the non-vitamin K–dependent oral anticoagulants (NOACs). The NOACs include dabigatran, which directly inhibits thrombin, and apixaban and rivaroxiban, which inhibit factor Xa. NOACs have not been adequately studied in the setting of STEMI.

Thrombin is a key protease of the coagulation system. Thrombin inhibitors (UFH and LMWH) prevent the formation of thrombin and inhibit the activity of already formed thrombin. UFH is a mixture of glycosaminoglycan chains that produces its anticoagulant effect by binding to antithrombin III, which inactivates factor IIa (thrombin), factor IXa, factor Ia, and factor Xa (see Fig. 12.1). UFH prevents growth of existing thrombus, but does not lyse clot.[178] LMWH produces more potent

TABLE 12.6 Duration of Antiplatelet and Anticoagulant Therapy Following ST Elevation Myocardial Infarction

Duration of Therapy	
Oral Antiplatelet Therapy	
Aspirin	Lifelong
Clopidogrel/ prasugrel/ ticagrelor	If patient had bare metal stent, minimum 1 month, or 1 year post-ACS
	If patient had drug-eluting stent, minimum 1 year, longer for select cases
	If patient has not been revascularized, can continue clopidogrel or ticagrelor for up to 1 year
Anticoagulant Therapy	
Unfractionated heparin (intravenous)	Up to 48 h, provided no other contraindications to discontinuation
	Can discontinue when patient has been revascularized by stenting
Low-molecular-weight heparin	Up to 8 d or duration of hospitalization, provided no other contraindications to discontinuation
	Can discontinue when patient has been revascularized by stenting
Fondaparinux	Up to 8 d or duration of hospitalization, provided no other contraindications to discontinuation
	Can discontinue when patient has been revascularized by stenting
Bivalirudin	Up to 3 days, provided no other contraindications to discontinuation
	Can discontinue when patient has been revascularized by stenting
Warfarin	If patient has left ventricular thrombus or aneurysm, 3 months to lifelong therapy

inactivation of factor Xa than thrombin, whereas UFH produces equal inhibition of factor Xa and thrombin. Fondaparinux is a synthetic heparin polysaccharide that binds to antithrombin with higher affinity than either UFH or LMWH and causes a conformational change that results in a preferential increase in the ability of the antithrombin–fondaparinux complex to inactivate factor Xa. Direct thrombin inhibitors, such as hirudin and bivalirudin, bind and inactivate thrombin without need for a cofactor, but have little effect on generation of thrombin. Bivalirudin is a synthetic analogue of hirudin that binds reversibly to thrombin and inhibits clot-bound thrombin.

In GUSTO-1,[152] in which intravenous and subcutaneous heparin and systemic alteplase and streptokinase were studied, an optimal activated partial thromboplastin time of between 60 and 70 seconds was associated with the lowest mortality, fewest bleeding complications, lowest reinfarction rate, and lowest frequency of hemorrhagic shock. Intravenous heparin should be given cautiously or not at all when streptokinase is used, unless it is specifically indicated. Prolonged heparin is effective in preventing LV thrombus after acute MI.[179]

One advantage of LMWH over UFH is that it does not require blood monitoring for titrating the dose to a therapeutic activated partial thromboplastin time. LMWH is renally cleared; thus it should be avoided in patients with renal failure. Side effects with

both types of heparin include bleeding, thrombocytopenia, and osteoporosis. Patients at high risk for bleeding include women, patients over 65 years of age, and patients with comorbid states such as peptic ulcer, liver disease, and malignancy. Intravenous protamine can be used to reverse UFH but only partially reverses LMWH.

Heparin-induced thrombocytopenia (HIT) is a well-known complication of UFH and LMWH therapy. Two types of HIT are recognized.[180] HIT type I occurs in the first 4 days with a platelet nadir of 100,000/mL, resolves even with continued therapy, and is not thought to be immune related. HIT type II occurs within 5 to 10 days in 1% to 3% of patients and is immune mediated. It should be suspected when the platelet count decreases more than 50%, if venous or arterial thrombosis develops, or if there is necrosis noted at heparin injection sites. LMWH is associated with lower rates of HIT than UFH, but should nevertheless still be avoided in patients with HIT.[181]

Monitoring of platelet counts is recommended for patients on heparin or LMWH. Patients exposed to heparin during the previous 3 months can develop early HIT type II mediated by circulating antibodies. Management of HIT type II includes immediate discontinuation of LMWH or UFH with careful attention to avoidance of routine heparin flushes and heparin-bonded catheters.[182] Patients who have a history of HIT type II should not be reexposed to either type of heparin because a recurrence can be expected 2 to 3 days after reexposure. STEMI patients with HIT or a history of HIT who require anticoagulation should be treated with a nonheparin anticoagulant, such as bivalirudin or argatroban.

Anticoagulant therapy in conjunction with thrombolytic therapy or primary PCI is addressed in detail elsewhere. For patients receiving fibrinolytic therapy, clinical trials support the use of unfractionated heparin, enoxaparin, and fondaparinux. For patients receiving primary PCI, evidence supports the adjunctive use of UFH and bivalirudin. Fondaparinux is not recommended in patients undergoing primary PCI owing to an increased risk of thrombotic procedural complications.

There have been no randomized controlled studies or new data to guide the management of STEMI patients who do not undergo reperfusion therapy. In ISIS-2, patients who were treated with aspirin and subcutaneous UFH did not show a survival advantage over those treated with intravenous heparin.[12] Although postlytic intravenous UFH increased bleeding in other trials, a statistically nonsignificant 18% decrease in mortality was also found.[183]

It is recommended that STEMI patients who require anticoagulation be given UFH as an intravenous infusion, with a bolus of 60 U/kg (maximum 4000 U) followed by infusion of 12 U/kg/hour (maximum 1000 U/hour). Weight-based initial dosing for intravenous heparin is preferred because of evidence that the effects of heparin are primarily mediated by weight.[184] A useful target is an activated partial thromboplastin time range of 50 to 70 seconds or 1.5 to 2 times control values based on data showing that values above this increase bleeding, stroke, and mortality, whereas lower values are associated with increased mortality. After thrombolytic therapy, anticoagulation can be continued for 48 hours or longer in patients at high risk for thromboembolism, such as those with anterior STEMI, severe LV dysfunction, CHF, history of systemic or pulmonary embolization, atrial fibrillation, or echocardiographic evidence of LV thrombus.[185] Anticoagulation is generally not continued after revascularization of the infarct-related artery by PCI unless there are specific indications (discussed later).

LMWH for the management of STEMI has also been studied. The Clinical Trial of Reviparin and Metabolic Modulation in Acute Myocardial Infarction Treatment Evaluation (CREATE)[186] randomly assigned 15,570 patients in India and China presenting with STEMI or new left bundle branch block, who had reperfusion therapy with either primary PCI or thrombolytic therapy, to LMWH (reviparin) or placebo. LMWH improved 30-day survival and reduced reinfarction regardless of whether the patient had primary PCI, lytic therapy, or no reperfusion therapy.

The effect of the factor Xa inhibitor fondaparinux (2.5 mg/day) was studied in the Organization for the Assessment of Strategies for Ischemic Syndromes (OASIS-6) trial of 12,092 STEMI patients.[187] The patients were divided into two strata. The first stratum, consisting of 5658 patients with no indication for heparin, was assigned to fondaparinux 2.5 mg daily for up to 8 days, or placebo; the second stratum, consisting of 6434 patients with an indication for heparin (e.g., fibrin-specific thrombolytic, primary PCI or no reperfusion), was assigned to fondaparinux for up to 8 days or UFH for 48 hours. Fondaparinux reduced 30-day mortality or reinfarction from 11.2% to 9.7% compared to control with benefits apparent at 9 days and driven primarily by reductions in stratum 1. In stratum 2, patients who were not managed with primary PCI, fondaparinux was superior to UFH in preventing death or reinfarction at 30 days. The overall findings indicated that in STEMI patients who are not managed with primary PCI, fondaparinux reduces mortality and reinfarction without increasing bleeding and strokes.[187]

There are some theoretical advantages in using a direct thrombin inhibitor over heparin. After thrombolytic therapy, a procoagulant state is induced by thrombin bound to soluble fibrin derivatives. In contrast to direct thrombin inhibitors, a heparin–antithrombin III complex is unable to inactivate thrombin within a clot because it cannot penetrate the clot.[188] The direct thrombin inhibitor, bivalirudin, has been studied in patients undergoing thrombolytic therapy[189] and in patients undergoing primary PCI.[190,191]

Oral Anticoagulation

Following acute MI, increased thrombin generation and increased activity of the coagulation system may persist for several months; this may account, at least in part, for a heightened risk of recurrent ischemic events.[192] The question of whether chronic oral anticoagulant reduces the risk of recurrent events after MI for patients with no other indications for anticoagulation has been evaluated in clinical trials that have included warfarin and NOACs.

Warfarin inhibits the vitamin K-dependent synthesis of biologically active forms of the clotting factors II, VII, IX, and X, as well as the regulatory factors protein C, protein S, and protein Z. Dosing of warfarin is highly variable between patients and should be titrated by assessing the patient's response through

the international normalized ratio (INR). The antithrombotic properties of warfarin do not occur for 72 to 96 hours after initiation of treatment. Its major side effect is bleeding related to its anticoagulant effect, which may be reversed with vitamin K or fresh frozen plasma. Warfarin-induced skin necrosis is a rare condition in which skin and subcutaneous tissue necrosis occurs owing to acquired protein C deficiency following treatment with warfarin.

The use of oral anticoagulation with warfarin for secondary prevention following MI has been studied in several randomized clinical trials. These trials were conducted before the common use of early invasive management with PCI and among select patients at relatively low risk for bleeding. In general, these trials showed modest benefit for warfarin with respect to reduction of composite ischemic endpoints, but none showed a reduction in mortality and all reported a 20% to 35% rate of drug discontinuation and a higher rate of bleeding with warfarin therapy. Two meta-analyses comparing warfarin plus aspirin to aspirin alone suggested that when the INR was maintained at 2.0 to 3.0, warfarin plus aspirin was associated with a reduction in the risk of ischemic events but there was no significant difference in the overall risk of major ischemic events and there was a significant increase in major bleeding.[193,194] Notably, none of the trials included patients treated with primary PCI or DAPT, limiting the applicability of warfarin for this indication in current practice.

Therefore, following STEMI, it is recommended that warfarin use be restricted to patients with other indications for anticoagulation, such as atrial fibrillation, documented LV thrombus, or a large akinetic or dyskinetic LV segment. There have been no randomized controlled studies of warfarin for LV thrombus. A meta-analysis of observational studies showed that anticoagulated patients had an 86% reduction in embolization rate.[185] Since most embolic events occur early, anticoagulation with warfarin for 3 months is recommended for STEMI patients with an LV thrombus.[10] When warfarin is combined with aspirin, the dose of aspirin should be kept low (75 to 81 mg) and the INR should be maintained in the range of 2.0 to 3.0.

LV aneurysm is a common complication of STEMI if reperfusion has not been attempted or achieved. Approximately 50% of LV aneurysms have a thrombus.[195] Patients with an LV aneurysm and thrombus after recent MI are at high risk of emboli—13% over a 6- to 15-month follow-up period—and should be anticoagulated. Chronic LV aneurysms have a lower risk of embolization—0.35% over a 5-year follow-up period—as the thrombus becomes organized. Warfarin is not warranted in these patients unless other indications are present.

The effects of two NOACs, apixaban and rivaroxaban, have also been studied in post-ACS populations with no other indications for anticoagulation. Apixaban is an oral factor Xa inhibitor approved for the treatment of deep vein thrombosis (DVT) and pulmonary embolism, prevention of DVT in postoperative patients, and for the prevention of systemic embolic events in patients with nonvalvular atrial fibrillation. In the Apixaban for Prevention of Acute Ischemic Events 2 (APPRAISE-2) trial,[196] 7392 patients with an ACS within the previous 7 days receiving DAPT were randomly assigned to apixaban 5 mg twice daily or placebo. The trial was stopped early owing to an increase in the rate of major bleeding in the apixaban group, while the rate of ischemic events at that time point (241 days) appeared similar in the 2 groups.

Rivaroxaban is an oral factor Xa inhibitor that is approved for reducing the risk of systemic embolic events and stroke in patients with nonvalvular atrial fibrillation as well as for the treatment of DVT and pulmonary embolism. It was studied in the setting of ACS in the Anti-Xa Therapy to Lower Cardiovascular Events in Addition to Standard Therapy in Subjects with Acute Coronary Syndrome–Thrombolysis in Myocardial Infarction 46 (ATLAS ACS–TIMI 46) trial,[197] which randomly assigned 15,526 patients within 7 days of hospitalization for ACS to twice-daily doses of either 2.5 mg (very low dose) or 5 mg (low dose) of rivaroxaban (one-quarter and one-half, respectively, of the full anticoagulation dose) or placebo. In this trial, approximately 50% of patients had STEMI, 25% had NSTEMI, 25% had unstable angina, 93% were also receiving DAPT, and patients with prior ischemic stroke or transient ischemic attack were excluded. At 13 months, the composite of death from cardiovascular causes, MI, or stroke and the rate of stent thrombosis were reduced by 16% by rivaroxaban (pooled dose groups vs. placebo); a lower rate of cardiovascular death was observed among patients receiving the very low 2.5 mg dose. Rivaroxaban also increased the rate of major bleeding and intracranial hemorrhage, but not fatal bleeding. Among the 7817 patients with STEMI in the trial, rivaroxaban significantly reduced the risk of recurrent ischemic events by 19% but also significantly increased major bleeding.[198]

Of note, rivaroxaban was approved in 2013 by the European Medicines Agency for the prevention of cardiovascular events in patients following an ACS. However, in the United States, an FDA advisory panel reviewed but voted against approval of an expanded indication for rivaroxaban to reduce the risk of secondary cardiovascular events in patients with ACS, citing incomplete safety data from the trial. Rivaroxaban is not recommended in current guidelines for treatment of patients following STEMI.

In some patients following STEMI or NSTE ACS, chronic oral anticoagulation may be indicated to lower the risk of thromboembolism or prosthetic valve dysfunction, such as those with atrial fibrillation, LV systolic dysfunction or thrombus, or prosthetic heart valves. Since such patients also have indications for DAPT, the use of chronic anticoagulation has raised challenging issues regarding managing bleeding risk and determining optimal regimens.

Among patients following PCI with stent implantation, observational studies examining the use of warfarin combined with both aspirin and clopidogrel ("triple therapy") have suggested a significantly increased risk of major bleeding. For this reason, for patients undergoing primary PCI who require anticoagulation, avoidance of a drug-eluting stent has been recommended to limit the required duration of triple therapy. When triple therapy is used, an INR targeted to a range of 2.0 to 2.5 is recommended with low-dose aspirin (75–81 mg) and no more than 75 mg/day of clopidogrel. Patients who have had PCI with stenting and are prescribed triple therapy after an ACS and who are without

recurrent events at 1 year may be considered to have stable disease and the P2Y$_{12}$ antagonist can be discontinued. Prasugrel and ticagrelor are not recommended as part of triple therapy. Based on a strategy examined in the What Is the Optimal Antiplatelet & Anticoagulant Therapy in Patients With Oral Anticoagulation and Coronary Stenting (WOEST) study,[199] some have advocated that, when warfarin is indicated following MI in patients who have received a drug-eluting stent, discontinuation of the aspirin from triple therapy and continuation of warfarin plus clopidogrel may reduce bleeding complications yet maintain a low risk of thrombotic events such as stent thrombosis. It should be recognized that a small minority of the patients in the WOEST trial presented with ACS and the risk of stent thrombosis may therefore have been lower than in a post-STEMI population.

Novel strategies using combinations of rivaroxaban at low dose and DAPT or a P2Y$_{12}$ antagonist alone were recently tested in the Open-Label, Randomized, Controlled, Multicenter Study Exploring Two Treatment Strategies of Rivaroxaban and a Dose-Adjusted Oral Vitamin K Antagonist Treatment Strategy in Subjects with Atrial Fibrillation who Undergo Percutaneous Coronary Intervention (PIONEER AF-PCI) study[200] and were compared to standard triple therapy. Rivaroxaban-containing regimens had lower bleeding rates than standard triple therapy but the trial was small and no firm conclusions on efficacy or safety to guide practice were possible. Further study is needed to guide the use of anticoagulants, when indicated, in combination with antiplatelet therapy among patients following MI and PCI.

Recommendations

Patients with STEMI who undergo primary PCI should be anticoagulated with UFH or bivalirudin; the choice may be based on the considerations and preference of the interventional operator in the context of an assessment of bleeding risk and interacting medications. Anticoagulation should generally be discontinued following revascularization, although continuation of bivalirudin for a limited period after stent implantation may be considered for select patients to reduce the risk of stent thrombosis. Patients with STEMI receiving fibrinolytic therapy should receive anticoagulation using UFH, enoxaparin, or fondaparinux for at least 48 hours or until revascularization.

At present, following STEMI, warfarin is recommended for patients with indications for continued oral anticoagulation, although caution is warranted for patients following primary PCI with stent implantation receiving warfarin in combination with DAPT (triple therapy), for whom the bleeding risk may be very high. Attention to using low-dose aspirin, clopidogrel at 75 mg daily and maintaining the INR in the range of 2.0 to 2.5 is recommended to reduce the bleeding risk in such patients. The ACC/AHA guidelines for anticoagulation in STEMI are summarized in the Appendix.

CONCLUSION

Adjunctive pharmacologic therapy is important for all STEMI patients whether they are treated with reperfusion therapy or not. This therapy can help minimize infarct size; reduce adverse ventricular remodeling; and reduce reinfarction, recurrent angina, and mortality. These agents can be used to widen the time frame for reperfusion therapy and to minimize reperfusion injury and ventricular dysfunction. Agents of proven benefit include aspirin, $P2Y_{12}$ antagonists, β-blockers, ACE inhibitors, ARBs, and aldosterone antagonists. Attention to early and comprehensive application of evidence-based therapies starting during the acute cardiac intensive care phase can significantly improve outcomes after MI.

Acknowledgment

I acknowledge the contributions of Drs. Jonathan Man, Wayne Tymchak, and Bodh Jugdutt, who were the authors of this chapter in the previous edition.

The full reference list for this chapter is available at ExpertConsult.com.

Postmyocardial Infarction Cardiogenic Shock

Eric R. Bates

Dramatic advances during the past several decades in diagnosing, monitoring, and treating patients with acute myocardial infarction (MI) have decreased hospital mortality rates by 50%. The organization of coronary care units in the 1960s to treat lethal arrhythmias[1] and the development of fibrinolytic therapy in the 1980s to reduce infarct size[2–5] were the biggest breakthroughs. Cardiogenic shock, not arrhythmia, is the most common cause of death in patients hospitalized with acute MI. Neither the incidence nor the mortality rate associated with cardiogenic shock has been reduced by modern cardiac intensive care unit interventions, including vasopressor and inotropic drug infusions, hemodynamic monitoring, and intraaortic balloon pump (IABP) counterpulsation (Table 13.1).[6–12] However, a survival advantage has been demonstrated for patients who undergo successful reperfusion with percutaneous coronary intervention (PCI) or coronary artery bypass graft surgery (CABG).[13–19] This chapter reviews the epidemiology, pathogenesis, clinical presentation, and current management of cardiogenic shock.

EPIDEMIOLOGY

Definition

Circulatory shock is characterized by the inability of multiorgan blood flow and oxygen delivery to meet metabolic demands.

Cardiogenic shock is a type of circulatory shock resulting from severe impairment of ventricular pump function rather than from abnormalities of the vascular system or blood volume. It is important to separate the shock state, in which tissue perfusion is inadequate, from hypotension, in which tissue metabolic demands may be met by increasing cardiac output or decreasing systemic vascular resistance. The diagnosis of cardiogenic shock should include the following:

1. Systolic blood pressure less than 80 mm Hg without inotropic or vasopressor support, or less than 90 mm Hg with inotropic or vasopressor support, for at least 30 minutes
2. Low cardiac output (<2.0 L/min per m^2) not related to hypovolemia (pulmonary artery wedge pressure <12 mm Hg), arrhythmia, hypoxemia, acidosis, or atrioventricular block
3. Tissue hypoperfusion manifested by oliguria (<30 mL/h), peripheral vasoconstriction, or altered mental status

The failure to consistently define cardiogenic shock or to hemodynamically confirm the presence of an elevated pulmonary capillary wedge pressure and low cardiac index have previously confused clinicians and confounded the literature.

Etiology

The most common cause of cardiogenic shock is acute MI.[20] Often, anterior MI due to acute thrombotic occlusion of the left

TABLE 13.1   Historical Milestones in Cardiogenic Shock

1934	Fishberg et al.[6] described the shock state as a peripheral complication of myocardial infarction.
1942	Stead and Ebert[7] attributed the shock state to extreme myocardial dysfunction.
1954	Griffith et al.[8] used L-norepinephrine as pressor support.
1967	Killip and Kimball[1] showed no survival advantage with coronary care unit monitoring.
1968	Kantrowitz et al.[9] described the clinical use of the IABP.
1972	Dunkman et al.[10] demonstrated successful treatment with CABG.
1973	Scheidt et al.[11] showed no survival advantage with IABP.
1976	Forrester et al.[12] defined hemodynamic subsets using the pulmonary artery catheter.
1980	DeWood et al.[13] showed a survival advantage with early CABG.
1980	Mathey et al.[14] demonstrated successful treatment with fibrinolytic therapy.
1982	Meyer et al.[15] demonstrated successful treatment with PTCA.
1988	Lee et al.[16] showed a survival advantage with PTCA.
1999	Hochman et al.[17–19] proved a survival advantage with revascularization in the SHOCK trial.

CABG, Coronary artery bypass graft surgery; *IABP,* intraaortic balloon pump; *PTCA,* percutaneous transluminal coronary angioplasty.

anterior descending artery results in extensive infarction. Alternatively, a smaller MI in a patient with borderline left ventricular function may be responsible for insufficient cardiac output. Large areas of ischemic nonfunctioning but viable myocardium occasionally lead to shock in patients with MI. The delayed onset of shock may result from reocclusion of a previously patent infarct artery, infarct extension, or metabolic decompensation of noninfarct-zone regional wall motion. Occasionally, right ventricular MI from occlusion of a proximal large right coronary artery in a patient with inferior MI is the cause.[21]

Mechanical complications unrelated to infarct size account for approximately 12% of cases. The papillary muscle of the mitral valve may infarct or rupture, causing acute, severe mitral regurgitation.[22] Rupture of the interventricular septum causing ventricular septal defect[23] or rupture of the left ventricular free wall producing pericardial tamponade[24] also needs to be considered.

Other causes of cardiogenic shock are not emphasized in this discussion. These include end-stage cardiomyopathy, myocardial contusion, myocarditis, hypertrophic cardiomyopathy, valvular heart disease, pericardial disease, right ventricular infarction, and post-cardiopulmonary bypass.

Incidence

Before the recent emphasis on time to treatment and primary PCI, the incidence of cardiogenic shock had remained unchanged for over 25 years, with approximately 8% of patients with ST elevation myocardial infarction (STEMI)[25,26] and 2.5% of patients with non-STEMI[27,28] developing cardiogenic shock. The latter group is more likely to have circumflex artery occlusion, comorbid disease, and severe three-vessel disease or left main disease.[28] Cardiogenic shock usually develops early after onset of symptoms, with approximately half of the patients developing shock within 6 hours and 72% within 24 hours.[29] Others first develop a preshock

state manifested by systemic hypoperfusion without hypotension.[30] These patients benefit from aggressive supportive therapy and revascularization; early intervention may abort the onset of cardiogenic shock.

PATHOGENESIS

Pathology

The early development of cardiogenic shock is usually caused by acute thrombosis of a coronary artery supplying a large myocardial distribution, with no collateral flow recruitment.[31] Frequently, this is the left anterior descending artery, although shock may result from coronary thrombosis in other sites if previous MI has occurred. Multivessel disease is present in two-thirds of patients.[32]

Autopsy studies have consistently shown that at least 40% of the myocardium is infarcted in patients who die of cardiogenic shock.[33] Various ages of infarction reflect previous infarction, reinfarction, or infarct extension.

The infarct border zone in patients without hypotension is clearly demarcated. In patients succumbing to shock, however, it is irregular, with marginal extension. Focal areas of necrosis remote from the infarct zone are also present. These findings result from progressive cell death due to poor coronary perfusion, are reflected by prolonged release of cardiac enzymes, and contribute to hemodynamic deterioration.[34]

Pathophysiology

Progressive hemodynamic deterioration resulting in cardiogenic shock results from a sequence of events (Fig. 13.1). A critical amount of ischemic or necrotic myocardium decreases contractile mass and cardiac output. When cardiac output is low enough that arterial blood pressure falls, coronary perfusion pressure decreases in the setting of an elevated left ventricular end-diastolic pressure. The resulting reduction in coronary perfusion pressure gradient from epicardium to endocardium exacerbates myocardial ischemia, further decreasing left ventricular function and cardiac output, perpetuating a vicious cycle. The speed with which this process develops is modified by the infarct zone, remote myocardial function, neurohumoral responses, and metabolic abnormalities.

The infarct zone can be enlarged by reocclusion of a previously patent infarct artery. Alternatively, infarct extension can result from side branch occlusion from coronary thrombus propagation or embolization or by thrombosis of a second stenosis stimulated by low coronary blood flow and hypercoagulability. Infarct expansion or aneurysm formation promotes left ventricular dilation, which increases wall stress and oxygen demand in the setting of decreased oxygen supply due to low cardiac output.

Preclinical and clinical studies[35] have demonstrated the importance of hypercontractility of remote myocardial segments in maintaining cardiac output in the setting of a large myocardial infarction. This compensatory mechanism is lost when multivessel disease is present and severe enough to produce ischemia in noninfarct segments.

A series of neurohumoral responses is activated in an attempt to restore cardiac output and vital organ perfusion. Decreased

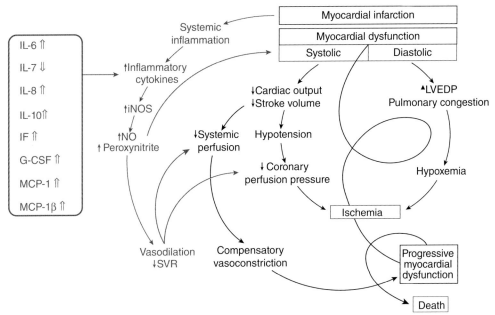

Fig. 13.1 Prognostically relevant components of cardiogenic shock complicating myocardial infarction. In addition to severe systolic and diastolic cardiac dysfunction compromising macrocirculation and microcirculation, systemic inflammatory response syndrome and even sepsis may develop, finally resulting in multiorgan dysfunction syndrome. The proinflammatory and antiinflammatory cytokines mentioned have prognostic significance, with either higher (↑) or lower (↓) serum levels in nonsurvivors compared with survivors. *G-CSF*, Granulocyte colony-stimulating factor; *IF*, interferon; *IL*, interleukin; *MCP*, monocyte chemotactic protein; *MIP*, macrophage inflammatory protein; *NO*, nitric oxide; *iNOS*, inducible macrophage-type nitric oxide synthase. (Modified from Hochman JS. Cardiogenic shock complicating acute myocardial infarction: expanding the paradigm. *Circulation.* 2003;107:2998–3002.)

baroreceptor activity due to hypotension increases sympathetic outflow and reduces vagal tone. This increases heart rate, myocardial contractility, venous tone, and arterial vasoconstriction. Vasoconstriction is most pronounced in the skeletal, splanchnic, and cutaneous vascular beds to redistribute cardiac output to the coronary, renal, and cerebral circulations. An increase in the ratio of precapillary to postcapillary resistance decreases capillary hydrostatic pressure, facilitating movement of interstitial fluid into the vascular compartment. Increased catecholamine levels and decreased renal perfusion lead to renin release and angiotensin production. Elevated angiotensin levels stimulate peripheral vasoconstriction and aldosterone synthesis. Aldosterone increases sodium and water retention by the kidney, raising blood volume. Release of antidiuretic hormone from the posterior pituitary by baroreceptor stimulation also increases water retention. Local autoregulatory mechanisms that decrease arteriolar resistance and increase regional blood flow are stimulated by hypoxia, acidosis, and accumulation of vasoactive metabolites (e.g., adenosine).

Enhanced anaerobic metabolism, lactic acidosis, and depleted adenosine triphosphate (ATP) stores result when compensatory neurohumoral responses are overwhelmed, further depressing ventricular function. Arrhythmias may reduce cardiac output and increase myocardial ischemia as well. Loss of vascular endothelial integrity because of ischemia culminates in multiorgan failure. Pulmonary edema impairs gas exchange. Renal and hepatic dysfunction results in fluid, electrolyte, and metabolic disturbances.

Gastrointestinal ischemia can lead to hemorrhage or entry of bacteria into the bloodstream, causing sepsis. Microvascular thrombosis due to capillary endothelial damage with fibrin deposition and catecholamine-induced platelet aggregation further impairs organ function.

A systemic inflammatory state with high plasma levels of cytokines (e.g., tumor necrosis factor-α, interleukin-6) and inappropriate nitric oxide production may also depress myocardial function or impair catecholamine-induced vasoconstriction, respectively. All of these factors, in turn, lead to diminished coronary artery perfusion and thus trigger a vicious cycle of further myocardial ischemia and necrosis. This results in even lower blood pressure, lactic acidosis, multiorgan failure, and ultimately death.[36]

CLINICAL PRESENTATION

History and Physical Examination

The diagnosis of acute MI must be confirmed. Noncardiac causes of shock need to be ruled out; these include aortic dissection, tension pneumothorax, massive pulmonary embolism, ruptured viscus, hemorrhage, and sepsis. Risk factors for developing cardiogenic shock include older age, anterior MI location, hypertension, diabetes mellitus, multivessel coronary artery disease, prior MI, prior congestive heart failure, STEMI, or left bundle branch block.[37,38]

Patients usually appear ashen or cyanotic, with cold and clammy skin. They may be agitated, disoriented, or lethargic from cerebral hypoperfusion. The pulses are rapid and faint, the pulse pressure narrow, and arrhythmias are common. Jugular venous distention and pulmonary rales are usually present in left ventricular shock, but may be absent. Jugular venous distention, Kussmaul sign (a paradoxic increase in jugular venous pressure during inspiration), and absent rales are found in right ventricular shock. Left ventricular dyskinesis may produce a precordial heave. A systolic thrill along the left sternal border is consistent with mitral regurgitation or ventricular septal defect. The heart sounds are distant. Third and fourth heart sounds or a summation gallop can be auscultated. The systolic murmur of mitral regurgitation is often present; ventricular septal defect also produces a systolic murmur. The absence of a murmur, however, does not exclude these complications. The extremities are usually vasoconstricted.

Electrocardiography and Laboratory Testing

A large anterior or anterolateral MI pattern is often present. Old anterior Q waves or new ST segment elevation in the right precordial leads consistent with right ventricular MI may be noted with acute inferior MI. Multiple lead ST segment depression without an injury current is another pattern that can occur with multivessel or left main disease. New left bundle branch block and third-degree atrioventricular conduction block are ominous findings. A relatively normal ECG should alert one to other causes of shock.

Troponin and creatine kinase levels are high, may peak late because of prolonged washout or ongoing necrosis, and can rise secondarily with infarct extension. Lactic acidosis, hypoxemia, and mixed venous oxygen desaturation are usually present.

Echocardiography

Echocardiography can be performed rapidly and offers valuable information on the extent of left ventricular dysfunction. A dilated, hypokinetic left ventricle suggests left ventricular shock, whereas a dilated right ventricle suggests right ventricular involvement. Normal ventricular function, low cardiac output, and mitral regurgitation are consistent with acute severe mitral regurgitation. Pericardial tamponade from hemorrhagic effusion or free wall rupture can quickly be detected. Doppler evaluation can easily confirm the presence of significant mitral regurgitation or ventricular septal rupture. Transesophageal echo is helpful in patients for whom image quality is inadequate or when a flail mitral leaflet is suspected but not seen on transthoracic echocardiography.

MANAGEMENT

General Measures

A number of supportive measures need to be instituted quickly (Fig. 13.2). If there is no clinical evidence for pulmonary edema, a fluid bolus should be given to exclude hypovolemia as a cause of hypotension. Patients with a history of inadequate fluid intake, diaphoresis, diarrhea, vomiting, or diuretic use may not have pump failure and will improve dramatically with fluid

---

> **BOX 13.1** **Conventional Therapy for Cardiogenic Shock**
>
> 1. Maximize volume (RAP 10–14 mm Hg, PAWP 18–20 mm Hg)
> 2. Maximize oxygenation (e.g., ventilator)
> 3. Correct electrolyte and acid-base imbalances
> 4. Control rhythm (e.g., pacemaker, cardioversion)
> 5. Sympathomimetic amines (e.g., dobutamine, dopamine, norepinephrine)
> 6. Phosphodiesterase inhibitors (e.g., milrinone)
> 7. Vasodilators (e.g., nitroglycerin, nitroprusside)
> 8. Intraaortic balloon counterpulsation

PAWP, Pulmonary artery wedge pressure; *RAP*, right atrial pressure.

administration. Because preload is critical in patients with right ventricular shock, fluid support and avoidance of nitrates and morphine are indicated (Box 13.1).

Oxygenation and airway protection are critical. Intubation and mechanical ventilation may be required, followed by sedation, and often muscular paralysis. These interventions also improve the safety of electrical cardioversion or cardiac catheterization, if needed, and decrease oxygen demand. Positive end-expiratory pressure (PEEP) decreases preload and afterload.

Hypokalemia and hypomagnesemia predispose patients to ventricular arrhythmias and should be corrected. Because metabolic acidosis decreases contractile function, hyperventilation should be considered, but sodium bicarbonate should be avoided given its short half-life and the large sodium load.

Arrhythmias and atrioventricular heart block have a major influence on cardiac output. Atrial and ventricular tachyarrhythmias should be electrically cardioverted promptly rather than treated with pharmacologic agents. Severe bradycardia due to excess vagotonia can be corrected with atropine. Temporary pacing should be initiated for high-degree heart block, preferably with a dual-chamber system. This is especially important in patients with right ventricular infarction who depend on the right atrial contribution to preload.

Aspirin and monitored unfractionated heparin should be administered to decrease the likelihood of reinfarction, ventricular mural thrombus formation, or deep venous thrombosis in the setting of low flow and hypercoagulability. Platelet P2Y$_{12}$ receptor inhibitors (clopidogrel, prasugrel, ticagrelor) are best withheld until cardiac catheterization has determined the need for emergency surgery because of their prolonged action and increased risk for perioperative bleeding. Morphine sulfate decreases pain and anxiety, excessive sympathetic activity, preload, and afterload, but should only be administered in small increments. Diuretics decrease filling pressures and should be used to control volume. Beta-blockers and calcium channel blockers should be avoided because they are negative inotropic agents. An insulin infusion may be required to control hyperglycemia.

Hemodynamic Monitoring

Central hemodynamic monitoring is critical for confirming the diagnosis and guiding pharmacologic therapy (Table 13.2). Urine output needs to be monitored hourly through catheter drainage. An arterial catheter allows constant monitoring of the blood pressure. A pulmonary artery catheter should be inserted as soon

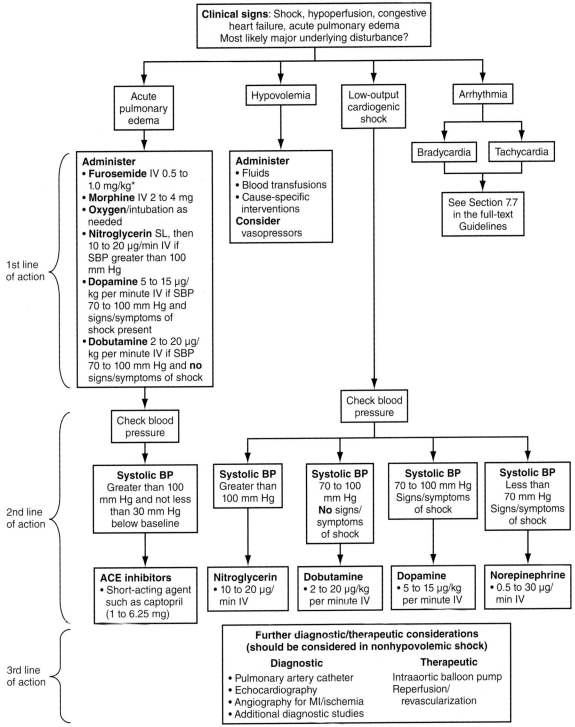

Fig. 13.2 Emergency management of complicated ST-elevation myocardial infarction. *ACE,* Angiotensin-converting enzyme; *BP,* blood pressure; *IV,* intravenous; *MI,* myocardial infarction; *SBP,* systolic blood pressure; *SL,* sublingual. (From Antman EM, Anbe DT, Armstrong PW, et al. ACC/AHA guidelines for the management of patients with ST-elevation myocardial infarction: a report of the American College of Cardiology/American Heart Association Task Force on Practice Guidelines. *Circulation.* 2004;110;e82.)

TABLE 13.2	**Hemodynamic Profiles**
Left ventricular shock	High PCWP, low CO, high SVR
Right ventricular shock	High RA
	RA/PCWP >0.8
	Exaggerated RA "y" descent
	RV square root sign
Mitral regurgitation	Large PCWP "v" wave
Ventricular septal defect	Large PCWP "v" wave, oxygen saturation step-up (>5%) from RA to RV
Pericardial tamponade	Equalization of diastolic pressures ~20 mm Hg

CO, Cardiac output; *PCWP*, pulmonary capillary wedge pressure; *RA*, right atrial; *RV*, right ventricular; *SVR*, systemic vascular resistance.

TABLE 13.3	**Pharmacologic Treatment for Cardiogenic Shock**	
Drug	**Dose**	**Side Effects**
Dobutamine	5–15 µg/kg/min IV	Tolerance
Dopamine	2–20 µg/kg/min IV	Increased oxygen demand
Norepinephrine	0.5–30 µg/min IV	Peripheral and visceral vasoconstriction
Nitroglycerin	10 µg/min, increased by 10 µg every 10 min, maximum 200 µg/min IV	Headache, hypotension, tolerance
Nitroprusside	0.3–10 µg/min IV	Hypotension, cyanide toxicity
Milrinone	50 µg/kg over 10 min IV, then 0.375–0.75 µg/kg/min	Ventricular arrhythmia
Furosemide	20–160 mg/IV	Hypokalemia, hypomagnesemia
Bumetanide	1–3 mg IV	Nausea, cramps

IV, intravenous.

as feasible to measure intracardiac pressures, cardiac output, systemic vascular resistance, and mixed venous oxygen saturation. Although use of the pulmonary artery catheter has not been associated with mortality benefit in patients without MI, it is very helpful in the titration of fluids and medications in patients with cardiogenic shock.

The hemodynamic profile of left ventricular shock, as defined by Forrester and coworkers,[12] includes pulmonary artery wedge pressure greater than 18 mm Hg and a cardiac index less than 2.2 L/min per m². Others have used a pulmonary wedge pressure of 15 or 12 mm Hg and a cardiac index of 2.0 or 1.8 L/min per m². The hemodynamic profile of right ventricular shock includes right atrial pressure of 85% or more of the pulmonary artery wedge pressure, steep Y descent in the right atrial pressure tracing, and the dip and plateau (i.e., square root sign) in the right ventricular wave form. Large V waves in the pulmonary artery wedge tracing suggest the presence of severe mitral regurgitation. An oxygen saturation step-up (>5%) from the right atrium to the right ventricle confirms the diagnosis of ventricular septal rupture. Equalization of right atrial, right ventricular end-diastolic, pulmonary artery diastolic, and pulmonary capillary wedge pressures occurs with severe right ventricular infarction or pericardial tamponade due to free wall rupture or hemorrhagic effusion. Cardiac power (mean arterial pressure × cardiac output/451) is the strongest hemodynamic predictor of hospital mortality.[39]

Pharmacologic Support

Vasopressor and inotropic drugs are the major initial interventions for reversing hypotension and improving vital organ perfusion (Table 13.3). Failure to improve blood pressure with these agents is an ominous prognostic sign. Continued hypotension results in progressive myocardial ischemia and deterioration of ventricular function. Although many patients temporarily respond to therapy, hospital mortality rates remain unchanged without successful reperfusion therapy.

Dobutamine, a synthetic catecholamine with predominantly β₁-adrenergic effects, is the initial inotropic agent of choice for patients with systolic pressures greater than 70 mm Hg. Cardiac output is increased and filling pressures are decreased. Dobutamine is particularly effective in right ventricular shock.

Dopamine, a natural catecholamine, is the initial vasopressor of choice when the systolic pressure is greater than 70 mm Hg. Low doses (2–5 µg/kg per minute) increase stroke volume and renal perfusion by stimulating dopamine receptors. Intermediate doses have a dose-dependent β₁-adrenergic receptor effect, increasing inotropy and chronotropy. High doses (15–20 µg/kg per min) activate α-adrenergic receptors, increasing vascular resistance.

Norepinephrine is a natural catecholamine with predominantly peripheral α-adrenergic effects. It is used when the systolic pressure is less than 70 mm Hg, because it is a potent venous and arterial vasoconstrictor. Many now prefer norepinephrine over dopamine as initial therapy.

Catecholamine infusions should be carefully titrated. A delicate balance must be obtained between increasing coronary perfusion pressure and increasing oxygen demand so that myocardial ischemia is not exacerbated. Moreover, excessive peripheral vasoconstriction decreases tissue perfusion, increased afterload increases filling pressures, and excessive tachycardia or arrhythmias can be stimulated. Extravasation of dopamine or norepinephrine can cause tissue necrosis.

Cardiac glycosides have no significant inotropic effect in patients with severe pump failure and they increase oxygen consumption. Ischemic myocardium is susceptible to the arrhythmogenic effects of digoxin, and intravenous administration causes coronary and peripheral vasoconstriction. Digitalis may be employed for supraventricular tachyarrhythmias to control heart rate.

Vasodilators are useful if adequate blood pressure and coronary artery perfusion pressure can be restored. Nitroprusside is an arterial dilator and a venodilator, whereas nitroglycerin is predominantly a venodilator. Afterload reduction increases stroke volume and is especially important when mitral regurgitation or ventricular septal rupture is present. Preload reduction decreases filling pressures and oxygen demand by reducing wall tension. The major hazard is that reduction in preload and afterload could decrease diastolic arterial pressure, compromising coronary artery perfusion pressure and resulting in extension of ischemic myocardial injury. Reflex tachycardia increases oxygen demand. Nitroglycerin and nitroprusside can be started at low-dose infusions and titrated against blood pressure and pulmonary capillary wedge pressure. Phosphodiesterase inhibitors (e.g., milrinone) are not indicated for acute cardiogenic shock but can be useful in low-output states when the patient is relatively stable by augmenting myocardial contractility and producing peripheral vasodilation.

Mechanical Support

When pharmacologic therapy provides insufficient hemodynamic support, mechanical circulatory assistance can be instituted, especially when revascularization or surgical repair of mechanical complications is planned (Figs. 13.3 and 13.4). IABP counterpulsation reduces systolic afterload and augments diastolic perfusion pressure. The usual result is a decrease in filling pressures, systolic blood pressure, heart rate, mitral regurgitation, and left-to-right shunting across a ventricular septal rupture,

along with an increase in diastolic and mean blood pressure, stroke volume, cardiac output, and urine output. Subendocardial blood flow is improved and, in contrast to vasopressor support, oxygen demand is decreased.

Kantrowitz and colleagues[9] first reported the use of IABP counterpulsation in treating cardiogenic shock. Mueller and coworkers[40] demonstrated improved hemodynamics and myocardial metabolism associated with IABP therapy. Improvement in infarct zone regional wall motion, but not adjacent noninfarct zone regional wall motion, was shown by Weiss and associates.[41] No improvement in coronary blood flow occurs distal to highly stenotic coronary arteries.[42] The IABP favorably influences systemic hemodynamics, but it does not improve ischemic zone blood flow or noninfarct zone wall motion.

The failure to improve ischemic myocardial blood flow probably explains why, despite temporary hemodynamic and clinical improvement in 75% of patients, no obvious difference in enzymatic infarct size or mortality rate with IABP counterpulsation has been noted in the literature.[10,11] The mortality rates in a large cooperative trial were 60% during IABP support, 77% during hospitalization, and 91% at 1 year for 87 patients.[11] The only

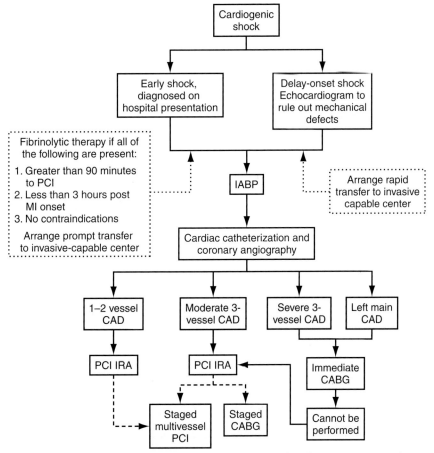

Fig. 13.3 Recommendations for initial reperfusion therapy. *CABG*, coronary artery bypass graft surgery; *CAD*, coronary artery disease; *IABP*, intraaortic balloon counterpulsation; *IRA*, infarct-related artery; *LBBB*, left bundle branch block; *MI*, myocardial infarction; *PCI*, percutaneous coronary intervention. (From Antman EM, Anbe DT, Armstrong PW, et al. ACC/AHA guidelines for the management of patients with ST-elevation myocardial infarction: a report of the American College of Cardiology/American Heart Association Task Force on Practice Guidelines. *Circulation.* 2004;110;e82.)

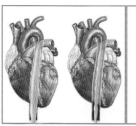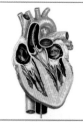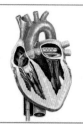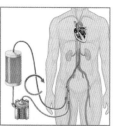

	IABP	IMPELLA	TANDEMHEART	VA-ECMO
Cardiac Flow	0.3-0.5 L/ min	1-5L/ min (Impella 2.5, Impella CP, Impella 5)	2.5-5 L/min	3-7 L/min
Mechanism	Aorta	LV → AO	LA → AO	RA → AO
Maximum Implant Days	Weeks	7 days	14 days	Weeks
Sheath Size	7-8 Fr	13-14 Fr Impella 5.0 - 21 Fr	15-17 Fr Arterial 21 Fr Venous	14-16 Fr Arterial 18-21 Fr Venous
Femoral Artery Size	>4 mm	Impella 2.5 & CP - 5-5.5 mm Impella 5 - 8 mm	8 mm	8 mm
Cardiac Synchrony or Stable Rhythm	Yes	No	No	No
Afterload	↓	↓	↑	↑↑↑
MAP	↑	↑↑	↑↑	↑↑
Cardiac Flow	↑	↑↑	↑↑	↑↑
Cardiac Power	↑	↑↑	↑↑	↑↑
LVEDP	↓	↓↓	↓↓	↔
PCWP	↓	↓↓	↓↓	↔
LV Preload	---	↓↓	↓↓	↓
Coronary Perfusion	↑	↑	---	---
Myocardial Oxygen Demand	↓	↓↓	↔↓	↔

Fig. 13.4 Comparison of mechanical support devices. *AO*, Aorta; *IABP*, intraaortic balloon pump; *LA*, left atrium; *LV*, left ventricle; *LVEDP*, left ventricular end-diastolic pressure; *MAP*, mean arterial pressure; *PCWP*, pulmonary capillary wedge pressure; *RA*, right atrium; *VA-ECMO*, venoarterial extracorporeal membrane oxygenation. (From Atkinson TM, Ohman EM, O'Neill WW, et al. A practical approach to mechanical circulatory support in patients undergoing percutaneous coronary intervention: an interventional persepective. *JACC Cardiovasc Interv.* 2016;9:871-883.)

randomized trial was performed by O'Rourke and colleagues.[43] No difference in enzymatic infarct size or mortality was observed.

IABP counterpulsation offers little support to shock patients with extensively scarred ventricles or after late presentation. The best use is in patients with ischemic, viable, but nonfunctioning myocardium that can be revascularized or with mitral regurgitation or ventricular septal rupture amenable to surgical repair. Dunkman and colleagues[10] showed that the addition of bypass graft surgery to IABP support decreased mortality from 84% to 60%.

Several reports have examined the use of IABP counterpulsation in conjunction with fibrinolytic therapy strategies.[44–48] There were some favorable trends but significantly more bleeding episodes. There has been only one randomized controlled trial comparing IABP counterpulsation plus fibrinolytic therapy to fibrinolysis alone. The Thrombolysis and Counterpulsation to Improve Cardiogenic Shock Survival (TACTICS) trial[48] sought to enroll 500 patients with acute STEMI complicated by shock, but only 57 patients were actually enrolled. Six-month follow-up showed a trend toward mortality reduction in the IABP group,

but this was not significant because of small sample size. The strategy of early fibrinolytic therapy and IABP counterpulsation, followed by immediate transfer for PCI or CABG, may be appropriate for hospitals that do not have revascularization capability.

The use of IABP therapy in patients undergoing primary or rescue PCI has also been evaluated. Early studies with balloon angioplasty suggested a reduction in infarct artery reocclusion rates and improvement in clinical outcome in patients without cardiogenic shock.[49,50] However, a recent trial in the stent era failed to demonstrate a survival benefit in cardiogenic shock.[51] In patients with cardiogenic shock, insertion of the IABP catheter before angiography provides optimal hemodynamic support during PCI and in the early treatment period even if it does not reduce mortality rates.

The American College of Cardiology/American Heart Association (ACC/AHA) STEMI guidelines have given a class IIa recommendation (can be useful) for use of IABP counterpulsation in patients with cardiogenic shock who do not quickly stabilize with pharmacologic therapy.[52]

Contraindications for IABP counterpulsation therapy include aortic regurgitation, aortic dissection, and peripheral vascular disease. Complications occur in 10% to 30% of patients with cardiogenic shock and include limb ischemia, femoral artery laceration, aortic dissection, infection, hemolysis, thrombocytopenia, thrombosis, and embolism.

Devices that offer greater circulatory support than IABP counterpulsation are available and have been used in cardiogenic shock as a bridge to recovery or to transplantation (see Fig. 13.4). These devices may be classified into those that can be placed percutaneously and those that require surgical placement. It is critical to recognize early which patients will require greater hemodynamic support than provided by IABP therapy.

Percutaneous cardiopulmonary bypass with venoarterial extracorporeal membrane oxygenation (VA-ECMO) can be initiated at the bedside via the femoral artery and vein and can provide 3 to 5 L/min of nonpulsatile flow and a mean aortic pressure of 50 to 70 mm Hg despite cardiac standstill.[53] A review of 52 studies (533 patients) suggested a mean survival to discharge of 51% (median 38%) among patients with cardiogenic shock treated with percutaneous bypass.[54] A single-center retrospective comparison of 219 patients treated with VA-ECMO versus a historical control of 115 patients without VA-ECMO supported a survival benefit (70% vs. 58%).[55] These results are encouraging since VA-ECMO is more commonly used emergently for cardiac arrest or near-arrest circumstances. Left ventricular decompression is not possible with these devices.

Another strategy has been to use ventricular assist devices (VADs) as a bridge to recovery or to transplant or even as destination therapy. These devices can be placed percutaneously or surgically. The TandemHeart device (CardiacAssist, Inc.) utilizes a 21 Fr femoral cannula placed across the interatrial septum into the left atrium, while a shorter 15 Fr or 17 Fr cannula is placed in the femoral artery, allowing left atrial to arterial assist pumping by an extracorporeal centrifugal continuous flow pump. Two small randomized trials compared IABP counterpulsation and the TandemHeart device in patients undergoing primary PCI for acute MI complicated by cardiogenic shock. While the TandemHeart device provided better hemodynamic support, the risk of complications was higher and there was no difference in 30-day mortality.[56,57]

The microaxial flow pump catheter (Impella; Abiomed, Inc.) is placed into the left ventricle across the aortic valve in retrograde fashion and pumps blood from the left ventricle into the aorta. The Impella EURO-SHOCK Registry included 120 patients treated with the Impella device: 30-day mortality was 64%.[58] A small randomized trial with 25 patients showed no difference in mortality compared with IABP counterpulsation.[59]

Surgically implanted VADs have also been used in cardiogenic shock. These devices require placement via thoracotomy but can be left in place long term. In a single-center series, the Thoratec biventricular assist device was used as a successful bridge to cardiac transplantation in 11 of 19 patients in cardiogenic shock.[60] Both percutaneous and surgical VADs are available only at select centers; early transfer of patients to these facilities should be considered for patients failing standard supportive measures.

REPERFUSION STRATEGIES

Fibrinolytic Therapy

Several multicenter randomized megatrials have demonstrated that fibrinolytic therapy reduces mortality from acute MI.[2–5] Moreover, the greatest survival benefit has been confirmed for patients with the most jeopardized myocardium (e.g., anterior infarction, new left bundle branch block). It is paradoxical and disappointing that no obvious survival benefit has been realized for the subset of patients with cardiogenic shock.[61]

Mathey and colleagues[14] first reported that the shock state could be reversed with successful reperfusion due to intracoronary streptokinase administration. However, a multicenter registry report on 44 patients treated with intracoronary streptokinase documented a 66% in-hospital mortality rate,[62] but the importance of successful reperfusion and outcome was first suggested by this report. Only 43% of the patients had successful reperfusion compared with 71% for the entire study, but their mortality rate was 42%, compared with 84% for unsuccessful reperfusion.

Compared with placebo, intravenous fibrinolytic therapy reduces the risk of subsequent cardiogenic shock in patients who initially present without shock.[3,4,63] Comparative trials of fibrinolytic agents have shown variable results. Those that show no difference in mortality between agents also do not show a reduction in the incidence of cardiogenic shock with any one agent.[64–66] In contrast, those comparative trials that show a mortality benefit in favor of one agent also showed a significant reduction in the incidence of cardiogenic shock in favor of that agent.[67–69] Thus one can conclude that therapy with fibrinolytic agents in acute MI significantly reduces the subsequent development of cardiogenic shock and that those agents that are associated with higher patency rates and improved survival in comparative studies also lead to lower rates of shock.

Fibrinolytic therapy for patients presenting in manifest cardiogenic shock is associated with relatively low reperfusion rates and no clear-cut treatment benefit.[61] Mean arterial pressure must be above 65 mm Hg for coronary blood flow to be maintained; flow ceases when mean arterial pressure is below 30 mm Hg. Furthermore, vasoconstriction and passive collapse of the arterial wall are additional factors that may limit the ability of the fibrinolytic agent to penetrate an intracoronary thrombus.[70] Canine studies demonstrated that restoration of blood pressure to normal ranges with norepinephrine infusion improved reperfusion rates, suggesting that coronary perfusion pressure, not cardiac output, is the major determinant of fibrinolytic efficacy.[71,72] Interestingly, the trials that compared streptokinase with alteplase showed mortality benefit for shock patients randomized to streptokinase, despite the fact that patients treated with alteplase fared better.[64,68] Streptokinase may be beneficial in this subset of patients because it causes a prolonged fibrinolytic state in the setting of low coronary blood flow (which may reduce the risk of reocclusion) and because it is less fibrin specific and may therefore penetrate the thrombus better because it does not bind preferentially to the surface of the clot. Because of the limitations of fibrinolytic therapy for cardiogenic shock, it should be considered as a secondary treatment option when revascularization therapy with PCI or CABG is not rapidly available. Viable patients should then be transferred to a hospital with revascularization capability as soon as possible so that the potential benefits of revascularization therapy might still be obtained.

Percutaneous Coronary Intervention

Meyer et al.[15] were the first to use PCI to treat cardiogenic shock. The first treatment series were reported in 1985. O'Neill and colleagues[73] obtained successful reperfusion in 24 (88%) of 27 patients, with an in-hospital mortality rate of 25%. Brown and coworkers[74] had a 61% successful reperfusion rate, associated with a 42% mortality rate; the mortality rate was 82% when reperfusion was unsuccessful. Multiple small observational reports since then have consistently shown a survival benefit for patients in whom PCI was successful compared with patients in whom PCI was unsuccessful or with historical controls.

There have been a few large observational reports on reperfusion therapy for cardiogenic shock. The Global Utilization of Streptokinase and Tissue Plasminogen Activator for Occluded Coronary Arteries (GUSTO-1) trial[75] included 2972 patients with cardiogenic shock treated with fibrinolytic therapy. There was a lower 30-day mortality rate for the 22% of patients who were subsequently treated with PCI compared with those receiving only medical therapy (43% vs. 61% with shock on arrival, 32% vs. 61% for those who developed shock after arrival). Another GUSTO-1 analysis included 2200 patients with cardiogenic shock.[76] Compared with a delayed strategy, angiography within 24 hours of shock onset with revascularization by PCI or CABG when deemed appropriate was independently associated with reduced 30-day mortality (38% vs. 62%).

A large registry evaluated the outcome of 1333 patients undergoing primary PCI for cardiogenic shock.[77] The in-hospital mortality in this cohort was 46%. The independent predictors of mortality were left main disease, thrombolysis in myocardial infarction (TIMI) less than grade 3 flow after PCI, older age, three-vessel disease, and longer time interval between symptom onset and PCI.

None of these reports represent randomized, controlled studies of PCI. A selection bias favoring PCI over historical controls could easily have resulted from excluding the elderly or patients in extremis or with comorbid disease. Hochman and colleagues[78] have documented that patients with cardiogenic shock who are selected for cardiac catheterization are younger and less likely to die (51% vs. 85%), even when not revascularized. Nevertheless, several studies and clinical experience clearly demonstrate the favorable impact that a patent infarct artery can have on reversing the shock state.

Two small randomized trials have been performed. The Swiss Multicenter trial of Angioplasty SHock (SMASH)[79] randomized 55 patients to either undergo emergency angiography and revascularization when indicated or initial medical management but was terminated prematurely because of poor enrollment. Mortality at 30 days was 69% in the invasive arm versus 78% in the medical arm. At 1 year, the mortality figures were 74% and 83%, respectively. Although the study failed to reach statistical significance because of sample size, the trend was clinically important. The Should We Emergently Revascularize Occluded Coronaries for Cardiogenic Shock (SHOCK) trial[17-19] randomized 302 patients to emergent revascularization or immediate medical stabilization. Concurrently, the 30 participating sites collected registry data on 1190 patients presenting with cardiogenic shock who were not randomized.[80] Medical stabilization included fibrinolytic therapy in over half the patients as well as inotropic and vasopressor agents. IABP counterpulsation was used in 86% of the patients. In the revascularization arm, 97% of patients underwent early angiography; 64% underwent PCI and 36% had CABG. There was no statistically significant difference in 30-day mortality between the revascularization and medical therapy groups (46.7% vs. 56.0%; $P = 0.11$), but by the 6-month endpoint, a significant survival advantage had emerged for patients randomized to revascularization (50.3% vs. 63.1%, $P = .027$) that was maintained at 1 year (53.3% vs. 66.4%).

Emergency PCI is recommended by the ACC/AHA STEMI guidelines for those who are suitable for revascularization unless further support is deemed futile (class I).[52] The best candidates for PCI are patients without prior MI who are younger than 75 years of age with fewer comorbidities and symptom duration less than 12 hours. The severity, distribution, and diffuseness of coronary artery disease and the degree of left ventricular dysfunction also influence outcome. Poor candidates because of very high mortality risk are those with rapidly progressive hemodynamic deterioration despite therapeutic interventions and elderly patients with comorbid disease. Additionally, patients with life-shortening illnesses, no vascular access, previously defined coronary anatomy that was unsuitable for revascularization, anoxic brain damage, and prior cardiomyopathy are poor candidates. Except for the elderly, all other subgroups had treatment benefit with revascularization in the SHOCK trial.[17]

Analysis of the elderly patient subgroup in the SHOCK registry[81] was performed to gain further insight in patients at least 75 years of age. Whereas the randomized trial included only 56 patients in that age group, the registry included 277 patients. Overall, in-hospital mortality in the elderly versus the younger age group was 76% versus 55% ($P < .001$). The 44 elderly patients selected for early revascularization, however, showed a significantly lower mortality rate than those who did not undergo revascularization (48% vs. 81%; $P = .0002$). Other reports[82-84] also support the use of primary PCI in selected elderly patients with cardiogenic shock complicating MI; thus, age alone should not be an exclusion for selecting patients for cardiac catheterization. Prior functional status, comorbidity, and patient and family preferences are important selection criteria.

Emergency angiography determines revascularization suitability. Angiographic exclusions for PCI include infarct artery stenosis less than 70% with TIMI grade 3 flow or lesion morphology that is high risk for no reflow or other complications. Emergency CABG surgery may be considered for patients with severe coronary anatomy unsuitable for PCI, multivessel disease, mechanical complications, or failed PCI if there is ongoing myocardial ischemia.

The procedure is most safely performed with the patient ventilated and sedated or paralyzed. Gas exchange is maximized, risk of aspiration is minimized, cardioversion can be performed easily, and patient movements do not interfere with the procedure.

Both femoral arteries and veins are cannulated with vascular sheaths. An IABP or Impella device is inserted through one femoral artery for hemodynamic support and a pulmonary artery catheter is inserted through a femoral vein. Interventions to control volume and pressure are titrated against the systemic and pulmonary artery wedge pressures. Electrolytes and blood gases are monitored and abnormalities are corrected. A temporary pacemaker is inserted if necessary.

PCI is best performed when the patient is maximally supported. Using a low osmolar ionic contrast medium, two orthogonal injections of the left coronary artery and one left anterior oblique injection of the right coronary artery are made in an attempt to identify the infarct artery. Left ventriculography should usually be avoided because of the contrast load. If PCI is to be attempted, it should be performed as quickly and efficiently as possible, with limited contrast injections. Although PCI for STEMI is usually limited to the infarct artery, patients in cardiogenic shock with multivessel disease may have the best survival chance with PCI of all proximal discrete lesions. Early resolution of arrhythmias, conduction blocks, or hypotension suggests an important therapeutic benefit. Conversely, failure to improve within the first 24 hours usually predicts mortality.

Coronary stents decrease restenosis rates in elective PCI compared with balloon angioplasty but have not reduced mortality rates in primary PCI.[85] Some observational studies in cardiogenic shock that have not completely corrected for confounding variables suggest lower mortality rates with stents than percutaneous transluminal coronary angioplasty (PTCA),[86-88] but others show no benefit[89] or higher mortality rates.[90] Randomized studies have not been performed. Most patients undergoing primary PCI for cardiogenic shock will receive stents because they improve the immediate angiographic result and decrease subsequent target vessel revascularization in survivors.

The use of platelet glycoprotein (GP) IIb/IIIa inhibitors may improve outcomes with primary PCI.[91] Observational studies suggested a benefit of abciximab in primary stenting for cardiogenic shock.[87,89,90,92] While there are no randomized controlled trials evaluating use of abciximab or other GP IIb/IIIa inhibitors in cardiogenic shock, they can be used as adjunctive therapy when unfractionated heparin is used instead of bivalirudin for anticoagulation. However, the use of GP IIb/IIIa inhibitors has greatly decreased since the introduction of oral platelet $P2Y_{12}$ receptor inhibitors.

Surgery

Dunkman and associates[10] were the first to report the use of CABG for cardiogenic shock. Emergency CABG is associated with mortality rates ranging from 25% to 60%. In the SHOCK trial,[17] one-third of the patients randomized to revascularization were treated with a surgical approach. Patients were more likely to have left main disease or three-vessel disease than those treated with PCI. Thirty-day mortality for patients undergoing surgery was equivalent to PCI mortality (42% vs. 45%). The high degree of surgical expertise required, inherent time delays, increasing hesitancy of surgeons to operate on patients with high operative mortality risk because of "scorecard" medicine, and favorable results with PCI make emergency CABG an increasingly rare

intervention. It is more often performed electively in survivors with multivessel disease.

Surgical repair of acute mitral regurgitation,[22] ventricular septal defect,[23] and free wall rupture[24] can be accomplished, although mortality rates are high. The use of emergency cardiac transplantation has been reported.[93]

NEW APPROACHES

New approaches to cardiogenic shock have focused on mechanisms beyond mechanical support and revascularization. A significant proportion of patients in the SHOCK trial exhibited a systemic inflammatory response syndrome (SIRS) marked by fever, leukocytosis, and low systemic vascular resistance.[36] Complement activation, release of inflammatory cytokines, expression of inducible nitric oxide synthase (NOS), and inappropriate vasodilation were deemed culpable and inhibition of NO production was explored as a therapeutic strategy. Early single-center clinical studies indicated a dramatic benefit from inhibition of NOS.[94,95] The phase 2, dose-ranging trial SHould we inhibit nitric Oxide synthase in cardiogenic shoCK 2 (SHOCK-2) demonstrated modest early changes in hemodynamic parameters, but no effect on survival.[96] The large multicenter Tilarginine Acetate Injection in a Randomized International Study in Unstable MI Patients with Cardiogenic Shock (TRIUMPH) trial was halted after no benefit was seen during an interim analysis.[97]

There is intense clinical and basic science activity exploring delivery of stem cells to the infarcted myocardium to improve left ventricular recovery. While the early studies remain inconclusive, it is likely that cardiogenic shock survivors will be enrolled in the pivotal trials once an effective strategy to salvage or revive the infarcted myocardium is discovered.

It is important to note that recent emphasis on reperfusion therapy for all patients with STEMI, the importance of time to treatment, and the increasing use of primary PCI as the reperfusion modality have dramatically decreased the number of patients developing cardiogenic shock as a complication of STEMI.[98] Because cardiogenic shock is usually an in-hospital complication of MI occurring hours after infarct artery occlusion, early restoration of infarct artery patency to prevent development of the shock state is the best approach to this complication.

PROGNOSIS

The historical early mortality rate for cardiogenic shock complicating acute MI treated with medical therapy was 65% to 80%. Current rapid reperfusion strategies and adjunctive therapies have reduced that rate to 40% to 50%. Rigorous observation of high-risk patients (e.g., age >75 years, history of prior MI, ejection fraction <35%, large myocardial infarction, diabetes, female gender); rapid diagnosis (e.g., careful physical examination, hemodynamic monitoring, echocardiography, cardiac catheterization); and prompt correction of arrhythmias, electrolyte and blood gas abnormalities, volume status, and hypotension may prevent the patient from spiraling into the shock state. When cardiogenic shock is present, early circulatory support to increase mean arterial pressure, reduction in left ventricular volume (preload) and pressure (afterload) to reduce myocardial oxygen demand, and coronary artery reperfusion decrease the risk of developing multiorgan dysfunction syndrome (MDS) and the SIRS.

In the SHOCK registry, in-hospital mortality rates rose from 34% to 51% as the number of diseased arteries increased from one to three.[99] After PCI, the mortality rate was 86% with absent reperfusion (TIMI grade 0/1 flow), 50% with incomplete reperfusion (TIMI grade 2 flow), and 33% with complete reperfusion (TIMI grade 3 flow). Similarly, final TIMI flow was a major predictor of outcome in a German registry with mortality rates of 78%, 66%, and 37% for TIMI grade 0/1, TIMI grade 2 and TIMI grade 3 flow, respectively.[77]

A total of 87% of the 1-year survivors in the SHOCK trial were in New York Heart Association (NYHA) functional class I or II.[100] The 13 lives saved per 100 patients treated with early revascularization in the SHOCK trial at 6 months and 1 year was maintained at 3 and 6 years.[19] Overall survival rates at 6 years were 32.8% in the early revascularization group and 19.6% in the initial medical stabilization group. The 6-year survival rates for the hospital survivors were 62.4% versus 44.4%, respectively.

At 30 days in the GUSTO-1 trial, 20,360 patients without shock (88.9%) and 953 (50.4%) patients with shock were alive.[101] After a median of 11 years, 69.4% without and 55.2% with shock remained alive. Patients receiving PCI were less likely to die (24.1% vs. 34.6%). Beginning in the second year, mortality rates were 2% to 4% per year for all patients regardless of shock status (Fig. 13.5).

CONCLUSION

Patients with cardiogenic shock complicating MI have a substantial survival benefit with PCI compared with no or late in-hospital

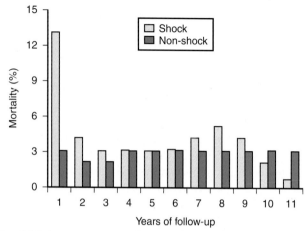

Fig. 13.5 Long-term mortality rate in 30-day survivors in the GUSTO-I trial (From Singh M, White J, Hasdai D, et al. Long-term outcome and its predictors among patients with ST-segment elevation myocardial infarction complicated by shock. *J Am Coll Cardiol.* 2007;50:1752.)

revascularization. These patients need to be directly admitted or transferred to tertiary care shock centers with expertise in acute revascularization and advanced intensive care unless further care is deemed futile. Novel therapies are needed to further decrease mortality rates in patients who develop cardiogenic shock, which remain high despite successful reperfusion therapy.

The full reference list for this chapter is available at ExpertConsult.com.

14

Right Ventricular Infarction

Jonathan D. Moreno, David L. Brown

Infarction of the right ventricle is now known to be a common clinical event, occurring in one-third of patients with inferior myocardial infarction (MI).[1-3] Right ventricular (RV) infarction confers a worse prognosis in patients with inferior wall MI.[2] Because of the requirement for different treatment strategies in right ventricular myocardial infarction (RVMI), prompt recognition and appropriate treatment require a thorough understanding of the unique anatomy and pathophysiology of the RV.

HISTORICAL PERSPECTIVE

In 1930, Sanders[4] reported the first clinical description of RVMI. During the following 4 decades, RVMI received attention mainly in autopsy series.[5] At that time, any shock syndrome was considered the result of MI.[6,7] This view was buttressed by evidence from open pericardium dog models in which destruction of the right ventricle was not associated with shock.[8,9] The development of surgical procedures that bypassed the right ventricle, such as the Glenn and Fontan procedures, furthered the belief that the right ventricle is mainly a volume conduit contributing little to cardiac output.[10,11]

In 1974, Cohn and coworkers[12] first called attention to RVMI as a unique clinical and hemodynamic syndrome characterized, in its extreme form, by shock, distended neck veins, and clear lung fields. During the ensuing 2 decades of intense investigation into the syndrome, the crucial role of ventricular interdependence through the pericardium and the septum was recognized.[13-16] Today, a rational approach to therapy of RVMI based on an understanding of its pathophysiology is possible.

CORONARY CIRCULATION AND THE RIGHT VENTRICLE

In the 85% of patients with right dominant coronary circulation, the RV receives its blood supply almost exclusively from the right coronary artery (RCA), with the septum and part of the posterior wall supplied by the posterior descending artery and the anterior and lateral RV walls supplied by acute marginal branches of the RCA.[17,18] The left anterior descending (LAD) artery supplies a small portion of the anterior wall of the right ventricle. In left dominant circulation, the left circumflex coronary artery supplies the posterior descending artery, and a nondominant RCA supplies the acute marginal branches. Isolated RV infarct without any LV involvement can occur with occlusion of a nondominant RCA.

The angiographic hallmark of RVMI is thrombotic occlusion of the RCA proximal to the origin of the acute marginal branches. Angiographic flow studies suggest that the status of RV branch perfusion is the critical determinant of RV ischemic dysfunction.[19] Proximal RCA occlusions typically limit RV branch perfusion in contrast to distal RCA occlusions.

Not every case of proximal RCA occlusion results in RV infarction.[18] This relative protection of the right ventricle from infarction is thought to be a consequence of its lower oxygen demand, its continued perfusion during systole, and the potential presence of collaterals from the LAD coronary artery, which, because of the lower systolic pressure on the right side, are more capable of supplying blood in the direction of the right ventricle than in the reverse direction. The LAD collaterals to the RV are mainly through the moderator band artery, a branch of the first septal perforator.[20] Prior severe stenosis or occlusions of the LAD coronary artery can limit the development of collaterals to the right ventricle with an acute RCA occlusion increasing the degree of acute ischemic RV dysfunction.[21]

VENTRICULAR INTERDEPENDENCE

The concept of ventricular interdependence in RVMI is central to understanding the pathogenesis of the resultant low cardiac output state. Ventricular interdependence is mediated through the common pericardium and shared septum. The septum is an integral component—both physically and functionally—to the RV and even under physiologic conditions, septal contraction contributes to RV performance.[22] In RVMI, acute RV dilation occurs.[15,16,23] Because the RV shares a relatively fixed space with the LV, the pericardial pressure abruptly increases, leading to impaired LV filling. In animal models with the pericardium removed, it is difficult to induce hypotension with RVMI.[8] When the pericardium is left intact,[16,24] however, RVMI is associated with the full syndrome, as originally described by Cohn and coworkers.[12] Incision of the pericardium leads to improvement in cardiac output, pressure equalization, and an increase in RV systolic pressure.[16]

The increase in right-sided diastolic pressure that occurs in RVMI leads to a reversal of the normal left-to-right transseptal diastolic gradient.[25] On echocardiography, the septum can be seen to flatten and encroach on the LV diastolic dimension. During systole, the septum can be seen to move paradoxically toward the RV, at times in a piston-like manner.[16]

Except in rare cases of isolated RVMI,[26,27] some degree of LVMI accompanies RVMI. The pericardial constraint and alterations in septal geometry lead to reduced LV filling; cardiac output is diminished further by the decrease in LV systolic function. Development of shock syndrome with isolated RV infarction[26] proves, however, that LV systolic dysfunction is not necessary for the development of shock. Echocardiographic assessment in cases of hemodynamically severe RVMI has confirmed that shock may be present with preserved LV systolic function.[16]

The hemodynamic hallmarks of RV infarction (Box 14.1) are a decrease in cardiac output, elevation of right atrial pressure

---

(>10 mm Hg), elevation of RV diastolic pressure, and decrease in RV systolic pressure.[28–30] There is diastolic equalization of RV and LV pressures, as in cardiac tamponade and the ratio between right atrial and pulmonary capillary wedge pressure increases. This ratio, which normally is less than 0.65, is usually greater than 0.8 in RVMI.[28] RV tracing reveals a delayed, depressed, and often bifid peak, indicating systolic RV failure.[16] RV diastolic failure is also manifested by a dip and plateau pattern on the RV pressure tracing. In most studies, hemodynamic tracings showed a blunted *x* descent with a prominent *y* descent, suggesting decreased compliance of the RV, as seen in pericardial constriction (Fig. 14.1).[18,28–32] Although the hemodynamic criteria for RVMI are usually present on admission, volume loading may increase the identification of these abnormalities in some patients.[29]

CLINICAL PRESENTATION

Clinically significant RVMI usually occurs in patients with concomitant inferoposterior infarction of the LV, and many of the symptoms overlap. Necropsy studies suggest that RVMI occurs almost exclusively in patients with transmural posteroseptal MI.[33] The size of the LV infarct does not correlate with RV infarct size. The size of the RV infarct influences the severity of RV dysfunction and presentation, however.[21] What is unique to RVMI is the occurrence of a syndrome of RV diastolic and systolic failure that, in its extreme form, is characterized by a triad of signs: hypotension that can progress to cardiogenic shock, elevated neck veins, and clear lung fields.[4,12,18,34]

When RVMI is hemodynamically significant, the physical examination is a sensitive method of detection. Dell'Italia and colleagues[34] found elevated jugular venous pressure to be 88% sensitive, with a specificity of 69% for inferior wall MI with RV involvement. Kussmaul sign, an inspiratory increase in the jugular venous pressure, was found to be 100% sensitive and specific in the same series; Bellamy and coworkers[35] found it to have a sensitivity of 59% and a specificity of 89%. Other associated findings include a high frequency of bradycardia, atrioventricular (AV) block, and atrial arrhythmias, including supraventricular tachycardias and atrial fibrillation or flutter. A right-sided fourth

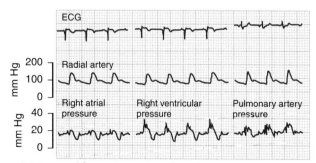

Fig. 14.1 Hemodynamic tracings in right ventricular myocardial infarction (RVMI). Noncompliant pattern of RVMI, with elevated right atrial pressure, a deep *y* descent in the atrial tracing, dip and plateau diastolic pattern in the right ventricle and relatively low pulmonary artery pressure. (From Lorrell B, Leinbach RC, Pohost GM, et al. Right ventricular infarction: clinical diagnosis and differentiation from cardiac tamponade and pericardial constriction. *Am J Cardiol.* 1979;43:465–471.)

BOX 14.1   Hemodynamic Findings in Cases of Right Ventricular Myocardial Infarction

Elevated right atrial pressure (>10 mm Hg)
Right atrial pressure/pulmonary wedge pressure ratio >0.8
Noncompliant jugular venous pattern (prominent *y* descent)
Dip and plateau right ventricular diastolic pressure pattern
Depressed and delayed (often bifid) right ventricular systolic pressure
Decreased cardiac output
Hypotension

heart sound was described in 11 of 16 patients in one series, with 4 of 16 having a right-sided third heart sound.[36] Tricuspid regurgitation may be audible. Pericardial friction rubs may be heard because infarction in the thin RV is usually transmural.[32]

The differential diagnosis includes tension pneumothorax, cardiac tamponade, constrictive pericarditis, pulmonary embolism, and, rarely, atypical RV-variant takotsubo cardiomyopathy.[37] When the full triad (hypotension, elevated neck veins, clear lungs) is present and ST segment elevations are observed in inferior leads, the diagnosis is straightforward. A potential pitfall is the occurrence of isolated RV branch infarction, which may manifest with the full clinical picture of RVMI but without evidence of MI on the standard 12-lead electrocardiogram (ECG)[26] or with ECG evidence of a presumed anterior infarct. Harnett et al.[38] recently presented a case series of two isolated RV branch MIs that were initially missed on angiography owing to an ECG pattern consistent with an anterior STEMI. Given the anatomic location, an isolated RVMI can mimic the clinical and ECG picture of an anterior LVMI. Consequently, anterior ST elevation in the precordial leads without reciprocal changes and lack of significant left coronary disease should prompt careful attention to the RV branch at time of angiography (Box 14.2).

Pulmonary embolism (PE) occasionally mimics RVMI and may predispose to occult RVMI.[39] Conversely, RVMI with secondary thrombus formation in the RV can lead to PE. Dyspnea is usually more severe in PE; RV systolic pressure, pulmonary artery pressure, and pulmonary vascular resistance are usually higher with PE than with RVMI. Cardiac tamponade may be acute and may manifest with a similar triad of elevated neck veins, hypotension, and clear lungs; it can be distinguished easily at the bedside with echocardiography, however. Pulsus paradoxus, a hallmark of tamponade, is unusual in RVMI, which tends to more closely resemble pericardial constriction.[32]

DIAGNOSIS

Electrocardiographic Diagnosis

ST Segment. The ECG remains the most useful tool for the diagnosis of RVMI.[40] The hallmark of acute RV ischemia is ST segment elevation in the right precordial leads, a finding first reported in 1976 by Erhardt and coworkers,[41] who used lead CR located in the fifth intercostal space at the right midclavicular line.[42] The importance of obtaining right-sided chest leads on presentation in patients with suspected acute MI, particularly with evidence of inferior wall involvement, cannot be overemphasized (Fig. 14.2).

Several studies have documented that ST segment elevation of 0.05 mV or greater (0.5 mm when using standard settings of 10 mm/mV) in lead V_{4R} in the setting of inferior MI is sensitive and specific for RV involvement, as documented by postmortem examination[42] or by radionuclide,[40,43,44] echocardiographic,[43] hemodynamic,[40] or angiographic studies.[32,44] Infrequently, ST segment elevation in V_{5R} or V_{6R} occurs in the absence of elevation in V_{4R}.[40,43] Zehender and colleagues[2,40] confirmed the utility of 0.1-mV ST segment elevation in any of the right precordial leads (V_{4R-V6R}) in a series of 200 patients, showing a sensitivity of 89% and a specificity of 83%.

The ECG findings in RVMI of right precordial ST segment elevations are the result of a rightward and anteriorly directed vector. Andersen and coworkers[45] showed that ST segment elevation in lead III exceeding that in lead II (i.e., ST segment vector directed rightward) is reasonably sensitive (68%) in diagnosing RVMI. This criterion had a specificity of only 11% and a positive predictive value of 58% in Zehender's series of 200 patients with inferior MI but had a sensitivity of 95%.[40]

Certain special situations with variant ECG findings that may cause confusion warrant mention. Geft and colleagues[46] described five patients with ST segment elevations in leads V_1 to V_5 who on catheterization were shown to have RCA occlusion and acute RVMI. All five patients had minimal or absent ST segment elevations in the inferior leads. The authors speculate that in the usual cases of RVMI, ST segment elevations in leads V_1 to V_5 are blocked by the dominant electrical forces of inferoposterior MI, resulting in isoelectric or even depressed ST segments in the left precordium. When these forces are absent, because of isolated RVMI[38,47] or with minimal posterior involvement, as may be seen in a patient with a codominant circulation,[46] ST segment elevation in the left precordial leads mimicking anterior wall MI may be seen. A distinguishing characteristic in RV infarction may be that the ST segment elevations are highest in leads V_1 or V_2 and decrease toward lead V_5, a pattern opposite that usually seen in anterior MI.[46]

If septal involvement can mimic RVMI, a left lateral wall infarction or a large true posterior infarction can be expected to cancel right precordial ST segment elevations. Such cases of false-negative findings have been described.[48,49]

Most studies of right precordial lead ST segment elevation have been limited to patients with evidence of inferior wall MI. In anterior MI, ST segment elevation in the right precordial leads has also been documented and has been found to be predictive of proximal LAD occlusion before the first septal branch, suggesting that the right precordial lead ST segment elevations are the result of a septal current of injury.[50] A distinguishing characteristic in cases of LAD occlusion is that the ST segment elevation has a leftward axis in contrast to the rightward ST segment in RV infarction, as emphasized by Hurst.[51] Other

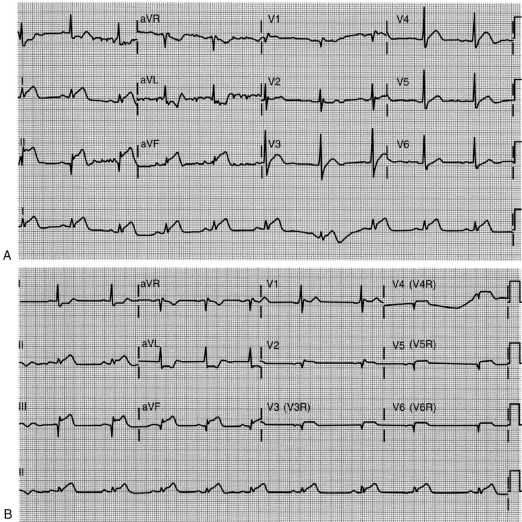

Fig. 14.2 (A) 12-Lead electrocardiogram from a 63-year-old man with chest discomfort after running on a treadmill, demonstrating ST elevation in lead III greater than in lead II; ST depression in leads I and aVL; and ST elevation in lead aVF greater than ST depression in lead V₂. Findings are suggestive of a right ventricular myocardial infarction. (B) 12-Lead electrocardiogram from the patient in (A) using right-sided precordial leads, demonstrating ST segment elevation in leads V₃R to V₆R, consistent with a right ventricular myocardial infarction. (From Nagam MR, Vinson DR, Levis JT. ECG diagnosis: right ventricular myocardial infarction. *Perm J.* 2017;21:16–105.)

causes of right precordial ST segment elevation in the absence of RVMI include pericardial disease, left anterior hemiblock, and PE.[52]

The time course of ST segment elevation in RVMI warrants emphasis. Braat and colleagues[43] reported that ST segment elevations in lead V₄R resolve within 10 hours after the onset of chest pain in half of patients. Similar findings were reported by Klein and colleagues.[48] Thus, it is important to obtain a right-sided ECG soon after the patient's presentation.

Q Waves in Right Ventricular Infarction. Because patients may present after the ST segments have returned to baseline, criteria using Q waves in the right precordial leads have been sought. In normal subjects, an rS pattern is always present in V₃R and usually (>90%) in V₄R. In one series[53] of patients with autopsy-documented RV infarction, the presence of a Q wave in these leads (as a QS or a QR pattern) was 100% specific and 78% sensitive. The high specificity (>90%) of Q waves was confirmed in Zehender's series of 200 patients with inferior wall MI.[40] Early in the course of infarction, Q waves are still absent and the sensitivity is low, particularly for patients presenting early. In patients admitted late (>12 hours after the onset of symptoms), the sensitivity increases to 95%.

Bundle Branch Block. RVMI, especially when extensive, has been shown to be associated with an incomplete and often transient right bundle branch block. The block is postulated to occur distally. Because there may also be precordial ST segment elevation in RV infarction, the right bundle branch block may be difficult to detect in lead V₁. Kataoka and coworkers[54] pointed to a cove-shaped ST-T elevation in lead V₁ as suggestive of an underlying right bundle branch block.

Atrioventricular Block. Significant AV block is more common in inferior wall MI with RV involvement.[55] The presence of ST segment elevation in V_{4R} was shown to predict the development of high-grade AV block, with 48% of patients in one series developing AV block during the first 3 days of infarction compared with only 13% without evidence of RVMI.[56] After AV block develops in the setting of RV infarction, it has important implications for therapy. Because cardiac output depends on preload and right atrial function, RV pacing alone may be inadequate to improve hemodynamics.

Arrhythmia. Atrial arrhythmias are common in RVMI. Because of the propensity for low cardiac output and preload dependence, these arrhythmias are poorly tolerated and should be treated aggressively. Early cardioversion and antidysrhythmic therapy for atrial fibrillation are recommended.[52] One study of patients with RVMI did not reveal an increase in ventricular arrhythmias compared with patients with inferior MI without RV involvement.[57]

Prognostic Implications. ECG findings for RV infarction have marked prognostic implications, even in the absence of hemodynamic abnormalities. In the series of 200 patients by Zehender and associates,[58] ST segment elevation in lead V_{4R} was shown on multiple logistic regression analyses to be the strongest predictor of in-hospital morbidity and mortality. Patients with inferior MI and ST segment elevation in V_{4R} had a mortality rate of 31% compared with 6% for patients without such evidence of RV involvement. Similarly, major complications (ventricular fibrillation, sustained ventricular tachycardia, cardiogenic shock, cardiac rupture, high-grade AV block, reinfarction) were markedly more common (64% vs. 28%; $P < .001$) in patients with ECG evidence of RV involvement. In one series, the presence of AV block in RV infarction was found to be associated with a mortality rate of 41%, whereas the mortality rate for patients with inferior wall infarction with RV infarction but without AV block and for patients with inferior MI with AV block but without RV infarction was only 11% to 14%.[59]

Echocardiography

Two-dimensional echocardiography is a fast, widely available, and inexpensive tool for assessment of RV function. It is also sensitive (80% to 90%) and specific (>90%) in the detection of hemodynamically significant RV infarction.[60–63] Key echocardiographic findings in RVMI include RV dilation, RV hypokinesis, abnormal (paradoxic) septal motion, septal flattening,[63] and reduced septal thickening (Video 14.1). Tissue Doppler imaging has also revealed that peak systolic velocity (S'_{TDI}) and peak early diastolic velocity (E'_{TDI}) are significantly reduced in RVMI.[64] Kidawa et al.[64] also utilized 3D echo to estimate RV ejection fraction (RVEF); while this performed no better than TDI in the diagnosis of RVMI, they found that an RVEF less than 51% has adequate specificity and sensitivity for RV infarct (Box 14.3).

Echocardiography is particularly useful in assessment of RVMI because it also provides information on LV function, associated valvular regurgitation, and possible alternative or concomitant

---

BOX 14.3 Echocardiographic Findings in Cases of Right Ventricular (RV) Myocardial Infarction

RV free wall dilatation and wall motion abnormalities (hypokinesis, akinesis)
Flattened interventricular septum (D-shaped septum) and paradoxic movement
Reduced septal wall thickening
Reduced tissue Doppler peak systolic velocity (S'), and early peak diastolic velocity (E')
Reduced RV ejection fraction (<51%)[64]

BOX 14.4 Treatment Strategies for Right Ventricular Myocardial Infarction

Volume resuscitation (goal: right atrial pressure 14 mm Hg)
Electrical stabilization and synchrony (may need atrial and ventricular sequential pacing)
Reperfusion therapy (early, primary percutaneous coronary intervention preferred)
Inotropic support for persistent hypotension with low output (dobutamine, dopamine, norepinephrine)
Right ventricular assist devices (Impella RP, intraaortic balloon pump, Tandem Heart)
Invasive hemodynamic monitoring

---

diagnoses such as cardiac tamponade. Echocardiography may also detect important complications, such as thrombus formation or pericardial effusion. Two-dimensional contrast echocardiography may help detect right-to-left shunting through a patent foramen ovale.[65] While echocardiography remains an indispensable tool for assessment of RV function, it remains technically challenging owing to the complex shape and structure of the RV, the need for multiple acoustic windows for complete visualization, and the transient nature of some echocardiographic abnormalities.[66]

Cardiovascular Magnetic Resonance Imaging

Late enhancement cardiovascular magnetic resonance imaging (MRI) has greater sensitivity at detecting RVMI than ECG, physical examination, or echocardiography. Late enhancement cardiovascular MRI findings of injury of the RV in the acute phase persist for 13 months, suggesting that this imaging modality can predict the extent of irreversible RV injury in the acute phase.[67]

TREATMENT

The goals of treatment for RV infarction are volume resuscitation to maintain arterial pressure, electrical stabilization, revascularization, and, if needed, mechanical or pharmacologic support and invasive hemodynamic monitoring. Box 14.4 summarizes treatment strategies for patients with RVMI.

Volume Resuscitation

Volume resuscitation in RVMI requires balancing the need for adequate RV preload and impaired LV diastolic filling. A key metric in the decision algorithm of volume resuscitation is involvement of the septum. The RV is preload dependent and, in the setting of ischemia with decreased diastolic compliance, it may benefit from an augmentation in preload. If hypovolemia is present, there may be a marked improvement with saline administration. When marked RV dilation has already occurred, however, further increases in RV preload do not result in an increase in RV stroke volume and may impair LV filling further through increased septal shift in combination with pericardial constraint.[14] Cardiac output and arterial blood pressure may not increase. In various studies,[68–70] an increase in mean right atrial pressure to 10 to 14 mm Hg was followed by an improvement in stroke volume and RV stroke work index, but further augmentation was associated with no improvement or even a decrease in stroke volume.[60–63] The optimal pulmonary capillary wedge pressure corresponding to maximum LV stroke work index was 16 mm Hg.[71] Given these narrow constraints, invasive hemodynamic monitoring is usually necessary to guide therapy.

Excessive volume loading can lead to elevation in pericardial pressure and shift the interventricular septum leftward, leading to impaired LV filling and a subsequent low-output state. In addition, LV septal involvement further impairs RV force generation. These patients tend to present with hypotension and low cardiac output and are more refractory to volume infusion. This subset of patients may benefit most from inotropic support.[66] Fig. 14.3 summarizes the detrimental effects of excessive volume loading.

Electrical Stabilization

Acute RVMI is often associated with bradyarrhythmias, including high-degree AV block, bradycardia, and AV dyssynchrony.[14,56,72] The mechanisms underlying bradycardia include excessive vagal tone, reflex-mediated bradycardia (e.g., Bezold-Harisch reflex), pharmacologic therapy (e.g.. β-blockers, calcium channel blockers), and AV node ischemia.[22] Bradyarrhythmias and hypotension are far more common with proximal RCA lesions and can also be induced in a relatively stable patient upon successful reperfusion.[73,74] Given a relatively fixed stroke volume of the ischemic RV, cardiac output in the preload-dependent LV is extremely sensitive to heart rate; maintaining chronotropic competence is therefore essential. Low-output RV failure can also be exacerbated by the loss of right atrial systole. Thus, while RV pacing may be of benefit, some patients require dual chamber pacing to restore AV synchrony.[75] Sequential pacing may have a marked salutary effect on cardiac output[52,75] and can lead to significant improvement and recovery from shock in patients refractory to RV pacing alone.[52] The clinician should be aware that, in practice, pacing can be complicated by improper placement of temporary pacing wires owing to right-sided chamber dilation, tricuspid regurgitation, and initiation of ventricular arrhythmias.[22] Further issues of impaired ventricular sensing and sustained impulse generation are common in the ischemic RV. A higher pacing threshold should

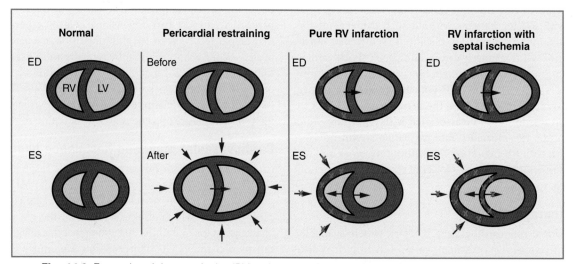

Fig. 14.3 Excessive right ventricular (RV) volume loading. Two physiologic concepts explaining the detrimental effects of excessive volume loading. *Normal ventricle:* At end systole (ES), the RV free wall moves toward the septum. *Pericardial restraining effects* (above, before volume loading; below, after excessive volume loading): RV dilatation, as a result of excessive volume loading, can lead to the elevation of intrapericardial pressure, increase in pericardial constraint (*red arrow*), and change of geometry due to interventricular septum shift. These changes contribute to the low-output state by decreasing left ventricular (LV) distensibility, preload, and ventricular elastance. *Role of the interventricular septum* (pure RV infarction, RV infarction with septal ischemia): At ES, the RV free wall moves toward the septum. At end diastole (ED), the RV dilates during diastole and the septum reverse curves toward the volume-reduced LV. At ES, the septum thickens but moves paradoxically into the RV, displacing the RV volume despite RV free wall dyskinesis. Septal ischemia depresses septal contraction and global LV function, resulting in LV dilatation. The septum stops thickening and there is increased systolic septal displacement into the RV. Pansystolic septal thinning and more extensive paradoxical displacement are associated with further depression of RV performance. (From Inohara T, et al. The challenges in the management of right ventricular infarction. *Eur Heart J Acute Cardiovasc Care.* 2013;2[3]:226–234.)

be anticipated.[59,76] Caution should be employed when placing a pacing wire in an area of infarction because the risk of rupture may be increased. If transvenous pacing fails, transcutaneous external pacing may be successful.[77]

Reperfusion Therapy

Proximal RCA occlusion can compromise both right atrial and RV branch perfusion, which can lead to both RV dysfunction and impaired atrial contraction. Thus patients with proximal RCA lesions are more unstable than those without.[66,78] Given the adverse prognosis of RVMI, establishing reperfusion by primary percutaneous coronary intervention (PCI) or thrombolytic therapy is particularly important in these patients. Meta-analyses have shown that PCI results in superior outcomes compared with thrombolysis when performed rapidly by an experienced team.[79] PCI should be the reperfusion modality of choice where available. If PCI is unavailable, thrombolysis is an appropriate alternative therapy that has been shown to reduce mortality.[2,80] Radionuclide studies have confirmed a marked reduction in the extent of RVMI in patients who achieved early reperfusion.[71,81] Other studies have suggested that complete RCA revascularization, especially when complicated by ventricular reperfusion arrhythmias, was associated with a better prognosis.[82,83] Thrombolytic therapy is relatively ineffective in the presence of cardiogenic shock, however. In the presence of shock not responsive to volume replacement and inotropic therapy, primary PCI is the preferable approach even if the patient requires transfer to another facility.

Inotropic Support

Dobutamine and dopamine have been evaluated in the setting of severe RVMI (defined by right atrial pressure >13 mm Hg) and have consistently been found to increase RV stroke work and cardiac output, while volume loading and nitroprusside were generally ineffective.[69] Dobutamine, which also has arteriolar vasodilating effects, usually does not increase mean arterial pressure significantly and has the least deleterious effect on afterload and oxygen consumption.[22] Dopamine (by activating dopaminergic and α-adrenergic receptors) and norepinephrine increase mean arterial pressure; they should be used when patients are severely hypotensive and require pressor support in addition to inotropy.[14] After the systolic blood pressure increases to greater than 90 mm Hg, dobutamine may be used, alone or in combination with dopamine or norepinephrine.

The use of milrinone,[84] a phosphodiesterase inhibitor, has been shown to be beneficial in chronic right heart failure, increasing myocardial contractility. While milrinone has the advantage of reducing pulmonary vascular resistance and unloading the right ventricle, it may exacerbate hypotension.[22] Its use in RVMI has not been systematically evaluated.

Right Ventricular Assist Devices

Recent reports of the use of percutaneous RV assist devices in patients with shock complicating RVMI are encouraging. There are currently three such devices in clinical practice: the Tandem Heart (CardiacAssist), the Impella RP (Abiomed), and the intraaortic balloon pump (IABP). For the Tandem Heart, two

21F cannulae are placed via both femoral veins, one in the right atrium and the other in the pulmonary artery with assist pumping using an extracorporeal centrifugal pump. The Impella RP utilizes a 22F catheter placed through the femoral vein and is positioned with the inlet valve in the RV and the outlet in the pulmonary artery (Video 14.2). It can deliver flow rates up to 4 L/min and can be placed for up to 14 days. It is indicated for acute right heart failure or decompensation. Data from the RECOVER-RIGHT trial indicate marked, immediate hemodynamic improvement with an average duration of use of 3 days. The overall survival at 30 days was 73.3%[85] (Fig. 14.4). Last, an IABP has recently been shown to improve hemodynamics in patients with cardiac shock secondary to RVMI.[86] The mechanism of beneficial effect for a left-sided device remains incompletely understood but likely stabilizes mean arterial pressure and improves coronary perfusion. Other postulated mechanisms include improved LV function through LV septal contraction. Thus, the temporary use of such invasive RV assistance is now a promising tool as a "bridge to recovery"; in all devices, the unloading of the RV reduces RV dilation and pericardial pressure while improving LV filling in the setting of shock from RVMI.[87,88]

Hemodynamic Monitoring

In a patient with hemodynamic instability in the setting of RVMI, the use of a pulmonary artery catheter often helps guide therapy. Extra caution should be employed in the placement of the catheter because a higher incidence of ventricular arrhythmias, including ventricular fibrillation, has been described in the setting of RVMI (4% vs. 0.3% in patients without RV infarction).[89] Flotation of the catheter under fluoroscopic guidance by a cardiologist or other intensivist may help minimize the risk.

Pulmonary Vasodilator Therapy

The use of selective pulmonary vasodilators might be expected to provide afterload reduction for the failing RV without concurrent systemic vasodilation and hypotension, potentially resulting in improved cardiac output. Inhaled nitric oxide acts as a selective pulmonary vasodilator, producing smooth muscle cell relaxation and vasodilation in the pulmonary circulation without systemic vasodilation owing to its active binding to hemoglobin and inactivation in circulating erythrocytes.[90] A few studies[91] have examined pulmonary vasodilator therapy with cautiously optimistic results, but further study and validation of these agents in RVMI is necessary.

Preload and Afterload Reduction

The RV is sensitive to preload, particularly in the setting of RVMI. Hypotension provoked by nitroglycerin, morphine sulfate, or diuretics in patients with an acute inferior MI should alert the clinician to the possibility of a preload-sensitive state, such as RVMI. The routine use of these agents should be discouraged in patients with acute inferior MI until RV involvement is ruled out. Sodium nitroprusside may result in marked afterload reduction which, if ineffective in increasing right-sided output, results in systemic hypotension.[69] In some clinical situations, such as combined right and left heart failure with severe LV dysfunction or when fluid administration has been overzealous, the cautious

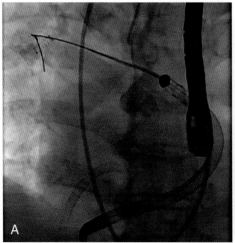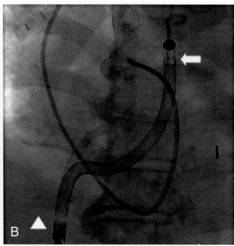

Fig. 14.4 Placement of the percutaneous right ventricular (RV) Impella right side percutaneous device (Abiomed). (A) Tracking the right-sided percutaneous device over an 0.018 stiff guidewire through the right ventricular outflow tract into the main pulmonary artery. The procedure was performed under general anesthesia with transesophageal echocardiography guidance. (B) Final position of the RV support device, with the device inflow located below the right atrial inferior vena cava junction *(arrow)* and the device outflow located in the main pulmonary artery *(arrowhead)*. Note the relationship of the device outflow to the pulmonary artery pulmonary artery catheter, a simple method to confirm device position on plain chest radiography. (From Margey R, et al. First experience with implantation of a percutaneous right ventricular Impella right side percutaneous support device as a bridge to recovery in acute right ventricular infarction complicated by cardiogenic shock in the United States. *Circ Cardiovasc Interv.* 2013;6[3]:e37–e38.)

BOX 14.5 Complications of Right Ventricular Myocardial Infarction

Atrioventricular block
Atrial tachyarrhythmias
Tricuspid regurgitation
Right-to-left shunting
Right ventricular thrombus
Pulmonary embolism
Paradoxical embolism
Septal rupture
Free wall rupture

---

use of vasodilators may be attempted.[14] Invasive hemodynamic monitoring should be used and right atrial pressure should be maintained at greater than 10 mm Hg.

COMPLICATIONS

Patients with inferior wall MI and accompanying RVMI have a much higher rate of complications than patients with inferior wall MI without RV involvement, accounting for part of the adverse prognostic implications of RVMI (Box 14.5). These include AV block, atrial arrhythmias, profound hypotension and bradycardia, and pericarditis. The cardiac intensivist should also be aware of several less common complications.[65,92–95]

Patent foramen ovale (PFO) is present in 25% of the population. In the setting of RVMI and elevated right-sided pressures, right-to-left shunting may occur, resulting in hypoxemia. Maneuvers that reduce LV pressures, such as afterload reduction, exacerbate this shunting. Percutaneous closure of the patent foramen may be necessary in extreme cases.[4]

As in LVMI, RVMI may predispose to thrombus formation in the infarcted ventricle with possible pulmonary embolism. In the presence of a PFO, paradoxical embolization may lead to systemic emboli. Thrombus has been identified in the RV of patients with RVMI (3 of 33; 9%) and in patients without RV infarction with posterior wall MI (4 of 106; 4%).[96]

Severe tricuspid regurgitation secondary to papillary muscle necrosis or severe RV dilation has been described in the setting of RVMI. In extreme cases, refractory heart failure has necessitated valve replacement.[97] Other complications include septal rupture,[95] RV free wall rupture,[97] and pericarditis, which is common in RV infarction because of the thinness of the RV wall.

Last, ventricular septal rupture in the setting of acute RVMI can be particularly disastrous, precipitating pulmonary edema, increased pulmonary pressures and resistance, and further decreasing cardiac output. Surgical repair is mandatory in most cases but is associated with significant mortality and morbidity.[22,98]

PROGNOSIS

RVMI is associated with markedly increased complication and mortality rates.[39] The reduction in mortality by reperfusion therapy is dramatic. Aggressive reperfusion therapy is indicated to maximize survival in the absence of severe mitigating circumstances.

After RVMI, RV function generally improves.[99] Long-term prognosis is determined, however, by residual LV rather than RV function, with similar posthospital courses for patients with and without RVMI.[39] A strong correlation exists between the outcome of RVMI and age.[33,100] In acute inferior MI, RV infarction substantially increases the risk of death and major complications in elderly patients.[33]

CONCLUSION

RVMI occurs mainly in the setting of inferior wall MI with proximal RCA occlusion. RV involvement in inferior MI has a marked adverse effect on complication rate and prognosis. Patients with RVMI benefit, however, from reperfusion therapy.

Complications such as hypotension, AV block, and atrial tachyarrhythmias should be treated aggressively. Although the short-term prognosis in RV infarction is poor, if the patient survives the acute illness, the long-term prognosis is good.

Acknowledgment

We acknowledge the contributions of Dr. Anil J. Mani to this chapter in the previous edition.

The full reference list for this chapter is available at ExpertConsult.com.

15

Mechanical Complications of Acute Myocardial Infarction

Adam Shpigel, David L. Brown

Early and effective reperfusion of acute myocardial infarction (MI) has resulted in a substantial decline in the incidence of mechanical complications, including free wall rupture, ventricular septal rupture, and papillary muscle rupture resulting in acute mitral regurgitation. However, mechanical complications remain important causes of morbidity and mortality in the peri-infarct setting. Mechanical complications are frequently associated with cardiogenic shock; approximately 12% of patients with cardiogenic shock have these complications. The critical care cardiologist must maintain a high degree of suspicion to identify and effectively treat these life-threatening and time-sensitive complications. In many patients, the MI may not be large.[1,2] Thus, if patients can be diagnosed early and treated effectively, they can often be discharged with reasonably preserved left ventricular (LV) function and have an acceptable quality of life. The mechanical complications of acute MI are described in this chapter and summarized in Box 15.1.

FREE WALL RUPTURE

Acute rupture of a cardiac free wall is a sudden, usually catastrophic complication of acute MI. It is the second most common cause of post-MI death after cardiogenic shock without mechanical defects.[3] Free wall rupture accounts for up to 20% of all deaths resulting from acute MI.[4] The overall incidence of free wall rupture is about 1% to 2%.[5] Risk factors for free wall rupture include female sex, advanced age, single-vessel disease, hypertension, transmural MI, and late reperfusion therapy.[4–8] The incidence of rupture for patients with successful reperfusion (0.9%) is less than that without reperfusion treatments (2.7%). The incidence

seems to be similar whether reperfusion is achieved by thrombolytic therapy or by percutaneous coronary intervention (PCI).

Pathophysiology

The most frequent site of post-MI cardiac rupture is the LV free wall (80% to 90%; Fig. 15.1).[2,9] Less commonly, the LV posterior wall, right ventricle (RV), or atria may rupture.[10,11] Rupture may rarely occur at more than one site[12] and occur in combination with papillary muscle[12] or septal rupture.[13]

Expansion of the infarct area seems to predispose to rupture.[14] When ruptures occur within 24 hours of onset of infarction, however, infarct expansion or infiltration by neutrophils does not seem to contribute to the pathogenesis.[15] The path of the rupture through the wall may be direct (through the center of the necrotic area) but is often serpiginous and frequently seen at an eccentric position, near the "hinge point" of mobility between the normally contracting and dyskinetic myocardium. These observations suggest that local shear forces contribute to the disruption of tissue.[16] It has been suggested that apoptosis of cardiomyocytes in the region of maximum wall strain contributes to rupture of the ventricular free wall.[17]

Infarct expansion and adverse ventricular remodeling have been suggested as contributors to subacute ventricular rupture.[18] Inappropriate changes in the extracellular matrix—in particular, collagen disruption and its degradation by dysregulation of matrix metalloproteinase metabolism—have been suggested to be important mechanisms in the pathogenesis of ventricular rupture after MI.[19] In experimental animal models, deficiency of local angiotensin type II receptor has been shown to cause decreased collagen deposition and an increased risk of cardiac rupture

BOX 15.1 Mechanical Complications of Acute Myocardial Infarction

Left ventricular free wall rupture
- Acute
- Subacute
- Pseudoaneurysm secondary to contained rupture

Right ventricular free wall rupture (very rare)

Interventricular septal rupture

Papillary muscle rupture
- Posteromedial
- Anterolateral (rare)
- Tricuspid (very rare)

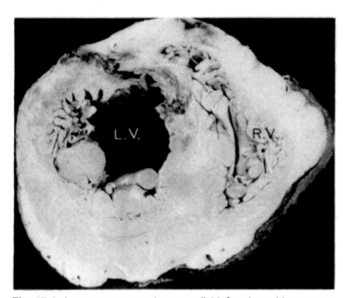

Fig. 15.1 Acute anteroseptal myocardial infarction with a rupture of the anterior wall of the left ventricle (L.V.) in a 72-year-old woman. Death from hemopericardium. *R.V.,* Right ventricle. (From Van Tasssel RA, Edwards J. Rupture of heart complicating myocardial infarction: analysis of 40 cases including nine examples of left ventricular false aneurysm. *Chest* 1972;61:104–116.)

after MI.[20] Angiotensin II induces transforming growth factor-β1, which promotes fibrogenesis.[21]

Clinical Features

Free wall rupture occurs within 24 hours in 25% to 35% of cases and within the first week in 87% of patients following the onset of the acute coronary syndrome.[22,23] Frequently, rupture occurs in patients with uncomplicated MI. There are no specific symptoms or signs of acute or subacute free wall rupture. Patients may present with syncope or signs and symptoms of cardiogenic shock.[6,10] Sudden onset of severe chest pain during or after some types of physical stress, such as coughing or straining at stool, may suggest the onset of free wall rupture. Some patients have premonitory symptoms, such as unexplained chest pains that are not typical of ischemia or pericarditis-related chest pains,[23] repeated emesis, restlessness, and agitation.[24]

Rapid onset of tamponade owing to hemopericardium, resulting in severe hypotension and electromechanical dissociation,

characterizes acute rupture; antemortem diagnosis is almost impossible in these patients. In patients with subacute rupture, relatively slower development of tamponade may allow antemortem diagnosis and corrective surgical therapy with salvage of these patients. In some patients, a pseudoaneurysm may develop. A pseudoaneurysm, in contrast to an aneurysm, is lined not by myocardium but by pericardium or fibrous tissue. It is a contained myocardial rupture. It most commonly occurs in the inferior or posterior walls. Elevated jugular venous pressure, pulsus paradoxus, muffled heart sounds, and a pericardial friction rub may indicate subacute rupture. A new systolic, diastolic, or "to-and-fro" murmur may be present in these patients with or without pseudoaneurysm.[25]

Diagnosis

In acute free wall rupture, the electrocardiogram (ECG) reveals electromechanical dissociation and terminal bradycardia.[8,26] In subacute rupture, several ECG findings have been described, including presence of Q waves; recurrent ST-segment elevation or depression; pseudonormalization of inverted T waves, particularly in the precordial leads; persistent ST segment elevation; and new Q waves in two or more leads.[5,22,24,26,27] None of the ECG findings are specific or sensitive enough to be of value for early diagnosis of impending rupture.

Transthoracic echocardiography should be performed as soon as the subacute rupture is suspected.[5–7,26] Color Doppler may be useful for the diagnosis of the rupture site.[28] The most frequent finding is pericardial effusion. The presence of echogenic masses in the fluid and detection of wall defects enhance diagnostic accuracy. If a pseudoaneurysm is present, in contrast to a true aneurysm, the "neck" of the aneurysm is narrow (Video 15.1). Although transesophageal echocardiography may provide a better delineation of these findings, because of the stress of the procedure, it should not be performed unless absolutely necessary. Contrast echocardiography may show extravasation of the contrast material into the pericardial space, confirming the diagnosis of free wall rupture.[28,29]

Determination of hemodynamics and contrast ventriculography are unnecessary for diagnosis and should be avoided. If a pulmonary artery (PA) catheter is already in place, determination of right heart hemodynamics reveals elevated right atrial (RA) and pulmonary capillary wedge pressures (PCWP) and equalization of the diastolic pressures.[5,26]

Management

Surgical repair is the definitive treatment for subacute rupture or pseudoaneurysm and salvage rates may be considerable. The operative mortality has been reported to be 24% to 35%, with a total in-hospital mortality rate of 50% to 60%.[5,7,26] Currently, conservative surgical techniques using simple sutures supported with felt or application of a patch to the epicardial surface with biologic glue are used.[24,30] Temporizing measures include pericardiocentesis, volume loading, inotropic support, and intraaortic balloon counterpulsation. In very-high-risk elderly patients, nonsurgical conservative treatment with adequate control of blood pressure with angiotensin inhibition and the use of β-blocking agents has been suggested.[31] The treatment approach of pseudoaneurysm is similar to that of subacute rupture without pseudoaneurysm.

MITRAL REGURGITATION

Although mild mitral regurgitation is common in patients with acute MI, severe mitral regurgitation owing to papillary muscle and LV wall dysfunction with or without rupture of the papillary muscle is much less frequent. The overall incidence of acute mitral regurgitation in patients receiving thrombolytic therapy was 1.7% in the Global Utilization of Streptokinase and Tissue Plasminogen Activator for Occluded Coronary Arteries (GUSTO-1) trial.[32] It has been reported that the incidence is significantly lower (0.31%) in patients undergoing primary PCI.[33] The reported incidence of mild and moderate mitral regurgitation is approximately 29% and 6%, respectively. The incidence of severe mitral regurgitation complicating MI is approximately 10%,[34] and the incidence of mitral regurgitation resulting from papillary muscle rupture is 1%.[1]

The risk factors for mitral regurgitation with and without papillary muscle rupture seem to be different, although advanced age and female sex are risk factors for both types.[35] In patients without papillary muscle rupture, prior MI, relatively large infarct size, multivessel coronary artery disease, recurrent myocardial ischemia, and heart failure on admission are more prevalent. In contrast, in patients with papillary muscle rupture, absence of previous angina, inferoposterior MI, absence of diabetes, and single-vessel disease are more common.

Pathophysiology

Several anatomic and functional derangements may cause mitral regurgitation in patients with acute coronary syndromes. Acute transient papillary muscle ischemia is associated with impaired shortening of the muscle, which usually causes only mild mitral regurgitation. Ischemic dysfunction of anterior and posterior papillary muscles may be associated with more severe mitral regurgitation.[36] Ischemia of only papillary muscles without involvement of the adjacent LV walls seldom results in severe mitral regurgitation.[37] The subendocardial position of the papillary muscles and their characteristic vascular anatomy (supplied by coronary end-arteries) predispose them to ischemia.[38] The posteromedial papillary muscle receives its blood supply from only the posterior descending coronary artery whereas the anterolateral papillary muscle receives its blood supply from the left anterior descending and left circumflex coronary arteries.[39] As a result, ischemia of the posteromedial papillary muscle is more common than ischemia of the anterolateral papillary muscle.

A large posterior MI that involves the anchoring area of the posteromedial papillary muscle may be associated with severe mitral regurgitation. The mechanism seems to be asymmetric annular dilation and misalignment of the papillary muscle and the leaflets during systole, causing severe leaflet prolapse.[40] A small inferior or inferoposterior MI with involvement of the posteromedial papillary muscle can also produce severe mitral regurgitation as a result of severe leaflet prolapse.

Rupture of the posteromedial papillary muscle is 6 to 12 times more frequent than rupture of the anterolateral papillary muscle, which explains the higher incidence of severe mitral regurgitation in patients with inferior MI.[34] In approximately 50% of patients with papillary muscle rupture, the infarct size is small.[41]

Mild to moderate mitral regurgitation usually does not induce any additional hemodynamic burden. Neither ejection fraction nor hemodynamics—such as PCWP, PA pressures, and cardiac output—are substantially influenced. In contrast, severe mitral regurgitation imposes sudden additional hemodynamic burden on LV dynamics and function. Sudden large-volume overload resulting from regurgitation to a left atrium (LA) with normal compliance and size causes a marked increase in LA and PCWP, causing severe pulmonary edema. Because of postcapillary pulmonary hypertension, which increases RV afterload, the RV also fails. LV forward stroke volume decreases, resulting in a reduction in cardiac output and systemic hypotension. The hemodynamic features of cardiogenic shock develop rapidly and, usually, abruptly. The ejection fraction is usually reduced due to dysfunctional ischemic or infarcted myocardium.

Clinical Features

Mitral regurgitation not resulting from papillary muscle rupture is detected at a median of 7 days (range, 5 to 45 days) after MI. Severe mitral regurgitation secondary to papillary muscle rupture occurs at a median of 1 day (range, 1 to 14 days) after the onset of the index infarction; approximately 20% of papillary muscle ruptures occur within 24 hours of onset of infarction.[1,25,42]

In patients with mild mitral regurgitation secondary to papillary muscle dysfunction, the only clinical indication may be the presence of a pansystolic (holosystolic) or more often a late systolic murmur. In patients with rupture of a papillary muscle, the clinical presentation is characterized by the abrupt onset of severe respiratory distress resulting from "flash" pulmonary edema. Hypotension and reflex tachycardia rapidly develop. Other clinical features of preshock or shock are also present. The sudden appearance of a pansystolic or early systolic murmur—radiating to the left axilla, to the base, or both—is a characteristic physical finding. A palpable thrill is uncommon. In some patients, the murmur may be abbreviated or absent. The abbreviation of the murmur results from a rapid decrease in the pressure gradient between the LA and LV.[25] "Bubbling" rales of pulmonary edema are present bilaterally and make cardiac auscultation difficult.

Diagnosis

The ECG most frequently reveals recent inferior or inferoposterior MI (55%); however, the location of the index infarction is anterior (34%) or posterior (32%) in patients with severe mitral regurgitation and cardiogenic shock.[34] In occasional patients, only ST-T abnormalities of a "shell infarct" are present. Radiographic evidence of acute severe pulmonary edema is invariably present.

Doppler and transthoracic echocardiography should be performed in all patients. Transthoracic echocardiography is less sensitive than transesophageal echocardiography for visualization of the disrupted mitral valve (45% to 50% vs. 100%),[43–45] but it is 100% sensitive for the detection by color Doppler of the resultant severe mitral regurgitation.[43,46]

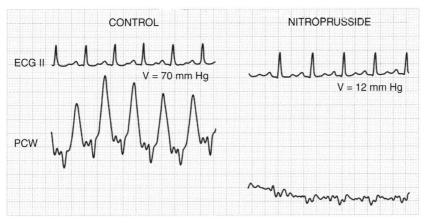

Fig. 15.2 Acute mitral regurgitation. *Left tracings:* Large "v" waves in the pulmonary capillary wedge *(PCW)* tracing. *Right tracings:* Reduction in magnitude of the v wave during sodium nitroprusside infusion. *ECG,* Electrocardiogram.

Echocardiography shows the underlying regional LV wall motion at the site of ischemia/infarction and excludes ventricular septal or free wall rupture.[43,47] A partial papillary muscle rupture may be detectable by two-dimensional echocardiography. A complete rupture is diagnosed when the head of the papillary muscle is seen as a freely moving mobile mass attached to the mitral valve chordae (Videos 15.2 and 15.3).[44,46,48–50]

PA catheterization is unnecessary for the diagnosis of severe mitral regurgitation. If it is undertaken, however, it reveals giant "v" waves in the PCWP tracing (Fig. 15.2). Giant v waves may also be present in patients with ventricular septal rupture. In ventricular septal rupture, increased pulmonary venous return owing to the large left-to-right shunt to an LA with normal size and compliance is associated with an accentuated v wave. The presence of a reflected v wave in a PA pressure tracing is diagnostic of acute or subacute severe mitral regurgitation.[51] In some patients with severe acute mitral regurgitation, reflux of the oxygenated pulmonary venous blood to the distal pulmonary artery branches occurs.

Management

Patients with mild mitral regurgitation do not require surgical intervention. After adequate reperfusion therapy, appropriate adjunctive treatments—such as angiotensin-converting enzyme inhibitors or angiotensin receptor blockers, β-blockers, aldosterone antagonists, antiplatelet agents, and lipid-lowering agents—should be employed to decrease the risk of development of heart failure, to minimize adverse ventricular remodeling, and to improve long-term prognosis. Even in patients with mild mitral regurgitation diagnosed during the acute phase of MI, the long-term prognosis is unfavorable, although the immediate prognosis is not affected.[52,53] Aggressive post-MI adjunctive therapies are essential.

Severe mitral regurgitation complicating acute MI with cardiogenic shock requires surgical intervention for mitral valve replacement or repair. In the Should We Emergently Revascularize Occluded Coronaries for Cardiogenic Shock (SHOCK) trial registry, in-hospital mortality without valve surgery was 71% versus 40% with surgery, indicating a significant improvement in the short-term prognosis.[34]

> **BOX 15.2 Suggested Management of Mitral Regurgitation Complicating Acute Myocardial Infarction**
>
> **Mild Mitral Regurgitation**
> Reperfusion treatments
> Adjunctive treatments
> Angiotensin-converting enzyme inhibitors or angiotensin receptor blockers, β-blockers, aldosterone antagonists, lipid-lowering agents, antiplatelet agents
>
> **Severe Mitral Regurgitation**
> Corrective valve surgery
> Stabilizing and supportive treatments
> Mechanical ventilation, diuretics, intraaortic balloon pump, vasodilators, vasopressors, inotropic agents
> Adjunctive treatments in survivors
> Angiotensin-converting enzyme inhibitors or angiotensin receptor blockers, β-blockers, aldosterone antagonists, lipid-lowering agents, antiplatelet agents

Supportive and stabilizing treatments consist of mechanical ventilation, diuretics, vasodilators, inotropic agents and, if possible, an intraaortic balloon pump. Vasodilator drugs, such as sodium nitroprusside, reduce regurgitant volume, decrease PCWP and PA pressures, and increase forward stroke volume and cardiac output.[54] Hypotension precludes the initial use of vasodilators, but they can be used after institution of intraaortic balloon pump. The intraaortic balloon pump reduces LV ejection impedance and maintains perfusion pressure concurrently. The therapeutic approach for mitral regurgitation complicating an MI is outlined in Box 15.2.

VENTRICULAR SEPTAL RUPTURE

The incidence of ventricular septal rupture complicating acute MI is approximately 0.2% in the reperfusion era.[55] Before the introduction of reperfusion therapy for MI, the incidence was 0.5% to 2%.[38,56] Patients with ventricular septal rupture tend to be older, more often female, and less often have previous MI, diabetes mellitus, or a smoking history.[57] Although it was previously thought that the incidence of septal rupture increased with thrombolytic therapy, placebo-controlled trials failed to confirm an increased risk of rupture with thrombolytic therapy.[58,59] Early occurrence of ventricular septal rupture has been observed, however, after thrombolytic therapy.[60] Whether a history of hypertension increases the risk of ventricular septal rupture remains controversial.[61]

Pathophysiology

Most commonly, ventricular septal rupture occurs after a first MI.[13,61] The rupture usually occurs in thin akinetic areas, and it may be direct or "complex." The complex rupture forms a dissection plane in a serpiginous path in the septum.[62] Complex ruptures may be associated with concurrent ruptures of other structures, such as the LV free wall or papillary muscle.[13] Lack of septal collateral flow, regional distortion, and infarct expansion seem to be important factors for the development of a ventricular septal rupture.[14,61] Ventricular septal rupture seems to occur with almost equal frequency in anterior and inferior MI;[63] single- or double-vessel disease is most common.[57]

Ventricular septal rupture usually produces a large, left-to-right shunt (pulmonary-to-systemic flow >3:1) that places a volume load on the RV, pulmonary circulation, LA, and LV. The LV performance, which is depressed by ischemia, is compromised further by the volume overload. In the SHOCK trial registry, the range of ejection fraction in patients with post-MI ventricular septal rupture was 25% to 40%.[57] LV forward stroke volume declines but RV stroke volume and pulmonary flow increase. There is a reflex increase in heart rate and systemic vascular resistance, which increases LV ejection impedance, further increasing the magnitude of left-to-right shunt. RV performance also declines because of the volume load and postcapillary pulmonary hypertension.

Clinical Features

In more than 70% of patients, the clinical presentation is characterized by circulatory collapse with hypotension, tachycardia, and low cardiac output along with other clinical features of shock that may develop abruptly or within a few hours after the occurrence of a new systolic murmur.[43] The murmur is best heard over the left lower sternal border and may be associated with a palpable thrill in approximately half of cases. Right-sided and left-sided S_3 gallops with an accentuated pulmonic component of S_2 are often present along with findings of tricuspid regurgitation. Pulmonary edema is less abrupt and fulminant than is seen with papillary muscle rupture. The chest radiograph shows a combination of pulmonary edema and increased pulmonary flow. The ECG shows evidence of MI with or without evidence of ischemia.

Diagnosis

Echocardiography with Doppler is mandatory in all patients with suspected ventricular septal rupture. Two-dimensional echocardiography reveals the septal defect in most cases (Video 15.4). Regional wall motion abnormalities and changes in RV and LV function are also visualized. Doppler echocardiography increases diagnostic yield by demonstrating transseptal flow.[43,47] Color flow imaging during echocardiography is very sensitive for diagnosing and characterizing ventricular septal rupture (Video 15.5).[28,43,47] Agitated saline can be used to identify the defect and may show negative contrast in the RV. Doppler echocardiography is also performed to estimate the magnitude of left-to-right shunt as well as RV and PA systolic pressures.

PA catheterization is not required for the diagnosis of ventricular septal rupture. If it is undertaken, however, it shows a step-up in oxygen saturation in the RV and PA compared with RA saturation (Fig. 15.3). The ratio of pulmonary to systemic flow can be calculated, and the hemodynamics can be determined.

Management

Urgent surgical repair of the ventricular septal rupture is a class I indication of the American College of Cardiology Foundation/American Heart Association guideline committee.[64] In the SHOCK trial registry,[57] surgical repair of ventricular septal rupture was undertaken in 31 of 55 patients with cardiogenic shock; 21 of these 31 patients also had concomitant coronary artery bypass graft surgery. Three of these patients also had aneurysmectomy.

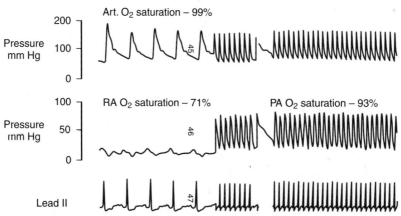

Fig. 15.3 Ventricular septal defect. Oxygen saturation step-up between the right atrium *(RA)* and pulmonary artery *(PA). Art.,* arterial.

Overall mortality in the surgical group was 81%. Only 1 of 24 patients not undergoing surgery survived. In the GUSTO-I trial, patients who presented with cardiogenic shock were excluded; mortality for surgical versus medical treatment was 47% versus 94%.[32] The results of these studies suggest that surgical repair should be considered if not absolutely contraindicated. In a few patients, catheter-based percutaneous closure of the ventricular septal rupture has been performed with success.[65] This technique is challenging given the necrotic ventricular septum at the site of rupture but may be considered for patients who cannot undergo surgery.

Survivors of surgery usually have improved functional class and a favorable late mortality rate.[66,67] A 10-year survival rate of 50% has been observed after surgical repair.[68] Medical therapy is required to stabilize patients before surgery. The goal of medical therapy is to reduce the magnitude of the left-to-right shunt, improve cardiac output and systemic perfusion, and decrease pulmonary congestion. The magnitude of the left-to-right shunt in ventricular septal defect is determined by the resistance at the defect and the relative resistances in the pulmonary and systemic vascular beds. When the size of the defect is large, as in patients with post-MI ventricular septal rupture, the magnitude of the left-to-right shunt is principally determined by the ratio of pulmonary to systemic resistance.

Vasodilators such as sodium nitroprusside may increase the magnitude of left-to-right shunt owing to vasodilation of the pulmonary artery. Vasodilators with less vasodilatory effects on the pulmonary vascular bed but significant systemic vasodilatory effect, such as hydralazine or phentolamine, may be more effective

---

BOX 15.3 Suggested Therapeutic Approach for Patients With Postinfarction Ventricular Septal Rupture

Corrective surgery as soon as feasible if not contraindicated

Intraaortic balloon pump to decrease magnitude of left-to-right shunt

Vasopressors and inotropic agents

Arteriolar dilators

Diuretics

Survivors—Angiotensin-converting enzyme inhibitors or angiotensin receptor blockers, β-blockers, aldosterone antagonists, lipid-lowering agents, antiplatelet agents

---

in reducing the magnitude of left-to-right shunt. The most effective nonsurgical treatment to decrease the magnitude of left-to-right shunt is intraaortic balloon counterpulsation, which selectively reduces LV ejection impedance. Inotropic agents and vasopressors are ineffective, although they are used frequently to maintain blood pressure. Diuretics are required to decrease pulmonary congestion. The therapeutic approach for the management of ventricular septal rupture is outlined in Box 15.3.

Acknowledgments

We acknowledge the contributions of Drs. Stuart J. Hutchinson, Tony M. Chou, Edward McNulty, and the late Kanu Chatterjee to this chapter in the previous edition.

The full reference list for this chapter is available at ExpertConsult.com.

16

Supraventricular and Ventricular Arrhythmias in Acute Myocardial Infarction

Dina M. Sparano, Judith A. Mackall

INTRODUCTION

Cardiac rhythm abnormalities occur in 72% to 95% of patients with acute myocardial infarction (MI) (Table 16.1).[1-3] Because arrhythmias tend to occur early and before the patient receives medical attention, the incidence may even be higher.[4] Mechanisms for the various arrhythmias seen in MI include reentry, automaticity, and triggered activity. These mechanisms may be exacerbated or caused by certain characteristics of the clinical course, such as infarct size, hemodynamic instability, electrolyte disturbances, use of inotropic agents, autonomic nervous system control and preexisting conduction system or rhythm disturbances.[2,5–7] Arrhythmias may be asymptomatic but can also result in symptoms of palpitations, angina, syncope, heart failure, or cardiac arrest. Whether supraventricular or ventricular in origin, they require treatment, particularly when they perturb hemodynamic stability, provoke myocardial ischemia, or threaten to degenerate into life-threatening arrhythmias. Timely recognition and treatment decreases morbidity and mortality associated with MI. However, preemptive antiarrhythmic treatment has not been shown to be effective.[5] This chapter reviews the mechanisms, diagnosis, and therapy for supraventricular and ventricular arrhythmias that occur in acute MI. Conduction disturbances in the setting of acute MI are discussed in Chapter 17.

SUPRAVENTRICULAR ARRHYTHMIAS

Sinus Tachycardia

Sinus tachycardia in the setting of acute MI usually occurs in response to an increase in sympathetic tone and can be seen in up to 30% of cases.[1–2] However, patients with isolated sinus tachycardia during acute MI fare more poorly than those without.[8,9] Acutely, MI patients with sinus tachycardia have higher levels of cardiac biomarker release, a larger proportion of anterior and diffuse infarcts, and a higher incidence of recurrent chest pain. Sinus tachycardia has also been shown to be an independent predictor of post-MI complications and in-hospital mortality. Sinus tachycardia may be an early manifestation of heart failure and, in this setting, is a poor prognostic sign. Sinus tachycardia that persists beyond 4 hours may be suggestive of another underlying cause, which should prompt further evaluation. Left untreated, these culprits, such as fever, pericarditis, pain, heart failure, and anemia, can lead to increased myocardial oxygen demand. Specific therapy to lower the heart rate and decrease

TABLE 16.1 Incidence of Arrhythmias in Acute Myocardial Infarction	
Arrhythmia	**Incidence (%)**
Sinus bradycardia	10–55
First-degree AV block	4–15
Second-degree AV block	
Mobitz type I	4–10
Multilevel AV block	2
Mobitz type II	Rare
Third-degree or complete AV block	
Inferior infarction	12–17
Anterior infarction	5
Asystole	1–10
Sinus tachycardia	30
Premature atrial contractions	54
Supraventricular tachycardia	<5
Atrial fibrillation	2.3–21
Atrial flutter	1–2
Premature ventricular contractions	90–100
Accelerated idioventricular rhythm	8–20
Ventricular tachycardia	10–40
Ventricular fibrillation	4–18

AV, Atrioventricular.

sympathetic tone, such as with β-blocker medications, may be helpful (Table 16.2).

Atrial Arrhythmias

Atrial arrhythmias occur in 20% to 54% of patients with acute MI overall and in about 11% to 20% of patients with acute MI and cardiogenic shock.[5,10–13] Patients with inferior MI in particular are more likely to develop atrial arrhythmias early in their clinical course, whereas patients with anterior MI tend to manifest atrial arrhythmias anywhere from 12 hours to days after MI onset.[14,15] Several factors have been implicated in the pathogenesis of atrial arrhythmias, including atrial distention from either left ventricular (LV) or right ventricular (RV) dysfunction, pericarditis, or atrial infarction.

In a small series of patients with documented inferior MI, Rechavia and colleagues found a significantly higher occurrence of premature atrial contractions and atrial fibrillation in patients with RV dysfunction.[15] It is unclear if this was because of atrial distention or atrial infarct; other studies have suggested that both factors may, in fact, play a role.[15] Atrial arrhythmias that occur late in the clinical course have been attributed to LV dysfunction. In these patients, treatment of congestive heart failure may prevent recurrences.[14,16]

Premature Atrial Contraction

Premature atrial contractions are the most common atrial arrhythmias, occurring in 54% of patients with acute MI.[10,13] They may result from heightened sympathetic tone exacerbated by pain or anxiety, atrial distention, pericarditis, atrial infarction, or atrial ischemia. Although premature atrial contractions may precipitate other atrial arrhythmias, they are usually of little clinical significance and are not associated with increased mortality. Thus suppressive treatment is not indicated.[13]

Paroxysmal or Persistent Supraventricular Tachycardia

Paroxysmal atrial tachycardia and reentrant supraventricular tachycardia are relatively rare in acute MI, occurring in less than 5% of patients.[14,17] Most of these arrhythmias are transient. However, a rapid ventricular response can be highly symptomatic and hemodynamically compromising. Management of these arrhythmias should first be directed at controlling the ventricular rate and initiated promptly, such as with intravenous β-blockers or calcium channel blockers (see Table 16.2). These agents or adenosine may also terminate persistent tachyarrhythmias if the atrioventricular (AV) node is an integral part of the reentry circuit. While adenosine may also terminate atrial tachycardia, it may result in atrial fibrillation (AF).[18] All of these agents should be administered with caution in acute MI, being mindful of associated hypotension or congestive heart failure.

In patients with hemodynamic instability, urgent synchronized direct current (DC) cardioversion is usually the safest and most expedient method to terminate the arrhythmia. Treating underlying heart failure may help to prevent recurrence.[14] Treatment of supraventricular tachycardia in the unstable patient is also reviewed in Chapter 25.

Atrial Fibrillation

AF occurs frequently in acute MI patients, affecting from 2.3% to 21% of hospitalized patients.[5,10,14,18–22] In approximately one-third of patients, AF is a preexisting condition, while new-onset AF occurs in the other two-thirds of these patients. Age, tachycardia at the time of clinical presentation, a history of AF, congestive heart failure, and both systolic and diastolic LV dysfunction are independent predictors for the development of AF in acute MI. Patients are also more likely to have had preexisting atrial arrhythmias, prior MI, or coronary artery disease, hypertension, diabetes mellitus, and more extensive myocardial damage at the time of presentation. The incidence of post-MI AF has declined markedly due in large part to the broad utilization of reperfusion strategies as well as commonly used medications, such as β-blockers, angiotensin-converting enzyme inhibitors, and angiotensin receptor blockers.[5]

AF impacts patient outcomes in the acute MI setting.[24–26] While some studies suggest a negative prognostic impact of AF,[15,24,25] other studies have disputed this. A meta-analysis of 43 studies that evaluated the impact of AF on mortality in MI patients found an increased odds ratio (OR) for mortality if patients developed new-onset (OR, 1.37) or had prior AF (OR, 1.28). The increased mortality risk was true even after controlling for age, diabetes mellitus, hypertension, prior MI, heart failure, and coronary revascularization in patients with new-onset AF. The increase in mortality held true for short-, mid- and long-term outcomes (out to 1 year) and included both sudden and nonsudden cardiac death.[23] Serrano and coworkers[14] investigated the short- and long-term outcomes of patients with supraventricular arrhythmias after MI. Although patients with arrhythmias during the late phase of MI (12 hours to 4 days) had significantly higher mortality rates at 1 month and 47 months, mortality was only shown to correlate with the extent of coronary artery disease.

TABLE 16.2   Antiarrhythmic Agents for Acute Myocardial Infarction[a]

Class	Drug	Indications	Dosage	Elimination Half-Life	Adverse Effects
IA	Procainamide	AVRT, VT	Intravenous: 15 mg/kg at 20 mg/min (load), then 1–6 mg/min (maintenance) Oral: 50 mg/kg/day in 4 divided doses	2.5–4.7 h	Hematologic: marrow suppression, lupus-like illness; proarrhythmia; hypotension (with intravenous infusion)
IB	Lidocaine	VT, PVCs, in setting of ischemia	Intravenous: 1 mg/kg bolus, then 1–4 mg/min (maintenance)	1.5–2 h	CNS: drowsiness, agitation, disorientation, tremulousness
II	Esmolol	Short-term rate control of AF, AFL; treatment of AVNRT, AVRT, MAT	Intravenous: 500 µg/kg over 1 min (load), then 50 µg/kg/min (maintenance)	2 min	Hypotension; CNS: dizziness, somnolence, headache; bronchospasm at higher doses
	Metoprolol	Rate control of AF, AF; treatment of AVNRT, MAT	Oral: 25–100 mg q6h Intravenous: 5 mg every 5–15 min up to 15 mg	3–4 h	As above
	Atenolol	As above	Oral: 25–200 mg qd[b]	6–7 h	As above
	Propranolol	As above	Intravenous: 0.5–3 mg, repeat in 2–5 min, then q4h Oral: 10–30 mg q6–8h	2 h (initial dose); 3, 4–6 h	As above; bronchospasm owing to β₂-antagonist activity
III	Amiodarone	VT, VF	Oral: 800–1600 mg/day for 1–3 wk (load), 200–400 mg qd (maintenance) Intravenous: 150 mg/min over 10 min, then 1 mg/min for 8 h, then reduce to 0.5 mg/min (maintenance)	9–11 days	Conduction disturbances: sinus bradycardia, heart block; abnormalities of thyroid function, liver function; pulmonary toxicity; hypotension more likely to occur with intravenous administration
IV	Diltiazem	Rate control of AF, AFL; treatment of AVNRT, MAT	Intravenous: 0.25 mg/kg over 2 min; if no response in 15 min, 0.35 mg/kg over 2 min, then 5–15 mg/h (maintenance) Oral: 30–125 mg tid, 120–300 mg CD qd	3.5–10 h	Hypotension; potentiation of sinus node dysfunction
	Verapamil	As above	Intravenous: 5–10 mg, may repeat in 15–30 min with 10 mg Oral: 80–120 mg q6–8h or 120–240 mg SR q12–24h	Intravenous: 2 h Oral: 4.5–12 h	Cardiac effects: congestive heart failure owing to negative inotropic effect, hypotension; gastrointestinal effects: constipation
Other	Digoxin	Rate control of AF, AFL; treatment of AVNRT	Intravenous/oral: 0.5 mg (initial), 0.25 mg q4–8h to total of 1 mg (load); 0.125–0.375 mg qd (maintenance)[b]	Intravenous: 30 min Oral: 34–44 h	Toxic side effects: nausea, accelerated functional rhythm, high-grade AV block
	Adenosine	Termination of AVNRT, AVRT, occasionally MAT, and exercise-mediated VT	Intravenous: 6 mg rapid bolus, may repeat with 12 mg in 1 min, then 18 mg	9.5 sec	Dyspnea, chest pain, flushing, sinus tachycardia
	Magnesium	Torsades de pointes	Intravenous: 1–2 g (load); 1–7.5 mg/min (maintenance)[b]		Hypotension

[a]Dosages and indications listed are based on current practice standards and therefore are subject to change in the future.
[b]Dosage should be adjusted in the presence of renal insufficiency.
AF, Atrial fibrillation; *AFL*, atrial flutter; *AT*, atrial tachycardia; *AV*, atrioventricular; *AVNRT*, atrioventricular nodal reentry tachycardia; *AVRT*, atrioventricular reentry tachycardia; *CD*, controlled delivery; *CNS*, central nervous system; *MAT*, multifocal atrial tachycardia; *PVCs*, premature ventricular contractions; *SR*, sustained release; *VF*, ventricular tachycardia; *VT*, ventricular tachycardia.

In another study, mortality was higher for patients with new-onset AF that developed 30 days or later after their MI (hazard ratio [HR], 2.58; 95% confidence interval [CI], 2.21–3.00 vs. HR, 1.81; 95% CI, 0.45–2.27 for AF between 3 and 30 days, and HR, 1.63; 95% CI, 1.37–1.93 for AF within 2 days).[73] AF is also associated with a higher rate of reinfarction, cardiogenic shock, heart failure, asystole, and recurrent AF.[22]

Patients with AF can develop symptoms from the loss of atrial contribution to cardiac output and impaired LV filling, as well as rapid ventricular rates. In patients with cardiogenic shock, increases in pulmonary capillary wedge pressure and left atrial pressure can contribute to the development of AF.[5] Other contributing factors can include atrial ischemia or infarction, LV dysfunction causing hemodynamic instability, and autonomic nervous system disturbances. In hemodynamically unstable patients, synchronized DC cardioversion can and should be utilized to promptly restore sinus rhythm. For stable patients, β-blockers or calcium channel blockers can be intravenously administered to control ventricular rates. Cardioversion may occur spontaneously; if not, synchronized DC cardioversion should be considered.

Atrial flutter is relatively rare in acute MI, occurring in only 1% to 2% of patients.[13,14] When it occurs, 2:1 conduction is often present and ventricular rate control may be difficult. DC cardioversion or pace termination, when available, can be utilized to terminate the tachycardia. Amiodarone may be used in an attempt to treat or prevent recurrence of atrial fibrillation or flutter, though it has the potential to cause hypotension. In patients with hemodynamic compromise, rate-lowering agents are often precluded by their negative inotropic effect.[5] Class IC antiarrhythmic medications, such as flecainide and propafenone, are contraindicated in acute MI patients and their use is to be avoided. Antiplatelet agents do not prevent or reduce the risk of thromboembolism in patients with AF. Therapeutic anticoagulation should be considered to reduce the long-term risk of thromboembolism in patients meeting current guideline criteria without contraindications.[27]

VENTRICULAR ARRHYTHMIAS

Ventricular tachyarrhythmias are potentially the most dangerous arrhythmias associated with acute MI, occurring in 10% to 50% of patients.[1,28] These arrhythmias are observed more frequently soon after the onset of MI. In experimental animals, factors that determine the occurrence of ventricular arrhythmias include the size of the ischemic area, psychological stress, preconditioning, increased heart rate, and autonomic nervous system influences.[29–34] The combination of ischemia and sympathetic stimulation is more arrhythmogenic than either factor alone.[35,36]

Considerable evidence indicates that factors that influence arrhythmias in experimental models also influence the occurrence of ventricular arrhythmias in humans. The incidence of ventricular tachyarrhythmias is related to infarct size and the presence of heart failure.[37–39] Patients with an absolute increase in sympathetic tone or decreased vagal efferent activity are at an increased risk of sudden cardiac death due to ventricular arrhythmias.[40–43] Acute MI causes several changes in the autonomic nervous system that may facilitate the initiation of ventricular arrhythmias. Activation of cardiac mechanoreceptors and cardiopulmonary and carotid baroreceptors results in increased circulating catecholamine levels and increased efferent sympathetic activity. Ischemic damage to cardiac adrenergic neurons results in the release of catecholamines as well. Transmural MI denervates viable myocardium distal to the infarct site. Ischemic and denervated viable myocardium is hypersensitive to circulating catecholamines.[43] Sympathetic stimulation also enhances automaticity in the Purkinje fibers. These effects result in inhomogeneities of repolarization and enhance automaticity.

Electrolyte abnormalities, including hypokalemia and hypomagnesemia, are potentially correctable causes of ventricular arrhythmias in acute MI.[44] Hypokalemia is an independent risk factor for ventricular arrhythmias early in MI. Hypomagnesemia often accompanies hypokalemia and may result in polymorphic ventricular tachycardia (VT). Coronary reperfusion may cause isolated premature ventricular contractions, accelerated idioventricular rhythm (AIVR), VT, or ventricular fibrillation (VF), presumably by enhancing automaticity of ischemic myocardium.[45] The severity of the arrhythmia induced by reperfusion is related to the duration of myocardial ischemia.

The circulating effects of certain antiarrhythmic drugs at the time of MI may also facilitate initiation and maintenance of ventricular arrhythmias. This proarrhythmic effect is thought to occur because of changes in the electrophysiologic action of the drugs in the setting of myocardial ischemia. In the Cardiac Arrhythmia Suppression Trial (CAST), the use of class IC antiarrhythmic drugs given to patients both early and late after prior MI (6 days to 2 years) for the treatment and suppression of premature ventricular beats ultimately lead to increased mortality and sudden cardiac death.[46]

Ventricular Premature Beats

Ventricular premature beats (VPBs) occur in almost all patients with acute MI and are rarely a cause of myocardial ischemia or systemic hypotension.[46] Previously, these beats were thought to potentially trigger VT or VF.[47,48] Data from animal models and human studies indicate that frequent and complex ectopy is neither a sensitive nor specific predictor for the development of sustained ventricular tachyarrhythmias early after MI.[28,49–53]

The incidence of frequent VPB and the R-on-T phenomenon is similar between patients who develop VF and those who do not.[28] Studies of animals and humans have shown that most VT episodes and 41% to 45% of VF episodes are initiated by late-coupled VPBs (after the T wave), suggesting that early beats are not required to initiate the arrhythmia.[49,50] VF occurs in the absence of preceding ventricular ectopy in 40% to 83% of patients.[49]

Ventricular Tachycardia

VT is defined as three or more consecutive ventricular ectopic beats at a rate greater than 100 beats/min. This arrhythmia may be classified as nonsustained (i.e., terminating spontaneously within 30 seconds) or sustained (i.e., requiring intervention or spontaneous termination >30 seconds after onset), monomorphic or polymorphic (pertaining to QRS complex morphology), and as early (occurring <24 hours) or late (>48 hours) after the onset of MI.

VT occurs in 10% to 40% of patients with acute MI; any wide QRS complex tachycardia associated with acute MI should be considered ventricular in origin until proven otherwise.[1,28] VT appears on the surface 12-lead electrocardiogram (ECG) as a wide QRS complex tachycardia. Although several criteria and algorithms have been proposed to differentiate this arrhythmia from supraventricular tachycardia with aberrant ventricular conduction, the diagnosis sometimes remains uncertain (Box 16.1).[54,55] The timing of VT has important implications regarding the mechanism and prognosis of the arrhythmia. VT that occurs late in the course of MI is more common in patients with transmural infarction and LV dysfunction.[1,56] Sustained, late-onset VT that results in hypotension is more likely to recur and is associated with increased in-hospital and long-term mortality rates.[56–58] VT that occurs early is more likely to have a reversible cause (e.g., ischemia, reperfusion, autonomic nervous system influences) and is less likely to recur.

Patients presenting with acute MI and cardiogenic shock are more likely to demonstrate VF (24% to 29%) than VT (17% to 21%). The mechanism of sustained monomorphic VT is often reentrant in nature.[59] Because monomorphic VT suggests an underlying stable reentrant circuit even when it occurs less than

48 hours after the onset of acute MI, a thorough electrophysiologic evaluation should be undertaken to determine the risk for recurrence and the need for therapy.[60] VT associated with reperfusion is often at a slower rate and is less likely to recur.

Polymorphic VT differs from monomorphic VT in that QRS complex morphology varies from beat to beat. This arrhythmia has been reported in 0.7% to 2% of patients hospitalized after acute MI.[59,61] Although the mechanism for the arrhythmia is unknown, polymorphic VT is not thought to be associated with a stable reentrant circuit. Polymorphic VT attributed to reperfusion, particularly early (within 6.5 hours of onset) in acute MI, is typically associated with a good prognosis. Late-onset polymorphic VT (2 to 13 days after acute MI) is more likely to be associated with recurrent ischemia and a poor prognosis.

Torsades de pointes is a specific type of polymorphic VT; it is usually caused by a proarrhythmic effect of antiarrhythmic drugs or metabolic derangements. Drugs that prolong refractoriness (class IA antiarrhythmic drugs and the class III drugs sotalol, dofetilide, ibutilide, and, rarely, amiodarone) may prolong the QT interval and predispose patients to this arrhythmia. In this situation, torsades de pointes is thought to result from triggered activity induced by early afterdepolarizations. Early afterdepolarization amplitude depends on heart rate; increased heart rate decreases the amplitude and the probability that the afterdepolarization will reach a threshold potential and "trigger" torsades de pointes. Faster heart rates also shorten repolarization and suppress early afterdepolarizations.

Ventricular Fibrillation

VF results in multiple electrical activation wave fronts that depolarize the ventricles in a disorganized and chaotic fashion. The absence of organized ventricular electrical activation results in the absence of QRS complexes and an irregular undulating baseline on the surface ECG. By definition, this arrhythmia does not terminate spontaneously and is lethal unless converted quickly.

VF is the leading cause of death early in the course of MI, occurring in 4% to 18% of hospitalized patients.[49,62] Arrhythmia is more likely to occur in patients with a large MI and may carry a genetic predilection.[63] The incidence of VF is lower among patients with a non-ST elevation MI. VF occurs with similar frequency, however, in patients with anterior or inferior MI.[28] Although VF that occurs early (<48 hours) is associated with increased in-hospital mortality, it does not increase long-term mortality and the overall incidence has decreased markedly over recent years due to aggressive early revascularization strategies.[5,64] Delayed treatment due to either late presentation by the patient or failed recognition of acute coronary syndrome by bystanders or medical personnel, insufficient access to centers equipped to manage acute MI with regard to prompt reperfusion, unsuccessful revascularization, and prior arrhythmogenic substrate all predispose patients to the development of unstable ventricular arrhythmias. Patients with a history of prior MI and LV dysfunction are at risk for sustained ventricular arrhythmias at the time they present with a new acute coronary event.

When associated with acute MI, VF has been classified as primary or secondary. Primary VF occurs early and unexpectedly in the absence of heart failure or other apparent causes. Approximately 50% of these episodes occur within 1 hour, 60% to 80% occur within 4 hours, and 80% occur within 12 hours of the onset of symptoms.[1,51,61] Secondary VF occurs as a result of severe heart failure or cardiogenic shock and can occur at any time during the course of MI.[1]

Whether VF occurs early or late, myocardial ischemia should be considered the underlying cause, particularly when the arrhythmia recurs frequently. VF may also result from coronary reperfusion and is related to the duration of myocardial ischemia. In animal models, the incidence of VF increases when ischemia is prolonged from 5 to 20 minutes but decreased when reperfusion is delayed beyond 30 minutes.

Sudden cardiac death and VF may be the presenting symptom in patients with acute MI. In these patients, the cause of the arrhythmia or the MI is often unclear. In many patients, VF may be the cause, rather than the result, of MI. In others, particularly patients with previous MI, VF may have occurred as a result of sustained VT. These are important considerations when evaluating the risk for recurrent VTs and the need for electrophysiologic testing and the role of long-term therapy.

Accelerated Idioventricular Rhythm

AIVR is defined by its rate, under 100 beats/min. AIVR occurs in 8% to 20% of patients, usually during the first 2 days after MI, and may be provoked by spontaneous or induced reperfusion.[65,66] AIVR may begin with a premature ventricular beat or may occur as a result of sinus slowing or an increase in the ventricular "escape" rate. Similarly, AIVR may terminate abruptly because the sinus rate increases or because the ventricular escape rate slows. Variation in the rate of this arrhythmia is common.

In humans, AIVR is the most common arrhythmia following coronary reperfusion.[57,67] Most cases of AIVR probably occur as a result of enhanced automaticity in Purkinje fibers on the endocardial surface near or within the infarction zone.[67] In vitro studies, using a model of coronary artery reperfusion, have shown AIVR caused by triggered activity associated with delayed afterdepolarizations.[68] Rapid VT with a rate twice that of the AIVR has been observed in some patients, suggesting reentry with episodic exit block as another possible mechanism for the arrhythmia.[69,70]

THERAPY

Ventricular Tachycardia

Ventricular tachyarrhythmias typically necessitate prompt treatment. Reversible causes should be sought and addressed in every patient. Acid-base status, arterial oxygen saturation, and serum electrolytes should be evaluated and corrected when appropriate. Certain antiarrhythmic medications may be proarrhythmic during an acute coronary syndrome and may require discontinuation.

Recognition of myocardial ischemia as the underlying cause for the ventricular arrhythmia is paramount as the rhythm disturbance may be the first or only manifestation of the ischemic event. Appropriate diagnostic measures and timely management geared mainly at restoring myocardial oxygenation as well as supportive care for patients with hemodynamic instability or cardiogenic shock is often the most effective and expedient way to quiet electrical instability and prevent recurrence. Mechanical circulatory support devices, by unloading the left ventricle, may be highly useful in treating incessant ventricular arrhythmias.

Cardioversion and Defibrillation

Rapid conversion of unstable VT is imperative because of its adverse hemodynamic effects and the potential for deterioration into VF. If possible, obtaining a 12-lead ECG prior to cardioversion can be helpful to further scrutinize the diagnosis and to guide future therapies, in particular, catheter ablation.

VT that is associated with hypotension should be treated promptly with a synchronized DC shock with defibrillator pads placed near the apex and base of the heart. The initial biphasic energy delivery should be 120 to 200 J for maximum efficacy.

Hemodynamically stable VT can sometimes be terminated chemically with antiarrhythmic drugs, though they are often more time consuming and less reliable than electrical cardioversion. Chemical cardioversion is appropriate as a first-line attempt to terminate the ventricular arrhythmia in hemodynamically stable patients who are not actively ischemic. However, it is prudent to have an external cardioverter defibrillator readily available.[71]

Antiarrhythmic drug therapy can be administered to treat stable VT or assist in the suppression of unstable VT after urgent cardioversion. Intravenous amiodarone can be given as a 150-mg infusion over 10 minutes with repeat boluses as necessary and then continuously at set infusion rates to achieve the desired loading dose. Amiodarone can cause hypotension; therefore, patients with unstable hemodynamics need to be closely monitored. Lidocaine is safe and can be an effective adjunct to amiodarone or given independently. It does not prolong the QT interval or cause hypotension and, thus, may be a more desirable agent. The initial infusion is given as a 50-mg to 100-mg intravenous bolus followed by a continuous infusion of 1 to 4 mg/min. Due to a significant first-pass effect in the liver, a second bolus may be administered 20 to 30 minutes after the initial dose to maintain a therapeutic serum drug level. Procainamide is also effective for cardioversion, though it requires a longer period to infuse and may not be a readily available agent in most cardiac intensive care units. Procainamide can be associated with hypotension due to its negative inotropic and vasodilatory effects. Procainamide prolongs refractoriness in atrial and ventricular myocardium and can be a very effective antiarrhythmic. It is administered intravenously and can be titrated to achieve the therapeutic effect. Procainamide undergoes acetylation in the liver to N-acetyl procainamide; both forms have antiarrhythmic activity. Serum concentrations of procainamide can be measured via a bioassay that correlates directly with efficacy and toxicity. Due to prolonged refractoriness in ventricular myocardium, procainamide can lead to QT prolongation. It can be tried in patients who cannot tolerate amiodarone, though it should be used cautiously in patients with recent amiodarone exposure. QTc prolongation beyond 550 ms is associated with an increased risk of torsades de pointes and may be an indication to decrease the dose or discontinue the drug. Sotalol, another class III agent, must be given orally and is often impractical because steady state is not achieved for several days.

Pacing, similar to antiarrhythmic drug therapy, may terminate VT. Pace termination of VT is effective in certain patients with relatively slow, hemodynamically tolerated monomorphic VT. Patients with temporary endocardial or epicardial ventricular pacing wires and patients with preexisting implantable cardioverter defibrillators are ideal candidates for this therapy. Synchronized pacing is performed at a cycle length that is 90% or less than that of the VT. Typically, 5 to 15 seconds of burst pacing is required to terminate the arrhythmia and can be repeated if the initial attempt is unsuccessful. Pacing should not be performed at a rate greater than 300 beats/min due to the increased risk of accelerating the rhythm or inducing VF. Pacing should not be performed unless a defibrillator is readily available for immediate use.

β-Blockers can be useful in preventing recurrent VT in the setting of ischemia. Typically, calcium channel blockers are to be avoided because they can provoke hemodynamic collapse as a result of their negative inotropic effect.

Ventricular Fibrillation

VF requires DC defibrillation administered as quickly as possible to improve patient outcome. Generally, 200 J of biphasic energy or greater is required for successful termination. Cardiopulmonary resuscitation (CPR) should be initiated whenever electrical countershock cannot be delivered immediately. Advanced Cardiac Life Support (ACLS) should be initiated with as little interruption as necessary for shock delivery.

Suppression

Ventricular Premature Beats and Nonsustained Ventricular Tachycardia.
Ventricular premature beats and nonsustained VT should be treated when the arrhythmia aggravates myocardial ischemia and/or adversely affects hemodynamics. Treatment of asymptomatic nonsustained VT is controversial because there is little evidence that this translates into improved mortality or morbidity.[72–74]

Ventricular Tachycardia. Antiarrhythmic therapy is usually not indicated when VT occurs early, particularly around the time of presentation, during or shortly after revascularization. VT is unlikely to recur when the underlying ischemia has been definitively addressed. Sustained VT should be suppressed, particularly when it occurs late or frequently in the patient's course.

Amiodarone can be given orally or intravenously to suppress recurrence of VT. An oral loading dose of 1200 to 1600 mg/day is usually administered until a 6- to 10-g loading dose is completed.[75–77] Intravenous amiodarone is usually administered for unstable VT or VF and has been shown to reduce the incidence of recurrence during the first 24 hours of infusion.[78] The recommended starting dose is 150 mg over 10 minutes followed by a 1 mg/min infusion rate for 6 hours, which is then lowered to 0. 5 mg/min for the following 18 hours or continued until the patient can tolerate oral therapy to complete the load. Lidocaine and procainamide are also effective intravenous antiarrhythmic drugs for the suppression of monomorphic VT. These drugs may be administered alone or in combination with each other. The utilization of pacing to increase the baseline heart rate may be an effective suppression tool, particularly for ventricular arrhythmias that are bradycardia mediated.

Catheter Ablation for Sustained Ventricular Arrhythmias

Catheter ablation may be considered for patients presenting with acute MI if the sustained ventricular arrhythmias are recurrent or incessant (i.e., electrical storm); not attributable to a reversible, treatable cause; and are drug refractory.[5] Sustained ventricular tachyarrhythmias in the acute MI patient, as previously discussed, can often cause or occur in the setting of profound hemodynamic instability and critical illness. Thus the timing of such procedures needs to be carefully considered. Furthermore, these complex ablations should only be performed by experienced operators in high-volume centers.

Torsades de Pointes

Suppression of this arrhythmia depends on increasing the heart rate and eliminating the offending agent. Increasing the heart rate (usually to 90 to 110 beats/min) shortens ventricular repolarization time and suppresses the arrhythmia. This may require the insertion of a temporary pacing wire. Intravenous atropine or isoproterenol (or both) can be administered. Magnesium, which also shortens ventricular repolarization, is an effective treatment for this arrhythmia when given intravenously (see Table 16.2).

Ventricular Fibrillation

Intravenous amiodarone is first-line suppressive therapy for this rhythm, with repeat boluses as necessary to treat frequent recurrence or incessant VF. Lidocaine can be administered when amiodarone is ineffective or associated with side effects. Pacing can be effective in preventing bradycardia-mediated VF. If VF is thought to be due to ongoing coronary ischemia, urgent cardiac catheterization should be considered. An intraaortic balloon pump may be necessary for refractory VT or VF, particularly in the setting of ongoing ischemia, severe LV dysfunction, or cardiogenic shock.

PREVENTION OF SUDDEN CARDIAC DEATH

Coronary Care Unit

The institution of coronary care units resulted in a significant decline in mortality for acute MI. These units eliminated primary arrhythmias as a cause of death, mainly due to timely recognition of both sustained arrhythmias and their precursors.[28,79] Also, because of the acute care provided to treat acute coronary syndrome and thereby limit infarct size, including rapid reperfusion strategies and mechanical circulatory support, the subsequent risk for arrhythmias is further reduced.

The duration of continuous telemetry monitoring depends on the risk for life-threatening arrhythmia. It may be prudent to monitor patients surviving relatively larger MIs complicated by heart failure, hemodynamic instability, or recurrent ischemia for 5 to 7 days.

Implantable Cardioverter Defibrillators

Implantable cardioverter defibrillators (ICDs) are generally not indicated in the peri-MI or immediate post-revascularization setting for the primary prevention of sudden cardiac death. Several large clinical trials evaluating this approach have failed to demonstrate a mortality benefit. The Coronary Artery Bypass Grafting–Patch trial (CABG–Patch) evaluated patients at the time of surgical revascularization and both the Defibrillator IN Acute Myocardial Infarction Trial (DINAMIT) and the Immediate Risk-Stratification Improves Survival (IRIS) trials evaluated patients in the immediate post-MI phase. The reduction of arrhythmogenic death in all three studies was offset by an increase in nonarrhythmic death with no impact on all-cause mortality.[80–82]

There are, however, certain cases when ICD implantation in the post-MI period is appropriate. In patients who have an indication for cardiac resynchronization therapy (CRT) or permanent pacing and who have depressed LV function, an ICD should be implanted.[83] An ICD should also be considered for the secondary prevention of sudden cardiac death in patients exhibiting VF or sustained hemodynamically significant VT more than 48 hours after the onset of an acute coronary event who have undergone complete revascularization, providing that a reversible cause (i.e., recurrent ischemia, loss of stent, or bypass graft patency) has been ruled out.[60] For patients with VF or polymorphic ventricular tachycardia within 48 hours of symptom onset who are not candidates for revascularization due to advanced disease, ICD implantation should also be considered.[83] For patients with asymptomatic nonsustained ventricular tachycardia who are more than 4 days post-MI, ICD should be considered if VT is inducible at the time of an electrophysiology (EP) study.[84] The EP study should be deferred until revascularization has been performed.

CONCLUSION

Cardiac arrhythmias are observed frequently in the setting of acute MI because of electrophysiologic alterations that result from myocardial ischemia and necrosis. These arrhythmias, whether supraventricular or ventricular, may precipitate hemodynamic collapse and death. Efforts should be made to identify and correct factors such as electrolyte disturbances, hypoxia, heart failure, and ongoing ischemia, which increase the risk of arrhythmia. The mortality associated with acute MI has been greatly reduced because of early recognition, timely treatment—including prompt application of resuscitative measures—revascularization techniques, and arrhythmia treatment and suppression.

Acknowledgment

We acknowledge the contributions of Dr. Mark Carlson, who was a coauthor of this chapter in the previous edition.

The full reference list for this chapter is available at ExpertConsult.com.

17

Conduction Disturbances in Acute Myocardial Infarction

David L. Brown

Infarction or ischemia of myocardial conduction tissue and/or autonomic imbalance that results in altered conduction through the heart can dramatically alter the presentation, management, and outcomes of patients presenting with an acute myocardial infarction (MI). Immediate recognition of conduction disturbances in the acute phase of MI is of prognostic and therapeutic significance. The nature of any conduction disturbance not only gives clues to the location of the infarct, but also aids in prioritizing the management of MI, including, but not limited to, the potential need for temporary pacemaker support.

ANATOMY

The sinus node, sinoatrial conduction system, atrioventricular (AV) node, bundle of His, right bundle, left bundle dividing into anterior and posterior fascicles and myocardial Purkinje fibers form the cardiac conduction system (Fig. 17.1). The bundle of His divides into the right and left bundle branches after leaving the AV node. The right bundle traverses the right side of the interventricular septum without giving off branches for most of its course. Ultimately, it branches near the base of the right anterior papillary muscle with fascicles supplying the septal and free wall of the right ventricle. The left bundle divides into several discrete branches after penetrating the membranous septum under the aortic valve. The anterior fascicle crosses the left ventricular outflow tract and terminates in the Purkinje system of the anterolateral wall of the left ventricle. The posterior fascicle courses inferiorly and posteriorly. The septum is activated earliest in all hearts by either a discrete septal fascicle or branches of the posterior fascicle.[1-4]

The sinoatrial node is supplied by the atrial branch of the proximal right coronary artery (RCA) in 55% of cases and by the proximal left circumflex coronary artery (LCX) in 45% of cases.[5] The RCA perfuses the AV node and the proximal portion of the His bundle in 90% of patients with perfusion originating from the LCX in the remaining 10%. The septal branches of the left anterior descending coronary artery (LAD) supply the distal part of the His bundle, the right bundle branch, and the anterior fascicle of the left bundle branch. The proximal portion of posterior fascicle of the left bundle is supplied by the AV nodal artery or by septal branches of the LAD. The distal portion is supplied by septal branches from the LAD coronary artery and RCA.

INCIDENCE

The overall incidence of new conduction disturbances, including bundle branch and fascicular block, during acute MI is difficult to accurately determine because these abnormalities may often be chronic and unrelated to the acute presentation. The National Registry of Myocardial Infarction 2 (NRMI-2) evaluated the incidence of bundle branch block in 297,832 patients admitted to a hospital in the United States with an acute MI between 1994 and 1997: 6.7% of patients had a left bundle branch block (LBBB) and 6.2% had a right bundle branch block (RBBB) on the initial electrocardiogram (ECG).[6] A similar rate of LBBB (9%) was noted in a prospective analysis of over 88,000 acute MI patients in Sweden.[7] Since both series only assessed the presence of a bundle branch block (BBB) on the initial ECG, these data provide no information on the incidence of new conduction disease in

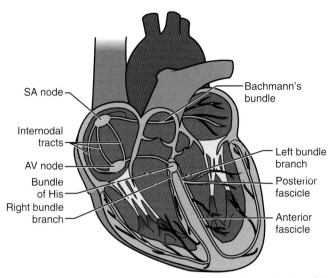

Fig. 17.1 Cardiac conduction system. *AV,* Atrioventricular; *SA,* sinoatrial.

acute MI. The development of BBB complicating acute MI after initial presentation appears to be rare, with only 0.73% and 0.15% of patients developing RBBB and LBBB, respectively, in the first 60 minutes after presentation.[8] However, this is likely an underestimate, as many patients probably develop an acute BBB prior to presenting to the hospital.

The largest experience with high-degree AV block in the fibrinolytic era comes from a review of almost 76,000 patients with ST-elevation MI (STEMI) enrolled in four large randomized trials.[9] The overall incidence of high-degree AV block was 6.9%: 9.8% associated with an inferior MI and 3.2% with an anterior MI.

In the thrombolytic era, the incidence of complete block has been reported in 3.2% of patients, 5.9% of patients with RCA occlusion, and 1.5% of patients with other infarct-related arteries.[10–14] These generally develop within the first 2 days. The incidence of complete heart block (CHB) in acute MI was about 4% to 5%,[15–19] with CHB or second-degree AV block occurring in 7% to 10% of patients.[9,18] Since the widespread use of primary PCI, the incidence of AV block appears to have declined. Among 2073 STEMI patients treated with primary PCI in the Danish National Patient Registry, only 3.2% presented with second- or third-degree AV block or developed it during hospitalization.[10]

Among 6662 STEMI patients enrolled in a French prospective registry between 2006 and 2013,[11] of whom 74% of patients underwent primary PCI and 90% had PCI at some point in the index hospitalization, 3.5% of patients developed Mobitz II or third-degree AV block—2.2% on admission and 1.3% later in the hospitalization. AV block was more common among those with RCA occlusion (5.9%) than those with other infarct-related arteries (1.5%). Rates of AV block developing during hospitalization were lower in patients who received primary PCI (1.2%) or thrombolysis (0.5%) than those with no reperfusion treatment (2.6%).

The Global Registry of Acute Coronary Events (GRACE) enrolled 59,229 patients with acute coronary syndromes (37% with STEMI, 33% with non-ST elevation MI [NSTEMI]) at 126 hospitals in 14 countries.[14] Second-degree Mobitz II or third-degree AV block occurred in 2.9% of patients (5% of STEMI patients, 1.9% of NSTEMI patients). AV block was noted on presentation in about half the patients and developed following admission in the other half. The RCA was the culprit vessel in 65% of patients with AV block and 31% of patients without AV block. A total of 35% of patients with AV block underwent temporary pacemaker placement and 5.9% required a permanent pacemaker.

Most reports that have assessed the incidence and prognostic significance of high-degree AV block after MI have not distinguished between STEMI and NSTEMI. In the Second Prevention Reinfarction Israeli Nifedipine Trial (SPRINT) of 610 patients with a first NSTEMI,[20] second- or third-degree AV block developed in 7% of patients. In the GRACE registry, 5% of STEMI patients developed Mobitz II second- or third-degree AV block compared to 1.9% of NSTEMI patients.[14]

SPECIFIC CONDUCTION ABNORMALITIES

Sinoatrial Node

Sinus Bradycardia. Sinus bradycardia is the most common arrhythmia in inferior MI and three times more common in inferoposterior than anterolateral MI.[21] Potential mechanisms include infarction or ischemia of the sinus node or the surrounding atrium, increased vagal tone (most commonly), and the Bezold-Jarisch reflex. The Bezold-Jarisch reflex consists of vasodilation and bradycardia, resulting in hypotension triggered by stimulation of cardiac inhibitory receptors during myocardial ischemia.

Stimulation of these inhibitory cardiac receptors increases parasympathetic activity and inhibits sympathetic activity. Paradoxically, reperfusion can also trigger this reflex.[22]

Sinoatrial Block and Sinus Arrest. Grade 2 or complete sinoatrial block suggests a proximal occlusion of the RCA or LCX and is often accompanied by atrial infarction. This is a sign of a large MI, potentially involving the right ventricle.[23]

ATRIOVENTRICULAR NODE

Prolongation of the PR interval (first-degree block) can arise in the AV node, the bundle of His, or the bundle branches. When the block is at the level of the AV node, it is caused by occlusion of the artery supplying the AV node (RCA or LCX). First-degree AV block from RCA occlusion is usually transient, resolving in 5 to 7 days with no treatment indicated. The mechanism of Wenckebach second-degree AV block (Mobitz type I) is similar to first-degree AV block. It is also transient and requires no specific treatment.

Infranodal Conduction Abnormalities

The various forms of conduction abnormalities known to occur below the AV node include Mobitz II second-degree AV block, 2:1 AV block, RBBB with or without left anterior fascicular block (LAFB) or left posterior fascicular block (LPFB), and LBBB.

RBBB is much more common than complete LBBB owing to the dual blood supply of various fascicles of the left bundle and a wide area of distribution within the myocardium. The clinical prognosis is worse when an MI results in RBBB with LAFB due to the large amount of myocardium involved.[6]

Complete heart block with inferior MI generally results from an intranodal lesion. It is associated with a narrow QRS complex and develops in a progressive fashion from first-degree to second-degree to third-degree block (Fig. 17.2). It often results in asymptomatic bradycardia (40 to 60 beats/min) and is usually transient, resolving within 5 to 7 days. LBBB occurs as a form of aberration during bradycardia—either sinus bradycardia or AV block with a junctional escape mechanism. Complete heart block with anterior MI generally occurs abruptly in the first 24 hours. It can develop without warning or may be preceded by the development of RBBB with either LAFB or LPFB (bifascicular or trifascicular block; Fig. 17.3).[24] The escape rhythm is wide and unstable, and the event is associated with a high mortality from arrhythmias and pump failure. Heart block in this setting is thought to result from extensive necrosis that involves the bundle branches traveling within the septum.

Inferior Wall Versus Anterior Wall Myocardial Infarction

High-degree (second- or third-degree) AV block associated with inferior wall MI is located above the His bundle in 90% of

patients.[25] For this reason, complete heart block often results in only a modest and usually transient bradycardia with junctional or escape rhythm rates greater than 40 beats/min (Fig. 17.4). It is common, however, for the junctional pacemaker that controls the ventricles to accelerate to greater than 60 beats/min. The QRS is narrow in this setting and the risk of mortality is low.

High-degree AV block associated with anterior MI is more often located below the AV node (more frequently within the His bundle or proximal bundle branches).[26] It is usually symptomatic and was historically associated with a mortality rate approaching 80% largely because of greater infarct size. Mortality rates may be lower in the current era because of improvements in the management of congestive heart failure and cardiogenic shock, but the risk remains substantial.

MORTALITY

High-degree AV block is associated with increased mortality in patients with inferior or anterior MI. Most of the increased risk is within the first 30 days.[27] High-degree AV block in patients with an anterior wall MI is associated with a greater increase in in-hospital and 30-day mortality than seen with an inferior wall MI, probably because of more extensive myocardial involvement and a higher incidence of hemodynamic complications.[9]

The presence of a fascicular or bundle branch block during an acute MI is associated with increased in-hospital and long-term

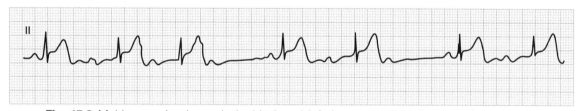

Fig. 17.2 Mobitz type I atrioventricular block and inferior myocardial infarction. (Courtesy Ary Goldberger, MD.)

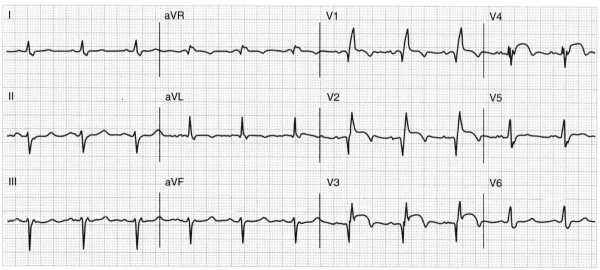

Fig. 17.3 12-Lead electrocardiogram from a patient with a history of an anteroseptal myocardial infarction (Q waves seen in leads V$_1$ to V$_3$) shows a typical right bundle branch block and left anterior fascicular block.

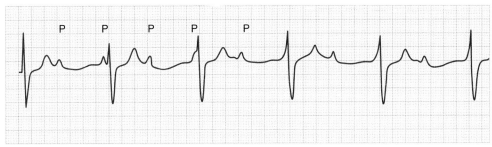

Fig. 17.4 Sinus rhythm with high-grade atrioventricular block. (Courtesy Ary Goldberger, MD.)

mortality. However, since it is usually impossible to know if these findings are chronic or acute, the increased mortality may represent increased comorbidity in the former and a larger infarct in the latter. Among 26,000 patients treated with thrombolytic therapy in the Global Use of Strategies to Open Occluded Coronary Arteries (GUSTO)-1 trial, in-hospital mortality was higher in patients with a BBB on initial ECG (18% vs. 11%). In addition, patients with a BBB were more likely to develop cardiogenic shock (19% vs. 11%), AV block or asystole (30% vs. 9%), and to require a pacemaker (18% vs. 11%). In the primary PCI era, RBBB or LBBB on baseline ECG remains associated with increased in-hospital and long-term mortality.[28–30] A post-hoc analysis of over 17,000 patients demonstrated that after adjustment for baseline characteristics, 30-day mortality was significantly increased only in patients with an RBBB at baseline and an anterior MI and in patients with a new LBBB or new RBBB with an anterior MI.[8]

MANAGEMENT

Patients with AV block may by asymptomatic or symptomatic. Even if asymptomatic, AV block associated with bradycardia may cause hypotension, reduced coronary perfusion pressure, and recurrent ischemia. In symptomatic patients, the most common therapies are atropine or transvenous right ventricular pacing. Transcutaneous pacing is painful and unreliable; thus, it should be avoided except when no alternatives exist.

Symptomatic bradyarrhythmias in the setting of an inferior MI may respond to atropine when they occur early in the course while those that occur more than 24 hours after presentation often do not. Atropine is administered intravenously in 0.5- or 1-mg doses to a maximum of 3 mg. Ventricular fibrillation has been described after atropine administration in the setting of BBB or Mobitz type II AV block. Refractory hypotension in an inferior MI after treatment of bradycardia with atropine should raise suspicion for volume depletion or right ventricular infarction.

Patients with two or more of the following new findings are at 25% to 36% risk of progression to complete heart block: PR prolongation, second-degree AV block, left anterior or posterior fascicular block, LBBB, and RBBB.[31]

Temporary Transvenous Pacing

The purpose of temporary transvenous pacemaker insertion is to maintain circulatory integrity by providing for standby pacing should sudden complete heart block ensue, to increase heart rate during periods of symptomatic bradycardia and occasionally to control sustained supraventricular or ventricular tachycardia.[32] Whether ventricular or AV sequential pacing should be used depends on hemodynamic considerations. An infarcted, preload-dependent right ventricle may require atrial filling achieved by AV synchronous pacing to maximize stroke volume and reverse shock. Performance of AV temporary pacing requires additional experience and can be considerably more difficult from a technical standpoint. Because temporary pacemakers are manufactured by many different vendors, physicians credentialed to insert temporary pacemakers should be familiar with the insertion equipment, leads, and external generators used in their own hospitals.

First-degree AV block does not require treatment. High-grade AV block with inferior STEMI usually is transient and associated with a narrow complex/junctional escape rhythm that can be managed conservatively. Prophylactic placement of a temporary pacing system is recommended for high-grade AV block and/or new bundle-branch (especially LBBB) or bifascicular block in patients with anterior MI.[33] Pacing can be considered in symptomatic bradycardia of any etiology if associated with hypotension and atropine administration is unsuccessful, Mobitz type II second-degree AV block, and bradycardia-induced tachyarrhythmias, such as torsades de pointes.

Guidelines for Permanent Pacemaker Placement

The American College of Cardiology/American Heart Association/Heart Rhythm Society (ACC/AHA/HRS) class I indications for placement of a permanent pacemaker after an acute MI are described in Box 17.1.[34] Indications for permanent pacing after STEMI in patients experiencing AV block are related in large measure to the presence of intraventricular conduction defects. In contrast to some other indications for permanent pacing, the criteria for patients with STEMI and AV block do not depend on the presence of symptoms. The requirement for temporary pacing in STEMI does not by itself constitute an indication for permanent pacing.

BOX 17.1 Permanent Pacing for Bradycardia or Conduction Blocks Associated With ST Segment Elevation Myocardial Infarction (STEMI)[34]

Class I

1. Permanent ventricular pacing is indicated for persistent second-degree AV block in the His-Purkinje system with alternating bundle branch block or third-degree AV block within or below the His-Purkinje system after STEMI (level of evidence: B).
2. Permanent ventricular pacing is indicated for transient advanced second- or third-degree infranodal AV block and associated bundle branch block. If the site of block is uncertain, an electrophysiologic study may be necessary (level of evidence: B).
3. Permanent ventricular pacing is indicated for persistent and symptomatic second- or third-degree AV block (level of evidence: C).

Class IIb

1. Permanent ventricular pacing may be considered for persistent second- or third-degree AV block at the AV node level, even in the absence of symptoms (level of evidence: B).

Class III

1. Permanent ventricular pacing is not indicated for transient AV block in the absence of intraventricular conduction defects (level of evidence: B).
2. Permanent ventricular pacing is not indicated for transient AV block in the presence of isolated left anterior fascicular block (level of evidence: B).
3. Permanent ventricular pacing is not indicated for new bundle branch block or fascicular block in the absence of AV block (level of evidence: B).
4. Permanent ventricular pacing is not recommended for persistent first-degree AV block in the presence of bundle branch block that is old or of indeterminate age (level of evidence: B).

Full guidelines are accessible in the Appendix at ExpertConsult.com.
AV, Atrioventricular.

Acknowledgment

I acknowledge the contribution of the late Mark Josephson, MD, to this chapter in prior editions.

The full reference list for this chapter is available at ExpertConsult.com.

PART IV

Noncoronary Diseases: Diagnosis and Management

18

Acute Heart Failure and Pulmonary Edema

Theo E. Meyer, Jeffrey A. Shih, Colleen Harrington

OUTLINE

INTRODUCTION

Acute heart failure (AHF) is a clinical syndrome of new or worsening signs and symptoms of heart failure (decompensated), often leading to hospitalization or a visit to the emergency department. Patients with AHF represent a heterogeneous population with high hospital readmission rates.[1-9] The most common reason for hospitalization is significant volume overload and, subsequently, congestive symptoms. Fewer patients present with hypotension and symptoms of reduced organ perfusion,[1,2] and some present with AHF due to "flash pulmonary edema," usually from uncontrolled hypertension or atrial fibrillation with a rapid ventricular response. In general, most patients have a slow progression of disease, resulting from cardiac ischemia, medication noncompliance, dietary indiscretion, or exacerbation of hypertension.[1] The average patient has had symptoms for about 5 to 7 days before seeking medical attention.[10,11]

AHF is the most common cause of hospital admission in patients older than 65 years, accounting for 1 million admissions annually.[12] AHF represents a period of high risk for patients, with a 20% to 30% mortality rate within 6 months after admission.[13–15] Early medical care of AHF and time to initiation of treatment are linked to outcome. These patients are generally cared for in telemetry units in the United States. Only 10% to 20% of these patients are admitted to intensive care units (ICUs).[8,9]

PATHOPHYSIOLOGIC CONSIDERATIONS

Integral to the understanding of the pathogenesis and treatment of AHF and pulmonary edema is a basic understanding of the forces involved in fluid retention, capillary–interstitial fluid exchange (Starling relationship), and myocardial pump performance.

Chronic Progressive Fluid and Water Retention

Renal sodium and water excretion normally parallels sodium and water intake so that an increase in plasma and blood volume is associated with increased renal sodium and water excretion. In patients with heart failure, sodium and water are retained despite an increase in intravascular fluid volume. Renal sodium and water retention in these patients may be regulated not by the total blood volume but rather by the degree of filling of the arterial compartment—the so-called effective blood volume. The dynamic equilibrium of the arterial circulation, as determined by cardiac output and peripheral vascular resistance or compliance, is the predominant determinant of renal sodium and water excretion.

Arterial underfilling is sensed by mechanoreceptors in the left ventricle, carotid sinus, aortic arch, and renal afferent arterioles.[16] Decreased activation of these receptors due to a decrease in systemic arterial pressure, stroke volume, renal perfusion, or peripheral vascular resistance leads to an increase in sympathetic outflow from the central nervous system, activation of the renin-angiotensin-aldosterone system, and the nonosmotic release of arginine vasopressin, as well as the stimulation of thirst.[16] These factors—together with increased release of vasoconstrictors, such as endothelin and vasopressin, and resistance to endogenous natriuretic peptides—contribute to sodium and water retention leading to decompensation of chronic heart failure.

Pulmonary Edema

The flux of fluid out of any vascular bed results from the sum of forces promoting extravasation of fluid from the capillary lumen versus forces acting to retain intravascular fluid. This concept of a dynamic equilibration between opposing forces in the lung is given mathematical expression in the Starling equation[17]:

$$Qf = Kf(Pv - Pint) - Kf(pV - pint)$$

where Qf is net transvascular fluid flow across the pulmonary capillary endothelium; Kf is the filtration coefficient of the microvascular endothelium (hydraulic conductivity of the capillary wall × surface area); Pv is hydrostatic pressure in the pulmonary capillaries; $Pint$ is hydrostatic pressure in the pulmonary interstitium; pV is plasma protein oncotic pressure; and $pint$ is protein oncotic pressure within the interstitial space.

Under normal conditions, the sum of the forces is slightly positive, producing a small vascular fluid flux into the precapillary interstitium of the lung that is drained as lymph into the systemic veins. The capillary coefficient (Kf) determines the effectiveness of the endothelial barrier to protein permeability, establishing the functionality of the oncotic gradient. Because the intravascular pressure in the pulmonary capillaries is always higher than plasma osmotic pressure, transcapillary fluid flux out of the pulmonary capillary is continuous. When the interstitial fluid exceeds the interstitial space capacity, fluid floods into the alveoli.[18] The interstitial space is drained by a rich bed of lymphatics. It is estimated that pulmonary lymph flow may increase threefold before fluid extravasates into the alveolar airspaces. The two most common forms of pulmonary edema are either initiated by an imbalance of Starling forces or caused by disruption of one or more components of the alveolar-capillary membrane. Box 18.1 lists the causes of pulmonary edema based on the initiating mechanism. Similar to the genesis of interstitial lung edema, pleural effusion occurs when lung interstitial pressure exceeds pleural pressure and fluid redistributes across the visceral pleura.

It has been shown experimentally that pulmonary edema occurs if the pulmonary capillary pressure exceeds the plasma colloid osmotic pressure, which is approximately 28 mm Hg in humans. The normal pulmonary capillary wedge pressure is approximately 8 mm Hg, which allows a margin of safety of about 20 mm Hg in the development of pulmonary edema.[19] Although pulmonary capillary pressure must be abnormally high to increase the flow of the interstitial fluid, these pressures may not correlate with the severity of pulmonary edema when edema is clearly present.[20] These pressures may have returned to normal when there is still considerable pulmonary edema because time is required for removal of interstitial and pulmonary edema.

The rate of increase in lung fluid at any given elevation of pulmonary capillary pressure is related to the functional capacity of the lymphatics, which may vary from patient to patient, and to variations in osmotic and hydrostatic pressures. Chronic elevations in left atrial pressures are associated with hypertrophy in the lymphatics, which then clear greater quantities of capillary filtrate during acute increases in pulmonary capillary pressure.[21] The removal of edema fluid from the alveolar and interstitial compartments of the lung depends on active transport of sodium and chloride across the alveolar epithelial barrier. Reabsorption of these electrolytes is mediated by the epithelial ion channels located on the apical membrane of alveolar epithelial type I and type II cells and distal airway epithelia. Water follows passively, probably through aquaporins that are found predominantly on alveolar epithelial type I cells.[22]

Clinical experience with patients who have chronically elevated atrial pressures suggests that these patients show minimal or no evidence of interstitial lung edema. The mechanisms by which pulmonary capillary pressure increases when the pumping ability of the ventricle is suddenly impaired are discussed later. When the alveolar-capillary membrane is injured, proteins leak from

---

BOX 18.1   Classification of Acute Pulmonary Edema

Cardiogenic Pulmonary Edema

A. Acute increase in pulmonary capillary pressure
   1. Increased LA pressure with normal LV diastolic pressure
      a. Thrombosed prosthetic mitral valve
      b. Obstructive left atrial myxoma
   2. Increased LA pressure due to elevated LV diastolic pressure
      a. Increased myocardial stiffness or impaired relaxation
         i. Myocardial ischemia
         ii. Acute myocardial infarction
         iii. Hypertrophic heart disease complicated by tachycardia or ischemia
         iv. Stress-induced cardiomyopathy
      b. Acute volume load
         i. Acute mitral or aortic regurgitation
         ii. Ischemic myocardial septal rupture
      c. Acute increases in LV afterload
         i. Hypertensive crisis
         ii. Thrombosed prosthetic aortic valve
B. Exacerbation of chronically elevated pulmonary capillary pressures
   1. Increase in elevated LA pressure with normal LV diastolic pressure
      a. Mitral stenosis and atrial fibrillation with rapid heart rate
      b. Left atrial myxoma
   2. Increase in elevated LA pressure due to a further increase in LV diastolic pressure
      a. Further increases in myocardial stiffness or impaired relaxation
         i. Cardiomyopathy complicated by myocardial ischemia or infarction
         ii. Hypertrophic heart disease complicated by tachycardia or ischemia

   b. Volume load imposed on preexisting LV diastolic dysfunction
      i. Worsening mitral regurgitation
      ii. Vigorous postoperative fluid administration
      iii. Dietary indiscretion
   c. Pressure load imposed on preexisting LV systolic dysfunction
      i. Accelerated hypertension

Noncardiogenic Pulmonary Edema

A. Altered alveolar capillary membrane permeability (adult respiratory distress syndrome)
   1. Infectious or aspiration pneumonia
   2. Septicemia
   3. Acute radiation or hypersensitivity pneumonitis
   4. Disseminated intravascular coagulopathy
   5. Shock lung
   6. Hemorrhagic pancreatitis
   7. Inhaled or circulating toxins
   8. Massive trauma
B. Acute decrease in interstitial pressure of the lung
   1. Rapid removal of unilateral pleural effusion
C. Unknown mechanisms
   1. High-altitude pulmonary edema
   2. Neurogenic pulmonary edema
   3. Narcotic overdose
   4. Pulmonary embolism
   5. After cardioversion
   6. After anesthesia or cardiopulmonary bypass

LA, Left atrial; *LV,* left ventricular.

---

the capillary into the interstitium, reducing the oncotic counterpressure tendency to oppose capillary filtration. Interstitial edema and the consequent alveolar edema formation can occur in the presence of low hydrostatic pressures.

Left Ventricular Pump Performance in Acute Heart Failure

The factors involved in regulating cardiac output are discussed in Chapter 5. The following discussion briefly reviews left ventricular (LV) pump performance in terms of the LV pressure-volume relationship as it pertains to a patient with AHF.

To appreciate fully the factors that contribute to AHF, it is appropriate to review briefly the pressure-volume relationships of normal and diseased hearts. The relationship between pressure and volume throughout the cardiac cycle can be presented as a pressure-volume loop (Fig. 18.1). The pressure-volume loop encapsulates the systolic and diastolic functions of the heart. Because these loops also circumscribe end-systolic and end-diastolic volumes, the stroke volume and ejection fraction can be derived. The bottom limb of the loop, also termed the diastolic pressure-volume curve, describes LV diastolic compliance. The pressure-volume loop can provide a simple, but comprehensive, description of LV pump function.

Progressive increases in systolic pressure produce a nearly linear increase in end-systolic volume. By matching the end-systolic pressure and volume coordinates from multiple, variably

loaded beats, a near-linear relationship is established. The slope of this relationship (E_{max}), determined by altering load, reflects LV contractility (see Fig. 18.1).[23] A positive inotropic intervention is associated with an increased end-systolic pressure and stroke volume and a decreased end-diastolic volume. This results in an increased E_{max} and a shift of the pressure-volume relationship to the left (Fig. 18.2A). Conversely, a negative inotropic intervention decreases end-systolic pressure and stroke volume and increases end-diastolic volume. This results in a decrease in E_{max} and a shift of the pressure-volume relationship to the right (see Fig. 18.2B).

In the intact human heart, an increase in systolic pressure is associated with an increase in end-systolic volume, and if the LV fails to dilate, stroke volume decreases (Fig. 18.3A). An increase in preload is accompanied by an increase in stroke volume and a modest increase in end-systolic pressure (see Fig. 18.3B). Acute and chronic changes in the pressure-volume relationship in the failing heart depend on the underlying myocardial structure and function, the type and extent of injury (e.g., infarction or myocarditis, regional or global myocardial depression), and the severity and nature of the hemodynamic load (pressure vs. volume).

Chamber Stiffness

Chamber stiffness is determined by analyzing the curvilinear diastolic pressure-volume relationships (Fig. 18.4). The slope of

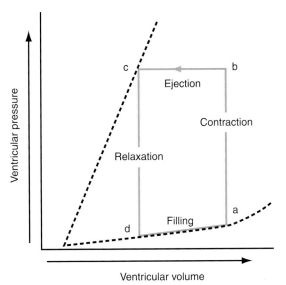

Fig. 18.1 Schematic representation of the left ventricular (LV) pressure-volume loop. The aortic valve opens at *b* and closes at *c*. The mitral valve opens at *d* and closes at *a*. The slope of the *broken line* through *c* represents the end-systolic pressure-volume relationship (E_{max}), and the *broken line* through *d* and *a* represents the end-diastolic pressure-volume relationship. As contractile force develops in the LV in systole, the pressure rapidly increases in the ventricular chamber (*a* → *b*) without changing its volume (i.e., isovolumic phase of systole). When the pressure exceeds the diastolic aortic pressure, the aortic valve opens and the ventricle ejects its contents into the arterial circulation (*b* → *c*, the ejection phase of systole). At the end of ejection (point *c*), LV pressure decreases and the aortic valve closes. Pressure rapidly declines at a constant volume (*c* → *d*, isovolumic relaxation) to levels below that of the left atrium. At this point, the mitral valve opens (point *d*), and the relaxing LV fills along the segment *d* → *a*. The trajectory *a* → *b* → *c* represents the contractile or inotropic function of the LV at any given end-diastolic volume, whereas the trajectory *c* → *d* → *a* represents the lusitropic function (relaxation and filling) of the heart at any given end-systolic pressure. The area within the loop graphically depicts the external work (i.e., stroke work) of the ventricle.

the tangent (dP/dV) to this curvilinear relationship defines the chamber stiffness at a given filling pressure. An increase in dP/dV due to an increase in volume, shown in Fig. 18.4 (A → B), has been called a preload-dependent change in stiffness. When the pressure-volume relationship shifts to the left (A → C), the tangent is steeper at the same diastolic pressure. The latter may be caused by an increase in myocardial mass or intrinsic myocardial stiffness or by changes in several extramyocardial factors. Chamber stiffness of the left ventricle is determined by static factors (e.g., chamber volume, wall mass, stiffness of the wall) and dynamic factors (e.g., pericardium, right ventricle [RV], myocardial relaxation, erectile effects of the coronary vasculature).[24,25] Most acute alterations in LV chamber stiffness result from a preload-dependent increase in chamber stiffness, a shift to a different pressure-volume curve, or a combination of the two. All can result in elevated left atrial pressures, pulmonary venous hypertension, and the signs and symptoms of AHF.

Compensatory Mechanisms in Acute Heart Failure

Rapid activation of neurohormonal systems occurs in the setting of decreased blood pressure and reduced cardiac output related to acute depression of LV pump performance. This causes an increase in heart rate and arterial resistance and a decrease in capacity of the venous system.[26,27] This decreased systemic vascular capacity after sympathetic activation is brought on predominantly by changes in the splanchnic vascular bed that result in a leftward shift of the venous pressure–volume relationship, causing a redistribution of blood from the unstressed to the stressed circulating pool (i.e., central blood pool).[28,29] In normal adults, sympathoadrenal stimulation can increase systemic blood volume by redistribution of up to 2 units of blood from the splanchnic venous reservoir.[29]

Mechanistic Considerations in Acute Heart Failure Syndromes

During the early phase of myocardial infarction (MI) or with acute ischemia, reduced ventricular ejection increases end-systolic volume (residual volume) and, together with reduced LV compliance, leads to rapid increases in LV filling pressures. It is thought that lusitropic dysfunction associated with ischemia is the result of an increase in stiffness in the ischemic myocardial segment (possibly caused by slowing and incompleteness of the relaxation process)[30] and dilation of the nonischemic segment, causing a preload-dependent increase in chamber stiffness.[31] The increase in LV filling pressure that occurs with acute infarction or ischemia is caused by the combination of a preload-dependent increase in chamber stiffness and a leftward shift of the diastolic pressure-volume curve. Increased diastolic pressures after an acute ischemic insult may also result from the redistribution of blood from the periphery to the central blood pool.[29] The effects of these changes on the pressure–volume relationship are shown in Fig. 18.5A.

In acute volume overload, as seen in patients with sudden and severe valvular regurgitation or after ischemic ventricular septal rupture, the LV dilates, causing the ventricle to operate on the steeper portion of the pressure-volume curve. Consequently, small increments in volume result in a marked increase in filling pressures. The effects of these changes on the pressure-volume relationship are shown in Fig. 18.5B.

The lusitropic abnormalities of LV hypertrophy secondary to aortic stenosis, severe hypertension, or hypertrophic cardiomyopathy are caused by abnormalities of the static and dynamic determinants of chamber stiffness. Increased passive stiffness of the hypertrophied heart results in part from the increased myocardial mass and the low volume-to-mass ratio; abnormal intrinsic myocardial stiffness also may contribute to increased chamber stiffness. Abnormalities of myocardial relaxation further impair filling in the hypertrophied heart. The effects of these changes on the pressure-volume relationship are shown in Fig. 18.5C.

Chronic heart failure is characterized by a compressed pressure-volume loop. This compressed loop, characterized by a decrease in end-systolic pressure and an increase in end-diastolic pressure, means that the work of the failing heart is reduced while

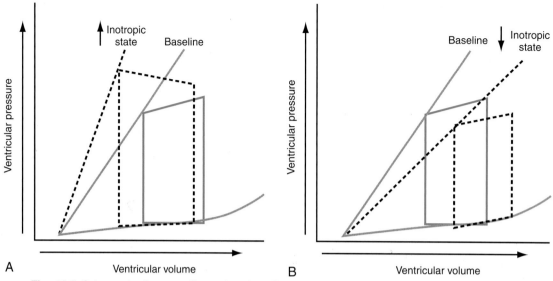

Fig. 18.2 Schematic diagrams illustrating the effects of inotropic interventions on the pressure-volume loop. (A) With a positive inotropic intervention, the pressure-volume loop *(broken line)* is shifted to the left and the slope of the end-systolic pressure-volume line is increased. (B) With a negative inotropic intervention, the pressure-volume loop is shifted to the right and the slope of the end-systolic pressure-volume line is decreased.

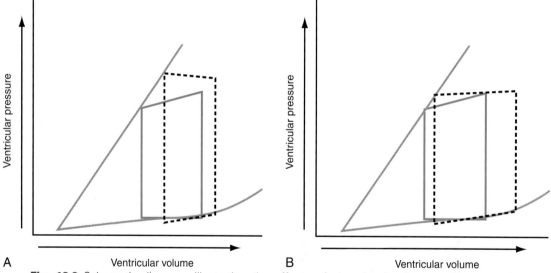

Fig. 18.3 Schematic diagrams illustrating the effects of changing loading conditions on the pressure-volume loop in the intact heart. (A) An increase in afterload shifts the pressure-volume loop *(broken line)* to the right, increasing the end-systolic and end-diastolic volumes and the end-systolic and end-diastolic pressures while decreasing the stroke volume. The slope of the end-systolic pressure-volume line is usually not affected by a pure change in afterload. (B) An increase in preload also shifts the pressure-volume loop *(broken line)* to the right, increasing the end-diastolic volume and end-diastolic pressure. The increase in preload may be associated further with a small increase in end-systolic volume and a modest increase in end-systolic pressure; in contrast to the case with an increase in afterload, however, the stroke volume increases. Similar to an increase in afterload, the slope of the end-systolic pressure-volume line is not affected by a change in preload.

maintaining a near-normal stroke volume. Comparable to the changes with ischemia, the elevated filling pressures in chronic heart failure is caused by a combination of a preload-dependent increase in chamber stiffness (i.e., the LV operates at higher end-diastolic volumes to optimize the Starling relationship) and

a preload-independent increase in chamber stiffness (see Fig. 18.5D). It should also be evident from the pressure-volume curve that these hearts operate near the limit of their preload reserve; therefore they are extremely vulnerable to any myocardial injury or insult. Even a minor perturbation, such as an arrhythmia,

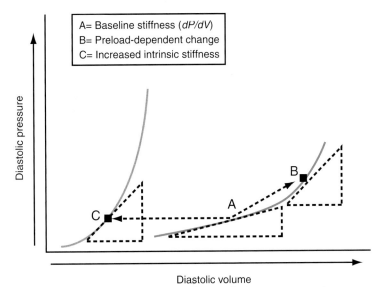

Fig. 18.4 Schematic diagram of the diastolic left ventricular pressure-volume curve. The slope of the tangent (dP/dV) to this curvilinear relationship defines chamber stiffness at a given filling pressure. An increase in dP/dV owing to an increase in volume, shown diagrammatically as $A \rightarrow B$, has been termed a preload-dependent change in stiffness. When the pressure-volume relationship shifts to the left, $A \rightarrow C$, the tangent is steeper (increased chamber stiffness) at the same diastolic pressure.

infection, or a small area of infarction, is likely to precipitate acute decompensation in these patients.

CLINICAL PRESENTATION OF ACUTE HEART FAILURE

The onset and severity of symptoms of AHF vary and depend to a great extent on the nature of the underlying cardiac disease and the rate at which the syndrome develops. The largest proportion of patients (70%) with AHF are admitted due to worsening chronic heart failure; up to 15% to 20% of patients present with heart failure for the first time and approximately 5% are admitted for advanced or end-stage heart failure. A few patients with AHF present with low blood pressure (<8%) or shock (<3%).[10,32] Most patients are elderly, with an average age of approximately 70 to 75 years. Patients with new-onset heart failure are more likely to present with pulmonary edema or cardiogenic shock. The heterogeneity of this patient population is evident when one considers that almost half of these patients have preserved LV ejection fraction. A history of coronary disease is present in 60% of patients, 45% of whom have had a prior MI, hypertension in 70%, atrial fibrillation in 30%, diabetes mellitus in 40%, and chronic obstructive pulmonary disease in 30%.[10,32] Secondary mitral regurgitation due to LV dilation is common.

For practical purposes, it is helpful to view the presentation of AHF according to the predominant clinical characteristics on admission. The European Society of Cardiology guidelines for the diagnosis and treatment of AHF classifies patients into 1 of 6 groups on the basis of the clinical and hemodynamic profiles.[5] These include (1) AHF, either new-onset or decompensated chronic heart failure, (2) hypertensive AHF, (3) AHF with pulmonary edema, (4) cardiogenic shock, (5) high output failure,

and (6) right heart failure. These syndromes are discussed here and are outlined in Table 18.1.

Group 1: Acute-on-Chronic Decompensated Heart Failure

This syndrome is seen in patients with an established diagnosis of heart failure who develop increasing signs or symptoms of decompensation after a period of relative stability. This scenario accounts for greater than 70% of all heart failure admissions. New-onset HF is seen much less frequently (15% to 20%) but may present with the same phenotype as chronic heart failure. Progressive dyspnea is the most common complaint of patients presenting with decompensated chronic heart failure. Patients may report lower extremity edema and epigastric tenderness or a sensation of abdominal fullness. Abdominal tenderness is often due to hepatic congestion and distention of the hepatic capsule. With severe hepatic congestion, the patient may also complain of nausea and anorexia. Other symptoms include nocturia and neurologic symptoms such as confusion, headaches, insomnia, anxiety, disorientation, and impaired memory.

Physical signs vary according to the severity of the volume overload. An elevated jugular venous pressure, positive hepato-jugular reflux test, and a tender, enlarged liver are frequent findings in these patients. Rales and wheezing are not common but may be heard in patients with significant pulmonary congestion. The absence of rales does not imply that the pulmonary venous pressures are not elevated. Diminished air entry at the lung bases is usually caused by a pleural effusion, which is often more frequent in the right pleural cavity than in the left. Leg edema is frequently evident in both legs, particularly in the pretibial region and ankles in ambulatory patients. Sacral edema can be detected in patients who are bedridden.

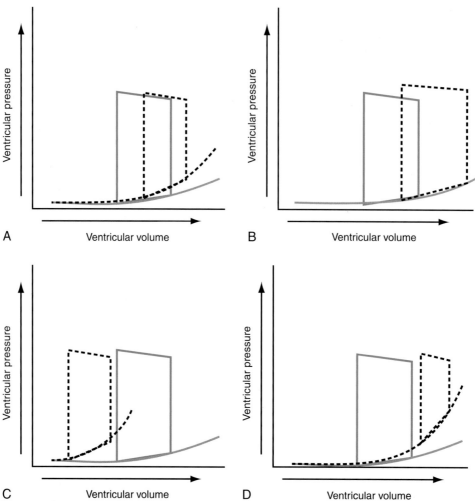

Fig. 18.5 Schematic diagrams of four different pathophysiologic states. In each diagram, the control pressure-volume loop and the diastolic pressure-volume relationship *(curve)* are shown in *solid lines*. The effects of different pathologic states on the pressure-volume relationship are depicted by the *broken lines* (A). With acute ischemia or infarction, the pressure-volume curve is shifted upward and to the right. (B) In a volume-overloaded heart (i.e., valvular regurgitation), the pressure-volume relationship is shifted to the right along the same diastolic pressure-volume curve. The increase in diastolic pressure is the result of the left ventricle operating on the steeper portion of the diastolic pressure-volume relationship. (C) With excessive hypertrophy, the pressure-volume relationship is shifted to the left, so that the heart operates at smaller end-diastolic and end-systolic volumes. The increase in chamber stiffness is reflected by the steep diastolic pressure-volume curve. (D) In chronic advanced heart failure, the pressure-volume loop is often compressed and shifted to the right. This compressed loop, characterized by a lower end-systolic and increased end-diastolic pressure, implies that the work of the heart is reduced, while maintaining a near-normal stroke volume. Comparable to the situation in (A), the elevated diastolic pressure is caused by preload-dependent and preload-independent increases in chamber stiffness.

The cardiac examination may be entirely normal in patients with heart failure with preserved ejection fraction, whereas many patients with advanced systolic dysfunction exhibit a third heart sound and a laterally displaced point of maximal impulse. A murmur of mitral regurgitation is often audible when the left ventricle is markedly enlarged, or a tricuspid regurgitation murmur is present when the RV is volume or pressure overloaded. These patients often do not have radiographic signs of marked interstitial lung edema.

Group 2: Hypertensive Acute Heart Failure

The syndrome of AHF is characterized by the rapid onset of symptoms or signs of heart failure. This phenotype is more common in females and the systolic blood pressure on admission usually exceeds 180 mm Hg.[33] There is usually predominant pulmonary rather than systemic congestion, as is manifest by minimal weight gain prior to admission. Virtually all patients have a preserved LV ejection fraction. Blood pressure elevation

TABLE 18.1 Acute Heart Failure Syndromes

Phenotype	Rate of Onset	Signs and Symptoms	Hemodynamic Profile	Diagnostics
1a. Acute-on-chronic HF	Gradual	Dyspnea and fluid overload	Normal or low normal BP	CR: normal or mild interstitial edema
		Adequate tissue perfusion	Possible pleural effusion	
1b. New-onset AHF	Gradual or rapid	Dyspnea, variable fluid overload	Normal or low BP	CR: normal or mild interstitial edema
		Variable tissue perfusion	Possible pleural effusion	
2. Hypertensive AHF	Rapid	Acute dyspnea	SBP >180 mm Hg	CR: interstitial lung edema
	Minimal fluid overload	Adequate tissue perfusion		
3. AHF and pulmonary edema	Rapid or gradual	Severe dyspnea, tachypnea	Low normal BP	Hypoxic on room air
	Tachycardia	Variable tissue perfusion		
4a. Cardiogenic shock (low output syndrome)	Usually gradual	Weakness/fatigue	Low normal BP	Echo shows severe LV dysfunction
		Alterered mental status		
		Poor tissue perfusion		
4b. Severe cardiogenic shock	Rapid	Weakness/fatigue	Low BP (< 90 mm Hg)	
		Oliguria/anuria		
5. High output HF	Rapid or gradual	Dyspnea; tachycardia and warm periphery	Normal BP	
6. Acute right HF	Rapid or gradual; marked fluid overload	Variable tissue perfusion	Severe dyspnea	Low normal BP

Modified from Nieminen MS, Bohm M, Cowie MR, et al. for the ESC Committee for Practice Guideline: Executive summary of the guidelines on the diagnosis and treatment of acute heart failure: The Task Force on Acute Heart Failure of the European Society of Cardiology. *Eur Heart J* 2005;26:384–416; and Joseph SM, Cedars AM, Ewald GA, et al. Acute decompensated heart failure: contemporary medical management. *Tex Heart Inst J.* 2009;36(6):510–20.
BP, Blood pressure; *CR*, chest radiograph; *HF*, heart failure; *SBP*, systolic blood pressure.

could develop rapidly, which is associated with increased filling pressures and enhanced sympathetic tone.

Group 3: Acute Heart Failure With Severe Pulmonary Edema

Severe pulmonary edema is seen in less than 3% of all patients admitted with AHF.[32] Patients typically experience a sudden and overwhelming sensation of suffocation and air hunger; this is invariably accompanied by extreme anxiety, cough, expectoration of a pink frothy liquid, and a sensation of drowning. The patient sits bolt upright, is unable to speak in full sentences, and may thrash about. The respiratory rate is increased, the alae nasi are dilated, and there is inspiratory retraction of the intercostal spaces and supraclavicular fossae. Respiration is often noisy, and there may be audible inspiratory and expiratory gurgling sounds. An ominous sign is obtundation, which may be a sign of severe hypoxemia. Sweating is profuse, and the skin tends to be cool, ashen, and cyanotic, reflecting increased sympathetic outflow.

The pulse rate is most often elevated secondary to an increased adrenergic drive. When the blood pressure is found to be markedly elevated, it is more likely to be the cause of, or an important contributing factor to, pulmonary edema rather than the consequence of the condition. The oxygen saturation is usually less than 90% on room air before treatment. Auscultation of the lung usually reveals coarse airway sounds bilaterally with rhonchi, wheezes, and moist fine crepitant rales that are detected first at the lung bases, but then extend upward to the apices as the lung edema worsens. Cardiac auscultation may be difficult in the acute situation, but third and fourth heart sounds may be present.

When valvular abnormalities or mechanical complications after MI result in AHF, the murmurs of mitral and aortic regurgitation and ischemic septal rupture are often audible, but detection requires a careful and skillful auscultator.

Group 4: Cardiogenic Shock and Low-Output Syndrome

Systolic blood pressure is less than 90 mm Hg in approximately 8% of patients with decompensated chronic heart failure.[5,10] Low-output heart failure is characterized by symptoms and signs that are related to decreased end-organ perfusion. A typical patient with this clinical syndrome has severely impaired LV function and usually presents with symptoms of fatigue, altered mental status, or signs of organ hypoperfusion, such as prerenal azotemia, abnormal hepatic enzymes, or elevated lactic acid. The patient may present with tachypnea at rest, tachycardia, and a cold and cyanotic periphery. The degree of peripheral hypoperfusion may be so advanced that the skin over the lower extremities is mottled and cool. A diminished pulse pressure, consistent with a reduced stroke volume, is often found in patients with AHF. Occasionally, the clinician may detect *pulsus alternans*—when a strong or normal pulse alternates with a weak pulse during normal sinus rhythm. This physical finding is rare but, when present, is a sign of severe LV dysfunction.

Group 5: High-Output Heart Failure

The phenotype is an uncommon cause of AHF and generally presents with warm extremities, pulmonary congestion, tachycardia, and a wide pulse pressure. Underlying conditions include anemia, thyrotoxicosis, advanced liver failure, and Paget disease.

Group 6: Right-Sided Heart Failure

This syndrome occurs commonly in patients with severe isolated tricuspid regurgitation; right ventricular dysfunction; chronic lung disease, such as those with chronic obstructive and/or insterstitial lung disease; or long-standing pulmonary hypertension. These patients are often oxygen dependent and present with signs and symptoms of right-sided volume overload.

DIAGNOSIS OF ACUTE HEART FAILURE

The rapid diagnosis of AHF is a necessary first step to initiate appropriate treatment. This is critical since early treatment is linked to outcome. The diagnosis of decompensated chronic heart failure is generally straightforward, especially when a patient presents with the triad of fluid retention, exertional dyspnea, and a history of heart failure. It is also essential to rule out alternate causes of the patient's signs and symptoms. Worsening exertional dyspnea could also be due to a range of other conditions, including pulmonary embolism, pneumonia, chronic obstructive pulmonary disease, asthma, pulmonary fibrosis, pleural effusion, anemia, hyperthyroidism, and musculoskeletal disorders.

For patients without a prior cardiac history, the diagnosis of AHF should be based primarily on signs and symptoms and supported by appropriate investigations, such as electrocardiogram (ECG), chest radiograph, biomarkers, and Doppler echocardiography according to the American Heart Association/American College of Cardiology and European Society of Cardiology Guidelines.[34,35] The electrocardiogram is rarely normal in AHF (resulting in a high negative predictive value).[35] The chest radiograph can be helpful for the diagnosis of AHF. The most specific findings in patients with AHF are pulmonary venous congestion, pleural effusions, interstitial or alveolar edema, and cardiomegaly. Up to 20% of patients with AHF may have normal chest radiographs.[36] Echocardiography is indicated early on only in patients with hemodynamic instability.

When the diagnosis is uncertain, determination of plasma B-type natriuretic peptide (BNP) or N-terminal pro-B-type natriuretic peptide (NT-proBNP) concentration should be considered in patients being evaluated for dyspnea who have signs and symptoms compatible with AHF. The natriuretic peptide concentration should not be interpreted in isolation but rather in the context of all available clinical data bearing on the diagnosis of AHF.

There is considerable overlap in BNP and NT-proBNP levels in patients with and without heart failure, which makes the test less robust in an individual patient with intermediate levels of BNP (~200 to 400 pg/mL). Because many conditions increase natriuretic pepide levels, low values of BNP (<100 pg/mL) or NT-proBNP (<300 pg/mL) are most useful because the diagnosis of decompensated heart failure is very unlikely as an explanation for dyspnea.[38] Decision analysis suggests that BNP or NT-proBNP testing is generally most useful in patients who have an intermediate probability of heart failure.[39] Unexpected low biomarkers are occasionally found in some patients with end-stage HF, acute pulmonary edema, constrictive pericarditis, and right-sided heart failure.[35] AHF remains a clinical syndrome that is characterized by a constellation of symptoms owing to a heterogeneous group of cardiac and vascular disorders; the diagnosis cannot be based on a single laboratory test. Results of BNP or NT-proBNP testing must be interpreted in the context of the overall clinical evaluation; such testing must support, rather than override, careful clinical judgment.

Differentiating Cardiogenic From Noncardiogenic Pulmonary Edema

It is crucial to establish whether respiratory failure (pulmonary edema) is due to cardiogenic or noncardiogenic causes. This distinction can invariably be made by assessment of the clinical context in which it occurs and through examination of the clinical data available (Table 18.2). The clinical data include tests that are routinely performed on all critically ill patients, such as ECG, blood gas analysis, blood count, electrolytes, and chest radiograph.

Noncardiogenic pulmonary edema (NCPE) is invariably associated with an underlying disease, which may or may not be readily apparent. The diagnosis of NCPE often depends on pretest probabilities: acute respiratory distress in a patient with documented sepsis (i.e., peritonitis) or pancreatitis should raise the strong possibility that the respiratory failure is due to NCPE. In contrast to cardiogenic pulmonary edema (CPE), NCPE is uncommonly associated with a well-defined acute cardiac event (i.e., MI). Subtle physical signs may also aid in differentiating NCPE from CPE. NCPE is usually a component of a hyperdynamic illness, clinically apparent as a warm, vasodilated periphery, whereas CPE is frequently associated with a cold and sweaty periphery. The findings of a third heart sound or murmurs of

---

TABLE 18.2 Differentiation of Noncardiogenic From Cardiogenic Pulmonary Edema Based on Clinical Data

	Noncardiogenic	Cardiogenic
History	Underlying disease (e.g., pancreatitis, sepsis)	Acute cardiac event (e.g., MI)
Physical examination	Warm periphery	Cool, mottled periphery
	Bounding pulses	Small-volume pulse
	Normal-sized heart	Cardiomegaly
	Normal JVP	Elevated JVP
	No S_3	S_3
	No murmurs	Systolic and diastolic murmurs
ECG	ECG usually normal	ST segment and QRS abnormalities
Chest radiograph	Peripheral infiltrates	Perihilar infiltrates
Laboratory test	Normal enzymes BNP <100 mg/mL	Elevated biomarkers
Ventilatory needs	Higher Fio_2 and PEEP to oxygenate	Lower Fio_2 and PEEP to oxygenate

Modified from Sibbald WJ, Cunningham DR, Chin DN. Non-cardiac or cardiac pulmonary edema? A practical approach to clinical differentiation in critically ill patients. *Chest.* 1983;84:452–61.
BNP, Brain natriuretic peptide; *Fio₂,* inspired oxygen concentration; *JVP,* jugular venous pressure; *MI,* myocardial infarction; *PEEP,* positive end-expiratory pressure.

aortic and mitral regurgitation and aortic stenosis may suggest a cardiogenic cause of pulmonary edema.

ST segment changes on ECG consistent with MI or myocardial ischemia would suggest an acute cardiac event as the cause of the pulmonary edema. Also, ECG evidence of LV strain, left bundle branch block, or other abnormalities of the QRS complex might indicate an underlying cardiac pathology. Unless there are major metabolic disturbances, the ECG is usually normal in patients with pure NCPE.

In NCPE and CPE, arterial hypoxemia is due to changes in the ventilation-perfusion ratio and intrapulmonary shunting. Patients with NCPE usually have a more pronounced defect in oxygenation than is seen in patients with CPE. This is largely due to the greater shunt fractions found in these patients. In the clinical setting, higher concentrations of inspired oxygen concentrations (FIO_2) and larger positive end-expiratory pressures are required to achieve acceptable oxygenation in NCPE compared with CPE.

Similar to other tests, the chest radiograph may be helpful in differentiating NCPE from CPE. With NCPE, the alveolar and interstitial disease might show a predominant peripheral distribution; in CPE, a perihilar distribution is more evident, often associated with Kerley lines or pleural effusions, or both. Heart size is more commonly increased in CPE than NCPE, but the lack of cardiomegaly does not exclude CPE. In most patients, the chest radiograph proves to be of little help. This is due partially to the fact that patients are often too ill to be examined by anything other than a portable unit and such films are usually of suboptimal interpretive quality. An example of acute CPE and less severe pulmonary congestion is shown in Fig. 18.6.

When the cause of pulmonary edema is clearly evident from the clinical data (i.e., MI), no further diagnostic tests are needed. If uncertainty remains regarding the etiology of the pulmonary edema, further diagnostic tests are appropriate. A BNP level of less than 100 pg/mL or NT-proBNP level of less than 300 pg/mL effectively rules out a cardiac cause for respiratory failure. Elevated BNP levels are found in patients with pulmonary hypertension, cor pulmonale, pulmonary emboli, and compensated heart failure. BNP levels are also higher in women, older patients, and patients with renal failure.[39] BNP and NT-proBNP values are also similarly elevated in patients with severe sepsis or septic shock and AHF independently of whether they present with or without shock.[40]

Clinical judgment is still required to differentiate CPE from NCPE. An echocardiogram should be obtained in all patients with pulmonary edema in whom the cause of pulmonary edema is unclear. Normal Doppler echocardiography assessments of systolic and diastolic function strongly point to a noncardiogenic cause of respiratory failure. If uncertainty persists, it is reasonable to obtain hemodynamic information via a pulmonary artery catheter to differentiate CPE from NCPE. With the availability of BNP levels and two-dimensional Doppler echocardiography, however, there seems to be less need to proceed with invasive monitoring.

Evaluation and Triage of Patients With Acute Heart Failure

After the diagnosis of AHF has been established, the initial focus is to ensure optimal oxygenation and hemodynamic stability. Several steps are necessary to comprehensively evaluate a patient with AHF.

Step 1: Define Clinical Severity of Acute Heart Failure. Several grading classifications of the severity of AHF have been in place for many years in coronary care units and ICUs. The Killip classification, based on clinical signs and chest radiography findings,[41] and the Forrester classification, based on clinical signs and hemodynamic characteristics,[42] are discussed elsewhere. These classifications have been validated in AHF after acute MI and are most applicable for patients with new-onset AHF. Other authors have proposed a straightforward clinical tool for classifying the severity of chronic decompensated heart failure. This classification is based on an assessment of adequacy of perfusion (warm perfused, cold hypoperfused) and of fluid overload/ congestion or filling pressures (wet congested, dry euvolemic).

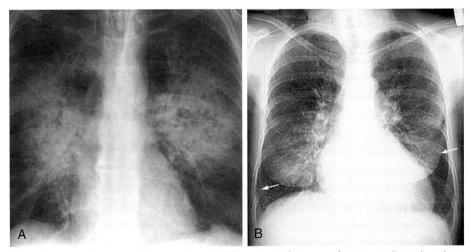

Fig. 18.6 Chest radiographs of two patients. (A) The classic features of acute cardiogenic pulmonary edema. Note the perihilar alveolar infiltrates. (B) Marked interstitial changes in the lung bases. Note the Kerley B lines *(arrows)*.

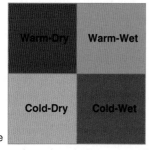

CONGESTION (–) CONGESTION (+)
Pulmonary edema
Peripheral edema
Jugular venous distension
Hepatomegaly
Ascites

HYPOPERFUSION (–)

Warm-Dry   Warm-Wet

HYPOPERFUSION (+)
Cold sweaty extremities
Oliguria
Mental confusion
Dizziness
Diminished pulse pressure

Cold-Dry   Cold-Wet

Fig. 18.7 Clinical phenotype based on the presence of congestion and/or hypoperfusion in acute heart failure.

Patients can be classified as warm and dry, warm and wet, cold and dry, and cold and wet (Fig. 18.7).[4,35] Such categorization permits attention to specific therapies and can provide prognostic information.

A pragmatic approach is simply to define the severity of AHF based on oxygen requirements and blood pressure. The most critical patient is the patient with the lowest blood pressure and highest oxygen requirement. A subset of patients with decompensated end-stage heart failure present to the emergency department in occult shock and are clinically indistinguishable from patients with mildly decompensated chronic heart failure and stable heart failure.[43] The only parameter differentiating occult shock patients from nonshock patients is a significantly elevated lactic acid level.[43]

In patients hospitalized with AHF, the risk of in-hospital mortality can be derived from admission clinical and laboratory variables. A blood urea nitrogen (BUN) level of 43 mg/dL or greater, serum creatinine level of 2.75 mg/dL or greater, and systolic blood pressure of less than 115 mm Hg are independent predictors of in-hospital mortality.[14,44] In addition, patients with AHF, the finding of a troponin I level of 1.0 μg/L or greater or troponin T of 0.1 μg/L or greater is associated with higher in-hospital mortality independent of other predictors.[45] Several other variables—such as age, heart rate, sodium, chronic obstructive pulmonary disease, and nonblack race—are also predictive of in-hospital mortality.[46]

Step 2: Establish Etiology of Acute Heart Failure. The most common causes of AHF are listed in Box 18.1. Echocardiography is an essential tool for the evaluation of the functional and structural cardiac changes underlying or associated with AHF.

Step 3: Identify Precipitating Causes of Acute Heart Failure. Precipitating causes are defined as factors that may precipitate acute decompensation in patients with underlying cardiac disease but are unlikely to cause cardiac decompensation in a patient with a normal heart. Patients with chronic heart failure are prone to infections. The most common are respiratory or urinary tract infections, septicemia, or nosocomial infections. Infections often manifest atypically in patients with AHF. Many patients are sick

BOX 18.2   Precipitants of Heart Failure

Dietary indiscretion
Vigorous fluid administration
Noncompliance to medical regimen
Worsening renal failure
Uncontrolled hypertension
Anemia
Systemic infection
Pulmonary embolism
Myocardial ischemia
Tachyarrhythmias and bradyarrhythmias
Electrolyte disturbances
Severe emotional or physical stress
Hyperthyroidism and hypothyroidism
Cardiodepressant and other drugs
- Antiinflammatory drugs
- Antiarrhythmic drugs
- Calcium channel blockers
- β-Adrenergic blocking agents

without a fever. Identifying the precipitating causes of acute hemodynamic decompensation has obvious therapeutic implications. Box 18.2 lists common precipitating causes.

Step 4: Decide on Disposition of Patient. Patients with severe respiratory failure and patients in shock or preshock should be admitted to the cardiac intensive care unit (CICU). Although no validated algorithms exist at this time to guide the clinician for triaging patients with decompensated chronic heart failure to regular floor beds or to the CICU, the European Society of Cardiology proposed the following criteria for admission to the CICU[35]:
- Need for intubation (or already intubated)
- Signs and symptoms of hypoperfusion
- Oxygen saturation (SpO$_2$ ≤90%) despite supplemental oxygen
- Use of accessory muscles and respiratory rate ≥25 breaths/ hour
- Heart rate less than 40 or more than 130 beats/min, systolic blood pressure less than 90 mm Hg

In North America, 10% to 12% of patients with AHF are managed in ICUs.[47]

Ongoing Evaluation of the Patient

Monitoring of a patient with AHF should be initiated as soon as possible after admission to the emergency department. The type and level of monitoring required for any individual patient vary widely depending on the severity of the cardiac decompensation and the response to initial therapy. Generally, the following parameters should be measured in all critically ill patients: mental status, blood pressure, temperature, respiratory rate, heart rate, and urine output. Some laboratory tests should be done repeatedly (i.e., electrolytes, creatinine, and glucose, or markers for infection or other metabolic disorders). Liver function tests and lactate levels should be measured when there is evidence of hypoperfusion. Routine arterial blood gas analysis is generally not needed. After admission to the ICU or step-down unit, patients with AHF

TABLE 18.3 Monitoring Patients With Acute Heart Failure

Goals	Parameters
Arterial oxygen saturation >95%	Pulse oximetry, arterial blood gas
	Consider placement of an indwelling radial artery catheter
Blood pressure	Automated blood pressure recordings
	Frequent assessments (every 5–10 min) early on to assess BP response to treatment
	BP via indwelling radial artery catheter
Normal sinus rhythm	Continuous ECG monitoring
Adequate diuretic response	Hourly urine production, daily weight
Adequate organ perfusion	Reversal of metabolic acidosis, lactic acid levels
	Liver function tests
	Adequate urine output
	Mean BP >65 mm Hg
	Central venous O_2 saturation >65%
Improved hemodynamics	Mean BP >65 mm Hg
	Assessment of JVP
	Central venous pressure line O_2 saturation
	Pulmonary artery catheter
Maintain calorie and nitrogen balance	Blood albumin concentrations
	Nitrogen balance
Control hyperglycemia	Glucose concentrations

BP, Blood pressure; *JVP*, jugular venous pressure.

should be carefully monitored to ensure that the treatment goals are met and continued progress is made toward a stable state. These goals are summarized in Table 18.3.

Pulmonary Artery Catheter. Controversy exists about the use of the pulmonary artery catheter in critically ill patients. The concern about pulmonary artery catheter use arose following prior studies that showed higher mortality for patients thought to require a pulmonary artery catheter during hospitalization. More recent data suggest that the routine use of pulmonary artery catheters in patients with AHF is unnecessary and unlikely to lead to a better outcome, although the use of inotropic or vasoactive support was discouraged in the clinical trial.[48] A pulmonary artery catheter may be of utility in select patients such as those with cardiogenic shock, rapidly decompensating heart failure, patients who are being considered for heart transplantation with significant pulmonary hypertension, obese patients who may be very difficult to assess and monitor clinically, and patients with severe LV and RV dysfunction for whom the response to vasodilator and other therapies may be difficult to predict.

TREATMENT OF ACUTE HEART FAILURE

The management of patients with AHF is primarily aimed at restoring perfusion of vital organs and relieving pulmonary and systemic congestion. In hemodynamic terms, the intention is to increase cardiac output and to decrease LV filling pressure while preserving adequate coronary perfusion.

General Measures

Several general measures are advisable for treating most patients with AHF. Bed rest should be enforced. Patients feel most comfortable in the semi-upright position, with legs dependent.

Oxygenation. Special attention should be paid to maintaining adequate oxygenation. When there is hypoxia (PaO_2 <60 mm Hg or SpO_2 <90%) without hypercapnia, oxygen-enriched inspired gas may suffice. This can be given through nasal prongs, Venturi masks, or reservoir bag masks, depending on the severity of gas exchange abnormality. Noninvasive ventilation by either continuous positive airway pressure breathing or bilevel positive airway pressure may become necessary when oxygenation cannot be maintained or there is evidence of progressive hypercapnia despite aggressive treatment. The use of noninvasive ventilation is associated with a significant reduction in the need for tracheal intubation and mechanical ventilation. Failing these interventions, intubation and mechanical ventilation may be needed to improve oxygenation and reverse hypercapnia. Intubation is generally recommended if respiratory failure cannot be managed noninvasively and blood gas demonstrates persistent hypoxemia (PaO_2 <60 mm Hg), hypercapnia ($PaCO_2$ >50 mm Hg), and respiratory acidosis (pH <7.35).

Deep Venous Thrombosis Prophylaxis. Patients with heart failure who are bedridden or with limited physical mobility are at high risk for developing deep venous thrombosis. Routine prophylactic treatment should be given unless there are contraindications to such therapy.

Diabetes. Hyperglycemia occurs commonly in patients with AHF owing to impaired metabolic control. Routine hypoglycemic drugs should be discontinued, and glycemic control should be obtained by using short-acting insulin titrated according to repeated blood glucose measurements. Intensive insulin therapy (blood glucose 81 to 108 mg/dL) in critically ill patients has been shown to increase 90-day mortality and should be avoided.[49,50]

Medications

The use of opiates in AHF should largely be avoided.[34,35] If morphine is used, the patient should be monitored for respiratory depression, which can be reversed by the narcotic antagonist naloxone. Morphine should be avoided if the pulmonary edema is associated with hypotension, intracranial bleeding, disturbed consciousness, bronchial asthma, chronic pulmonary disease, or reduced ventilation, specifically in patients with an increased arterial PCO_2.

Treatment of Triggers of Decompensation

Acute Coronary Syndrome. The coexistence of an acute coronary syndrome and AHF identifies a very-high-risk group in which early revascularization is recommended.

Rapid Arrhythmias and Severe Bradycardia. Unstable tachycardic and or bradycardic rhythm disturbances should be treated promptly with either cardioversion or temporary pacing.

Acute Mechanical Instability. Patients usually require circulatory support with surgical or percutaneous interventions when the structural integrity of the heart is compromised by acute and sudden valvular regurgitation, free wall or septal wall rupture following ischemic injury, or severely compromised myocardial function secondary to fulminant myocarditis.

Hemodynamic Goals of Treatment

Reduction of LV preload is highly desirable in patients with AHF and CPE. It is primarily intended to shift central blood volume to the periphery, reducing LV diastolic volume and pressure. When AHF is associated with an expanded circulating volume, as with acute decompensation of chronic heart failure, substantial preload reduction can be achieved without a significant decline in arterial pressure. In the setting of hypertension and normovolemia, aggressive reduction in preload may lead to a substantial decrease in blood pressure. It is important to decide in advance whether a patient who presents with AHF is likely to be at increased risk of developing hypotension with reductions in LV preload.

Ventricular afterload is increased in most patients with heart failure; the detrimental effects of afterload excess are proportional to the degree of LV systolic dysfunction. Afterload reduction with vasodilator therapy is directed at reducing excessive LV wall stress, with a resultant increase in stroke volume and a decrease in end-diastolic pressure. A reduction in afterload provides the greatest hemodynamic benefit for patients with the most advanced heart failure; a far greater increase in stroke volume and decrease in end-diastolic pressure are achieved with similar reductions in wall stress in patients with severe LV systolic dysfunction compared with patients with milder forms of heart failure (Fig. 18.8). Although there are no robust randomized data to support the use of vasodilators and diuretics in AHF, the consensus among experts is that these agents are first-line therapy in most patients with AHF. A simple treatment algorithm for the management of AHF according to the different hemodynamic phenotypes is outlined in Fig. 18.9.

Specific Interventions

Vasodilators. The endpoints of vasodilator therapy can vary from patient to patient, but reasonable hemodynamic endpoints include a reduction in LV filling pressure to 15 mm Hg or less and an increase in cardiac output that would ensure adequate tissue oxygen delivery (usually a cardiac index >2.5 L/min/m^2) while maintaining a systemic blood pressure of 90 mm Hg or greater.

Nitroglycerin

Actions. Nitroglycerin causes vasodilation by stimulating guanylate cyclase within the vascular smooth muscle of arterial resistance and venous capacitance vessels.[51] The predominant site of action depends on the dose being administered. At lower doses, nitroglycerin acts principally on the peripheral veins and reduces RV and LV filling pressures. At higher doses, nitroglycerin causes modest arterial vasodilation; consequently, it may improve cardiac output. Nitroglycerin can reduce the degree of mitral regurgitation[52,53] and decreases the preload-dependent chamber stiffness by redistributing blood from the central blood pool (heart and lungs) to the periphery (mesenteric bed),[54,55] decreasing LV volumes, which decreases the pericardial constraint.[56]

Nitrates reduce subendocardial ischemia by coronary vasodilation and by reducing myocardial oxygen requirements through unloading effects. One disadvantage of nitrates is the rapid development of tolerance, especially when given intravenously in high doses, limiting their effectiveness to 16 to 24 hours only. Nitrates should be given at doses aimed at achieving

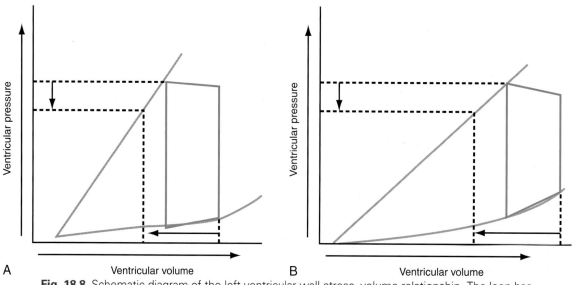

Fig. 18.8 Schematic diagram of the left ventricular wall stress–volume relationship. The loop has the same configuration as the pressure-volume relationship. (A) With mild heart failure, a decrease in wall stress *(arrows)* results in an increase in stroke volume. (B) With more advanced heart failure, a similar decrease in wall stress is accompanied by a marked increase in stroke volume. Vasodilator therapy (i.e., afterload reduction) produces a larger increase in stroke volume in advanced heart failure than in mild heart failure.

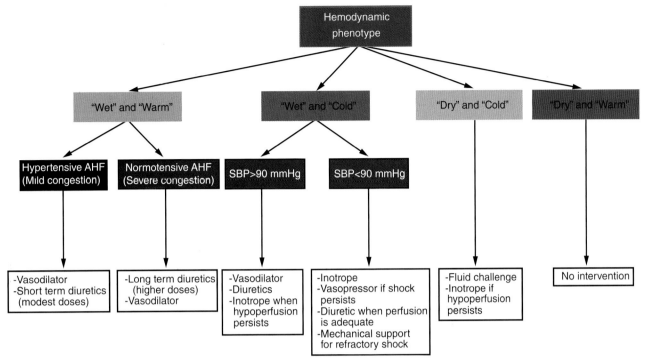

Fig. 18.9 Management of acute heart failure based on the clinical phenotype. (Modified from Ponikowski P, Voors AA, Anker SD, et al. 2016 ESC Guidelines for the diagnosis and treatment of acute and chronic heart failure: The Task Force for the diagnosis and treatment of acute and chronic heart failure of the European Society of Cardiology (ESC). Developed with the special contribution of the Heart Failure Association (HFA) of the ESC. *Eur J Heart Fail.* 2016;18:891–975.)

optimal vasodilation, leading to an increase in cardiac index and decrease in pulmonary wedge pressure.

Use in acute heart failure. Randomized trials in AHF have established the efficacy of intravenous nitrates in combination with furosemide and have shown that titration to the highest hemodynamically tolerable dose of nitrates with low-dose furosemide is superior to high-dose diuretic treatment alone.[57] Nitroglycerin is effective in relieving the symptoms of acute pulmonary edema and is often the vasodilatory agent of choice in patients with underlying ischemic heart disease.[58] Nitroglycerin should be administered in a manner to ensure the fastest onset of action. The intravenous route generally is preferred. The initial infusion rate is 5 µg/min, and the rate may be increased to 200 µg/min to achieve desired effects. The dose of nitroglycerin should not be increased when the systolic arterial pressure is less than 90 mm Hg. From a practical perspective, a reduction of 10 mm Hg in mean arterial pressure should be achieved.

Nitroglycerin can be administered orally or by inhalation (glyceryl trinitrate spray, 400 µg [2 puffs] every 5 to 10 minutes), or buccally (isosorbide dinitrate, 1 or 3 mg), while monitoring blood pressure. Buccal absorption may be erratic. One should be particularly cautious when administering nitrates to a patient with aortic stenosis or hypertrophic obstructive cardiomyopathy.

Nitroprusside

Actions. Nitroprusside infusion improves ventricular performance by decreasing all the major components of LV afterload: systemic vascular resistance, arterial stiffness, arterial wave reflectance, and LV size.[59] Proper dose selection achieves a reduction in afterload and preload with little change in systemic blood pressure. An often overlooked aspect of afterload reduction is the reduction of RV load. Vasodilators that are associated with a decrease in LV filling pressures invariably unload the right heart.[60] Within the confined space of the pericardium, interventions that reduce the excessive volume of the RV have a favorable hemodynamic effect on the septal interaction between the right and left ventricles, which consequently may improve LV filling and diastolic pressures. Nitroprusside is likely to achieve some of its favorable effects through this mechanism of ventricular interaction.

The incidence of side effects and toxicity is directly related to the dose and duration of administration. Cyanide may accumulate with prolonged high doses of nitroprusside and contribute to lactic acidosis. Toxicity can be avoided by monitoring blood lactate and thiocyanate levels.

Use in acute heart failure. Intravenous nitroglycerin is usually the vasodilator of choice for most patients with AHF, especially if a patient has underlying ischemic heart disease, but nitroprusside is the vasodilator of choice when a substantial reduction in LV afterload is required. Although both vasodilators affect vascular smooth muscle, nitroprusside and nitroglycerin differ in important ways. Because the magnitude of arterial vasodilation achieved with nitroprusside is greater than that with nitroglycerin, nitroprusside has the greater potential to produce hypotension. Such hypotensive action may lead to more neurohormonal activation, which may be the reason why rebound hemodynamic effects after abrupt withdrawal of the drug occur more frequently with nitroprusside than with nitroglycerin.[61]

Nitroprusside is reserved for clinical situations requiring acute, short-term afterload reduction. Nitroprusside is most beneficial for hypertensive patients or patients with an elevated LV filling pressure (≥20 mm Hg) and a systemic arterial pressure of 100 mm Hg or greater. This clinical picture is commonly encountered in patients with a large MI, with decompensated chronic heart failure, with acute valvular regurgitation, or after cardiopulmonary bypass. The use of nitroprusside in those with low-output, advanced heart failure (classified in the cold and wet profile) has been demonstrated to be safe when titrated for a mean arterial pressure of 65 to 70 mm Hg and appears to benefit both hemodynamic measurements and, possibly, all-cause mortality.[62] Nitroprusside usually represents a stabilizing pharmacologic bridge to more definitive interventions (e.g., valve replacement or coronary revascularization). The optimally effective and safe administration of nitroprusside often requires hemodynamic monitoring by means of intraarterial catheters. The initial dose of 5 to 10 μg/min is gradually increased as needed (up to 300 μg/min) to attain the desired clinical and hemodynamic effects.

Nesiritide

Actions. Nesiritide is a recombinant human BNP that is identical to the endogenous hormone. Nesiritide has venous, arterial, and coronary vasodilatory properties that reduce preload and afterload, and increase cardiac output without direct inotropic effects.[63]

Use in acute heart failure. Nesiritide was compared with intravenous nitroglycerin and resulted in improvement in hemodynamics more effectively and with fewer adverse effects, although this did not translate into improvement in clinical outcome.[64] In a randomized clinical trial, nesiritide had no significant impact on co-primary endpoints of dyspnea and the composite endpoint of rehospitalization for heart failure or death within 30 days in patients with AHF, although it did not worsen renal failure.[65] Nesiritide may cause hypotension, and some patients are nonresponders. The role of this agent is uncertain in the context of AHF. In most hospitals, nesiritide is not given as a first-line agent, but this medication may be considered when a patient does not respond rapidly to conventional treatment. The recommended dose of nesiritide is an intravenous bolus of 2 μg/kg followed by a continuous infusion of 0.01 μg/kg/min.

Other Vasodilators.

The intravenous use of direct-acting vasodilators such as hydralazine has a very limited or no role in the management of AHF and CPE. Other vasodilators, such as calcium antagonists or α-adrenergic blockers, cannot be recommended as first-line therapy for patients with AHF. Angiotensin-converting enzyme inhibitors are not indicated in the early stabilization of patients with AHF. Novel agents such as serelaxin (a recombinant form of relaxin-2) appear to significantly improve dyspnea, although their impact on mortality requires further investigation.[66]

Decongestive Therapy

Interventions that target congestion or fluid overload are the principal focus in the management of AHF in the vast majority of patients. Despite our best efforts, persistent congestion remains at discharge in more than a quarter of patients.[67,68] Recognition and avoidance of incomplete decongestion is important since residual congestion at discharge is associated with increased risks of rehospitalization and mortality.[69]

Diuretics

Actions. Loop diuretics block the $Na^+/2Cl^-/K^+$ transporter, resulting in increased urine volume by enhancing the excretion of water, sodium chloride, and other ions.[70] This, in turn, leads to a decrease in plasma and extracellular fluid volume, total body water, and sodium. These effects result in a reduction in RV and LV filling pressures and a decrease in peripheral and pulmonary congestion. In patients with decompensated chronic heart failure, the diuretic dose-response curve shifts downward and to the right to the extent that higher doses are required to achieve a therapeutic effect.[71,72] Intravenous administration of loop diuretics also exerts a vasodilating effect, manifested by an early (5 to 30 minutes) decrease in right atrial and pulmonary wedge pressure and pulmonary resistances. These hemodynamic effects result from the direct peripheral arterial and venodilating actions. It is thought that vasodilation rather than diuresis is the principal early mechanism by which diuretics alleviate symptoms of pulmonary edema.[73] High bolus doses (>1 mg/kg) of diuretics may lead to reflex vasoconstriction. As opposed to long-term use of diuretics, in severe decompensated heart failure, the use of diuretics improves loading conditions and may reduce neurohormonal activation in the short term.[74]

Use in acute heart failure. Intravenous loop diuretics (furosemide, bumetanide) are the most widely used diuretics in the treatment of AHF and CPE; they should be initiated in the emergency department without delay. The dose should be titrated according to the diuretic response and relief of congestive symptoms. Administration of a loading dose followed by continued infusion of furosemide has been thought to be more effective than bolus alone.[75,76] However, data from the recent Diuretic Optimization Strategies Evaluation (DOSE) trial suggest that there is no significant advantage to continuous furosemide over the diuretic given as intermittent boluses.[77] Thiazides and spironolactone can be used in association with loop diuretics; the combination in low doses is more effective and has fewer secondary effects than the use of higher doses of a single drug. Combination of loop diuretics with inotropes or nitrates is another therapeutic approach that is more effective and produces fewer secondary effects than increasing the dose of the diuretic. The diuretic doses for patients with mild congestion and new-onset AHF are generally much lower than doses for patients with advanced fluid overload or patients with renal dysfunction. The doses of diuretics as they relate to severity of AHF are summarized in Table 18.4.

Diuretic resistance. This is defined as the clinical state in which diuretic response is diminished or lost before the goal of treatment has been achieved. Such resistance is associated with a poor prognosis.[78] Mechanisms underlying diuretic resistance include the "braking phenomenon," "rebound" effect, and hyperaldosteronism.[79] The braking phenomenon occurs when long-term diuretic use results in a reduced natriuretic response due, in part, to nephron adaptations that leads to avid sodium

TABLE 18.4 Diuretic Dosing

Clinical Scenario	Diuretic	Dose
Moderate fluid overload	Furosemide	20–40 mg IV q12h[a]
	Bumetanide	0.5–1 mg IV q12h[a]
Severe fluid overload	Furosemide	40–80 mg IV q12h[b,c] or Bolus of 60 mg IV + continuous infusion at 10–20 mg/h
	Bumetanide	1–2 mg IV q12h[b] or bolus of 2 mg IV + continuous infusion at 0.25–0.5 mg/h
Severe fluid overload *and* renal dysfunction (GFR < 30 mL/min)	Furosemide	80–200 mg IV q12h or bolus + continuous infusion at 20–40 mg/h
Diuretic resistance	Add hydrothiazide or metolazone	25 mg or 50 mg 5 mg or 10 mg 30 min prior to loop diuretic

The IV loop diuretic dose should be equal to or double the outpatient oral dose for patients with decompensated chronic HF.
[a]Double dose if goal not attained.
[b]If goal not attained, add a thiazide (see diuretic resistance).
[c]Lower dose if systolic blood pressure <100 mm Hg.
GFR, Glomerular filtration rate; *HF*, heart failure; *IV*, intravenous.
From Ponikowski P, et al. 2016 guidelines for the diagnosis and treatment of acute and chronic heart failure: the Task Force for the Diagnosis and Treatment of Acute and Chronic Heart Failure of the European Society of Cardiology (ESC) developed with the special contribution of the Heart Failure Association (HFA) of the ESC. *Eur Heart J.* 2016;37(27):2129–2200.

reabsorption at more distal sites.[80] This phenomenon argues for the use of sequential nephron blockade with combinations of loop and thiazide diuretics in patients who do not have adequate responses to optimal doses of a loop diuretic. However, their use has been associated with increased arrhythmia risk due to hypokalemia. The rebound effect involves postdiuretic sodium retention, typically in the setting of inadequate dosing frequency and insufficient sodium restriction.[81]

To overcome inadequate response to diuretics, it is important to adhere to the following principles (also see Table 18.4):

1. Diuretics should be used in moderation; excessive bolus doses of any single drug should be avoided.
2. A loop diuretic is the diuretic of choice in patients with renal insufficiency and in patients with more than mild fluid retention.
3. The diuretic response of loop diuretics is not increased by giving larger bolus doses, but it may be enhanced by giving moderate doses more frequently or using continuous infusion at higher doses (≥20 mg/h).
4. Sodium restriction (<1.5 to 2 g/day) and fluid restriction (1.5 to 2 L/day) may be helpful.
5. The clinician can make use of synergism by adding a thiazide when there is apparent tolerance to loop diuretics. This diuretic regimen can be used to achieve euvolemia. Hydrochlorothiazide combined with spironolactone should be considered to prevent excessive potassium wasting. Metolazone, a potent thiazide, could be added to a loop diuretic when hydrochlorothiazide

seems to be ineffective in promoting sodium excretion. This combination often causes severe electrolyte disturbances.

6. In patients who have poor responses to intermittent doses of a loop diuretic, a continuous intravenous infusion could be entertained. A continuous infusion allows for the administration of higher diuretic doses with less risk of ototoxicity. It may also be reasonable to consider inotropes if diuretic resistance is thought to be related to low cardiac output.

Worsening renal failure (WRF). Decongestive therapy with diuretics is complicated by WRF (defined as an increase in serum creatinine of ≥0.3 mg/dL during hospitalization) in one-third of heart failure admissions and is associated with increased length of stay, increased readmission rate, and decreased short- and long-term survival.[82–84] However, recent data have suggested that transient WRF during AHF therapy may not affect postdischarge outcomes.[85] It seems reasonable to conclude that transient WRF may be a reasonable trade-off for decongestion given that persistent congestion is associated with WRF and adverse events. Progressive WRF can be avoided in patients with persistent congestion by decreasing the rate of volume removal with diureses.[86] In some patients, as stated earlier, inotropic support may be warranted if WRF is deemed to be a manifestation of end-organ hypoperfusion. The differential diagnosis of WRF should include the possibility of inadequate decongestion and progressive cardiorenal syndrome. These two ends of the volume spectrum should be easily distinguishable by history and physical examination. The overdiuresed patient with WRF will frequently complain of orthostatic symptoms, have low jugular venous pressure (JVP) and no or minimal peripheral edema. The underdiuresed patient with WRF will not be orthostatic, will have persistent elevations in JVP, and persistent peripheral edema.

Vasopressin Antagonists.
Elevations of arginine vasopressin (AVP) in HF promote water retention, with resultant congestive symptoms and hyponatremia.[87] AVP antagonists have been developed to block the action of AVP at the V2 receptor in renal tubules to promote aquaresis. Currently, two vasopressin antagonists are available for clinical use: conivaptan and tolvaptan. It may be reasonable to consider a vasopressin antagonist to treat symptomatic hypervolemic or normovolemic hyponatremia in patients with HF.[34] Vasopressin antagonists such as tolvaptan enhance fluid loss, appear safe, and provide moderate benefits with dyspnea relief in randomized trials, but do not appear to impact mortality or hospitalization for heart failure.[88–90]

Ultrafiltration.
Conventional ultrafiltration requires central venous access and the typical volume of water removed per ultrafiltration session is 3000 to 4000 mL. In general, the hemodynamic changes produced by ultrafiltration are modest. The reduction in water with ultrafiltration is accompanied by decreases in right atrial and pulmonary venous pressures. Cardiac output and stroke volume are unchanged or increase slightly. In the Ultrafiltration versus Intravenous Diuretics for Patients Hospitalized for Acute Decompensated Congestive Heart Failure (UNLOAD) trial, the weight loss was more sustained when contrasted with the weight loss achieved with furosemide

treatment.[91] However, the enthusiasm for this strategy as a routine intervention has waned after the results of the Cardiorenal Rescue Study in Acute Decompensated Heart Failure (CARRESS-HF) trial.[92] This randomized trial, involving patients hospitalized for acute decompensated heart failure, worsened renal function, and persistent congestion, showed that the use of a stepped pharmacologic therapy algorithm was superior to a strategy of ultrafiltration for the preservation of renal function at 96 hours, with a similar amount of weight loss with the two approaches. Ultrafiltration was associated with a higher rate of adverse events. Recent guidelines indicate that in patients for whom diuretic strategies have been unsuccessful or with severe renal dysfunction and/or refractory fluid retention, continuous ultrafiltration may become necessary.[34,35]

Circulatory Support

Inotropic Agents. These agents are indicated in the presence of hypotension and end-organ hypoperfusion (decreased renal function) with or without congestion or pulmonary edema refractory to diuretics and vasodilators at optimal doses. Anecdotal experience suggests that positive inotropic agents may be especially useful in these patients when LV and RV systolic function are markedly depressed. Their use is potentially harmful because they increase oxygen demand and calcium loading; thus they should be used with caution.[93] More recent data do not support the routine intravenous use of these agents as an adjunct to standard therapy in the treatment of patients hospitalized for decompensated chronic heart failure.[94] The choice of agent depends on the predominant hemodynamic abnormality. Inotropes are not indicated in patients with preserved systolic function.

Dopamine

Actions. Physiologically, dopamine is the precursor of norepinephrine and releases norepinephrine from the stores of the nerve endings in the heart. Dopamine has the valuable property in severe heart failure of specifically increasing renal blood flow by activating postjunctional dopaminergic receptors.[95] This vasodilatory effect is observed at doses of 1 to 2 μg/kg per minute and peaks at a dose of 7.5 μg/min: the vasoconstrictive effect begins at a dose of 10 μg/kg per minute. Because the inotropic effects of dopamine result primarily from its indirect effects, its use in advanced heart failure is limited by the neurotransmitter depletion present in the failing heart.[96] In milder forms of heart failure, dopamine may have similar effects to dobutamine except for the greater tendency to increase heart rate and a tendency to increase systemic vascular resistance and ventricular filling pressures at medium and higher doses.

Use in AHF. Dopamine should be infused through a long, indwelling catheter because of the risk of extravasation, which may cause necrosis and sloughing of the surrounding tissue because of the vasoconstrictive effects of the agent. Infusion with dopamine should be started at doses of 2 to 5 μg/kg per min and should not be increased beyond 5 μg/kg per minute in patients with blood pressures of 100 mm Hg or greater. This agent may be deleterious in patients with AHF because it may augment the LV afterload, pulmonary artery pressure, and pulmonary resistance. It has been proposed that dopamine may improve renal function in patients with severe heart failure by increasing renal blood flow and possibly by reducing renal venous pressure, but data supporting such a potential benefit are limited. Specifically, the addition of low-dose dopamine to diuretic therapy was not found to enhance decongestion or improve renal function.[97] In markedly hypotensive patients with peripheral hypoperfusion, large doses of dopamine can be used to support systemic blood pressure. Recent data, however, showed that there was no significant difference in the rate of death between patients with shock who were treated with dopamine as the first-line vasopressor agent and those who were treated with norepinephrine, but the use of dopamine was associated with a greater number of adverse events.[98]

Dobutamine

Actions. Dobutamine is a β-adrenergic agonist that stimulates β_1-adrenergic, β_2-adrenergic, and α_1-adrenergic receptors.[99] Cardiac contractility is increased by virtue of its β_1 and α_1 effects, but because the α_1-adrenergic effects are generally counterbalanced by the β_2 actions, there is generally little change in blood pressure. Dobutamine markedly increases cardiac output but produces only modest changes in LV filling pressures and virtually no increase in blood pressure.[100] Heart rate generally increases only when doses greater than 10 μg/kg per minute are used. Compared with dobutamine, dopamine is a better vasoconstrictor[100] and milrinone is a better vasodilator.[101] The elimination of the drug is rapid after cessation of infusion, making it a convenient inotropic agent.

Use in AHF. The usual dose of dobutamine is 2.5 to 20 μg/kg per minute. Short-term infusions are often extremely effective in the treatment of unstable AHF, especially when systolic pressures are preserved. Long-term infusion should be avoided because of the development of hemodynamic tolerance.[102] Dobutamine is likely to increase myocardial oxygen consumption and can cause serious arrhythmias. There are no controlled trials on dobutamine in AHF patients, and some trials show unfavorable effects with increased untoward cardiovascular events.

Milrinone

Actions. Milrinone is a type III phosphodiesterase inhibitor that produces dose-dependent increases in cardiac output and decreases in LV filling pressures as a result of the interaction of its positive inotropic, positive lusitropic, and peripheral vasodilator actions.[103,104] The net result is a hemodynamic profile similar to that of the combination of nitroprusside and dobutamine. Because of its vasodilating effects, milrinone is less likely than dobutamine to increase heart rate and myocardial oxygen consumption. Despite these theoretical advantages, myocardial ischemia has been provoked by these agents, and marked hypotensive episodes have been observed.

Use in AHF. Milrinone requires a loading dose of 25 to 75 μg/kg over 10 minutes followed by a maintenance infusion of 0.375 to 0.75 μg/kg per minute. The dose should be adjusted in patients with decreased renal clearance. This agent may be preferred to dobutamine in patients receiving concomitant β-blocker therapy, or with an inadequate response to dobutamine, or both. The data regarding the effects of milrinone administration on the outcome of patients with AHF are insufficient but raise concerns about safety.[105] The routine administration of milrinone in AHF is to be discouraged due to adverse effects on heart failure, arrhythmias, and blood pressure.[106]

Digitalis. Digitalis generally has no role in the treatment of AHF unless the patient has been taking digitalis for chronic heart failure or if digitalis is given to control a rapid ventricular response in atrial fibrillation.

Vasopressors. Vasopressors are largely used to treat cardiogenic shock and are discussed in Chapter 37. Norepinephrine is an endogenous α_1-adrenergic vasoconstrictor and a β_1-adrenergic agonist that is stored in the sympathetic nerve terminal. This agonist is now more commonly used as the preferred vasopressor over dopamine to support AHF patients with refractory hypotension.[98]

Mechanical Support

When cardiogenic shock persists despite optimization of the patient's volume status and treatment with inotropic drugs and vasopressors, and if it is considered to be potentially reversible, a reasonable treatment option is mechanical circulatory support. The only mechanical modality evaluated by a randomized trial is the use of an intraaortic balloon pump (IABP) to treat cardiogenic shock due to MI. However, the IABP-Shock-II trial showed that this intervention did not reduce mortality among patients with an acute MI who were destined for percutaneous coronary intervention.[107] Several other percutaneous and surgical LV and right ventricular assist devices are now available at many hospitals to stabilize patients as either a bridge to recovery or bridge to decision. These advanced interventions are discussed in detail in Chapters 47 and 48.

CONTINUED THERAPY FOR CHRONIC HEART FAILURE

Patients who are admitted with normotensive AHF should be maintained on oral disease-modifying heart failure therapy. Outpatient doses of β-blockers can be safely continued in the absence of cardiogenic shock.[34,35] Patients with newly diagnosed AHF secondary to a reduced LV ejection fraction should be started on guideline-directed medical therapy before leaving the hospital.[34,35]

Choice of Therapeutic Regimen

In choosing the appropriate medical regimen, it is helpful to revisit the different AHF syndromes. These are outlined in Table 18.5. Two special scenarios warrant mention.

Hypertensive Acute Heart Failure. LV systolic function is normal in patients hospitalized with pulmonary edema and hypertension. Vasodilator therapy should aim for an initial rapid (several minutes) reduction of systolic blood pressure of 30 mm Hg, followed by a more measured decrease of blood pressure to the values obtained during stable periods. No attempt should be made to restore normal values of blood pressure because this may cause deterioration in renal function. The initial blood pressure reduction may be achieved by intravenous loop diuretics, particularly if the patient is clearly fluid overloaded with a long history of chronic heart failure, combined with intravenous nitroglycerin or nitroprusside.

Acute Heart Failure With Preserved Ejection Fraction. The most effective treatment of patients with AHF with preserved ejection fraction is to address the underlying cause. The treatment is similar to hypertensive AHF. In this regard, blood pressure control and the treatment of underlying ischemia are important

TABLE 18.5 Treatment for Acute Heart Failure Syndromes

Acute Heart Failure Syndrome	Systolic Blood Pressure	First-Line Treatment	Second-Line Treatment	Third-Line Treatment
Hypertensive	>140 mm Hg	Oxygen CPAP if needed IV loop diuretic IV nitroglycerin	Increase doses of nitroglycerin or diuretic or both	Intravenous nitroprusside
Normotensive	100–140 mm Hg	Oxygen CPAP if needed Loop diuretic Vasodilators	Increase doses of nitroglycerin or diuretic or both Add thiazide diuretic	Milrinone when there is evidence of prerenal azotemia
Preshock	85–100 mm Hg	Oxygen CPAP Vasodilator and diuretics	Dobutamine or milrinone	Add norepinephrine
Cardiogenic shock	<85 mm Hg	Oxygen CPAP Volume-loading Norepinephrine	Norepinephrine Vasopressin	Mechanical support IABP Consider LVAD

CPAP, Continuous positive airway pressure; *IABP,* intraaortic balloon pump; *IV,* intravenous; *LVAD,* left ventricular assist device.
Modified from Nieminen MS, Bohm M, Cowie MR, et al. Executive summary of the guidelines on the diagnosis and treatment of acute heart failure: Task Force on Acute Heart Failure of the European Society of Cardiology. *Eur Heart J.* 2005;26:384–416.

goals. A major goal of therapy is to reduce the left atrial and pulmonary venous pressures. Diuretics, vasodilators, and other preload-reducing agents are used as discussed previously. The steep or stiff diastolic pressure volume curve (see Fig. 18.4) can be responsible for a substantial decrease in filling pressure with little change in volume; as a result, hypotension often occurs with the usual doses of diuretics. Cautious administration of lower than usual doses of diuretics is advisable.

The full reference list for this chapter is available at ExpertConsult.com.

19

Acute Fulminant Myocarditis

Bettina Heidecker, Leslie T. Cooper Jr

DEFINITION AND EPIDEMIOLOGY

Myocarditis is defined as inflammation of the myocardium generally following an injury such as infection, ischemia, or trauma.[1] Approximately 2.5 million cases of myocarditis and cardiomyopathy were diagnosed globally in 2015.[2] Most cases of acute myocarditis present with chest pain or mild left ventricular (LV) dysfunction. Fulminant myocarditis refers to a specific clinicopathologic form of recent-onset myocarditis requiring inotropic or mechanical circulatory support to maintain tissue perfusion. The most commonly identified trigger of fulminant myocarditis is a viral infection; however, giant cell myocarditis, hypersensitivity, and toxic drug reactions can present with identical clinical features.

This chapter focuses on myocarditis requiring cardiac intensive care unit (CICU) management. This includes myocarditis complicated by severe LV or right ventricular (RV) failure as well as myocarditis associated with sustained and symptomatic arrhythmias. Fulminant myocarditis presenting in this manner is uncommon, probably accounting for less than 10% of all cases. The frequency of fulminant myocarditis is more commonly described in case series of children than adults, possibly due to a less robust immune response or different pathogens with older age.[3]

Etiology

Most commonly, fulminant myocarditis is caused by a viral infection.[4] While enteroviruses—in particular, coxsackievirus strains in North America and Western Europe[5,6]—were the most frequently identified strains until the 1990s, parvovirus B19 has become the most common cause in recent years.[7] Although many other viruses have been identified in endomyocardial biopsies (EMBs), their role in fulminant disease is not yet established.

Hypersensitivity myocarditis associated with dobutamine is relevant to the CICU patient population.[8,9] Occasionally, cardiomyopathy related to methamphetamine can require inotropic support. In the setting of acute physical or emotional stress, typical or atypical takotsubo or stress-induced cardiomyopathy should be considered. Giant cell and necrotizing eosinophilic myocarditis are rapidly fatal causes of acute cardiomyopathy of particular importance to the CICU physician as they frequently respond to early immunosuppression in addition to guideline-directed medical management.

PATHOPHYSIOLOGY OF FULMINANT MYOCARDITIS

The transitions from acute viral infection through active inflammation to chronic dilated cardiomyopathy can be conceptualized as a multiphase model recently reviewed by Heymans et al.[10] The initial acute injury can be caused by direct cytotoxicity to the myocardium by pathogens such as viruses, while cytokines released during the immune response lead to further cell death and remodeling.[11] Multiple cellular and extracellular components of the myocardium and the immune system contribute to effector and regulatory influences that shape the clinical presentation.

In models of fulminant myocarditis, cytokines with negative inotropic influence, such as tumor necrosis factor α (TNF-α), are expressed at high levels.[12] T effector cells and proinflammatory macrophages predominate in the inflammatory infiltrates and contribute to myocardial depression. Within weeks, the regulatory immune elements increase and downregulate the acute response in model systems. In clinical practice, the purpose of mechanical circulatory support is to bridge patients through the acute period of fulminant disease to the phase in what healing factors predominate.

TABLE 19.1	Etiologies of Myocarditis
Infectious Myocarditis	
Bacterial	*Staphylococcus, Streptococcus, Pneumococcus, Meningococcus, Gonococcus, Salmonella, Corynebacterium diphtheriae, Haemophilus influenzae, Mycobacterium* (tuberculosis), *Mycoplasma pneumoniae, Brucella*
Spirochaetal	*Borrelia* (Lyme disease), *Leptospira* (Weil disease)
Fungal	*Aspergillus, Actinomyces, Blastomyces, Candida, Coccidioides, Cryptococcus, Histoplasma, Mucormycoses, Nocardia, Sporothrix*
Protozoal	*Trypanosoma cruzi, Toxoplasma gondii, Entamoeba, Leishmania*
Parasitic	*Trichinella spiralis, Echinococcus granulosus, Taenia solium*
Rickettsial	*Coxiella burnetii* (Q fever), *R. rickettsii* (Rocky Mountain spotted fever), *R. tsutsugamushi*
Viral	RNA viruses: coxsackieviruses A and B, echoviruses, polioviruses, influenza A and B viruses, respiratory syncytial virus, mumps virus, measles virus, rubella virus, hepatitis C virus, dengue virus, yellow fever virus, Chikungunya virus, Junin virus, Lassa fever virus, rabies virus, human immunodeficiency virus–1
	DNA viruses: adenoviruses, parvovirus B19, cytomegalovirus, human herpes virus–6, Epstein-Barr virus, varicella-zoster virus, herpes simplex virus, variola virus, vaccinia virus
Immune-Mediated Myocarditis	
Allergens	Tetanus toxoid, vaccines, serum sickness
	Drugs: penicillin, cefaclor, colchicine, furosemide, isoniazid, lidocaine, tetracycline, sulfonamides, phenytoin, phenylbutazone, methyldopa, thiazide diuretics, amitriptyline
Alloantigens	Heart transplant rejection
Autoantigens	Infection-negative lymphocytic, infection-negative giant cell
	Associated with autoimmune or immune-oriented disorders: systemic lupus erythematosus, rheumatoid arthritis, Churg-Strauss syndrome, Kawasaki disease, inflammatory bowel disease, scleroderma, polymyositis, myasthenia gravis, insulin-dependent diabetes mellitus, thyrotoxicosis, sarcoidosis, Wegener granulomatosis, rheumatic heart disease (rheumatic fever)
Toxic Myocarditis	
Drugs	Amphetamines, anthracyclines, cocaine, cyclophosphamide, ethanol, fluorouracil, lithium, catecholamines, hemetine, interleukin-2, trastuzumab, clozapine
Heavy metals	Copper, iron, lead (rare, more commonly cause intramyocyte accumulation)
Miscellaneous	Scorpion sting, snake, and spider bites; bee and wasp stings; carbon monoxide; inhalants; phosphorus, arsenic, sodium azide
Hormones	Pheochromocytoma, vitamins: beri-beri
Physical agents	Radiation, electric shock

From Caforio AL, Pankuweit S, Arbustini E, et al. Current state of knowledge on aetiology, diagnosis, management, and therapy of myocarditis: a position statement of the European Society of Cardiology Working Group on Myocardial and Pericardial Diseases. *Eur Heart J.* 2013;34:2636–2648.

The close temporal link between a well-defined viral prodrome and the onset of fulminant myocarditis led to the hypothesis that a robust immune response could clear viral infection at the price of short-term myocardial depression and lead within weeks to a high rate of recovery.[13] Most recent clinical data support this concept in that adults and children with fulminant myocarditis can frequently be bridged to recovery with mechanical circulatory support.[14,15]

Other causes of fulminant myocarditis, such as giant cell myocarditis and necrotizing eosinophilic myocarditis, have ill-defined triggers and unclear pathogenesis. Nonetheless, case series support the use of mechanical circulatory support (MCS) as a bridge to recovery or transplant in these scenarios, often in combination with some form of immunosuppression.[16,17]

DIAGNOSTIC EVALUATION OF A PATIENT WITH SUSPECTED MYOCARDITIS

Laboratory Tests

Myocarditis should be suspected in all cases of acute nonischemic cardiomyopathy according to the criteria suggested in the current European Society of Cardiology (ESC) position statement on the management of myocarditis (Table 19.1).[18] Cardiac troponins and creatine kinase levels are elevated in many cases of acute myocarditis; however, cardiac enzymes are not specific for cardiac inflammation and, in a large multicenter trial, troponin I was elevated in only about a third of the subjects with histologically active or borderline myocarditis.[19] The greater sensitivity of third-generation troponin assays will improve the detection rate for myocyte injury compared to the historical literature. The current American Heart Association (AHA) scientific statement and ESC position statements on the management of myocarditis recommend that biomarkers of cardiac injury be drawn if myocarditis is suspected.[18,19]

Natriuretic peptides and soluble ST2[21] can be useful to assess heart failure in patients with myocarditis.[22] Transcriptomic biomarkers of total[23–27] and microribonucleic acids[10,28,29] have shown promise to improve diagnostic and prognostic assessment of myocarditis in the future (Fig. 19.1).

Electrocardiographic Findings

The current AHA scientific statement and ESC position statements on the management of myocarditis recommend that an electrocardiogram (ECG) be obtained in patients with suspected

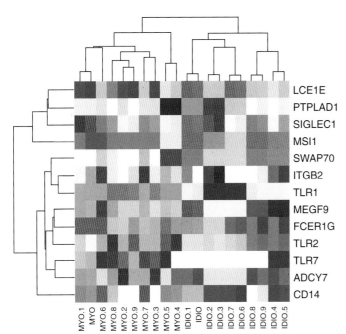

Fig. 19.1 Transcriptomic biomarker that accurately distinguished patients with lymphocytic myocarditis from idiopathic dilated cardiomyopathy. The heatmap was created with an unsupervised clustering approach based on euclidean distance using gene expression levels from quantitative real-time polymerase chain reaction (RT-PCR). RT-PCR was used as a confirmatory test for a subset of genes or molecular signature that was discovered with microarray analysis. Columns represent samples and rows represent genes labeled with their corresponding symbol. This biomarker identified lymphocytic myocarditis with greater accuracy than standard histology. (From Heidecker B, Kittleson MM, Kasper EK, et al. Transcriptomic biomarkers for the accurate diagnosis of myocarditis. *Circulation*. 2011;123:1174–84.)

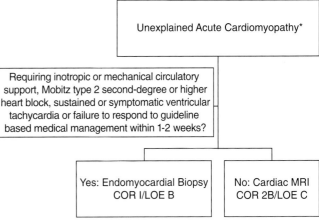

Fig. 19.2 Algorithm for the evaluation of suspected myocarditis in the setting of unexplained acute cardiomyopathy. *Usually a dilated cardiomyopathy. Fulminant myocarditis may have normal end-diastolic diameter with mildly thickened walls. Exclude ischemic, hemodynamic (valvular, hypertensive), metabolic, and toxic causes of cardiomyopathy, as indicated clinically. *COR*, Class of recommendation; *LOE*, level of evidence; *MRI*, magnetic resonance imaging. (From Bozkurt B, Colvin M, Cook J, et al. Current diagnostic and treatment strategies for specific dilated cardiomyopathies: a scientific statement from the American Heart Association. *Circulation*. 2016;134:e579-e646.)

myocarditis despite relatively low sensitivity. ECG changes suggestive of myocarditis are diffuse concave ST-T segment elevations (rather than convex in myocardial ischemia) without reciprocal changes.[30] Conduction disturbances in the presence of LV cardiomyopathy should raise suspicion for Lyme disease, cardiac sarcoidosis, or giant cell myocarditis.[30] Prolongation of the QRS for 120 ms or longer is an independent predictor of death or transplantation in case series from Europe and Asia.[31]

Echocardiography

Echocardiography is useful to exclude pericardial and valvular causes of heart failure and to define LV and RV function.[32,33] Myocarditis may present with dilated, hypertrophic, or restrictive cardiomyopathy. Regional wall motion abnormalities may mimic ischemic heart disease.[32,33] A thicker left ventricle with diminished systolic function is more typical of fulminant myocarditis as compared to acute disease without hemodynamic compromise.[34]

Indications for Endomyocardial Biopsy

EMB should be performed in patients with new onset of unexplained cardiomyopathy with the following clinical risk factors: (1) Heart failure requiring inotropic or mechanical circulatory support, (2) Mobitz type 2 second-degree or higher heart block,

(3) sustained or symptomatic ventricular tachycardia, or (4) failure to respond to guideline-based medical management within 1 to 2 weeks (Class I, level of evidence B; Fig. 19.2).[19,35] Histologic evaluation is required to categorize myocarditis into clinically important subtypes with specific treatment algorithms: eosinophilic, lymphocytic, giant cell, and sarcoid (idiopathic granulomatous). If these additional risk factors are absent, further diagnostic evaluation may be pursued with magnetic resonance imaging (MRI; Class IIB, level of evidence C; see Fig. 19.2).[19] Immunohistology with cell-specific secondary antibodies has a greater sensitivity than histology with hematoxylin and eosin for the diagnosis of myocarditis. Because of sampling error, a mean of 17 samples per patient has been estimated to obtain a sensitivity of 79% using blind RV septal biopsy and the Dallas criteria, which is not feasible in clinical practice.[36]

The right internal jugular vein or right femoral vein are commonly used to access the interventricular septum of the right ventricle. In the setting of isolated LV disease, EMB of the left ventricle increases the sensitivity of EMB.[37] Major complications occur in 0.64% of LV EMBs and 0.82% of RV EMBs. Minor complications (including postprocedural pericardial effusion) occurred in up to 2.89% of LV EMBs and 5.10% of RV EMBs.[37] A subsequent study in an animal model suggested that the diagnostic sensitivity of EMBs may be improved if combined with real-time MRI.[38] Therefore, MRI-guided EMB may be considered but is not currently a standard procedure.

Magnetic Resonance Imaging

The AHA scientific statement recommends that in patients with suspected myocarditis, MRI may be useful (Class IIBB, level of evidence C; see Fig. 19.2). Patients with hemodynamic compromise

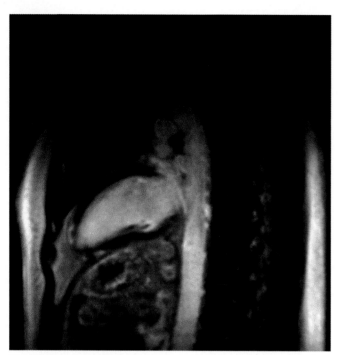

Fig. 19.3 T1-weighted magnetic resonance imaging of patient with myocarditis. Apical and inferior late gadolinium enhancement are consistent with myocarditis (1.5 T scan). (Courtesy Robert Manka, MD, University Hospital Zurich.)

are frequently too unstable to lie flat and hold their breath for the required sequences. As mentioned earlier, if patients also meet criteria for EMB, cardiac MRI prior to biopsy may help target the left ventricle.[37,38] Non–contrast-enhanced T2-weighted sequences and early post-gadolinium T1-weighted sequences have been used separately and in combination to diagnose myocarditis.[19] An international consensus group for cardiovascular MRI in myocarditis has established the Lake Louise criteria to define the diagnosis of myocarditis on MRI.[39] Diagnostic findings of delayed gadolinium enhancement (DGE) can evolve from a focal to a more diffuse pattern (Fig. 19.3) and then resolve over the course of 2 to 4 weeks after symptom onset.[40] The MyoRacer Trial suggested that cardiac mapping techniques with T1- and T2-weighted imaging outperform the Lake Louise criteria, and that T1-weighted imaging was more accurate in acute myocarditis versus T2-weighted imaging, which was better for chronic myocarditis.[41] The presence of late gadolinium enhancement, particularly in the anteroseptal region, is associated with a more than doubled risk of major adverse cardiac events.[41a,41b]

THERAPY

Fulminant myocarditis should be managed in accordance with the current guidelines for systolic heart failure (HF), as outlined by the AHA/American College of Cardiology (ACC) and the ESC.[19,30,42] These recommendations are based on clinical experience, as clinical trials of heart failure therapy specifically in myocarditis have not been done. Patients with fulminant myocarditis require hemodynamic support with vasopressors or MCS, such as intraaortic balloon pump, extracorporeal membrane oxygenation, or percutaneous or surgically placed ventricular

assist devices. Early transfer of those patients to a tertiary care center with expertise in heart transplantation and destination mechanical circulatory support is essential.

Intravenous amiodarone has been shown to be effective for the management of ventricular arrhythmias.[43] Digoxin is contraindicated, as the risk for atrioventricular (AV) block is increased in myocarditis. Temporary pacing may be required if complete AV block develops; some patients may require a Lifevest during the acute phase if severe ventricular arrhythmias (ventricular tachycardia or fibrillation) persist until the patient is otherwise ready for discharge.[30,44] Implantation of an implantable cardioverter defibrillator should be deferred, as there is a significant rate of LV recovery.

In myocarditis related to systemic autoimmune disease—such as sarcoidosis, systemic lupus erythematosus, or a specific vasculitis—treatment is based on the underlying disorder and often includes immunosuppression.[30,45] The role of immunosuppressive, antiviral, and intravenous immunoglobulin therapies in myocarditis patients requiring MCS has not been systematically investigated. The major treatment trials of immunosuppression either excluded patients on MCS or enrolled very few of these patients.[45] Treatment of mild to moderately severe acute myocarditis with immunosuppressive drugs is not recommended in adults, as immunosuppression with prednisone and either azathioprine or cyclosporine has been shown to lead to similar changes in LV ejection fraction and transplant-free survival as placebo.[46] Two randomized trials of immunosuppression in chronic (>6 months' duration) inflammatory cardiomyopathy without an identifiable pathogen showed favorable results with prednisone and combinations of prednisone and azathioprine or cyclosporine.[45,47–49]

Nonsteroidal antiinflammatory drugs (NSAIDs) should be avoided because of the risk of increased inflammation and mortality in experimental models.[50] Interferon, high-dose immunoglobulin, and immunoadsorption are currently not recommended in adults with myocarditis due to limited data.[30]

Giant cell myocarditis can deteriorate rapidly into cardiogenic shock and multiorgan failure, with a rate of death or cardiac transplantation of 89%.[51] Retrospective and prospective studies have shown relatively favorable outcome at 1 year in patients treated with prednisone and cyclosporine with or without anti-T-cell antibodies.[46] Repeat EMB may be considered in select cases to monitor the histologic response if the clinical response is incomplete. If a transplant is required, the recurrence rate of giant cell myocarditis is approximately 20% to 25% in the allograft.[52]

Eosinophilic necrotizing myocarditis is the most fulminant form of eosinophilic myocarditis and is characterized by rapidly progressing heart failure. Eosinophilic myocarditis can be a manifestation of hypersensitivity to certain medications, such as sumatriptans.[53] Case reports describe success with high-dose steroid therapy in addition to guideline-directed medical management.[53,54] In summary, the clinical trajectory of myocarditis requiring CICU care is variable. Approximately 50% of patients improve within 2 to 4 weeks, 25% develop persistent cardiac dysfunction, and about 12% to 25% will potentially require a transplant or long-term MCS. The average rate of survival after cardiac transplantation for adults with myocarditis is similar to survival after transplantation for other types of cardiomyopathy. However, recent data in children suggest that the post-transplantation risk is higher if active myocarditis was detected in the explanted heart, raising the possibility that preexisting inflammation or viral infection may adversely affect graft survival.[55]

In those patients who recover, competitive sport participation should be avoided for a minimum of 3 to 6 months after the diagnosis of myocarditis. Reassessment with clinical evaluation and functional testing is indicated before competitive sport participation is resumed.

The full reference list for this chapter is available at ExpertConsult.com.

20

Stress (Takotsubo) Cardiomyopathy

Abhiram Prasad

Stress cardiomyopathy (SCM) is a generally reversible acute cardiac syndrome that was originally described in the Japanese population over 30 years ago.[1] Hence, the Japanese term takotsubo (an octopus trap with a narrow neck and round bottom, Fig. 20.1) cardiomyopathy/syndrome has gained favor, as it describes the appearance of the left ventricle during systole. SCM is also known as apical ballooning syndrome (ABS), broken heart syndrome, and ampulla cardiomyopathy.[2,3] The clinical features mimic an acute myocardial infarction (MI); therefore, patients with this syndrome frequently present to the cardiac intensive care unit (CICU). SCM should be considered in the differential diagnosis of patients presenting with an acute coronary syndrome.[4] The typical patient is a postmenopausal woman presenting with symptoms of myocardial ischemia that is temporally related to a physical or emotional stressful event, with positive cardiac biomarkers and/or an electrocardiogram (ECG) that has evidence of ischemia or injury.

EPIDEMIOLOGY

SCM is the final diagnosis in approximately 1% to 2% of all patients initially suspected of either an acute coronary syndrome or MI.[5,6] The proportion may be as high as 12% in women with ST elevation myocardial infarction.[7] The incidence of SCM among patients in intensive care units has been estimated at 1.5% and 8% among those with cardiogenic shock.[8] However, an accurate incidence is difficult to ascertain because of underdiagnosis. Over time, there has been increasing recognition of this entity, as highlighted by data from the Nationwide Inpatient Sample in which the mean number of patients with a discharge diagnosis of SCM from a group of community hospitals increased from 315 per year in 2006 to 6,230 per year in 2012.[9] Approximately 90% of all reported cases are in postmenopausal women[10] and 5% of the patients are younger than 50 years.[11]

PATHOPHYSIOLOGY

The pathophysiology of SCM remains to be established; however, several observations suggest that the sympathetic nervous system plays an important role.[12] These include the temporal relationship with preceding emotional or physical stressful triggers, hyperadrenergic states, such as pheochromocytoma and subarachnoid hemorrhage causing a transient cardiomyopathy that is similar to SCM, documentation of high levels of circulating catecholamines,[13] SCM being precipitated by inadvertent administration of supratherapeutic doses of catecholamines,[14] animal models of stress immobilization and exogenous catecholamine administration inducing left ventricular apical hypokinesis,[15] and the presence of contraction band necrosis on endomyocardial biopsies,[16] a feature of catecholamine toxicity. However, elevation in circulating catecholamines and contraction band necrosis are not always present.

Early reports of cases with SCM were associated with multivessel epicardial coronary spasm, which was initially proposed as a potential mechanism for the myocardial stunning. However, this has not been supported in large case series and is unlikely to be the underlying cause of SCM in the vast majority of patients. Aborted MI due to left anterior descending artery plaque rupture and thrombosis with spontaneous thrombolysis has also been proposed but seems unlikely to be the underlying mechanism.[17] Conversely, microvascular dysfunction can be detected in at least two-thirds of the patients at the time of presentation and its severity correlates with the magnitude of troponin elevation and ECG abnormalities.[18] The microvascular dysfunction may be a primary mechanistic feature or an epiphenomenon. Abnormal glucose and fatty acid metabolism is frequently present, colocalizing with the wall motion abnormality.[19,20]

A preceding stressful trigger is present in over two-thirds of patients. The list of potential emotional triggers is extensive, but

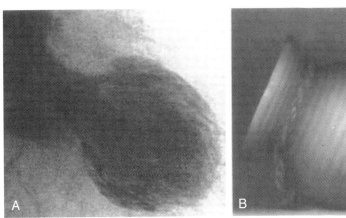

Fig. 20.1 (A) Ventriculogram. (B) An octopus pot ("tako-tsubo"). (Courtesy #FOAMed Medical Education Resources, LITFL.)

most often relates to experiences of significant grief or personal loss, fear or anxiety, anger and frustration, and interpersonal conflicts. Common physical triggers include acute medical conditions (e.g., severe exacerbation of obstructive airways disease, sepsis), neurologic conditions (e.g., subarachnoid hemorrhage, seizures), falls and other trauma, noncardiac surgery (e.g., orthopedic, major abdominal), malignancy, and experiencing severe pain.[21] The absence of such triggers does not exclude the diagnosis.

Patients who are conscious typically have symptoms that are similar to that associated with MI,[10,22,23] the most common being angina-like chest pain, present in approximately 50% of cases. Other presenting symptoms include dyspnea and, less frequently, syncope or out-of-hospital cardiac arrest. Among patients presenting primarily with SCM, it is those with ST segment elevation and severe left ventricular dysfunction who most often are admitted to the CICU. Typically, the ejection fraction is reduced to 30% to 40%,[10] which may be accompanied by significant diastolic dysfunction with elevation in left ventricular filling pressure.[24] Myocardial relaxation is impaired due to the ischemia related to microvascular dysfunction and myocardial edema. Acute heart failure is a frequent complication, but major hemodynamic decompensation is uncommon, with cardiogenic shock developing in approximately 10% to 15% of patients.[10] These patients should be particularly assessed for the presence of transient left ventricular outflow obstruction and clinically significant mitral regurgitation, which can be exacerbating factors,[25] each being present in approximately 10% to 20% of cases. The mechanisms for regurgitation appear to be papillary muscle displacement leading to tethering and impaired coaptation of the leaflets, and/or systolic anterior motion.[25,26] Outflow tract obstruction likely occurs owing to a combination of factors, including hyperdynamic basal function, systolic anterior motion of the mitral valve, and a sigmoid-shaped ventricle.

Additional complications that may lead to admission to the CICU include arrhythmias. Atrial fibrillation occurs in approximately 5% of cases,[27] whereas ventricular tachycardia, torsade de pointes, and ventricular fibrillation have been reported in 3% to 4% of patients and asystole in 0.5%.[28] Other rare

complications of SCM include left ventricular thrombus, thromboembolism, and cardiac rupture.[29]

Patients who develop SCM secondary to a noncardiac illness or other physical trigger may not have the typical symptoms described earlier but instead present with ischemic changes on the ECG, elevated cardiac biomarkers of myonecrosis, pulmonary edema, and hypotension. Hypotension may due to the reduction in stroke volume and, in some cases, dynamic left ventricular outflow tract obstruction.[30]

The ventricular dysfunction resolves over days to weeks, with complete recovery of global systolic function by 4 to 8 weeks. The prognosis of SCM is good in the absence of significant underlying comorbid conditions. In-hospital mortality is approximately 3% to 5%. Among those who are discharged, long-term survival appears to be similar to that of the general age-matched population. The subgroup of patients in whom there is a physical trigger—such as major surgery, malignancy, and fractures—appear to have a worse prognosis, likely related to the underlying condition. The recurrence rate of SCM is approximately 1% to 2% per year.[31]

DIAGNOSIS

There are no diagnostic ECG or biomarker findings that can differentiate SCM from an acute coronary syndrome or myocarditis; hence, it is a diagnosis of exclusion. The characteristic features of the syndrome have been incorporated into several proposed diagnostic criteria.[32,33] Box 20.1 provides the Mayo Clinic criteria that can be applied at the time of presentation. All four criteria must be present.[34]

Electrocardiogram

Between 30% to 50% of patients have ST segment elevation at presentation. The precordial leads are most commonly involved, but ST segment elevation may also occur in the limb leads. The electrocardiographic findings do not reliably distinguish SCM from an acute MI.[35] Pathologic Q waves may be present transiently. Some patients present with deep T-wave inversion, nonspecific T wave abnormality, and the ECG may be normal in some cases. ST segment depression is infrequently present. Characteristic evolutionary changes during hospitalization include resolution of ST segment elevation and diffuse and often deep T-wave inversion associated with prolongation of the corrected QT interval (Fig. 20.2). The electrocardiographic abnormalities usually resolve gradually over weeks to months but may persist even after systolic function has recovered.

BOX 20.1 Proposed Mayo Clinic Criteria for Apical Ballooning Syndrome

1. Transient hypokinesis, akinesis, or dyskinesis of the left ventricular mid-segments with or without apical involvement. The regional wall motion abnormalities extend beyond a single epicardial vascular distribution. A stressful trigger is often present, but not always.[a]
2. Absence of obstructive coronary disease or angiographic evidence of acute plaque rupture.[b]
3. New electrocardiographic abnormalities (either ST segment elevation and/or T-wave inversion) or modest elevation in cardiac troponin.
4. Absence of pheochromocytoma, myocarditis.

From Prasad A, Lerman A, Rihal CS. Apical ballooning syndrome (tako-tsubo or stress cardiomyopathy): a mimic of acute myocardial infarction. *Am Heart J.* 2008;155:408–417.

[a]There are rare exceptions to these criteria, such as those patients in whom the regional wall motion abnormality is limited to a single coronary territory.

[b]It is possible that a patient with obstructive coronary atherosclerosis may also develop apical ballooning syndrome (ABS). However, this is very rare in our experience and in the published literature, perhaps because such cases are misdiagnosed as an acute coronary syndrome.

In both of the above circumstances, the diagnosis of ABS should be made with caution and a clear stressful precipitating trigger must be sought.

Cardiac Biomarkers

Cardiac troponin levels, using contemporary assays, are invariably elevated on admission and generally peak within 24 to 48 hours. Creatine kinase MB fraction is elevated in the great majority of cases. The levels are lower compared to patients with ST segment elevation MI, but similar to that of patients with non ST elevation MI and relatively low for the extent of acute left ventricular systolic dysfunction. Blood level of brain natriuretic peptide (BNP) or N-terminal pro-BNP, markers of ventricular dysfunction, are elevated in the majority of patients and may correlate with left ventricular end-diastolic pressure.[36–39]

Left Ventricular Imaging and Coronary Angiography

Transthoracic echocardiography can be readily performed in the intensive care setting and hence is the preferred mode of imaging to detect systolic dysfunction and potential complications that accompany SCM. In the classical form of the cardiomyopathy, basal left ventricular function is preserved and may even be hyperdynamic, but there is hypokinesis or akinesis of the mid- and apical segments leading to the "ballooning" appearance (Fig. 20.3, Video 20.1). The wall motion abnormality virtually always extends beyond the distribution of a single coronary artery. In a significant proportion of patients, apical contraction is preserved and the wall motion abnormality is restricted to the mid-segments (apical-sparing variant; Video 20.2).[40] The least common variant is known as inverted or reverse takotsubo in which there is hypokinesis of the basal segment of the left ventricle with preserved apical function. The variant forms of SCM have similar clinical characteristics and prognosis as the typical form. The right ventricle also develops a similar pattern

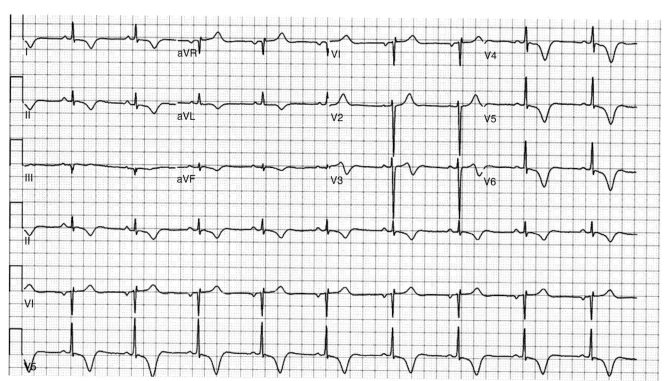

Fig. 20.2 Twelve-lead electrocardiogram with T-wave inversion in the precordial and limb leads associated with prolongation of the QT interval.

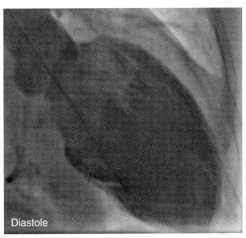
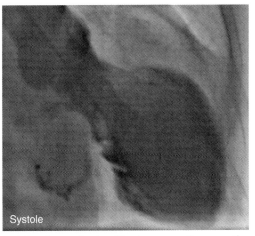

Diastole

Systole

Fig. 20.3 Left ventriculogram in diastole and systole of a patient with stress cardiomyopathy with hyperdynamic basal contraction and akinesis of the mid- and apical segments.

of regional wall motion abnormality in approximately one-third of cases.[41] Biventricular dysfunction SCM is associated with a worse hemodynamic profile and the patients are often sicker and more likely to develop acute heart failure.

Cardiac magnetic resonance may be a useful imaging modality for documenting the extent of regional wall motion abnormality and differentiating SCM (virtually always characterized by the absence of delayed gadolinium hyperenhancement) from myocarditis and MI in which delayed hyperenhancement is present.[42]

Patients with SCM either have angiographically normal coronary arteries or mild atherosclerosis. Obstructive coronary artery disease is infrequent despite most patients being in their seventh and eighth decade of life.[43] When present, the extent and distribution of obstructive plaque is generally insufficient to account for the widespread regional wall motion abnormality. Coronary angiography, either invasive or noninvasive, should be performed in patients suspected of SCM in order to exclude an acute coronary syndrome. In contemporary treatment pathways, the presence of ST segment elevation typically leads to emergency angiography to exclude coronary thrombotic occlusion that requires revascularization prior to admission to the CICU.

MANAGEMENT

The recommendations for SCM management are based on expert opinion as clinical trials have not been conducted owing, in part, to the low incidence and the fact that supportive therapy leads to spontaneous recovery in the great majority of patients. The initial therapy is frequently directed toward treating myocardial ischemia with aspirin, anticoagulants, statins, and β-blockers since an acute coronary syndrome is the presumed diagnosis in the majority of cases. Aspirin, anticoagulants, and statins can be discontinued once the diagnosis of SCM has been made unless there is coexisting coronary atherosclerosis. In the absence of contraindications, a β-blocker or a combined α- and β-blocker may be initiated because excess catecholamines have been implicated in the pathogenesis. Long-term therapy should be

considered with the aim of reducing recurrence even though observational data has not supported this recommendation.[10] Initiation of angiotensin-converting enzyme inhibitor or angiotensin receptor blocker therapy for acute ventricular dysfunction is recommended, especially as the diagnosis may not be certain at the time of discharge. Inhibitors of the renin angiotensin system may be discontinued once there is complete recovery of systolic function, though there are observational data that suggest that they may have long-term benefits.[10]

Mild to moderate acute heart failure responds to diuretic therapy. Severe cases with pulmonary edema may require intubation and mechanical ventilation. If present, left ventricular outflow tract obstruction may be treated with phenylephrine with the goal of increasing afterload and left ventricular cavity size. Phenylephrine use requires close monitoring due to the presence of systolic dysfunction. In the absence of heart failure, β-blockers and/or intravenous fluids may be effective.

Inotropes are often used with good effect in cardiogenic shock, although there are theoretical reasons for avoiding them because of the potential role of catecholamine toxicity in precipitating the syndrome. Intraaortic balloon pump counterpulsation or other mechanical support devices may be preferable. The former has the potential to exacerbate outflow tract obstruction and should therefore be used cautiously.

The acute treatment of atrial and ventricular arrhythmias is similar to other clinical situations. Although torsade de pointes is rare, patients should be on continuous ECG monitoring until the QTc is less than or equal to 500 msec. If pause-dependent torsade occurs, β-blocker therapy should be withheld and temporary pacing considered. Implantable cardioverter-defibrillator therapy is not routinely indicated for ventricular tachycardia or fibrillation as the cardiomyopathy is reversible. In cases of recurrent aborted sudden cardiac death or life-threatening ventricular arrhythmia, the role of implantable cardioverter-defibrillator therapy is unclear.

The full reference list for this chapter is available at ExpertConsult.com.

Distributive Shock

Joyce Ji, David L. Brown

The range of care covered by cardiac intensive care units (CICUs) has expanded drastically since they were originally developed as coronary care units (CCUs) for the management of acute myocardial infarction (MI) in the early 1960s.[1] In addition to the rising complexity of cardiovascular diseases seen in the CICUs, other critical conditions such as respiratory failure, renal failure, and sepsis have become increasingly more prevalent as well.[2] The overlap in populations between the CICU and other ICUs continues to grow (Fig. 21.1). Given the expansive breadth of diseases now seen in contemporary CICUs, it is important to broaden the knowledge base and training for cardiac intensivists. This chapter explores the epidemiology, pathogenesis, clinical presentation, and current management of distributive shock.

EPIDEMIOLOGY

Definition

Shock can be classified into four states: hypovolemic, cardiogenic, obstructive, and distributive. Of the four, distributive shock is the most common condition encountered in the critical care setting. Distributive, or vasodilatory, shock is characterized by the shunting of oxygen transport to the tissues, resulting in abnormal distribution of tissue perfusion and impaired regional oxygen extraction. In contrast to the other categories of shock, this classically occurs in the presence of normal or increased cardiac output.

The diagnosis of distributive shock should include the following:

1. Systolic blood pressure less than 90 mm Hg or mean arterial pressure (MAP) less than 65 mm Hg for at least 30 minutes.
2. Normal or high cardiac index (≥ 2.0 L/min per m^2). It is important to note that although distributive shock is typically characterized by high cardiac output, it is a state that may result in transient myocardial depression or may occur in a patient with underlying left ventricular dysfunction.
3. Tissue hypoperfusion manifested by oliguria (<0.5 mL/kg per hour), altered mental status, elevated lactate (>2 mmol/L).

Etiology

Distributive shock can be further categorized into its different causes. Septic shock is the classic form of distributive shock, as it is the most prevalent type of shock encountered in the ICU. Septic shock occurs as a result of an infection that induces circulatory dysfunction in the host. Neurogenic shock is a form of distributive shock that occurs in patients with severe traumatic brain injury and spinal cord injury that result in autonomic dysfunction. Anaphylactic shock results from a serious immunoglobulin E (IgE)-mediated reaction to an allergen. Distributive shock may also occur as a component of the systemic inflammatory state encountered in patients with a large acute MI.[3,4] Other less common causes of distributive shock include postcardiac arrest, pancreatitis, drug or toxin reactions, burns, air or fat embolism, adrenal crisis, and thyrotoxicosis.

Incidence

Of the different types of shock, septic shock is most commonly encountered in the ICU. In an analysis of 1600 patients who

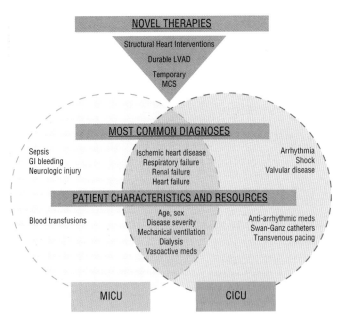

Fig. 21.1 Overlap between contemporary medicine intensive care units (MICU) and cardiac intensive care units (CICU). *GI*, Gastrointestinal; *LVAD*, left ventricular assist device; *MCS*, mechanical circulatory support. (From Katz JN, Minder M, Olenchock B, et al. The genesis, maturation, and future of critical care cardiology. *J Am Coll Cardiol.* 2016;68:69.)

presented with shock, septic shock occurred in 62%, cardiogenic shock in 16%, hypovolemic shock in 16%, other types of distributive shock in 4%, and obstructive shock in 2%.[5] Rates of sepsis and septic shock have continued to increase over the years, likely due to the advancing age of the population, multidrug-resistant organisms, and the increased use of immunosuppressive agents.[6–8] An emphasis on the earlier detection of sepsis may contribute to this increase as well. While four discrete classifications of shock are described, it is important to recognize that a substantial number of patients may present with "mixed" or multifactorial states of shock. The overlapping features of these presentations make it challenging to determine the definitive diagnosis and subsequent management.

PATHOGENESIS

Pathophysiology

Circulatory shock is characterized by a severe deficiency in oxygen delivery and failure of tissue perfusion. Depending on the etiology of the shock state, this can occur through a variety of mechanisms. The end result is the critical impairment of oxidative metabolism, ultimately leading to organ failure and death. It is important to identify the etiology of the shock and its underlying pathophysiology in order to manage it rapidly and effectively.

The microcirculation may be considered its own organ system, consisting of a complex network of vessels involved in the delivery of oxygen to cells. A variety of factors influence the microcirculatory system. In distributive shock, abnormalities in the microcirculation lead to significant peripheral vasodilatation and impairment of autoregulatory mechanisms required to maintain adequate tissue perfusion.[9–12] Multiple mechanisms contribute

to the microcirculatory derangements (Fig. 21.2). Endothelial cells become more leaky and less responsive to vasoactive agents. Inflammatory activation leads to upregulation of the nitric oxygen (NO) system, resulting in shunting of blood flow within the microcirculation. An imbalance of vasoactive substances also contributes to alterations in blood flow and, thus, a regional mismatch in oxygen supply and demand. Additionally, both the activation of the coagulation cascade and the reduced deformability of erythrocytes and leukocytes lead to microvascular plugging, further compromising capillary flow. Blood flow is shunted away from the vital organs, resulting in tissue hypoxia. The uneven distribution of microcirculatory blood flow can result in impaired oxygen delivery even when patients are normotensive.

The prototype of distributive shock is septic shock. In septic shock, the interaction between the microorganism and the host immune system creates an exaggerated inflammatory response. The systemic overexpression of inflammatory mediators, such as tumor necrosis factor-α (TNF-α) and interleukin-1β (IL-1β), lead to microcirculatory dysfunction and ineffective distribution of blood flow away from vital organs.[13] Aside from deficient oxygen delivery, mitochondrial dysfunction within the cells—that is, cytopathic hypoxia—contributes to inadequate oxygen utilization as well.[14] In addition, inflammatory cytokines activate the coagulation cascade, inducing a procoagulable state that may subsequently lead to disseminated intravascular coagulation (DIC). While septic shock typically manifests as a hyperdynamic state with high cardiac output, the cytokines and endotoxins activated in sepsis cause myocardial depression.[15,16] This sepsis-induced cardiomyopathy is characterized by ventricular dilatation, reduction in contractility, and depressed ejection fraction. The cardiomyopathy is typically reversible and resolves within 7 to 10 days.[16]

Anaphylactic shock is mediated by a systemic IgE-mediated allergic reaction.[13] This occurs when the patient is sensitized to a particular antigen, resulting in the production of IgE specific to that antigen. Upon reexposure to the allergen, IgE on mast cells and basophils recognizes the antigen and activates a cascade of inflammatory mediators. These mediators cause endothelial injury, cellular edema, and smooth muscle contraction. This is manifested by excessive peripheral vasodilatation and capillary leakage. Properties of other types of shock may contribute as well, such as cardiogenic shock from decreased myocardial contractility and obstructive shock from pulmonary vasospasm.

In neurogenic shock, injury to the spinal cord or brain that affects the sympathetic nervous system leads to severe autonomic dysregulation.[13] Peripheral vasodilatation results, manifesting as hypotension. This is classically accompanied by bradycardia, as there is unopposed parasympathetic activation in the setting of sympathetic denervation.

CLINICAL PRESENTATION

History and Physical Examination

The clinical presentation depends on the etiology of the distributive shock. Features common to patients presenting with shock include hypotension (i.e., systolic blood pressure <90 mm Hg;

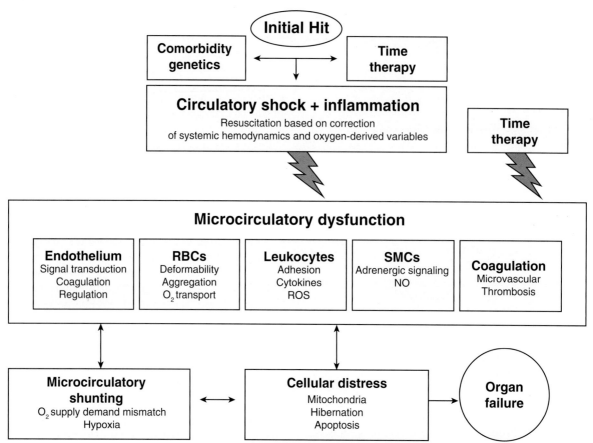

Fig. 21.2 Microcirculatory dysfunction plays a key role in the pathophysiology of distributive shock through the interaction of multiple complex pathways. *NO,* Nitric oxide; *RBCs,* red blood cells; *ROS,* reactive oxygen species; *SMCs,* smooth muscle cells. (From Ince C. The microcirculation is the motor of sepsis. *Crit Care.* 2005;9:S14.)

TABLE 21.1	Modified Early Warning Score						
	3 Points	**2 Points**	**1 Point**	**0 Points**	**1 Point**	**2 Points**	**3 Points**
SBP (mm Hg)	≤70	71–80	81–100	101–199		≥200	
Respiratory rate (breaths/min)		<9		9–14	15–20	21–29	≥30
Heart rate (beats/min)		≤40	41–50	51–100	101–110	111–129	≥130
Temperature (°C)		≤35	35.1–36	36.1–38	38.1–38.5	>38.5	
Level of consciousness			Confused	Alert	Responds to voice	Responds to pain	No response

SBP, Systolic blood pressure.

mean arterial pressure <65 mm Hg; vasopressor dependence), tachycardia (except in the case of neurogenic shock), tachypnea, oliguria, and altered mental status.[17–19] Cool, clammy, and mottled skin with poor capillary refill classically represents poor peripheral perfusion in shock states and portends a poor prognosis.[20–23] However, warm and hyperemic skin does not preclude the diagnosis of shock, as it is often present in early distributive shock secondary to the systemic peripheral vasodilatation or in terminal shock when compensatory peripheral vasoconstriction fails.

The history and physical examination is crucial to revealing the etiology of shock and thus guiding management. There are multiple clinical and physical examination signs that help predict

the development of shock. The modified early warning score[24] utilizes four major vital signs (systolic blood pressure, heart rate, respiratory rate, temperature) and mental status to determine the severity of the patient's condition (Table 21.1). Deviation of these parameters from normal values predicts the risk of hospital mortality and, therefore, determines which patients would benefit from more intensive monitoring and aggressive resuscitation.

Examination of the patient's volume status, such as evaluation of the jugular venous pulse, can help in distinguishing between distributive and cardiogenic shock in particular. Using the method of Lewis to evaluate the jugular venous pulse, the detection of a central venous pressure (CVP) of 5 cm H_2O or less has a fairly high sensitivity (90%) and specificity (89%).[25] Patients with septic shock often have other features concerning for infection, such as fever or hypothermia. History and physical examination will often point toward potential sources of infection. In anaphylaxis, hemodynamic instability is often accompanied by nausea/vomiting, respiratory distress, wheezing, diaphoresis, flushing, urticaria, and/or pruritus. Allergic reactions usually occur within minutes of exposure to the allergen, although occasionally delayed reactions may occur hours after exposure. Biphasic anaphylactic reactions may develop as well, and patients can experience recurrence of anaphylaxis after 4 to 8 hours. Neurogenic shock typically occurs after a severe traumatic injury to the spinal cord or brain. Classically, hypotension is accompanied by bradycardia. In severe cases, patients may eventually progress to complete heart block or cardiac arrest.

Clinicians typically rely heavily on hemodynamic parameters such as blood pressure to determine suitability for circulatory support. However, arterial blood pressure alone is not a sensitive marker of tissue perfusion.[26,27] The microcirculation, rather than macrocirculation, is a more important determinant of vital organ perfusion in distributive shock. The underlying microcirculatory system may be severely impaired even when arterial blood pressure is adequate.[28,29] Therefore, it is important to find other methods of diagnosing and monitoring distributive shock.

Laboratory Testing

The key prognostic laboratory marker in shock is the lactate level, as it is an indicator of impaired microcirculatory flow. Although it is a nonspecific marker of anaerobic metabolism, elevated levels of lactate are highly predictive of mortality, especially when increased above 4 mmol/L.[30–33] Early detection of elevated lactate leads to rapid management of critically ill patients, even if they appear to be hemodynamically stable.

Abnormalities in other laboratory markers—such as serum creatinine, liver function tests (e.g., bilirubin), and the coagulation system (e.g., platelet count)—are indicators of poor end-organ perfusion as well. These parameters are used in the Sequential (sepsis-related) Organ Failure Assessment (SOFA) score that was primarily designed to evaluate the severity of organ failure in patients with sepsis[34,35] (Table 21.2). This score may be used to predict mortality in patients in the ICU with shock.

Invasive Hemodynamic Monitoring

An intraarterial catheter may be placed in the ICU in order to continuously monitor MAP, which is the gold standard measurement of blood pressure. MAP is used as a representation of end-organ perfusion and is more accurate than sphygmomanometer measurements, especially in patients with shock.[36]

Central venous catheters can be helpful in several ways. CVP, which may be measured from the right atrium or superior vena cava, reflects intravascular volume status and filling pressures in the right side of the heart. Low CVP is an indication of volume depletion, while an elevated CVP is an indication of right ventricular volume overload. However, CVP can be influenced by a multitude of factors, including right ventricular function, intrathoracic pressure, intraabdominal pressure, and venous compliance. Overall, CVP is an unreliable estimate of volume status and a poor predictor of fluid responsiveness.[37,38]

Mixed venous oxygen saturation (or SvO_2) is a measurement of the oxygen saturation of pooled blood from the entire postcapillary venous system in the body and, therefore, represents the balance between oxygen supply and demand. As SvO_2 requires more invasive monitoring with a pulmonary artery catheter, central mixed venous oxygen saturation ($ScvO_2$) is often used as a substitute.[39] It is measured from superior vena cava blood drawn through a central venous catheter. It is less accurate than SvO_2 (typically 3% to 5% higher) as it only reflects oxygen saturation of venous blood from the upper half of the body. Mixed venous saturation is decreased in patients with low cardiac output or other low flow states, but is usually normal or elevated (>65%) in distributive shock.[40] Elevated mixed venous saturation is an indication of underlying cytopathic hypoxia and microcirculatory shunting.[14,41]

A pulmonary artery (PA) catheter is often used in patients with cardiogenic shock but is rarely used for those in distributive shock. In addition to the measurement of SvO_2, multiple useful parameters can be collected from the PA catheter, including PA pressures, pulmonary capillary wedge pressure (PCWP), cardiac output/cardiac index, and systemic vascular resistance (SVR). It can be particularly helpful in situations in which the etiology of shock is unclear (i.e., distinguishing between cardiogenic and

TABLE 21.2 Sequential Organ Failure Assessment (SOFA) Score

Variables/Scores	0	1	2	3	4
Respiratory (PaO₂/FiO₂, mm Hg)	>400	≤400	≤300	≤200	≤100
Coagulation (platelets × 10³/µL)	>150	≤150	≤100	≤50	≤20
Liver (bilirubin, mg/dL)	<1.2	1.2–1.9	2–5.9	6–11.9	>12
CNS (Glasgow Coma Scale)	15	13–14	10–12	6–9	<6
Renal (creatinine, mg/dL, or urine output, mL/d)	<1.2	1.2–1.9	2–3.4	3.5–4.9 or UOP <500	>5 or UOP <200
Cardiovascular	MAP ≥70 mm Hg	MAP <70 mm Hg	Dopamine ≤5 or dobutamine (any dose), µg/kg/min	Dopamine >5, epinephrine ≤0.1, or norepinephrine ≤0.1, µg/kg/min	Dopamine >15, epinephrine >0.1, or norepinephrine >0.1, µg/kg/min

CNS, Central nervous system; *MAP*, mean arterial pressure; *UOP*, urine output.

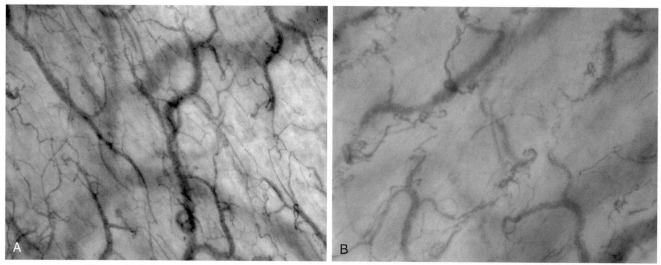

Fig. 21.3 Sidestream dark-field videos of sublingual microcirculation from (A) a healthy patient with well-perfused capillaries and (B) a septic patient with diminished capillary density and increased perfusion heterogeneity. (Courtesy Michael Massey, PhD, and Nathan Shapiro, MD, Beth Israel Deaconess Medical Center, Harvard Medical School.)

distributive shock) or mixed. In distributive shock, the expected PCWP is normal or low, SVR is low, and cardiac output is normal or high. While PA catheters may provide additional information, they have not been shown to improve survival or other outcomes in ICU patients.[42,43]

Assessment of Microcirculation

As discussed previously, microcirculatory blood flow may be compromised even in the setting of normal blood pressures.[28,29] Therefore the current standard measurements of end-organ perfusion may be inadequate. Imaging techniques have been developed to evaluate microcirculation more directly, such as orthogonal polarization spectral (OPS), sidestream dark field (SDF), and incident dark field (IDF) imaging[44] (Fig. 21.3, Video 21.1). These noninvasive techniques use videomicroscopy in order to determine vascular density and heterogeneity of perfusion. Laser Dopplers can also be used to evaluate tissue perfusion as well as microvascular reactivity to transient ischemia by measuring dynamic tissue blood flow.[44]

In addition, tissue perfusion can be indirectly evaluated by near-infrared spectroscopy (NIRS), which uses near-infrared light to measure tissue oxygen saturation.[44] Another method is to utilize tissue carbon dioxide partial pressure (PCO_2), which reflects the balance between tissue metabolism and tissue perfusion. An elevated gap between tissue PCO_2 and arterial PCO_2 is an indication of tissue hypoxia.[44]

While management directed by microcirculatory abnormalities would be helpful in theory, these techniques are not yet widely available or practical in application.

MANAGEMENT

While the majority of the literature pertaining to management of distributive shock focuses on septic shock, many of the same principles can be applied to other types of distributive shock.

Early goal-directed therapy (EGDT) refers to the protocol of early fluid resuscitation and use of vasopressors within the first 6 hours of presentation.[45] This was developed for the management of septic shock. The evidence for optimal targets of therapy is conflicting, but the goal is to target MAP of 65 mm Hg or greater, urine output 0.5 mL/kg per hour or greater, CVP 8 to 12 mm Hg, ScVO_2 70% or greater, or SVO_2 65% or greater. The implementation of this protocol was based on a single randomized, controlled trial that showed mortality benefit in patients assigned to EGDT compared to those assigned to standard care.[46] However, subsequent trials have failed to demonstrate mortality benefit with the EGDT protocol.[47–49]

Fluid Resuscitation

Fluid resuscitation is essential in the initial management of distributive shock. The goal is to improve tissue perfusion and cardiac output in the case of reduced left ventricular preload. Prolonged hypotension is associated with increased mortality in septic shock.[50,51] Two main types of fluids are used in shock: crystalloids and colloids. Crystalloid solutions, usually saline solutions or Ringer's lactate, are widely available and relatively inexpensive. Therefore they are typically the first choice for fluid resuscitation. Colloid solutions, such as albumin, have the theoretical advantage of more effective intravascular volume expansion and a decreased risk of pulmonary edema. More colloid solution remains in the intravascular space than crystalloid solution. However, there has been no evidence that using colloid over crystalloid solutions improves mortality.[52–54] Rapid infusion of fluids is important for volume repletion, but this must be monitored carefully as patients with sepsis are at risk of developing acute respiratory distress syndrome (ARDS).

Pharmacologic Support

Treatment with vasopressors should not be delayed in patients with distributive shock, especially if they are not fluid responsive

TABLE 21.3 Vasopressors and Inotropes in Shock

Vasopressor/Inotrope	Dose	Effects
Norepinephrine: strong α_1, β_1 agonist, weak β_2 agonist	0.02–3 µg/kg/min	Vasoconstriction, ↑MAP, ↑CO, ↑SVR
Epinephrine: strong α_1, β_1, β_2 agonist	0.05–2 µg/kg/min	↑MAP, ↑SVR, ↑HR, ↑CO
Dopamine: dopamine agonist, β_1 agonist (low doses), α_1 agonist (high doses)	2–20 µg/kg/min	Dose-dependent ↑HR, ↑CO, ↑MAP
Phenylephrine: strong α_1 agonist	0.5–4 µg/kg/min	Vasoconstriction, ↑MAP, ↑SVR
Vasopressin	0.04 U/min	Vasoconstriction, ↑MAP, ↑SVR
Dobutamine: strong β_1, weak β_2 agonist	2.5–20 µg/kg/min	↑CO, ↑HR, ↓SVR
Milrinone: phosphodiesterase inhibitor	0.125–0.75 µg/kg/min	↑CO, ↑HR, ↓SVR, ↓PVR
Levosimendan: calcium sensitizer	0.05–0.2 µg/kg/min	↑CO, ↓SVR

CO, Cardiac output; *HR,* heart rate; *MAP,* mean arterial pressure; *PVR,* pulmonary vascular resistance; *SVR,* systemic vascular resistance.

(Table 21.3). The goal is to maintain MAP at 65 mm Hg or greater[45] for preservation of end-organ perfusion. Multiple studies have investigated the efficacy of different blood pressure targets; there is no evidence that targeting higher MAP goals (75 to 85 mm Hg) is superior to lower MAP goals (65 to 70 mm Hg).[55–57] In a randomized controlled trial, the efficacy of low-target MAP (65 to 70 mm Hg) versus high-target MAP (80 to 85 mm Hg) on mortality was studied in 776 patients with septic shock.[58] There were no significant differences in mortality at either 28 or 90 days. Of note, a subgroup analysis of patients with chronic hypertension demonstrated that the high MAP target was associated with better renal function. However, the high MAP group also had higher incidences of atrial fibrillation, likely related to the higher doses of vasopressors required.

The vasoactive agent of choice is norepinephrine, which has predominantly α_1-adrenergic properties resulting in potent vasoconstriction along with modest β_1-adrenergic effects that assist in maintaining cardiac output. Dopamine is a vasopressor that has predominantly β-adrenergic activity at lower doses and α-adrenergic activity at higher doses. It also acts on dopamine-1 receptors, which selectively dilate splanchnic and renal blood supply, although there is no clear clinical evidence of renal protection. Epinephrine has both α- and β-adrenergic activity, with predominantly β_1-adrenergic stimulation at lower doses. Phenylephrine is a pure α-adrenergic agonist and therefore mainly causes vasoconstriction without significant effect on cardiac output.

A multicenter, randomized trial comparing dopamine versus norepinephrine as the first-line vasopressor in patients with shock showed no significant differences in mortality, but dopamine was associated with more adverse events.[5] A recent meta-analysis including 11 randomized trials comparing norepinephrine to dopamine demonstrated that the use of norepinephrine led to decreased mortality and decreased risk of major adverse events and arrhythmias.[59] In the comparison of norepinephrine to epinephrine, there was no mortality difference but there was evidence of increased adverse events with epinephrine use.[59,60] Phenylephrine is rarely used in distributive shock, as there is sparse literature on its benefits.

In patients with septic shock, there is often a relative vasopressin deficiency,[61,62] although the significance of this unclear. Vasopressin or terlipressin may be added as an additional agent to norepinephrine. It may be particularly beneficial in patients

with significant tachycardia or tachyarrhythmias, as it spares β-adrenergic activation. However, it should be avoided in patients with evidence of end-organ ischemia, as it causes splanchnic vasoconstriction. Clinical trials have not demonstrated any benefit in the outcomes of vasopressin compared to norepinephrine.[63,64] Subgroup analysis in the Vasopressin and Septic Shock Trial (VASST) indicated that the addition of vasopressin to the regimens of patients receiving less than 15 µg/min of norepinephrine appeared to improve survival.[63]

As discussed previously, myocardial depression occurs in certain patients with septic shock, although cardiac output is usually preserved by compensatory mechanisms. Dobutamine is an inotropic agent with predominantly β_1-adrenergic activity and vasodilatory effects. The use of dobutamine to augment cardiac output has not been demonstrated to improve outcomes in septic shock.[65,66]

Levosimendan, a calcium sensitizer, is a potential alternative to dobutamine in sepsis-induced cardiomyopathy. Myocardial desensitization to calcium plays an important role in the pathophysiology of myocardial depression in the setting of septic shock. There is evidence that levosimendan is more efficacious than dobutamine in these patients,[67,68] although large randomized controlled trials are still required to confirm its enhanced efficacy.

Targeted Therapies

Septic Shock. Antibiotics should be administered immediately when septic shock is suspected. Every hour of delay in initiation of antibiotic therapy is associated with a significant increase in mortality.[69] Cultures should be drawn before antibiotics when possible in order to guide therapy. In addition to antibiotic treatment, source control of the infection is essential, such as debridement of infected tissues, drainage of abscesses, and removal of infected devices. Early source control within the first 6 to 12 hours is critical in improving the chances of survival.[70–72]

"Stress-dose steroids" are routinely used in patients with septic shock (usually 50 mg IV hydrocortisone every 6 hours), based on the concept that patients in septic shock have relative adrenal insufficiency. However, evidence of clinical benefit is conflicting and it is unclear what levels of cortisol production would be considered optimal in these conditions. The Corticosteroid Therapy of Septic Shock (CORTICUS) study demonstrated no mortality benefit from stress-dose steroids compared to placebo in patients either with or without response to adrenocorticotropic hormone (ACTH) stimulation tests.[73] While there appeared to be more rapid reversal of shock in the hydrocortisone group, increased rates of superinfection occurred in this group. Systematic reviews of stress-dose steroids have revealed conflicting data in terms of mortality benefit.[74,75] The current guidelines recommend the use of intravenous hydrocortisone at a dose of 200 mg/day only if unable to achieve hemodynamic stability with adequate fluid resuscitation and vasopressor therapy.[45]

The rationale behind using intravenous immunoglobulin (IVIG) is that it binds endotoxin. Most trials investigating IVIG are small. The Score-based Immunoglobulin G Therapy of Patients with sepsis (SBITS) trial showed no evidence of mortality benefit at 28 days.[76] Meta-analyses have found conflicting evidence on the outcomes of IVIG in septic shock.[77–80] Any mortality benefit that was shown disappeared when low-quality trials were excluded. The prevailing recommendation is against the use of IVIG.[45]

Other adjunctive treatments under investigation for septic shock include blood purification, interferon-γ, and granulocyte-macrophage colony-stimulating factor (GM-CSF). These and other alternative therapies that have shown potential benefits in animal studies are purely experimental at this time in humans and require further investigation.[45]

Anaphylactic Shock.

In a study of fatal anaphylactic reactions, the median time to respiratory or cardiac arrest was 30 minutes for foods, 15 minutes for venom, and 5 minutes for iatrogenic reactions.[81] Airway, breathing, and circulation need to be assessed promptly and managed accordingly. Immediate recognition of anaphylaxis and rapid infusion of epinephrine is crucial. Intramuscular (IM) preparation is most commonly used, administered as 0.3 to 0.5 mg of the 1 mg/mL preparation. This can be repeated every 5 to 15 minutes as needed. If symptoms are severe and the patient is unresponsive to IM injections, IV epinephrine (0.1 mg/mL) infusion can be initiated at 0.1 μg/kg per minute and uptitrated as needed. Treatment also includes rapid infusion of IV fluids, as severe intravascular volume depletion is common in anaphylactic shock due to significant fluid shifts from increased vascular permeability.

Adjunctive therapies include inhaled albuterol for the treatment of bronchospasm. Antihistamines, both H_1- and H_2-blockers, may provide relief for pruritus and urticaria but do not alleviate airway obstruction or shock. The onset of action is typically 30 to 40 minutes and, thus, not immediately helpful. Usual dosing is 25 to 50 mg IV diphenhydramine and 50 mg IV ranitidine. Similarly, glucocorticoids have a long onset of action (up to several hours) and are not beneficial in the immediate setting. Glucocorticoids are typically administered in order to theoretically help prevent biphasic reactions, although this has not been confirmed.[82-83] A dose of 125 mg IV methylprednisolone may be administered as an adjunct to a total of 1 to 2 mg/kg per day for 1 to 2 days.

For patients with refractory anaphylaxis, IV epinephrine infusion may be initiated as discussed. These patients may also require the addition of a second vasoactive agent. Patients who are on

β-blockers may be resistant to epinephrine administration. This subset of patients may be given glucagon, which has inotropic and chronotropic properties that are not dependent on β-receptors.[84] Glucagon is administered as a 1- to 5-mg IV bolus, which may be followed by infusion of 5 to 15 μg/min. An alternative therapy is methylene blue, which inhibits nitric oxide synthase and guanylate cyclase and, in turn, induces vasoconstriction. Methylene blue may be administered as a bolus of 1 to 2 mg/kg, although dosing is not standardized. The rationale for this therapy is largely based on anecdotal evidence and case reports.[85] Finally, in severe refractory cases, extracorporeal membrane oxygenation (ECMO) can be used as supportive care.

Neurogenic Shock.

Fluid resuscitation and vasopressor therapy are the mainstay of initial management in patients with neurogenic shock. Blood pressure goals are different than those recommended for septic shock, although the supporting data are not strong. Guidelines recommend a target MAP of 85 to 90 mm Hg or greater.[86–88] IV fluids should be initiated but monitored closely, as fluid overload can lead to exacerbation of brain or spinal cord swelling. Neurogenic shock may be accompanied by bradycardia, for which atropine can be administered. Phenylephrine should be avoided, as it could result in significant reflex bradycardia. Dopamine and epinephrine may be favored due to their chronotropic effects. In severe cases of bradycardia or complete heart block, patients may require a pacemaker.

In addition to surgical intervention, glucocorticoids may be considered. Empiric data on the benefits of glucocorticoid therapy are limited.[89–92] Their use remains controversial; the potential risks versus benefits must be weighed before considering administration. The usual dose is IV methylprednisolone 30 mg/kg bolus, followed by infusion of 5.4 mg/kg per hour for 23 hours. Therapy should only be initiated within 8 hours of injury.[89]

Modulation of Microcirculation

Microcirculatory abnormalities are central to the pathophysiology of distributive shock. There are multiple potential points along the microcirculatory pathways that may be targeted during the management of distributive shock (Fig. 21.4). The use of vasodilator agents to manipulate microcirculatory blood flow has not been extensively studied. Theoretically, vasodilator therapy can enhance recruitment of the microcirculation and minimize shunting, resulting in improved local tissue perfusion. Potential agents include prostacyclin, nitroglycerin, and dobutamine. Both prostacyclin and nitroglycerin have demonstrated improvement in microcirculatory blood flow along with oxygen delivery (DO_2) and oxygen consumption (VO_2) in patients with septic shock who have been adequately resuscitated.[93–98] The trials are small and administration of these agents is limited by the potential worsening of arterial hypotension. Dobutamine has also been shown to improve both DO_2 and VO_2 in small clinical studies.[93,99–101]

The exact clinical significance of using vasodilator agents in distributive shock has yet to be elucidated. While microcirculatory flow is important, modulation with vasodilators is restricted by macrocirculatory and hemodynamic parameters. Further research is necessary to evaluate the impact of novel therapies that target the microcirculation in distributive shock.

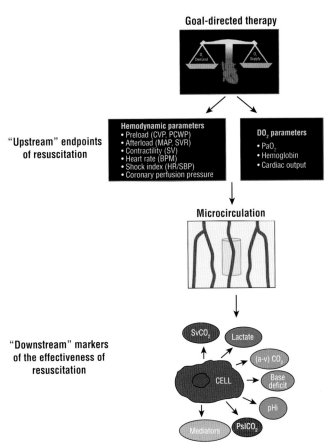

Fig. 21.4 Multiple upstream endpoints of resuscitation may be targeted in the modulation of microcirculation. The efficacy of management can be monitored by various downstream markers of tissue perfusion. *BPM*, Beats per minute; *CVP*, central venous pressure; *DO₂*, oxygen delivery; *HR*, heart rate; *MAP*, mean arterial pressure; *PCWP*, pulmonary capillary wedge pressure; *pHi*, gastric intramucosal pH; *SBP*, systolic blood pressure; *PslCO₂*, sublingual pCO₂; *SV*, stroke volume; *SvO₂*, mixed venous oxygen saturation; *SVR*, systemic vascular resistance. (From Trzeciak S, Rivers EP. Clinical manifestations of disordered microcirculatory perfusion in severe sepsis. *Crit Care.* 2005;9:S23.)

PROGNOSIS

Severe sepsis and septic shock are commonly encountered in patients in the ICU, which result in significant morbidity and mortality. Mortality rates can be anywhere from 10% to 52% depending on the study.[6–8,102–112] Studies have also demonstrated that increased severity of the sepsis corresponds with increased rates of mortality, especially in the presence of shock.[113–115] Recently, several epidemiologic studies have shown a trend of declining mortality among patients with septic shock.[7,8,104–106] While some of the evidence suggests that this trend is at least in part due to improved therapeutic strategies, it is difficult to confirm that correlation.

There are multiple scoring systems used to predict outcomes in patients in the ICU. The Acute Physiologic and Chronic Health Evaluation (APACHE) scoring system is widely recognizable and standardized for general ICU patients in the United States. The most updated version, the APACHE-IV, uses 129 variables collected within the first 24 hours of admission. The ability of APACHE-IV to predict mortality and length of ICU stay has been validated, and appears to be superior to other ICU scoring systems.[116–119]

The SOFA scoring system was originally developed to assess organ failure in patients with sepsis in the ICU.[34] The multiorgan system variables are collected 24 hours after ICU admission and every 48 hours afterward. The mean, peak, and increase in scores are all predictive of mortality. Patients in septic shock, defined as a SOFA score greater than or equal to 2 with vasopressor requirement and elevated lactate (>2 mmol/L) despite adequate fluid resuscitation, have a predicted mortality of approximately 40%.[114,120]

CONCLUSION

The range of diseases treated in the CICU has significantly broadened over the 50 years since the initiation of the original CCUs. The prevalence of distributive shock, specifically septic shock, is increasing in the CICU. Early treatment has significant impact on outcome. Therefore, it is important for physicians to promptly recognize and treat these conditions. Mortality continues to be high in patients with distributive shock despite well-established guidelines of management. Novel therapies, including those directed at addressing microcirculatory abnormalities, require further investigation in order to improve the outcomes in patients with distributive shock.

The full reference list for this chapter is available at ExpertConsult.com.

Cardiorenal Syndrome Type 1

David L. Brown

Various organ systems within the body are intimately connected to each other and communicate via organ crosstalk, the complex biologic communication and feedback between organ systems mediated by soluble and cellular messengers. In the normal state, this crosstalk helps to maintain homeostasis and optimal function of the body and all its component systems. However, during disease, this crosstalk can transfer signals from the diseased organ that initiate and perpetuate dysfunction in other organs.[1,2]

DEFINITION AND CLASSIFICATION

Combined disorders of the heart and kidney are referred to as cardiorenal syndromes (CRSs) and have been defined as "a complex pathophysiological disorder of the heart and the kidneys whereby acute or chronic dysfunction in one organ may induce acute or chronic dysfunction in the other organ."[3] The CRSs are classified into four subtypes based on the primary organ that is dysfunctional, either "cardiorenal" syndromes (types 1 or 2) or "renocardiac" syndromes (types 3 or 4) and whether the organ dysfunction is acute (types 1 and 3) or chronic (types 2 and 4). A fifth subtype is characterized by simultaneous cardiac and renal dysfunction in the setting of a systemic illness. The five subtypes are summarized in Table 22.1.[3] The temporal sequence of the organ dysfunction and which problem predominates can also be used to distinguish types 1 or 2 (cardiac first) from types 3 or 4 (renal first).[4] Furthermore, the classification is not static, as patients may transition between different CRS subtypes both in and out of the hospital.[5] For example, a patient with chronic congestive heart failure (CHF) and chronic kidney disease (CKD) who is considered to have CRS type 2 may develop acute decompensated heart failure (ADHF) requiring hospitalization complicated by acute kidney injury (AKI); the patient would then be diagnosed with CRS type 1. Successful treatment of the ADHF with resolution of the AKI will return the patient to CRS type 2. Likewise, the same patient could progress to end-stage renal disease and develop acute pulmonary edema requiring

emergent dialysis, in which case the diagnosis would be CRS type 3. In the cardiac intensive care unit (CICU) environment, the most commonly encountered CRS is type 1, which will be the focus of this chapter.

CRS type 1 is characterized by an acute deterioration in cardiac function that then leads to a reduction in glomerular filtration rate (GFR) and AKI (Fig. 22.1). The most common precipitants of acute cardiac dysfunction in the CICU that result in AKI are cardiogenic shock, ADHF, acute myocardial infarction (MI), acute mitral or aortic regurgitation, pericardial tamponade, constrictive pericarditis, or prolonged arrhythmias with associated hypotension or cardiogenic shock. For any given patient, there are four patterns of CRS type 1: (1) de novo cardiac injury leading to de novo kidney injury; (2) de novo cardiac injury leading to acute-on-chronic kidney injury; (3) acute on chronic cardiac decompensation leading to de novo kidney injury; and (4) acute-on-chronic cardiac decompensation leading to acute-on-chronic kidney injury.[4]

PREVALENCE

CRS type 1 has been described in 27% to 45% of hospitalized patients with ADHF[6–12] and in 9% to 54% of patients with acute coronary syndromes (ACS).[13–19] Of patients with preexisting CKD who present with ADHF, approximately 60% will develop AKI.[4] AKI can be present on admission or can develop after admission. Approximately 20% to 30% of heart failure patients develop an increase in serum creatinine of more than 0.3 mg/dL[9,20–23] following admission. The rise in serum creatinine usually occurs in the first 3 to 5 days of hospitalization for ADHF.[24]

PROGNOSIS

The development of CRS type 1 is associated with worse clinical outcomes, more rehospitalizations, and greater health care expenditures.[11,12,15,25] The mortality risk associated with CRS type

TABLE 22.1	Classification of the Cardiorenal Syndromes		
Class	**Type**	**Description**	**Examples**
1	Acute cardiorenal syndrome	Acute worsening of cardiac function resulting in AKI	ADHF Cardiac surgery Acute coronary syndromes CIN
2	Chronic cardiorenal syndrome	Chronic abnormalities of cardiac function leading to CKD	Hypertension CHF
3	Acute renocardiac syndrome	Abrupt worsening of renal function leading to acute cardiac dysfunction	Acute pulmonary edema in AKI Arrhythmia due to acidosis or electrolyte abnormalities or volume overload CIN leading to CHF
4	Chronic renocardiac syndrome	CKD leading to chronic cardiac dysfunction	Left ventricular hypertrophy in CKD
5	Secondary cardiorenal syndrome	Systemic disorders causing cardiac and renal dysfunction	Sepsis Systemic lupus erythematosus Diabetes

ADHF, acute decompensated heart failure; *AKI,* acute kidney injury; *CHF,* congestive heart failure; *CIN,* contrast-induced nephropathy; *CKD,* chronic kidney disease.
Modified from Cruz DN. Cardiorenal syndrome in critical care: the acute cardiorenal and renocardiac syndromes. *Adv Chronic Kidney Dis.* 2013; 20:56–66.

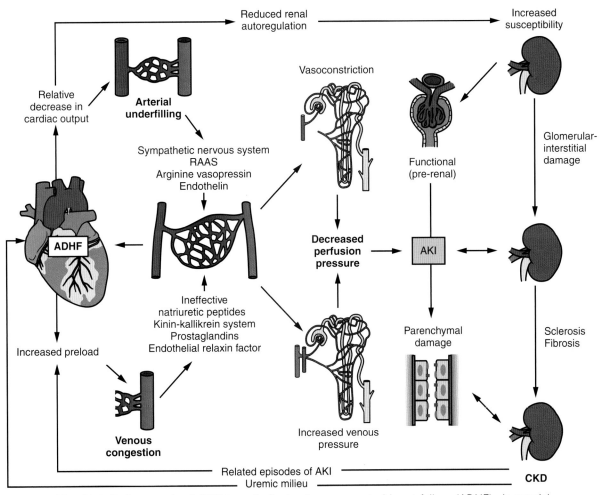

Fig. 22.1 Pathogenesis of CRS type 1. Acute decompensated heart failure (ADHF) via arterial underfilling and venous congestion sets off a series of changes in neurohormonal and hemodynamic factors that culminate in acute kidney injury (AKI). *CKD,* Chronic kidney disease; *CRS,* cardiorenal syndrome; *RAAS,* renin-angiotensin-aldosterone system. (Modified from Ronco C, Cicoira M, McCullough PA. Cardiorenal syndrome type 1. Pathophysiological crosstalk leading to combined heart and kidney dysfunction in the setting of acute decompensated heart failure. *J Am Coll Cardiol.* 2012;60:1031–1042.)

1 is most pronounced early[25] but an increased risk of death has been observed 10 years after the index hospitalization for acute MI patients who develop AKI.[18] Furthermore, a biologic gradient has been observed between the severity of CRS type 1 and mortality risk.[17,25]

In ADHF, any reduction in GFR is generally associated with a worse prognosis, whether it is present at baseline or develops during treatment. A systematic review of 16 studies including more than 80,000 patients with heart failure[20] categorized renal function as normal (estimated GFR [eGFR] 90 mL/min or higher), mildly impaired (eGFR 53 to 89 mL/min), or moderately to severely impaired (eGFR <53 mL/min). The mortality rate at a follow-up of 1 year or more was 24% in those with a normal eGFR compared with 38% and 51% in patients with mild and moderate to severe reductions in eGFR, respectively (adjusted hazard ratios, 1.6 and 2.3, respectively). It is estimated that mortality increases by approximately 15% for every 10 mL/min reduction in eGFR. However, the relationship between change in GFR and prognosis is complex. Patients with improving renal function may also experience worse outcomes. Fluctuating renal function may reflect a sicker cohort of patients with significantly worse survival than those with stable renal function. An analysis of 401 patients enrolled in the Evaluation Study of Congestive Heart Failure and Pulmonary Artery Catheterization Effectiveness (ESCAPE) trial found that patients with an improvement or a decline in estimated GFR during treatment of ADHF had similar outcomes.[26] Compared to patients with a stable GFR, those with either an improvement or a decline in GFR were significantly more likely to have a reduced cardiac index and to require intravenous inotrope and vasodilator therapy. These patients also experienced a significantly higher rate of all-cause mortality.

Additionally, the mechanism of worsening renal function in heart failure impacts its prognostic significance. An analysis of 6337 subjects enrolled in the Studies of Left Ventricular Dysfunction (SOLVD) trial showed that early worsening of renal function was associated with increased mortality in the overall population.[27] However, in the enalapril group, early worsening of renal function was not associated with increased mortality, while in the placebo group, the association with mortality was significant. A significant survival benefit from enalapril therapy was observed in patients who continued enalapril despite early worsening renal function. These findings suggest that worsening renal function is not always a marker of adverse clinical outcome. On the contrary, in the case of angiotensin-converting enzyme (ACE) inhibitor administration, it is a manifestation of the agent's pharmacologic properties, which exert a favorable effect on long-term outcome.

RISK FACTORS

Several predisposing risk factors for CRS type 1 have been identified. Nonmodifiable risk factors include a history of diabetes, prior admissions for ADHF or MI, and more severe cardiac dysfunction at the time of presentation (pulmonary edema, tachyarrhythmias, worse Killip class or lower ejection fraction).[10,13,14,28] Impaired kidney function on admission has consistently been associated with higher risk for CRS type 1. Modifiable risk factors include

high doses of diuretics (e.g., daily furosemide dose >100 mg/day or in-hospital use of thiazides) and/or vasodilator therapy as well as higher contrast volumes (e.g., contrast media volume-to-creatinine clearance ratio [V/CrCl] >3.7) during cardiac catheterization and intervention.[6,7,10,12,24,29,30]

DIAGNOSIS

Among patients with heart failure who have an elevated serum creatinine and/or a reduced estimated GFR, it is important to distinguish between underlying kidney disease and impaired kidney function due to CRS type 1.[31] This distinction may be difficult since many patients have both. Findings suggestive of underlying kidney disease include significant proteinuria (usually >1000 mg/day), an active urine sediment with hematuria with or without pyuria or cellular casts, and/or small kidneys on radiologic evaluation. However, a normal urinalysis, which is typically present in CRS without underlying kidney disease, can also be seen in variety of renal diseases, including nephrosclerosis and obstructive nephropathy.[31] Ultimately, the diagnosis of CRS type 1 is made retrospectively after treatment to improve cardiac performance results in improvement in renal function.

PATHOPHYSIOLOGY

ADHF may reduce GFR by several mechanisms, including neurohumoral adaptations, reduced renal perfusion, increased renal venous pressure, and right ventricular (RV) dysfunction[32–35] (see Fig. 22.1). In addition, exposure to nephrotoxins may precipitate CRS type 1. The pathophysiology of CRS type 1 may vary at different time points during a single hospitalization. For example, early in a CICU admission, AKI may be related to a low cardiac output state and/or marked increase in central venous pressure (CVP). However, later in the hospital course, exposure to nephrotoxins—such as contrast media or medications that impair renal perfusion, including nonsteroidal antiinflammatory drugs (NSAIDs) or ACE inhibitors—may contribute to the development of CRS type 1. Iatrogenic causes of CRS type 1 are presented in Fig. 22.2.

Impaired LV function leads to several hemodynamic derangements, including reduced stroke volume and cardiac output, arterial underfilling, elevated atrial pressures, and venous congestion.[36] These hemodynamic derangements trigger a variety of compensatory neurohormonal adaptations, including activation of the sympathetic nervous system and the renin-angiotensin-aldosterone system and increases in the release of vasopressin and endothelin-1, which promote salt and water retention as well as systemic vasoconstriction. These pathways lead to the disproportionate reabsorption of urea compared with that of creatinine.[37–39] In the setting of ADHF, blood urea nitrogen therefore represents a surrogate marker of neurohormonal activation.[40,41] These adaptations overwhelm the vasodilatory and natriuretic effects of natriuretic peptides, nitric oxide, prostaglandins, and bradykinin.[11,34,42]

In the short term, neurohumoral adaptations contribute to preservation of perfusion to vital organs (the brain and heart) by maintenance of systemic pressure via arterial vasoconstriction

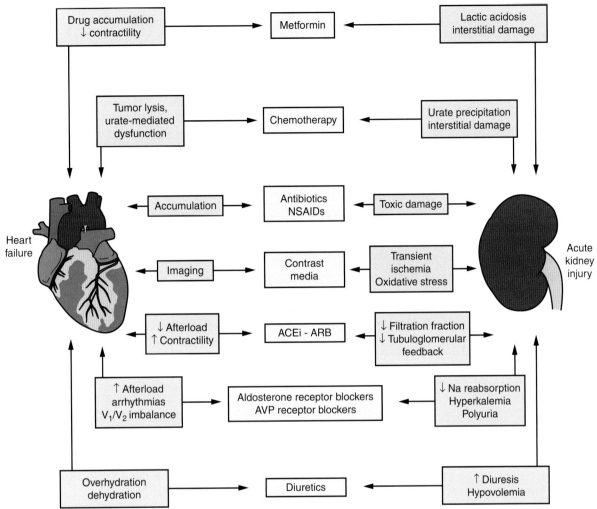

Fig. 22.2 Iatrogenic causes of CRS type 1. Multiple sources of iatrogenic injury, some of which may be unavoidable, can result in either cardiac, renal, or cardiorenal impairment and kidney damage in patients with acutely decompensated heart failure (ADHF). *ACEi,* Angiotensin-converting enzyme inhibitor; *ARB,* angiotensin receptor blocker; *AVP,* arginine vasopressin; *NSAIDs,* nonsteroidal antiinflammatory drugs. (Modified from Ronco C, Cicoira M, McCullough PA. Cardiorenal syndrome type 1. Pathophysiological crosstalk leading to combined heart and kidney dysfunction in the setting of acute decompensated heart failure. *J Am Coll Cardiol.* 2012;60:1031–1042.)

in other circulations, including the renal circulation, and by increasing myocardial contractility and heart rate. However, over the long term, systemic vasoconstriction increases cardiac afterload and reduces cardiac output, which can further reduce renal perfusion. The maladaptive nature of these adaptations is evidenced by the slowing of disease progression and reduction in mortality with the administration of ACE inhibitors and β-blockers in patients with heart failure and reduced ejection fraction.

In the absence of shock, impaired renal perfusion is an uncommon cause of CRS type 1 in ADHF. Hypotension is an uncommon finding in patients hospitalized for ADHF. In the Acute Decompensated Heart Failure National Registry (ADHERE) of over 100,000 patients, 50% had a systolic blood pressure of 140 mm Hg or higher, while less than 2% had a systolic blood pressure below 90 mm Hg.[22] ADHF patients with reduced ejection fraction have little or no reduction in cardiac output with loop diuretic therapy because they are on the flat part of the Frank-Starling curve, where changes in left ventricular end-diastolic pressure (LVEDP) have little or no effect on cardiac performance. Furthermore, the ESCAPE trial of 433 patients with ADHF[6] found no correlation between the cardiac index and either the baseline GFR or worsening kidney function. Increasing the cardiac index did not improve renal function after discharge. In contrast, patients with ADHF and preserved systolic function are on a steep Starling curve such that, for every unit reduction in LVEDP induced by diuresis, there is a significant fall in stroke volume. These patients are more sensitive to diuresis; excessive diuresis can reduce preload and cardiac output, leading to hypotension, a reduction in renal perfusion, and CRS type 1 (Fig. 22.3).

Increased intraabdominal or central venous pressure, which increases renal venous pressure, reduces GFR.[32,43] Raising the intraabdominal venous pressure to about 20 mm Hg reduces renal plasma flow and GFR of 24% and 28%, respectively, in

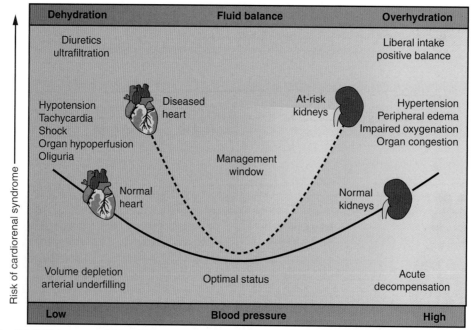

Fig. 22.3 Volume and blood pressure management window. Patients at risk for cardiorenal syndrome type 1 have a narrow window for management of both blood pressure and volume; extremes in either parameter can be associated with worsened renal function. (Modified from Ronco C, Cicoira M, McCullough PA. Cardiorenal syndrome type 1. Pathophysiological crosstalk leading to combined heart and kidney dysfunction in the setting of acute decompensated heart failure. *J Am Coll Cardiol*. 2012;60:1031–1042.)

normal adults.[44] Studies in heart failure patients demonstrate an inverse relationship between venous pressure and GFR when the central venous pressure was measured directly[45–47] or elevated jugular venous pressure was diagnosed on physical examination.[48]

RV dilation and dysfunction may adversely affect kidney function through at least two mechanisms[31]: (1) the associated elevation in CVP elevation can lower the GFR; and (2) RV dilation impairs LV filling and, therefore, forward output, via ventricular interdependence (the reverse Bernheim phenomenon).[49] Increased pressure within a distended RV increases LV extramural pressure, reducing LV transmural pressure for any given intracavitary LV pressure and inducing leftward interventricular septal bowing, thereby diminishing LV preload and distensibility and reducing stroke volume and forward flow.[50,51] An intact pericardium plays a role in ventricular interdependence but is not critical to the interaction.[52] Thus, a reduction in RV filling pressure during treatment of ADHF may lead to an increase in GFR, both by reducing renal venous pressure and by diminishing the impairment of LV filling.[53]

Some drugs commonly prescribed for the treatment of ADHF can also contribute to development of AKI by disturbing systemic and renal hemodynamics (see Fig. 22.2). Diuretics are recommended in ADHF to reduce dyspnea and edema, but their overuse may result in excessive intravascular volume depletion and further compromise kidney perfusion (see Fig. 22.3).[54,55] Diuretic resistance may also complicate the clinical picture of CRS type 1 by acutely or chronically increasing sodium retention.[56] ACE inhibitors, angiotensin receptor blockers (ARBs), and aldosterone receptor antagonists are guideline-directed therapies for heart failure[57] because these drugs have been shown to significantly improve survival of these patients.[58–64] However, they affect renal hemodynamics, and their use must be carefully monitored to avoid the development of AKI in decompensated patients.

Another important iatrogenic nephrotoxin in ADHF and ACS is iodinated contrast media commonly used for vascular imaging procedures (see Fig. 22.2). These agents induce intense and prolonged vasoconstriction at the corticomedullary junction of the kidney and directly impair the autoregulatory capacity of the kidney through a reduction in nitric oxide synthesis.[65,66] These effects, coupled with direct tubular toxicity of iodinated radiocontrast, can lead to overt acute tubular necrosis and AKI.

PREVENTION

CRS type 1 is a result of the interaction between complex pathogenic factors; once it becomes clinically apparent, it is difficult to abort and is often irreversible. Most important, CRS type 1 is associated with adverse outcomes, even if the AKI resolves.[11,15] Thus, prevention of CRS is paramount in clinical practice with an aim to identify and avoid precipitating factors as well as to use measures to maintain optimal functioning of the heart and kidneys. This may involve multimodality and multidisciplinary preventive strategies, working via diverse therapeutic targets. Although evidence-based guidelines currently exist for management of ADHF,[67,68] ACS,[69–71] and AKI,[72] there are no clear recommendations for the management of CRS type 1.[73] The multitude of pathophysiologic interactions and their complexity render the management of CRS challenging.

BOX 22.1 Renoprotective Strategies in the Cardiac Intensive Care Unit

- Regular monitoring of fluid intake/output, urine output, renal function, blood pressure
- Accurate and frequent monitoring of volume status
- Hold ACE inhibitors/ARBs in patients with worsening renal function
- Optimize volume status
- Adjust diuretic doses based on volume status
- Pharmacovigilance (drug monitoring, avoid nephrotoxins, attention to drug interactions)
- Initial use of vasodilators (nitrates, hydralazine) in ADHF if blood pressure is adequate
- Avoid unnecessary use of iodinated contrast agents
- Optimize volume status before use of iodinated contrast agents
- Minimize volume of iodinated contrast agents

ACE, Angiotensin-converting enzyme; *ADHF,* acute decompensated heart failure; *ARBs,* angiotensin receptor blockers.
Modified from Cruz DN. Cardiorenal syndrome in critical care: the acute cardiorenal and renocardiac syndromes. *Adv Chronic Kidney Dis.* 2013;20:56–66.

Improving the natural history of heart failure and avoiding acute decompensation are the cornerstones of prevention of CRS type 1.[74] Strategies for prevention in these patients should follow those recommended by the American College of Cardiology/American Heart Association (ACC/AHA) for stage A and stage B heart failure.[75] These include coronary artery disease risk factor modification and avoidance of medications that may precipitate salt and water retention, including NSAIDs and thiazolidinediones. More important, use of renin-angiotensin-aldosterone system antagonists and β-blockers should be optimized. In patients with CKD, efforts must be made to cautiously introduce these cardioprotective agents with close monitoring of kidney function.

Another mainstay of prevention is to recognize patients at risk for CRS. Patients who develop CRS type 1 are generally older, have a history of previous hospitalizations for heart failure or MI, and often have baseline kidney dysfunction and hypertension. Risk prediction scores for AKI have been published for ADHF[24] for contrast-induced AKI after percutaneous coronary intervention,[76] after cardiac surgery,[77] and in hospitalized patients.[78] Such scoring systems can be used to recognize preemptively the patients at a high intrinsic risk of developing AKI. Renoprotective measures can then be selectively instituted in high-risk patients to reduce the risk of acute CRS[79] (Box 22.1).

MANAGEMENT

No medical therapies directly increase the GFR (manifested clinically by a decline in serum creatinine) in patients with heart failure. On the other hand, improving cardiac function can result in increases in GFR, indicating that CRS type 1 has substantial reversible components.[80]

AKI induced by primary cardiac dysfunction implies inadequate renal perfusion until proven otherwise.[81] Inadequate perfusion may be a consequence of a low cardiac output state, increased CVP leading to renal congestion, or both. Elevated CVP leading to renal venous hypertension is a product of right

heart function, blood volume, and venous capacitance—all of which are heavily influenced by neurohormonal systems.[4] A careful history and physical examination can usually differentiate a volume-depleted patient from one who is severely volume overloaded. Diuretics, typically beginning with a loop diuretic, are first-line therapy for managing volume overload in patients with ADHF as manifested by peripheral and/or pulmonary edema. In patients with heart failure, an elevated BUN/creatinine ratio should not deter diuretic therapy if clinical evidence of congestion is present.[80] That aggressive diuresis improves outcomes is suggested in two studies, ESCAPE[82] and Efficacy of Vasopressin Antagonism in Heart Failure Outcome Study with Tolvaptan (EVEREST),[83] in which hemoconcentration, an indicator of aggressive diuresis, was found to be associated with worsening of renal function in the hospital but an improvement in survival after discharge. These findings provide support for the recommendation included in the 2013 ACC/AHA heart failure guidelines that the goal of diuretic therapy is to eliminate clinical evidence of fluid retention, such as an elevated jugular venous pressure and peripheral edema.[84] The rapidity of diuresis can be slowed if the patient develops hypotension or worsening renal function. However, the goal of diuretic therapy is to eliminate fluid retention even if this leads to asymptomatic mild to moderate reductions in blood pressure or renal function.

The optimal diuretic regimen has not been determined in randomized controlled trials. Continuous intravenous infusion of diuretics has traditionally been considered more effective than bolus in severe ADHF.[85,86] However, in the recent Diuretic Optimization Strategies Evaluation (DOSE) randomized trial, there were no significant differences in patients' symptoms or in the change in kidney function when diuretic therapy was administered by bolus as compared with continuous infusion or at a high dose (2.5 times the previous outpatient oral dose) as compared with a low dose (equivalent to the previous oral dose).[87] The high-dose strategy was associated with greater diuresis and more favorable outcomes in some secondary measures but also with transient worsening of kidney function (23% vs. 14% in low dose, $P = .04$). It is frequently overlooked that the median hourly dose of furosemide by continuous infusion in the DOSE trial was only 5 mg in the low-dose arm and 10.7 mg in the high-dose arm. These doses are significantly below the 20- to 40 mg/h doses frequently required in CRS type 1 patients. In addition, ADHF patients with serum creatinine greater than 3 mg/dL were excluded from the DOSE trial. Those patients are more likely to need higher doses of furosemide and are more susceptible to develop CRS type 1 during hospitalization for ADHF.

Intravenous administration of inotropic drugs—such as dobutamine, dopamine, and milrinone—has a role in the treatment of patients who develop cardiogenic shock. However, both routine use of short-term intravenous therapy in patients with ADHF and prolonged therapy with oral inotropic drugs other than digoxin has been associated with an increase in mortality. As a result, the main role of inotropic drugs other than digoxin is in the management of cardiogenic shock. The role of inotropes in patients with CRS is uncertain and the routine use of inotropes is not recommended given their lack of proven efficacy and their association with adverse events when used in patients other than those with cardiogenic shock or ADHF who are deteriorating toward cardiogenic shock.[80]

Ultrafiltration is an alternative to loop diuretics for the management of fluid overload in patients with ADHF and worsening kidney function. The Ultrafiltration versus Intravenous Diuretics for Patients Hospitalized for Acute Decompensated Congestive Heart Failure (UNLOAD) trial randomized 200 ADHF patients to ultrafiltration or intravenous diuretics and found that ultrafiltration safely produced greater weight loss and fluid removal than intravenous diuretics and reduced readmissions for heart failure.[88] However, in the Cardiorenal Rescue Study in Acute Decompensated Heart Failure (CARRESS-HF) trial,[89] the use of a stepped pharmacologic-therapy algorithm was superior to a strategy of ultrafiltration for the preservation of renal function at 96 hours, with a similar amount of weight loss with the two approaches. Ultrafiltration was associated with a higher rate of adverse events. Thus, although ultrafiltration may be helpful for fluid removal in ADHF in patients unresponsive to diuretic therapy, the available evidence does not establish ultrafiltration as first-line therapy for ADHF or as an effective therapy for CRS type 1. The 2009 ACC/AHA guidelines state that ultrafiltration is reasonable for patients with refractory congestion not responding to medical therapy.[68]

Intravenous vasodilators used in the treatment of ADHF include nitroglycerin, nitroprusside, and nesiritide. In the ADHERE database of almost 100,000 patients, worsening of renal function was significantly more common when intravenous diuretics were given with nitroglycerin or nesiritide compared with intravenous diuretics alone (relative risk, 1.20 and 1.44, respectively).[90] However, a causal effect could not be distinguished from patients requiring combination therapy because they had worse heart failure.

There are no randomized trials of nitroglycerin or nitroprusside. Randomized trials have yielded conflicting results on the effect of nesiritide therapy on renal function in the treatment of ADHF. The largest trial, the Acute Study of Clinical Effectiveness of Nesiritide in Decompensated Heart Failure (ASCEND-HF), nesiritide was not associated with a worsening of renal function but was associated with increased rates of hypotension.[91] Similarly, the Renal Optimization Strategies Evaluation (ROSE) trial found that low-dose nesiritide did not enhance decongestion or alter renal function when added to diuretic therapy.[92] Overall, nesiritide has not been found to be of benefit in ADHF and it is not currently recommended for the prevention of AKI.[72]

SUMMARY

In summary, CRS type 1 is a complex and multidimensional entity that is commonly encountered in the CICU and has a significant effect on morbidity and mortality. Preventive strategies in general for all patients at risk for CRS type 1 will help decrease the incidence of AKI. The management of CRS type 1 is challenging because of the many complex pathophysiologic interactions between the heart and kidney. Although evidence-based guidelines currently exist for management of ADHF, ACS, and AKI, at present there are no clear recommendations for the management of CRS type 1.

The full reference list for this chapter is available at ExpertConsult.com.

23

Sudden Cardiac Death

Jodi Zilinski, Masood Akhtar

Cardiovascular disease is one of the most common causes of death, accounting for approximately 1 of every 2.9 deaths in the United States[1] and approximately 17 million deaths worldwide each year.[2] Of deaths due to a cardiovascular cause, more than 50% occur suddenly, making sudden cardiac death (SCD) one of the most common causes of death in the United States.[3] Despite advances in the understanding of cardiac pathophysiology, the implementation of primary and secondary prevention of sudden cardiac death, and improvements in resuscitation and postresuscitation care, SCD remains a major clinical and public health concern.

DEFINITION

There are multiple purported definitions for SCD; however, it is generally defined as the sudden cessation of cardiac activity associated with rapid hemodynamic collapse within 1 hour of the onset of symptoms in the absence of an apparent extracardiac cause.[4] Although sudden cardiac arrest (SCA) is used to describe a nonfatal cardiac event, SCD is conventionally used in the literature to define both fatal and nonfatal cardiac arrests. A limitation of this definition is that events are rarely witnessed, thus the duration of symptoms is not known in approximately one-third of cases. If the death is not witnessed, the term SCD still applies when the victim was observed to be in his or her usual state of health 24 hours before the event.[2]

EPIDEMIOLOGY

Estimates of the incidence of SCD vary widely depending on the source of data, definition used, and methods for extrapolation, ranging from 180,000 to greater than 450,000.[5,6] Low autopsy rates further limit the ability to determine the true incidence and cause of SCD. As the majority of out-of-hospital SCAs occur in individuals not monitored, the exact mechanism leading to a cardiovascular collapse is often difficult to establish. A cause is thus assigned on the basis of presentation and the earliest available rhythm recordings. In monitored victims and cases with a short

delay between the time of collapse and rhythm identification, ventricular fibrillation (VF) or ventricular tachycardia (VT) historically have been identified as the most common initial rhythms (observed approximately 75% to 80% of the time).[7] With advances in the treatment of coronary artery disease (CAD) and an increase in the use of prophylactic implantable cardioverter defibrillators (ICDs), VT/VF presently account for less than 30% of the initial rhythms identified during out-of-hospital cardiac arrests (OHCA). Rather, pulseless electrical activity (PEA) is increasingly identified as the initial rhythm, with some series observing PEA in 25% of OHCA events.[8] Another proposed explanation for the declining rates of VF being identified as the initial rhythm is that the aging population has increased comorbidities and modern treatments have increased the prevalence of end-stage cardiovascular disease. This results in older, sicker patients who are more likely to have acute triggers for PEA (i.e., metabolic, respiratory) and are less likely to sustain VT/VF until emergency medical services (EMS) arrival.[9] In the setting of unmonitored collapse, asystole is the most common initial rhythm. However, the initial rhythm correlates with the duration of the event as VF is seen early after collapse and degenerates to asystole as time passes (Fig. 23.1).

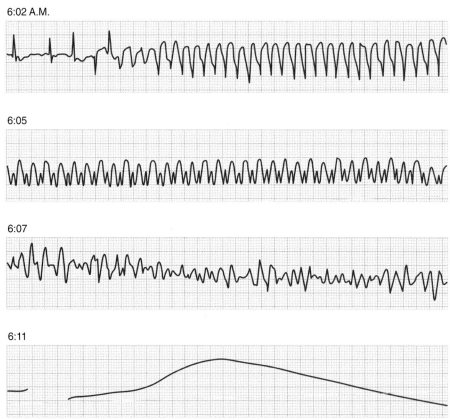

Fig. 23.1 Fortuitous Holter recording from a patient who experienced sudden cardiac death outside the hospital documents the usual and typical sequence of events. The initial rapid ventricular tachycardia continues into the second panel with widening of the QRS, probably owing to myocardial metabolic changes. Subsequent degeneration to ventricular fibrillation is shown in the third panel, followed by asystole in the fourth panel. The prognosis depends on the initial documented rhythm and how soon emergency personnel arrive to treat the individual. (Modified from National Heart, Lung, and Blood Institute. *What Is An Implantable Cardioverter Defibrillator?* https://www.nhlbi.nih.gov/health/health-topics/topics/icd.)

Recent advances in cardiopulmonary resuscitation (CPR) and postresuscitation care have improved survival rates from OHCA. A prospective clinical registry of OHCA survivors in the United States reported an increased survival rate to hospital discharge from 5.7% in 2005 to 8.3% in 2012.[10] Even with advances in the treatment of cardiovascular disease and improvements in the performance and availability of CPR, the long-term outcome of SCA victims remains poor, with the prognosis strongly influenced by the initial rhythm at the time of cardiac arrest. Survival rates are higher for individuals in whom VF is the initial rhythm, with approximately 30% surviving to hospital discharge. Nonshockable rhythms—such as PEA, bradycardia, or asystole—have been associated with poor long-term survival rates (8% for PEA).[7]

DEMOGRAPHICS

The risk of suffering an SCA varies with a number of factors, increases dramatically with age, and is overwhelmingly more common in the setting of underlying structural heart disease. The majority of SCDs occur in adults, with approximately 1% occurring in individuals younger than age 35 years.[5] However, the proportion of deaths that are sudden is elevated in younger age groups. The presence of underlying structural heart disease results in a 6- to 10-fold increase in the risk of SCA. Furthermore, SCD is the mechanism of death in approximately 60% of patients with known coronary heart disease (CHD)[11,12] and SCA is the initial clinical manifestation of CHD in 15% of patients.[13] Autopsy studies suggest that 21% to 45% of victims of SCD have a normal cardiac postmortem examination.[14,15]

The incidence of SCD also varies by sex and race. Men are 2 to 3 times more likely to experience SCA than women, even when adjusting for predisposing conditions.[16] Compared to men, women who experience a cardiac arrest are more likely to be older, to present with PEA, and to have a cardiac arrest at home.[17] In regard to survival from SCA, women—especially younger women—have increased rates of successful resuscitation and survival from shockable rhythms than men.[17,18]

Variations in rates of SCD and survival from SCA have been observed in different racial and ethnic populations. African Americans, as opposed to whites, have been documented to have higher rates of SCD and worse rates of survival from SCA, in part owing to their increased likelihood of suffering an unwitnessed cardiac arrest or documentation of PEA as the initial rhythm at the time of cardiac arrest.[19–21] However, this does not completely account for worsened survival rates, as the rate of survival to hospital discharge in African-American SCA victims with VT/VF documented as the initial rhythm is 27% lower than the survival rate in white patients.[22] Possible contributing factors for worsened survival rates include African-American patients receiving treatment at hospitals with worse outcomes and a decreased likelihood that patients in low-income African-American neighborhoods will receive bystander-initiated CPR than victims in high-income, white neighborhoods.[22,23]

PATHOPHYSIOLOGY

The epidemiology of SCD is intertwined with the pathophysiology underlying the event. SCD may be considered as the outcome of an interaction between an abnormal cardiac substrate and a transient functional disturbance that triggers the arrhythmia at a specific point in time. In the absence of demonstrable structural heart disease, inheritable arrhythmic conditions are more commonly being identified as potential substrates for SCA. With the increased availability of genetic testing, genetic mutations are increasingly demonstrated as the etiology for SCA, with a decreasing proportion of SCA being classified as idiopathic.

Mechanisms of Ventricular Fibrillation

VF has been postulated to be the result of multiple localized areas of microreentry in the absence of any organized electrical activity[24] and is often depicted as rotating spiral waves.[25] It has also been proposed that in the setting of structural heart disease or abnormal depolarization and/or repolarization from a channelopathy, there is diffuse, heterogenous myocardial depolarization and dispersion of electrical activity that creates the electrophysiologic substrate for reentry. Although the structure to accommodate reentry may be present in a heart, a trigger event is typically required to initiate an arrhythmia in the vulnerable heart.[26]

The aforementioned myocardial heterogeneity results in fragmentation of impulse conduction with multiple focal spiral wavelets of myocardial activation. On the electrocardiogram (ECG), this localized reentry is depicted by high-frequency undulating waves that are irregular in amplitude, morphology, and cycle length. These uncoordinated localized wavelets do not result in organized electrical activity; thus no myocardial depolarization or contraction is generated, resulting in an absence of cardiac output and presence of global ischemia. With prolonged VF, there is worsened ischemia and acidosis, which is manifested on the ECG by an increase in fibrillation cycle length, and the fibrillation waves may ultimately become so fine that electrical activity is not apparent.[27,28]

Pathologic Substrates

The common thread to the underlying mechanism of VT/VF is the concept of heterogeneity in myocardial structure resulting in abnormal depolarization and/or repolarization. There are multiple different etiologies that result in heterogeneous myocardial structure and function, creating a potential pathologic substrate for SCA. When a person experiences SCD, especially in the setting of preexisting structural heart disease, the presumed mechanism is electrical instability with a trigger of ischemia or some other arrhythmogenic stimulus that induces a lethal arrhythmia that leads to hemodynamic collapse. However, as PEA has become increasingly identified as the initial rhythm at time of OHCA,[8] a proportion of SCDs may be the result of abrupt hemodynamic collapse without a preceding lethal arrhythmia.

While variations in the reporting of SCD events and the rarity of autopsy limits the reliability of estimates on the etiology of SCD, CHD remains the most common contributing factor in SCA cases (present in 70% to 75%).[3] Other structural cardiac abnormalities, such as dilated cardiomyopathy (DCM) and hypertrophic cardiomyopathy (HCM), are responsible for the second largest proportion of SCA cases. Despite extensive clinical evaluation in SCA survivors or autopsy in SCD victims, no significant cardiac abnormality is identified in approximately 5% of SCA cases.[29,30]

Coronary lesions have been identified in up to 90% of SCD victims,[31] although CHD may present as an acute, chronic, or acute-on-chronic process. Acutely, in the setting of plaque erosion, platelet aggregation, and thrombosis, individuals with the rapid onset of ischemia may present with a lethal arrhythmia. Only 20% of SCD victims are identified as suffering from an acute myocardial infarction (MI) at the time of cardiac arrest.[32] In the setting of chronic CHD, myocardial scars from previous MIs are more reflective of the source pathology in SCA.[33]

DCM represents the underlying pathology in approximately 10% to 19% of SCD victims depending on the population evaluated. In DCM, interstitial patchy fibrosis, myocyte degeneration, and necrosis contribute to the formation of heterogeneous areas of electrical conduction involved in the mechanism of reentry in VT/VF. Left ventricular hypertrophy (LVH) is an independent risk factor for SCD and the majority of SCA victims with CHD have coexisting LVH. The pathophysiology underlying this increased risk is related to altered membrane electrophysiology (EP) with delayed inactivation of slow inward Ca^{2+} currents and delayed activation of K^+ rectifier currents affecting the action potential in hypertrophied ventricular myocytes. Furthermore, transient ischemia increases the susceptibility of hypertrophied myocytes to delayed afterdepolarizations and triggered arrhythmias. In HCM, pathologic examination demonstrates myofibrillar disarray that also contributes to myocardial heterogeneity.

Infiltrative, inflammatory valvular diseases and congenital cardiac lesions account for a minority of SCA events in patients with structural heart disease. Infiltrative diseases, such as sarcoidosis and amyloidosis, are associated with an increased risk of SCD due to both arrhythmia and pump failure. In the case of sarcoidosis, EP studies in patients with cardiac sarcoidosis have demonstrated multiple inducible VTs. The mechanism is felt to be consistent with scar-mediated reentry, with possible contributions from inflammation triggering ventricular ectopy or slowed conduction in granulomatous scar.[34] In young adults, acute viral myocarditis is among the more common causes of SCD,[35] with high-grade inflammatory processes in the myocardium contributing to diffuse fibrosis[36] that acts as a substrate for arrhythmia. Congenital cardiac lesions, such as anomalous coronary arteries, are associated with an increased risk of SCD. In addition, SCD is also one of the leading causes of death in adults with congenital heart disease, accounting for 7% of all deaths in one series.[37]

Structural abnormalities of the cardiac conducting tissue are best exemplified by the Wolff-Parkinson-White (WPW) syndrome and diseases of the His-Purkinje system. Patients with WPW syndrome who have pathways with short refractory periods are susceptible to VF during atrial fibrillation/flutter. There is an increased risk of SCD in individuals with disease within the His-Purkinje system related to an increased risk of VT rather than bradyarrhythmic events.[38]

While genetically determined disorders account for a small proportion of SCDs (1%–3%),[35] they are more likely than CHD to be the cause of SCD in young adults. Some of the inheritable arrhythmic disorders include long QT syndrome, short QT syndrome, Brugada syndrome, arrhythmogenic right ventricular cardiomyopathy (ARVC), HCM, and catecholaminergic

polymorphic ventricular tachycardia (CPVT).[39] Identification of these inheritable arrhythmic conditions is important in the event of SCA or SCD, as it can provide valuable information and affect clinical management of the survivor of an SCA plus prevent future events in family members.

Functional Modulators

While a pathologic substrate is typically required to sustain an arrhythmia, the initiation of a fatal arrhythmia often is the result of the interaction between the underlying structural abnormality and a functional modulator converting stable abnormalities in electrical conduction to an unstable state. Functional modulators, such as transient ischemia or acquired long QT, can even initiate a fatal arrhythmia in the absence of structural heart disease, particularly in the setting of an intense stimulus or profoundly abnormal disturbances. While possible, clinically fatal arrhythmias less commonly present in the structurally normal heart. Some of the functional abnormalities that can contribute to initiation of a potentially fatal arrhythmia are described next.

Transient Ischemia. Ischemia plays a major role in producing fatal arrhythmias. Some of the contributing factors at the cellular level resulting from acute ischemia include dispersion of both conduction patterns and refractoriness, providing the environment for reentrant arrhythmias and generating abnormal automatic activity. Ischemia contributes to heterogeneity in the myocardium by preferentially opening the ATP-sensitive K^+ channels in the epicardial cells as opposed to the endocardial cells. The resulting heterogeneous refractoriness increases the susceptibility of the myocardium to arrhythmias. Reperfusion events also may contribute to arrhythmias as, during reperfusion, an inward flux of calcium results in calcium overload and correlates with a burst of spontaneous ventricular ectopy, possibly resulting from automaticity or triggered activity.

Hemodynamic Deterioration. A cardiac arrest may be precipitated by acute hemodynamic deterioration, possibly as a result of ischemia and/or alteration of metabolic substrates. In the setting of hemodynamic deterioration, cardiac arrest carries a high short-term mortality rate. Hypoxemia can also result in ischemia and alteration of metabolic substrates contributing to SCD. Furthermore, a hypoxemic event often precedes a bradycardic and/or asystolic arrest.

Metabolic Disturbances. Hypokalemia and hyperkalemia have been implicated in an increased risk of SCD and total cardiovascular mortality. Both hypokalemia and hypomagnesemia play a role in the genesis of torsades de pointes (TdP) and other polymorphic VT. Similarly, acidosis has been shown to be a contributing factor to SCD and correction of acidosis is one of the central tenets in the resuscitation of PEA.

Altered Systemic Autonomic Balance. Structural abnormalities, particularly those resulting in cardiomyopathy and systolic heart failure, affect the neurohormonal milieu generating autonomic disturbances that result in altered β-adrenergic receptor content, coupling proteins, and adenylate cyclase activity. The resulting dispersion of quantitative and qualitative responses to sympathetic stimulation predisposes the structurally abnormal heart to arrhythmias. Clinically, altered systemic autonomic balance is manifested as a loss of the normal diurnal variation of heart rate variability, which is considered a marker for risk of SCA among MI and SCA survivors.[40]

Drug Toxicity. Drug toxicity as a cause of SCA has been documented in connection with a variety of both cardiac (antiarrhythmic) and noncardiac drugs, particularly those resulting in QT prolongation (e.g., psychotropic drugs and antibiotics, such as erythromycin and fluoroquinolones). However, a variety of electrophysiologic mechanisms are operative in the genesis of lethal ventricular tachyarrhythmias induced by various drugs. There may be concurrent structural and functional abnormalities that act in concert to initiate a potentially fatal arrhythmia. Combination of drugs and toxins may also predispose an individual to SCA. Recent reports have demonstrated an increased risk of SCA with concomitant use of cocaine and alcohol, possibly as a result of the generation of a cardiotoxic metabolite, cocaethylene.[41]

ETIOLOGIES

To predict SCA, it is important to recognize the conditions described in greater detail later that can potentially lead to abrupt cessation of cardiac output. Fig. 23.2 shows data derived from various studies demonstrating the predominant pathologic substrates of SCD. The relative risk of SCD is dependent on the underlying substrate and is graphically demonstrated for various populations in Fig. 23.3. These substrates are outlined in greater detail later.

Coronary Artery Disease

CAD is the most common underlying substrate in SCD events, accounting for 60% to 75% of all cases.[3,11,12] SCD in the setting of a coronary event is more common in men than women as well as in African Americans than whites. The majority (40% to 75%) of SCA events attributed to CAD occur in individuals with evidence of a prior MI; however, approximately 15% of SCA victims initially present during a new ST elevation myocardial infarction (STEMI).[13] Many of the risk factors for CAD are also predictors for SCA, including, but not limited to, hypertension, diabetes, smoking, obesity, and left bundle branch block on ECG.[2]

Nonatherosclerotic Coronary Artery Disease

Nonatherosclerotic CAD also poses a significant risk for SCA, especially in the younger population. Common nonatherosclerotic coronary artery abnormalities include congenital anomalies, embolism, vasculitis, myocardial bridging, vasospasm, and dissection.

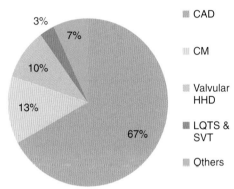

Fig. 23.2 Prevalence of underlying heart disease in adult patients who have experienced sudden cardiac death, based on data derived from several studies.[9,198–202] The predominant substrates are coronary artery disease *(CAD)*, cardiomyopathies *(CM)*, valvular and hypertensive heart disease *(HHD)*, and inheritable arrhythmia syndromes. *LQTS,* Long QT syndrome; *SVT,* supraventricular tachycardia. (Modified from Deshpande S, Vora A, Axtell K, Akhtar M. Sudden cardiac death. In Brown DL, editor. *Cardiac Intensive Care.* Philadelphia: Saunders, 1998, 391–404.)

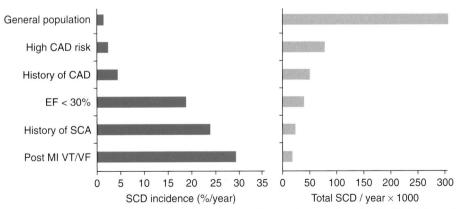

Fig. 23.3 The incidence and number of patients with sudden cardiac death (SCD) in various subgroups of patients. *Left,* SCD incidence percent per year in each subgroup. *Right,* Total number of SCDs per year (n × 1000). *CAD,* Coronary artery disease; *EF,* ejection fraction; *MI,* myocardial infarction; *SCA,* sudden cardiac arrest; *VT/VF,* ventricular tachycardia/ventricular fibrillation. (Modified from Myerburg RJ, Kessler KM, Castellanos A. Sudden cardiac death: structure, function and time-dependence of risk. *Circulation.* 1992;85[Suppl I]:I-2–I-10.)

Coronary Artery Anomalies. Although hemodynamically significant coronary artery anomalies are uncommon (prevalence ranging from 0.21% to 5.79%),[42] they are the second most common cause of SCD in young adults.[43] The anomaly most commonly associated with SCD occurs when an anomalous coronary artery originates from the opposite sinus of Valsalva and the course of the artery traverses between the aorta and the pulmonary trunk. However, other coronary artery anomalies with an interarterial course as well as variants of coronary artery anatomy (e.g., hypoplastic right coronary or anomalous origin from pulmonary trunk) have also been implicated in SCD.[44] SCD events that occur in individuals with this anomaly typically occur during or shortly after vigorous exercise, with the proposed mechanism entailing compression of an acutely angulated proximal coronary artery (possibly with a slit-like ostium) and/or compression of the left main as it courses against the root of the pulmonary trunk during exercise when the great vessels dilate, compromising coronary blood flow, resulting in myocardial ischemia.[45] Antemortem diagnosis of this coronary artery anomaly is rare despite a significant number of patients experiencing prodromal symptoms (e.g., syncope, exertional chest pain). The index of suspicion for a coronary artery anomaly in patients, especially athletes who present with exertional syncope, needs to be high so that the diagnosis can be made with appropriate diagnostic imaging, such as a cardiac computed tomography (CT) scan that can identify not only the origin of the artery but also its course.

Vasculitis. During the acute phase of Kawasaki disease, coronary artery aneurysms and ectasia develop in 10% to 25% of patients.[46] In later years, shrinkage of the aneurysm, intimal proliferation, and coronary calcification contribute to stenosis, which may result in SCD from cardiac arrhythmia and acute MI.[47] Other vasculitides, such as polyarteritis nodosa[48] and syphilitic aortitis,[49] can affect the coronary circulation and SCA may be a rare sequelae.

Myocardial Bridging. Myocardial bridging is a rare (0.5% to 4.5% of the general population) congenital variant in which a segment of an epicardial coronary artery traverses through the myocardium during a portion of its course, with a typically affected region being the mid-portion of the left anterior descending coronary artery.[50] During exertion, a critical degree of systolic compression on the tunneled segment may occur, resulting in myocardial ischemia. SCA has been reported to occur, especially during exertion, in patients with severe myocardial bridging.[51]

Coronary Artery Spasm. Coronary artery vasospasm is a sudden narrowing of the coronary artery caused by the contraction of smooth muscle tissue in the vessel wall. Coronary artery spasm can occasionally trigger ventricular arrhythmias and culminate in SCA, possibly as a result of abrupt reperfusion after a period of ischemia.[52,53] Vasospastic angina may also occur as a result of cocaine abuse.[41]

Coronary Artery Dissection. Another rare cause of acute coronary syndrome and, potentially, SCA is a spontaneous dissection of the coronary arteries that results from separation of the media layer of the artery wall by hemorrhage with or without an associated intimal tear.[54] Coronary artery dissection is associated with a variety of conditions, including Marfan syndrome,[55] the peripartum period of pregnancy,[56] coronary involvement with any type I aortic dissection from other causes, or a rupture of the sinus of Valsalva aneurysm involving the coronary ostia, all of which can potentially cause SCA.[57]

Myocardial Disease

Hypertrophic Cardiomyopathy. Despite a relatively low incidence in the general population, HCM is the most common cause of SCD in young adults and the second largest cause of SCD overall,[58] with an annual mortality rate ranging from less than 1% in asymptomatic patients to 6% in patients with multiple risk factors.[59,60] Unlike most other heart diseases, the risk of SCA in HCM declines with age.[61] HCM is inherited as an autosomal-dominant condition. Patients with HCM have asymmetric, diffuse LV hypertrophy without compensatory dilatation of the LV chamber and in the absence of any known cardiac or systemic cause. On histologic examination, there is gross disorganization of muscle bundles and myofibrillar architecture, altered gap junctions, increased basal membrane thickness, and interstitial fibrosis.[62] These microscopic abnormalities manifest in patients as both electrical instability and myocardial hypertrophy with altered hemodynamics.

Possible mechanisms for SCA in HCM include malignant ventricular arrhythmias arising within the hypertrophied LV, syncope from abrupt hemodynamic deterioration with LV outflow tract obstruction, and ischemia, most commonly manifested as VT/VF.[63–66] The genesis of these arrhythmias is found in a complex interplay of electrophysiologic and hemodynamic abnormalities, primarily from electrophysiologic derangement of hypertrophied and heterogeneous muscle.

SCA may often be the first manifestation of heart disease in HCM patients; thus, it is implicated as the substrate explaining lethal arrhythmias in young adults or athletes. Major risk factors for SCD include LV maximum wall thickness greater than or equal to 30 mm, previous episode of SCA, left ventricular outflow tract gradient of 30 mm Hg or greater at rest or 50 mm Hg or greater with provocation, nonsustained VT, and inducible VT at EP study.[58] Additional incremental risk factors include young age, LV dilatation with depressed EF, presence of fibrosis (delayed enhancement on cardiac magnetic resonance imaging), and reduced functional flow reserve.[63,67,68]

Ventricular hypertrophy secondary to systemic or pulmonary hypertension or owing to valvular or congenital heart disease is also associated with an increased risk for SCA.[69] The risk is proportionate to the level of severity of the hypertrophy.[70]

Nonischemic Dilated Cardiomyopathy. Nonischemic dilated cardiomyopathy (NIDCM) is defined by the presence of LV or biventricular dilatation and impaired systolic function in the absence of any ischemia or abnormal loading conditions. Primary causes include familial cardiomyopathies, myocardial injuries from infections, autoimmune disorders, metabolic conditions, or exposure to toxins (e.g., alcohol, chemotherapy, heavy metals, or other drugs).[71] In many patients with NIDCM, no causative agent is identified; thus, the cause is labeled as idiopathic. Genetic mutations are identified in up to 40% of patients with no other identifiable etiology, with mutations in genes encoding titin (TTN), myosin heavy chain (MYH7), sarcomere of cardiac troponin T (TNNT2), and lamin A/C (LMNA) among the most commonly reported.[9]

A phenotypically distinct form of NIDCM is defined by noncompaction of the ventricular myocardium (NVM) and is presumed to be caused by the arrest of normal embryogenesis of the endocardium and myocardium. Three major clinical manifestations include heart failure, embolic events, and arrhythmias.[72] Both atrial and ventricular tachyarrhythmias have been observed with VT in 47% of patients. SCD accounted for 50% of deaths in some reported series of NVM patients.[73,74]

Overall survival is poor following a clinical diagnosis of NIDCM: approximately 70% survival at 1 year and 50% survival at 2 years, with the majority of deaths being sudden in nature.[75] NIDCM is responsible for 10% of all adult SCD cases[76] and SCD can be the initial presentation of NIDCM. Risk factors for SCD in the setting of NIDCM include reduced left ventricular ejection fraction (EF), prior sustained VT, syncope, symptomatic heart failure, and family history of SCD. Syncope is a poor prognostic factor and is associated with a 44% incidence of SCD in 4-year follow-up.[77] Ventricular tachyarrhythmias[78] are the most common mode of death, but bradyarrhythmias[79] also occur, especially in patients with severe LV dysfunction. The arrhythmia most commonly implicated in SCA is primary polymorphic VT or VF. Furthermore, rapidly sustained monomorphic VT, in some cases resulting from bundle branch reentry, has been observed.[38] The recognition of bundle branch reentry is critical because these patients can be successfully cured by catheter ablation of the right bundle branch.[38] Monomorphic VT, unrelated to bundle branch reentry, is likely associated with the presence of smaller reentrant circuits within the myocardium. In most instances, the triggering mechanism for the onset of primary polymorphic VT or VF is unclear. In some cases, triggers such as electrolyte abnormalities or the use of antiarrhythmic medications are more easily identifiable.

Arrhythmogenic Right Ventricular Cardiomyopathy. ARVC is an inherited cardiomyopathy with the characteristic histologic appearance of transmural loss of right ventricular (RV) myocytes with replacement by adipose and fibrous tissue. The hallmark on ECG is the presence of epsilon (ε) waves, although inverted T waves, notched S wave, and widening of QRS (>110 ms) in the right precordial leads have also been observed (Fig. 23.4).[80] Often, the signal-averaged ECG is markedly abnormal, with late potentials being commonly seen in ARVC.[81] Diagnostic findings on imaging include regional RV akinesia, dyskinesia, or aneurysmal dilatation on echocardiography or cardiac magnetic resonance (CMR) imaging. Intramyocardial fat, RV wall thinning, and delayed enhancement on CMR imaging are complementary radiologic findings but are no longer considered diagnostic.[82]

The estimated prevalence of ARVC is 1 in 2000 to 5000 and it is typically inherited in an autosomal dominant fashion, although due to incomplete penetrance the disease occurs in only 30% to 50% of offspring. Multiple genetic mutations have been discovered that result in ARVC, with more than 60% of mutations occurring in genes encoding desmosomal proteins (e.g., plakoglobin, plakophilin 2, desmoglein 2, desmocollin 2, and desmoplakin), which anchor intermediate filaments to the cytoplasmic membrane in adjoining cells in the gap junction.[83]

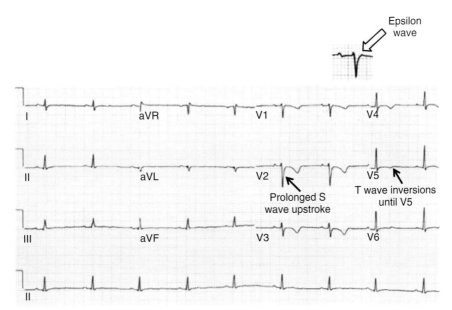

Fig. 23.4 Electrocardiograph morphology of arrhythmogenic right ventricular dysplasia with inverted T waves, ε waves, notched S wave, and widening of QRS (>110 ms) in the right precordial leads (V$_1$–V$_3$). (From Nasir K, Bomma C, Tandri H, et al. Electrocardiographic features of arrhythmogenic right ventricular dysplasia/cardiomyopathy according to disease severity: a need to broaden diagnostic criteria. *Circulation*. 2004;110:1527–1534.)

Patients are generally asymptomatic; unexplained syncope or SCD may be the initial clinical manifestation, with SCD being the first arrhythmic event in up to 50% of cases.[84] In ARVC patients treated with an ICD, the annual rate of death or VF ranges from 1.5% to 4% in observational studies. Predictors of delivery of ICD therapy include prior SCA or hemodynamically significant VT, younger age, LV involvement, unexplained syncope, presence of nonsustained VT, and VT induced during an electrophysiologic study (EPS).[85,86]

Valvular Heart Disease. Disease of the heart valves poses an increased risk for future SCA, usually as a result of LV dilatation and/or hypertrophy. In 1% and 5% of victims of SCD, the cause of death is attributed to valvular heart disease.[5,6] Rheumatic valvular heart disease can, in rare cases, result in SCD due to arrhythmias, ball valve thrombosis in the left atrium obstructing the mitral orifice, embolization to the coronary arteries, or acute low output circulatory failure. In aortic stenosis (AS), hypertension and low cardiac output in the setting of LVH provoke coronary hypotension and contribute to VT that leads to SCD.[87] Prior to aortic valve replacement (AVR), asymptomatic patients with severe AS have an annual SCD rate of 13%.[88,89] However, this risk is not completely mitigated by surgery, as SCD is one of the most common modes of death in AS patients after AVR (especially within the first 2 years), primarily attributable to arrhythmias and thromboembolism.[90] Although mitral valve prolapse (MVP) is often described as a risk factor for SCD, there is no well-defined mechanism for MVP causing SCD. While MVP is typically benign, certain characteristics—such as leaflet thickness, redundancy, fibrosis of the papillary muscles and inferobasal wall, and LV dilation—are associated with increased ventricular tachyarrhythmias.[91,92] Although VT is associated with these characteristics, this may not contribute to SCD risk.[93]

Inflammatory and Infiltrative Disorders. Inflammatory disorders, such as myocarditis, are an important cause of SCD in the young. Myocarditis can be acute or chronic and is defined by inflammation of the myocardium that has an infectious origin (e.g., viral, bacterial, or parasitic infections). Patients are typically asymptomatic and SCD (resulting from either lethal ventricular arrhythmias or damage to the specialized conduction system) can be the only presenting sign in up to 12% of adult myocarditis patients.[94] Initially, there is direct myocardial injury producing edema, necrosis, and contractile dysfunction. Scarring after the acute myocarditis has resolved may contribute to SCA.

Noninfectious inflammatory conditions—such as collagen vascular diseases, progressive systemic sclerosis, and granulomatous disorders (i.e., sarcoidosis)—can also cause SCA.[95] Cardiac sarcoidosis is defined by the development of sarcoid granulomas in the heart muscle that can affect the conduction system, causing complete heart block; create granulomatous scar, contributing to the development of macro-reentrant ventricular arrhythmias; or impair myocardial contractility, resulting in heart failure.[96,97] Patients with cardiac sarcoidosis are at risk for SCD and limited data are available to aid in risk stratification. ICDs are generally indicated when the patient has experienced sustained VT or survived SCA; when the EF remains less than or equal to 35% despite optimal medical therapy and immunosuppression; and when the patient has an indication for a permanent pacemaker, unexplained syncope presumed to be arrhythmic in etiology, or sustained VT induced at EP study.[96] Compared to other patients with NIDCM, patients with cardiac sarcoidosis appear to receive more frequent appropriate ICD therapies.[98,99]

Infiltrative diseases, such as hemochromatosis and amyloidosis, also can increase a patient's risk of SCA. Amyloidosis cardiomyopathy results from the deposition of amyloid protein in the myocardial interstitium, ultimately contributing to diffuse myocardial thickening with impaired ventricular contractility and/or diastolic dysfunction with restrictive physiology.[100] In the setting of cardiac amyloidosis, SCD can result from pump failure owing to progressive diastolic and subsequent systolic biventricular dysfunction, ventricular tachyarrhythmias, or embolization of intracardial thrombus.[101,102] Prognosis for patients with cardiac amyloidosis in the presence of symptomatic heart failure is extremely poor, with a median survival of approximately 4 to 6 months.[100] In cardiac amyloidosis patients with ICDs, appropriate ICD therapies for ventricular arrhythmias are common (27% in one series).[103]

Congenital Heart Disease. SCD is a major cause of mortality in adults with congenital heart disease (ACHD), affecting 7% to 19% of the population.[37,104] The underlying cardiac lesions can be mild but the majority of cases involve complex congenital heart disease. Arrhythmias are the most common cause of SCD in the ACHD population; aortic dissection, cerebrovascular accident, pulmonary embolus/hemorrhage and MI also contribute to SCD in this population, however. Factors that were associated with SCD in adults with congenital heart disease include supraventricular tachycardia (SVT), moderate to severe dysfunction of the systemic ventricle, and increased QRS duration.[104]

Various congenital lesions have been associated with SCA. Congenital aortic stenosis[105] can predispose to SCA. The risk for SCA correlates with the severity of the stenosis; AVR does not eliminate the risk but has been shown to reduce it. Both cyanotic and noncyanotic Eisenmenger syndrome[106] can predispose to SCA. Patients who have undergone surgical procedures for correction of transposition of the great arteries (TGA) may be at increased risk for SCA resulting from bradycardia (e.g., sick sinus syndrome) and tachycardias (e.g., atrial flutter).[107] Longstanding right ventricular strain, abnormal electrophysiologic architecture secondary to general and physical stress, and sequelae of the surgical corrective procedure all contribute to the increased risk of SCD in TGA patients.[108] The incidence of late SCD is approximately 50% but has been reduced with the arterial switch operation.[107] Up to 5% of patients with surgically repaired tetralogy of Fallot (ToF) may experience potentially fatal arrhythmias as a late complication. Some of the risk factors in adults with ToF include LV systolic or diastolic dysfunction, nonsustained VT, QRS duration greater than 180 ms, extensive RV scarring (particularly in the right ventricular outflow tract [RVOT]) or inducible sustained VT at EP study. The mechanism for sustained monomorphic VT in ACHD patients is generally macro-reentrant with a critical isthmus located within an extensively scarred RVOT or ventriculotomy incision.[109] Polymorphic VT or VF affect a subset of ACHD patients, especially those with evidence of extensive myocardial hypertrophy, diffuse fibrosis, myocardial ischemia, and/or reduced EF in the systemic ventricle.

Wolff-Parkinson-White Syndrome. The prevalence of WPW syndrome is 0.1% to 0.3%[110] of the general population; the incidence of sudden death in asymptomatic individuals is as high as 1 per 100 patient years of follow-up.[111] In symptomatic patients, the estimated risk of a malignant arrhythmia resulting in SCD is approximately 0.25% per year or a lifetime risk of 3% to 4%.[112] SCA occurs as a result of atrial fibrillation with a very rapid ventricular response over an accessory pathway with short refractory periods, leading to VF.[113] Patients with preexcited R-R intervals of less than or equal to 250 ms during induced atrial fibrillation are at increased risk of SCD.[114] Patients with multiple accessory pathways, a family history of WPW syndrome with SCD, and, obviously, those with concomitant heart disease are at a higher risk for SCA.

Cardiac Conduction System Abnormalities. Patients with congenital atrioventricular (AV) block or nonprogressive intraventricular block have a lower risk for SCA. Abnormalities of the specialized cardiac conduction system are a rare cause of SCA and are usually noted in young, otherwise healthy individuals without a prior history of arrhythmia. Unless an exhaustive and elaborate autopsy analysis is made, the underlying abnormality may never be discovered in the postmortem examination, leading to the belief that no such abnormality existed. Both acquired AV nodal and His-Purkinje disease, owing to CAD and primary fibrosis, can also uncommonly cause SCA.

Inherited Arrhythmic Disorders

In individuals younger than age 35 years who suffered SCD, an autopsy fails to demonstrate a cause in 27% to 29%[115,116] of cases, although this percentage decreases when detailed histologic examination is performed.[117] Approximately 50% of patients with no identifiable etiology on autopsy will have an inherited arrhythmic syndrome, such as long QT syndrome, short QT syndrome, Brugada syndrome, or catecholaminergic polymorphic VT. Table 23.1 describes the known mutation, chromosome locus, mode of inheritance, and effect on the ion channel for the inherited arrhythmia disorders or channelopathies.

Long QT Syndrome. Long QT syndrome (LQTS) is an inherited channelopathy, with a prevalence of 1 to 2 per 10,000,[118] which results in abnormally delayed myocardial repolarization in the absence of structural heart disease, leading to characteristic prolongation of the QT interval on the ECG. As a result of QT prolongation, patients with LQTS are predisposed to TdP, which may subsequently degenerate into VF. Clinically, patients with LQTS may present with syncope, aborted cardiac arrest, or SCD, with SCD being the initial and only symptom in 10% to 15%.[119] Among symptomatic patients with LQTS, the young are primarily affected, with 50% of individuals experiencing their first cardiac event before the age of 12 years and 90% before the age of 40 years.[120]

Approximately 60% of patients with LQTS will have a pathogenic mutation identified on genetic testing. Over 15 genetically distinct types of LQTS have been reported. All of these genotypes have similar phenotypic presentation (long QT) but different clinical profiles regarding T-wave patterns, arrhythmia triggers, prognosis, and response to therapy. Even within the same mutation, there may be incomplete penetrance and/or variable expressivity, meaning that the same mutation may have different phenotypic manifestations in different individuals. Of genotype-positive LQTS patients, 90% of the mutations are found in three genes: KCNQ1, KCNH2, and SCN5A, causing LQT1, LQT2, and LQT3, respectively.[121] These three genotypes can be characterized by their ECG appearance (Fig. 23.5) and by specific triggers that provoke events (Fig. 23.6). LQT1 is the most common (40% to 50%) with an ECG appearance of broad-based T-wave morphology. Sympathetic hyperactivity, associated with exercise (especially swimming) or emotional stress are typical triggers for cardiac arrhythmia. Catecholamine increases the function of the slowly activating delayed-rectifier potassium channel (IKs) to shorten the QT interval during tachycardia. However, due to "loss of function" of the IKs channel in LQT1, the QT interval is prolonged and causes TdP, leading to SCD. LQT2 is the second most common (35% to 50%), with characteristic ECG appearance of low-amplitude, notched, or biphasic T waves and arrhythmic events typically occurring during sleep or rest or with sudden auditory stimuli. It results from mutations in two genes (KCNH2 "HERG" and KCNE2 "MiRP1"), causing loss of function of the rapidly activating delayed-rectifier potassium channel (IKr) and leading to QT interval prolongation, then to TdP and SCD. Finally, LQT3 accounts for 10% of LQTS and manifests with an ECG that has a long isoelectric segment followed by a narrow-based T wave. Cardiac arrhythmias typically occur at rest or during sleep. The SCN5A encoded defect causes "gain of function," leading to production of persistent, noninactivating inward sodium current (INa) during the plateau phase of the action potential and prolongation of the QT interval.[122] The remaining pathogenic mutations are rarer and are found in genes encoding for other ion channels or ion channel interacting proteins (see Table 23.1).

Extracardiac manifestations in LQTS are uncommon but have been observed in the setting of two clinical syndromes. One is the Jervell and Lange-Nielsen syndrome, an autosomal recessive disease caused by mutations that encode for the IKs channel (KCNQ1 and KCNE1), which affects both the cardiac cell membrane and the production of endolymph in the inner ear, thus it manifests as severe QT prolongation and sensorineural deafness. Andersen-Tawil syndrome is the other, caused by mutations in KCNJ2 (LQT7), and is characterized by potassium-sensitive periodic paralysis, neuromuscular manifestations, facial dysmorphic features, a variable degree of QT interval prolongation with giant U waves, bidirectional or polymorphic tachycardia, and—rarely—SCD.[122]

The risk of arrhythmic events and SCD in LQTS is related to the degree of QT prolongation with corrected QT (QTc) greater than or equal to 500 ms being an established risk factor. Patients with a history of syncope are also at increased risk. Genotype can affect risk as well, with LQT1 being the lowest risk genotype. The incidence of cardiac arrest or SCD in untreated patients under age

TABLE 23.1	**Characteristics of Ion Channelopathies**						
Type	Gene Mutation	Mode of Inheritance	Locus	Effect on Ion Current	Frequency	Arrhythmia Trigger	Syndrome
Long QT							
LQT1	KCNQ1	AD/AR	11p15.5	↓ IKs	30%	Exercise or emotion	Jervell and Lange-Nielsen type I (AR)
LQT2	KCNH2	AD	7q35-q36	↓ IKr	46%	Auditory, emotion, or rest/sleep	
LQT3	SCN5A	AD	3P21	↑ INa	42%	Rest/sleep	
LQT4	ANK2	AD	4q25-q27	↓ Coordination of Ncx, Na/K ATPase	Rare	Exercise	Severe SB and episodes of AF
LQT5	KCNE1	AD/AR	21q22.1-q22.2	↓ IKs	2%–3%		Jervell and Lange-Nielsen type II
LQT6	KCNE2	AD	21q22.1	↓ IKr	Very rare		
LQT7	KCNJ2	AD	17q23.1-24.2	↓ IK1	Rare		Andersen-Tawil
LQT8	CACNA1C	AD	12p13.3	↑ ICa-L	Rare		Timothy
LQT9	CAV3	AD	3p25	↑ INa	Rare		
LQT10	SCN4B	AD	11q23	↑ INa	Rare		
LQT11	AKAP9	AD	7q21-q22	↓ IKs	Very rare		
LQT12	SNTA1	AD	20q11.2	↑ INa	Very rare		
LQT13	KCNJ5	AD	11q24	↓ IK1	Very rare		
Short QT							
SQT1	KCNH2	AD	7q35-q36	↑ IKr			
SQT2	KCNQ1	AD	11p15.5	↑ IKs			
SQT3	KCNJ2	AD	17q23.1-24.2	↑ IK1			
Brugada							
BrS1	SCN5A	AD	3p21	↓ INa	25%–30%		
BrS2	GPD1L	AD	3p24	↓ INa			
BrS3	CACNA1C	AD	12p13.3	↓ ICa-L			
BrS4	CACNB2b	AD	10p12.33	↓ ICa-L			
BrS5	SCN1B	AD	19q13.1	↓ INa			
BrS6	KCNE3	AD	11q13-q14	↑ IKs/Ito			
BrS7	SCN3B	AD	11q23.3	↓ INa			
BrS8	KCNJ8	AD	12p11.23	↑ Ik-ATP			
BrS9	HCN4	AD	15q24.1	—			
BrS10	RANGRF	AD	17p13.1	↓ INa			
BrS11	KCNE5	AD	Xq23	—			
BrS12	KCND3	AD	1p13.2	↑ Ito			
BrS13	CACNA2D1	AD	7q21.11	↓ ICa			
BrS14	SLMAP	AD	3p14.3	—			
BrS15	TRPM4	AD	19q13.33	—			
BrS16	SCN2B	AD	11p23.3	↓ INa			
BrS17	SCN10A	AD	3p22.2	—			
CPVT							
CPVT1	RYR2	AD	1q42.1-q43	↑ SR Ca^{2+} release	60%	Exercise or emotion	
CPVT2	CASQ2	AR	1p13.3-p11	↑ SR Ca^{2+} release	~3%		
CPVT3	KCNJ2	AD	17q23.1-24.2	↓ IK1	Rare		
CPVT4	TRDN	AR	6q22-q23	↓ SR Ca^{2+} release	Rare		
CPVT5	CALM1	AD	14q31-q32	↓ SR Ca^{2+} release	Rare		

Characteristics include gene mutation, mode of inheritance, chromosomal location, the effect on the ion current, the frequency of the mutation in patients, triggers for arrhythmia, and the name of the syndrome if present.
AD, Autosomal dominant; *AF,* atrial fibrillation; *AR,* autosomal recessive; *BrS,* Brugada syndrome; *CPVT,* catecholaminergic polymorphic ventricular tachycardia; *LQT,* long QT; *Ncx,* sodium-calcium exchanger; *SB,* sinus bradycardia; *SQT,* short QT; ↑, gain of function; ↓, loss of function.

40 years is estimated to be 0.30% per year, 0.60% per year, and 0.56% per year in LQT1, LQT2, and LQT3, respectively.[122] The risk of cardiac events has also been associated with gender, with the risk in men being mitigated after adolescence, a finding that has not been observed in women. Exercise should be restricted in all patients to prevent cardiac events. The mechanism of LQTS is related to the amplification of transmural dispersion of repolarization because of preferential prolongation of the action potential duration of M cells. The development of early afterdepolarization-induced triggered activity underlies

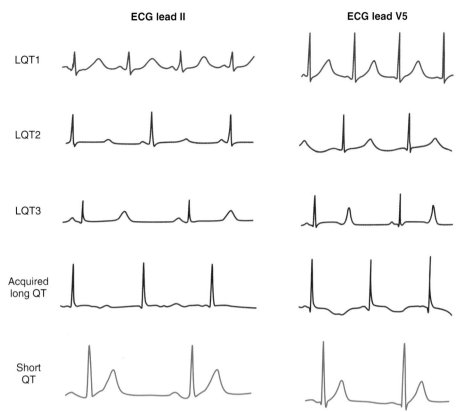

Fig. 23.5 Electrocardiographs (ECGs) demonstrating the typical QT morphology of the three most common long QT syndromes as well as an ECG characteristic of acquired long QT and an ECG characteristic of short QT syndrome. *LQT,* Long QT syndrome. (Modified from Mortada ME, Akhtar M. Sudden cardiac death. In Jeremias A, Brown DL, editors. *Cardiac Intensive Care.* Philadelphia: Saunders, 1998; and Giustetto C, Di Monte F, Wolpert C, et al. Short QT syndrome: clinical findings and diagnostic-therapeutic implications. *Eur Heart J.* 2006;27:2440–2447.)

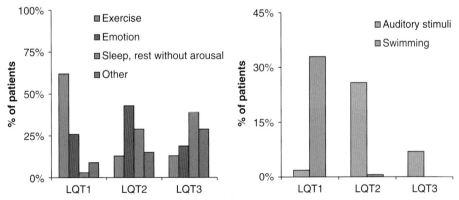

Fig. 23.6 Gene-specific triggers for life-threatening arrhythmias in the three most common long QT (LQT) syndromes. *Left,* Exercise, emotion, sleep, or other triggers. *Right,* Swimming versus auditory stimulus as a trigger for cardiac events in patients with the most common LQT syndromes. (Modified from Schwartz PJ, Priori SG, Spazzolini C, et al. Genotype-phenotype correlation in the long-QT syndrome: gene-specific triggers for life-threatening arrhythmias. *Circulation.* 2001;103:89–95.)

the substrate and acts as a trigger for the development of life-threatening ventricular arrhythmias.[123]

Acquired QT prolongation is more commonly encountered in clinical practice than congenital long QT and can result in marked QT prolongation (see Fig. 23.5). Recent studies have demonstrated that up to one-third of patients with acquired long QT carry a mutation for a gene causing congenital long QT, with *KCNH2* being the most common mutation identified.[124] Some of the triggers or conditions associated with acquired long QT include hypokalemia, hypomagnesemia, hypothermia, or bulimia/anorexia nervosa. Often, acquired long QT occurs as a side effect of medications, including, but not limited to, antiarrhythmic agents, antibiotics, psychotropic medications, methadone, and alternative chemotherapeutic agents (e.g., arsenic trioxide, cesium chloride).

Short QT Syndrome. Short QT syndrome (SQTS) is a rare condition inherited as an autosomal-dominant syndrome characterized by a QTc of 330 ms or less in the absence of tachycardia or bradycardia and tall peaked symmetrical T waves on ECG (see Fig. 23.5). Patients are at increased risk of atrial fibrillation, VF, and SCD from increased transmural dispersion of repolarization.[123,125] EP studies demonstrate very short atrial and ventricular refractory periods and easily inducible VF.[126] Gain-of-function mutations in genes encoding potassium channels—*KCNH2* in IKr channel (SQT1), *KCNQ1* in IKs channel (SQT2), and *KCNJ2* in IK1 channel (SQT3)—and loss-of-function mutations in the α_1 and β_2b-subunit of the L-type calcium channel have been associated with SQTS.[122,126]

Brugada Syndrome. Brugada syndrome (BrS) is a rare condition in which symptomatic patients have syncope or SCA due to rapid polymorphic VT or VF. The characteristic type 1 Brugada ECG has a coved-type ST segment with at least 2 mm J-point elevation in the right precordial leads (V_1 to V_3), typically followed by negative T waves.[127] Arrhythmias typically occur while at rest, during sleep, or after large meals, possibly due to high vagal tone. Fever is an additional risk factor for inducing a Brugada pattern on ECG and subsequently leading to arrhythmic events. The mean age of patients with Brugada syndrome and arrhythmic events is 41 ± 15 years, with a clear male predominance (70% to 95%).[127]

According to the most recent guidelines, a spontaneous type 1 pattern on ECG is sufficient for the diagnosis of BrS.[127] Some experts recommend that clinical features (i.e., prior SCA, unexplained syncope, documented VT/VF, agonal nocturnal respirations or positive family history of SCD in first-degree relatives <45 years) should also be present for the diagnosis of BrS. The type 1 ECG pattern is dynamic; up to 50% of patients with Brugada syndrome may have a transient normalization of the ECG or a saddleback-type ST elevation, that is, a type 2 ECG pattern[122,123,127] (Fig. 23.7). In patients with suspected BrS (based on clinical features) and a nondiagnostic ECG, a drug challenge can be performed using a sodium channel blocking agent to induce the type 1 ECG pattern. The role of EP study for risk stratification is controversial. All patients with BrS are recommended to aggressively treat febrile illnesses with antipyretics and avoid drugs that block sodium channels that can provoke the type 1 ECG pattern and lead to arrhythmias.

Brugada syndrome is inherited as an autosomal-dominant trait with incomplete penetrance in 20% to 50% of patients. A causal mutation is identified in up to 35% of patients with Brugada syndrome, with the most common mutation involving the *SCN5A* gene. The *SCN5A* mutation leads to a loss of function in the INa channel.[127] The arrhythmogenic substrate is the amplification of heterogeneity intrinsic to the early phases (Ito) of the action potential cells residing in different layers of the RV, leading to loss of the action potential dome at some epicardial

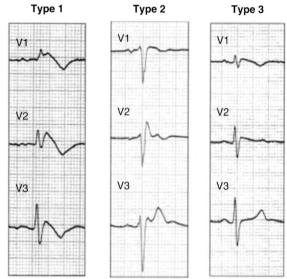

Fig. 23.7 Types of electrocardiographic (ECG) morphology for Brugada syndrome. A spontaneous type I appearance *(left)* with coved-type ST segment elevation in right precordial leads followed by inverted T waves is diagnostic for Brugada syndrome. If the saddleback-type ST elevations as noted in type 2 ECG appearance *(middle)* or type 3 ECG *(right)* appearance is noted in a patient with clinical suspicion of Brugada syndrome, a drug challenge with a sodium channel blocker may be performed to observe for conversion to type 1 ECG pattern. (From Napolitano C, Priori SG. Brugada syndrome. *Orphanet J Rare Dis.* 2006;1:35.)

sites but not others, creating phase 2 reentry and coupled extrasystoles.[128] A marked transmural dispersion of repolarization develops as a consequence of the heterogeneity, creating a vulnerable window that, when captured by a premature extrasystole, can trigger a circus movement reentry in the form of VT/VF and subsequently SCD.[123]

Catecholaminergic Polymorphic Ventricular Tachycardia. CPVT is a rare inherited disorder (prevalence 1 in 10,000) characterized by physical or emotional stress-induced bidirectional VT, polymorphic VT, and a high risk of SCA in the setting of a structurally normal heart and normal resting ECG.[122] Affected individuals usually develop arrhythmic events (syncope, aborted SCA, or SCD) during sympathetic stimulation in the first or second decade of life, with an SCA event rate of 30% to 50% in untreated CPVT patients by age 20 years.[129] While several mutations have been identified, two mutations account for the majority of cases. A mutation in the cardiac ryanodine receptor 2 (*RYR2*) results in gain of function in ryanodine release and is identified in approximately 65% of index cases.[130] A loss-of-function mutation in calsequestrin 2 (*CASQ2*) has also been reported.[131] The net result of both the *RYR2* and *CASQ2* mutation is leakage of calcium and delayed afterdepolarizations arising from the epicardium, endocardium, or M region. Alternation and migration of the source of ectopic activity is responsible for the bidirectional VT and slow polymorphic VT, leading to amplification of transmural dispersion of repolarization, giving rise to reentrant VT/VF and SCA.[123]

CLINICAL PRESENTATION

It is estimated that only 30% to 40% of SCD victims can be identified as being at risk for SCA before the event. Approximately half of all SCD victims will have warning symptoms during the 4 weeks preceding their SCA event, but the majority of symptoms are transient. The other 50% are completely asymptomatic before experiencing SCD.[7] Of the symptoms experienced during the weeks preceding the event, 46% complain of chest pain and approximately 20% report dyspnea.[132] Other symptoms—including palpitations, weakness, or fatigue—have also been reported. Approximately 80% of patients experience symptoms within 1 hour of the SCA event.[7,13,14] Symptoms occurring a few hours or minutes before the episode are more specific for the underlying heart disease and are usually secondary to arrhythmias, ischemia, or congestive heart failure.

Cardiac arrest itself is characterized by the abrupt loss of consciousness that leads to death without active resuscitation; spontaneous reversions do occur rarely, however. Survival after SCA is strongly influenced by the documented initial rhythm and the time elapsed since the collapse. Survival is most likely when the initial rhythm is shockable (VT/VF) with an overall survival of approximately 30%. Victims with PEA have worse outcomes, with an overall survival rate of 8% (7.5% for home cardiac arrests and 14.9% for public cardiac arrests).[7] Only a small subset of patients with bradyarrhythmias, owing to some electrolyte or pharmacologic abnormality, respond well to acute interventions. Young patients with less severe cardiac disease and without coexisting multisystem disease have a higher probability of survival. Mortality is higher in patients with associated noncardiac disease, such as renal failure, pneumonia, diabetes, sepsis, and malignancy.

Time to initiation of high-quality CPR and prompt defibrillation when a shockable rhythm is present are keys to survival with a favorable neurologic outcome. The survival rates decrease by 7% to 10% for every minute between collapse and first defibrillation.[133] The development of the automated external defibrillator (AED) has played a role in early defibrillation by allowing minimally trained first responders to deliver defibrillation and restore spontaneous circulation.[134] Early initiation of high-quality CPR is essential to extending the successful defibrillation window and delaying degeneration of VT/VF into asystole.[133] More recently, studies in compression-only CPR have shown improvement in neurologically intact survival to more than 30%.[135] High-quality CPR (chest compression at a depth of 2 inches and at a rate of 100 to 120 chest compressions per minute in adults) can deliver up to one-third of normal cardiac output, aiding in the preservation of neurologic function.[134]

INITIAL MANAGEMENT OF THE SCA SURVIVOR

Following SCA, survival—particularly neurologically intact survival—does not depend solely on timely and effective cardiac resuscitation. The initial management and stabilization after return of spontaneous circulation (ROSC) as well as treatment of the underlying etiology are also critical. SCA survivors are usually cared for in a cardiac intensive care unit (CICU) with continuous rhythm monitoring. A significant proportion of these patients succumb to cardiogenic shock, congestive heart failure, respiratory complications, and sepsis, accounting for an in-hospital mortality of up to 60%.[136] The most immediate threat after resuscitation is recurrent cardiovascular collapse as myocardial function in the early phase post-ROSC is usually depressed and many patients require transient interventions (e.g., IV fluid boluses, vasopressors, inotropes) for hemodynamic stabilization to prevent secondary injury from hypotension. Additionally, normalization of any electrolyte abnormalities and optimization of oxygenation and ventilation are essential in the initial hours after resuscitation.

During the past decade, improvements in survival and neurologically intact survival are, in large part, due to early revascularization for ischemic events and therapeutic hypothermia. As the majority of SCA events in adults have an underlying substrate of CHD, rapid 12-lead ECG is critical following ROSC to identify patients that will benefit from emergent revascularization. Current guidelines strongly recommend emergent coronary angiography for patients with STEMI and prompt reperfusion has been associated with improved survival and neurologic outcomes.[137] In 27% to 58% of patients with ischemic VF, there is no evidence of ST elevation on post–cardiac arrest ECG, yet these patients are found to have acute coronary occlusion on cardiac catheterization. Early revascularization in this subset of patients has also been associated with improved survival and favorable neurologic outcomes[138,139]; per guidelines, emergent coronary angiography is reasonable in patients with VT/VF arrest without evidence of ST elevation but with suspicion of acute ischemia.[137] Early reperfusion may also be essential to hemodynamic management and maintaining end-organ perfusion following ROSC.

Therapeutic hypothermia has also contributed to recent improvements in survival to hospital discharge and favorable neurologic outcomes. Initial studies[140,141] in therapeutic hypothermia (target temperature 32°C to 34°C) in comatose post–cardiac arrest patients demonstrated marked improvement in overall survival and neurologic function. Although these trials were limited to patients with shockable rhythms, guidelines extended the indication for therapeutic hypothermia to all comatose cardiac arrest victims following ROSC. More recently, a large prospective randomized study[142] has resulted in a modification to these recommendations, suggesting that hypothermia to 33°C did not confer any benefit in neurologic status or survival as compared to a targeted temperature of 36°C. Current recommendations are for targeted temperature management between 32°C and 36°C in comatose adult patients initiated as soon as possible after hospital admission for at least 24 hours after achieving target temperature.[137] The degree of hypoxic brain injury following SCA is variable. However, coma persisting 72 hours after the event (or 72 hours after return to normothermia in the absence of sedation or paralytics) is usually associated with poor prognosis.[143,144]

EVALUATION OF THE SCA SURVIVOR

Following the initial period of stabilization and neurologic improvement, all patients should undergo a complete cardiac evaluation unless it is contraindicated by the presence of terminal illness. Evaluation of the SCA survivor includes: assessment of potentially reversible causes, evaluation for structural heart disease, evaluation for primary electrical disorders when structural heart disease is not apparent (increasingly this includes genetic assessment), and cascade screening of family members if an inherited arrhythmia disorder is identified. The etiology of SCA in these patients can usually be categorized as being associated with either ischemic or nonischemic heart disease or as occurring in the absence of overt cardiac disease. This approach is helpful in determining the direction to proceed for further evaluation and in determining management strategies. Both noninvasive and invasive laboratory evaluations, including electrophysiologic studies, are performed in these patients and have variable yields and implications depending upon the underlying substrate.

Immediate Evaluation

History and Physical. A detailed history from the patient (if awake) and witnesses may offer possible clues for triggering mechanisms (e.g., ischemia and proarrhythmia) and a family history may suggest underlying heart disease. It is important to establish the presence of any prior diagnosis of structural heart disease, any medication use (especially antiarrhythmic drugs, diuretics, and drugs that prolong the QT interval), and/or ingestion of toxins or substance abuse. Knowledge of prodromal symptoms and the nature of activity or stressful events at the time of the SCA are also important. The clinical examination is focused on determining the nature of the underlying heart disease or systemic disease, if any, and the extent of its involvement, particularly with reference to ventricular function.

Electrocardiogram. An initial resting ECG is essential as part of the immediate evaluation in determining the presence or absence of underlying structural or functional abnormalities, both acute and chronic. It is important to assess for ongoing ischemia as part of an acute MI. Other conditions that may be diagnosed via the ECG include prior MI, conduction system disease, ARVC, LQTS, SQTS, BrS, HCM, or WPW syndrome. Repolarization abnormalities after cardiac arrest and resuscitation are common, transient, and nonspecific.[145] These ECG abnormalities are possibly caused by electrical cardioversion, electrolyte abnormalities, or hypothermia.[146] Thus it is recommended that the ECG be repeated as the patient's cardiac, hemodynamic, and metabolic conditions stabilize.

Laboratory Testing. Immediate laboratory evaluation is aimed at determining the presence of triggering agents (electrolyte abnormalities, ischemia, acidosis, metabolic disturbances, and screening for toxic substances). If antiarrhythmic medications had been prescribed previously, it is useful to draw plasma samples to determine drug levels.

Evaluation for Structural Heart Disease

Cardiac Catheterization. A complete cardiac catheterization—including coronary angiography, left and right heart hemodynamics, and left ventriculography—is usually performed early in the evaluation of cases of SCA. Even in young patients, there is a role for cardiac catheterization in order to rule out coronary anomalies. Patients with a STEMI after ROSC following SCA should undergo urgent cardiac catheterization and revascularization, as appropriate.[137] In the absence of an acute coronary syndrome, coronary angiography is often still performed (unless another etiology has been identified) to exclude stable, chronic coronary heart disease. Long-term outcomes appear to be improved in individuals who have successful urgent revascularization for total occlusion of a coronary artery or unstable coronary lesions even if the initial ECG did not demonstrate ST elevation.[147,148] In patients with new-onset heart failure and new ventricular arrhythmias, in which myocarditis or a cardiomyopathy is suspected, a right ventricular endomyocardial biopsy performed during the catheterization procedure may provide additional diagnostic information to guide management.[149]

Echocardiography. Evaluation of LV function is critical because it is the strongest independent predictor for recurrence and long-term survival following OHCA.[150] The transthoracic echocardiogram (TTE) with color Doppler is also used to identify structural abnormalities of wall motion or myocardial contractility, valvular abnormalities, infiltrative myocardial disorders, coronary artery anomalies, and abnormalities of the aortic root. As global LV dysfunction from myocardial stunning can be seen following cardiac arrest, CPR, or electrical cardioversion, evaluation of LVEF is recommended to be performed at least 48 hours after ROSC.[151] Potential etiologies of SCD that can be identified on TTE include CHD (based on wall motion abnormalities or the presence of an aneurysm), HCM, ARVC, AS, NIDCM, and cardiac amyloidosis.

Cardiac Magnetic Resonance Imaging. When standard evaluation with ECG, laboratory evaluation, catheterization, or echocardiogram fail to elucidate a diagnosis, CMR imaging can be useful in the evaluation of possible structural heart disease. In certain conditions, CMR imaging can aid in establishing the diagnosis due to characteristic features of a disease on CMR imaging. In HCM, delayed enhancement is a risk factor for SCD[152] and wall thickness may be more accurately quantified, especially in certain subtypes such as apical HCM, given the limitations of ultrasound windows in echocardiography.[153] Diagnostic features of myocarditis on CMR imaging include myocardial edema in T2-weighted images, hyperemia/capillary leak in T1-weighted sequences, and necrosis/fibrosis in delayed enhanced sequences.[154] In patients with ARVC, CMR imaging may allow for more accurate assessment of regional and global RV dysfunction, evaluation of intramyocardial fat, and myocardial fibrosis on delayed enhancement imaging.[153]

Evaluation for a Primary Electrical Disorder

In approximately 5% to 10% of SCD survivors, there is no evidence of structural heart disease or a noncardiac etiology. In these patients, additional diagnostic testing is aimed at identifying an inherited arrhythmia disorder or WPW syndrome.

Signal-Averaged Electrocardiography. Low-amplitude, high-frequency potentials recorded in the terminal portion of the filtered QRS signal-averaged electrocardiography (SAECG) complex are thought to represent electrical activity from the anatomic arrhythmogenic substrate. Their presence, especially in patients with CAD, is thought to predict spontaneous future arrhythmic events, mainly in patients in whom no revascularization is performed and particularly when combined with assessment of LV function. SAECG is an excellent negative predictor for SCA in patients with CAD (negative predictive value, 89% to 99%). It is important to recognize that the prognostic value of the SAECG is less well defined in patients with nonischemic heart disease, except for ARVC and HCM. The SAECG may be abnormal in 15% to 20% of patients with HCM, but its predictive value for SCA remains unproven. In ARVC, the presence of late potentials on an SAECG is a minor Task Force criterion for diagnosis; the filtered QRS duration, low-amplitude signal and root mean square amplitude of the last 40 ms of the QRS on an SAECG are markedly abnormal in ARVC patients as compared to controls.[81]

Exercise Stress Testing. Exercise stress testing is not usually part of the evaluation for CAD in SCD survivors, as the majority of patients undergo coronary angiography. However, the provocation of ischemia with exercise, independent of coronary anatomy, is useful as VT/VF provoked during exercise predicts a higher recurrence rate of SCA. In patients without structural heart disease, exercise testing can be used in the diagnosis of LQTS or CPVT. In LQTS, evidence of QT prolongation with sympathetic stimulation and increased heart rate is suggestive of LQT1. In CPVT patients, the pathognomonic finding of bidirectional VT may be seen rarely during exercise testing, but polymorphic VT that is provoked with exercise may also be suggestive of CPVT in the appropriate patient. Exercise stress testing can also be useful in risk stratification in patients with WPW syndrome, as resolution of the delta wave with exercise and increased heart rate generally correlates with decreased likelihood of preexcited atrial fibrillation with rapid ventricular response degenerating to VF.

Pharmacologic Challenge. In patients with a normal resting ECG, echocardiogram, coronary angiogram, and CMR, a drug challenge can be used to elicit diagnostic ECG changes suggestive of inherited arrhythmia disorders, as the ECG abnormalities in inherited arrhythmic conditions such as LQTS or BrS may be intermittent or latent and genetic testing may not yet be comprehensive enough to exclude all possible disorders. Infusion of epinephrine (0.025 to 0.3 µg/kg per minute) is used to induce polymorphic VT suggestive of CPVT. Challenge with low-dose epinephrine can also be used to assess for LQTS (specifically, LQT1) due to the paradoxical increase of the QT interval with increased heart rate and sympathetic stimulation; the negative predictive value of low-dose epinephrine for LQT1 is 96%.[155] Procainamide challenge (10 mg/kg IV over 10 minutes) can also be used to induce the characteristic ECG abnormalities of Brugada syndrome. In one report of survivors of SCA with structurally normal hearts and no diagnosis based on standard evaluation, a diagnosis was established with pharmacologic provocative testing in two-thirds of patients.[156]

Ambulatory ECG Monitoring. Ambulatory ECG monitoring is of limited value for the noninvasive evaluation of cardiac arrest survivors. Although monitoring may or may not document complex ventricular ectopy after cardiac arrest, it has little or no utility in assessing the ability to suppress ventricular ectopy by antiarrhythmic agents or predicting reduction in risk for future SCA. Complex ventricular ectopy, therefore, appears to be a marker of underlying cardiac disease rather than the cause of increased mortality. The majority of SCA survivors will have an ICD placed prior to discharge capable of recording and storing ventricular tachyarrhythmias, which may preclude the need for ambulatory ECG monitoring.

Electrophysiology Study. Electrophysiologic testing is not usually performed in patients with an established etiology for their SCD. The practice of assessing antiarrhythmic drug efficacy with an EPS has largely been abandoned. In SCA survivors, there is no indication for an EPS owing to the strong evidence of ICD benefit in these patients. In patients with specific high-risk conditions (e.g., ischemic cardiomyopathy, NIDCM, BrS, HCM, and ARVC) who are not candidates for an ICD implantation, EPS may be useful. The study should be performed in the absence of antiarrhythmic therapy since the results may be influenced by the drug. The likelihood of inducing a sustained ventricular arrhythmia depends on the underlying heart disease (coronary vs. noncoronary), LV function, the presenting clinical arrhythmia (VT/VF) and the aggressiveness of the programmed stimulation protocol. Data suggest that the use of triple versus double extrastimuli yields a higher number of patients who are inducible. However, aggressive stimulation protocols can induce polymorphic VT or VF in some individuals without cardiac disease. Although VF may occasionally be induced, it may be a clinically irrelevant arrhythmia. However, there is evidence that inducible VF, particularly when induced repeatedly with nonaggressive protocols, suggests the diagnosis of idiopathic VF and may predict recurrent arrhythmic events.[157]

EPS is warranted for risk stratification in patients with nonsustained VT, remote MI, and LV dysfunction (EF ~40%), and in patients with symptoms suggestive of VT/VF (e.g., palpitations, presyncope, or syncope).[2] It is a valid diagnostic tool for the investigation of wide QRS complex tachycardias of unknown origin or in conjunction with ablation of ischemic or nonischemic VT (e.g., RVOT) or supraventricular tachycardia (e.g., WPW syndrome). In the setting of BrS, the utility of EPS is controversial.[158] It has not been proven useful as a diagnostic tool for other ion channelopathies.[2]

Genetic Testing. Even after a comprehensive clinical evaluation has been performed in survivors of SCA, there may be no identifiable etiology for the cause. Performing genetic testing in survivors or postmortem (a "molecular autopsy") results in identification of an inheritable arrhythmic syndrome in up to 35% of cases of SCD.[159] Identification of the genetic basis of the disease is important for both identification of cause for the proband (initial person in family who experienced symptoms) and for "cascade screening" of all first-degree relatives, which can allow for identification of affected individuals before they demonstrate symptoms, potentially preventing future SCA events. In the case of some inheritable conditions (i.e., LQTS), identification of the specific mutation may affect treatment of individuals who are genotype positive and phenotype negative.

With improvements in genetic sequencing, genetic testing for cardiac channelopathies has advanced rapidly as extended gene panels can now be screened more rapidly and with less cost. Limitations in genetic testing do exist as next-generation sequencing has also increased the yield of genetic testing, leading to an increased number of variants of unknown significance. Further workup in the context of a variant of unknown clinical significance depends on both the clinical context and genetic testing result. In addition, genetic conditions may exhibit incomplete penetrance and, therefore, may not affect all individuals that carry the genetic variant. There may be genetic conditions underlying an unexplained SCA that associate with variable expressivity, meaning that the same mutation may have different phenotypic manifestations in different individuals. Genetic testing for unexplained SCA is probabilistic and may not predict future clinical manifestations of the condition. In some cases, the results of genetic testing are either inconclusive or negative. Among the causes of negative or inconclusive testing are that the current annotation of variants is imperfect and the causal variant lies in a gene that was not sequenced, that the causal variant lies in a noncoding region, that a deletion or duplication mutation not well captured by existing technology is responsible for the condition, or that the condition does not actually have a genetic basis.

THERAPY

Selection of therapy for SCA survivors should be individualized. Before initiating specific therapy, the underlying substrate, ventricular function, and hemodynamic state should be well established.

Pharmacologic Therapy

The selection of pharmacologic therapy as an option for cardiac arrest survivors depends on the underlying cause. Pharmacologic therapy is an important adjunct to ICD therapy to reduce the frequency of ventricular and supraventricular arrhythmias that may cause symptoms and result in ICD shocks (both appropriate and inappropriate).

All post-MI trials and LV dysfunction trials show significant survival benefit associated with the use of a β-blocker. In addition, angiotensin-converting enzyme inhibitors, angiotensin-receptor blockers, and HMG-CoA reductase inhibitors (statins) are essential in post-MI patients to reduce risk for future acute coronary syndromes and mortality. In general, β-blockers are first-line therapy in the management of ventricular arrhythmias in the prevention of SCD. Amiodarone has a broad spectrum of antiarrhythmic activity that may inhibit or terminate ventricular arrhythmias by influencing automaticity and reentry, making it useful as an adjunct therapy to ICD to reduce the frequency of ventricular arrhythmias and ICD shocks. While a survival benefit compared to placebo has not been demonstrated for the use of amiodarone in patients with reduced LVEF,[160] it can

be used without increasing mortality in patients with heart failure as compared to the class Ic antiarrhythmics that have been shown to be harmful and are contraindicated in the presence of ischemia or structural heart disease.[161] Antiarrhythmic medications such as sotalol, dofetilide, mexiletine, ranolazine or quinidine (alone or in combination) may also be useful as an adjunct therapy to an ICD in reducing the frequency of ventricular arrhythmia.[162]

In SCA survivors with normal heart structure, pharmacologic therapy may be helpful in reducing the risk of VT/VF and recurrence of SCA. β-Blockers, calcium channel blockers, sotalol, and flecainide have been used in RVOT tachycardias. The β-blocker sotalol is the drug of choice in ARVC to treat frequent ventricular ectopy or nonsustained VT.[163] However, recent registry data suggest that amiodarone may be superior in preventing ventricular arrhythmias in ARVC patients.[164] In patients with LQTS (and some carriers of a causative LQTS mutation with normal QT interval) β-blockers are the drug of choice to prevent dysrhythmia.[2] The predictors of failure of β-blockade include QTc greater than 500 ms, LQT2 or LQT3, and early age of episode of SCD (<7 years). In patients with LQT3, sodium channel blockers (mexiletine, flecainide, or ranolazine) may be considered as add-on therapy to shorten the QT interval less than 500 ms.[2] In contrast, sodium channel blockers increase the risk of arrhythmia and SCA in BrS. Quinidine is highly effective in reducing the frequency of VF in BrS, especially in VT storm. Quinidine and disopyramide are effective in reducing the frequency of VT/VF in SQTS type I patients. Either disopyramide or β-blockers may be used in patients with HCM. In CPVT, β-blockers, but not calcium channel blockers, are recommended in all patients and flecainide should be considered when patients experience recurrent syncope or polymorphic/bidirectional VT while on β-blockers to minimize ICD shocks.[2]

Correcting the secondary causes of SCA may be accomplished with a pharmacologic approach or with oxygen supplementation (e.g., hypoxia). Drug toxicity, leading to arrhythmias and SCA, can be managed by stopping the medication. Cardiac arrhythmias due to electrolyte imbalance (e.g., hypomagnesemia, hypokalemia, hyperkalemia) can be addressed by specific electrolyte supplementation or dialysis.

Myocardial Revascularization and Arrhythmia Surgery

Acute myocardial ischemia is considered a contributing factor to SCA based on several clinical observations.[32] It is therefore likely that prevention or reduction of myocardial ischemia can consequently decrease the incidence of SCA in those patients with CAD with either symptomatic or silent myocardial ischemia. In addition, myocardial revascularization has been shown to reduce the incidence of SCA in patients who have been successfully resuscitated from a previous episode related to acute MI.[165] The induction of VF in the preoperative EPS may be suppressed in more than half of the patients who undergo myocardial revascularization. Furthermore, early revascularization for survivors of SCA in the setting of STEMI and/or SCA survivors with no evidence of ischemia on ECG but suspicion for acute ischemia has been shown to improve survival and neurologic outcomes.[147,148]

Approaches to ischemia reduction include using optimal pharmacologic therapy, percutaneous coronary intervention, or coronary artery bypass graft surgery. All of these techniques are associated with reduction in the risk for SCD.[2]

Revascularization alone is unlikely to eliminate clinical or inducible monomorphic VT, especially in patients with a fixed anatomic substrate (myocardial scar/ventricular aneurysm). Thus an ICD will be indicated, with the possible need for an EPS-guided excision[166] or ablation[167] of this tissue. This technique is fairly complicated, however, and should be performed by a team with experience in these procedures.

Catheter Ablation

Catheter ablation is considered a state-of-the-art approach for the potentially curative management of VT and as adjunctive therapy to an ICD. In a minority of patients, the underlying etiology for SCA may be supraventricular in origin (e.g., WPW syndrome). Ablation of a rapidly conducting accessory pathway likely reduces SCD by preventing rapid conduction of atrial fibrillation that can degenerate to VF. Data from the WPW registry have confirmed that RF ablation in WPW patients is safe and successful, with no further recurrence of malignant arrhythmia causing SCD.[168] Patients with bundle branch reentry VT, those with idiopathic VT originating in the RVOT or LVOT, and patients with fascicular VT may also have SCA. The utility of performing a detailed EPS in an SCA survivor is highlighted by the fact that the majority of idiopathic VTs (with the exception of rare locations, such as the anterior papillary muscle, moderator band, and epicardial VT that have higher rates of recurrence)[169] can be cured by radiofrequency catheter ablation, thus obviating the need for further therapy and possibly eliminating future risk.[169]

Despite improvements in mapping techniques and ablation catheter technology, the outcomes for ablation in patients with structural heart disease remain poor, with less than a 50% success rate and excess risk of major complications, including stroke and death.[169] Nonetheless, catheter ablation has an important role in controlling incessant VT and reducing recurrent ICD shocks in patients with scar-related heart disease.[170,171] Catheter ablation of scar-related VT involves the identification of potential reentry circuit isthmi and exit sites based on substrate, pace, and entrainment mapping.[172] Substrate ablation has been used in the setting of unmappable VT to create scar homogenization by RF ablation of all sites with abnormal electrograms and has been shown to increase freedom from VT in patients with structural heart disease.[173,174] Most of these sites can be approached endocardially using vascular catheters or, if that fails, a percutaneous epicardial approach may be used.[175]

Automated External Defibrillator

Only about 10 % of out-of-hospital SCA victims survive because of the brief window for resuscitation available from the initial onset of VT/VF to the point of death. However, nearly one in three victims survive when the cardiac arrest is witnessed by a bystander.[176] The chance of successful resuscitation falls by 7% to 10% each minute after collapse.[133] Thus the development and widespread distribution of the AED has been an important advance in the prevention of SCD and in improving the rates

of survival.[177,178] The AED has now been accepted as a standard tool during resuscitation of OHCA.[134]

Public access to defibrillation has been shown to be an important part of the successful chain of survival program. Placement of AEDs has been most cost-effective in select locations with significant public traffic or density, including casinos, airports, sports stadiums, corporate offices, shopping malls, schools, community centers, high-risk homes, and senior centers. The United States Food and Drug Administration (FDA) has approved the use of AEDs in public areas. Some AEDs can now be purchased over the counter. However, most need a physician's prescription. The average price for a single AED unit is between $1150 and $1600. In August 2002, the FDA gave approval to the first home-use AED. Since then, most states have passed liability immunity legislation for the use of an AED in a not grossly negligent manner. Audible and/or visual prompts guide the user through the process of defibrillation, making AEDs easy to use. Most AEDs require that the operator initiate the delivery of the shock in some way, such as by pushing a button. AEDs have been shown to be accurate in diagnosis of shockable rhythms with overall sensitivity in detecting VF reported to range from 76% to 96%. Specificity (correctly identifying non-VF rhythms) is reported to be nearly 100%.[179] Both bystander CPR and AED use have been positively correlated with improvements in rates of survival and survival with functional recovery.[180]

Implantable Cardioverter Defibrillator

The ICD has emerged as one of the most revolutionary therapies developed to treat patients with life-threatening ventricular arrhythmias. Over the past 3 decades, it has evolved from its more primitive form to a sophisticated device capable of tiered therapy and data storage. The basic premise behind the effectiveness of the ICD is that the majority of SCDs result from malignant ventricular tachyarrhythmias. Furthermore, survivors of arrhythmic SCA are at increased risk of recurrent VT/VF with rates of recurrent arrhythmia nearing 43% at 5 years.[181] The ICD system consists of sensing and defibrillation electrodes connected to a generator that houses the battery and integrated circuitry. VT arrhythmias are detected by rate, duration, onset, and morphologic criteria. Programmed therapies are then automatically delivered based on the detection criteria of the arrhythmia sensed. In addition, all transvenous ICD generators now provide backup ventricular bradycardia pacing, providing a safety net for primary or secondary bradycardia arrhythmic events. Initially, the ICD was implanted surgically and connected to leads fixed to the ventricles via a thoracotomy. Currently, the preferred approach is the nonthoracotomy approach using transvenous lead(s) inserted into the right heart for both pacing and for defibrillation with a defibrillation vector between an intracavitary right heart coil and the can of the implanted defibrillator located in the pectoral region (Fig. 23.8). Perioperative mortality associated with ICD implantation has now been reduced to less than 1%. Long-term studies have demonstrated the efficacy of ICDs over a mean follow-up of 8 years.[182] There are long-term complications associated with defibrillators, including an approximate 6% rate of device-related infection and 17% rate of lead failure over 12 years.[183]

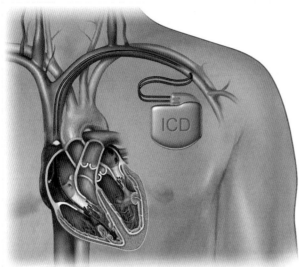

© medmovie.com

Fig. 23.8 Schematic representation of a current transvenous implantable cardioverter defibrillator *(ICD)* and lead system. A right ventricular endocardial rate-sensing/defibrillation lead is shown inserted via the left subclavian vein with its tip in the right ventricular apex. This lead is connected to a pulse generator overlying the left pectoralis major muscle. (Courtesy medmovie.com: https://www.hrsonline.org/Patient-Resources/Treatment/Implantable-Cardioverter-Defibrillator.)

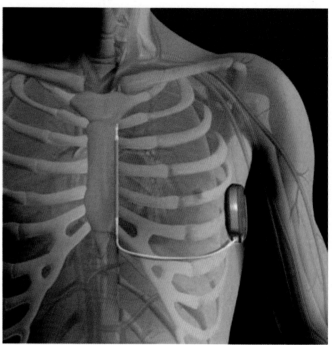

Fig. 23.9 Schematic representation of a current subcutaneous implantable cardioverter defibrillator (S-ICD) and lead system. The electrodes on the lead system are tunneled from the pocket in the midaxillary line to an incision at the xiphoid process and then tunneled to the superior incision along the left sternal border. This lead is connected to a pulse generator overlying the serratus muscle in the vicinity of the fifth to sixth intercostal spaces along the midaxillary line. (From Hauser RG. The subcutaneous implantable cardioverter-defibrillator—should patients want one? *J Am Coll Cardiol.* 2013;61[1]:20–22.)

The therapeutic options for treatment of ventricular tachyarrhythmias include antitachycardia pacing, low-energy synchronized cardioversion, and high-energy cardioversion/defibrillation. A detection algorithm allows differentiation of sinus tachycardia or supraventricular arrhythmias from ventricular tachyarrhythmias to obviate unnecessary delivery of therapy. However, inappropriate shocks may still occur in up to 20% of delivered therapies.[183] Noninvasive interrogation of the device using an external wand allows the review of ventricular electrograms stored from detected episodes, affording confirmation of device effectiveness. Furthermore, the majority of ICDs are now capable of remote patient monitoring (RPM) as well as wireless RPM. This allows for closer monitoring of the patient between office visits as well as the potential for early intervention if device malfunction or clinical deterioration is detected. Evidence suggests that RPM is associated with a significantly lower risk of mortality and rehospitalization.[184]

In addition to the conventional transvenous ICD system, an entirely subcutaneous ICD (SICD) system is now available that may be useful as an alternative to transvenous ICDs in patients who do not require bradycardia pacing, cardiac resynchronization therapy, or those who suffer from ventricular tachyarrhythmias that can be easily terminated by antitachycardia pacing. The system consists of three electrodes: an ICD can be implanted in the midaxillary line over the fifth intercostal space; a defibrillator lead is tunneled subcutaneously to the xiphoid process (proximal electrode) and then superiorly along the left parasternal edge (distal electrode), as shown in Fig. 23.9. Potential advantages of the SICD include decreased risk for lead-related complications, easier reintervention, lack of systemic dissemination in the case

of device infection, and obviating the need for intravascular access in patients with limited vascular access (e.g., patients on dialysis or with prior indwelling venous catheters). Available data suggest that the SICD is safe and effective at preventing sudden death[185] (with a rate of inappropriate shock of ~11% at 3 years),[186] but prospective randomized trials are ongoing.

Although SCA is the result of the complex interaction of functional disturbances with an underlying structural abnormality, the ICD effectively terminates VT/VF regardless of its mechanism (Fig. 23.10). In this regard, it provides unsurpassed protection against arrhythmic SCD because it does not attempt to modulate the structural or functional abnormalities as antiarrhythmic drugs do. The beneficial effect of these drugs, even when chosen after they have been demonstrated to effectively suppress VT/VF, may be mitigated by alterations in the functional state of the individual (e.g., acute ischemia, hypokalemia, catecholamine surge).

Indications for ICD. Trials evaluating the use of ICD as compared to antiarrhythmic therapy in the secondary prevention of SCD have consistently supported the implantation of an ICD in all patients surviving SCA that was not due to transient or reversible causes.[187–189] A meta-analysis of these trials has demonstrated that ICD therapy is associated with a 50% relative risk reduction in arrhythmic mortality and a 28% relative risk reduction for overall

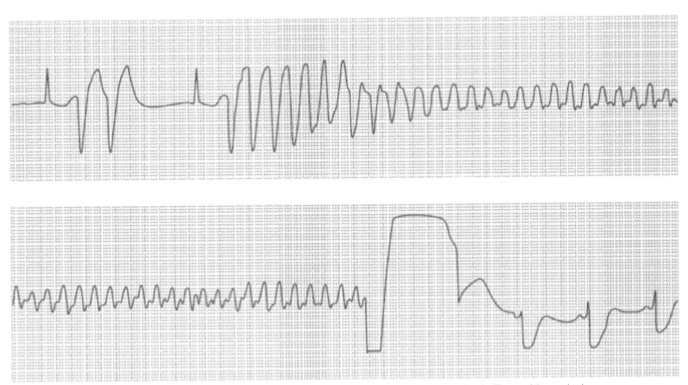

Fig. 23.10 A clinically documented implantable cardioverter defibrillator shock. The rapid ventricular tachycardia is promptly detected and effectively terminated by a single shock with restoration of sinus rhythm *(lower panel)*. (From Tchou PJ, Kadri N, Anderson J, et al. Automatic implantable cardioverter defibrillators and survival of patients with left ventricular dysfunction and malignant ventricular arrhythmias. *Ann Intern Med.* 1988;109:529–534.)

mortality.[190] An ICD is superior to any antiarrhythmic therapy, although if antiarrhythmic therapy is warranted, amiodarone is the most effective choice to reduce the recurrence of VT/VF. In patients with spontaneous or EPS-induced sustained VT, an ICD is strongly recommended for secondary prevention of SCD.

Furthermore, recent studies and updated guidelines consider an ICD essential in the primary prevention of SCD in high-risk patients.[2,191] All patients with ischemic or nonischemic LV dysfunction (EF <35%) and congestive heart failure despite optimized medical therapy are considered at high risk for SCD.[160] If such a patient has ischemic cardiomyopathy and has undergone revascularization therapy, LV dysfunction may improve, resulting in a decreased risk for SCD. LV function must be reevaluated in 90 days; if the EF remains 35% or less, the risk for SCD still exists and an ICD is recommended.[192] In medically treated acute MI patients with LV dysfunction, an ICD must be deferred for at least 40 days after the MI since studies showed no difference in outcome between patients with or without ICD during this period.[193] An exception to the 90- or 40-day waiting period would be if the patient developed nonsustained VT and had inducible sustained VT on EPS.[194] Some patients with LV dysfunction are candidates for cardiac transplantation; the ICD may also be used as a "bridge to cardiac transplantation" for SCD prevention in selected individuals.[195]

Patients with normal LV function can still be at high risk for SCD in some circumstances, requiring an ICD for the primary prevention of SCD. For example, indications for an ICD in patients with HCM include history of prior resuscitation from VT/VF, presence of a very thick intraventricular septum (>3 cm), history of failure to raise blood pressure on exercise testing, nonsustained VT or inducible sustained VT on an EPS and a strong family history of SCD.[58] ICD implantation is recommended for patients with congenital heart disease who are survivors of an aborted SCA, have symptomatic sustained VT, have an EF less than 35% in the systemic ventricle despite optimal medical therapy, have syncope with advanced ventricular dysfunction or inducible sustained VT/VF on EPS, have ToF with multiple risk factors (LV dysfunction, nonsustained VT, QRS duration >180 ms, or inducible sustained VT on EPS), or have advanced single or systemic RV dysfunction and multiple risk factors (nonsustained VT, New York Heart Association [NYHA] Class II to III heart failure symptoms, or severe systemic atrioventricular valvular regurgitation).[2]

Patients with a structurally normal heart can also be at high risk for SCA if they have an inherited arrhythmia disorder, although these cases are rare. An ICD is recommended[2,191] in the following high-risk subgroups:

1. ARVC: Recommended in patients who have a history of aborted SCD or sustained VT that is not hemodynamically tolerated or with depressed LV function or inducible sustained VT on EPS, and may be considered in patients with hemodynamically tolerated sustained VT

2. LQTS: Recommended in patients resuscitated from cardiac arrest, syncope, and/or VT while receiving adequate dose of

β-blockers; and may be considered in asymptomatic carriers of a pathogenic mutation in *KCNH2* (LQT2) or *SCN5A* (LQT3) when the QTc is greater than 500 ms

3. Brugada: Recommended in patients who are survivors of an aborted SCA or have documented sustained spontaneous VT or a spontaneous type 1 ECG and a history of syncope, and may be considered if VF is seen during EPS with two or three extrastimuli at two sites

4. SQTS: Recommended in survivors of an aborted SCA or documented sustained spontaneous VT

5. CPVT: Recommended in survivors of SCA, recurrent syncope, or polymorphic/bidirectional VT despite optimal therapy

There are a few conditions for which ICD implantation is contraindicated. They include the following[2,191]:

1. VT/VF resulting from arrhythmias amenable to surgical or catheter ablation (e.g., WPW syndrome, RVOT VT, fascicular VT)

2. VT/VF due to a transient irreversible disorder (e.g., AMI, blood electrolyte imbalance, drugs, or trauma)

3. Terminal illnesses with projected life expectancy of less than 6 months (e.g., metastatic cancer, drug refractory advanced heart failure in a patient who is not a candidate for cardiac transplantation)

4. Noninducible VT on EPS in cases for which a complex EPS is indicated

5. Significant psychiatric illnesses that may be aggravated by device implantation or may preclude systematic follow-up

6. Incessant VT or VF

In summary, the results of EPS, the degree and type of underlying heart disease, and LV function are critical determinants in guiding management.

Wearable Automatic Defibrillator

An external defibrillator attached to a wearable vest has been shown to successfully identify and terminate VT/VF,[196] and has been approved by the FDA for patients with a transient, high risk for VT/VF, such as those awaiting cardiac transplantation, as a bridge until the ICD is implanted (during the 40-day waiting period after recent MI or 90-day waiting period after revascularization), or in patients who are candidates for ICD but who are at high risk for infection during antibiotic therapy. No prospective randomized control trials evaluating the wearable defibrillator have been reported, but registry data have demonstrated that the rate of sustained VT/VF within 3 months was 3% in patients with ischemic cardiomyopathy and congenital/inherited disease and 1% among nonischemic cardiomyopathy patients; the rate of inappropriate therapy was 0.5%.[197]

CONCLUSION

SCA is a major public health concern worldwide, with a substantial proportion occurring outside the hospital. CAD is overwhelmingly the most common underlying pathology. Noncoronary cardiac diseases are less common but may occur in otherwise healthy individuals in whom an antemortem diagnosis is often difficult. A substantial risk of recurrence persists in these patients and mandates secondary prevention measures. Any significant reduction in the incidence of SCD in the community will require accurate identification of potential victims, training and implementation of bystander CPR and AEDs, and effective primary and secondary preventive interventions.

Acknowledgments

We gratefully acknowledge the assistance of Brian Miller and Brian Schurrer, Aurora Research Institute, in the preparation of illustrations, and Susan Nord and Jennifer Pfaff, Aurora Cardiovascular Services, in editing the manuscript.

The full reference list for this chapter is available at ExpertConsult.com.

24

Electrical Storm and Incessant Ventricular Tachycardia

David L. Brown

Ventricular tachycardia (VT) accounts for 5% to 10% of admissions to cardiac intensive care units (CICUs).[1] With the successes of modern reperfusion therapy to reduce mortality in ST elevation myocardial infarction (STEMI), of pharmacotherapy and implantable cardioverter defibrillators (ICDs) to prolong survival in heart failure, and of implantable left ventricular assist devices (LVADs) to sustain life in end-stage cardiomyopathy, the number of patients with the substrate for ventricular arrhythmias continues to increase. In addition, an increasing number of genetic arrhythmia syndromes and proarrhythmic medications are being identified. This chapter will focus on patients who present with the life-threatening syndromes of electrical (or VT) storm and incessant VT.

DEFINITION

Although there are multiple definitions, electrical storm is commonly defined by three or more episodes of VT, ventricular fibrillation (VF) or appropriate ICD shocks in a 24-hour period.[2] This definition does not capture ICD patients with VT that is slower than the programmed detection rate of the device or VT that is terminated by antitachycardia pacing. Incessant VT is defined as hemodynamically stable VT that lasts for more than 1 hour. These events may develop during acute coronary syndromes (ACS), including acute myocardial infarction (MI), in patients with pre-existing structural heart disease or in patients with structurally normal hearts, such as those with Brugada or long QT syndromes (LQTS). Causes of electrical storm are presented in Box 24.1.[3]

INCIDENCE

The incidence of electrical storm is a function of the population described and the definition used. In patients with ICDs, when electrical storm is defined by more than two VT/VF episodes requiring device therapy within a 24-hour period, the incidence is 2% to 10% per year of follow-up.[4–14] Patients with ICDs placed for primary prevention develop electrical storm less frequently than those in whom they were placed for secondary prevention. The incidence of electrical storm when ICDs are placed for primary prevention in the setting of ischemic cardiomyopathy is about 4% over 20.6 months.[15] In contrast, the incidence of electrical storm is approximately 28% in dilated cardiomyopathy patients with ICDs implanted for secondary prevention during a mean follow-up of 33 ± 23 months.[16]

TRIGGERS

Although it has been estimated that only 10% to 25% of patients have reversible factors triggering the electrical storm episode,[10] correctable triggers should be considered in all patients presenting with electrical storm or incessant VT. Potential triggers are listed in Box 24.2.[17] If an apparently responsible trigger can be found, it should be treated aggressively.

PROGNOSIS

The development of electrical storm frequently heralds a downward deflection in the natural history of patients with structural heart disease. It is associated with reduced short- and long-term survival, especially in patients with severely reduced left ventricular (LV) function. In the Antiarrhythmic Versus Implantable Defibrillators (AVID) secondary prevention trial, 34 of 90 (38%) electrical storm patients died during follow-up compared to 15% of those without electrical storm. Electrical storm was a significant independent risk factor for subsequent death independent of ejection fraction (EF) and other prognostic variables (relative risk [RR], 2.4; $P = .003$), but VT/VF unrelated to electrical storm were not. The risk of death was greatest within the first 3 months after electrical storm (RR, 5.4) and diminished beyond this time.[6] In a study of 32 electrical storm patients who had an ICD for secondary prophylaxis, 17 (53%) died during

---

BOX 24.1   Causes of Electrical Storm

Structural heart disease
Ischemic heart disease
    Acute or recent myocardial infarction/acute coronary syndrome
    Prior myocardial infarction
Nonischemic heart disease
    Dilated cardiomyopathy
    Hypertrophic cardiomyopathy
    Arrhythmogenic right ventricular dysplasia/cardiomyopathy
    Valvular heart disease
    Corrected congenital heart disease
    Myocarditis
    Cardiac sarcoidosis
    Chagas disease
    Metastatic cardiac tumor
Structurally normal hearts (abnormal electrical substrate)
    Primary causes
        Idiopathic
        Brugada syndrome
        Early repolarization syndrome
        Long QT syndrome
        Short QT syndrome
        Catecholaminergic polymorphic ventricular tachycardia
    Secondary causes
        Electrolyte abnormalities
        Toxic/drug related
        Endocrinologic
        Perioperative
        Iatrogenic (T wave pacing)

From Maruyama M. Management of electrical storm: the mechanism matters. *J Arrhythmia.* 2014;30:242–249.

BOX 24.2   Reversible Triggers of Electrical Storm

Acute myocardial ischemia
Electrolyte abnormalities (hypokalemia and hypomagnesemia)
Decompensated heart failure
Hyperthyroidism
Infections, fever
QT prolongation
Drug toxicity
Electrolyte imbalance

---

3 years of follow-up, compared with 19 of the 137 (14%; *P* < .001) ICD patients without electrical storm, suggesting that electrical storm was a strong independent predictor of poor outcome in ICD patients.[18] Among patients who have received an ICD for primary prophylaxis, electrical storm has also been associated with higher mortality. In the Multicenter Automatic Defibrillator Implantation Trial II (MADIT-II),[7] patients who experienced electrical storm had a significantly higher risk of death. The hazard ratio for death in the first 3 months was 17.8 compared with those with no VT/VF. After the 3 months, the hazard ratio decreased to 3.5.

Electrical storm also increases the need for hospitalization and adversely impacts quality of life. In an analysis of the Shock Inhibition Evaluation with Azimilide (SHIELD) trial,[10] electrical storm led to a 3.1-fold increase in arrhythmia-related hospitalization (*P* < .0001) compared with patients with isolated VT/VF. ICD therapies, especially repeated frequent shocks, have significant psychological effects on both patients and their families.[19] In the AVID trial, the development of at least one ICD shock in the initial year of follow-up was associated with significant declines in both physical functioning and mental well-being and increased patient concerns.[20] Although electrical storm is associated with higher mortality, higher hospitalization, and worse quality of life, it remains unclear if the development of electrical storm directly causes the subsequent poor outcomes due to the detrimental effects of VT, VF, or ICD shocks on LV function[21,22] or is merely a marker of end-stage structural heart disease.[5,18]

CLINICAL PRESENTATION

The clinical presentation of patients with electrical storm is variable and depends on the ventricular rate, presence and degree of underlying heart disease, LVEF, and the presence or absence of an ICD or LVAD.[23] Patients without an ICD may present with no symptoms, palpitations, presyncope, or syncope if the ventricular arrhythmia is hemodynamically well tolerated. When the arrhythmia is not tolerated, patients may develop cardiac arrest. Patients with an ICD usually present with multiple ICD therapies, including antitachycardia pacing or ICD shocks. If the VT rate is below the threshold for delivering ICD therapy, patients may present in the same way as patients without an ICD. LVAD patients who present with electrical storm are generally hemodynamically stable but those with ICDs may also present with multiple episodes of antitachycardia pacing or shocks.

Patients with incessant VT may present with chest pain, new or worsening dyspnea, palpitations, presyncope, or syncope depending on the VT rate and their hemodynamic tolerance of it. Patients with hemodynamically well-tolerated VT may present days after its onset complaining of new heart failure symptoms from the development of a tachycardia-mediated cardiomyopathy.[23]

Unless a patient with electrical storm or incessant VT is admitted to the CICU before definitive treatment, the 10 seconds captured on a standard 12-lead electrocardiogram (ECG) is unlikely to demonstrate the inciting arrhythmia. However, it may give important clues to the predisposing substrate, including evidence of STEMI or prior MI, other findings suggestive of ACSs, conduction abnormalities, and prolonged or shortened QT intervals. Assessment of the QT interval is especially important for patients with electrical storm from polymorphic VT, as the approach to patients with prolonged QT interval is different than in patients with a normal QT interval.

In cases in which the initial ECG or telemetry monitoring demonstrate a regular wide-complex tachycardia, VT must be distinguished from ventricular preexcitation, rate-related aberrancy, or preexisting bundle branch block in the setting of supraventricular tachycardia (SVT). The hemodynamic tolerance of the arrhythmia is not helpful in making the distinction. The only finding with 100% positive predictive value for the diagnosis of VT is the demonstration of atrioventricular dissociation manifested by fusion or capture beats. In their absence, various

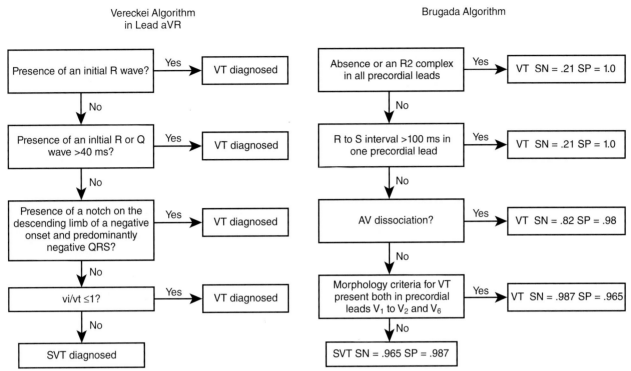

Fig. 24.1 The Vereckei and Brugada algorithms for differentiation of ventricular tachycardia from supraventricular tachycardia. *SN*, Sensitivity; *SP*, specificity; *SVT*, supraventricular tachycardia with aberrancy; *vi/vt*, initial (vi) and terminal (vt) ventricular activation velocity ratio; *VT*, ventricular tachycardia. (From Baxi RP, Hart KW, Vereckei A, et al. Vereckei criteria as a diagnostic tool amongst emergency medicine residents to distinguish between ventricular tachycardia and supra-ventricular tachycardia with aberrancy. *J Cardiol.* 2012;59:307–312.)

algorithms are available to help differentiate VT from SVT. Two algorithms are presented in Fig. 24.1.[24] Since no algorithm is perfect, a wide-complex tachycardia in patients with underlying structural heart disease should be assumed to be VT until proven otherwise. The administration of treatments for SVT, such as adenosine or calcium channel blockers, can precipitate cardiac arrest in patients with VT who were otherwise hemodynamically tolerating the arrhythmia. In most cases, continuous telemetry monitoring or ICD interrogation of intracardiac electrograms are required to document the VT. On interrogation of ICDs of patients with electrical storm, 86% to 97% have monomorphic VT, 1% to 21% have primary VF, 3% to 14% have combined VT/VF, and 2% to 8% have polymorphic VT.[5–7,9,10,12,13,16,18,25,26] Patients with these arrhythmias can be further divided into those with and without structural heart disease to facilitate diagnosis and treatment (Fig. 24.2).[3]

Monomorphic VT storm (Fig. 24.3) is usually associated with structural heart disease and is due to electrical wavefront reentry around a fixed anatomic barrier, most commonly scar tissue following a prior MI, fibrosis in nonischemic cardiomyopathies, arrhythmogenic right ventricular cardiomyopathy/dysplasia, sarcoidosis, amyloidosis, Chagas disease, or a prior surgical incision. Surviving myocytes within the dense scar lead to a zone of slow conduction and, combined with areas of anatomic or functional conduction block, give rise to electrical reentry circuits for reentry that can be triggered by a premature ventricular depolarization.[3]

When monomorphic VT occurs in structurally normal hearts, it is referred to as idiopathic VT. The characteristics of idiopathic VT depend on the origin of the VT. VT arising from the outflow tract is the most common form of idiopathic VT and characteristically will present with a left bundle branch block and inferior axis (Fig. 24.4). The usual mechanism involves triggered activity due to cyclic adenosine monophosphate (cAMP)-mediated delayed afterdepolarizations. β-Adrenergic stimulation increases intracellular cAMP and intracellular calcium levels, resulting in spontaneous calcium release from the sarcoplasmic reticulum, delayed afterdepolarizations, and triggered activity.[3] Fascicular (or idiopathic) VT is the second most common cause of monomorphic VT in the absence of structural heart disease. The mechanism is thought to involve macro-reentry involving the Purkinje fiber network, which connects to the left fascicle.[3,27,28] Fascicular VT is classified according to the ECG morphology (right bundle branch pattern and superior or inferior QRS axis) and corresponding fascicle coupled to the reentrant circuit: left posterior fascicular VT, left anterior fascicular VT, and left upper septal VT. Left posterior fascicular VT is most common (Fig. 24.5). The fascicular VTs have characteristic ECGs demonstrating a relatively narrow QRS that results from rapid spread of depolarization using the specialized conduction system. Other less common causes of monomorphic VT storm in structurally normal hearts include nonreentrant focal Purkinje VT, papillary muscle VT, and mitral/tricuspid annular VT. It is important to realize that these patients may have depressed LV function when they

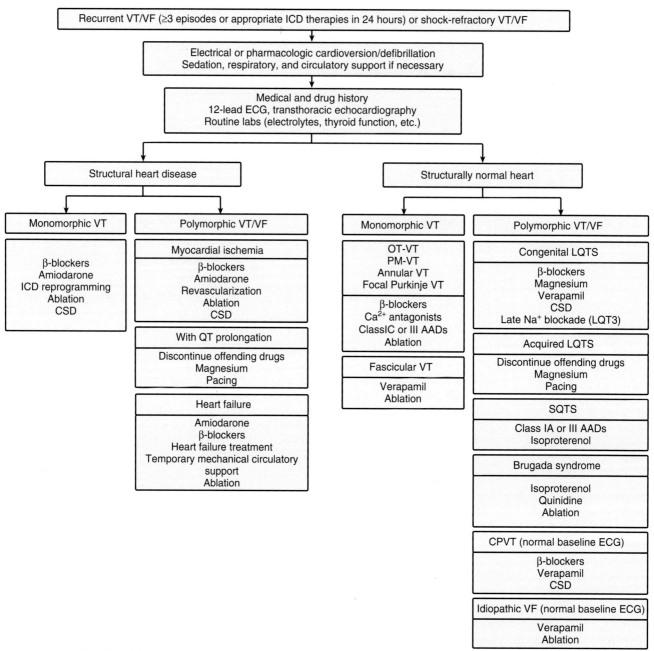

Fig. 24.2 Management of electrical storm. *ADDs*, Antidysrhythmic drugs; *CPVT*, catecholaminergic polymorphic ventricular tachycardia; *CSD*, cardiac sympathetic denervation; *ICD*, implantable cardioverter defibrillator; *LQTS*, long QT syndrome; *OT-VT*, outflow ventricular tachycardia; *PM-VT*, papillary muscle ventricular tachycardia; *SQTS*, short QT syndrome; *VF*, ventricular fibrillation; *VT*, ventricular tachycardia. (Modified from Maruyama M. Management of electrical storm: the mechanism matters. *J Arrhythmia*. 2014;30:242–249.)

come to medical attention that is due to the detrimental impact of incessant VT on LV function rather than an indication of structural heart disease. The LV dysfunction in such situations tends to be global as opposed to segmental[3] and usually recovers after the VT is terminated.

VF is fatal if not treated immediately. Following defibrillation, VF may recur repeatedly and present as electrical storm. Mortality rates in this setting are 85% to 97%.[29,30] Since ischemia is the primary mechanism of VF storm, patients should be emergently triaged to coronary angiography and revascularization. Patients

with a structurally normal heart can develop VF storm triggered by closely coupled monomorphic PVCs. Brugada syndrome, an inherited arrhythmia syndrome caused by mutations in the cardiac sodium channel gene, can present as recurrent VF or electrical storm and a characteristic ECG pattern of right bundle branch block and ST segment elevation in leads V_1 to V_3 (Fig. 24.6).[31]

Polymorphic and monomorphic VT reflect different arrhythmogenic mechanisms. For polymorphic QRS complexes to be present on the surface ECG, multiple wavefronts must propagate throughout the heart or appear simultaneously in different areas

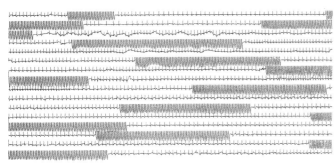

Fig. 24.3 Monomorphic ventricular tachycardia storm. Continuous electrocardiographic strips in a patient with recurrent syncopal episodes are shown. (From Maruyama M. Management of electrical storm: the mechanism matters. *J Arrhythmia*. 2014;30:242–249.)

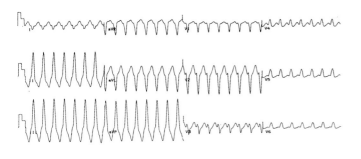

Fig. 24.4 A 12-lead electrocardiogram (ECG) of right ventricular outflow tract (RVOT) ventricular tachycardia demonstrating a left bundle branch block pattern in the precordial leads with transition from a small r wave to a large R wave at V_3 to V_4 consistent with a right-sided site of origin. Also consistent with the outflow tract site is the inferior ECG axis. (From Prystowsky EN, Padanilam BJ, Joshi S, Fogel RI. Ventricular arrhythmias in the absence of structural heart disease. *J Am Coll Cardiol*. 2012;59:1733–1744.)

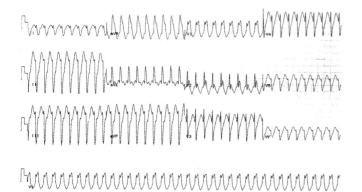

Fig. 24.5 A 12-lead electrocardiogram of left posterior fascicular ventricular tachycardia demonstrating a right bundle branch block pattern with a superior axis. This type of tachycardia has a site of origin near the left posterior fascicle. (From Prystowsky EN, Padanilam BJ, Joshi S, Fogel RI. Ventricular arrhythmias in the absence of structural heart disease. *J Am Coll Cardiol*. 2012;59:1733–1744.)

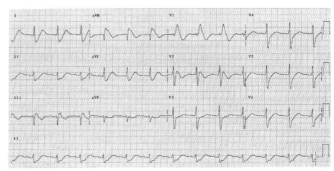

Fig. 24.6 A 12-lead electrocardiogram of Brugada syndrome demonstrating coving of the ST segment in the early precordial leads and right bundle branch block pattern. (From Prystowsky EN, Padanilam BJ, Joshi S, Fogel RI. Ventricular arrhythmias in the absence of structural heart disease. *J Am Coll Cardiol*. 2012;59:1733–1744.)

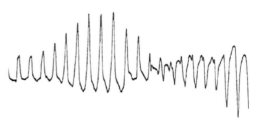

Fig. 24.7 Drug-induced torsades de pointes following quinidine treatment. (From Schwartz PF, Woosley RL. Predicting the unpredictable. Drug-induced QT prolongation and torsades de pointes. *J Am Coll Cardiol*. 2016;67:1639–1650.)

of the heart.[32] Polymorphic VT, which can occur with a normal or prolonged QT interval (Fig. 24.7), is most often encountered in patients with acute coronary syndromes. As such, electrical storm can be the initial manifestation of acute ischemia. In acute MI, polymorphic VT can be caused by ischemia, altered membrane potentials, triggered activity, necrosis, or scar formation. Ischemia may cause dispersion of electrical refractory periods between the endocardium and epicardium, which is required for multiple waves of reentry.[33] Ischemia increases Purkinje cell automaticity, leading to spontaneous firing of these fibers, which triggers polymorphic VT or VF.[34] However, patients without acute ischemia, such as those with acute myocarditis or hypertrophic cardiomyopathy, can also develop polymorphic VT storm.

Polymorphic VT storm is rare in structurally normal hearts but can occur in patients with primary genetic abnormalities, due to secondary causes or with no discernible cause, referred to as *idiopathic VF*. The treatment strategies differ greatly among patients with polymorphic VT storm. The baseline ECG is of critical importance in making the diagnosis. If the QT interval is markedly prolonged, the polymorphic VT is most likely torsades de pointes due to congenital or acquired LQTS.

The congenital LQTS is an ion channel disorder characterized by abnormally prolonged QT intervals (corrected QT interval >440 ms in men and >460 ms in women) with or without morphologic abnormalities of the T waves[35] (Fig. 24.8). A decrease in outward potassium currents or an increase in inward sodium currents prolongs the repolarization phase of the cardiac action potential, resulting in prolongation of the QT interval and

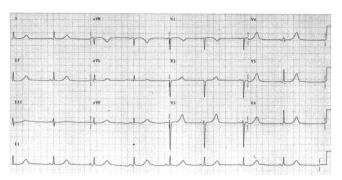

Fig. 24.8 A 12-lead electrocardiogram of long QT syndrome demonstrating a QT interval of 580 ms and a corrected QT interval of 513 ms. Genetic testing revealed an LQT1 syndrome. (From Prystowsky EN, Padanilam BJ, Joshi S, Fogel RI. Ventricular arrhythmias in the absence of structural heart disease. *J Am Coll Cardiol.* 2012;59:1733–1744.)

predisposition to early afterdepolarizations and torsade de pointes. At least 15 different genes involved in inherited LQTS have been described. The first 3—LQT1, LQT2, and LQT3—account for 60% to 75% of the genotyped LQTS cases.[3] The remainder involve mutations related to other channel subunits or their regulator proteins. Approximately 25% of affected patients have no identifiable gene mutations.

Acquired LQTS is caused by QT-prolonging drugs. As of 2016, 48 medications were on the list of drugs known to cause torsades de pointes (including 10 removed from the United States market but which may still be available in other countries). Another 72 were on the list for possible risk and 32 were on the list for conditional risk. A list of drugs that have a risk of QT prolongation and/or torsades des pointes can be found on the CredibleMeds website (https://www.crediblemeds.org/).[36] Electrolyte abnormalities or drugs that induce hypokalemia, hypocalcemia, or hypomagnesemia can also lead to torsades de pointes in patients with or without genetic susceptibility.

Short QT syndrome is rare but should be considered if the QT interval is markedly truncated with a nearly absent ST segment along with peaked and symmetrical T waves.[3] Brugada syndrome—which is characterized by a distinct ECG pattern, the absence of structural heart disease, and a high risk of polymorphic VT/VF and sudden death—can present as electrical storm.[3] In addition to over 100 different mutations of the sodium channel itself, mutations of genes that modulate sodium channel function are also associated with Brugada syndrome.[37] Hypokalemia, high vagal tone, and fever are predisposing factors for electrical storm. Three different types of ECG changes have been associated with Brugada syndrome based on the morphology in V1 and V2.[37] Type 1 ECG is characterized by a 2 mm or greater J-point elevation, coved type ST-T segment elevation, and inverted T wave in leads V_1 and V_2 (see Fig. 24.6). Type 2 ECG is characterized by a 2 mm or greater J-point elevation, 1 mm or greater ST segment elevation, saddleback ST-T segment, and a positive or biphasic T wave. Type 3 ECG is the same as type 2, except that the ST segment elevation is less than 1 mm. Among these three types of ECGs, only type 1 is diagnostic of Brugada syndrome.[38]

In patients with a normal ECG and a structurally normal heart who present with polymorphic VT/VF storm, the possible diagnoses include catecholaminergic polymorphic VT (CPVT)

and idiopathic VF.[3] CPVT is an inherited abnormality of intracellular calcium handling and is commonly seen in young patients with stress- or exertion-induced syncope. The hallmark of CPVT is alternating left bundle branch and right bundle branch QRS complexes. Idiopathic VF presents as syncope or aborted sudden cardiac death in young people with normal hearts and no identifiable genetic syndrome. The events are typically unrelated to stress or activity but may occur in clusters characterized by frequent ventricular ectopy and short episodes of VF or polymorphic VT. The spontaneous VF or polymorphic VT events are triggered by premature ventricular contractions (PVCs), generally with a short coupling interval, often referred to as *short coupled torsade*. The PVCs triggering the events may arise from the Purkinje fibers or the myocardium; the former generally has shorter coupling intervals. Isoproterenol may be effective in suppressing VF storms in the acute setting.[35]

MANAGEMENT

Patients with electrical storm or incessant VT should be rapidly assessed for hemodynamic instability. Pulseless patients or those with clinical evidence of hemodynamic compromise manifested by hypotension, chest pain, dyspnea, or altered mental status should be immediately treated according to advanced cardiac life support (ACLS) protocols with electrical cardioversion.

PHARMACOLOGIC THERAPY

In hemodynamically stable patients with electrical storm or incessant VT, urgent pharmacologic therapy is indicated to both terminate the ventricular arrhythmia and to interrupt the detrimental effect of the associated intense adrenergic stimulation on the heart. Intravenous amiodarone is the most commonly used agent to treat patients with electrical storm or incessant VT in patients with structural heart disease (see Fig. 24.2). The usual dose is 150 mg by IV bolus followed by 1 mg/min IV infusion for 6 hours, followed by 0.5 mg/min for an additional 18 hours. Rapid intravenous infusion of amiodarone blocks fast sodium channels in a use-dependent fashion, meaning there is more channel blockade at faster heart rates. It also inhibits norepinephrine release and blocks L-type calcium channels without prolonging ventricular refractoriness.[34] Amiodarone has minimal negative inotropic effects and is therefore safe in patients with depressed LVEF. In addition, despite the potential for causing QT prolongation, the incidence of torsades de pointes is low. About 60% of patients will have their electrical storm terminated by intravenous amiodarone.[34]

Because of the adrenergic stimulation associated with electrical storm, incessant VT, or ICD shocks, β-blockers should be administered along with amiodarone. Although metoprolol is the more commonly used agent, propranolol may suppress electrical storm that is refractory to metoprolol.[39] In patients with congestive heart failure, propranolol decreases sympathetic outflow more than metoprolol. Furthermore, the lipophilic nature of propranolol enables penetration of the central nervous system, allowing blockade of central and prejunctional receptors in addition to peripheral β receptors.[40,41] The dose of intravenous propranolol is 1 to 3 mg every 5 minutes to a total of 5 mg. The dose of intravenous metoprolol is 2.5 to 5 mg over 5 minutes, which can be repeated to a maximum dose of 15 mg over 15 minutes. Oral amiodarone and β-blockers should be initiated once the patient is stable.

Lidocaine binds to fast sodium channels in a use-dependent fashion.[34] However, outside of the setting of ischemia, lidocaine has relatively weak antiarrhythmic properties. Conversion rates from VT are 8% to 30% and a randomized trial has demonstrated that survival is significantly greater with amiodarone than lidocaine for treatment of out-of-hospital, shock-resistant VT or VF.[42] Thus, amiodarone has replaced lidocaine as first-line therapy for refractory VT and VF. The 2017 American College of Cardiology/American Heart Association guidelines gives a IIa recommendation for intravenous lidocaine as a less effective alternative to amiodarone in the treatment of polymorphic VT associated with no reversible causes.[2] If lidocaine is used, it is administered as an IV bolus of 1 to 1.5 mg/kg followed by an initial bolus of 0.5 to 0.75 mg/kg that can be repeated every 5 to 10 minutes as needed to a total dose of 3 mg/kg. A continuous IV infusion of 1 to 4 mg/min is used to maintain therapeutic levels.

In patients without structural heart disease, the treatment should be tailored to the specific underlying cause. Outflow tract VT can be suppressed by β-blockers that lower stimulated levels of cAMP and thus decrease intracellular calcium. Alternatively, nondihydropyridine calcium channel blockers, such as verapamil or diltiazem, may be effective at suppressing outflow tract VT by directly reducing intracellular calcium. The distinctive feature of fascicular VT is its sensitivity to intravenous verapamil, which is the preferred therapy. The response to class I antidysrhythmic drugs or β-blockers is variable.[3]

The initial treatment of polymorphic VT storm in patients with LQTS is discontinuation of QT-prolonging medications and/or rapid correction of electrolyte abnormalities. β-Blockers are primary pharmacologic therapy for congenital long QT syndromes types 1 and 2. Intravenous verapamil effectively suppresses polymorphic VT in patients who are refractory to β-blockers. Intravenous magnesium may facilitate termination of polymorphic VT associated with LQTS. If the long QT syndrome genotype is known to be type 3, drugs with late sodium current blocking effects—such as mexiletine, ranolazine, and propranolol—are helpful. However, in patients with acquired LQTS, β-blockers may promote VT by inducing bradycardia. Temporary pacing is the treatment of choice in patients with bradycardia-dependent polymorphic VT in LQTS. Isoproterenol can be used while awaiting pacemaker insertion. In patients with short QT syndrome, class I and class III antidysrhythmic drugs—such as quinidine, disopyramide, and amiodarone—are effective at prolonging the QT interval. Isoproterenol suppresses VT storm in Brugada syndrome. Quinidine may also prevent VT/VF in Brugada syndrome.[3]

The trauma that patients with electrical storm or incessant VT experience from multiple electrical cardioversions can have short-term and long-term physical and emotional consequences. Thus, all patients with electrical storm should be sedated. Short-acting agents—such as propofol, benzodiazepines, and some general anesthetics—have been shown to convert or suppress VT.[43] Left stellate ganglion blockade and thoracic epidural anesthesia have been reported to suppress electrical storm that was refractory to multiple antidysrhythmic therapies.[44,45] General anesthesia may also be helpful.

NONPHARMACOLOGIC THERAPIES

For patients with electrical storm and incessant VT in whom acute myocardial ischemia is thought to be an inciting factor, coronary angiography and percutaneous revascularization should be urgently performed as restoration of coronary perfusion may terminate arrhythmias.[46,47] An intraaortic balloon pump or other temporary percutaneous LV mechanical support device may also be placed while in the catheterization laboratory. These devices may suppress ventricular arrhythmias by increasing coronary perfusion pressure or unloading a failing LV. Balloon counter-pulsation has been reported to terminate electrical storm even in the absence of ischemia,[48] presumably by reducing afterload, LV size, and wall tension. In extreme cases of refractory arrhythmias, extracorporeal membrane oxygenation can be considered but should be implemented early in the course before irreversible end-organ damage has occurred.[34] Ultimately, recurrent refractory ventricular arrhythmias may be an indication to place an LVAD or list a patient for cardiac transplantation.

Catheter ablation is effective therapy for many patients with electrical storm or incessant VT refractory to or intolerant of medical therapy.[49–51] In one series, radiofrequency (RF) ablation completely suppressed drug-refractory electrical storm in 95 of 95 patients, many of whom were hypotensive and required hemodynamic support. Long-term suppression of electrical storm was achieved in 92% of patients and 66% were free of VT at 22 months.[49] Notably, the endpoint of ablation was the elimination of all clinical VTs. Of the 10 patients who continued to have inducible VT, eight had recurrent electrical storm and four died despite ICD therapy. RF ablation is also indicated in recurrent polymorphic VT when specific triggers such as monomorphic PVCs can be identified and targeted.[34] This approach has been successful in suppressing electrical storm in patients with both ischemic and nonischemic cardiomyopathies.[52–55] Antiarrhythmic therapy should be continued in CICU patients who have undergone RF ablation. Withdrawal of antidysrhythmic medications may be considered later.

CONCLUSION

Electrical storm and incessant VT are increasingly common life-threatening syndromes characterized by poor short- and long-term outcomes. A diagnostic approach based on the ECG morphology of the ventricular arrhythmia (monomorphic versus polymorphic) and the presence or absence of structural heart disease facilitates selection of the most appropriate therapies for these patients. The initial management consists of identifying and treating underlying ischemia, electrolyte imbalances, or other inciting factors. Amiodarone and β-blockers are appropriate initial therapy in most, but not all, patients. RF ablation may be helpful in patients who are refractory to appropriate antidysrhythmic medications.

The full reference list for this chapter is available at ExpertConsult.com.

25

Diagnosis and Treatment of Unstable Supraventricular Tachycardia

Nimesh Patel, Mark S. Link

INTRODUCTION

Supraventricular tachycardias (SVTs) occur frequently in critically ill patients and are associated with increased morbidity and mortality. Immediate exact diagnosis is not necessary and initial management should focus on ensuring hemodynamic stability. Tachycardias should be characterized by QRS complex width, rate, regularity, and rapidity of onset, as initial treatment can be guided by these characteristics rather than a precise diagnosis.[1] Hemodynamically stable regular tachycardias should initially be treated with vagal maneuvers or adenosine, as these are generally safe and short-acting interventions that not only terminate many tachycardias but also may provide important diagnostic information. Hemodynamically unstable SVT should be treated with synchronized direct current cardioversion (DCCV). After initial stabilization, focus should transition to establishing the etiology of SVT and considering the need for antiarrhythmic drugs or ablation.

EPIDEMIOLOGY

SVT occurs in up to 10% to 20% of critically ill intensive care unit (ICU) patients.[2] While not usually life threatening, SVT is associated with increased morbidity and mortality, especially in patients who are critically ill. Several medical conditions frequently encountered in the ICU are associated with SVT, including sepsis, acute coronary syndrome, decompensated heart failure, hemorrhagic shock, pulmonary embolism, respiratory failure, and thyrotoxicosis. Any medical condition that stimulates a sympathetic response will enhance cellular automaticity and trigger premature ventricular or atrial contractions that promote arrhythmogenesis. In addition, atrial and atrioventricular (AV) nodal conductions are enhanced, which allows for reentrant arrhythmias.

DIAGNOSIS

Although the precise diagnosis of SVT is not necessary in its initial management, a differential can be generated by assessing the QRS width, rate, regularity, and rapidity of onset (Table 25.1).

Wide complex tachycardias (WCTs) may be ventricular in origin (i.e., ventricular tachycardia [VT] or ventricular fibrillation [VF]) or SVTs with left or right bundle aberrancy, preexcitation, or pacemaker tracking. If there is underlying heart disease, WCT is much more likely ventricular in origin and should be treated as such. In stable WCT, adenosine is useful diagnostically and therapeutically.[3] It will terminate many of SVTs and idiopathic VTs, but will not perturb reentrant VT.

Sinus tachycardia is characterized by a gradual onset of a regular tachycardia and generally reaches a maximum rate of around 220 beats/min minus the patient's age (Fig. 25.1). The rhythm originates from the sinus node and the ventricular rate is proportional to the degree of hemodynamic stress. Sinus tachycardia is treated by addressing the underlying condition and is not considered to be pathologic itself; thus patients should not be given pharmacologic agents to control sinus tachycardia.

Atrial fibrillation (Fig. 25.2) is the most common tachyarrhythmia encountered in critically ill patients. It is seen particularly in men, older patients, and in patients with underlying hypertension or cardiopulmonary disease. It occurs secondary to simultaneous depolarization of multiple wavelets within the atria, with variable conduction to the ventricle via the AV node and His-Purkinje system. Acute onset atrial fibrillation is characterized by a rapid rise in ventricular rate and an irregular ventricular response. In patients who have chronic atrial fibrillation, the ventricular rate rises gradually proportional to the degree of sympathetic activation from physiologic stress. In the absence of severe systolic left ventricular dysfunction or disorders that severely impair left ventricular filling, such as hypertrophic cardiomyopathy or severe left ventricular hypertrophy, atrial fibrillation rarely causes hemodynamic instability. The surface electrocardiogram (ECG) shows an absence of discernable P waves and an irregular ventricular rhythm.

Atrial flutter (Fig. 25.3) is the second most common pathologic SVT and, in its typical form, involves a reentry circuit around the tricuspid valve in the right atrium. Atypical atrial flutters

TABLE 25.1 Differential Diagnosis of the Supraventricular Tachycardias (SVTs), Arranged by Regularity

SVT	Underlying Conditions	Regularity	Rate (beats/min)	Onset	P:QRS Ratio	Adenosine Response	ECG
Atrial fibrillation (AF)	Cardiac disease, pulmonary disease, pulmonary embolism, hyperthyroidism, postoperative	Irregular	100–220	Acute gradual (if in chronic AF)	None	Transient slowing of ventricular rate	
Multifocal atrial tachycardia (MAT)	Pulmonary disease, theophylline	Irregular	100–150	Gradual	Changing P morphology prior to QRS	None	
Frequent atrial premature contractions (APC)	Caffeine stimulants	Irregular	100–150	Gradual	P prior to QRS	None	
Sinus tachycardia (ST)	Sepsis, hypovolemia, anemia, pulmonary embolism, pain, fear, fright, exertion, myocardial ischemia, hyperthyroidism, heart failure	Regular	Up to 220 – Age	Gradual	P prior to QRS	Transient slowing	
Atrial flutter (Aflutter)	Cardiac disease	Regular (occasionally irregular if variable AV conduction)	150	Acute	Flutter waves	Transient slowing of ventricular rate	
Atrioventricular (AV) nodal reentrant tachycardia (AVNRT)	None	Regular	150–250	Acute	No apparent atrial activity or R' at termination of QRS	Terminate	
AV reentrant tachycardia (AVRT)	Rarely, Epstein anomaly	Regular	150–250	Acute	Orthodromic AVRT: retrograde P wave / Antidromic AVRT: P wave usually not seen / AF with WPW: no P waves present	Terminate	Orthodromic AVRT Antidromic AVRT AFib with WPW
Atrial tachycardia (AT)	Cardiac disease, pulmonary disease	Regular	150–250	Acute	P prior to QRS	Terminates 60%–80%	

From Link MS. Clinical practice. Evaluation and initial treatment of supraventricular tachycardia. *N Engl J Med.* 2012 Oct 11;367(15):1438-1448.
ECG, Electrocardiogram; *WPW,* Wolff-Parkinson-White syndrome.

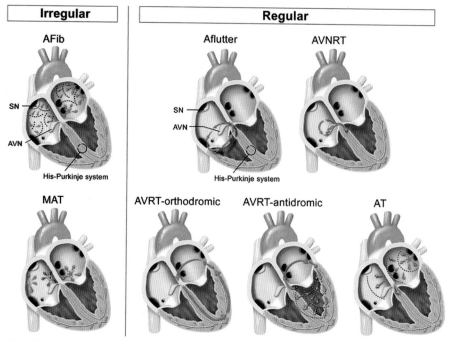

Fig. 25.1 Basic mechanisms of supraventricular tachycardia *(SVT)*. Typical atrial flutter *(Aflutter)* is a reentrant circuit around the tricuspid valve in the right atrium. Atrioventricular nodal reentry tachycardia (AVNRT) is reentry within the atrioventricular node (AVN) and perinodal tissue. Orthodromic AVNRT is a reentry circuit that traverses down the AVN and up a bypass tract, leading to a narrow QRS. In antidromic atrioventricular reentry tachycardia *(AVRT)*, conduction is first down the bypass tract and then up the AVN, leading to a wide QRS complex. Atrial tachycardia *(AT)* is an ectopic focus of atrial activity at a faster rate than the sinus node. Atrial fibrillation *(AFib)* is several simultaneous wavelets in the atrium with variable conduction through the AVN. Multifocal atrial tachycardia *(MAT)* involves at least three distinct ectopic atrial foci. (From Link MS. Clinical practice: evaluation and initial treatment of supraventricular tachycardia. *N Engl J Med.* 2012;367[15]:1438–1448.)

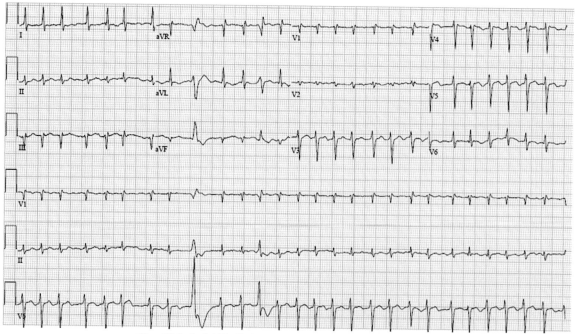

Fig. 25.2 Atrial fibrillation with rapid ventricular response.

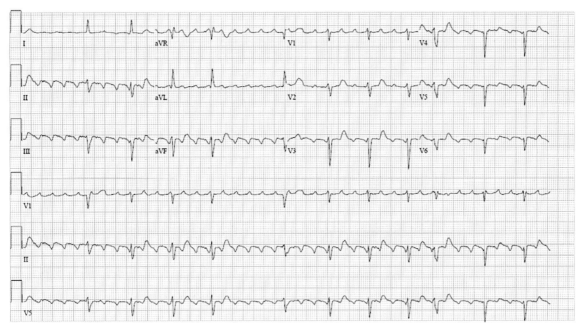

Fig. 25.3 Typical atrial flutter with variable conduction. Typical negatively deflected flutter waves are seen in the inferior leads with positive flutter waves in V₁. 2∶1 atrial flutter can sometimes be difficult to distinguish from atrioventricular nodal reentry tachycardia; adenosine can be used to increase the degree of atrioventricular block and unmask the flutter waves.

occur in different locations within either atrium, are less common, and are typically observed in patients with prior atrial fibrillation ablations or cardiac surgeries. The flutter rate is usually around 300 beats/min, with the ventricular rate determined by the degree of AV node block. Acute atrial flutter presents with a rapid rise in ventricular rate to about 150 beats/min, consistent with 2∶1 AV node block. The ventricular rate can be irregular if there are varying degrees of AV node block. Typical sawtooth-appearing flutter waves can be seen on the surface ECG.

Atrioventricular nodal reentry tachycardia (AVNRT; Fig. 25.4) is a reentry circuit within the AV node or perinodal tissue characterized by a rapid-onset, regular tachycardia with a rate typically between 150 and 250 beats/min. There are two pathways within the AV node with different conduction properties. The difference in conduction allows for a premature atrial contraction (PAC) or premature ventricular contraction (PVC) to stimulate conduction down one pathway while the other is refractory. At the right timing, conduction can then propagate retrograde up the previously refractory pathway, thereby initiating a continuous circuit within the AV node. Conduction of the atria (retrograde) and ventricle (anterograde) occur almost simultaneously in this setting; this is reflected in an ECG that shows a P wave that is either buried in the QRS complex or occurs just shortly after it (pseudo S wave in inferior leads).

Atrioventricular reentry tachycardia (AVRT) is a reentry circuit involving the AV node and an atrioventricular bypass tract some distance from the AV node. Like AVNRT, it is precipitated by a PAC or PVC and is characterized by a rapid onset with a ventricular rate between 150 and 250 beats/min. If conduction occurs initially down the AV node and then retrograde up the bypass

tract, depolarization of the His-Purkinje system and synchronized ventricular contraction occur and the QRS complex is narrow (orthodromic AVRT). A retrograde P wave is typically seen further after the QRS than in AVNRT. If conduction occurs down the bypass tract first, there is slow myocyte-to-myocyte ventricular depolarization with subsequent retrograde conduction through the AV node, leading to a wide QRS complex on surface ECG (antidromic AVRT). A prior ECG can be helpful in establishing the diagnosis, as it may identify preexcitation down a bypass tract characterized by a short PR interval with a delta wave (Wolff-Parkinson-White syndrome).

Atrial fibrillation with conduction down an accessory pathway (Fig. 25.5) is of concern, as it can lead to ventricular fibrillation. Rapid irregular depolarization of wavelets within the atrium can conduct directly down the bypass tract into the ventricle without protection by the AV node, leading to a wide complex irregular tachycardia with a ventricular rate that can be greater than 250 beats/min.

Atrial tachycardia (Fig. 25.6) involves an ectopic atrial pacemaker that can overtake the rate of the sinus node. These tachycardias are more likely to occur under a state of sympathetic activation and thus are more common in the ICU. Atrial tachycardia is characterized by an acute-onset, regular tachycardia with a ventricular rate generally less than 220 beats/min. There is often a slow increase in rate (warm up) over the first 5 to 10 seconds. Atrial tachycardia is also characterized by frequent short bursts. The ECG is characterized by a regular ventricular rate and a P wave morphology distinct from the P wave in sinus rhythm that depends on the anatomic origin of the ectopic atrial activity.

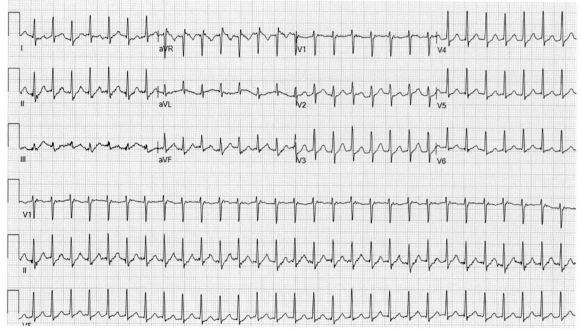

Fig. 25.4 Typical atrioventricular nodal reentry tachycardia. Regular narrow complex tachycardia with pseudo–S wave pattern seen in inferior leads and retrograde P wave seen shortly after the QRS in lead V₁.

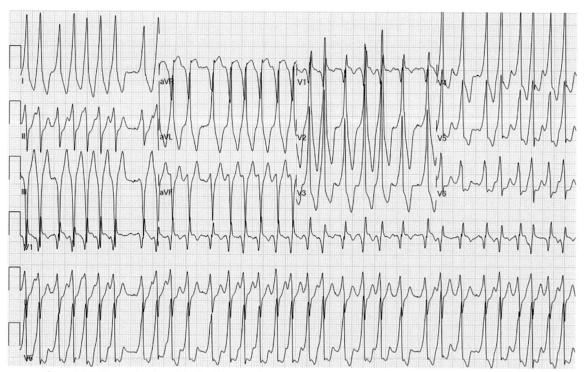

Fig. 25.5 Preexcited atrial fibrillation characterized by a bizarre, wide complex irregular tachycardia.

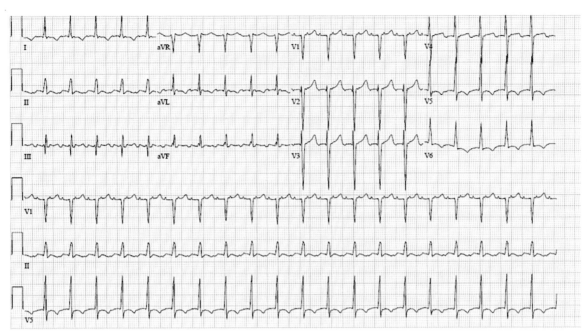

Fig. 25.6 Atrial tachycardia with 2:1 atrioventricular block. Note the P waves in lead III that do not appear to be sinus P waves. The 2:1 atrioventricular pattern is most clearly seen in lead V₁.

Multifocal atrial tachycardia (MAT) involves the presence of multiple ectopic atrial pacemakers with a faster rate than the sinus node. The ECG shows an irregular ventricular rhythm with at least three distinct P wave morphologies and variable PR intervals. MAT is associated with severe pulmonary disease, often during an acute exacerbation. Thus MAT is not uncommon in the ICU.

THERAPY

The therapy for SVT outlined is largely consistent with the 2015 American Heart Association (AHA) Advanced Cardiac Life Support (ACLS)[4] guidelines and the 2015 American College of Cardiology (ACC)/AHA/Heart Rhythm Society (HRS) SVT guidelines.[5] Patients with SVT should be initially evaluated for hemodynamic instability. This includes assessment of blood pressure, cardiopulmonary status, mental status, and peripheral perfusion by physical examination.

If it is clear that the SVT is causing hemodynamic instability, it should be immediately treated with synchronized DCCV, regardless of the exact rhythm. Adequate sedation should be provided during the procedure if tolerated hemodynamically. Pads should be placed on the chest with the heart between the pads. The initial voltage of cardioversion depends on the suspected arrhythmia based on QRS width and regularity of the tachyarrhythmia. Cardioversion can be repeated at a higher voltage if initially unsuccessful. A second set of pads may be applied to the patient's chest to increase the voltage, especially for patients with a large body habitus. Repeated recurrence of SVT should prompt consideration for the use of an antiarrhythmic drug (AAD) and consultation with an electrophysiologist.

For patients who have a regular tachycardia that causes symptoms but are hemodynamically stable, vagal maneuvers should be performed to temporarily block AV node conduction. Vagal maneuvers include carotid massage, having the patient bear down, and application of ice-cold water to the face. Performed appropriately, vagal maneuvers can terminate AV node–dependent reentrant arrhythmias (AVNRT, AVRT) in up to 20% of patients.[6] A modified Valsalva maneuver with transition from a sitting to supine position with passive leg raise after Valsalva strain was shown to improve the success rate for cardioversion to about 43% in the REVERT trial.[7] For SVT due to enhanced automaticity or due to non-AV node–dependent reentrant arrhythmias (atrial fibrillation, atrial tachycardia, atrial flutter, MAT), vagal maneuvers may temporarily block AV node conduction to unmask atrial activity. This can be useful diagnostically, especially during 2:1 atrial flutter when typical flutter waves may not be easily discerned without increasing the degree of AV node block.

For patients who do not respond to vagal maneuvers, adenosine should be administered. Adenosine is a short-acting endogenous nucleotide that blocks AV node conduction for a few seconds. Its half-life is very short, as it is metabolized by red blood cells; the drug should be administered rapidly via a large-bore IV and flushed with saline. Like vagal maneuvers, adenosine is useful therapeutically and diagnostically, as it can terminate AV node–dependent reentry SVT or unmask atrial activity with increased AV node block. Caution should be taken in administering the drug to patients with significant reactive airway disease, as it can cause bronchospasm. Patients who have undergone heart transplantation are particularly sensitive to adenosine and should receive a smaller dose. Adenosine can precipitate atrial fibrillation in up to 10% to 15% of patients after administration.[8] This is of consequence with antidromic AVRT, as conversion to atrial fibrillation in this setting can cause rapid conduction down the atrioventricular bypass tract and lead to hemodynamic instability.

In addition to adenosine, β-blockers and nondihydropyridine calcium channel blockers (diltiazem, verapamil) can also be used to block the AV node and suppress node-dependent reentrant tachycardias. Caution should be exercised with the use of these agents in a critically ill patient given a longer half-life and more potently negative inotropic effects than adenosine. AV nodal blockers are also effective in controlling the ventricular rate of atrial tachyarrhythmias.

An AAD can be administered to cardiovert patients with SVT, to facilitate DCCV, or to promote maintenance of sinus rhythm. The most commonly used AAD used in the acute setting by intensivists is the class III drug amiodarone. The drug has properties of all the major classes in the Vaughan Williams–Singh antiarrhythmic classification and is less likely to be proarrhythmogenic than other AADs. Amiodarone is frequently used to control the rate of atrial fibrillation and to prevent recurrence after spontaneous or DC cardioversion. Use of amiodarone long term should be limited given its toxicities (thyroid, pulmonary, liver, skin). Other AADs may be used in consultation with and electrophysiologist depending on the clinical scenario.

Unlike most other SVTs, preexcited atrial fibrillation frequently causes hemodynamic instability. Vagal maneuvers, adenosine, or other nodal-blocking agents should not be used as they have no effect on the conduction of the bypass tract. Prompt DCCV or administration of procainamide or ibutilide are reasonable initial management options, with subsequent consideration of accessory pathway ablation. Procainamide is a class Ia antiarrhythmic that blocks sodium channels; it causes decreased conduction velocity manifested on the ECG with a widening of the QRS complex. It works primarily by modifying the accessory pathway conduction and decreasing the degree of preexcitation. Ibutilide is an intravenous class III antiarrhythmic that terminates preexcited atrial fibrillation by cardioverting it to sinus rhythm. It can cause potent QTc prolongation; thus pads should be placed on the patient's chest and potassium and magnesium levels should not be low. Ibutilide should be avoided if the patient has significant hypokalemia or hypomagnesemia.

After conversion of SVT to sinus rhythm or after achievement of hemodynamic stability, attention should shift to potential precipitating causes of SVT and ongoing arrhythmia management. Consultation with an electrophysiologist should be considered, especially for AV node reentrant arrhythmias, accessory pathways, or atrial flutter, as these arrhythmias are readily amenable to ablation. Ablation should be performed when the patient is hemodynamically stable and the underlying factors predisposing to SVT have been addressed.

The full reference list for this chapter is available at ExpertConsult.com.

26

Acute Presentations of Valvular Heart Disease

Ruth Hsiao, Daniel Blanchard, Barry Greenberg

OUTLINE

Acute deterioration in valvular function represents a tremendous challenge to the practicing clinician. The presentation of valvular emergencies is usually dramatic; a thorough knowledge of predisposing etiologies, hemodynamic abnormalities, and therapeutic modalities is essential to making appropriate management decisions. Despite an increasing population of patients with prosthetic valves, a resurgence of rheumatic fever, and the continued rise in intravenous drug use–associated infective endocarditis, the overall incidence of valvular emergencies in cardiac intensive care unit (CICU) settings is low. However, the consequences of a missed diagnosis or a delay in therapy can be devastating. Therefore, an important guideline is to always entertain the possibility of acute valvular dysfunction in a patient presenting with hemodynamic instability or acute congestive heart failure.

This review focuses primarily on acute dysfunction of the aortic and mitral valves leading to severe regurgitation and aortic valves leading to acute stenosis. The unique valvular complications associated with prosthetic valves and acute tricuspid regurgitation will also be discussed. Finally, valvular complications associated with mechanical assist devices will be addressed.

ACUTE AORTIC REGURGITATION

Etiology

Aortic regurgitation occurs as a result of either dilation of the aortic root and annulus or disruption of the valve leaflets. The most common etiologies of acute aortic regurgitation are infective endocarditis and aortic dissection.[1] Infective endocarditis is more likely to occur in a congenitally abnormal or rheumatically involved valve; it results in acute aortic regurgitation through a process of endothelial damage, development of nonbacterial thrombotic vegetation, adherence of circulating organisms to the vegetation, proliferation of infection within the vegetation, and progressive valve destruction.[2] Acute, type A, aortic dissection is complicated by some degree of aortic regurgitation in approximately 50% of cases.[3,4] Aortic dissection can lead to aortic regurgitation by direct extension of the dissection to the base of the aortic valve leaflets, dilation of the sinuses with incomplete coaptation of the leaflets at the center of the valve, involvement of a valve commissure leading to inadequate leaflet support, and/or prolapse of the dissection flap across the aortic valve into

BOX 26.1   Etiologies of Acute Aortic Regurgitation

Infective endocarditis
Aortic dissection—predisposing and associated conditions
    Hypertension
    Marfan syndrome
    Congenital bicuspid aortic valve
    Coarctation of aorta
    Ehler-Danlos syndrome
    Turner syndrome
Chest trauma
Rupture of a myxomatous valve
Systemic connective tissue disorders
    Ankylosing spondylitis
    Systemic lupus erythematosus
Granulomatous diseases
    Tertiary syphilis
    Giant cell arteritis
    Takayasu arteritis

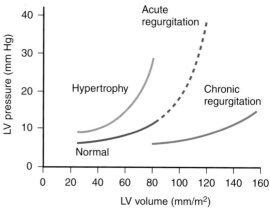

Fig. 26.1 Diastolic pressure-volume relationships in the left ventricle. *Acute regurgitation* is sudden volume loading of the left ventricle without the benefit of adaptive ventricular remodeling. It results in the left ventricle functioning on the steep portion of the normal curve *(dotted line)*. *Chronic regurgitation* is volume loading in the presence of a remodeled ventricle. It shifts the curve to the left and allows normalization of left ventricular (LV) filling pressure at significantly increased LV volumes. *Hypertrophy* (e.g., aortic stenosis) shifts the curve to the right and results in a noncompliant ventricle that is highly dependent on atrial booster pump function for LV filling. (From Hall RJ, Julian DG. *Diseases of the Cardiac Valves.* New York: Churchill Livingstone, 1989; 291.)

the left ventricular outflow tract in diastole, impeding leaflet closure. Other etiologies of acute aortic regurgitation are listed in Box 26.1.

Pathophysiology

The presentation of acute, severe aortic regurgitation differs significantly from that of chronic aortic regurgitation owing to the dramatic hemodynamic changes that occur when the unadapted left ventricle (LV) is suddenly required to augment total stroke volume in order to maintain normal forward flow while simultaneously being exposed to a substantial increase in volume overload. The basic function of the heart is to maintain cardiac output commensurate with body demands. In the normal setting, it does so while operating on the flat portion of the curvilinear LV diastolic pressure-volume relationship and filling pressures remain low. Cardiac output is the product of heart rate and forward stroke volume. Forward stroke volume is the total stroke volume minus the regurgitant volume. Under normal circumstances, the latter is negligible so that total and forward stroke volumes are synonymous.

In acute, severe aortic regurgitation, the large regurgitant volume imposed on the unprepared LV markedly reduces forward stroke volume and shifts the LV diastolic pressure–volume relationship to the steep ascending portion of the curve. Because the LV and its surrounding pericardium have limited distensibility, acute increases in LV end-diastolic volume due to regurgitant flow result in an abrupt rise in LV end-diastolic pressure (LVEDP) (Fig. 26.1). This leads to a rapid increase in the ventriculoatrial gradient, which can cause the mitral valve to close prematurely before the onset of the next systole. This is beneficial in that the high LVEDP is not transmitted to the pulmonary venous system and it offers a degree of protection against the development of pulmonary edema. However, protection owing to premature mitral valve closure can be lost if a further rise in the ventriculoatrial gradient reopens the mitral valve in late diastole, leading to diastolic mitral regurgitation. Systolic mitral regurgitation

can also manifest from the persistent ventriculoatrial gradient as a result of extension of the high LVEDP level to the isovolumic contraction period during early systole, causing mitral valve opening. This mitral regurgitation is usually effective in lowering the LVEDP and the left atrium (LA) essentially serves as a reservoir for blood that has regurgitated from the aorta to the LV. However, left atrial pressure may rise further, leading to pulmonary edema.[5]

Coronary ischemia can complicate acute aortic regurgitation as a reduction in diastolic coronary flow leads to a decrease in myocardial perfusion, while elevated LVEDP and tachycardia increase myocardial oxygen demand. Diastolic coronary flow may be reduced by a reduction in diastolic blood pressure in the aorta, elevation of diastolic pressures in the LV, and by the adverse effects of regurgitant flow on forward flow into the coronary vessels owing to the Venturi effect. The supply-demand mismatch that develops in the setting of acute aortic regurgitation is worsened further if obstructive coronary lesions are present or when aortic dissection impairs coronary flow.[6]

To further complicate the picture, reflex sympathetic activation, in response to a reduction in cardiac output and systemic blood pressure, produces tachycardia and increases systemic vascular resistance (SVR). This rise in SVR further worsens regurgitant flow and impedes ejection of blood from the LV to the aorta so that a rise in aortic systolic pressure is inhibited. In some cases, the LV and aortic diastolic pressures are equalized. As opposed to chronic aortic regurgitation, aortic diastolic pressure usually does not fall significantly in the acute setting for two reasons: (1) the rapid increase in LVEDP reduces the driving gradient between the aorta and LV and (2) peripheral runoff is limited by an increase in SVR.[7,8]

Clinical Presentation

The clinical features of aortic regurgitation are profoundly different in the acute compared to the chronic setting. These differences include the presence of markedly elevated LVEDP and absence of a wide pulse pressure in patients with acute severe aortic regurgitation. Because compensatory structural changes in the LV develop gradually over time, the presentation of an additional volume load imposed by acute aortic regurgitation on the unprepared LV may lead to the rapid onset of severe congestive heart failure or cardiogenic shock.[9,10] Detection of aortic regurgitation can be difficult in the acute setting; it is often misdiagnosed as another acute condition, such as sepsis, pneumonia, or nonvalvular heart disease.[5]

Patients with acute aortic regurgitation typically present with severe dyspnea, weakness, or hypotension. They are often tachycardic. The LV impulse may be normal in both location and duration. Owing to early mitral valve closure from the rapid elevation of LVEDP and consequent reversal of pressures between the LV and LA in late diastole, the first heart sound is often soft or inaudible. Occasionally, mitral valve closure may be heard during diastole and accompanied by diastolic mitral regurgitation.[11,12] The Austin-Flint murmur, which is thought to represent turbulent flow from the LA to the LV because of partial mitral valve closure from the aortic insufficiency jet, is either absent or brief and ceases when LV pressure exceeds LA pressure in diastole.[13,14] An accentuated pulmonic closure sound suggests elevated pulmonary arterial pressure. A third heart sound (S_3) is frequently heard. A fourth heart sound (S_4), however, is usually not present because the mitral valve is either closed before atrial systole occurs or LVEDP is already so high that there is little flow to the ventricle during this period. The acute aortic regurgitation murmur is characteristically short, early, and of medium pitch, unlike the long, high-pitched murmur of chronic aortic regurgitation. In tachycardic patients, this diastolic murmur can easily be overlooked. Edema and weight gain are not often seen in severe acute aortic insufficiency because there is inadequate time for substantial secondary salt and water retention. The extremities may be cool and mottled owing to both poor cardiac output and elevated SVR. Peripheral manifestations characteristic of chronic aortic regurgitation, such as wide pulse pressure and others (e.g., Quincke's pulse, water hammer pulse), are uncommon in the acute setting. Clinical features seen in acute and chronic aortic regurgitation are listed in Table 26.1.

Diagnosis

The diagnosis of acute aortic regurgitation should be considered in the differential of any patient presenting with acute pulmonary edema or circulatory collapse. A history of known valvular disease, evidence of infective endocarditis, long-standing hypertension, Marfan syndrome, or chest trauma should make one particularly suspicious. Initial diagnostic testing in patients suspected of having acute aortic regurgitation includes an electrocardiogram (ECG), chest radiograph, blood cultures (if infective endocarditis is suspected or if the patient has a prosthetic valve), and a transthoracic echocardiogram (TTE).

TABLE 26.1	Clinical Features of Severe Aortic Regurgitation	
Feature	**Acute**	**Chronic**
Congestive heart failure	Rapid and sudden	Insidious
Rhythm	Sinus tachycardia	Regular rate
Point of maximal impulse	Not hyperdynamic and nondisplaced	Hyperdynamic and shifted inferolaterally
Pulse pressure	Normal	Widened
Heart sounds		
S_1	Soft or absent	Soft
S_2	Soft A2, accentuated P2	Normal P2
S_3	Present	Absent
S_4	Absent	Usually absent
Aortic regurgitation murmur	Soft, early	Holodiastolic
Cardiac output	Decreased	Normal
LVEDP	Increased	Normal
LV size	Normal	Increased

LV, Left ventricle; *LVEDP,* left ventricular end-diastolic pressure.

An ECG is required in all patients with pulmonary edema, primarily to rule out acute myocardial infarction (MI). The ECG can also be helpful in the patient with acute aortic regurgitation to identify evidence of myocardial ischemia or injury that results from the hemodynamic perturbations that adversely affect the myocardial supply and demand ratio. The ECG in acute aortic regurgitation may be normal with a left axis deviation. With early LV volume overload, there can be Q waves in leads I, aVL, and V_3 to V_6. As disease progresses, the prominent initial forces decrease but total QRS amplitude increases.

In the absence of preexisting heart disease, the chest radiograph generally reveals a normal cardiac silhouette with evidence of pulmonary edema (Fig. 26.2). A widened aortic root suggests the presence of dissection. Noninvasive imaging by TTE provides crucial information regarding the presence, severity, and etiology of the valve lesion. With severe aortic regurgitation, in addition to visualizing the regurgitant jet with color Doppler, quantitative measurements, such as jet or vena contracta (narrowest portion of regurgitant jet immediately distal to valve orifice) width, can be obtained (Fig. 26.3, Video 26.1). A jet width greater than 65% of LV outflow tract and vena contracta greater than 0.6 cm are consistent with severe aortic regurgitation.[5] Continuous wave Doppler is used to calculate the pressure half-time, which reflects the equilibration between aortic and LV diastolic pressure. With acute, severe aortic regurgitation, the rapid equilibration of pressures results in a short pressure half-time of less than 300 msec.[15] Other echocardiographic findings supportive of severe aortic regurgitation include premature closure of the mitral valve, detected best by M-mode echocardiography and holodiastolic flow reversal in the descending aorta (Fig. 26.4). Transesophageal echocardiography (TEE) may be required in individuals in whom transthoracic echo windows are limited. In addition, TEE has increased sensitivity for evaluating the underlying etiology of aortic regurgitation, such as endocarditis (vegetations or aortic root abscess; Fig. 26.5, Video 26.2) or aortic dissection (dissection flap).[16,17]

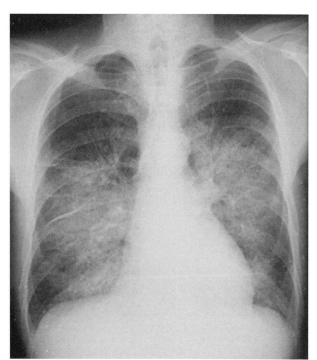

Fig. 26.2 Chest radiograph from a patient with acute aortic insufficiency secondary to pneumococcal endocarditis. Note the classic findings of acute pulmonary edema with a normal cardiac silhouette.

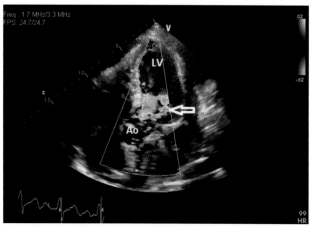

Fig. 26.3 Five-chamber transthoracic echocardiogram shows the presence of severe aortic regurgitation on color Doppler (arrow; see also Video 26.1). Ao, Aorta; LV, left ventricle.

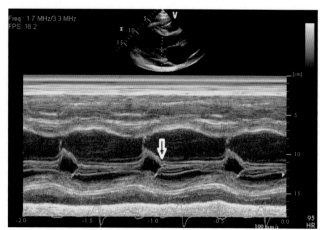

Fig. 26.4 M-mode transthoracic echocardiogram demonstrates the presystolic mitral valve closure (arrow) from the increased left ventricular pressure compared with left atrial pressure.

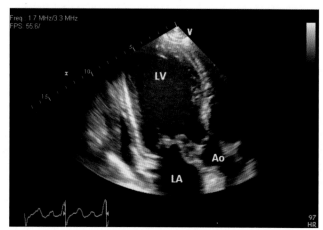

Fig. 26.5 Apical three-chamber transthoracic echocardiogram shows the presence of a mitral valve and aortic valve vegetation (see also Video 26.2). Ao, Aorta; LA, left atrium; LV, left ventricle.

Aortic dissection should be considered in the differential diagnosis of any patient having acute aortic regurgitation. This diagnosis can be confirmed either by computed tomography (CT), TEE, or magnetic resonance imaging (MRI). These imaging modalities have largely replaced aortography, the previous gold standard. TTE can be a very useful and quick tool for identifying aortic valve dysfunction and may screen for abnormalities in the proximal 4 to 8 mm of the ascending aorta and a short segment of the descending aorta. The sensitivity for diagnosing aortic dissections with a TTE is only 59% to 83% and the specificity is 63% to 93%. Its sensitivity is higher for type A aortic dissection at 78% to 100%, but for type B, the sensitivity

is only 31% to 55%.[18] Thus, TTE should be used to evaluate complications of acute aortic syndrome—such as valve dysfunction, pericardial tamponade, or wall motion abnormalities—and not for diagnosis in suspected acute aortic syndromes. Alternatively, TEE is highly accurate in detecting acute aortic syndromes due to the close proximity of the esophagus to the thoracic aorta and its ability to visualize both the ascending and descending aortas. A true dissection flap features random mobility, constant echo intensity along its course, and margination of flow on color flow imaging, which can be identified by a skilled and experienced operator. TEE can reach a sensitivity of 99% and a specificity of 89%.[18,19] However, owing to its requirement for a skilled operator and adequate sedation to prevent a hypertensive response in the patient, CT is the preferred modality for evaluation of aortic dissection in the emergency department (Fig. 26.6). A contrast study is highly accurate, with a sensitivity and specificity about 95% to 98%, and is able to provide the site(s) of dissection and extent of involvement.[18] MRI is also highly accurate, with a sensitivity and specificity of about 94% to 98%. However, it

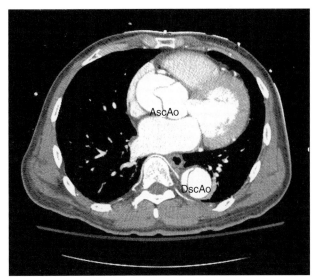

Fig. 26.6 Computed tomographic angiogram reveals a type A aortic dissection with the presence of an intimal flap in the ascending aorta *(AscAo)* and descending aorta *(DscAo)*. *LA,* Left atrium; *LV,* left ventricle.

is time consuming and often not readily available in the emergency setting and is probably most useful in the follow-up of aortic dissection after surgical repair.[18]

Treatment

Patients with acute severe aortic regurgitation are often desperately ill with both systemic hypoperfusion and pulmonary edema; not surprisingly, many of these patients require urgent surgery. However, medical therapy has an important role in optimizing hemodynamics perioperatively. In the presence of severe hemodynamic compromise, admission to the CICU is clearly indicated. The principles of management include recognizing the degree of hemodynamic impairment, reducing pulmonary venous pressure, maximizing cardiac output, and initiating therapy for any underlying disorder.[20] Invasive hemodynamic monitoring by placement of a Swan-Ganz pulmonary artery catheter is extremely helpful in critically ill patients in that it allows the clinician to assess the response to therapy and gauge the tempo of the illness.

Medical therapy for congestive heart failure owing to acute aortic regurgitation includes both loop diuretics and intravenous vasodilators. The objectives are to maximize cardiac output while reducing intracardiac filling pressures. The hemodynamic response to medical therapy in large part determines the urgency of surgical intervention.

In patients with acute aortic regurgitation, intravenous vasodilator therapy can significantly reduce pulmonary artery pressures and increase forward cardiac output. Nitroprusside is the vasodilator of choice. The drug is started at 0.25 μg/kg per minute given intravenously and gradually uptitrated by increments of 0.25 to 0.5 μg/kg per minute with the goal of achieving optimal hemodynamics or until systemic hypotension supervenes.[21] The speed of uptitration is dictated by the degree of hemodynamic compromise. In severely ill patients, the nitroprusside dose

can be increased every 5 minutes; in stable patients, a more gradual approach is often used. During maintenance therapy, one needs to be alert for signs and symptoms of both cyanide and thiocyanate toxicity (e.g., tinnitus, altered mental status, nausea, and abdominal pain). These breakdown products of nitroprusside accumulate with prolonged use, especially in the presence of renal insufficiency. Diuretics should be initiated in sufficient doses to induce a brisk sustained urine output, using pulmonary capillary wedge pressure as a guide to therapy. Titrating the intravenous doses of furosemide (start 40 to 80 mg every 6 to 12 hours; maximum 600 mg/day), bumetanide (start 0.5 to 2 mg every 12 to 24 hours; maximum 10 mg/day), or torsemide (start 10 to 20 mg daily; maximum 200 mg/day) with or without oral metolazone (2.5 to 20 mg/day in divided doses) or intravenous chlorothiazide (500 to 1000 mg/day in divided doses) 30 minutes before administering the loop diuretic is extremely effective in decongesting patients.

In general, inotropic agents do not play a significant role in management of acute aortic regurgitation because most cases occur in the setting of normal or even accentuated LV contractile function. However, if preexisting myocardial dysfunction exists, agents such as dobutamine at a dose of 5 to 15 μg/kg per minute may assist in maintaining cardiac output.[22] Intraaortic balloon pumps (IABPs) are contraindicated with aortic regurgitation because balloon inflation during diastole would increase regurgitant flow, thereby increasing LV diastolic pressure and further compromising forward cardiac output. Additional medical therapy includes appropriate antibiotics in suspected infective endocarditis.[23] In the case of aortic dissection, intravenous β-blockers are thought to be useful in reducing the velocity of LV ejection, thereby minimizing aortic wall stress. However, when aortic dissection is complicated by acute aortic regurgitation, β-blockers should be used cautiously, if at all, as the compensatory tachycardia that occurs in this setting would be blunted, further reducing forward cardiac output.

If, despite medical therapy, hemodynamic instability persists, emergent surgical valve repair or replacement represents the only definitive option for cure. Indications for surgery in the presence of infective endocarditis are outlined in Box 26.2. Even in the presence of active infective endocarditis, valve surgery should not be delayed in order to achieve a bacteriologic cure. In a prospective, multinational cohort study, early surgical repair of native valve endocarditis including aortic, mitral, and tricuspid was associated with a significant mortality reduction from 21% to 12% compared to medical therapy. Survival benefits in the early surgery group were seen in patients with perivalvular complications, systemic embolization, stroke, and *Staphylococcus aureus* native valve endocarditis but not in patients with valve perforation or congestive heart failure.[24]

Based on the recent International Registry of Acute Aortic Dissection (1995–2013) analysis, there has been a decline in overall mortality for type A aortic dissection from 31% to 22% driven mostly by a reduction in surgical mortality from 25% to 18%.[25] The majority of type A dissections are managed surgically (86% overall), with an overall increase in rates of operative intervention from 79% to 90% in the later time periods. If managed medically, the in-hospital mortality remained high at

---

BOX 26.2 Indications for Surgery in Infective Endocarditis of Native or Prosthetic Valve

Early Surgery (During Initial Hospitalization Before Completion of Full Antibiotic Course)

Valve dysfunction causing heart failure symptoms (class I)

Left-sided infective endocarditis caused by highly resistant organism (*S. aureus,* fungi) (class I)

Heart block, abscess, or destructive penetrating lesion (class I)

Persistent infection (persistent bacteremia or fevers lasting longer than 5–7 days despite appropriate therapy; class I)

Recurrent emboli and persistent vegetations despite appropriate antibiotic therapy (class IIa)

Large (>10 mm) mobile vegetation on native valve (class IIb)

Indication for surgery but with complication of a stroke with no evidence of intracranial hemorrhage or extensive neurologic damage (class IIb)

Surgery

Relapsing prosthetic valve endocarditis (recurrence of bacteremia after completion of antibiotic course with subsequent negative blood cultures (class I)

Complication of major ischemic stroke or intracranial hemorrhage and hemodynamically stable, delay surgery for at least 4 weeks (class IIb)

From Nishimura RA, Otto CM, Bonow RO, et al. 2017 AHA/ACC Focused Update of the 2014 AHA/ACC Guideline for the Management of Patients With Valvular Heart Disease. *J Am Coll Cardiol.* 2017;70:252–289.

57%. Endovascular repair alone was associated with a high mortality rate (71%).

AORTIC STENOSIS

Etiology

Aortic stenosis presents as a slowly progressive disorder characterized by narrowing of the aortic valvular orifice resulting in dyspnea, angina, or syncope.[26] The etiology varies from a degenerative, calcific process of the aortic leaflets due to age or chronic rheumatic heart disease to congenital abnormalities in valve structure (e.g., bicuspid valve) that predispose to accelerated degenerative changes over time.

Several conditions may lead to an acute deterioration in aortic stenosis patients. To discern the inciting events leading to acute decompensation in valvular aortic stenosis, it is important to understand the underlying pathophysiologic state. Progressive valvular aortic stenosis leads to increasing LV systolic pressure and wall stress. In an effort to normalize this afterload mismatch, the LV hypertrophies. Initially, this normalizes wall stress, but it also results in a shift of the LV pressure-volume curve upward and to the left. This necessitates higher filling pressures for a given ventricular volume, leading to elevated pulmonary venous pressures with consequent dyspnea on effort. Because of this abnormal LV pressure-volume relationship, any diminution in preload will seriously impair stroke volume. Therefore, conditions that lead to acute volume shifts (e.g., dehydration or acute blood loss) will result in a significant impairment of cardiac output. The altered LV pressure-volume relationship reduces passive LV filling, making LV preload critically dependent on atrial contraction.[27]

Any impairment in the contribution of diastolic filling by atrial systole, such as atrial fibrillation or atrioventricular dyssynchrony, can lead to acute decompensation. In addition to atrial arrhythmias and conduction abnormalities, increasing heart rate may also impair LV filling simply by decreasing the diastolic filling period. It is also important to realize that a markedly reduced heart rate will impair forward cardiac output because stroke volume may be compromised in patients with severe aortic stenosis and overall cardiac output becomes increasingly dependent on heart rate. This is particularly true when LV systolic function is impaired. Any condition that further impairs LV relaxation (e.g., acute coronary ischemia) will also have a significant impact on diastolic filling. Relative ischemia may also occur in the setting of normal coronary arteries or nonobstructive coronary artery disease when myocardial oxygen demands have exceeded coronary reserve.[28]

Physical examination of the patient with aortic stenosis reveals a small-volume, slowly rising, sustained pulse. The apical impulse of the heart may be displaced downward and to the left with a marked presystolic impulse or "a" wave. The harsh ejection systolic murmur of aortic stenosis is best heard at the base and is transmitted to the carotids but may also be heard at the apex, particularly in patients with age-related calcification of a tricuspid valve (Gallavardin phenomenon). In general, late peaking murmurs of longer duration signify more severe stenosis.[29,30] However, it is important to remember that with decreasing cardiac output, there is a fall in the gradient with an associated diminution in the intensity of the murmur. The authors have encountered several patients with severe aortic stenosis who have had low-intensity murmurs occurring early in systole.

Treatment

The treatment of patients who present with acute manifestations of aortic stenosis is targeted toward correcting the underlying problem that led to acute decompensation. In cases of volume depletion due to dehydration or blood loss, volume replacement must be judicious to avoid precipitating pulmonary edema. Cautious use of an inotrope that can also constrict peripheral resistance vessels, such as dopamine, may be useful in volume-depleted hypotensive patients. If pulmonary congestion occurs, loop diuretics can be used cautiously to decrease pulmonary capillary pressure.

Atrial fibrillation should be treated with urgent synchronized cardioversion, particularly if systemic hypotension or pulmonary congestion has been precipitated by the arrhythmia. Atrioventricular conduction abnormalities should be managed with temporary pacing followed by a dual chamber permanent pacemaker if the conduction disturbance persists. Once the patient is stabilized, urgent valve replacement should be undertaken. If there is a question of coronary artery disease, cardiac catheterization should be performed to define coronary anatomy. Occasionally, when the patient is gravely ill from LV failure, it may be necessary to proceed directly to valve replacement without preoperative coronary angiography.

Valve replacement for aortic stenosis includes surgical or transcatheter aortic valve replacement (TAVR). Based on the updated 2017 American Heart Association/American College of

Cardiology (AHA/ACC) guidelines for severe and symptomatic (stage D) aortic stenosis, surgical AVR is a class I recommendation for low-risk and intermediate surgical risk patients. TAVR is a class IIa recommendation for intermediate surgical risk patients. For patients with high surgical risk, surgical AVR and TAVR are both class I recommendations. For patients with a prohibitive risk for surgical AVR, TAVR is a class I recommendation.[31]

Mechanical circulatory support approaches have emerged as a rescue therapy in critical aortic valve stenosis with or without cardiogenic shock or as a bridge to TAVR. Currently, the use of mechanical therapies has a class IIb recommendation for cardiogenic shock in ST elevation MI; however, there have been case reports and small institutional studies in which the use of TandemHeart (CardiacAssist) and Impella (Abiomed) has been tried in patients with critical aortic stenosis. The TandemHeart is an extracorporeal left ventricular assist device that is placed in the femoral vein with the cannula traversing across the atria septum into the LA, where oxygenated blood is aspirated and pumped into the femoral arterial system at a rate of 4.0 L/min. The Impella is a percutaneous ventricular assist device that is inserted via the femoral artery and passed across the aortic valve. Blood is aspirated from the LV and pumped into the systemic system. The Impella 2.5 can generate 2.5 L/min of cardiac output; a larger device, Impella 5.0, can maintain a cardiac output of 5.0 L/min. In 2009, Gregoric et al.[32] published a retrospective review of 10 patients in which TandemHeart was used as a rescue therapy for patients with critical aortic stenosis with cardiac arrest or severe refractory cardiogenic shock. Of the eight patients who underwent percutaneous ventricular assist device placement before surgical aortic valve repair, seven were long-term survivors. In 2012, Martinez et al.[33] published a retrospective study describing the use of the Impella 2.5 in patients with chronic aortic stenosis and LV dysfunction requiring percutaneous interventions, such as coronary interventions or balloon valvuloplasty, prior to TAVR placement. There were no periprocedural deaths, and the 30-day mortality was 14.2%.

Post–Transcatheter Aortic Valve Replacement Aortic Regurgitation. The recent increase in percutaneous valve replacement has been accompanied by an increase in complications that lead to acute valvular disease. TAVR is now a well-established procedure performed for patients with surgically intermediate or high-risk or inoperable severe aortic stenosis. Because the heart valves are implanted without the use of sutures and use oversizing to anchor the prosthetic stent frame at the level of the aortic annulus, incomplete circumferential apposition can lead to perivalvular aortic leak or regurgitation. This is different from central aortic regurgitation, which is most commonly seen in diseased native valves or damaged prosthetic valves. Conversely, perivalvular aortic regurgitation (PAR) is a complication only of aortic valve prostheses and occurs most commonly following TAVR.

Several studies have shown that up to 85% of all patients after TAVR have PAR after the procedure. Approximately 12% have PAR graded moderate or severe at discharge.[34] After surgical aortic valve repair, the incidence of moderate or severe residual aortic regurgitation is 4%.[35] More than mild PAR has significant impact on prognosis after TAVR, with a twofold to fourfold

increased 1-year mortality risk compared with patients without clinically significant PAR. There are conflicting results regarding the impact of mild PAR on survival; further studies are needed to evaluate the direct causal relationship between PAR and mortality in patients with milder degrees of regurgitation. To date, there has not been a direct comparison of the rate of PAR after TAVR between the two most frequently used heart valves, the Edwards balloon-expandable valve (Edwards Lifesciences) and the self-expandable CoreValve (Medtronic). Based on the French Aortic National CoreValve and Edwards 2 Registry, the 1-year data demonstrated that the balloon-expandable valve is associated with a moderate to severe PAR in 12.2% of patients at discharge compared with 19.8% for the self-expandable valve.[35,36]

PAR develops by three main mechanisms: (1) suboptimal placement of the prosthesis that leads to incomplete sealing of the annulus by the skirt; (2) incomplete apposition of the prosthesis owing to calcification of the annulus, native leaflets, or LV outflow tract; (3) and/or mismatch between the size of the annulus and the size of the prosthesis owing to undersizing of the replacement aortic valve. Valve sizing is one of the strongest predictors of PAR. Appropriate sizing using multidetector CT is the gold standard and has been associated with reduced rates of significant PAR. Risk factors for PAR include degenerative calcification of the native aortic valve or cusp and functional bicuspid aortic valve with heavy calcification of the fused commissures.

Intraprocedural imaging with a TEE is useful for detection and assessment of acute PAR. Using the biplane mode or a single-plane, short-axis view, the valve deployment, stent positioning, shape, leaflet motion, and presence and severity of AR can be quickly evaluated. For PAR, the short-axis plane of imaging should be just below the valve stent and skirt and just within the LV outflow tract. To evaluate PAR, recent TAVR studies have shown that qualitative assessment with angiography of PAR correlated well with echocardiography.

Intraprocedural imaging is important in establishing the diagnosis and severity of PAR and can be used to help guide the management of PAR when it occurs. Corrective techniques include using balloon post-dilation for frame underexpansion, valve-in-valve implantation for a malpositioned transcatheter heart valve or central regurgitation, and snare technique for valves implanted too deeply. In cases of properly placed valves with good expansion, if a localized AR jet can be identified, transcatheter device closure can be attempted to close the perivalvular leak.

Acute circulatory collapse is a very rare but serious complication that may develop during or after TAVR. Causes include coronary ischemia, severe aortic regurgitation, cardiac tamponade, valve embolization, and LV failure. For mild hemodynamic disturbances related to PAR, medical therapy may be sufficient. However, for refractory cardiogenic shock due to severe valvular regurgitation, mechanical support may be required. Use of an IABP is contraindicated when severe PAR is the cause of shock. The TandemHeart has been placed successfully in a case report study in which the left main stem was occluded after a TAVR.[37] The Impella is advantageous because it requires a single arterial access and can be quickly implanted as it does not require a transseptal puncture that the TandemHeart requires. Two cases of successful use of the Impella post-TAVR have been reported: one for cardiac tamponade and the other for acute aortic regurgitation. In both cases, the Impella assisted in stabilizing patients from their post-TAVR complications until definitive surgical therapy was performed.[38] It is important to note that moderate to severe native aortic valve regurgitation and severe aortic valve calcifications are contraindications to the use of the Impella.

Post–Left Ventricular Assist Device Aortic Regurgitation. The use of mechanical circulatory support (MCS) is increasing rapidly as both bridge to transplant or as destination therapy. As many patients fall into a gray zone in which their candidacy for transplant is uncertain, MCS devices are increasingly being used as a bridge to decision. During implantation of LV assist devices (LVADs), an incompetent aortic valve is treated by oversewing, repairing, or replacing the valve. This strategy is employed to prevent formation of a circulatory loop where a portion of the LVAD output is immediately returned to the pump. The development of de novo aortic valvular disease, however, may occur in LVAD patients. The clinical significance of AR in this setting and its optimal treatment is still being defined.

Based on observational study, de novo development of aortic regurgitation is common and can occur early after LVAD placement.[39] The exact mechanism is not clearly understood. It is hypothesized that aortic blood flow dynamics and prolonged aortic valve closure contribute to postimplantation aortic regurgitation. The aortic outflow conduit is smaller than the aorta and can lead to significant changes in aortic blood flow dynamics and kinetics, which contribute to changes in the sheer stress and diastolic luminal pressures experienced by the aortic wall.[39] At 90 days postimplantation, microscopic examination of the aorta demonstrates evidence of aortic wall atrophy; it has been postulated that this promotes aortic root dilation and wall insufficiency, leading to valve malcoaptation and development of aortic regurgitation.[40] Additionally, patients whose aortic valves do not open regularly with each beat have a greater risk of progression of aortic regurgitation. These patients may require a higher amount of LVAD support as the ventricle is unable to generate the LV systolic pressure to open the aortic valve. Because the aortic valve remains closed during systole due to the LVAD support as opposed to being open in normal systole, it is subjected to an unaccustomed high systolic pressure due to the retrograde flow from the aortic outflow conduit, leading to valve degeneration. Because the aortic outflow conduit is smaller in diameter than the aorta, there is an associated higher velocity required to deliver the same volume. The valve trauma from high-velocity and pressure blood flow and intermittent aortic valve opening leading to progressive valve degeneration allows for de novo aortic regurgitation to develop and progress. The clinical significance of progressive de novo aortic regurgitation has not been well defined, but it appears to be associated with an increase in number of heart failure admissions and arrhythmias.[39]

The management of aortic regurgitation post-LVAD implantation is mostly anecdotal. Medical therapy targeting afterload and preload with vasodilators and diuretics to reduce volume overload is the mainstay of treatment. Inotropic support can be used

when there is refractory heart failure or cardiogenic shock. There have been case reports regarding the use of TAVR to treat patients with impending hemodynamic collapse from progressive aortic regurgitation. Both the CoreValve and SAPIEN (Edwards Lifesciences) transcatheter aortic valves have been successfully implanted to improve cardiac hemodynamics in this setting.[41–43]

ACUTE MITRAL REGURGITATION

Etiology

The presentation of acute severe mitral regurgitation is not unlike acute aortic regurgitation as both valve lesions result in sudden, severe LV volume overload. To better understand the underlying pathophysiologic states leading to acute mitral regurgitation, it is important to first recognize the functional components of the mitral valve apparatus. These components include the LA, mitral annulus, mitral valve leaflets, network of chordae tendineae, papillary muscles, and the subjacent LV wall. All these structures must work in concert to produce effective mitral valve leaflet apposition during systole, and abnormalities of any one can be the cause of mitral regurgitation. Not surprisingly, given the multiplicity of moving parts, there are numerous etiologies of acute mitral regurgitaton, listed in Box 26.3.

Infective endocarditis may cause acute mitral regurgitation by mechanisms including leaflet perforation, alteration of mitral valve annulus secondary to abscess formation, or chordae tendineae rupture. Coronary artery disease is another common cause of acute mitral regurgitation. The onset of myocardial ischemia/injury due to coronary artery disease can affect valvular function in a number of ways: (1) papillary muscle rupture after myocardial infarction,[44] (2) ischemic papillary muscle dysfunction,[45] (3) papillary muscle fibrosis,[45] (4) dyssynergy of the LV segment that anchors what may be a normally functioning papillary muscle,[46] and (5) diffuse LV enlargement that causes mitral annular dilation and changes in the normal geometry of the subvalvular apparatus. The posteromedial papillary muscle has only one vascular supply arising from either the right coronary or left circumflex artery and is, therefore, more susceptible to ischemic dysfunction or infarction. Etiologies of chordal pathology and rupture include myxomatous degeneration associated with mitral valve prolapse or Marfan disease, spontaneous rupture, trauma, or rheumatic disease.[47,48] With the increasing use of percutaneous balloon valvotomy for rheumatic mitral stenosis,

---

BOX 26.3　Etiologies of Acute Mitral Regurgitation

Myocardial infarction
Chordal or papillary muscle rupture
Myxomatous disease
Infective endocarditis
Rheumatic heart disease
Acute cardiomyopathy
Prosthetic valve dysfunction
Trauma
Iatrogenic

iatrogenic mitral regurgitation requiring valve replacement is more frequent as compared with closed surgical valvotomy.[49–51] Finally, degeneration of a bioprosthetic valve, impaired closure of a mechanical mitral valve by pannus ingrowth, or perivalvular regurgitation from suture disruption may lead to acute prosthetic valve mitral regurgitation.

Pathophysiology

The severity of mitral regurgitation depends on the volume of regurgitant flow, LA compliance, and preexisting LV function. The volume of regurgitant flow is a function of the size of the incompetent valve orifice and the pressure gradient between the LV and LA.[52] In the presence of a relatively noncompliant LA, the abrupt increase in pressure is transmitted to the pulmonary circulation with resultant pulmonary edema.[53] With continuing acute regurgitation, the LV begins to fail as a result of elevated wall stress from the mismatch between abrupt elevations in LV end-diastolic volume and pressure and that between development of compensatory LV thickness and mass, which increases only slowly over time. In the presence of mitral regurgitation, there are two outlets to flow from the LV: (1) the relatively high-impedance systemic circulation and (2) the low-impedance LA. In this setting, forward stroke volume is highly dependent on SVR. As SVR increases, a greater proportion of the total LV stroke volume is directed to the LA and the regurgitant fraction increases ([Total stroke volume − Forward stroke volume]/Total stroke volume).[54] A reduction in forward cardiac output increases SVR as neurohormonal systems that cause vasoconstriction are activated in order to maintain blood pressure. The unwanted consequence of rising SVR is a worsening in the severity of mitral regurgitation. As regurgitant flow increases further, cardiac output continues to decline and pulmonary congestion gets progressively worse. This leads to a vicious cycle of further neurohormonal activation and intense peripheral vasoconstriction with even more deleterious consequences on hemodynamics.

Clinical Presentation

The clinical features of acute mitral regurgitation reflect both the pathophysiology and pathoanatomy of the mitral valve apparatus as described earlier. A wide spectrum of clinical illness may be seen, ranging from complete papillary muscle rupture with cardiovascular collapse to mild dyspnea after rupture of a secondary or tertiary chordae.

The general appearance of the patient may provide important diagnostic clues regarding the underlying etiology of mitral regurgitation. A specific phenotype, such as that associated with Marfan or Ehlers-Danlos syndrome, may suggest a diagnosis of chordal rupture. Alternatively, peripheral manifestations of vascular (emboli, Janeway lesions) or immunologic (Osler nodes, Roth spots) findings consistent with the diagnosis of infective endocarditis may be present. Finally, the presence of anginal-type chest pain leads one to suspect myocardial ischemia or infarction, with resulting papillary muscle disease as the underlying etiology of acute mitral regurgitation.

Most patients with acute mitral regurgitation demonstrate tachycardia, which represents a compensatory mechanism to maintain cardiac output in the presence of declining forward stroke volume. The jugular venous pulse may be elevated, with 50% of patients having a prominent "a" wave.[55] Precordial examination often reveals a hyperdynamic, nondisplaced apical impulse with a prominent presystolic expansion, suggesting LV overload with increased atrial systole. A left parasternal lift is also common, as filling from the combination of pulmonary venous and regurgitant flow into the LA (which is the posterior portion of the heart) lifts the entire organ anteriorly. Presence of a parasternal lift is an indication of severe mitral regurgitation, often occurring in association with elevated right ventricular (RV) systolic pressures. A systolic apical thrill may be felt in up to 75% of patients with ruptured chordae tendineae.[55] The presence of a thrill is less common in papillary muscle dysfunction or rupture.[56]

Cardiac auscultation reveals a normal S_1 because in most cases of acute mitral regurgitation the mitral valve leaflets are normal. This is in contradiction to chronic mitral regurgitation, in which S_1 is soft secondary to intrinsically abnormal mitral valve leaflets. Accentuated pulmonary valve closure suggests pulmonary hypertension[55] and, because the LV empties rapidly, the aortic component may close early, giving rise to a widened split of the second heart sound.[57] The presence of an S_4 is common. An S_3 gallop is almost universally heard with severe mitral regurgitation and is related to LV volume overload. The murmur of acute mitral regurgitation differs according to the underlying pathophysiology. In papillary muscle dysfunction, a crescendo-decrescendo murmur may be heard during mid-to-late systole, while papillary muscle rupture results in a pansystolic murmur. Acute chordal rupture results in an ejection murmur that begins in the apex and radiates to the base of the heart.[58] Chronic mitral regurgitation, on the other hand, gives rise to a soft blowing holosystolic murmur heard throughout systole that begins at the apex and radiates to the axilla and back. Early termination of the murmur in acute mitral regurgitation results from rapid equalization of LA and LV pressures and suggests a greater degree of regurgitation.[59] The intensity of the murmur may not reflect the severity of the valve malfunction as widely incompetent valves through which flow may be less turbulent or low flow due to LV dysfunction may give rise to low-grade murmurs despite the presence of severe valvular incompetence.[60] A summary of the differences in clinical presentation between acute and chronic mitral regurgitation is listed in Table 26.2.

Diagnosis

As in the case of acute aortic regurgitation, accurate assessment of intracardiac filling pressures becomes critical, especially in the patient who is hemodynamically unstable. Initial noninvasive diagnostic tests include a chest radiograph, which typically reveals a normal cardiac silhouette with pulmonary venous congestion or edema.[61] However, with preexisting valvular or myocardial disease, there may be radiographic evidence of cardiac enlargement. Occasionally, an unusual pattern of right upper lobe pulmonary edema[62] may result that can be confused with pneumonia (Fig. 26.7). However, prompt resolution with diuretic and vasodilator therapy rapidly clarifies the diagnosis. TEE has demonstrated that this radiologic finding is related to the regurgitant jet being directed toward the right superior pulmonary vein.[63]

The ECG often reveals sinus tachycardia; however, atrial fibrillation with a rapid ventricular response is another common presenting rhythm. A large negative terminal deflection of the P wave in lead V_1 and broadened P wave in lead II suggest LA volume overload. Nonspecific ST segment and T wave abnormalities are quite common; however, if acute mitral regurgitation occurs as a result of ischemia or infarction, the ECG becomes essential for both diagnosis and treatment.

TABLE 26.2   Clinical Features of Severe Mitral Regurgitation

Feature	Acute	Chronic
Congestive heart failure	Rapid and sudden	Insidious
Rhythm	Sinus tachycardia	Atrial fibrillation
Point of maximal impulse	Hyperdynamic and nondisplaced	Hyperdynamic and shifted inferolaterally
Right ventricular lift	Present	Absent
Precordial thrill	Usually present	Absent
Jugular venous pressure	Prominent "a" wave	Normal tracing
Heart sounds		
S_1	Normal	Soft
S_2	Accentuated P2 with wide split	Normal P2 with wide split
S_3	Present	Present
S_4	Present	Absent
Mitral regurgitation murmur	Loud, decreasing in late systole	Blowing holosystolic
Radiation of mitral regurgitation murmur	Toward base	Toward axilla
Mitral diastolic flow murmur	Present	Absent
Cardiac output	Decreased	Normal
Ejection fraction	Normal to reduced	Normal to increased
LVEDP	Increased	Normal
LV size	Normal	Increased

From Depace NL, Nestico PF, Morganroth J. Acute severe mitral regurgitation: pathophysiology, clinical recognition and management. *Am J Med.* 1985;78:293.
LV, Left ventricle; *LVEDP,* left ventricular end-diastolic pressure.

Because the underlying pathoanatomy of the mitral valve influences prognosis and determines the type of therapeutic intervention, rapid assessment of the mitral valve apparatus is an essential component of the management approach. Echocardiography is the most commonly used imaging modality in patients with acute mitral regurgitation. In the presence of good echocardiographic windows, transthoracic imaging can be performed quickly and safely at the bedside to accurately determine the underlying etiology and severity of mitral regurgitation. In addition, overall LV function and wall motion abnormalities indicative of ischemia or infarction can be assessed. Finally, structural cardiac disorders that mimic mitral regurgitation, such as ventricular septal rupture, can be ruled out.[64]

Depending on the etiology of acute mitral regurgitation, a variety of echocardiographic abnormalities may be seen. There may be an obvious flail leaflet, chordal rupture, or vegetation (Fig. 26.8, Video 26.3). Papillary muscle rupture is often directly visualized as a mass attached to the involved leaflet with discontinuity of the base of the muscle.[65] Despite the accuracy of transthoracic imaging, technical difficulties may impair visualization and limit interpretation. In these circumstances, TEE is a useful alternative modality for assessing acute mitral regurgitation. Compared with TTE, TEE has superior resolution and a significant advantage in terms of visualizing the mitral valve apparatus, especially when a prosthetic mitral valve is present. Doppler imaging provides both qualitative and quantitative assessment of mitral regurgitation severity (Fig. 26.9). A color Doppler jet width at the vena contracta of more than 6 mm by multiplane TEE detects angiographically severe mitral regurgitation with a sensitivity and specificity of 95% and 98%, respectively.[66] If systolic retrograde flow into the pulmonary veins is detected, mitral regurgitation is at least moderate in severity (Fig. 26.10, Video 26.4). Finally, echocardiography clearly distinguishes acute mitral regurgitation from ventricular septal rupture, which can have a very similar clinical presentation (Fig. 26.11, Table 26.3).

If diagnostic studies, including ECG and echocardiography, suggest that ischemia or infarction is the underlying etiology of acute mitral regurgitation, then urgent cardiac catheterization should be considered, with the timing dependent on the

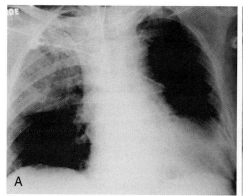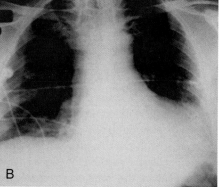

Fig. 26.7 Unusual radiographic appearance of acute mitral regurgitation mimicking lobar pneumonia. (A) Prominent right upper lobe alveolar infiltrate. (B) Rapid resolution occurred in 48 hours with diuretic therapy. (Courtesy Steve Primack, MD, Department of Radiology, Oregon Health Sciences University, Portland.)

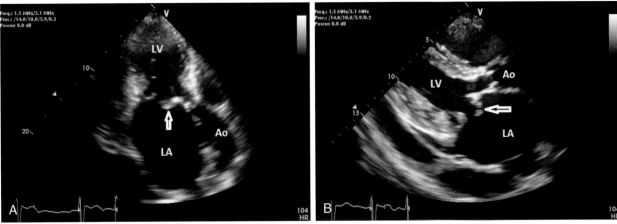

Fig. 26.8 (A) Apical three-chamber transthoracic echocardiogram shows a flail mitral valve leaflet *(arrow)*. (B) Parasternal long-axis transthoracic echocardiogram view of the flail mitral valve leaflet *(arrow;* see also Video 26.3). *Ao,* Aorta; *LA,* left atrium; *LV,* left ventricle.

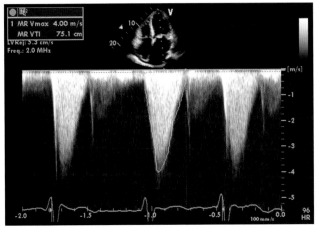

Fig. 26.9 Doppler image from a transthoracic echocardiogram shows the right-angle triangle appearance rather than the normal symmetric parabola owing to the transmitted left ventricular (LV) pressure to the left atrium (LA) from a wide-open mitral regurgitation and consequently the narrowed gradient between the LA and LV pressures.

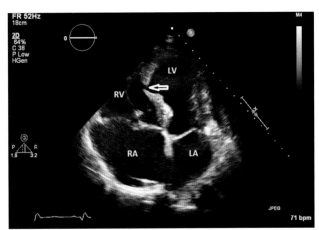

Fig. 26.11 Four-chamber transthoracic echocardiogram shows a ventricular septal defect *(arrow)*. *LA,* Left atrium; *LV,* left ventricle; *RA,* right atrium; *RV,* right ventricle.

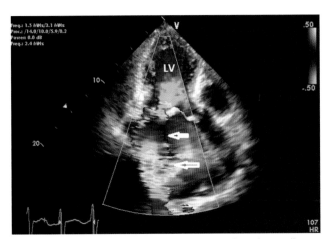

Fig. 26.10 Apical three-chamber transthoracic echocardiogram shows a flail mitral valve leaflet and Doppler demonstrating systolic retrograde flow into the pulmonary veins (see also Video 26.4). *LV,* Left ventricle.

hemodynamic stability of the patient. Coronary angiography defines coronary anatomy and may delineate a culprit lesion amenable to catheter-based or surgical intervention.

Treatment

The management of acute severe mitral regurgitation is similar to that of acute aortic regurgitation. The principles of treatment focus on reducing LVEDP, decreasing aortic impedance to LV ejection so that blood flow can be directed in a forward rather than retrograde direction, and initiating specific therapy for the precipitating etiology. As with acute aortic regurgitation, right heart catheterization is an integral component in the management of acute mitral regurgitation. The clinical severity of the regurgitation and the tempo of the illness, as evidenced by serial hemodynamic measurements, determine the urgency of emergent valve surgery. In the case of papillary muscle rupture, which is the cause of death in 1% to 5% of fatal MIs, urgent surgical intervention is mandatory if the patient cannot be quickly stabilized with medical therapy.[67]

TABLE 26.3 Differentiation of Papillary Muscle Rupture and Ventricular Septal Rupture

Feature	Papillary Muscle Rupture	Ventricular Septal Rupture
Age (mean, years)	65	63
Days after myocardial infarction	3–5	3–5
Anterior myocardial infarction	25%	66%
Murmur	Variable systolic	Pansystolic at lower sternal border
Palpable thrill	Rare	Yes
"v" wave in pulmonary capillary wedge tracing	++	++
Oxygen step-up from right atrium to pulmonary artery	±[a]	++
Echocardiographic findings	Flail or prolapsing leaflet	Visualize defect
Doppler	Regurgitant jet in LA	Detect shunt
Mortality rate		
Medical	90%	90%
Surgical	40%–90%	50%

From Antman EM. ST-elevation myocardial infarction: management. In: Zipes DP, Libby P, Bonow RO, et al, eds. *Braunwald's Heart Disease: A Textbook of Cardiovascular Medicine.* 7th ed. Philadelphia: Elsevier; 2005:1204.

[a]Oxygen step-up may occasionally be seen in papillary muscle rupture as a result of the regurgitant "v" from left atrium contaminating the mixed venous sample from the pulmonary artery.

+, occasionally present; ++, invariably present; ±, rarely present.

Vasodilator therapy is the key component of medical management and the preferred agent is intravenous nitroprusside (for dosage, see section on treatment for aortic regurgitation).[68] Its rapid onset and offset of action allow careful titration to optimize the hemodynamic response. Nitroprusside improves forward stroke volume directly by decreasing aortic impedance and also indirectly by decreasing LV volume, which reduces the area of the incompetent mitral valve orifice, thereby minimizing regurgitant flow.[69] Reduction of mean LA pressure and the regurgitant "v" wave reduce pulmonary congestion. Optimal therapy is defined as the maximal increase in cardiac output and reduction in pulmonary capillary wedge pressure that can be obtained without provoking evidence of organ hypoperfusion due to systemic hypotension. An additional degree of afterload reduction may be provided by placing an IABP.[70] Improvement in diastolic coronary flow that occurs in response to an IABP may also have some salutary effects on LV function, especially in the presence of myocardial ischemia. If significant hypotension is present, dopamine (starting at 2.5 to 5 µg/kg per minute to a maximum of 10 to 20 µg/kg per minute) may be useful in stabilizing the patient and maintaining systemic blood pressure. However, at doses greater than 5 µg/kg per minute, α-adrenergic-induced peripheral vasoconstriction may actually worsen the degree of regurgitation by increasing afterload. If LV contractility is impaired and cardiac output is significantly reduced, the addition of

dobutamine (start at 2 to 5 µg/kg per minute to a maximum 10 to 15 µg/kg per minute) or milrinone (start at 0.25 µg/kg per minute to a maximum of 1.0 µg/kg per minute with or without a loading dose) can be beneficial. Finally, diuretics (as outlined in the section on treatment for aortic regurgitation) are useful to reduce pulmonary congestion.

Infective endocarditis complicated by chordal rupture or leaflet perforation should be treated with appropriate antibiotics in addition to medical therapy to optimize the hemodynamics of acute mitral regurgitation. The decision to proceed with emergent valve surgery is based on the hemodynamic response to medical management of acute congestive heart failure and other factors. Recurrent systemic emboli despite appropriate antimicrobial therapy and infection with resistant organisms or fungi are additional indications for valve replacement. Finally, more complex infections, such as those involving valve ring abscess or fistula formation, also require surgical intervention. Indications for surgery are listed in Box 26.2.

Ischemic Mitral Regurgitation

Significant ischemic mitral regurgitation occurs in 3% of patients with acute MI[71] and 8% of those having cardiogenic shock.[72] Patients with ischemic mitral regurgitation have a worse prognosis than those with other etiologies of mitral regurgitation. In addition, despite the significantly improved survival after acute MI with thrombolytic therapy or percutaneous intervention, 1-year mortality for patients with concomitant severe ischemic mitral regurgitation is 52% compared with 11% in a cohort without mitral regurgitation.[71]

Papillary muscle rupture in the setting of MI represents the most dramatic presentation of ischemic mitral regurgitation and is a surgical emergency. Although this occurs in only 1% to 3% of patients with acute MI, it accounts for up to 5% of infarct-related deaths.[67] Despite aggressive medical management, previous studies have documented the dismal prognosis of these patients, with an up to 70% mortality rate in the first 24 hours without surgical intervention.[73,74] Acute mitral regurgitation occurs more frequently in patients with inferior or posterior MIs and often leads to cardiogenic shock. In a series of 54 patients from the Mayo Clinic, the overall surgical mortality for mitral valve replacement or repair and concomitant revascularization with CABG decreased from 16% to 8.7% after 1990. Operative mortality was similar in delayed and nondelayed cases. The longer-term outcomes if surgical correction was performed were similar to that of MI without papillary muscle rupture. This illustrates the importance of pursuing surgical repair for patients with acute mitral regurgitation from papillary muscle rupture.[75] Although the MitraClip (Abbott) is generally implanted in patients with chronic mitral regurgitation, a few case reports have described the promising alternative of using transcatheter mitral valve repair with the MitraClip device for patients with acute severe mitral regurgitation with associated papillary muscle rupture who are not surgical candidates.

Ischemic mitral regurgitation may also be secondary to papillary muscle dysfunction without rupture. The mechanism involves ischemic apical and posterior papillary muscle displacement and wall motion abnormalities, which result in tethering of mitral valve leaflets and systolic tenting with incomplete valve closure. This condition can occur intermittently or continuously. Intermittent papillary muscle dysfunction classically presents as recurrent episodes of dyspnea associated with pulmonary edema. There have been conflicting results regarding whether mitral valve surgery is warranted as opposed to medical therapy alone and whether revascularization of the coronary arteries with percutaneous coronary interventions or surgery improves acute mitral regurgitation. A 2014 meta-analysis aimed to review the medical literature regarding mitral valve surgery with medical therapy compared to medical therapy alone in patients with acute ischemic mitral regurgitation without papillary muscle rupture.[76] The review was inconclusive, as there was insufficient literature regarding optimal intervention for treatment of acute mitral regurgitation after an MI. There is no clear consensus regarding the standard of treatment; current therapy is mainly guided by expert opinion.

A proposed algorithm for the management of patients with acute ischemic mitral regurgitation includes emergent surgery for acute ischemic mitral regurgitation with papillary muscle rupture, surgery or medical therapy for moderate to severe mitral regurgitation, and medical therapy for mild to moderate mitral regurgitation. The role of mechanical circulatory support has not been well studied in acute mitral regurgitation, but these devices may be useful in cases of decompensated heart failure that does not respond to medical therapy.

ACUTE PROSTHETIC VALVE DYSFUNCTION

Prosthetic heart valves have been in use for over half a century. They are primarily implanted for hemodynamically significant valvular stenosis or regurgitation. A tremendous amount of experience with these devices has been gained over the past several decades. What has become apparent is that prosthetic valves, despite their obvious benefit, constitute another type of valvular heart disease due to the risk of prosthetic valve dysfunction. As this may occur rapidly, compensatory changes that could mitigate the effects of prosthetic valve dysfunction do not have time to develop. As a result, cardiac decompensation can be both severe and abrupt in patients who develop prosthetic valve dysfunction.

Etiology and Clinical Presentation

Acute prosthetic valve complications, which affect both mechanical and bioprosthetic valves, may be classified as either structural or nonstructural leading to prosthetic valve obstruction or regurgitation; refer to Box 26.4.

Mechanical valves have an extremely low risk of structural failure and usually last at least 20 to 30 years.[77] On the contrary, bioprosthetic valves have a higher rate of failure within 10 to 15 years of implantation. The fact that the rate of structural failure with bioprosthetic valves increases dramatically as the valve ages raises concerns about the selection of this type of prosthesis in younger patients. Structural dysfunction due to progressive tissue deterioration from cusp calcification is the main cause of bioprosthetic valve failure. This mineralization process may result in pure stenosis, abnormal coaption of the valve

---

BOX 26.4 Acute Complications of Prosthetic Valves

Structural Valve Dysfunction
Bioprosthesis
Valve degeneration—usually associated with leaflet calcification and tear

Mechanical Prosthesis
Ball or disk variance—change in ball or disk size and function due to infiltration by lipid
Strut fracture (particularly with the older Bjork-Shiley valves)

Nonstructural Valve Dysfunction
Perivalvular leak
Thrombosis or pannus formation
Embolization
Hemolysis
Prosthetic valve endocarditis
Early (≤60 days postsurgery)—occurs before endothelialization of valve, usually caused by *Staphylococcus epidermis* or *S. aureus;* occasionally gram-negative organisms or fungi may be implicated.
Late (≥60 days postsurgery)—occurs after endothelialization of valve; caused by typical endocarditis organisms (viridans streptococci, enterococci, etc.)

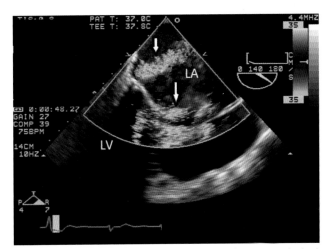

Fig. 26.12 Transesophageal echocardiogram shows a perivalvular jet of mitral regurgitation *(arrow). LA,* Left atrium; *LV,* left ventricle.

---

leaflets, or secondary tears. Progressive collagen deterioration is another common cause for prosthetic valve dysfunction. Although bioprosthetic valves sustain a high structural failure rate within 15 years, mechanical prosthetic valves are more thrombogenic, with caged-ball valves having the highest thrombogenicity and bileaflet-tilting disk valves the lowest. Formation of tissue overgrowth, thrombus, or perivalvular leaks contribute to nonstructural valve dysfunction in both bioprosthetic and mechanical valves (Fig. 26.12).

The usual clinical presentation of acute prosthetic valve dysfunction is that of rapidly progressive heart failure with evidence of either prosthetic valvular regurgitation or stenosis. The mechanisms of aortic bioprosthetic dysfunction are equally distributed between predominantly stenotic, regurgitant, or mixed stenosis/regurgitation. In patients with a mitral bioprosthesis, regurgitation is the predominant mechanism of valve dysfunction

(49%), followed by stenosis (21%) and combined regurgitation/stenosis (30%). The incidence of both aortic and mitral bioprosthesis deterioration requiring reintervention is 20% to 30% at 10 years and over 50% at 15 years, although it is important to note that the clinical manifestations are more often chronic than acute. Acute prosthetic valve dysfunction due to thrombosis or endocarditis can also manifest as thromboembolism (cerebral or peripheral).

Diagnosis

Normally functioning prosthetic valves are associated with various opening and closing clicks and systolic and occasionally diastolic flow murmurs. A new or changing murmur may therefore signal a pathophysiologic alteration in prosthetic valve function. In addition, the absence or damping of normal valve clicks that are characteristic of mechanical prostheses also suggests abnormalities in valve function.

As part of the initial evaluation, identification of the class, type, and model of the implanted valve and the date of implantation is extremely important. The chest radiograph can be invaluable in assessing for the presence of heart failure and may provide confirmatory radiologic evidence as to the type of valvular prosthesis that is in place.[78] The ECG may show signs of LV overload but these findings are not specific in detecting prosthetic valve dysfunction, as they may antedate valve replacement. Anemia in association with an elevated serum lactic dehydrogenase level greater than 600 IU, suggesting hemolysis is virtually never found in a normal functioning prosthesis and should always raise the suspicion of a perivalvular leak and destruction of red blood cells due to increased shear stress.[79]

Echocardiography is an essential tool in the evaluation of prosthetic valve dysfunction.[80] It serves the dual purpose of identifying the etiology of the valve abnormality and assessing LV function. Doppler echocardiography to assess the color flow, pulsed wave, and continuous wave Doppler imaging should be performed to further interrogate the prosthesis. Measurements should be taken from the average of three consecutive cardiac cycles for patients in sinus rhythm or a minimum of five cardiac cycles if the patient is in an irregular rhythm. Some caveats with the use of echocardiography include the familiarity of the echocardiography reader with normal prosthetic jets and the real-time hemodynamics of the patient that may affect Doppler-derived values. A skilled echocardiography reader should be familiar with the appearance of normal transprosthetic jets that arise due to the design of the prostheses to prevent an erroneous diagnosis of pathologic regurgitation or stenosis. Additionally, Doppler-derived hemodynamic parameters, such as mean gradient and peak velocity, are dependent on the flow state. For example, these hemodynamic parameters may be elevated in high flow states—such as tachycardia, hyperthyroidism, or renal disease—rather than from pathologic obstruction or regurgitation.

Color Doppler flow mapping has several important applications in prosthetic valve disease: (1) directing continuous-wave Doppler cursor parallel to the stenotic flow jet, allowing more accurate estimation of transprosthetic velocities and gradients[81]; (2) semiquantitative evaluation of prosthetic valve regurgitation, which has been shown to correlate well with angiographically

derived measurements[82,83]; and (3) differentiating valvular from perivalvular leaks.[81] The evaluation for prosthetic valve dysfunction uses Doppler-derived variables, including velocity, acceleration time, pressure gradient, time velocity integral (TVI), Doppler velocity index (DVI), and effective orifice area (EOA). The normal values for velocities and pressures vary based on the prosthetic valve location, type, and size. Expected values for different valve types can be found in the 2009 American Society of Echocardiography (ASE) Prosthetic Valve guidelines.[84]

Continuous-wave Doppler imaging is effective in assessing valvular stenosis by virtue of the modified Bernoulli equation:

$$Pressure = 4 \times Velocity^2$$

The transvalvular velocities measured by Doppler echocardiography correlate well with invasive measures in patients with native valve disease and after valve replacement.[85] When the valve orifice is smaller or more stenotic, the acceleration and velocity increases to maintain the same stroke volume. Using the Doppler-measured velocities proximal and distal to the valve, the pressure gradient or difference can be calculated. Although transvalvular pressure differences are proportional to the degree of stenosis, variables such as heart rate, contractility, cardiac output, and the size and type of prosthesis can alter the measured gradient.[86]

The dynamic flow velocities can also be plotted against the ejection time axis to provide the TVI, a representation of the distance the blood travels with each cardiac cycle. The DVI is a dimensionless ratio of proximal velocity in the LV outflow tract to that of flow velocity through the prosthesis. It is not dependent on the flow conditions through the valve, whereas the gradient and velocity are. In addition, the DVI is less dependent on the valve size. A DVI less than 0.25 is highly suggestive of significant valve obstruction.[84] The EOA can be calculated by dividing the left ventricular stroke volume by the TVI using the continuity equation. Since it is dependent on the size of the prosthetic valve, there are different reference values for the type of valve. In general, an EOA less than 0.8 cm^2 is concerning for significant stenosis. In patients with normal or low EOA, prosthetic-patient mismatch or a pathologic valve obstruction is highly suspected, particularly if the mean gradient is elevated. Prosthesis-patient mismatch refers to the condition in which the effective prosthetic valve area is less than the normal human valve after insertion into the patient. Obstruction is often due to a pannus ingrowth, thrombus, or vegetation. If the EOA index is elevated with a high mean gradient, the concern for prosthetic valve regurgitation is heightened. Although prosthetic valves are generally inherently stenotic, physiologic regurgitation can also be seen in mechanical valves. Pathologic regurgitation that is central valvular may be secondary to degeneration, vegetation, or leaflet malfunction; perivalvular regurgitation is concerning for dehiscence, abscess, or improper seating of the prostheses. Various cutoffs have been proposed for the location and type of prostheses.[84]

An important phenomenon to be mindful of when evaluating mean gradients in prosthetic valves is pressure recovery. When blood is pumped through the aortic prosthetic valve, the lowest pressure and highest velocity is at the vena contracta, which is a few millimeters from the prosthesis outflow orifice. As the blood is propelled forward through the aorta, the pressure recovers as the velocity decreases. Thus, the pressure gradient (LV pressure–aortic pressure) is dependent on where the velocity is interrogated in reference to the vena contracta. For smaller mechanical bileaflet valves, a higher mean gradient is often considered to be normal owing to pressure recovery. Clinically, it is the net pressure gradient rather than the maximal pressure gradient that correlates with the true hemodynamic burden on the LV.[87]

It should also be remembered that there is a wide variation in valvular gradients depending on the class, type, and model of the valve. Therefore patients with newly implanted valves should have a full TTE study, including comprehensive Doppler assessment, to evaluate the prosthesis as a baseline for future follow-up. The 2014 American Heart Association/American College of Cardiology (AHA/ACC) guidelines recommend that the initial TTE be obtained 6 weeks to 3 months after valve implantation.[88] Repeat TTE is recommended in patients with prosthetic heart valves if there is a change in clinical signs or symptoms suggesting valve dysfunction. Compelling evidence to support a particular strategy in timing of echocardiographic follow-up for asymptomatic patients with prosthetic heart valves is lacking. Current guidelines do not recommend further echocardiographic testing after the initial postoperative period in asymptomatic patients with mechanical valves. Annual TTE in asymptomatic patients with a bioprosthetic valve after the first 10 years even in the absence of a change in clinical status is reasonable, as the likelihood of valve dysfunction is more common at this time. In cases in which valve function is difficult to visualize owing to artifact or acoustic shadowing on a TTE, TEE, fluoroscopy, and/or gated CT imaging may be warranted.[89]

When transthoracic imaging is limited secondary to reverberatory artifacts caused by metallic components of a mechanical valve or technically difficult echocardiographic windows, TEE is a useful adjunctive tool.[90–96] Because imaging is performed without intervening cardiac structures, excellent delineation of valvular anatomy and function may be obtained. This is particularly true in the case of the mitral valve because the esophageal window is not obstructed by the metallic valve components. In addition, several studies have suggested that TEE may, in fact, be more sensitive and specific than TTE in the evaluation of partial valve thrombosis,[97–99] prosthetic valve endocarditis with aortic ring abscess,[100] perivalvular leaks,[95] Starr-Edwards prosthesis function,[94] and bioprosthetic valve degeneration.[96] TEE may also be appropriate when TTE findings are not consistent with the observed clinical syndrome. However, it should be emphasized that the combined approach of using TTE with TEE facilitates a more complete evaluation of LV function.

In the case of acute prosthetic valve dysfunction with heart failure, right heart catheterization is essential for continuous hemodynamic monitoring and for helping to define therapeutic interventions. Because echocardiography has, in large part, replaced traditional catheterization measurements for valvular insufficiency and stenosis, cardiac catheterization is withheld unless the available echocardiographic data are inconclusive or there is a suspicion of significant coronary artery disease. In some cases, simple fluoroscopy may be used to identify prosthetic valve dysfunction and assess the effects of thrombolytic therapy on abnormalities caused by clots that affect valve function.[101–103]

Treatment

Congestive Heart Failure. Therapy for acute prosthetic valve dysfunction depends on the type and severity of hemodynamic abnormality, the valve involved, and the underlying etiology. If the valve becomes obstructed acutely, the clinical presentation is likely to be dramatic, with syncope and death in the absence of immediate surgical intervention. On the other hand, stenotic lesions that develop more gradually present as progressive heart failure and a low cardiac output state. Medical management consists of reducing LA pressure and maximizing ventricular performance with inotropic agents. Acute regurgitant lesions are managed according to the guidelines outlined in the sections on treatment for aortic, mitral, and tricuspid regurgitation. Usually, this will involve a combination of vasodilators, diuretics, and inotropic support. Definite therapy usually involves reoperation and replacement of the dysfunctional valve. The mortality risk for reoperation will depend primarily on the preoperative functional class, the underlying etiology of the valve dysfunction (endocarditis and valve thrombosis carrying the highest risk) and the need for emergency surgery. Valve surgery is recommended in severe prosthetic valve stenosis and severe prosthetic valve or paraprosthetic valve regurgitation with heart failure or intractable hemolysis. For high operative risk yet symptomatic patients with bioprosthetic aortic valve stenosis or regurgitation, a transcatheter valve-in-valve procedure is now included as a class IIa recommendation in the focused update of the 2017 AHA/ACC Valvular Heart Disease guidelines. Percutaneous repair is suggested for patients with severe perivalvular regurgitation with intractable hemolysis and New York Heart Association (NYHA) class III or IV heart failure who are at high risk from surgery.

Prosthetic Valve Endocarditis. Specific management of prosthetic valve endocarditis (PVE) includes obtaining blood cultures and initiating empiric antibiotic therapy. Because there is a fairly well-defined difference between the pathophysiology and type of organisms responsible for early and late PVE, the initial choice of antibiotics will depend on the time of presentation relative to the date of surgical valve replacement. In early infection within 2 months of implantation, the new valve apparatus has not endothelialized, allowing microorganisms direct access to the new structures either from direct intraoperative contamination or hematogenous spread. Most common pathogens are nosocomial, including *S. aureus* and coagulase-negative staphylococci. In late infections, defined as 2 months or more after implantation, the valve apparatus has become endothelialized; thus, the pathogenesis of endocarditis is similar to that of native valve endocarditis. The most common pathogens in late infections are streptococci and *S. aureus*.

In addition to progressive heart failure, PVE may also be complicated by embolic phenomena or perivalvular leak (with or without hemolytic anemia). As progressive damage may advance rapidly in patients with prosthetic valves who have these complications, it is appropriate to obtain blood cultures and initiate empiric antibiotic therapy. In the setting of aortic prosthetic valvular endocarditis, the development of new atrioventricular conduction delay is specific for the presence of a valve ring abscess.[79] Invariably, the vast majority of patients with PVE will require valve replacement. Based on the 2015 AHA scientific statement regarding infective endocarditis, early surgery during the initial hospitalization for antibiotic therapy is recommended for patients with PVE with one or more of the following: signs or symptoms of heart failure from valvular dysfunction, heart block or valve abscess due to perivalvular invasion, PVE caused by fungi or a highly resistant organism, such as *S. aureus*, or persistent bacteremia despite appropriate therapy.[104]

Transcatheter heart valve endocarditis is an emerging complication of percutaneous valve replacement. Early TAVR-related PVE has been reported at a rate of 0.3% to 0.4% per patient year.[105] Complications include heart failure, perivalvular invasion of the infection, embolic events, and valvular dysfunction, such as stenosis or regurgitation. There is limited evidence regarding optimal treatment for TAVR-related PVE and surgical indications that is often adapted from PVE on surgically placed valves and made on an individual basis.

Prosthetic Valve Thrombosis. Although valvular obstruction may occasionally be secondary to bacterial vegetations, they are more commonly the result of pannus ingrowth or thrombus formation. Subclinical asymptomatic prosthetic valve thrombosis (PVT) is likely more common than symptomatic PVT; however, there are limited data on the incidence and clinical significance of subclinical PVT. The incidence of PVT with currently available mechanical devices varies from 0.3% to 1.3% with a higher rate of approximately 6% in patients with mechanical prostheses who have had subtherapeutic anticoagulation. Mitral mechanical PVT is more common than aortic mechanical PVT. The incidence of bioprosthetic PVT is less well defined. Although a major risk factor for PVT is inadequate anticoagulation, approximately 40% of patients have adequate prothrombin times at the time of presentation.[106] This may be explained by the fact that PVT is a complex process that consists of a significant component of fibrous tissue ingrowth with associated secondary thrombosis.

PVT may present acutely with heart failure or more indolently with slowly progressive symptoms of dyspnea and fatigue. A high level of suspicion must be maintained in any patient with a valvular prosthesis with nonspecific cardiac symptoms. TTE provides assessment of hemodynamic severity, whereas CT imaging or fluoroscopy is often used to delineate valve motion and clot burden. TEE is useful in measuring thrombus size (Videos 26.5 and 26.6). Although the mortality rate for reoperation is variable between reports, ranging from 4.5% to 35%, it tends to be high; there is a correlation between risk and advanced functional class.

Options for the management of PVT include medical or surgical therapy. The 2017 focused update of the AHA/ACC valvular heart disease guidelines now includes a class IIa recommendation for initiation of vitamin K antagonist agents in patients with suspected or confirmed bioprosthetic valve thrombosis who are hemodynamically stable based on case series data. According to the 2014 AHA/ACC valvular heart disease guidelines, emergent

surgery is a class I recommendation for patients with left-sided prosthetic valve thrombosis with NYHA class III to IV symptoms. Surgery is a class IIa recommendation for left-sided prosthetic valve thrombosis that is mobile or large (>0.8 cm). This is mostly based on a meta-analysis of seven observational studies that demonstrated that surgery for left-sided PVT with severe functional impairment was associated with significantly lower rates of thromboembolism, major bleeding, and recurrent PVT compared to fibrinolytic therapy. Mortality rates and complete restoration of valve function was not significantly different.[107] Fibrinolytic therapy for persistent valve thrombosis despite intravenous heparin therapy is a class IIa recommendation for right-sided prosthetic valve thrombosis or left-sided prosthetic valve thrombosis with recent onset of symptoms (<14 days), stable thrombus (<0.8 cm^2), and/or NYHA class I/II symptoms. Streptokinase or tissue plasminogen activator (tPA) is recommended for fibrinolytic therapy; urokinase is less effective. Complications of left-sided PVT fibrinolysis include major bleeding, systemic embolization, recurrent PVT, and death. The degree of risk for thromboembolism and bleeding is directly related to thrombus size, with thrombus areas greater than 0.8 cm^2 associated with a higher risk.

TRICUSPID REGURGITATION

In general, the hemodynamic impact of acute tricuspid regurgitation is less significant than that of acute left-sided valvular lesions. More commonly, persistent, severe, chronic tricuspid regurgitation results in salt and water retention leading to peripheral edema, ascites, and congestive hepatomegaly. However, acute tricuspid regurgitation can lead to massive RV volume overload, causing significant reduction in LV ejection fraction due to paradoxic early systolic septal motion that results from the severe volume overload of the RV.[108] Although hemodynamic instability may be pronounced at the time of initial presentation, many patients with the onset of acute severe tricuspid regurgitation can be effectively managed with a combination of diuretics and inotropic agents, provided that pulmonary arterial pressure remains normal and RV function is preserved. Once stabilized, the long-term prognosis of these patients tends to be favorable. In general, the clinical presentation, response to medical therapy, and underlying pathology determine the need for surgical intervention.

Etiology

It should be emphasized that isolated, acute tricuspid regurgitation is a relatively uncommon medical emergency. The chronic form of tricuspid regurgitation predominates and usually results from annular dilation secondary to left-sided valvular pathology, severe LV dysfunction, or pulmonary hypertension. In the current era, infective endocarditis remains the most common cause of acute tricuspid regurgitation and is almost exclusively a disease of intravenous drug users.[109] Despite antibiotic sterilization of the valve lesion, these individuals frequently develop ruptured chords or leaflet perforation. Occasionally, tricuspid regurgitation can be caused by a large, healed vegetation that impairs leaflet apposition. Rarer causes of acute tricuspid regurgitation include nonpenetrating chest trauma[110,111] and RV infarction.[112,113] With the growing number of cardiac transplant recipients, an iatrogenic form of tricuspid regurgitation has been recognized with increasing frequency.[114–117] Transplant patients undergo repeated endomyocardial biopsies for evaluation of cardiac allograft rejection and, occasionally, the bioptome may inadvertently damage the tricuspid valve chordae or leaflet, resulting in acute tricuspid regurgitation.

Clinical Presentation

The physical findings in acute tricuspid regurgitation are dependent, in part, on the severity of the RV volume overload. In the case of papillary muscle rupture or RV infarction, there may be hypotension and cardiovascular collapse. Most patients, however, maintain blood pressure within the normal range and typically demonstrate findings consistent with right-sided heart failure. There is usually a prominent "v" wave visible in the jugular venous pulse and a holosystolic murmur along the left sternal border. The tricuspid regurgitation murmur increases in intensity with inspiration, a finding that differentiates it from mitral regurgitation. An S_3 gallop originating from the RV can be heard; abdominal examination may reveal a large and pulsatile liver. In general, peripheral stigmata of infective endocarditis are absent when the tricuspid valve is affected and, if present, suggest paradoxic emboli or additional, left-sided valvular lesions. In the case of intravenous drug users, track marks and evidence of "skin popping" may be seen.

Diagnosis

The diagnostic modality of choice for evaluating acute tricuspid regurgitation is two-dimensional and Doppler echocardiography.[118] The echocardiogram provides structural information about the tricuspid valve, including detection of vegetations. In addition, the severity of tricuspid regurgitation and RV dysfunction can be assessed. Most important, pulmonary artery pressures can be estimated using the modified Bernoulli equation:

$$PAS = RAP + 4 \times V^2$$

where *PAS* is pulmonary artery systolic pressure, *RAP* is right atrial pressure measured by physical examination [5 cm + jugular venous pressure (cm above clavicle)], and *V* is the peak velocity of the tricuspid regurgitation jet measured by continuous-wave Doppler.[119] In general, transthoracic echocardiography is satisfactory for assessing tricuspid valve structure and RV function (Figs. 26.13 and 26.14). An important caveat, though, is that when the RV fails, flow directed into the pulmonary artery and backwards into the right atrium may be reduced so that the severity of pulmonary hypertension or tricuspid regurgitation may be underestimated. TEE may not offer any significant diagnostic advantage over TTE. In a prospective study by San Román and colleagues, TTE was equivalent to TEE in the diagnosis of tricuspid valve infective endocarditis; however, the relationship of the vegetation to the leaflet was better characterized by TEE.[120]

The ECG in cases of trauma may show right bundle branch block. If the tricuspid regurgitation has been long standing, there may be ECG criteria for RV hypertrophy. RV infarction with acute tricuspid regurgitation rarely occurs in isolation and typically presents in conjunction with inferior MI, which can be diagnosed

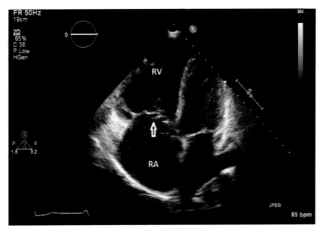

Fig. 26.13 Four-chamber transthoracic echocardiogram shows a flail tricuspid valve *(arrow)*. *RA*, Right atrium; *RV*, right ventricle.

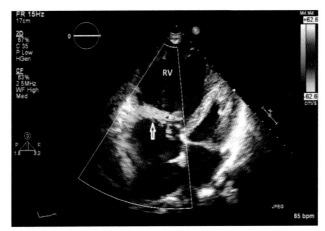

Fig. 26.14 Apical transthoracic echocardiogram with color Doppler, a flail tricuspid valve, and associated tricuspid regurgitation *(arrow)*. *RV*, Right ventricle.

by the characteristic ST segment elevation in leads II, III, and aVF. The presence of ST segment elevation in the right-sided lead V_4R confirms the diagnosis of an RV infarct and suggests that the patient may be at high risk for complications.[121]

The chest radiograph may show signs of cardiomegaly that represent RV and right atrial (RA) enlargement. The presence of cavitary septic pulmonary emboli may also be seen with tricuspid valve endocarditis. As noted, blood cultures are an essential component of the diagnostic workup for patients with suspected infective endocarditis. In patients with a history of intravenous drug use, staphylococcal organisms are the predominant isolate.

Right heart catheterization can be extremely helpful in confirming the diagnosis of pure tricuspid regurgitation and ruling out significant LV abnormalities. The presence of a large "v" wave in the RA tracing with concomitant elevation in mean RA pressure usually signifies the presence of significant tricuspid regurgitation. In addition, if the pulmonary artery and capillary wedge pressures are normal, the tricuspid regurgitation is likely to be related to primary dysfunction of the valvular apparatus and not secondary to left-sided heart dysfunction or pulmonary hypertension.

Treatment

The management strategy for acute tricuspid regurgitation should be focused primarily on medical therapy. Most patients can be effectively treated with a diuretic alone or in combination with an inotropic agent, such as dobutamine. Milrinone, another inotropic agent, may be used as well, particularly in patients who have evidence of pulmonary hypertension. In rare instances of acute massive tricuspid regurgitation, the patient who is refractory to medical therapy may require immediate surgical intervention. Whenever possible, tricuspid valve repair, often with ring annuloplasty, is preferred over valve replacement. However, when valve replacement is required, a bioprosthetic valve is often used as there is a high incidence of valve thrombosis when mechanical valves are implanted in the tricuspid position.[122] In the case of tricuspid regurgitation related to infective endocarditis, the decision to implant a prosthetic valve becomes even more complex. Because many of these patients are young, noncompliant, and often return to intravenous drug use, their risks for adverse events—whether self-induced or iatrogenic—are significant. The operative mortality for reoperation, particularly for recurrent prosthetic valve endocarditis, can be extremely high. Furthermore, if a bioprosthesis is used, the risk of valve failure over time is higher because of the younger age of the intravenous drug–using population. The choice of a mechanical valve for durability is also fraught with complications from both the inherently higher thrombotic risk despite anticoagulation and the general trend of medication noncompliance among these patients. Although treatment cannot be generalized for the intravenous drug–use population, these recurring problems have fostered the development of several unique surgical approaches. These options include complete valve excision with no prosthetic replacement,[123] valve repair after sterilization of the infection,[124] and "vegectomy,"[125] which refers to isolated resection of the bacterial vegetation with preservation of the valvulochordal apparatus. Even with complete valve excision, many of these patients may continue to do well, with minimal symptoms of right-sided heart failure. This is particularly true when the pulmonary vascular resistance is normal and RV function is preserved. Naturally, any management plan for infective endocarditis must include appropriate antibiotic coverage for an adequate period of time.

The treatment of tricuspid regurgitation secondary to an inferior MI with RV involvement is revascularization. The type of revascularization procedure will depend on the nature of the coronary anatomy, extent of atherosclerotic disease, myocardial territory at risk, and LV function.

CONCLUSION

Acute heart failure secondary to valvular dysfunction remains an extremely difficult clinical dilemma from the standpoint of both diagnosis and treatment. Since the underlying pathophysiology determines the clinical course, expeditious treatment with appropriate diagnostic testing is of paramount importance. In most cases of acute heart failure secondary to valvular disease, both echocardiography and pulmonary artery catheterization are invaluable tools that allow the clinician to determine the severity of the lesion as well as underlying cardiac function, assess the patient's hemodynamic status, and reach decisions regarding the best management strategy. Providers treating patients with acute valvular dysfunction must not only understand the pathophysiology of the disease but also be cognizant of the limitations of medical therapy. As surgical intervention represents the most definitive intervention, early cardiothoracic surgical consultation is a critical step in the management algorithm of these often desperately ill individuals.

The full reference list for this chapter is available at ExpertConsult.com.

27

Hypertensive Emergencies

Brigitte M. Baumann, Richard M. Pescatore II

DEFINITION

Hypertensive emergencies are characterized by severe elevations in blood pressure (BP) (>180/120 mm Hg) complicated by impending or progressive target organ dysfunction.[1] Targeted organs typically include the aorta, brain, eyes, heart, and kidneys. Immediate (minutes to hours) BP reduction is essential to prevent further morbidity. This contrasts with *hypertensive urgencies*, in which severe elevations in BP are *not* accompanied by target organ dysfunction. In these cases, BP reduction may occur in an outpatient setting with oral medication over 24 to 48 hours. The terms *malignant hypertension* and *accelerated hypertension* are older, less commonly used, and have been replaced by these newer terms in national guidelines. Collectively, hypertensive emergencies and urgencies are referred to as *hypertensive crises*.[1] Table 27.1 outlines definitions and management goals of hypertensive emergencies.[1-6]

INCIDENCE AND PREVALENCE

Approximately 1 billion individuals have hypertension worldwide; by 2025, 1.6 billion will be affected.[7] The prevalence in developing countries is rapidly increasing, with 16% of the adult population in sub-Saharan Africa and 27% in mainland China categorized as hypertensive. Mass migrations from rural to urban settings and changes in lifestyle and diet are considered major contributing factors.[8,9] In the United States, the prevalence has also increased from 24% to 29% from the 1990s to 2008.[10] In France, Germany, Italy, Spain, and the United Kingdom, the total population is projected to grow by only 6% from 2010 to 2025 but the prevalence of hypertension is anticipated to increase by 15%. This increase is due primarily to aging of the populations.[11]

Although worldwide prevalence of hypertension is increasing, the proportion of patients who will experience a hypertensive emergency remains quite low. Of emergency department (ED) patients, 1% to 6% will present with severe hypertension (>180/120 mm Hg); of those, between one-third to one-half will have target organ damage.[12-16] A more recent estimate places this risk at 2 per 1000 ED visits.[17]

Risk factors for development of hypertensive emergency include male sex, older age, greater mean diastolic BP (DBP), and medication nonadherence.[13,15,18] Nonadherence is likely multifactorial: lack of health insurance or primary care physician, insufficient funds to pay for medications, and treatment ambivalence (lower hypertension knowledge, medication side effects and feeling that the medications do not help) may all play a role.[19]

PATHOPHYSIOLOGY

Although the pathophysiology of hypertensive emergencies is incompletely understood, an initial abrupt rise in vascular resistance appears to be an initiating step.[20,21] When accompanied by disruption or deactivation of the arterial baroreflex, BP continues

TABLE 27.1	Definitions of Hypertensive Emergency With Management Recommendations					
	2003 JNC 7 HTN Guideline[1]	2013 ESH HTN Guideline[2]	2013 ACCF/ AHA STEMI Management Guidelines[3]	2013 AHA/ASA Ischemic Stroke Guidelines[4]	2010 ACCF/AHA Aortic Dissection Guidelines[5]	2015 ACOG Acute, Severe HTN Guidelines in Pregnancy and the Postpartum Period[6]
Definition	BP >180/120 mm Hg Associated with impending or progressive target organ damage	BP >180/120 mm Hg Associated with impending or progressive organ damage				SBP ≥160 or DBP ≥110 mm Hg In pregnancy or postpartum period
Management	Immediate BP reduction: <25% decrease in MAP within first hour. If stable, to 160/110–100 in the next 2–6 h; gradual reductions over next 24–48 h to a normal BP[a]	Prompt, but partial (<25%) BP reduction in the first few hours; proceed cautiously thereafter	Reduce BP to <180/110 mm Hg if fibrinolytic therapy is planned	Reduce BP if >220/120 mm Hg; If tPA planned, use IV antihypertensive medications to bring BP <185/110 mm Hg prior to tPA administration	Goals: heart rate <60 beats/min and SBP <120–100 mm Hg in acute abdominal or thoracic aortic dissection	Initiate fetal surveillance and if BPs remain severely elevated >15 min, begin intravenous antihypertensive therapy; delivery of the fetus may be necessary

[a]Exceptions include pregnant patients and patients with ischemic stroke or aortic dissection.
ACCF, American College of Cardiology Foundation; *ACOG*, American Congress of Obstetrics and Gynecology; *AHA*, American Heart Association; *ASA*, American Stroke Association; *BP*, blood pressure; *DBP*, diastolic blood pressure; *ESH*, European Society of Hypertension; *JNC 7*, The Seventh Report of the Joint National Committee on Prevention, Detection, Evaluation, and Treatment of High Blood Pressure 7; *MAP*, mean arterial pressure; *SBP*, systolic blood pressure; *STEMI*, ST elevation myocardial infarction; *tPA*, tissue plasminogen activator.

to escalate.[21,22] While the degree of BP elevation does not correlate closely with the severity of organ damage, the rate of change of BP increases the likelihood of target organ damage.[23] Individuals with long-standing hypertension have adaptive vascular changes that protect organs from changes in BP, lowering the probability of hypertensive emergency.[20,23] Conversely, normotensive individuals may develop hypertensive emergency at substantially lower BPs, in part because this adaptive measure is absent. For example, a DBP of 140 mm Hg in a chronic hypertensive patient may not result in organ dysfunction, whereas a DBP of 110 mm Hg may be devastating in a previously normotensive woman with eclampsia or in a perioperative cardiac patient. Certain underlying conditions also predispose patients (Box 27.1).[20]

The biochemical mechanisms leading to hypertensive emergencies involve a confluence of endothelial injury, neurohormonal imbalance, and autoregulatory dysfunction (Fig. 27.1).[20,22,24] Endothelial injury and the release of hormonal vasoconstrictors from the blood vessel wall are thought to be precipitants. During the initial rise in BP, the endothelium maintains homeostasis through increased release of vasodilator molecules such as nitric oxide and prostacyclin.[25] When hypertension is sustained or severe, these responses are overwhelmed, leading to endothelial decompensation, promoting further rises in BP and endothelial damage.[20] Endothelin, endothelium-derived contracting factors, (EDCF) and proinflammatory cytokines—such as interleukin-1 (IL-1), IL-6, and tumor necrosis factor-α (TNF-α)—are released. Local activation of the clotting cascade also ensues with platelet and fibrin deposition, as well as fibrinoid necrosis of the arterioles. This leads to a vicious cycle of further vascular injury, tissue ischemia, and release of vasoconstrictor substances.[24,26]

Increased levels of catecholamines, angiotensin II, vasopressin, and aldosterone also contribute to the pathophysiology of hypertensive crisis.[20,21,27] Activation of the renin-angiotensin-aldosterone system (RAAS) via catecholamine surge, endothelial vasoconstrictor release, or relative hypovolemia from pressure natriuresis leads to further vasoconstriction.[26] Increased activity of the RAAS also induces expression of proinflammatory cytokines and vascular cell adhesion molecules, compounding vascular injury and vasoreactivity.[20]

The arterial baroreflex is the alteration in sympathetic and parasympathetic cardiovascular activity in response to acute changes in arterial pressure detected by baroreceptors in the carotid sinuses and aortic arch. Aging, deconditioning, and chronic hypertension have all been implicated in baroreflex dysfunction.[22] In a hypertensive crisis, the normal negative feedback loop in the arterial baroreflex is impaired or disrupted.[21] The anticipated sympathetic inhibition (decreased peripheral resistance) and an increase in parasympathetic output (decreased heart rate and contractility) in response to an acute rise in BP never occur. When coupled with acute endothelial damage, hypertensive emergencies ensue.

EVALUATION AND MANAGEMENT

Patients with severely elevated BP (>180/120 mm Hg) should be screened for a hypertensive emergency. If a patient has no prior history of hypertension, do not discount the diagnosis. Up to 16% of hypertensive emergencies occur in such patients[13]: previously normotensive patients who experience an abrupt rise in BP are at risk, such as children (acute renal disease), young

---

BOX 27.1   Underlying Causes of Hypertensive Emergencies

Essential hypertension
Renal parenchymal disease
   Acute glomerulonephritis
   Vasculitis
   Hemolytic-uremic syndrome
   Thrombotic thrombocytopenic purpura
   Polycystic kidney disease
Renovascular disease
   Renal artery stenosis (atheromatous or fibromuscular dysplasia)
Pregnancy
   Preeclampsia
   Eclampsia
Endocrinopathy
   Pheochromocytoma
   Cushing syndrome
   Renin-secreting tumors
   Mineralocorticoid hypertension
   Primary aldosteronism (adrenal aldosteronoma or adrenal hyperplasia)
   Hypo or hyperthyroidism
   Hyperparathyroidism

Drugs
   Sympathomimetics: cocaine, amphetamines, phencyclidine hydrochloride, lysergic acid diethylamide, diet pills, tricyclic antidepressants
   Erythropoietin, cyclosporine, antihypertensive withdrawal
   Monoamine-oxidase inhibitor interactions (tyramine pressor response)
   Herbal supplements: ginseng, licorice, and ephedra (*ma huang*)
   Lead intoxication
Autonomic hyperreactivity
   Autonomic hyperactivity in presence of Guillain-Barré, Shy-Drager, or other spinal cord syndromes
   Acute intermittent porphyria
Central nervous system disorders
   Head trauma, cerebrovascular accident, brain tumors
Coarctation of aorta
Perioperative
   Post coronary artery bypass grafting
   Post carotid artery repair

Modified from Vaughan CJ, Delanty N. Hypertensive emergencies. *Lancet*. 2000;356:411–417.

---

women (eclampsia) and perioperative patients. The spectrum of hypertensive emergencies based on the prevalence of target organ damage is presented in Table 27.2.

The physician evaluating the patient should inquire about the duration, severity, and level of control of preexisting hypertension, antihypertensive drug treatment, and the extent of preexisting end-organ damage. The presence of concomitant illnesses (see Box 27.1) and medications—including prescription drugs, over-the-counter preparations such as sympathomimetic agents, and illicit drugs such as cocaine or methamphetamines—should be noted. Patients should be asked about immunosuppressive drugs, as these agents may predispose patients to hypertensive encephalopathy with only mild elevations in BP.[30,31]

Excess sodium intake and alcohol and benzodiazepine use and abrupt cessation should also be assessed. Women should be asked about pregnancy status to exclude preeclampsia. Family history may reveal inherited conditions that may predispose the patient to a hypertensive crisis.

Presenting complaints should be elicited from patients, with special attention given to chest pain, back pain, dyspnea, and neurologic complaints. The most common presenting complaints of hypertensive emergency patients are presented in Table 27.3; Table 27.4 provides additional guidance for history taking.

The physical examination should start with serial BP measurements measured in both arms while the patient is resting quietly. Measurements should be taken with the patient both supine and upright to ascertain volume status. BP differences between arms can result from aortic dissection, coarctation, peripheral vascular disease, and some unilateral neurologic and musculoskeletal abnormalities. While inter-arm BP differences occur in "normal" individuals, a between-arm difference greater than 10 to 20 mm Hg is considered meaningful since, in the outpatient setting, each 10 mm Hg difference carries an increasing mortality

hazard.[32,33] When a BP difference is detected, treat the higher BP and obtain subsequent measurements on the same (higher BP) arm.[32]

The ocular fundi should be examined for acute hypertensive retinopathy. A third heart sound, elevated jugular venous pressure, and crackles on lung examination suggest pulmonary edema. New-onset mitral regurgitation murmur may signify papillary muscle rupture during an acute myocardial infarction (MI). An abdominal bruit suggests renal artery stenosis and an aortic aneurysm may be palpated on the abdominal examination. Discrepancies in peripheral pulses and the murmur of aortic regurgitation suggest aortic dissection. Focal neurologic findings, including visual field deficits and subtle cerebellar findings, are suggestive of a cerebrovascular accident or a mass lesion. Delirium or depressed level of consciousness are found in patients with hypertensive encephalopathy.

The basic diagnostic evaluation for patients with hypertensive crisis includes a basic chemistry panel and complete blood count with a peripheral blood smear to look for microangiopathic anemia. A bedside glucose check should be done in patients with altered sensorium or neurologic deficits to exclude acute hypoglycemia and to identify concomitant diabetes.[20,34] Urine studies may reveal proteinuria or hematuria in patients with renal damage. Additional studies include pregnancy testing and a urine drug screen to help identify illicit substance use if the history is unavailable. An electrocardiogram is needed to exclude acute myocardial ischemia and associated arrhythmias, such as atrial fibrillation. Imaging should be directed by the clinical presentation. A chest radiograph may demonstrate pulmonary edema from left ventricular failure or widening of the mediastinum due to thoracic aortic dissection.[20,34] Bedside ultrasound conducted by an experienced clinician can be used to help identify acute aortic dissection, depressed myocardial function, and bladder

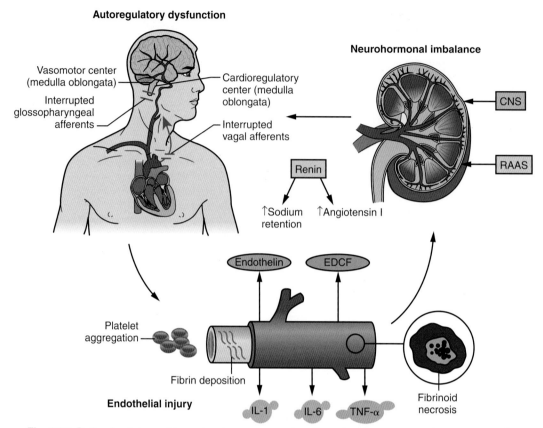

Fig. 27.1 Pathophysiology of hypertensive emergencies. Hypertensive emergencies are a complex consequence of biochemical vasoreactivity. Cerebral autoregulation is disrupted, as afferent feedback from the vagus and glossopharyngeal nerves to the medullary cardioregulatory and vasomotor centers is interrupted and vasomotor inhibition from descending general visceral efferents shifts toward sympathetic predominance. Endothelial control of vascular tone is overwhelmed as fibrin deposition and arteriolar fibrinoid necrosis contribute to increased endothelial permeability, platelet aggregation, and autocrine and paracrine release of vasoconstrictors. Endothelin-1, endothelium-derived contracting factor (EDCF), and inflammatory cytokines including interleukin 1 (IL-1) and interleukin 6 (IL-6) and tumor necrosis factor-α (TNF-α) further compound systemic vasoconstriction and renal hypertensive damage. Acute changes in vascular resistance occur in response to excess aldosterone, antidiuretic hormone, and catecholaminergic influence on renal physiology, leading to increased renin production, sodium reuptake, and angiotensin II activity, causing potent vasoconstriction and further neurohormonal imbalance. *CNS*, Central nervous system; *RAAS*, renin-angiotensin-aldosterone system.

outlet obstruction (Videos 27.1 and 27.2). Computed tomography (CT) or magnetic resonance imaging (MRI) may be needed to identify neurologic or vascular hypertensive emergencies. In select patients, measurement of plasma renin activity and aldosterone drawn at the time of admission can be useful in making a retrospective diagnosis. Table 27.4 provides additional guidance for patient evaluation.

Management of patients with hypertensive emergency begins with appropriate monitoring—including serial, automated BP assessments, cardiac telemetry, and intravenous access. BP reduction (usually with an intravenous drug) should not be deferred while arrangements for admission or transfer to the intensive care unit are being made. An arterial line for continuous BP monitoring should be established no later than the initiation of intravenous antihypertensive medications. This will facilitate identification and avoidance of further elevations and sudden drops in BP. Precipitous drops in BP to normotensive or hypotensive levels must be avoided as they may aggravate target organ ischemia or infarction.

The goal in BP management is a rapid but controlled reduction in BP to prevent further end-organ damage. In general, the goal of therapy is to lower the mean arterial pressure (MAP) by approximately 25% over several minutes to 1 hour depending on the clinical situation. If the patient remains stable, then BP should be reduced to 160/100 to 110 mm Hg over the next 2 to 6 hours.[1] If this BP is tolerated, further gradual reductions toward a normal BP can be implemented in the next 24 to 48 hours.[1] Exceptions to these guidelines include aortic dissection and hypertensive encephalopathy, both of which require more expeditious BP reductions. Finally, most hypertensive emergency patients are volume depleted; therefore BP reduction should be accomplished via a decrease in peripheral vascular resistance, not volume

TABLE 27.2 Prevalence of Target Organ Damage in Patients With Hypertensive Emergency

Study	Inclusion Criteria: BP (mm Hg)	HTN Crisis, HTN Emergency, n (%)	MI/UA (%)	Acute Pulmonary Edema/Heart Failure (%)	Total CVA, Ischemic, Hemorrhagic (%)	Hypertensive Encephalopathy (%)	Acute Aortic Dissection (%)	Acute Renal Failure (%)	Eclampsia (%)
Pinna et al.,[a] 2014[15]	≥220/120	1546 crisis 391 (25) emergency	70 (18) MI	121 (31)	86 (22) 60 (15) 26 (7)	19 (5)	31 (8)	23 (6)	–
Salkic et al., 2014[28]	>180/120	85 crisis 14 (17) emergency	13 (93)	1 (7)	0	0	0	0	0
González et al., 2013[29]	>180/120	538 crisis 412 (77) emergency	245 (60)	104 (25)	21 (5)	–	26 (6)	16 (4)	–
Martin et al., 2004[13]	Diastolic ≥120	452 crisis 179 (40) emergency	14 (8) MI 9 (5) UA	45 (25)	104 (58) 70 (39) 34 (19)	0	0	0	7 (4)
Rodriguez et al., 2002[14]	≥220/120	118 crisis 26 (22) emergency	15 (58)	4 (15)	5 (19) 4 (15) 1 (4)	2 (8)	0	0	0
Zampaglione et al., 1996[12]	Diastolic ≥120	449 crisis 108 (24) emergency	13 (12) MI or UA	39 (36) 0	31 (29) 26 (24) 5 (5)	18 (17)	2 (2)	0	5 (5)
Total HTN emergencies[a,b]		1130 (100)[a]	379/1130 UA	314/1130 (28)	247/1130 (22)	37/718 (5)	59/1130 (5)	39/1130 (4)	12/327 (4)

[a]In the Pinna et al. 2014 study, 391 patients were noted to have hypertensive emergencies but only 350 are accounted for in their breakdown of target organ damage. This results in a shortfall of 10% in the sum of hypertensive emergencies (first row) and a shortfall of 5% in the sum of total hypertensive emergencies (last row).

[b]Studies that did not include these patients or target organ damage (denoted by –) were not included in the total HTN emergencies denominator.

CVA, Cerebrovascular accident; HTN, hypertension; MI, myocardial infarction; UA, unstable angina.

TABLE 27.3 Presenting Signs and Symptoms in Patients With Hypertensive Emergency[12-15,28]

Presenting SIGN or symptom	N	%
Neurologic deficit[12-15]	202/718	29
Chest pain[12-14,28]	89/327	27
Dyspnea[12-14,28]	81/327	25
Headache[12-14,28]	65/327	20
Vertigo/dizziness[12-14,28]	38/327	12
Nausea/vomiting[12,13,28]	26/692	9
Syncope/faintness[12,13]	16/287	6
Epistaxis[12,13,28]	0/301	0

contraction. Diuretics should be reserved for patients with fluid overload.

After BP has been controlled for 12 to 24 hours, oral antihypertensive agents may be initiated while the patient is weaned off intravenous agents.[35] During hospitalization, patients should be evaluated for secondary hypertension (see Box 27.1), if indicated, and those noncompliant with antihypertensive medications should be interviewed for root causes. Social work intervention is indicated if lack of a primary care physician, lack of health insurance, or insufficient funds for medications are factors in noncompliance. For patients who are noncompliant owing to adverse side effects, alternative medications should be explored and offered. Counseling about lifestyle changes and patient education should also be provided to better ensure outpatient compliance.[19]

PROGNOSIS

Untreated hypertensive emergency has a very poor prognosis, with 1-year mortality rates as high as 79%.[36] In the 1930s, the mean survival of hypertensive emergency patients was 10.5 months, with no survivors at 5 years.[36] Currently, mortality rates range between 2% and 4% in European studies and 5% and 10% in US cohorts.[17,37,38] In developing countries, mortality rates are much higher, ranging from 15% (Thailand) to 22% (Nigeria).[39,40] This discrepancy is thought to be due to patients presenting with advanced hypertensive disease and limited diagnostic testing and delayed or absent intravenous antihypertensive therapy in health care settings.

The major factor in prognosis is not the level of BP elevation but rather the degree of renal impairment and other target organ damage.[41] The most common cause of death in a study of 315 patients with hypertensive emergency was renal failure (40%)

TABLE 27.4   Pathogenesis, Presentation, and Evaluation of Hypertensive Emergencies

Condition	Pathophysiology/Risk Factors	Symptoms and Signs	Diagnostic Evaluation
Cardiovascular Emergencies			
Acute aortic dissection	Hypertension or congenital abnormality Intimal tear with dissection into media	Chest pain, back pain Unequal blood pressures (>20 mm Hg difference) in upper extremities	Widened mediastinum on chest radiograph Abnormal CT angiogram of chest and abdomen/pelvis or transesophageal echocardiogram of the aorta
Acute coronary syndrome/myocardial infarction	Thrombus or ruptured plaques in the coronary arteries leading to ischemia or infarction	Chest pain, nausea, vomiting, diaphoresis	Changes on ECG or elevated levels of cardiac biomarkers
Acute heart failure/pulmonary edema	Activation of the neurohormonal cascade, salt and water retention, increased vascular resistance, decreased cardiac output, increased pulmonary pressures	Dyspnea, chest pain or pressure Signs of heart failure on exam, including raised jugular venous pressure, crackles on chest auscultation, third heart sounds or gallop	Interstitial edema on chest radiograph
Neurologic Emergencies			
Hypertensive retinopathy	Vasoconstriction and choroidal ischemia results in optic disc edema Rupture of microaneurysms in retina (developed in response to chronic hypertension)	Blurred vision	Retinal hemorrhages and cotton wool spots (exudates), and sausage-shaped veins
Hypertensive encephalopathy/PRES	Hypertension leading to endothelial dysfunction, hydrostatic leakage across capillaries and cerebral edema	Headache, altered mental status, nausea, vomiting, visual disturbance, altered level of consciousness, seizures (late)	May see papilledema or arteriolar hemorrhage or exudates on funduscopic examination, may note cerebral edema with a predilection for the posterior white matter of the brain on MRI
Subarachnoid hemorrhage	Hypertension causing pseudoaneurysms and microbleeds	Headache, focal neurologic deficits	Abnormal CT of the brain; red blood cells on lumbar puncture
Intracerebral hemorrhage	Bleeding due to autoregulatory dysfunction with excessive cerebral blood flow, aneurysm rupture, arteriopathy due to chronic hypertension	Headache, new neurologic deficits	Abnormal CT of the brain
Acute ischemic stroke	Hypertension and atherosclerosis Thrombosis, embolism, or hypoperfusion	New neurologic deficits	Abnormal MRI or CT of the brain
Other Hypertensive Emergencies			
Acute renal failure	Hypertension causing benign nephrosclerosis Vascular, glomerular, and tubulointerstitial changes	Oliguria, hematuria (late) May have systolic or diastolic abdominal bruit	Urinalysis: proteinuria, microscopic hematuria, red blood cells or hyaline casts Chemistry panel: elevated BUN and creatinine, hyperkalemia or hypokalemia,[a] hyperphosphatemia, acidosis, hypernatremia
Severe preeclampsia, HELLP syndrome, eclampsia	Primarily a disorder of first pregnancies Possibly related to incomplete trophoblastic invasion and alterations in immune responses Can occur up to 8 wk postpartum	Headache, visual disturbances, seizures, altered level of consciousness, congestive heart failure, right upper quadrant pain, oliguria	Proteinuria, normal or slightly elevated serum creatinine, thrombocytopenia, microangiopathic hemolytic anemia, elevated liver function tests
Acute perioperative hypertension	Sympathetic activation during induction of anesthesia Exaggerated blood pressure and heart rate response as anesthesia wears off (immediate postoperative period)	Bleeding unresponsive to direct pressure	Clinical diagnosis; manifestations of other hypertensive emergencies—such as myocardial ischemia, heart failure, renal insufficiency, and stroke
Sympathetic crisis[b]	Either direct or indirect effects on the sympathetic system	Anxiety, palpitations, tachycardia, diaphoresis, paresthesias	Clinical diagnosis in the setting of sympathomimetic drug use (e.g., cocaine, amphetamines) or pheochromocytoma (24-h urine assay for catecholamines and metanephrine or plasma fractionated metanephrines)

[a]Hyperaldosteronism (a secondary cause of hypertension) promotes renal potassium wasting.
[b]In this syndrome, acute end-organ dysfunction may not be measurable, but complications affecting the brain, heart, or kidneys may occur in the absence of acute treatment.
BUN, Blood urea nitrogen; *CT,* computed tomography; *ECG,* electrocardiogram; *HELLP,* hemolysis, elevated liver enzymes, low platelets; *MRI,* magnetic resonance imaging; *PRES,* posterior reversible encephalopathy syndrome.

followed by stroke (24%) and MI (11%).[42] A 2009 registry report of 1588 patients presenting with hypertensive emergency demonstrated similar target organ complications, including renal insufficiency (44%), MI (26%), acute heart failure (22%), and stroke (19%).[43]

SPECIFIC HYPERTENSIVE EMERGENCIES

Cardiovascular Emergencies

Acute Coronary Syndrome. BP goals for patients presenting with acute coronary syndrome (ACS: myocardial ischemia, MI, or unstable angina) have not yet been established.[44] This is due, in part, to conflicting results from recent trials of hypertensive ST elevation myocardial infarction (STEMI) and non-STEMI (NSTEMI) patients. Specifically, there is an approximately 20% increase in in-hospital mortality for every 10 mm Hg BP decrease at patient presentation.[45] A SBP of <100 mm Hg is associated with increased mortality risk, yet, elevated BP (>140 mm Hg) is not.[46,47] One trial even demonstrated a *protective* effect in patients with systolic BP (SBP) as high as 200 mm Hg.[45]

The anticipated U-shaped mortality curve at BP extremes has not been shown in the ACS population. This may be because myocardial perfusion primarily occurs in diastole and, in patients with occlusive coronary disease, a low DBP further impedes coronary perfusion. In hypertensive ACS patients with concomitant left ventricular hypertrophy, this perfusion deficit is exacerbated. Thus, the only recommendation for BP control is for patients about to undergo thrombolytic therapy to decrease the risk of intracerebral hemorrhage.[48]

Patients with ACS should be given aspirin and oxygen (if oxygen saturation is <90% or the patient is dyspneic). Nitroglycerin should be given to patients with ongoing chest pain or hypertension and heart failure.[3] Nitroglycerin promotes coronary dilation, improves coronary perfusion, and reduces chest pain symptoms. Given that BP may fluctuate in the early phase of ACS, the focus should be on patient stabilization and a reduction in symptoms. For patients whose BP is refractory to nitroglycerin or who are experiencing ongoing ischemia or tachyarrhythmias (atrial fibrillation), intravenous β-blockers such as metoprolol, esmolol, or labetalol may be used. β-Antagonists reduce heart rate and myocardial oxygen consumption and are useful in combination with nitrates.[3,44] Of note, intravenous β-antagonists are contraindicated in patients with hemodynamic instability or borderline hemodynamics owing to an increased risk of cardiogenic shock, particularly in the first two days of hospitalization.[49] Other agents with demonstrated risk reduction for patients with ACS, independent of BP lowering, include angiotensin-converting enzyme (ACE) inhibitors or angiotensin receptor blockers (ARBs) and, in select patients, aldosterone antagonists. Titrate these agents to full doses before other agents that are not evidence based are used (Tables 27.5 and 27.6).[44] At discharge, a BP goal of less than 130/80 mm Hg is appropriate. Higher target BPs are indicated in elderly patients with wide pulse pressures.[44]

Aortic Dissection. Aortic dissection is discussed in Chapter 28. Management recommendations are given in Table 27.5.

Acute Pulmonary Edema. Until recently, acute pulmonary edema in patients with severe hypertension was believed to be due to transient left ventricular systolic or diastolic dysfunction, acute dyssynchrony, or ischemic mitral regurgitation.[50] However, limited data suggest that acute pulmonary edema in hypertensive emergency patients may primarily be due to transient diastolic dysfunction.[50,51] Given this uncertainty, there are no clear evidence-based guidelines for treatment. Current recommendations include vasodilators and intravenous diuretics.[52] Intravenous, sublingual, and topical nitrates reduce BP, decrease myocardial oxygen consumption, and improve coronary blood flow.[52,53] Diuretics improve symptoms within 6 hours of administration but have not been shown to improve mortality rates.[54]

When hypertensive pulmonary edema is a result of ACS, nitrates are first-line agents. β-Antagonists should be reserved for patients with pulmonary edema due to atrial fibrillation with rapid ventricular response.[55] If acute systolic dysfunction is still suspected, intravenous nicardipine increases both stroke volume and coronary blood flow, which should help alleviate symptoms (see Table 27.5).

Neurologic Emergencies

Hypertensive Encephalopathy/Posterior Reversible Encephalopathy Syndrome. The constellation of headache, altered mental status, restlessness, nausea, and sometimes seizures and coma in association with severely elevated BP has been recognized as the syndrome of hypertensive encephalopathy for almost 100 years.[56] In 1996, Hinchey et al. described a reversible encephalopathy, now commonly known as posterior reversible encephalopathy syndrome (PRES).[30] PRES is a disorder of reversible subcortical vasogenic edema, which appears to be along the continuum of hypertensive encephalopathy.[31,57,58]

The pathophysiology of PRES is poorly defined and largely based on animal models. PRES appears to be the consequence of disordered cerebral autoregulation leading to endothelial injury as well as the direct effects of cytokines on the endothelium. This leads to breakdown of the blood-brain barrier, focal transudation of fluid (brain edema), and petechial hemorrhages of the brain (Fig. 27.2).[30,57,59] The posterior brain regions are most susceptible to subsequent perfusion abnormalities due to minimal sympathetic innervation in the posterior fossa, which limits any residual autoregulation or adaptation.[59]

Manifestations include encephalopathy (50% to 80%), seizures (60% to 70%), headache often nonlocalized and unresponsive to analgesics (50%), visual disturbances (33%), and focal neurologic deficits in the setting of acute hypertension or in patients receiving cytotoxic or immunosuppressant therapies.[31,57,58] The onset is typically gradual but some patients initially experience a seizure. At presentation, up to 20% of patients with PRES are normotensive or hypotensive, suggesting that the proportional rise and rapidity of BP rise are more important than absolute BP.[60] A large percentage of patients, particularly children, have a history of an autoimmune disorder, lending further support to theories of endothelial disruption.[31,58,59,61] The diagnosis is made with T2-weighted FLAIR MRI. Findings include vasogenic edema in the parieto-occipital or posterior frontal regions of

Text continued on p. 286

TABLE 27.5 Hypertensive Emergencies: Specific Therapeutic Agents

Hypertensive Emergency	Agents to Use	Comments/Risks	Agents to Avoid
Cardiovascular Emergencies			
Acute coronary syndrome (ACS)	**Nitroglycerin** continuous IV infusion **Metoprolol, bisoprolol,** or **labetalol** IV bolus[44] **ACE I** and **ARBs** IV bolus[44] For cocaine-associated ACS, see hyperadrenergic states	Avoid nitrates in patients who have taken phosphodiesterase inhibitors for erectile dysfunction ≤24 h (48 h for tadalafil). Do not give β-antagonists in HF, low-output states, prolonged first-degree or high-grade AV block, or in patients with asthma/RAD or in those who use cocaine. ACE inhibitors may reduce infarct expansion/remodeling and chamber dilatation.[44] Avoid ACE I and ARBs in patients who are volume depleted.	Avoid nondihydropyridine CCB (verapamil, diltiazem) in patients with left ventricular dysfunction or in combination with β-antagonists.[44] Avoid carvedilol in patients with reactive airway disease due to β₂ antagonism. Avoid nitroprusside and hydralazine (coronary steal). Avoid other diuretics.
Aortic dissection	**Labetalol**[5] IV continuous infusion or **esmolol**[5] IV, bolus, then continuous infusion **Propranolol** 1–10 mg IV bolus, then continuous infusion **Verapamil, diltiazem** IV **Nicardipine**[5] IV continuous infusion (after β-blocker) **Nitroprusside**[5] continuous infusion (after β-blocker)	Possible respiratory distress in COPD and asthma patients given β-blockers; test dose of esmolol recommended; switch to diltiazem if esmolol intolerant.[5] Always use β-blocker prior to vasodilators (nicardipine or nitroprusside). Avoid β-blockers, verapamil, and diltiazem in patients with aortic dissection complicated by aortic regurgitation: increased risk of reflex tachycardia.[5]	Nitroprusside alone increases wall stress from reflex tachycardia; cyanide and thiocyanate toxicity in patients with reduced renal function or therapy >24–48 h. Avoid hydralazine: it increases wall shear stress and provides less accurate BP control.
Acute pulmonary edema	**Nitroglycerin**[52,53] SL, topical, or IV continuous infusion **Enalaprilat**[53] IV **Nicardipine**[52,53] IV continuous infusion **Nitroprusside**[52,53] IV continuous infusion **Nesiritide**[52,53] IV	IV nitrates dilate capacitance vessels at low doses, higher doses dilate arterioles and lower BP. ACE inhibitors can worsen renal function, especially in volume-depleted patients. Use nicardipine with caution; some patients experience a negative inotropic effect. Nesiritide: Mixed outcomes; most recent ASCEND-HF trial showed no difference in dyspnea and mortality when compared to placebo.[54]	Caution with nitroprusside: cyanide and thiocyanate toxicity in patients with reduced renal function or therapy >24–48 h.
Neurologic Emergencies			
Hypertensive encephalopathy/PRES	**Clevidipine**[63] continuous IV infusion **Nicardipine**[64] continuous IV infusion **Labetalol**[65] continuous IV infusion **Fenoldopam**[66] continuous IV infusion	Decrease MAP 10%–15% in the first hour of presentation. Some recommend a target <160/100 mm Hg. Caution in the elderly and those with preexisting hypertension.[59] Withdraw all immunosuppressive and cytotoxic drugs.[31]	Cerebral perfusion autoregulation may be significantly impaired; avoid rapid reductions in BP. Avoid nitroglycerin, as it may worsen cerebral dysautoregulation.[7]
Subarachnoid hemorrhage	**Nicardipine**[70] IV continuous infusion **Labetalol**[72] IV bolus 10–20 mg or continuous infusion **Esmolol**[74] IV bolus 500 µg/kg, then continuous infusion **Clevidipine**[73] IV continuous infusion	All patients should receive nimodipine 60 mg PO q4h for vasospasm prophylaxis.[75] The magnitude of blood pressure control to reduce the risk of rebleeding has not been established, but current guidelines recommend that a decrease in systolic blood pressure to <160 mm Hg is reasonable.[68]	Avoid nitroprusside, as it requires more frequent titrations and increases the risk of iatrogenic hypotension and cerebral hypoperfusion.[71]
Intracerebral hemorrhage	**Nicardipine**[81,82] IV continuous infusion **Labetalol**[83,84] IV bolus or continuous infusion	For ICH patients presenting with SBP >220 mm Hg and without contraindication to acute BP treatment, acute lowering of SBP to 140 mm Hg is safe and can be effective for improving functional outcome.[79]	Treatment with candesartan in the first week following intracerebral hemorrhage has been associated with worse functional outcomes.[85]

TABLE 27.5   Hypertensive Emergencies: Specific Therapeutic Agents—cont'd

Hypertensive Emergency	Agents to Use	Comments/Risks	Agents to Avoid
Acute ischemic stroke	**Labetalol**[4,93] 10 mg IV bolus, followed by IV continuous infusion or PO **Nicardipine**[4] IV continuous infusion **Lisinopril**[4] PO or SL	Antihypertensive treatment not recommended unless blood pressure elevations are extremely high (SBP >220 mm Hg or DBP >120 mm Hg) or if the patient is eligible for thrombolysis.[4] It is likely that the fate of the vulnerable ischemic penumbra has been determined by 10 h post–stroke onset. Once this period of vulnerability has lapsed, a benefit may be gained from BP reduction.	Caution with BP control efforts in patients taking oral β-blockers or clonidine; antihypertensive withdrawal syndrome may occur. Avoid ACE inhibitors and ARBs in patients who are volume depleted, as hypoperfusion may occur.
Renal insufficiency	**Fenoldopam**[99] IV continuous infusion **Nicardipine**[99] IV continuous infusion **Clevidipine** IV continuous infusion	Fenoldopam considered first line, as it improves natriuresis and creatinine clearance in these patients.[99,100] Caution with ACE inhibitors and ARBs, as they may cause hypotension and worsen renal function.[101]	Avoid β-antagonists, which reduce blood flow and GFR. Avoid nitroprusside owing to increased risk of cyanide and thiocyanate toxicity and no improvement in renal perfusion.[102]
Preeclampsia/eclampsia	**Labetalol**[6,107] 20 mg IV bolus followed by 40 mg, then 80 mg **Hydralazine**[107,118] 5–10 mg IV bolus **Nifedipine**[107] 10–20 mg PO	Maximum 1 h IV labetalol dose of 220 mg. Hydralazine lowers MAP more than labetalol; however, labetalol has a more rapid onset of action. Labetalol may cause fetal bradycardia. Women who receive oral nifedipine have faster BP reduction than those receiving intravenous labetalol or hydralazine.[6]	Avoid labetalol in patients with greater than first-degree heart block, bradycardia, or asthma. Avoid ACE inhibitors and ARBs, as these are contraindicated in pregnancy. Avoid nitroprusside, as it may cause maternal hypotension and is associated with fetal cyanide toxicity.
Perioperative hypertension	**Clevidipine**[134] IV continuous infusion **Nicardipine**[128] IV continuous infusion **Labetalol**[130] IV bolus **Esmolol**[5] IV infusion	Caution with IV β-antagonists in setting of myocardial ischemia or left ventricular dysfunction. Caution with nitrates in cardiac and vascular patients, as a tachycardia may develop.	Avoid ACE inhibitors and ARBs, as their mechanism of action may be unpredictable and prolonged in a perioperative patient.
Hyperadrenergic state due to sympathomimetic drugs	**Benzodiazepine**[143,144] IV bolus **Nitroglycerin**[144] SL, topical, or IV continuous infusion **Phentolamine** IV bolus or IM **Dexmedetomidine**[133,134] IV infusion	Benzodiazepines are first-line agents; observe for respiratory depression. Dexmedetomidine adverse effects include hypotension, bradycardia, and sinus blockade.	Use of mixed α-antagonists, β-antagonists (labetalol and carvedilol) is controversial; if given, administer along with a nitrate. Avoid all other β-adrenergic receptor antagonists owing to the potential of unopposed α-adrenergic stimulation, causing coronary vasoconstriction and BP increase.[133,144]
Hyperadrenergic state due to abrupt cessation of antihypertensive agents	**Restart original agent** **Labetalol** IV bolus	Calcium channel blockers, phentolamine, nitrates may also be used.	
Hyperadrenergic state due to pheochromocytoma and paraganglioma	**Phentolamine**[152] IV bolus or IM	α-Receptor blockade is the cornerstone of blood pressure control. There is a risk of reflex tachycardia with phentolamine, which can be treated with esmolol.[153,154]	Avoid labetalol, as paradoxic episodes of hypertension thought to be secondary to incomplete α blockade may occur.
Hyperadrenergic state due to autonomic dysreflexia	**Nitroglycerin** SL, topical, or IV continuous infusion **Labetalol**[157] IV bolus **Nicardipine** IV infusion	Sit patient upright. First, address the underlying problem: pain, abdominal distension. **Dexmedetomidine has been used with some success in refractory cases.**[158,159]	

ACE, Angiotensin-converting enzyme; *ARB,* angiotensin receptor blocker; *AV,* atrioventricular; *BP,* blood pressure; *CCB,* calcium channel blocker; *COPD,* chronic obstructive pulmonary disease; *GFR,* glomerular filtration rate; *HF,* heart failure; *ICH,* intracranial hemorrhage; *IM,* intramuscular; *IV,* intravenous; *MAP,* mean arterial pressure; *RAD,* reactive airway disease; *PRES,* posterior reversible encephalopathy syndrome; *SBP,* systolic blood pressure; *SL,* sublingual.

TABLE 27.6	**Therapeutic Agents for Hypertensive Emergency**		
Drug	**Dosing (Intravenous)**	**Mechanism of Action**	**Adverse Effects/Risks**
ACE Inhibitors			
Enalaprilat Onset: 15 min Duration: 6 h	0.625–1.25 mg q4–6h Titrate at increments of 1.25 mg q12–24h. Maximum of 5 mg q6h	Active metabolite of oral enalapril It blocks the formation of angiotensin II and causes a reduction in systemic vascular resistance and arterial BP.	Contraindicated in pregnancy. Patient's response may be unpredictable. First-dose hypotension is common, especially in high renin or volume-depleted patients. If first dose yields unsatisfactory results, use a second agent. Common side effects: angioedema, rash
β-Receptor Antagonists			
Esmolol Onset: 1–2 min Duration: 10–20 min	Loading dose: 250–500 µg/kg over 1 min, then 50 µg/kg for 4 min, then increase dose by 50 µg/kg every 5 min up to 300 µg/kg/min	$β_1$ receptor antagonist Metabolized by bloodborne esterases Used primarily for short-term BP control (perioperative setting).	Avoid in patients with bradycardia, heart block, cardiogenic shock, decompensated heart failure, reactive airway disease. Avoid concomitant use of verapamil or diltiazem. Anemic patients will have prolonged half life.
Labetalol Onset: 2–5 min Duration: 3–6 h Peak effect: 15 min	Bolus 10–20 mg (0.25 mg/kg for an 80-kg patient) over 2 min May administer 20–80 mg as IV bolus every 10 min. Up to 300 mg total dose or 2 mg/min continuous infusion	Nonselective β-antagonist with modest $α_1$-antagonist effects Has an α- to β-blocking ratio of 1:7.[148]	Avoid in patients with bradycardia, heart block, cardiogenic shock, decompensated heart failure, reactive airway disease. Avoid concomitant use of verapamil or diltiazem. Prolonged effect in patients with liver impairment. Elderly may have a less predictable response, increased risk of hypotension and adverse effects.
Calcium Channel Antagonists			
Clevidipine Onset: 2–4 min Duration: 5–15 min	Continuous infusion: start at 1–2 mg/h. Dose titration: double dose at short (90-sec) intervals initially. As BP approaches goal, increase dose by less than doubling and lengthen time between dose adjustments to every 5–10 min. Maximum dose: 16 mg/h	Dihydropyridine L-type calcium channel antagonist Highly selective for vascular smooth muscle, reducing mean arterial BP by decreasing systemic vascular resistance. Has little or no effect on myocardial contractility or cardiac conduction. Metabolized by esterases in the blood and extravascular tissues; safe in patients with renal and liver dysfunction. Ideal for patients with labile BP.	Contraindicated in patients with egg or soy hypersensitivity Avoid in patients with advanced aortic stenosis. Avoid in patients receiving IV β-antagonists and in patients with decompensated heart failure. Lipid intake restrictions may be needed for patients with lipid metabolism disorders. Common side effects: headache, hypotension, vomiting, and tachycardia Very limited data on doses at 32 mg/h
Nicardipine Onset: 5–10 min Duration: 1–4 h	Continuous infusion: start at 5 mg/h, increase by 1–2.5 mg/h every 15 min. Maximum dose: 15 mg/h	Dihydropyridine calcium channel antagonist Relaxes cardiac and smooth muscle cells and causes decrease in systemic vascular resistance, afterload, and arterial BP. Minimal negative inotropic effect	Avoid in patients with advanced aortic stenosis. Avoid in patients receiving IV β-antagonists and in patients with decompensated heart failure. Dosing adjustment may be needed in patients with hepatic insufficiency. May cause worsening of GFR in patients with renal insufficiency. Common side effects: headache, hypotension, vomiting, and tachycardia
Vasodilators			
Hydralazine Onset: 10–20 min Duration: 2–8 h	Bolus: 10–20 mg IV or 10–40 IM; repeat q4–6h In pregnancy: bolus 5–10 mg IM or IV, then 5–10 mg every 20–40 min PRN or 0.5–10 mg/h infusion Maximum total dose of 20–25 mg in pregnancy	Preferentially relaxes arterial smooth muscle cells with little effect on veins, which reduces peripheral vascular resistance, afterload, and arterial BP with little or no change in preload or venous capacitance. Increases cardiac output, myocardial work, and myocardial oxygen demand.	Contraindicated in patients with acute aortic dissection. Avoid in patients with mitral valve disease (increases pulmonary artery pressure), renal impairment, volume depletion, CAD/ACS (reflex tachycardia), SLE and neurologic emergencies (increases ICP). Common side effects: reflex tachycardia, angina, fluid retention, headache, nausea, flushing, rash, dizziness

TABLE 27.6 Therapeutic Agents for Hypertensive Emergency—cont'd

Drug	Dosing (Intravenous)	Mechanism of Action	Adverse Effects/Risks
Nitroglycerin Onset: 2–5 min Duration: 5–10 min	Continuous infusion: start at 5 μg/min. Increase by 5 μg/min every 3–5 min to 20 μg/min. If no response at 20 μg/min, increase by 10 μg/min every 3–5 min, up to 200 μg/min (many clinicians initiate with a higher infusion rate).	**Nitroglycerin** is converted by mitochondrial aldehyde dehydrogenase to nitric oxide, a potent venodilator. It causes venous capacitance vessel dilatation at low doses (5 μg/min) and arterial dilatation only at very high doses.	Avoid in cases of compromised cerebral and renal perfusion. Avoid concurrent use (within past 24–48 h) with phosphodiesterase 5 inhibitors (sildenafil, tadalafil, or vardenafil). Methemoglobinemia may occur. Common side effects: hypotension (especially in volume-depleted patients), reflex tachycardia, headache, nausea, vomiting
Nitroprusside Onset: within seconds Duration: 1–3 min	Continuous infusion: start at 0.5 μg/kg/min. Increase in increments of 0.5 μg/kg/min every 5–10 min; titrate to desired effect. Maximum dosage is 10 μg/kg/min IV for 10 min. For infusions 4–10 μg/kg/min, institute a thiosulfate infusion.	Nitric oxide donor, which reduces both preload and afterload Can cause dose-related decreases in coronary, cerebral, and renal perfusion.	Avoid in patients with kidney or hepatic failure, atriovenous shunts, hereditary optic nerve atrophy (increases nerve ischemia), elevated ICP, or patients who are pregnant. Risk of cyanide and thiocyanate toxicity in patients with reduced renal function or therapy >24–48 h or at rates >2 μg/kg/min. Greater variability in BP response; needs more titrations than patients receiving nicardipine.[71] Greater cardiac surgery mortality rates than with clevidipine.[128] Nitroprusside is recommended only when other agents fail. Common side effects: hypotension, nausea, vomiting, cyanide, and thiocyanate toxicity
Other Agents			
Dexmedetomidine Onset: 4–6 min Duration: 2–4 h	Loading dose: 1 μg/kg over 10 min, then 0.2–0.7 μg/kg/h (≤24 h)	**Centrally acting α₂-adrenergic agonist that is 8–10 times more selective to α₂-adrenergic receptors than clonidine.** **It decreases BP via a decrease in peripheral vascular resistance.**	Primarily used for light to moderate sedation in ICU settings; second agent for sympathomimetic hypertensive emergencies.[133,134] Slight increase in blood pressure at the onset of infusion, lasting approximately 5–10 min. Common side effects: hypotension, bradycardia
Fenoldopam Onset: 5–10 min Duration: 10–15 min	Continuous infusion: 0.03–0.1 μg/kg/min Titrate no more than every 15 min by 0.05–0.1 μg/kg/min. Fenoldopam is approved for short-term use in adults (≤48 h) and children (≤4 h).	Peripheral dopaminergic-1 receptor agonist, which raises intracellular cyclic AMP and leads to vasodilation of most arterial beds, including renal, mesenteric, and coronary arteries.[148]	Avoid in patients with concomitant β-antagonist use and with elevated intraocular pressure or ICP. Avoid in patients with CAD (reflex tachycardia). May cause hypotension in patients receiving concomitant β-antagonist therapy. May cause hypokalemia or anaphylactic reactions in patients sensitive to sodium metabisulfite. Associated with hypokalemia (<3 mEq/L). Common side effects: headache, dizziness, reflex tachycardia, excessive hypotension, flushing
Phentolamine Onset: 1–2 min Duration: 10–30 min Peak effect: 10–20 min	Bolus 2–5 mg every 5–10 min (normally given IV but also can be given IM)	Competitive α-adrenergic receptor antagonist α₁ > α₂ effects α₁ leads to relaxation of systemic vasculature, which leads to activation of the baroreceptor reflex, norepinephrine release, which is attenuated by phentolamine's effects on α₂-receptors, and a decrease in BP, which is accompanied by a rise, sometimes dramatic, in heart rate.	Contraindicated in patients with MI or CAD. Avoid in patients with neurologic hypertensive emergencies—has been associated with CVA owing to cerebral artery occlusion. Common side effects: hypotension, tachycardia, arrhythmias, angina, headache, nausea, vomiting

ACS, Acute coronary syndrome; *BP,* blood pressure; *CAD,* coronary artery disease; *CVA,* cerebrovascular accident; *GFR,* glomerular filtration rate; *ICP,* intracranial pressure; *ICU,* intensive care unit; *IM,* intramuscular; *IV,* intravenous; *MI,* myocardial infarction; *SLE,* systemic lupus erythematosus.

both hemispheres and occasionally hemorrhage (Fig. 27.3).[31,59] PRES is a reversible form of hypertensive encephalopathy. In cases in which neurologic deficits remain, the majority are believed to be due to intracerebral hemorrhage.[56]

The treatment goal of PRES is to reduce the SBP by 10% to 15% within the first hour and by 25% within the first few hours, with some recommending a target of less than 160/100 mm Hg.[59,62] Few therapeutic trials of PRES treatment are available; thus, the choice of antihypertensive agent is left to the discretion of the treating physician and may include calcium channel antagonists, labetalol, and fenoldopam.[63–66] Clevidipine, a dihydropyridine calcium channel blocker, has gained favor due to its rapid action and ease of titration (see Table 27.5).[63,64,67]

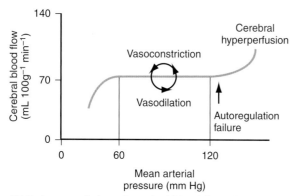

Fig. 27.2 Autoregulation of cerebral blood flow. (From Vaughan CJ, Delanty N. Hypertensive emergencies. *Lancet.* 2000;356: 411–417.)

Subarachnoid Hemorrhage. Subarachnoid hemorrhage (SAH) is a significant cause of morbidity and carries a mortality rate as high as 67%. Roughly half of survivors experience persistent neurologic deficits.[68] The classic presentation of SAH involves an awake patient who describes the "worst headache of my life" often characterized as reaching maximal intensity within the first hour of onset (thunderclap headache). Noncontrast head CT remains the cornerstone for diagnosis of SAH with a negative predictive value of 99.9% if performed within 6 hours from symptom onset.[69] The sensitivity of CT falls sharply as time progresses and, to ensure a diagnosis, a lumbar puncture is required. Xanthochromia or red blood cells in the cerebrospinal fluid are highly suggestive of an SAH.

Acute BP reduction in the setting of SAH has not been shown to improve patient morbidity or mortality. There is, however, general agreement that acute hypertension should be controlled after aneurysmal SAH and prior to aneurysm obliteration, but parameters for BP control have not yet been defined. Titratable infusions are preferred, such as nicardipine, clevidipine, labetalol, and esmolol.[70–74]

The feared delayed complication of aneurysmal SAH, cerebral vasospasm, occurs most frequently 7 to 10 days following aneurysm rupture. The cascade of events culminating in arterial narrowing is initiated when oxyhemoglobin comes in contact with the abluminal side of the vessel.[68] To prevent cerebral artery vasospasm, all patients should receive oral nimodipine, a dihydropyridine calcium channel blocker, which was originally developed for the treatment of hypertension. As such, it modestly decreases BP as well as vasospasm and subsequent cerebral infarction rates.[68] Clinical trials have demonstrated a reduction

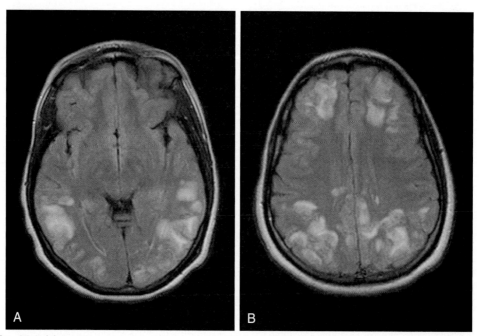

Fig. 27.3 Magnetic resonance brain axial fluid-attenuated inversion recovery images showing radiographic features of posterior reversible encephalopathy syndrome. There is vasogenic edema resulting in a symmetrical high signal within subcortical white matter of predominately occipital and parietal lobes. These MRIs were obtained on a 16-year-old, postpartum female who presented with intractable headache and depressed sensorium.

in mortality by 74% and marked improvements in neurologic disability in patients receiving nimodipine prophylaxis.[75] Clazosentan, an investigational endothelin receptor antagonist that can be given intravenously, also decreases the incidence of vasospasm and has similar BP lowering effects as nimodipine but its effects on morbidity and long-term disability remain unclear.[76] Nonsteroidal antiinflammatory drugs (NSAIDs) have shown some promise in patients with aneurysmal SAH, with reduced mortality rates, shorter duration of intensive care unit and total hospital stays, as well as better functional outcomes in patients treated with NSAIDs compared to controls.[77] If seizure prophylaxis is initiated, use caution with intravenous phenytoin and benzodiazepines, as these can further lower BP (see Table 28.5).

Intracerebral Hemorrhage. Intracerebral hemorrhage (ICH) affects more than 1 million people worldwide annually and is the least treatable of all stroke syndromes.[78] Elevated BP is extremely common in acute ICH, likely owing to a confluence of factors—including stress, pain, increased intracranial pressure, and premorbid hypertension.[79] Current evidence indicates that early intensive BP lowering is safe and feasible and that surviving patients show modestly better functional recovery.[79] Although the largest trial to date, the second Intensive Blood Pressure Reduction in Acute Cerebral Hemorrhage Trial (INTERACT II),

demonstrated no statistically significant difference in the primary outcome of death or disability among patients randomized to an SBP target of less than 140 mm Hg compared to standard treatment (SBP <180 mm Hg), functional improvements among subgroups were noted.[80] For ICH patients presenting with SBP greater than 140 mm Hg, the American Heart Association (AHA) recommends consideration of antihypertensive therapy for improving functional outcome (Fig. 27.4).[79] Antihypertensive therapy should be individualized, with consideration of pharmacologic profile, potential side effects, and cost. Nicardipine and labetalol have consistently been demonstrated to be safe and effective in this population (see Table 27.5).[81–85]

Ischemic Cerebrovascular Accident. The acute hypertensive response in the setting of ischemic stroke is poorly understood. Because it occurs in patients with transient ischemic attack as well as stroke patients, the Cushing reflex is likely not responsible, except in cases of massive cerebral infarction.[86] Up to 80% of patients with acute ischemic stroke are hypertensive on presentation.[87] The elevated BP usually spontaneously resolves and, 10 days after the event, approximately two-thirds of patients are normotensive. In some, the response reflects poorly treated or long-standing hypertension. In others, it appears to be due to other transient and stroke-specific mechanisms, including anxiety surrounding the event or an abnormal autonomic response

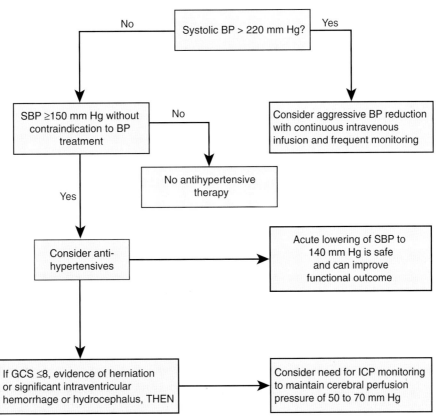

Fig. 27.4 Blood pressure management algorithm for patients with intracerebral hemorrhage. *GCS,* Glasgow Coma Scale; *ICP,* intracranial pressure. (Modified from Hemphill JC 3rd, Greenberg SM, Anderson CS, et al. Guidelines for the management of spontaneous intracerebral hemorrhage: a guideline for healthcare professionals from the American Heart Association/American Stroke Association. *Stroke.* 2015;46[7]:2032–2060.)

induced by the ischemic insult and direct injury to areas of the brain involved in cardiovascular regulation.[86,88] Hypertension during acute ischemic stroke is an independent indicator of poor neurologic prognosis.[4]

Optimal management of BP in ischemic stroke remains unclear. Aggressive lowering of BP may reduce cerebral perfusion pressure, aggravating brain ischemia and threatening the vulnerable ischemic penumbra. Conversely, very high BP may worsen cerebral edema and increase the risk for hemorrhagic transformation.[88,89] Furthermore, there is evidence that controlling hypertension immediately poststroke confers no benefit on short-term mortality or morbidity.[90] Current guidelines recommend against lowering the BP unless BP elevations are extremely high (SBP >220 mm Hg or DBP >120 mm Hg) or if the patient is eligible for thrombolysis.[4] Both US and European guidelines recommend BP reduction if thrombolysis is planned (goal <185/110 mm Hg).[4,91] Observational studies have demonstrated a strong association between postthrombolysis hypertension and poor outcome, prompting strong recommendations for careful BP management in patients treated with tissue plasminogen activator (tPA).[92]

For the treatment of ischemic stroke, labetalol and nicardipine are the recommended agents. However, the route and degree of BP reduction depend on whether the patient is a candidate for reperfusion therapy (Table 27.5).[4,90,93]

Acute Renal Insufficiency

Patients with acute renal insufficiency may present with peripheral edema, oliguria, loss of appetite, nausea and vomiting, orthostatic changes, or confusion. However, some patients have few or no specific symptoms. A patient with severely elevated BP with either new hematuria (microscopic or gross) or a decline in renal function is experiencing a hypertensive emergency. Physicians should inquire about past kidney and urologic issues, including renovascular disease, renal parenchymal disease, autoimmune diseases (for possible vasculitis), renal artery stenosis and anatomic abnormalities, such as horseshoe kidney, solitary kidney, and prior renal transplantation.[94–96] Patients should be asked about the use of diuretics, nephrotoxic drugs, and sympathomimetic agents. In renal transplant patients, stenosis of the graft site and the use of cyclosporine, steroids, and other immunosuppressants can predispose patients to a hypertensive emergency.[97] Excessive renin secretion by the native kidney may also precipitate a hypertensive crisis.

Evaluation of these patients includes a basic chemistry panel to reveal electrolyte abnormalities, the degree of creatinine elevation, and the patient's bicarbonate level. Current values should be compared to prior values to see if the decline in renal function is acute.[34] A bedside, postvoid residual sonogram may identify bladder outlet obstruction, in which case a urinary bladder catheter should be placed. This should be followed by a renal sonogram to evaluate kidney size and higher urinary tract obstructions because obstruction of the urinary tract at any level can raise BP.[98] BP management in renal hypertensive emergency patients includes fenoldopam, nicardipine, and clevidipine, as they reduce systemic vascular resistance while preserving renal blood flow.[99–102] In patients presenting with severe hypertension

owing to renal vasculitis, such as scleroderma renal crisis and Takayasu arteritis, enalaprilat has been shown to work well and preserve renal function.[103,104]

Preeclampsia or Eclampsia

Hypertensive disorders of pregnancy, including preeclampsia and eclampsia, complicate up to 10% of pregnancies worldwide and account for up to 80,000 maternal and 500,000 perinatal deaths annually.[105,106] HELLP syndrome (hemolysis, elevated liver enzymes, low platelets) is considered to be a variant of preeclampsia and presents within the same time period. The three are not separate entities but rather related diseases along a continuum.

From 1987 to 2004, the incidence of preeclampsia in the United States increased 25%.[107] This may be due to the increased prevalence of obesity (a strong risk factor for preeclampsia), changes in the diagnostic criteria, or earlier symptom identification.[108,109] Preeclampsia is characterized by severe hypertension (typically ≥160/110 mm Hg) in patients who have progressed beyond the 20th week of gestation. Current diagnostic criteria for the diagnosis no longer require the presence of proteinuria and instead incorporate other features of target organ damage (Fig. 27.5).[6,107]

Risk factors for the development of preeclampsia and eclampsia include maternal age 30 years or greater, high body mass index, nulliparity, absence of antenatal care, chronic hypertension, gestational diabetes, cardiac or renal disease, pyelonephritis or urinary tract infection, and severe anemia.[110] Patients often complain of headache, visual changes, and nausea or vomiting. Since preeclampsia can rapidly become fulminant, health care providers need to remain vigilant when mild disease has been diagnosed.[111] When seizures occur in the setting of elevated BP, this indicates progression to eclampsia. Eclamptic patients can present from 20 weeks of gestation to 8 weeks postpartum.[112]

The cause of preeclampsia is unclear; however, leading hypotheses summarize the syndrome as a failed interaction between two genetically different organisms.[111] Impaired placentation of the trophoblast and incomplete vascular remodeling result in ischemia-reperfusion injury, oxidative stress, and a systemic inflammatory response.[113] Endothelial dysfunction results with decreased release of nitric oxide and prostacyclin, causing more vasoconstriction, BP elevation, and eventually end-organ damage (Fig. 27.6).[114]

Definitive treatment of preeclampsia and eclampsia is delivery. However, there are risks with this approach: for preeclamptic women remote from term (<34 weeks), there is evidence that expectant management confers perinatal benefit with a minimum of additional maternal risk.[115] In a study of women of 34 to 37 weeks gestation with nonsevere hypertensive disorders, immediate delivery resulted in only minimal improvement in maternal outcome and it was at the expense of significant increases in neonatal morbidity and neonatal health care costs.[116,117]

For preeclamptic women with severe hypertension (≥160/110 mm Hg) or elevated BP with target-organ damage, antihypertensive therapy is recommended with labetalol, hydralazine, and oral nifedipine considered first-line agents (see Table 27.5).[6,107,118] Patients with severe preeclampsia or eclampsia should be given

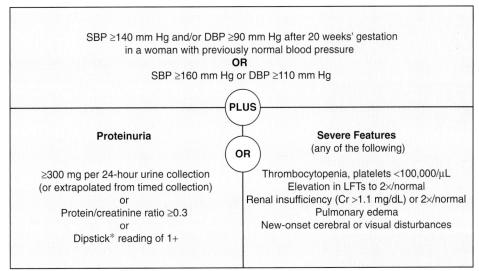

SBP ≥140 mm Hg and/or DBP ≥90 mm Hg after 20 weeks' gestation
in a woman with previously normal blood pressure
OR
SBP ≥160 mm Hg or DBP ≥110 mm Hg

PLUS

Proteinuria

OR

≥300 mg per 24-hour urine collection
(or extrapolated from timed collection)
or
Protein/creatinine ratio ≥0.3
or
Dipstick* reading of 1+

Severe Features
(any of the following)

Thrombocytopenia, platelets <100,000/μL
Elevation in LFTs to 2×/normal
Renal insufficiency (Cr >1.1 mg/dL) or 2×/normal
Pulmonary edema
New-onset cerebral or visual disturbances

Fig. 27.5 Diagnostic criteria for preeclampsia. *Use only if other methods are not available. *Cr,* Creatinine; *DBP,* diastolic blood pressure; *LFTs,* liver function tests; *SBP,* systolic blood pressure. (Modified from Hypertension, Pregnancy-Induced—Practice Guideline. ACOG Task Force on Hypertension in Pregnancy. 2013;1–100. http://www.acog.org/Resources-And-Publications/Task-Force-and-Work-Group-Reports/Hypertension-in-Pregnancy.)

intravenous magnesium sulfate for seizure prophylaxis and treatment.[107]

Perioperative Hypertension. Hypertensive emergencies typically occur in perioperative patients with preexisting hypertension who are either untreated or inadequately treated.[119] The mechanism of action for elevated BP in perioperative patients is thought to be multifactorial, including cessation of antihypertensive medications (often the previous day), sympathetic activation during induction of anesthesia and endotracheal intubation, loss of vasodilation as anesthetic agents are weaned and further sympathetic discharge, especially in patients with postoperative pain.[120,121] Management of these patients can be difficult owing to hemodynamic instability that may occur during the operative state: sudden changes in BP may be owing to release of catecholamines, rapid intravascular volume shifts, blunted baroreceptor response, renin-angiotensin activation, and reperfusion injury.[122–124] The proinflammatory and hypercoagulable state of operative patients further contributes to vascular injury, platelet activation, and endothelial dysfunction.[119] Complications include bleeding from surgical sites, cardiovascular events (myocardial ischemia and infarction and cardiac arrest), stroke, and death. These complications are significant, as bleeding, MI, and cerebral ischemia owing to acute hypertension occur in 5% to 35% of perioperative patients and carry a fourfold higher mortality risk.[119,125,126] While it is generally accepted that preoperative and operative hypertension are predictive of poor postoperative outcomes, there is increasing evidence that postoperative hypertension may also lead to adverse events, including increased mortality, longer length of hospital stay, and higher incidence of renal dysfunction.[127]

BP control in perioperative patients is complex and depends on the condition being managed operatively, whether the patient has preexisting hypertension or was previously normotensive,

and what target organs are being affected or are at risk.[119] BP goals must be individualized and tailored to these factors while taking into consideration patient comorbidities, analgesia or anxiolytic requirements, the need for fluid resuscitation, and the potential for hemodynamic instability.

The greatest experience in BP control has been in cardiac and vascular surgery patients. After coronary artery bypass graft (CABG) surgery or carotid endarterectomy, bleeding from vascular anastomoses is a significant concern. Perioperative BP control is associated with increased mortality in cardiac surgery patients. In a recent study of cardiac surgery patients, clevidipine was compared to nitroglycerin, sodium nitroprusside, and nicardipine. The composite safety endpoint of 30-day death, MI, stroke, or renal dysfunction did not differ among treatment groups. Clevidipine, however, was more effective than nitroglycerin or sodium nitroprusside in maintaining BP control and there was a trend for lower mortality in the clevidipine group.[128] In a meta-analysis comparing clevidipine to other antihypertensive agents for the management of BP in the perioperative setting, similar results were found: clevidipine was more effective in maintaining BP within prespecified ranges and demonstrated a reduction in treatment failure rates when compared to other agents. There was also no difference in adverse events.[129] Other agents that have been used with success in cardiovascular surgical patients include nicardipine and labetalol (see Table 27.5).[119,130]

A unique consideration for BP control is following carotid endarterectomy or carotid artery stent procedures. These patients frequently suffer from labile BPs that can last for days. Possible causes include the disruption of the baroreceptor reflex from trauma or damage to the carotid sinus or vagus nerve during surgery. Hypertension in this period can lead to hyperperfusion syndrome, in which resolution of the stenosis leads to hyperperfusion distal to the site. This syndrome is commonly seen in patients with high-grade carotid artery stenosis, especially with bilateral

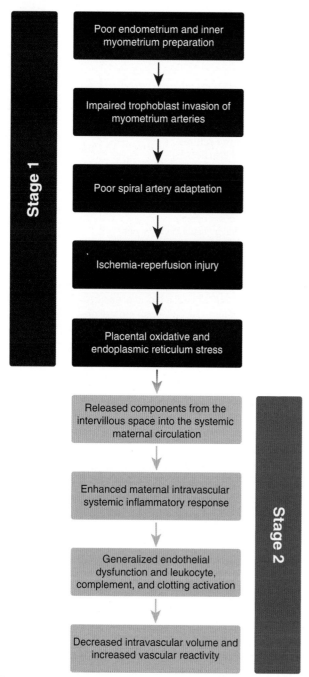

Stage 1

Poor endometrium and inner myometrium preparation

↓

Impaired trophoblast invasion of myometrium arteries

↓

Poor spiral artery adaptation

↓

Ischemia-reperfusion injury

↓

Placental oxidative and endoplasmic reticulum stress

Stage 2

Released components from the intervillous space into the systemic maternal circulation

↓

Enhanced maternal intravascular systemic inflammatory response

↓

Generalized endothelial dysfunction and leukocyte, complement, and clotting activation

↓

Decreased intravascular volume and increased vascular reactivity

Fig. 27.6 Two-stage pathogenesis of preeclampsia. The first stage begins with poor preparatory remodeling and spiral artery adaptation, while the second stage is associated with exaggerated endothelial activation and a generalized inflammatory state. (Modified from Steegers EA, von Dadelszen P, Duvekot JJ, et al. Pre-eclampsia. *Lancet.* 2010;376[9741]:631–644.)

disease, presumably because of a maximal dilation of the arteries distal to the stenosis to maintain perfusion in a situation in which autoregulatory mechanisms are lost. These patients present with a range of neurologic complaints, including headache, seizure, intracranial hemorrhage, altered mental status, and focal neurologic changes.[131] Intensive management of BP, with intravenous β-antagonists or nitrates titrated to resolution of symptoms, has been shown to decrease the incidence of

hyperperfusion syndrome and intracerebral hemorrhage from 29% to 4%.[132]

Management of other perioperative hypertensive emergencies—such as myocardial ischemia, aortic dissection, left ventricular failure, and stroke—can be found in Table 27.5.

Hyperadrenergic States

Sympathomimetic Agents. Sympathomimetic drugs—such as cocaine, amphetamines, phencyclidine hydrochloride (PCP), and lysergic acid diethylamide (LSD)—can precipitate a hypertensive emergency.[44,133–136] Cocaine hypertensive emergencies have been documented in patients with illicit use and patients suffering from iatrogenic complications due to epistaxis treatment or when cocaine is used as a topical anesthetic for laryngoscopy.[137,138] Cocaine blocks the presynaptic reuptake of norepinephrine and dopamine, releases norepinephrine from sympathetic nerve terminals, and stimulates adrenal gland catecholamine release. Patients present with agitation, tachycardia, hypertension, mydriasis, and hyperthermia. Other agents that can precipitate a hypertensive emergency include dietary supplements such as *Ephedra sinica*, also known as *ma-huang*. This supplement contains ephedrine, a chemical that stimulates the nervous and endocrine systems to generate an acute rise in BP and has been temporally associated with stroke, MI, and sudden death.[139] Although banned by the U.S. Food and Drug Association in 2006, it can still be obtained outside the United States and via Internet sources.[140] Patients receiving monoamine oxidase inhibitor therapy who consume tyramine-containing foods may develop a hyperadrenergic state and resultant hypertensive crisis.[141] Patients present with tachycardia, elevated BP, diaphoresis, chest pain, and—depending on the agent—mental status changes. Licorice can also cause acute elevations in BP and complications may include PRES. The active agent, glycyrrhic acid, inhibits 11β-hydroxysteroid dehydrogenase, causing mineralocorticoid excess. Most commercial preparations do not have enough of this compound to cause adverse effects, but some "original" or "old time" formulations may and, if consumed in large amounts, can lead to hypertensive crisis.[142]

Patients with monoamine oxidase inhibitor toxicity often benefit from intravenous benzodiazepine. Phentolamine, nitroglycerin, and calcium channel blockers may also be used. These patients should be closely monitored, as the hypertensive phase is often followed by a hypotensive phase. Therapeutic options for these patients are presented in Table 27.5.[143,144]

Abrupt Cessation of Antihypertensive Drugs. An acute catecholaminergic syndrome may occur with abrupt discontinuation of oral or transdermal clonidine. This "rebound hypertension" often yields BP elevations higher than pretreatment levels and is exacerbated by concomitant β-blocker therapy due to unopposed α-mediated vasoconstriction.[145] Elevations in BP have also been noted with acute cessation of β-antagonists, but to a lesser degree than with clonidine withdrawal.[146] This is thought to be owing to increased sympathetic activity related to adrenergic receptor upregulation during the period of sympathetic blockade.[147] Patients with underlying coronary artery disease are at risk of myocardial ischemia and death with abrupt cessation of β-blockers.

In both settings, reinstitution of the original agent is preferred and will typically have the greatest effect on BP. In patients with rebound hypertensive emergency owing to abrupt clonidine withdrawal, BP may be difficult to control unless clonidine is reinstituted. Clonidine may be given orally at the patient's normal dose or, if unknown, 0.1 to 0.2 mg initially. A reduction in BP will occur within 30 to 60 minutes and peak at 2 to 4 hours.[148] Less ideal is the use of a clonidine patch for patients who are unable to take oral medications. Here, the onset of action may be delayed by 2 to 3 days and titration is challenging. For maximum absorption, apply the patch to the chest or upper arm.[148] If additional BP control is needed, labetalol may be added.

Pheochromocytoma and Paraganglioma. Tumors arising from chromaffin cells of the adrenal medulla and the sympathetic ganglia are referred to as pheochromocytomas and paragangliomas (extra-adrenal pheochromocytomas), respectively. Both secrete catecholamines, have similar presentations, and are managed in a comparable fashion. The main difference between them is the risk for malignancy. Pheochromocytoma is rare, occurring in less than 0.2% of patients with hypertension; between 5% and 20% of tumors are malignant. Patients may experience life-threatening hypertension, particularly in times of stress, that is, acute trauma, surgery, infection, or pregnancy.[149] There have been several reports of pheochromocytoma patients presenting with ACS, prompting the term "the great imitator"; the diagnosis should be considered, especially in patients with normal coronary arteries on angiography.[150,151] Symptoms and signs of pheochromocytoma include headache, alternating periods of normal and elevated BP, tachycardia, and flushed skin, punctuated by asymptomatic periods. Patient evaluation includes measurement of 24-hour urinary fractionated catecholamines and metanephrines in patients with a low suspicion of pheochromocytoma. In patients for whom there is a higher suspicion of a catecholamine-secreting tumor, free plasma metanephrines (drawn supine with an indwelling cannula for 30 minutes) is the best screening test owing to its high sensitivity (99%). This is also considered the best test for high-risk children, given its relative ease of collection compared to a 24-hour urine collection.[152] Elevated metanephrines should prompt a search for the catecholamine-secreting mass, with CT as the initial diagnostic test. In patients for whom metastatic disease is suspected, MRI is preferred. Iodine[173] metaiodobenzylguanidine (MIBG) scintigraphy can be done if suspicion is high but no tumor is found with CT or MRI. MIBG is a compound that resembles norepinephrine and is taken up by adrenergic tissue. An MIBG scan is also helpful in identifying multiple tumors when the CT or MRI is positive.[152]

In patients with pheochromocytoma and a hypertensive emergency, intravenous phentolamine, a nonselective α-receptor blocker, is recommended (or intramuscular if venous access is impaired).[153] A short-acting β-antagonist, such as esmolol, may be needed to control reflex tachycardia.[153,154] Definitive treatment is open surgical resection for large or invasive pheochromocytomas and for most paragangliomas and laparoscopic resection of isolated adrenal gland masses or small, noninvasive paragangliomas.[152]

In the preoperative setting, patients who are hypertensive but not in crisis may be managed and prepared for resection with oral phenoxybenzamine, a long-acting (irreversible), nonselective, α-receptor blocker for 7 to 14 days to allow adequate time to normalize heart rate and BP.[152] Phenoxybenzamine forms a permanent bond with α-receptors, preventing the binding of adrenaline and noradrenaline. The α_1-receptor blockade in the walls of blood vessels leads to vasodilatation and a decrease in BP. Since this is a nonselective α-receptor blocker, it also blocks α_2-receptors, which can lead to a reflex tachycardia. Even with this pretreatment, patients will often require additional BP control perioperatively with additional agents.

Autonomic Dysfunction. Autonomic dysfunction due to acute spinal cord or head trauma, intracerebral hemorrhage, or abnormalities such as spina bifida may also present as a hypertensive emergency. Autonomic dysreflexia is well documented in chronic spinal cord patients, but it can also occur in the acute phase (<1 month after spinal cord injury).[155] Typically, this occurs in patients with injuries above T6, where exaggerated sympathetic responses to noxious stimuli below the level of the injury lead to diffuse vasoconstriction and hypertension. The parasympathetic response results in bradycardia and vasodilation above the level of the lesion and patients may complain of headache, flushing, and diaphoresis. This response, however, is insufficient to reduce elevated BP and may cascade into hypertensive emergency and even cardiac arrest. Spinal cord injuries below T6 do not produce this complication, because intact splanchnic innervation allows for compensatory dilatation of the splanchnic vascular bed.[156] Immediate interventions include sitting the patient upright and addressing causative factors—such as somatic pain (bed sores, fracture pain), fecal impaction, and abdominal distension (often due to incomplete bladder emptying)—before initiating pharmaceutical therapy.[155] Agents for BP control include nitroglycerin, labetalol, and nicardipine.[157] Several cases of paroxysmal autonomic instability with dystonia (PAID) with BP control refractory to the aforementioned agents were successfully managed with dexmedetomidine, a central acting α_2 agonist.[158,159]

For additional guidance with pharmaceutical management of hypertensive emergencies, see Table 27.6.

Acknowledgment

We acknowledge the contributions of Drs. Eduardo Pimenta, David A. Calhoun, and Suzanne Oparil, authors of this chapter in the previous edition.

The full reference list for this chapter is available at ExpertConsult.com.

28

Acute Aortic Syndromes: Diagnosis and Management

Peter C. Spittell

INTRODUCTION

Acute thoracic aortic syndromes comprise a spectrum of medical and surgical emergencies, including acute aortic dissection, penetrating aortic ulcer, and aortic intramural hematoma. All of these conditions are potentially life threatening and warrant prompt diagnosis and emergent management. The clinical presentation of acute aortic syndromes is highly variable, ranging from occult disease to classic clinical presentations. Numerous etiologic factors, acting singly and in combination, have been identified. Diagnosis is possible by noninvasive imaging in the majority of patients, but in some patients complementary noninvasive tests (transesophageal echocardiography [TEE], computed tomography [CT], and magnetic resonance imaging [MRI]) are required for diagnosis. The management of acute aortic syndromes continues to be a therapeutic challenge, while diverse surgical and percutaneous strategies for the treatment of aortic syndromes are continuously evolving. As a result of increasing knowledge and better management strategies in this area, the outcomes of patients treated for acute aortic syndromes have improved. Therefore, awareness of the clinical features of acute aortic syndromes and familiarity with currently available diagnostic techniques is basic to their effective treatment.

ACUTE AORTIC DISSECTION

Acute dissection of the thoracic aorta is one of the most common catastrophic aortic conditions encountered in clinical practice. The incidence of aortic dissection has been reported to be approximately 2.9 per 100,000 per year.[1] The variable clinical presentations of aortic dissection, in combination with a mortality rate in untreated cases as high as 1% per hour during the first 48 hours after the onset of symptoms, underscore the importance of a high index of suspicion and prompt diagnosis and therapy.[2–4] Noninvasive testing (TEE, CT, and MRI) allows an accurate diagnosis to be made in the majority of patients.[5,6] Effective treatment exists so that future improvements in initial and long-term survival in acute aortic dissection depend on increased clinical awareness, rapid noninvasive diagnosis, and the early institution of appropriate medical and/or surgical therapy.

Pathogenesis

Aortic dissection originates at the site of an intimal tear in more than 95% of patients.[2] The resultant intimal tear exposes the media to pulsatile aortic flow, creating a second or "false" aortic lumen that then dissects in the outer layer of aortic media, propagating distally and, occasionally, proximally.

Ascending aortic dissections are almost twice as common as descending dissections. Some 50% to 65% of aortic intimal tears originate in the ascending aorta and approximately 20% to 30% of intimal tears originate in the vicinity of the left subclavian artery.[7]

Once initiated, the dissection usually extends distally and, occasionally, proximally for a variable distance. As the dissecting process encounters branches of the aorta, it may pass around their origins, extend into their walls, or occlude them.[2] Reentry of the dissection through a second, more distal intimal tear may occur, usually in one of the iliac arteries. External rupture of

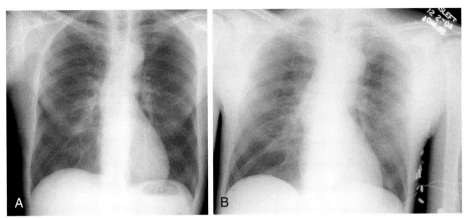

Fig. 28.2 Chest radiographs in a patient with aortic dissection. (A) Baseline anteroposterior chest radiograph before presentation with aortic dissection. (B) Chest radiograph 1 year later when the patient presented with acute aortic dissection. Note the increased diameter of the ascending aorta and aortic arch and new widening of the superior mediastinum.

separating a false lumen from the true lumen. Currently available noninvasive imaging modalities that are accurate in the diagnosis of acute aortic dissection include multiplane TEE, CT angiography, and MR angiography.

Transthoracic echocardiography (TTE) can be very useful in some patients with suspected aortic dissection (Video 28.1). When the findings of a dilated aortic root (end-diastolic diameter >42 mm), widening of the aortic walls (16 to 20 mm for the anterior wall and 10 to 13 mm for the posterior wall), and a linear undulating echo representing the intimal flap are present, the positive predictive value for TTE is 100%.[58–60] Advantages of TTE are its portability; real-time diagnosis; ability to identify associated aortic regurgitation; and to assess left ventricular function, regional wall motion abnormalities, pericardial effusion, and cardiac tamponade. The diagnosis of cardiac tamponade in a patient suspected of having aortic dissection deserves special mention. **Echocardiographically guided pericardiocentesis should be avoided in this setting, as the rapid withdrawal of pericardial fluid can result in a prompt improvement in left ventricular systolic function, left ventricular dP/dT, and systolic blood pressure, producing aortic rupture.**[61,62] The patient with aortic dissection complicated by cardiac tamponade should be taken emergently to surgery for institution of cardiopulmonary bypass followed by evacuation of blood from the pericardial space. Disadvantages of TTE in the diagnosis of aortic dissection include difficulty in adequately visualizing the descending thoracic aorta[5] and suboptimal echocardiographic windows in patients with obesity or chronic obstructive pulmonary disease. Overall, the sensitivity and specificity of TTE are inferior to TEE, CT, and MRI in the diagnosis of aortic dissection. Intravenous contrast agents improve the diagnostic accuracy of TTE in patients with aortic dissection, achieving a sensitivity and specificity similar to TEE in type A dissection.[63] It should be remembered that a negative TTE does not exclude aortic dissection.

Multiplane TEE has a sensitivity of 99% and a specificity of 98% in the diagnosis of aortic dissection.[64] TEE is portable, minimally invasive, and can accurately determine the type and extent of dissection safely in an emergent setting, allowing rapid triage of patients to either surgical or medical therapy[65,66] (Video

28.2). Color flow Doppler imaging significantly improves the sensitivity of TEE by allowing visualization of the intimal flap, dissection entry site, the true and false lumens, presence of thrombus, mechanism and degree of aortic regurgitation, and the proximal coronary arteries[66] (see Fig. 28.2). In addition, multiplane TEE provides a comprehensive assessment of left ventricular systolic function, regional wall motion, pericardial effusion, and cardiac tamponade. The overall sensitivity of TEE is comparable with CT,[67] MR,[5,68,69] and aortography[70] in the diagnosis of aortic dissection. Current multiplane TEE probes have largely overcome impediments in the ascending aorta, although artifacts in this region continue to be a diagnostic challenge.

CT with intravenous iodinated contrast enhancement is an accurate noninvasive screening test in patients with suspected aortic dissection.[71] Advantages of CT include ready availability at most hospitals and improved accuracy with spiral (helical) CT and electron beam (ultrafast) or multidetector (multislice) CT.[72] CT can reliably demonstrate the intimal flap, pericardial and pleural effusion, associated mediastinal hemorrhage, and involvement of the aortic arch vessels and branches of the abdominal aorta, as well as coronary artery disease[5] (Fig. 28.3). Disadvantages of CT include the need for iodinated contrast exposure and nonportability, limiting its use in patients with significant renal insufficiency and in hemodynamically unstable patients, respectively. In addition, the site of entry is rarely identified.

Although less commonly used,[7] MRI is a highly accurate noninvasive technique in the evaluation of patients with suspected aortic dissection.[73] MRI is superior to TEE and CT in detecting arch vessel involvement and in identifying the anastomosis in patients managed with surgical therapy and may facilitate comparison of serial studies.[5,68,74] Gated spin-echo MRI accurately demonstrates the entry site and intimal flap[75] and may be the optimal method for demonstrating thrombus formation and entry site location within all segments of the aorta[76] (Fig. 28.4). The ability to obtain oblique and longitudinal planes of a section makes MRI especially valuable in demonstrating dissection without intimal tear.[5,69,77] Disadvantages of MRI include cost,

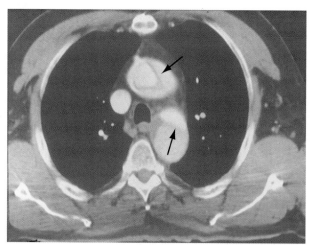

Fig. 28.3 Computed tomographic scan in a patient with type A aortic dissection. Note the complex intimal flap seen within the distal ascending aorta and descending thoracic aorta *(arrows)*, and differential opacification of the true and false lumens.

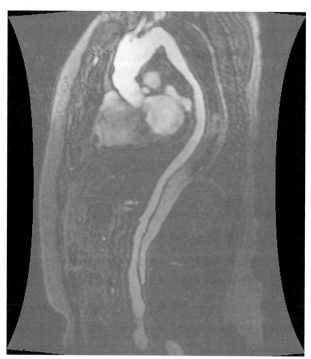

Fig. 28.4 Magnetic resonance imaging in the sagittal plane shows type A aortic dissection with an intimal flap extending into the distal abdominal aorta.

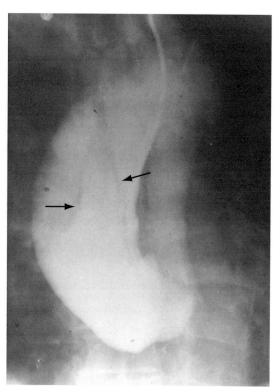

Fig. 28.5 Aortogram shows a spiraling intimal flap *(arrows)* in the ascending aorta and aneurysmal dilation of the ascending aorta.

examination time, reduced availability, nonportability, and standard contraindications to MRI.

Of the definitive noninvasive imaging modalities in suspected acute aortic dissection (TEE, CT, MRI), a systematic review of the diagnostic accuracy of these imaging techniques has demonstrated a pooled sensitivity (98% to 100%) and specificity (95% to 98%) that is comparable between the three imaging techniques. Therefore the choice of test depends upon which imaging modality is readily available at a particular institution and the hemodynamic stability of the patient.

Aortography, the traditional definitive diagnostic method in aortic dissection, is able to localize the site of origin of the dissection and delineate the extent of the dissection and circulation to vital organs. Diagnostic aortographic features include opacification of the false lumen, deformity of the true lumen by the false lumen, dilation of the aorta, narrowing or occlusion of branches of the aorta, and the presence of an intimal flap[78] (Fig. 28.5). Disadvantages of aortography include nonportability, invasive technique, exposure to ionizing radiation, the use of intravenous iodinated contrast agents, and an inherent delay in diagnosis. False-negative aortogram results can occur if there is simultaneous and equal opacification of the true and false lumina or if the false channel is very faintly opacified.[79] For these reasons, aortography has generally been replaced by noninvasive imaging tests in the diagnosis of acute aortic dissection. However, for patients in whom the suspicion for ascending aortic dissection is very strong but noninvasive imaging is unavailable or inconclusive, digital subtraction aortography should be performed. Intravascular ultrasound, in combination with standard aortographic technique, greatly improves the accuracy of aortography, can be performed rapidly and safely, and could serve as an accessory diagnostic procedure in selected patients with suspected aortic dissection.[80,81]

In view of the increased early mortality of untreated acute aortic dissection, the screening test chosen depends on which test is most readily available at a particular institution and the patient's hemodynamic status. Noninvasive diagnosis of acute aortic dissection by TEE, CT, or MR, if readily available, is

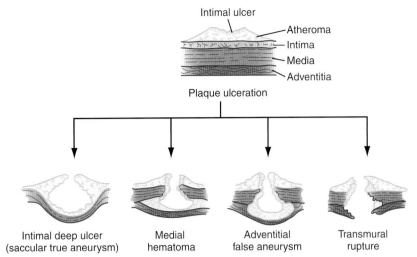

Fig. 28.6 Pathologic consequences of penetrating atherosclerotic ulcer of the aorta. Atheromatous ulceration that burrows deeply into an atheroma can result in one of four potential outcomes: true saccular aneurysm, medial hematoma, adventitial false aneurysm, or transmural rupture. An intramural (medial) hematoma is the most commonly observed consequence of a penetrating aortic ulcer.

preferred as it avoids the risks and delays inherent in invasive angiography.[82]

Management

Treatment for acute aortic dissection is initiated when the diagnosis is first suspected clinically. After initial patient stabilization, the diagnosis is pursued with expedited noninvasive imaging (Fig. 28.6). Treatment recommendations (discussed later) are generally in agreement with multidisciplinary cardiovascular guidelines.[83–85]

The initial treatment objectives in suspected aortic dissection are to control pain and provide anti-impulse therapy to reduce systemic blood pressure, lower the rate of change of pressure development (dP/dT) to decrease aortic shear stress, and limit propagation of the dissection. In hypertensive patients, treatment consists of an intravenous (IV) β-adrenergic blocking agent, often in combination with IV sodium nitroprusside. β-Blockade before nitroprusside therapy is essential because the latter increases the velocity of left ventricular ejection, increases aortic shear stress, and may promote propagation of the dissection.[86] Intravenous labetalol in place of a β-blocker and sodium nitroprusside is an alternative, but it has the potential for hepatotoxicity with long-term therapy.[87] In normotensive patients, an IV β-adrenergic blocking agent may be used alone. Intravenous verapamil or diltiazem is an alternative in patients who cannot tolerate β-blockers. To assist in monitoring blood pressure and renal perfusion, an intraarterial cannula and indwelling bladder catheter are advisable. Following initial patient stabilization, expedited noninvasive aortic imaging is pursued (as discussed in the previous section). If the patient continues to require close monitoring and support, an emergency bedside TEE is the test of choice.

Patients with acute type A aortic dissection should undergo emergent surgical repair, unless significant comorbidities that limit survival to 1 year or less are present.[8,88,89] **Coronary angiography before surgery is not indicated because it does not improve survival and it results in a delay in surgical intervention.**[90,91] Resection of the ascending aorta and replacement with Dacron is the usual procedure in type A aortic dissection.[88,89] The objectives of surgery include excision of the intimal tear, obliteration of the entrance into the false lumen, repair of aortic regurgitation (if present), and restoration of patency to any major arteries occluded by the dissection. With associated aortic regurgitation, resuspension of the valve, if possible, is preferred. Intraoperative TEE can define the severity and mechanisms of aortic regurgitation and can assist the surgeon in identifying patients in whom valve repair is likely to be successful.[92] If there is associated annuloaortic ectasia or destruction of the aortic wall, a valved conduit may be used. The coronary arteries are reimplanted or, if they are involved by the dissection, they are reattached using vein bypass grafts anastomosed proximally to the aortic graft and distally to the uninvolved coronary arteries.[89,93,94] If compromise of a branch of the aorta supplying a vital organ is present and is not relieved by closing the false channel, then direct repair or surgical replacement of that branch is indicated. Aortic fenestration may be indicated in patients with severe organ or limb ischemia complicating either acute or chronic aortic dissection. Fenestration, by either surgical or percutaneous techniques, can effectively relieve the ischemia and can be performed safely in chronic aortic dissection.[95,96] Operative mortality for type A dissection at experienced centers varies from 7% to 36%, which is well below the more than 50% mortality with medical therapy.[7,56,97,98] In-hospital mortality is approximately 14% to 27%, patients with cardiogenic shock and those requiring concomitant coronary artery bypass grafting being the highest-risk subgroup.[97,98]

There is limited experience with endovascular stent grafts in patients with type A dissection, although preliminary studies suggest that endovascular repair can be performed with minimal adverse effects on aortic valve function and sustained survival.[99] Larger studies are needed to confirm the durability of endovascular therapy and to more accurately identify those patients most likely to benefit from this approach.

With acute type B (type III) aortic dissection, urgent surgical intervention is reserved for patients who have a complicated course (rupture, acute expansion or impending rupture, or vascular occlusion).[100] Independent predictors of surgical mortality include those 70 years and older, and hypotension or stroke on admission.[101] The optimal treatment for uncomplicated type III aortic dissection is less well defined, but the majority of patients are best treated with medical therapy.[102] Overall in-hospital mortality for these patients is approximately 10%.[103] Long-term medical therapy emphasizes control of blood pressure, using a β-blocker if possible, and periodic evaluation for evidence of any progression of dissection, patency of the false lumen, progression of aortic diameter to greater than 5 cm, or development of saccular aneurysm.[104-106] The reported long-term survival rate with medical therapy is approximately 60% to 80% at 4 to 5 years and approximately 40% to 45% at 10 years.[103] Survival is best in patients with noncommunicating and retrograde dissections. The proximal descending thoracic aorta is the major site of aneurysm development; an enlarged false lumen in this region predicts poor outcome and subsequent aneurysm development.[107] Furthermore, partial false lumen thrombosis (34% of patients) predicts a significantly worse 3-year mortality rate.[108] An alternate approach is 2 to 3 weeks of pharmacologic therapy followed by surgical repair if the dissection becomes stable and the patient's general condition does not contraindicate surgery.[109,110] Endovascular intervention in type B aortic dissection is being successfully performed with increasing frequency and may provide an alternative to surgery in highly selected patients in the future.[111-113] Randomized trials comparing endovascular intervention and conventional medical management have not demonstrated a significant difference in overall survival at 2 years, although remodeling with thrombosis of the false lumen and reduction of its diameter was evident in the stent graft group.[114-116]

Postoperatively, continuation of β-blockade is essential, if possible, as hypertension and left ventricular ejection velocity play an important role in the recurrence of aortic dissection. Following hospital dismissal, noninvasive testing is performed at periodic intervals to detect the development of an anastomotic aneurysm or saccular aneurysm, extension of the dissection, patency of the false lumen, or progressive aortic dilation.[117,118] Initial follow-up noninvasive imaging at 3, 6, and 12 months is warranted. Subsequent follow-up is performed every 1 to 2 years if there is no evidence of disease progression. MRI is generally preferred for follow-up (a baseline MRI before hospital discharge should be performed).

PENETRATING AORTIC ULCER

Penetrating aortic ulcer shares several clinical features with aortic dissection, especially type B aortic dissection, but the absence of certain clinical signs favors a diagnosis of penetrating aortic ulcer. Results of noninvasive imaging studies are usually diagnostic, allowing differentiation of penetrating aortic ulcer from typical aortic dissection.[119,120] Differentiation between the two disorders is important in view of the fact that the natural history of penetrating aortic ulcer is less well defined; therefore, treatment may differ from that currently used for classic aortic dissection.[119,120]

Pathogenesis

Penetrating aortic ulcer refers to an atherosclerotic lesion of the thoracic aorta that undergoes ulceration, which penetrates the internal elastic lamina of the thoracic aorta, resulting in formation of one of the following: intramural hematoma within the media of the aortic wall, a true saccular aneurysm, a pseudoaneurysm, or transmural aortic rupture[121] (Video 28.3).

Predisposing Factors

Risk factors for penetrating aortic ulcer are similar to those for aortic dissection, the most common being advanced age, chronic systemic hypertension, and evidence of advanced atherosclerotic disease.[122] In contrast to aortic dissection, men and women are equally affected. Long-standing hypertension is present in the majority of patients and likely contributes to the advanced atherosclerotic disease that is universally evident. More than one-half of the patients with penetrating aortic ulcer have advanced atherosclerotic disease in other locations, including coronary artery disease, peripheral arterial occlusive disease, and cerebrovascular disease. An increased association of penetrating aortic ulcer and abdominal aortic aneurysm, and aneurysms in other locations, has also been reported.[121,123]

Clinical Features

The clinical presentation of penetrating aortic ulcer and acute aortic dissection is similar, the most common presentation being an elderly patient with systemic hypertension and the sudden onset of severe pain in the chest, back, and—less commonly—epigastrium. Unlike aortic dissection, the pain is rarely migratory. Since the most common site of penetrating aortic ulcer is in the descending thoracic aorta, a new murmur of aortic regurgitation, pericardial friction rub, and peripheral pulse deficits are not seen. In addition, visceral vessel involvement has not been reported. Neurologic deficits are very rare, but acute lower extremity paraplegia may occur.[121] In a patient with a history compatible with aortic dissection, it is the *absence* of physical findings that suggests the diagnosis of penetrating aortic ulcer. Asymptomatic penetrating aortic ulcer does occur and is usually incidentally discovered as enlargement of the descending thoracic aorta or a hilar mass on routine chest radiography or on CT done for another indication.[121,123]

Laboratory Findings

Routine laboratory studies are nonspecific with penetrating aortic ulcer. Chest radiography is the most helpful of the routine laboratory tests because it is often abnormal. It may demonstrate mediastinal widening, focal or diffuse enlargement of the descending thoracic aorta, a hilar mass, left apical mass, bilateral pleural effusion, or isolated left pleural effusion.[119,120] However, normal chest radiographic findings do not exclude penetrating aortic ulcer. The most common electrocardiographic abnormality is left ventricular hypertrophy from chronic systemic hypertension.

Diagnosis

The findings on CT, MRI, TEE, and aortography in patients with penetrating aortic ulcer are characteristic, allowing for differentiation of penetrating aortic ulcer from classic aortic dissection. In contrast to aortic dissection, an intimal flap or false lumen is not present; in addition, significant, often advanced atherosclerotic disease of the aorta, most commonly the descending thoracic aorta, is evident. An echolucent intramural hematoma with overlying advanced atherosclerotic disease is the most common TEE finding in patients with acute penetrating aortic ulcer. Careful evaluation may demonstrate a crater-like ulceration with surrounding atheroma. When the intramural hematoma undergoes thrombosis, it becomes echogenic, creating the appearance of an increase in aortic wall thickness. The intramural hematoma may extend proximally or distally for a variable distance from the entry site. Additional findings in patients with penetrating aortic ulcer include aortic pseudoaneurysm or saccular aneurysm. Using CT, penetrating atherosclerotic ulcer manifests as focal involvement with adjacent subintimal hematoma and is often associated with aortic wall thickening or enhancement. Magnetic resonance imaging is superior to conventional CT in differentiating acute intramural hematoma from atherosclerotic plaque and chronic intraluminal thrombus and allows unenhanced multiplanar imaging (Fig. 28.7). Spiral CT involves shorter examination times and allows high-quality two- and three-dimensional image reconstruction. CT angiography can demonstrate complex spatial relationships, mural abnormalities, and extraluminal pathologic conditions. It should be noted that penetrating aortic ulcer is strongly associated with abdominal aortic aneurysm, which is seen concomitantly in 42% of patients. Therefore imaging of the abdominal aorta should be included in the initial evaluation.[122]

Management

The optimal treatment for penetrating aortic ulcer is not well defined. Treatment is individualized, as the natural history of penetrating aortic ulcer and indications for surgery are evolving. Although careful follow-up is necessary, many penetrating aortic ulcers involving the descending thoracic aorta can be managed nonoperatively in the acute setting. The natural history of an intramural hematoma involving the descending thoracic aorta has been shown by serial noninvasive imaging studies to follow a course of resorption of the hematoma and compensatory aortic dilation in the region of the involved aorta in 85% of patients over 1 year.[120,121] Patients with an intramural hematoma should be treated medically initially, with special emphasis placed on impulse control therapy, preferably with a β-adrenergic blocking agent.[123] Ascending aortic involvement, progressive aortic dilation, persistent symptoms, or hypertension that is difficult to control are indications for surgery. When saccular or pseudoaneurysm is the result of a penetrating atherosclerotic ulcer of the aorta, surgery is also recommended. Thoracic endograft technology is being applied to patients with penetrating aortic ulcer involving the descending thoracic aorta with high procedural success and a low perioperative morbidity and mortality.[124–127]

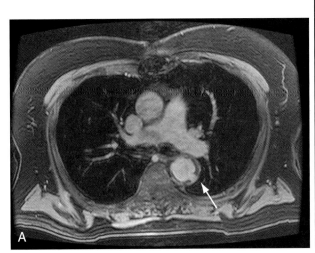

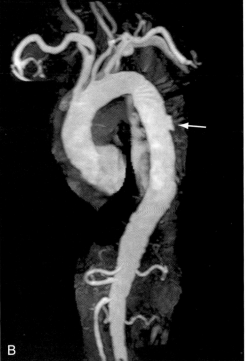

Fig. 28.7 Magnetic resonance (MR) imaging in a patient with multiple penetrating aortic ulcers. (A) Transverse imaging plane shows a penetrating aortic ulcer in the proximal descending thoracic aorta *(arrow)*. (B) MR angiogram with gadolinium enhancement shows severe atherosclerotic changes of the descending thoracic aorta and a penetrating aortic ulcer in the proximal descending thoracic aorta *(arrow)*.

AORTIC INTRAMURAL HEMATOMA

Aortic intramural hematoma (IMH) is an acute, potentially lethal disorder that is similar to but pathologically distinct from acute aortic dissection. Although hemorrhage into the aortic media occurs in both disorders, an intimal tear with resultant false lumen is not present in IMH. The prevalence of IMH among patients with acute aortic syndromes has been reported to be 5% to 20%.[62,128,129] The clinical presentation and noninvasive diagnosis of IMH are similar to aortic dissection, as are the classification scheme and general principles of management.

Pathogenesis

Although hemorrhage into the aortic media occurs in both acute aortic dissection and IMH, an intimal tear with resultant false lumen is not present in IMH. Although the mechanism is not certain, two mechanisms have been described: hemorrhage within the aortic wall owing to rupture of the vasa vasorum or rupture owing to an atherosclerotic penetrating aortic ulcer.[130] IMH evolves very dynamically in the short term to regression, dissection, or aortic rupture.[131] The most frequent long-term outcome of IMH is the development of aortic aneurysm or pseudoaneurysm. Lesions of the ascending aorta appear to represent the early stage of a classic dissection in some patients.[132] Complete regression without changes in aortic diameter is observed in one-third of cases, and progression to classical dissection is less common (between 8% and 16%).[128,133] A normal aortic diameter in the acute phase is the best predictor of IMH regression without complications, and absence of echolucent areas and atherosclerotic ulcerated plaque are associated with evolution to aortic aneurysm.[131] IMH is most often associated with long-standing hypertension (50% to 84% of patients) but has also been reported in association with trauma (e.g., auto accident or iatrogenic) in 6% of cases in a meta-analysis.[128,129,134]

Classification

The classification scheme for IMH is the same as is used for classic aortic dissection (see earlier section on aortic dissection). Patients with IMH are more likely to have type B lesions than those with classic aortic dissection (e.g., 60% vs. 35%).[128]

Clinical Features

Clinically, patients with acute IMH have a similar presentation to those with acute aortic dissection. Sudden, severe chest and/or back pain, as occur in classic aortic dissection, are common in IMH.[129] Although not specific, anterior chest pain is more common with ascending (type A) lesions, whereas interscapular back pain is more common with descending (type B) lesions.[135] In contrast to aortic dissection, manifestations associated with aortic branch vessel disease (e.g., myocardial infarction, stroke, aortic regurgitation, visceral vessel compromise, and paraplegia) are relatively uncommon with type A IMH.

Diagnosis

The noninvasive imaging methods used to diagnose IMH are the same as those used in the diagnosis of acute aortic dissection (TEE, CT, MRI). Exclusion of a dissecting intimal flap is a

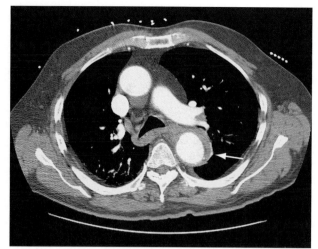

Fig. 28.8 Computed tomographic scan with contrast enhancement in a patient with sudden and severe chest pain shows a circumferential intramural hematoma involving the mid-descending thoracic aorta *(arrow)*.

prerequisite for the diagnosis of IMH. Specific findings on TEE for IMH include crescentic or circumferential regional thickening of the aortic wall exceeding 7 mm, echolucent areas within the involved aortic wall, displaced intimal Ca^{2+}, and absence of an intimal flap (Video 28.4). CT and MRI will typically demonstrate a crescentic or circular high attenuation area along the aortic wall that does not enhance with contrast[136] (Fig. 28.8).

Management

In general, the acute management of IMH and acute aortic dissection are similar. Initial treatment places emphasis on impulse control therapy (see section on management of acute aortic dissection). β-Blockade is indicated in all patients without absolute contraindications to their use. Patients with ascending aortic involvement have a reduction in early mortality with surgical intervention as compared with medical management (14% vs. 36%).[129] Patients with type B lesions have a similar mortality with medical or surgical management (14% vs. 20%). Therefore, surgical intervention is usually recommended in patients with type A IMH, whereas aggressive medical therapy is the most common course for patients with type B IMH.

Progression of disease in patients who are managed medically and survive the acute phase of the illness often occurs, although the rate of progression can be reduced in patients treated with β-blocker therapy acutely.[135] Aortic diameter at the time of initial presentation may also predict which patients are most likely to have disease progression (aortic diameter >5 cm predicting progression), potentially identifying a high-risk group that would benefit from early surgical intervention. Interestingly, in patients with ascending aortic IMH managed medically (due to advanced age and comorbid medical conditions), the mortality rate is much lower as compared with patients with type A aortic dissection who do not undergo surgery.[132]

The full reference list for this chapter is available at ExpertConsult.com.

29

Acute Pericardial Disease

Jacob Luthman, Brian D. Hoit

Pericardial disease is encountered less frequently than myocardial disease in the cardiac intensive care unit (CICU). However, its ability to mimic ischemic heart disease and congestive heart failure can make the diagnosis of pericardial disease challenging at times. While many patients with pericardial disease have a subacute or chronic presentation, the astute clinician must always consider pericardial disease in patients who present with hemodynamic embarrassment and shock in the CICU, for the failure to recognize cardiac tamponade can have dire consequences. This chapter will provide clinicians with the tools to recognize, diagnose, and manage patients with pericardial disease in the CICU setting.

ANATOMY AND PHYSIOLOGY OF THE NORMAL PERICARDIUM

The normal pericardium consists of a double-layered membranous sac that envelops the heart and proximal portions of the great vessels. The outer layer, or parietal (fibrous) pericardium, serves to anchor the heart within the thorax, and becomes contiguous with the adventitia of the great vessels. The inner layer, or visceral pericardium, is a serosal monolayer that adheres firmly to the myocardium as the epicardium, reflects over the origin of the great vessels creating the oblique and transverse sinuses and pericardial recesses (major contributors to the pericardial reserve volume), and fuses with the tough, fibrous parietal layer. Under normal physiologic conditions, there is typically less than 50 mL of pericardial fluid (largely an ultrafiltrate of plasma) between the layers of the pericardium.

While not essential for survival, the pericardium and fluid within serves many important yet subtle functions. Briefly, the pericardium limits distention of the cardiac chambers, facilitates ventricular interaction and coupling of the atria and ventricles, equalizes physical forces across the entire myocardial surface, minimizes friction with surrounding structures, and provides an anatomic barrier from the spread of infection.[1]

CLINICAL PRESENTATION OF PERICARDIAL DISEASE

Although there are relatively few disease processes that primarily affect the pericardium, the pericardium can be affected by many disease states (e.g., trauma, rheumatologic, infectious, metabolic, neoplastic, and congenital disease). As such, the clinical presentation of pericardial disease varies from acute to chronic, and from benign to life threatening, depending on the underlying etiology. This propensity for varying clinical presentation and an ability to mimic life-threatening disease processes (e.g., chest pain and ST segment elevation seen with acute pericarditis mimicking acute myocardial infarction [MI]) make the diagnosis of acute pericardial disease challenging, particularly when time is of the essence. Therefore, the astute intensivist must understand which patients require evaluation for pericardial disease, be able to rapidly and accurately diagnose pericardial disease, and facilitate timely management. The major ways in which pericardial disease may simulate ischemic syndromes are listed in Box 29.1.

Clinically, diseases of the pericardium present in several ways. Acutely, pericarditis, pericardial effusion (without hemodynamic compromise), and cardiac tamponade remain the primary concern in the CICU setting. Chronic and subacute presentations—including chronic pericardial effusion, constrictive pericarditis, and effusive-constrictive pericarditis—are less commonly observed in the CICU and will not be discussed in any detail.

ACUTE PERICARDITIS

Acute pericarditis is the most common disorder involving the pericardium, occurring in up to 0.2% of hospitalized patients and in 5% of patients admitted to the emergency department for nonischemic chest pain.[2,3] While idiopathic/viral pericarditis remains the most common etiology in the immunocompetent host in developed countries (80% to 90% of cases), radiation therapy, cardiac surgery (postpericardiectomy syndrome), and invasive procedures have become important causes.[4,5] In contrast, *Mycobacterium tuberculosis* pericarditis is more common in underdeveloped countries and immunocompromised hosts.[4]

In the CICU setting, pericarditis is most often related to MI and less commonly to cardiac or coronary interventions. Early post-MI pericarditis occurs during the first few days after MI and is caused by transmural necrosis with inflammation affecting the adjacent pericardium. Pericardial involvement is related to infarct transmurality and size and is associated with a poor prognosis. It is often asymptomatic and is identified only by the presence of a friction rub on physical examination. When patients are symptomatic, it is essential to distinguish between recurrent ischemic pain and pericardial pain. Late post-MI pericarditis (Dressler syndrome) is one of the postcardiac injury (autoimmune) syndromes, occurring from a week to a few months after MI; it is less commonly seen in the modern era of early revascularization. Patients may present with pleuritic chest pain, friction rub, fever, leukocytosis, and sometimes pleural effusion or pulmonary infiltrates. The diagnosis is clinical, although objective findings—such as elevated inflammatory markers, electrocardiographic changes, and pericardial effusion on echocardiogram (ECG)—can be helpful.

Clinical Diagnosis

The diagnosis of acute pericarditis can be made in the presence of at least two of the following criteria: (1) typical chest pain, (2) a pericardial friction rub on auscultation, (3) changes on the ECG, and (4) new or worsening pericardial effusion. Elevation of inflammatory markers or evidence of pericardial inflammation on other imaging modalities can help support the diagnosis in atypical cases but are not part of the diagnostic criteria. Modest elevations of troponin reflect concurrent myocardial inflammation. All patients suspected of having acute pericarditis should have the following studies: an ECG, chest radiograph, complete blood count, troponin level, serum C-reactive protein level, renal function panel, blood cultures (if fever >38°C or signs of sepsis), and a transthoracic echocardiogram.[5]

Chest pain is the most common presenting symptom and typically has a sudden onset, variable severity and intensity, and may radiate to the trapezius ridge. The pain is generally pleuritic, becoming worse with inspiration, and is alleviated by sitting up and leaning forward. The pericardial friction rub, auscultated best at the left sternal border with the patient seated and leaning forward, is considered pathognomonic for pericarditis.[6] While highly specific, its absence does not exclude pericarditis, as it may be evanescent, and is heard in only one-third of patients with acute pericarditis.[4] Notably, the pericardial friction rub can be monophasic, biphasic, or triphasic in nature and does not vary with the respiratory cycle, which helps differentiate pericardial from pleural friction rubs. While the friction rub remains an accurate means of diagnosis, all patients presenting to the CICU with chest pain deserve a thorough clinical examination, including assessment of vital signs, jugular venous pressure (JVP) and pulsation, blood pressure determination in each upper extremity, auscultation for cardiac murmurs, and the evaluation for pulsus paradoxus in order to alert the clinician to complications of pericarditis (e.g., tamponade), or suggest alternate pathology (e.g., MI or aortic dissection).

ECG changes are common in pericarditis and typically progress through four stages: stage I, diffuse ST segment elevation and PR segment depression; stage II, normalization of the ST and PR segments; stage III, T-wave inversion that occurs after normalization of the ST segment; and stage IV (which is variably present), normalization of the T waves. These "classic" ECG changes of diffuse ST segment elevation and PR segment depression are seen in the first hours to days of the disease process and have been shown to be present in only approximately 60% of cases of pericarditis[5] (Fig. 29.1). Distinguishing the ECG changes of acute pericarditis from those of acute myocardial ischemia can be challenging. In differentiating the two conditions, it should be remembered that the ST segment elevation seen in pericarditis starts at the J-point, is concave upwards and distributed throughout nearly all leads on the ECG (i.e., in multiple vascular territories), and is associated with PR depression and an absence of Q-waves. In contrast, the ST segment change seen in ST elevation MI (STEMI) originates at the J-point, is convex (dome-shaped), generally occurs in a single coronary vascular territory, does not have associated PR segment changes, and may have reciprocal ST segment changes in other vascular territories of the myocardium. Sustained dysrhythmia is also more common with myocardial ischemia as compared to acute pericarditis (provided that the pericarditis is not the result of a transmural infarction), although atrial arrhythmias complicate 5% to 10% of cases of acute pericarditis. When pericarditis is associated with an acute MI, the degree of ST elevation may be exaggerated, the reciprocal ST segment changes of infarction masked, and atypical T wave evolution or early normalization of inverted T waves may be seen.

While transthoracic echocardiography has little utility in evaluating the pericardium itself, it is invaluable for diagnosing acute pericarditis and its complications (pericardial effusion and tamponade) and for recognizing alternative diagnoses. Because of its noninvasive nature and widespread availability, both the European Society of Cardiology (ESC) and the American Society

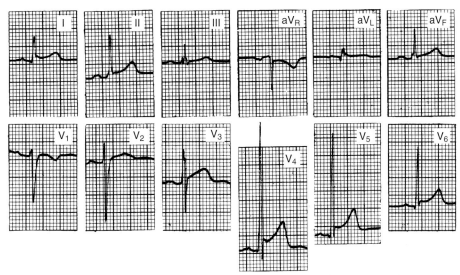

Fig. 29.1 Echocardiogram of a patient with acute viral pericarditis. Characteristic features include ST segments elevated concave upward and not localized. T waves are upright in leads with ST segment elevation. Reciprocal repolarization changes are seen in aVR and V₁. PR segments are depressed.

of Echocardiography recommend that a transthoracic ECG be performed in all patients with suspected acute pericarditis.[6]

Leukocytosis and elevations in the erythrocyte sedimentation rate and C-reactive protein are nonspecific indicators of inflammation and therefore are not useful for the diagnosis of pericarditis; however, they do have prognostic value. For example, in an Italian study of 156 consecutive patients with idiopathic or viral pericarditis, hs-CRP elevation at 1 week was a significant independent risk factor for recurrence of disease (hazard ratio [HR], 2.36).[7] Cardiac troponin has also been evaluated in acute idiopathic or viral pericarditis as a marker for myocardial involvement. In one study, 38 of 118 consecutive patients with pericarditis were found to have troponin elevations. However, after a mean follow-up of 24 months, a similar rate of recurrent pericarditis and constrictive pericarditis was noted among those with positive and negative troponin values and no cases of tamponade were detected in the cohort with positive troponin values.[8]

An exhaustive diagnostic evaluation is not recommended in the immunocompetent patient owing to the diminished value of testing compared to the cost incurred and the low probability of any result having a significant impact on management. However, following a basic evaluation, patients with fever greater than 38°C, subacute onset of symptoms, immunosuppression, trauma, oral anticoagulation therapy, evidence of myopericarditis, moderate or large pericardial effusion, or cardiac tamponade are considered high risk and should be admitted to the hospital (and, if appropriate, to the CICU) for further evaluation of a specific etiology of the pericarditis.[9]

Treatment of Acute Pericarditis

Aspirin and nonsteroidal antiinflammatory drugs (NSAIDs) are a mainstay of therapy for idiopathic acute pericarditis. The open-label Colchicine for Acute Pericarditis (COPE) trial prospectively studied aspirin monotherapy compared to aspirin plus colchicine for acute idiopathic pericarditis. The addition of

colchicine to aspirin led to a statistically significant reduction in symptom persistence at 72 hours (11.7% vs. 36.7%) and a significant reduction in the recurrence rate at 18 months (10.7% vs. 32.2%), with the number needed to treat to prevent one recurrence being five.[10] Multiple subsequent randomized controlled trials and systematic reviews have documented similar efficacy of colchicine in acute idiopathic pericarditis.[11–13]

Treatment for early post-MI pericarditis is generally supportive, as most cases are self-limiting. Symptomatic patients may be treated with high-dose acetylsalicylic acid (ASA) for 1 to 2 weeks. The addition of colchicine may be helpful in reducing inflammation and reducing the risk for recurrent pericarditis. NSAIDs and glucocorticoids should be avoided because of the possibility of harmful effects in the early post-MI setting and the increased risk of recurrent pericarditis. Patients with an associated pericardial effusion generally do not need to have antiplatelet therapy or anticoagulation withheld. However, those with large or enlarging pericardial effusions or signs of tamponade may need cessation of anticoagulation to avoid hemorrhagic conversion of the pericardial effusion. An exhaustive review of specific regimens is beyond the scope of this chapter. The interested reader is referred to the excellent review by Schwier and Tran.[14]

Pericardial Effusion

While the presence of a pericardial effusion can be suggested by the history and physical examination, ECG, and chest radiograph, many are discovered incidentally during the evaluation for other cardiopulmonary processes, as there are no symptoms directly attributed to the effusion until it produces hemodynamic effects. In contrast, patients with a hemodynamically significant pericardial effusion usually present with chest pain and fullness along with signs and symptoms related to impaired cardiac function—such as fatigue, dyspnea, hypotension, pulsus paradoxus, elevated JVP, and edema—all of which can also be present in cardiomyopathy or disease processes affecting the right heart.[2] Less commonly,

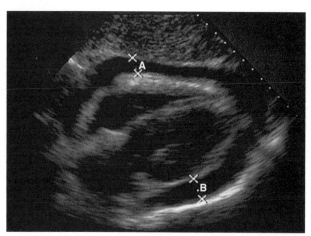

Fig. 29.2 Echocardiogram showing a large circumferential pericardial effusion. Anterior *(A)* and posterior *(B)* aspects of the effusions are shown. (From Shabetai R. Pericardial disease. In: Brown DL, ed. *Cardiac Intensive Care.* Philadelphia: Saunders; 1988:469–475.)

compression of adjacent intrathoracic structures results in hoarseness, hiccough, and nausea.[15] Therefore clinicians must maintain a high index of suspicion for pericardial effusion, particularly in the intensive care setting, where it is common for many patients to have undergone percutaneous cardiac procedures that can be complicated by perforation of coronary arteries, the coronary sinus, or the cardiac chambers.

On the ECG, pericardial fluid appears as an echolucent space between the pericardium and the epicardium (Fig. 29.2). Pericardial effusions are classified according to their onset, size, distribution, hemodynamic impact, and composition.[15] The detection of a pericardial effusion often has important implications for diagnosis (e.g., acute pericarditis after MI), prognosis (e.g., patients with cancer), or both (e.g., acute aortic dissection). Rapidly accumulating blood in the pericardial space may be seen in CICU patients with blunt trauma, ascending aortic dissection, cardiac rupture that may complicate MI, or after invasive cardiac procedures. After cardiac surgery, pericardial effusions are common but are typically not large and usually resolve without medication by 1 month; late (>1 week) tamponade is unusual (1 to 2%) and the effusions appear not to be responsive to NSAIDs or colchicine.

Pericardial effusion should be suspected in patients with any systemic disorder known to involve the pericardium, elevated JVP, chest pain consistent with pericarditis or aortic dissection, unexplained cardiomegaly (especially with a flask-shaped cardiac silhouette) without pulmonary congestion on chest radiograph, persistent fever with or without an obvious source of infection, the presence of an isolated left pleural effusion and a fever, or hemodynamic deterioration in a patient with another disease process (or after an invasive cardiac procedure) that can involve the pericardium.[15]

CARDIAC (PERICARDIAL) TAMPONADE

The potential hemodynamic impact of an effusion ranges from none to mild compromise to the most extreme clinical

manifestation, cardiac tamponade. Factors that determine the degree of hemodynamic compromise include the size of the effusion; its rate of accumulation; and whether the pericardium is inflamed, scarred, or adherent. Localized pericardial adhesions or organization of the pericardial fluid can result in localized tamponade, which is most common after cardiac surgery and may be difficult to recognize. Diffuse pericardial inflammation and/or scarring with effusion can result in effusive-constrictive pericarditis, which has features of both cardiac tamponade and pericardial constriction.[6]

If fluid accumulation is gradual, pericardial pressure remains low because the pericardium can increase its compliance by undergoing stretch. However, with continued accumulation of fluid, the pericardial reserve volume (the difference between unstressed pericardial volume and cardiac volume that accommodates physiologic changes in ventricular filling) is exceeded and the intrapericardial pressure eventually increases; once this becomes high enough to impede cardiac filling, cardiac output falls.[1,2]

Cardiac tamponade is a hemodynamic condition characterized by equal elevation of atrial (pulmonary capillary wedge and right atrial) and pericardial pressures, an exaggerated (>10 mm Hg) inspiratory decrease in aortic systolic pressure (pulsus paradoxus) and arterial hypotension (Fig. 29.3). The pathophysiology of cardiac tamponade and pulsus paradoxus readily explains findings on clinical examination, Doppler echocardiography, and at cardiac catheterization. The primary abnormality is compression of the cardiac chambers owing to increased pericardial pressure that is exerted throughout the cardiac cycle. While the pericardium has some degree of elasticity (part of the pericardial reserve volume), once the elastic limit is reached, the heart must compete with the intrapericardial fluid for a fixed intrapericardial volume.[2] As the total pericardial volume reaches the stiff portion of its pressure–volume relation, tamponade rapidly ensues. As cardiac tamponade progresses, the cardiac chambers become smaller, transmural chamber pressures (i.e., preload) decrease, and diastolic chamber compliance and ventricular filling decrease owing to enhanced ventricular interdependence, which lead to the characteristic elevation and equalization of diastolic filling pressures and decreases in stroke volume and blood pressure.

It is important to realize that the clinical presentation and diagnostic findings associated with tamponade physiology are not all-or-none phenomena. Rather, the clinical presentation—echocardiographic and catheterization features present in tamponade—lie on a spectrum of severity that is dependent as much on the acuity of presentation and etiology as the patient's underlying comorbidities (e.g., ventricular dysfunction, volume status, valvular disease) and the ability to sustain a compensatory physiologic response.

Patients with acute tamponade may present with chest pain, tachypnea, or altered consciousness owing to decreased cardiac output. On examination, the classic triad of hypotension, elevated JVP, and diminished heart sounds (one of Beck's triads) is present in only a minority of patients.[16] A recent systematic review of patients with known tamponade suggested that five features were present in a majority of patients: dyspnea (87% to 89% sensitive), tachycardia (77% sensitive), pulsus paradoxus (82% sensitive),

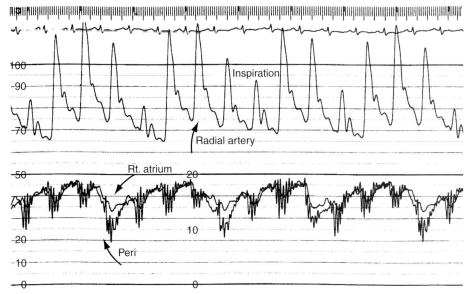

Fig. 29.3 Hyperacute cardiac tamponade caused by penetration of a saphenous vein graft during angioplasty of the graft. The radial arterial tracing shows tachycardia and extreme pulsus paradoxus. The right atrial and pericardial pressures are equilibrated at a very high level. The volume of blood in the pericardium was small.

elevated JVP (76% sensitive), and cardiomegaly on chest radiograph (89% sensitive), while another review suggests that the presence of pulsus paradoxus greater than 10 mm Hg in patients with effusion increases the likelihood of tamponade (likelihood ratio, 3.3).[17]

Echocardiography is the preferred diagnostic modality for identifying the hallmarks of tamponade physiology, that is, cardiac chamber collapses (most often right atrial and right ventricular), exaggerated respiratory variation of cardiac chamber dimensions, and transvalvular flow velocities and inferior vena cava (IVC) dilation with reduced respiratory change in dimension (vena caval plethora; see Videos 29.1 to 29.4). Cardiac chamber collapse occurs when the intrapericardial pressure exceeds the intracardiac pressure in a given chamber; the right ventricular (RV) free wall buckles or invaginates in early diastole when RV pressure is at a minimum. This is often best visualized in the subcostal view with an M-mode cursor through the affected chamber wall to determine timing within the cardiac cycle.[2] Early-diastolic RV collapse is highly specific for tamponade, although other conditions can reproduce this finding in the absence of a hemodynamically significant effusion.[18] At end-diastole when right atrial pressure is at its nadir, pericardial fluid pressure exceeds right atrial pressure, resulting in right atrial collapse, often best appreciated in four-chamber imaging (Fig. 29.4). If persistent for longer than one-third of diastole, the sensitivity, specificity, and positive predictive values approach 100% in patients with tamponade.[19] The degree of invagination has no predictive value for the presence of tamponade. It is important to note that the absence of any chamber collapse has a nearly 90% negative predictive value for clinically significant tamponade.[20] Collapse of the left atrium and the left ventricle are less common; the latter is usually in the presence of right ventricular pressure and volume overload or when tamponade is regional (e.g., after cardiac surgery).

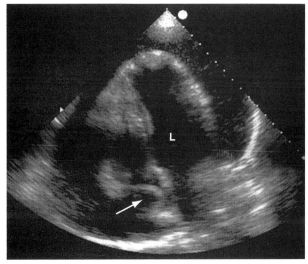

Fig. 29.4 Echocardiogram showing severe right atrial compression *(arrow)* in a patient whose pericardial effusion had caused cardiac tamponade. *L,* Left ventricle. (From Shabetai R. Pericardial disease. In: Brown DL, ed. *Cardiac Intensive Care.* Philadelphia: Saunders; 1988:469–475.)

In normal individuals, there is minimal variation in flow velocity during normal respiration. In tamponade, exaggerated respiratory variation in transvalvular velocities results from enhanced ventricular interdependence and suggests the presence of pulsus paradoxus. With inspiration, tricuspid flow velocity increases markedly, with a concomitant decrease in mitral flow velocity. By recent consensus, the percentage of respiratory variation for mitral and tricuspid inflow is calculated as: $100 \times$ (expiration – inspiration)/expiration.[6] In tamponade, tricuspid flow variance usually exceeds 60%, while mitral flow exceeds

30%. It is important to note that transvalvular flow velocity should not be the sole criterion used for the diagnosis of tamponade.[6] IVC plethora is present in many patients with tamponade. In one study, up to 92% of patients with an effusion requiring drainage were found to have dilation and less than 50% inspiratory decrease in the diameter of the IVC during inspiration, findings suggestive of elevated central venous pressure.[21] While this finding is highly sensitive, it lacks specificity, as many other conditions are associated with increased right atrial pressure and have the same echocardiographic finding.

LOW PRESSURE TAMPONADE

Patients who are severely hypovolemic because of traumatic hemorrhage, hemodialysis and ultrafiltration, excessive GI losses, or excessive diuresis may have low pressure tamponade, in which the intracardiac and pericardial diastolic pressures are only 6 to 12 mm Hg (Fig. 29.5).[22] In 143 patients with cardiac tamponade (equal pericardial and right atrial pressures before pericardiocentesis), 29 had an initial pericardial pressure less than 7 mm Hg; the spectrum of etiologies and the frequency and severity of echocardiographic findings were similar to patients with classic cardiac tamponade.[22] However, clinical findings associated with classic cardiac tamponade—including increased heart rate, elevated JVP, and pulsus paradoxus—were significantly less common. As such, clinicians should maintain a high index of suspicion for tamponade in patients with confounding conditions that may affect the hemodynamic response to elevated intrapericardial pressure. Treatment consists of intravenous fluid replacement and pericardiocentesis.

Causes of Tamponade in the CICU

While the majority of cases of tamponade in the CICU are likely to be related to MI and coronary/cardiac interventions, cases of

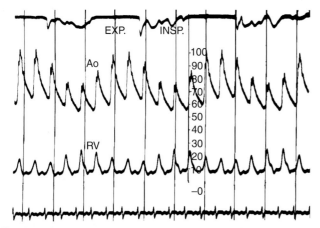

Fig. 29.5 Low-pressure cardiac tamponade. The right ventricular pressure was only 10 mm Hg, but otherwise the characteristic hemodynamic abnormalities of severe tamponade were present, including pulsus paradoxus, which was out of phase between the right ventricle (RV) and the aorta (Ao), and absence of an early diastolic dip. *EXP,* Expiration; *INSP,* inspiration. (From Shabetai R. Cardiac tamponade. In: Shabetai R, ed. *The Pericardium.* Norwell, MA: Kluwer Academic Press; 2003:122–166.)

cardiac tamponade owing to a variety of causes may be admitted to the CICU for monitoring and treatment. After MI, cardiac tamponade may complicate both early post-MI pericarditis, Dressler syndrome, and cardiac rupture. While the latter is often immediately fatal, the rate of intrapericardial hemorrhage may be slow enough or contained to allow detection (usually by echocardiography with contrast) and surgical repair of the rupture and any resultant pseudoaneurysm.

Treatment of Cardiac Tamponade

The 2015 ESC Guidelines treatment recommendations include targeting the therapy of pericardial effusion to the specific etiology whenever possible, the use of ASA/NSAID/colchicine when effusion is associated with systemic inflammation, pericardiocentesis or cardiac surgery for cardiac tamponade or symptomatic moderate to large effusions that are not responsive to medical therapy, and for suspicion of unknown bacterial or neoplastic pericarditis (all IC recommendations).[15]

The choice between pericardiocentesis (see Chapter 44 and open surgical drainage is based on local preference and experience, the etiology of the effusion, hemodynamic status of the patient, and characteristics of the pericardial fluid/contents. Generally, for a majority of free-flowing or uncomplicated effusions, echo-guided percutaneous drainage is preferred in the hands of a skilled operator. Conversely, the presence of loculated or organized fluid, hemopericardium, a traumatic etiology of the effusion, or concern for aortic dissection may be best served with surgical evacuation of the pericardium.[15]

Pericardiocentesis can be performed under fluoroscopic or echocardiographic guidance. The latter allows the operator to select the shortest route to the effusion and the puncture site with the largest collection of fluid. In the largest published series, the para-apical location was utilized in two-thirds, while the subxiphoid location was ideal in only 15%.[23] An indwelling pericardial catheter with intermittent or continuous suction is left in the pericardial space until the rate of fluid return is negligible (<25 mL/d). Following drainage, whether percutaneous or surgical, patients should remain on telemetry for at least 24 hours, with a two-dimensional Doppler echocardiogram completed prior to hospital discharge to evaluate for fluid reaccumulation. Early follow-up echocardiography 1 to 2 weeks after discharge to evaluate for recurrence or early constriction should be considered in the appropriate setting.[15]

Surgical pericardiectomy with drainage, though less commonly performed than pericardiocentesis, is often preferred when the pericardial effusion has reaccumulated, is loculated, biopsy of the pericardium is desired, or the patient has a coagulopathy. For both chronic and recurrent effusions, the 2015 ESC Guidelines recommend surgical pericardiectomy only in patients with symptomatic effusions in whom medical therapy and repeated pericardiocenteses were not successful.[15]

Patients who are diagnosed with a large pericardial effusion with minimal or no evidence of hemodynamic compromise may be treated conservatively with careful hemodynamic monitoring, serial echocardiographic studies, avoidance of diuretics and vasodilators (a IIIC recommendation), and therapy aimed at the underlying cause of the pericardial effusion. Effusions that progressively enlarge, lead to worsening symptoms suggesting cardiac tamponade, or that are otherwise refractory to a conservative approach should be treated with pericardial fluid drainage. There is no role for medical therapy of cardiac tamponade, but fluid resuscitation may be helpful while preparing for pericardial drainage. Mechanical ventilation should be avoided whenever possible.

CONSTRICTIVE PERICARDITIS

Constrictive pericarditis can occur following virtually any cause of pericarditis but most commonly occurs after idiopathic/viral, postcardiac surgery, and following radiation therapy. It may present transiently (i.e., either spontaneous resolution or response to medical therapy), subacutely, or chronically. Constrictive pericarditis is seldom an indication for admission to the CICU, but intensivists might manage patients with transient or subacute presentations that may clinically resemble cardiac tamponade. Patients with chronic constriction often present with exertional dyspnea, lower extremity edema, fatigue, or abdominal distention and, in rare instances, congestive hepatopathy. Distinguishing constrictive pericarditis from cardiac tamponade, acute decompensated heart failure, and disorders such as restrictive cardiomyopathy and chronic liver disease is essential, as treatments are markedly different. The critical pathophysiologic features of constrictive pericarditis—which are responsible for the physical examination, hemodynamic, and imaging findings—are enhanced ventricular interaction (interdependence) and dissociation of intracardiac and intrathoracic pressures.

The physical exam in constriction is notable for elevated jugular venous pressure (reported in as many as 93% of patients with surgically confirmed constrictive pericarditis), hepatomegaly, splenomegaly, ascites, and edema. The jugular venous waveform demonstrates prominent x and y descents. The Kussmaul sign (failure of the JVP to decrease with inspiration) is an examination finding relatively specific to constriction but does not distinguish constrictive pericarditis from severe tricuspid valve disease or right-sided heart failure. In contrast, pulsus paradoxus is rare and, if present, should raise suspicion for effusive-constrictive disease (pericardial constriction with a concomitant effusion). A pericardial knock, an accentuated heart sound that occurs slightly earlier than an S_3, is distinctive but reported in only approximately 50% of cases.

Patients with suspected constrictive pericarditis should undergo initial evaluation with ECG, chest radiograph, and echocardiography. Unlike patients with cardiomyopathy, B-type natriuretic peptide (BNP) and N-terminal pro-BNP levels are usually only mildly elevated in constriction. Two-dimensional Doppler echocardiography is critical in the diagnosis of constriction and in differentiating constriction from tamponade, effusive-constrictive disease, and restrictive cardiomyopathy.[24]

The most specific echocardiographic sign of constriction is a septal bounce with abrupt transient rightward movement of the interventricular septum. Doppler echocardiography demonstrates elevated early diastolic tissue Doppler velocities (é) with the septal e' often greater than the lateral é tissue velocity (annulus paradoxus) and an expiratory increase in early mitral inflow velocity greater than 25% and an expiratory decrease of tricuspid inflow greater than 40%.[6] Computed tomography, magnetic resonance imaging, and cardiac catheterization are useful to confirm the diagnosis, particularly in patients with nondiagnostic echocardiographic findings, and to assist in perioperative management. Delayed enhancement cardiac magnetic resonance is valuable to assess the extent of pericardial inflammation and the response to antiinflammatory medications in patients with increased inflammatory biomarkers or a short duration (<3 months) of constrictive symptoms.[6]

For patients with newly diagnosed constrictive pericarditis who are hemodynamically stable and do not have evidence of chronic constriction, a trial of conservative management rather than pericardiectomy is warranted. Pericardiectomy is the only definitive treatment option for patients with chronic symptomatic constrictive pericarditis.

CONCLUSION

While the spectrum of pericardial disease varies from benign to life threatening, failure to recognize pericardial disease, particularly in the setting of shock, can have devastating consequences. Often, a simple ECG and two-dimensional Doppler echocardiography, in the hands of a skilled clinician, will provide both a diagnosis and assist in facilitating timely management of patients with hemodynamic embarrassment due to pericardial disease.

The full reference list for this chapter is available at ExpertConsult.com.

30

Acute Respiratory Failure

Holly Keyt, Jay I. Peters

Respiratory failure is defined as the inability to maintain either the normal delivery of oxygen to tissues or the normal removal of carbon dioxide from the tissues. From a physiologic perspective, respiratory failure can be caused by diffuse pulmonary dysfunction (ventilation/perfusion [$\dot{V}/\dot{Q}$] mismatch or pulmonary shunt), neurologic dysfunction (depression of the respiratory drive), cardiac dysfunction (low cardiac output or pulmonary edema), or a lack of hemoglobin to transport gases. Clinically, this is seen as arterial hypoxemia leading to tissue hypoxia and/or arterial hypercapnia. Acute respiratory failure (ARF) may evolve over a period of minutes to hours to days depending on the clinical situation. ARF, therefore, is a generic term that encompasses a heterogeneous spectrum of diseases that eventually end with the same pathophysiologic outcomes: arterial hypoxemia (usually with partial pressure of O_2 [PaO_2] of <60 mm Hg) or hypercapnia (partial pressure of CO_2 [$PaCO_2$] of >45 to 50 mm Hg).

PHYSIOLOGY OF GAS EXCHANGE

In the lung, gas exchange occurs at the capillary-alveolar interface. Microscopic examination of septal capillaries reveals that they are significantly thinner on the side that bulges into the air space. This conformation enhances the diffusion of oxygen from the air space into the blood and the elimination of carbon dioxide from the blood into the air space. Equilibration of partial pressures of gases between the two compartments occurs rapidly. Oxygen in the blood is carried by hemoglobin. Only a small percentage is transported as dissolved gas. The following equation describes the arterial oxygen content (CaO_2):

$$C_aO_2 = (1.36 \times Hgb \times SaO_2) + (0.003 \times PaO_2)$$

where CaO_2 is the oxygen content of arterial blood in milliliters of O_2 per deciliter of blood; Hgb is the hemoglobin concentration in grams per deciliter of blood; SaO_2 (oxygen saturation) is the fraction of hemoglobin sites bound by oxygen; and PaO_2 is the arterial partial pressure of oxygen.

Because the amount of dissolved oxygen is small in comparison to the amount transported by hemoglobin, in most clinical situations, CaO_2 depends primarily on the hemoglobin concentration and the oxygen *saturation* of the arterial blood, not on PaO_2. Even in severe anemia, the contribution of dissolved oxygen in the overall CaO_2 is negligible despite very high PaO_2. This principle is important clinically in patients with ARF for whom increasing CaO_2 can be accomplished by increasing hemoglobin concentration and SaO_2, but not necessarily by increasing PaO_2. This follows from the sigmoid shape of the oxygen-hemoglobin dissociation curve, in which significantly higher PaO_2 is needed to increase the SaO_2 beyond 90% as the curve plateaus.

Carbon dioxide is transported in the blood mostly in the form of carbonic acid. Only approximately 5% is transported by binding with hemoglobin. Ten percent is transported as dissolved gas.[1] As the tissues extract an increasing amount of oxygen from the blood, the deoxygenated hemoglobin increases its ability to carry carbon dioxide (Haldane effect). Similarly, as an increasing amount of oxygen becomes available in the arterial and venous blood, less carbon dioxide may be carried by the oxidized hemoglobin. This effect has been implicated in the pathogenesis of worsening hypercapnia after oxygen supplementation in patients with baseline hypercapnia.

To achieve optimal gas exchange, local matching of ventilation and perfusion has to occur. The interrelationships between ventilation and blood flow are shown schematically in Fig. 30.1, in which imbalance (B) is typified by bronchospasm, shunt (C) is typified by dense pneumonia or severe acute respiratory distress syndrome (ARDS), and dead space (D) is typified by destruction of the capillaries in emphysema.

Normally, both ventilation and perfusion exhibit a gradient from the top to the bottom of the lung. However, the gradient is more pronounced in blood flow than in ventilation, such that in the upper portions of the lung there are predominantly high $\dot{V}/\dot{Q}$ areas and in the lower portions of the lung there are low $\dot{V}/\dot{Q}$ areas. The overall $\dot{V}/\dot{Q}$ ratio of the normal lung is 0.8.[2]

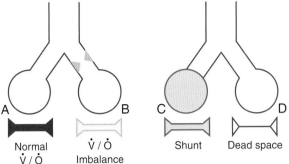

Fig. 30.1 Schematic representation of various patterns of ventilation ($\dot{V}$) and perfusion ($\dot{Q}$). *A*, Normal $\dot{V}/\dot{Q}$ ratio in which the PVO_2 = 40 mm Hg and PCO_2 = 46 mm Hg. After equilibration, the capillary PO_2 = 101 mm Hg, PCO_2 = 40 mm Hg, and $P(A - a)O_2$ = 0 mm Hg. *B*, $\dot{V}/\dot{Q}$ imbalance caused by airway obstruction would decrease the PO_2. This could be corrected with supplemental oxygen. *C*, A shunt allows mixed venous blood to traverse the capillary without any gas transfer. *D*, Dead space, the ventilated area of the lung that does not participate in gas exchange. (From Greene KE, Peters JI. Pathophysiology of acute respiratory failure. *Clin Chest Med.* 1994;15:1–11.)

TABLE 30.1	Berlin Definition of Acute Respiratory Distress Syndrome
Timing	Within 1 week of a known clinical insult or new or worsening respiratory symptoms.
Chest imaging (radiograph or computed tomography)	Bilateral opacities not fully explained by effusions, lobar/lung collapse, or nodules.
Origin of edema	Respiratory failure not fully explained by cardiac failure or fluid overload. Need objective assessment (e.g., echocardiography) to exclude hydrostatic edema if no risk factor present.
Oxygenation	Mild: PaO_2/FIO_2 ratio of 200–300 mm Hg with PEEP or CPAP ≥5 cm H_2O
	Moderate: PaO_2/FIO_2 ratio of 100–200 mm Hg with PEEP or CPAP ≥5 cm H_2O
	Severe: PaO_2/FIO_2 < 100 mmg Hg with PEEP or CPAP ≥5 cm H_2O

CPAP, Continuous positive airway pressure; *FIO₂*, fraction of inspired oxygen; *PaCO₂*, partial pressure of arterial carbon dioxide; *PEEP*, positive end-expiratory pressure.

The overall efficiency of gas exchange can be assessed in terms of maintenance of normal PaO_2 and $PaCO_2$. The assessment can be performed by calculating the alveolar-arterial partial pressure oxygen difference ($P_AO_2 - PaO_2$), which is also known as the A-a gradient. The mean alveolar oxygen tension (PaO_2) is calculated by using the alveolar gas equation as follows:

$$P_AO_2 = FIO_2(PB - PH_2O) - PaCO_2/R$$

where PB is the barometric pressure of the atmosphere, which changes with altitude; FIO_2 is the fraction of inspired oxygen (approximately 0.21 in room air); $PaCO_2$ is the partial pressure of arterial carbon dioxide; and R is the respiratory quotient. This equation gives an estimation of PaO_2, which changes with altitude (PB), with inspired oxygen concentration, and with $PaCO_2$. PaO_2 not only changes with changes in P_AO_2 but also decreases with age in normal individuals. Therefore P_AO_2-PaO_2 increases with age and can be estimated in most adults breathing room air to be approximately 4 mm Hg for each decade of life until the maximum of the seventh decade. This estimation is not valid for patients receiving oxygen supplementation. For these patients, assessment of efficiency of gas exchange can be obtained using the ratio of PaO_2 to FIO_2 (PaO_2/FIO_2 ratio normally is >400 mm Hg). Although it is not as accurate as the P_AO_2-PaO_2 difference, it is useful clinically because most patients with ARF receive supplemental oxygen at the time that blood gas analysis is performed. This ratio also forms one of the basic criteria for the diagnosis of ARDS. By consensus, ARDS is defined by PaO_2/FIO_2 ratio less than or equal to 300 mm Hg when respiratory failure is present and not otherwise explained by cardiac failure or fluid overload (Table 30.1).[3] This ratio is most helpful when used serially or when the ratio changes significantly with a therapeutic maneuver.

PATHOPHYSIOLOGY OF ACUTE RESPIRATORY FAILURE

The three most important pathophysiologic mechanisms that cause ARF are hypoventilation, $\dot{V}/\dot{Q}$ mismatch, and shunt. Diffusion abnormalities, which occur with mild pulmonary edema or early interstitial lung disease, may cause exercise-induced hypoxemia but rarely cause clinically significant hypoxemia. Reduction of inspired PO_2 and venous admixture are other potential but less common causes of hypoxemia.

Hypoventilation can be defined as the inadequate movement of fresh alveolar gas necessary for maintaining a normal $PaCO_2$. Pure hypoventilation is a relatively uncommon clinical event. In most cases, hypoventilation occurs along with other causes of hypoxemia. When pure hypoventilation does occur, it is usually caused by depression of the respiratory center by sedative-hypnotic drugs or by neuromuscular diseases that affect the respiratory muscles.

The increase in $PaCO_2$ that accompanies pure alveolar hypoventilation invariably affects PaO_2 as predicted in the alveolar gas equation, causing a decrease in PaO_2. This results in hypoxemia with a normal P_AO_2-PaO_2 gradient. In patients on room air, the PaO_2 will fall 5 mm Hg for every 3 mm Hg rise in $PaCO_2$. If the P_AO_2-PaO_2 gradient is abnormally increased, then other mechanisms may also be involved in the pathogenesis of hypoxemia. Hypoxemia resulting from pure alveolar hypoventilation usually responds adequately to increasing FIO_2.

By far, the most common cause of clinically important hypoxemia is $\dot{V}/\dot{Q}$ mismatching, which is present as a continuum from pure shunt ($\dot{Q}$, without $\dot{V}$) to pure dead space ventilation ($\dot{V}$ without $\dot{Q}$) and unlimited patterns of $\dot{V}/\dot{Q}$ mismatching in between. In young normal individuals, $\dot{V}/\dot{Q}$ ratios range from 0.6 to 3.0 and usually center around 1.0.[4] Low $\dot{V}/\dot{Q}$ lung units can result from compromised ventilation, such as obstructed airways or from partial alveolar filling with pneumonia or pulmonary edema. High $\dot{V}/\dot{Q}$ lung units most often occur with obstruction of blood flow owing to pulmonary vascular disease or from a lack of capillaries owing to lung parenchymal destruction, such as that seen in emphysema.

$\dot{V}/\dot{Q}$ mismatching causes hypoxemia and hypercapnia. However, in most cases, an increase in minute ventilation stimulated by hypercapnia results in normalization of $PaCO_2$ with persistent hypoxemia. This is possible because the CO_2 dissociation curve is linear, allowing well-ventilated areas to compensate. The O_2 dissociation curve is sigmoid shaped; therefore, the increase in minute ventilation, despite producing higher end-capillary PO_2, results in very modest changes in oxygen saturation, which in most cases is inadequate to reverse the hypoxemia (Fig. 30.2). Hypoxemia due to $\dot{V}/\dot{Q}$ mismatching is usually correctable by increasing the FIO_2. Local hypoxia in low $\dot{V}/\dot{Q}$ areas triggers reflex hypoxic pulmonary vasoconstriction in an attempt to correct the $\dot{V}/\dot{Q}$ imbalance. This reflex vasoconstriction can be abolished by a number of vasodilators, including nitroprusside, nitroglycerin, calcium channel blockers, and inhalational anesthetics. When compensatory mechanisms fail in a patient with severe lung disease, the body may set a new steady-state $PaCO_2$ and pH as an adaptive response to conserve the work of breathing.

Right-to-left shunt occurs when there is no ventilation into a lung unit while perfusion is preserved. It is one of the extreme ends in the spectrum of $\dot{V}/\dot{Q}$ mismatches. In a normal lung, the amount of shunt present is less than 5%. Shunt in the lung results from atelectasis, severe pulmonary edema, and air space consolidation, such as pneumonia. In addition, right-to-left shunt can also occur as a consequence of arteriovenous malformation and intracardiac shunts from a patent foramen ovale, patent ductus arteriosus, or ventricular septal defect. Shunts cause significant hypoxemia owing to the mixture of oxygenated blood with shunted, poorly oxygenated venous blood. Hypercapnia is usually not present until the shunt is greater than 50%. In contrast to other mechanisms of respiratory failure, hypoxemia owing to shunting is not responsive to increases in FIO_2. This feature of shunt can be conveniently used to separate it from other causes of hypoxemia. Calculation of shunt ($\dot{Q}s/\dot{Q}t$) is easily done by administering 100% oxygen for 15 minutes and then analyzing arterial blood gases. Percent shunt can be estimated using a nomogram or by using the following formula:

$$\dot{Q}s/\dot{Q}t = \frac{(CcO_2 - CaO_2)}{(CcO_2 - C\overline{v}O_2)} \times 100$$

In this equation, C denotes content, and the lowercase letters c, a, and v denote end-capillary, arterial, and venous blood, respectively. A simplified shunt equation assumes that the Cvo_2 is normal and that the shunt is less than 25%. This simplified shunt equation states that

$$\dot{Q}s/\dot{Q}t = \frac{PAO_2 - PaO_2}{20}$$

When the FIO_2 used is less than 1.0, the resulting calculation is called venous admixture instead of shunt. This reflects the contribution of severe $\dot{V}/\dot{Q}$ mismatching, including very low $\dot{V}/\dot{Q}$ ratios that approach zero, which may act like shunts when alveoli are not ventilated with 100% oxygen. The hypoxemia of shunts is remarkably resistant to correction by increasing the FIO_2. Patients with significant shunts may have the same arterial oxygen saturation when maintained on a relatively toxic FIO_2 (near 1.0) or when titrated down to relatively safe FIO_2 (0.6 to 0.7).

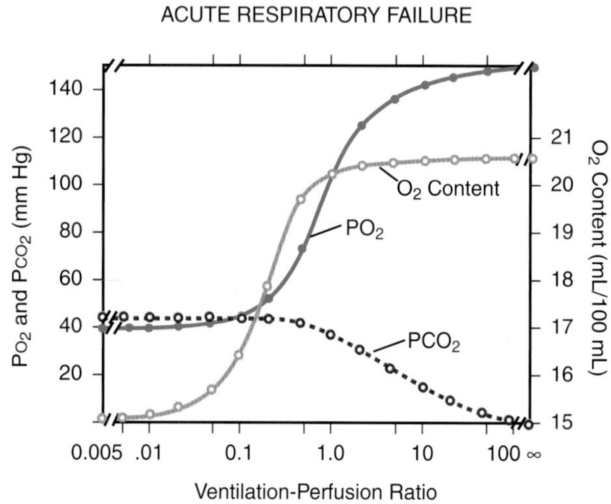

CLINICAL ASSESSMENT

Patients with ARF commonly have dyspnea. For those with underlying lung disease, dyspnea may be present chronically. Therefore, mild changes in the degree of dyspnea may or may not be perceived. In the presence of significant hypoxemia and acidosis, patients may have symptoms of central nervous system depression ranging from irritability to coma. Patients may also have evidence of the effects of hypoxemia or acidosis on the cardiovascular system, such as arrhythmias, angina, or myocardial infarction. Depending on the underlying disease, other symptoms may also be present. Although they may be important and helpful in evaluating the underlying process causing the respiratory failure, they are not that helpful in evaluating the degree of respiratory dysfunction. For example, the additional symptoms of cough, sputum production, and fever may suggest pneumonia, whereas pleuritic chest pain with certain characteristics may suggest pneumothorax or pulmonary embolism as the cause of the respiratory distress.

Initial physical examination of patients with ARF should focus on overall appearance, vital signs, and the ABCs (airway, breathing, and circulation). In general, patients with ARF have tachypnea, tachycardia, and variable mental status. The degree of alteration of mental status may reflect the severity of the respiratory failure. Confusion or disorientation in the presence of dyspnea and tachypnea may reflect profound hypoxemia or hypercapnia with its attendant respiratory acidosis. Pulsus paradoxus, a decrease in arterial systolic pressure of greater than 10 mm Hg with

Fig. 30.2 Variations in PO_2, PCO_2, and O_2 content in a gas exchange lung unit as its ventilation-perfusion ratio is progressively increased. This lung is assumed to be breathing air, and the mixed venous blood PO_2 and PCO_2 are 40 mm Hg and 45 mm Hg, respectively. (From West JB. Ventilation-perfusion relationships. *Am Rev Respir Dis.* 1977;116:919–943.)

TABLE 30.2 Radiographic Approach to Acute Respiratory Failure

Radiograph	Clinical Characteristics	Responses to Oxygen[a]
"White" Chest Radiograph		
Pneumonia	Fever, leukocytosis, sputum production	+ to + + +
Acute respiratory distress syndrome	Predisposing risk factors, bilateral infiltrates on imaging	+ to + +
Cardiogenic edema	Paroxysmal nocturnal dyspnea, orthopnea, edema	+ + + to + + + +
Interstitial lung disease	Prior chest radiographic abnormalities	+ + + to + + + +
"Black" Chest Radiograph		
Chronic obstructive pulmonary disease/asthma	Reduced flow on bedside spirometry	+ + to + + +
Pulmonary emboli	Acute dyspnea, pleuritic pain	+ + + to + + + +
Right-to-left shunt	History and physical examination consistent with pulmonary hypertension	+
Microatelectasis	Postoperative or rib fracture, bronchial breath sounds	+ + to + + +

[a]Range from +, which is shuntlike (Po_2 increases 1 mm Hg for 1% rise in FIO_2), to + + + +, which is $\dot{V}/\dot{Q}$ imbalance (Po_2 increases 5 mm Hg for 1% rise in FIO_2).

inspiration, also suggests severe airway obstruction associated with significant negative intrathoracic pressures. Patients with severe respiratory distress are usually unable to speak in full sentences. Likewise, the presence or absence of adventitious breath sounds may assist the clinician in evaluating the degree and acuity of the respiratory distress. Crackles suggest alveolar flooding or early bronchopneumonia, whereas rhonchi often herald an increase in mucus production or an inability to clear secretions. Wheezing suggests airway obstruction, whereas wheezes located over the neck suggest upper airway stridor that may be associated with respiratory collapse. Decrease in breath sounds may be seen in patients with chronic obstructive pulmonary disease (COPD) or those with severe airway obstruction. The absence of wheezing and breath sounds in a patient with underlying obstructive lung disease and respiratory distress may suggest impending respiratory collapse as a result of very limited air movement. Absence of breath sounds may also be associated with pneumothorax. Subcutaneous emphysema usually indicates pneumomediastinum with or without accompanying pneumothorax.

Despite advances in noninvasive technologies in oxygenation assessment, arterial blood gas analysis remains the best and most accurate test in the initial assessment of patients with ARF. Pulse oximetry is acceptable as a method for following oxygenation once it has been calibrated to true blood gas co-oximetry saturation and the arterial PaO_2 is known. Pulse oximetry (SpO_2) carries plus or minus 4% error in measuring oxygen saturation. In patients with carbon monoxide poisoning, SpO_2 does not reflect true PaO_2, and profound hypoxemia may be missed. With methemoglobinemia, the SpO_2 may falsely read the oxygen saturation at around 85%, irrespective of the true saturation. Furthermore, pulse oximetry does not give information on $PaCO_2$ and pH, which may be crucial in the differential diagnosis and management of the patient with ARF. The presence of hypercapnia is a marker of the severity of disease. Hypercapnia is more likely to complicate hypoxemic failure when the disease is superimposed on significant underlying lung or neuromuscular disease.

The presence of hypoxemia, hypercapnia, and respiratory acidosis can be used to define ARF; however, it is difficult to set specific levels of PaO_2 or $PaCO_2$ because patients with underlying lung disease may have markedly abnormal baselines. Given these qualifications, patients with ARF generally have a PaO_2 less than 55 mm Hg or a $PaCO_2$ more than 50 mm Hg. The pH is very helpful in assessing the acuity of the hypoventilation. In cases of subacute or chronic hypoventilation, the patient usually has an elevated serum bicarbonate level and a mild depression of the pH. In acute respiratory acidosis without renal compensation, the pH drops by 0.08 for each 10 mm Hg rise in $PaCO_2$.

Compensatory bicarbonate retention or wasting by the kidneys to buffer the pH changes usually takes 2 to 3 days to occur. After renal compensation, a change of 10 mm Hg of $PaCO_2$ will produce a 0.03 change in pH in the opposite direction.

The chest radiograph is extremely useful in sorting out the differential diagnosis of ARF during the initial presentation. The causes of hypoxemia can be classified based on radiographic appearance. Table 30.2 shows examples of diseases associated with "white" chest radiographs showing diffuse or patchy infiltrates and diseases associated with "black" chest radiographs showing normal or clear lung fields.

Differential Diagnosis

The clinical classification of ARF based on chest radiographic appearance provides a convenient algorithm in evaluating hypoxemic patients. Posteroanterior and lateral radiographs or computed tomography (CT) of the chest provide better quality than portable films and can help visualize the retrocardiac space. Patients having a "white" chest radiograph usually have pneumonia, ARDS, cardiogenic pulmonary edema, or progressive interstitial lung disease. Patients having a "black" chest radiograph usually have obstructive lung disease, pulmonary emboli, a right-to-left shunt, or microatelectasis. Most patients with hypoxemic respiratory failure have radiographic infiltrates.

The presence of additional compatible history and physical examination findings often allows the clinician to narrow the differential diagnosis. With fever, cough, sputum production, and lobar or patchy infiltrate, pneumonia is a likely possibility. Pneumonia often presents in an atypical fashion in patients older than 65 years old.[5] Up to 50% of older patients do not have a fever or specific respiratory complaints; confusion or mild hypotension may be the primary findings on examination. Cardiogenic pulmonary edema superimposed on abnormal lung parenchyma, such as in emphysema, will often give bilateral patchy radiographic infiltrates and not necessarily the classic central batwing distribution. In such cases, a history of underlying heart disease and compatible physical examination may aid in arriving at the presumptive diagnosis of congestive heart failure. In recent years, an increase in the use of brain natriuretic peptide (BNP) levels have been used to support the diagnosis of heart failure. A review by Korenstein et al. pooled over 3,000 patients and determined that BNP of less than 100 pg/mL essentially rules out the diagnosis of heart failure, whereas a BNP greater than 400 pg/mL has a sensitivity and specificity of 81% and 90%, respectively.[6] Elevated levels do not distinguish between right and left ventricular failure and may be seen in patients having pulmonary emboli and cor pulmonale. BNP levels have also been noted to be elevated in patients with septic shock without evidence of clinical heart failure.

The most helpful feature in separating these disorders is the radiographic response to therapy. Radiographically, pneumonia resolves over 3 to 12 weeks, whereas cardiogenic pulmonary edema may clear over days. In the absence of supportive clinical evidence for left ventricular failure, diffuse infiltrates may represent noncardiogenic pulmonary edema, pulmonary hemorrhage, or interstitial pneumonitis. Noncardiogenic pulmonary edema (presenting in ARDS) most often occurs in hospitalized patients. If a patient presents to the hospital with ARDS, a diagnosis of severe bilateral pneumonia should strongly be considered. Most patients with ARDS have one of the common precipitating factors leading to this disorder. The common predisposing events include sepsis, hypotension, massive aspiration, severe pneumonia, and massive trauma or transfusions. Less common precipitating events include pancreatitis, drug overdose, and recent cardiopulmonary bypass. The diagnostic criteria for ARDS were updated in 2012 (see Table 30.1) and replaced with the Berlin Definition.[3] Major changes from the prior consensus definition include elimination of the term "acute lung injury," removal of the pulmonary capillary wedge pressure criterion, and addition of minimal ventilator settings.[3] Mechanical ventilation strategies with low tidal volumes of 6 to 8 mL/kg of ideal body weight and plateau pressures less than 30 to 32 cm H_2O have been shown to significantly reduce mortality in patients with ARDS.[7] Comprehensive reviews of ARDS have been published[8] and therapeutic trials and protocols are maintained on the ARDSNet website (www.ARDSNet.org).

In a patient with a history of joint complaints, an undiagnosed rash or unexplained renal insufficiency, a diagnosis of vasculitis or collagen vascular disease should be considered. In the presence of an acute drop in hematocrit, pulmonary hemorrhage syndrome may be entertained, in which case a definitive diagnosis may require bronchoscopy to allow proper treatment and management. In some cases, pulmonary hemorrhage is not accompanied by hemoptysis.

The Infectious Diseases Society of America (IDSA) in conjunction with the American Thoracic Society (ATS) has published consensus guidelines on the management of community-acquired pneumonia in adults. The antibiotic regimen chosen by the IDSA/ATS mainly relies on macrolides (with or without a β-lactam) or respiratory fluoroquinolones (e.g., levofloxacin or moxifloxacin) for outpatient therapy. Respiratory fluoroquinolones or cephalosporins plus macrolides are recommended for hospitalized patients. The IDSA and ATS also published guidelines in 2016 to distinguish between hospital-acquired pneumonia (HAP) and ventilator-associated pneumonia (VAP). A prior category of health care–associated pneumonia (HCAP) was removed from the guidelines due to increasing evidence that many of these patients are not at risk for multidrug-resistant pathogens and treating them as such may have implications for antibiotic stewardship.[9] Management of severe pneumonia emphasizes early, appropriate antibiotics in adequate doses. Initial broad-spectrum therapy is narrowed based on microbiologic cultures and clinical response.[9] If patients receive an initially appropriate antibiotic regimen, efforts should be made to shorten the duration of therapy from the traditional 14 to 21 days to periods as short as 7 days if the patient has a good clinical response with resolution of clinical features of infection and the etiologic pathogen is not *Pseudomonas aeruginosa*.[10]

Pneumonia may be difficult to distinguish from atelectasis presenting as a localized infiltrate. Atelectasis can be seen with pulmonary embolism (PE), diaphragmatic dysfunction with volume loss, splinting from rib fracture or pleuritis, and in mechanically ventilated patients. The presenting signs and symptoms including dyspnea, chest pain, and fever, and leukocytosis may overlap in many instances. High clinical suspicion is needed to prevent missing the diagnosis of PE. Mortality of untreated PE has been reported to be about 30% compared to 8% with appropriate treatment.[11] High-probability $\dot{V}/\dot{Q}$ scans carry a positive predictive value for PE of 88%.[12] With the addition of strong clinical suspicion, the positive predictive value is as high as 96%. About 12% of patients with low-probability $\dot{V}/\dot{Q}$ scan may have angiographically proven PE. Therefore, if PE is clinically suspected, further evaluation after a low-probability scan is needed. Evaluation of the lower extremities for deep venous thrombosis (DVT) with Doppler ultrasonography is noninvasive and, if positive, obviates the necessity to perform pulmonary angiography. If the patient does not have a high pretest probability of PE, some advocate repeating Doppler ultrasonography after 72 hours. If both Doppler studies are negative, there is a very low probability of significant PE. Pulmonary angiography has been shown to be safe in the 755 patients enrolled in the Prospective Investigation of Pulmonary Embolism Diagnosis (PIOPED) study. The diagnostic utility of $\dot{V}/\dot{Q}$ scans for acute PE persists even in the presence of preexisting cardiac or pulmonary disease.[13,14] In recent years, there has been an increased use of D-dimer testing in patients presenting to the emergency department. D-dimer is formed from the degradation products of cross-linked fibrin by plasmin. It is very sensitive but nonspecific (elevated in almost all patients with carcinoma and most seriously ill hospitalized patients) for either DVT or PE. A negative D-dimer using enzyme-linked immunosorbent assays (ELISA) has a negative predictive value of 95%.[15]

Righini and colleagues[16] showed that a diagnostic strategy that included clinical probability, D-dimer, Doppler ultrasonography, and helical chest CT was highly cost-effective. A negative D-dimer in the setting of a negative Doppler ultrasound may obviate the need for further testing. Helical chest CT with a PE protocol has virtually replaced pulmonary angiography. The great benefit of chest CT is in providing additional diagnoses to explain the patient's symptoms; sensitivity and specificity ranges from 78% to 100%. Its accuracy drops in the areas of atelectasis and segmental or subsegmental vessels. Multidetector scanning increases the sensitivity to 89% and can visualize thrombi up to the sixth pulmonary artery branch. The Prospective Investigative Study of Acute Pulmonary Embolism Diagnosis (PISAPED) investigators published diagnostic algorithms based on their 40 years of experience that relies heavily on ventilation/perfusion lung scanning and used multidetector scanning in only 16% of the cases when there was discordance between pretest probability and lung scanning. This option may be very useful in patients who cannot tolerate intravenous iodinated contrast dye owing to renal insufficiency.[17]

Exacerbation of underlying obstructive lung disease is the most common cause of hypoxemic respiratory failure in patients who do not have infiltrates on chest radiography. The most important precipitants of ARF in patients with COPD are airway infection, congestive heart failure, anatomic interference with chest wall function (e.g., pleural effusion, pneumothorax, or rib fracture), and medication noncompliance.[18] Additionally, PE and oversedation can precipitate respiratory distress. The most common bacteria isolated from the airway and lungs of patients with COPD are *Haemophilus influenzae*, *Streptococcus pneumoniae*, and *Moraxella catarrhalis*.[19] Antibiotics have been shown to be beneficial in patients having at least two of the following: dyspnea, increased sputum production, and sputum purulence.[20] Therefore, a β-lactam antibiotic (e.g., amoxicillin, oral cephalosporin) or trimethoprim-sulfamethoxazole is frequently given during exacerbations of COPD. Studies have documented the benefit of oral corticosteroids in acute exacerbations of COPD. A large randomized, controlled study of 271 patients with COPD exacerbation who were randomly assigned to receive either systemic corticosteroids or placebo for up to 2 weeks demonstrated that systemic corticosteroids reduced the 30-day treatment failure rate (23% vs. 33%), 90-day treatment failure rate (37% vs. 48%), and hospital stay (8 vs. 10 days) while improving lung function. A dose of 40 mg of prednisone per day for 5 days is recommended by the most recent Global Initiative for Chronic Obstructive Lung Disease (GOLD) guidelines, which are available online at www.goldcopd.org.[21]

Another cause of respiratory failure with a normal chest radiograph is a right-to-left shunt. The presence of a significant shunt can be suspected when arterial hypoxemia is resistant to improvements with higher FIO_2. An acute rise in right-sided cardiac pressures from PE or from right ventricular myocardial infarction (MI) may cause a right-to-left shunt through a patent foramen ovale. An echocardiogram with a bubble study may be used to detect a cardiac shunt. Finding radio-macroaggregated albumin in the brain or kidney after a lung perfusion scan is a sensitive and specific way of identifying the presence of a pulmonary or cardiac right-to-left shunt.

Microatelectasis is another cause of respiratory failure with a normal chest radiograph. This disorder almost always occurs in the setting of inadequate ventilation and is frequently seen in postoperative patients or in the setting of splinting secondary to chest wall pain. Diffuse alveolar collapse leads to bronchial breath sounds at the base of the lung without the infiltrate that is seen with obstructive atelectasis. The use of analgesics for pain, incentive spirometry, and the addition of positive pressure to the airway leads to resolution of this process. In hospitalized patients, inspiratory positive pressure breathing devices with nebulized therapy is often beneficial, especially in postoperative patients.

Hypercapnia may develop in patients with either a "black" (normal) chest radiograph or "white" (infiltrative) chest radiograph. Hypercapnic respiratory failure results usually from alveolar hypoventilation, severe $\dot{V}/\dot{Q}$ mismatching, or a combination of the two. In patients with normal lungs, it generally occurs in the setting of reduction in central nervous system respiratory drive or acute neuromuscular weakness. In both cases, alveolar hypoventilation is the predominant mechanism. In patients with preexisting lung disease, hypercapneic respiratory failure usually occurs in the setting of severe lung disease and $\dot{V}/\dot{Q}$ mismatching. Whatever the triggering event may be, the patient is generally incapable of increasing the minute ventilation needed to compensate for the increased ventilatory workload requirements.

Reduction in central nervous system respiratory drive may be caused by sedative-hypnotic medications or depressed mental status from organic and metabolic or hypoxic encephalopathy. Although patients with stroke or brain hematoma rarely have clinically significant depression of respiratory drive, hypercapnia may still occur if the breaths are shallow with small tidal volumes, increasing dead space ventilation and resulting in alveolar hypoventilation. Acute hypoxemia that results in global brain hypoxia may then lead to depression of mental status and alveolar hypoventilation.

Neuromuscular weakness is a less common cause of clinically significant alveolar hypoventilation. Typically, the tidal volume is reduced secondary to shallow breathing, with an increased respiratory rate in an attempt to restore minute ventilation. This type of shallow and rapid breathing increases dead space ventilation and, given the same minute ventilation, alveolar ventilation will be reduced. Amyotrophic lateral sclerosis, high cervical spinal cord injury, Guillain-Barré syndrome, myasthenia gravis, phrenic nerve paralysis, and muscular dystrophy may result in both hypercapneic and hypoxemic respiratory failure. Hypercapnia may also result from respiratory muscle fatigue after a period of sustained rapid breathing as seen in the later stages of acute exacerbations of asthma or COPD.

Hypercapnic respiratory failure that occurs in the absence of respiratory drive depression or neuromuscular weakness is usually caused by severe $\dot{V}/\dot{Q}$ mismatching and often associated with conditions that increase CO_2 production. For example, fever increases VCO_2 by 13% for each degree Celsius.[22] Patients with severe preexisting $\dot{V}/\dot{Q}$ abnormality, in particular those with large low $\dot{V}/\dot{Q}$ areas, may not be able to compensate for the increased workload. Therefore, when compensatory efforts fail in a COPD patient with pneumonia and fever, hypercapnia ensues. Patients with severe lung disease, baseline hypoxemia, and hypercapnia are also at risk of worsening hypercapnia when they receive oxygen supplementation. When these patients require oxygen therapy for hypoxemic exacerbation, extreme caution must be exercised to prevent providing too much oxygen. Low-flow oxygen (1 to 2 L/min nasal cannula or 24% to 28% FIO_2 by mask) should be started and titrated up until the saturation is approximately 90%. If acute severe hypercapnia occurs, assisted ventilation is the treatment of choice. The pathophysiology of this process is still being debated and may involve three mechanisms.[23–25] Worsening of $\dot{V}/\dot{Q}$ mismatching is believed by many to be the major mechanism. Additionally, displacement of CO_2 molecules from hemoglobin (the Haldane effect) has been proposed but probably plays only a small role. Finally, suppression of hypoxic ventilatory drive has long been debated and remains controversial.

MANAGEMENT

The initial approach to managing patients in acute respiratory failure is supportive. The essential first steps remain assessment of airway patency, presence of breathing, and adequacy of circulatory function. Once this is ensured, specific treatments must be directed at the underlying disease that initiated respiratory failure. Specific therapy for each of these disorders is beyond the scope of this chapter but has been reviewed.[26]

In most cases, administration of supplemental oxygen is required. The ultimate goal of oxygen therapy is to provide adequate oxygen to the tissues to preserve tissue and organ function. Because there is no clinically useful measure of cellular oxygen tension, tissue hypoxia can only be indirectly predicted from overall organ function and oxygen transport. The critical level of hypoxemia that compromises organ function varies depending on the organ system and local factors. Clinical studies in patients without adaptive mechanisms suggest that short-term memory is adversely affected at PaO_2 less than 55 mm Hg.[27] Generally, PaO_2 of about 60 mm Hg, usually corresponding to SaO_2 of about 90%, is considered to be an adequate target. Further increase in PaO_2 offers little additional benefit because of the shape of the oxygen–hemoglobin dissociation curve and may potentially increase the risk of hypercapnia in some patients. Therefore, hypoxemic patients with severe lung disease, especially those with baseline hypercapnia, must be monitored closely with serial blood gases for correction of hypoxemia and prevention of worsening hypercapnia. The use of pulse oximetry to follow the adequacy of oxygenation may be appropriate if the pulse oximetry saturation (SpO_2) has been properly calibrated to accurately reflect co-oximetry saturation (SaO_2) of the patient when hypercapnia is not a concern.

Once the decision for oxygen supplementation has been made, the next step is to choose the method of delivery. In patients who are intubated, delivery of oxygen can be accomplished through a ventilator or through a T-piece, the latter if mechanical breaths are not needed. For patients who are not intubated, there are several choices of oxygen delivery systems. A nasal cannula is the most commonly used low-flow system. It delivers pure (100%) oxygen at various rates up to 5 to 6 L/min and is able to achieve an FIO_2 reported as high as 48%. High-flow nasal cannula (HFNC) devices deliver oxygen at rates up to 60 L/min in adults, or 8 L/min in infants. At these rates, HFNC can provide an FIO_2 up to

100% with constant delivery due to dead space washout creating an oxygen reservoir. In adults with acute hypoxemic respiratory failure without hypercapnia, high-flow oxygen therapy is a reasonable alternative to standard oxygen therapy or noninvasive positive pressure ventilation.[28] These systems are simple to use and comfortable, allowing the patient to speak, eat, and drink without much interference. However, as is true with all low-flow systems, the FIO_2 is not accurate, depending on several factors, including total minute ventilation.[29,30]

A simple face mask also delivers low-flow oxygen with a somewhat higher FIO_2 than a simple nasal cannula because of the presence of 100 to 200 mL of reservoir space between the mask and the patient's face. It must be removed transiently when the patient eats or drinks. Face masks with reservoir bags come in two varieties. A partial rebreather mask has a reservoir that is filled with pure oxygen mixed with a small amount of early exhaled gas that mainly comes from high oxygen tension dead space. This mask is able to achieve FIO_2 of 0.6 to 0.8. A nonrebreather mask has a reservoir containing pure oxygen and is not mixed with exhaled gas. In addition, there are one-way exhalation valves allowing exhaled gas to leave the mask without inhaling air. This mask allows the achievement of FIO_2 close to 0.9, but not quite 1.0, because of the presence of small amounts of exhaled gas in the space between the mask and the face.

Venturi masks are low-flow masks that use the Bernoulli principle to entrain room air when pure oxygen is delivered through a small orifice, resulting in a large total flow at predictable FIO_2. The size of the orifice determines the FIO_2. This oxygen delivery system is useful in patients with ARF who require oxygen supplementation, but in whom there is substantial risk for development of or worsening hypercapnia because the FIO_2 does not fluctuate significantly even with considerable changes in the patient's minute ventilation. Venturi masks or a Venturi device in a humidifier-mixer is accurate only to 40% to 50% FIO_2; above this range, many patients overbreathe the system. When a higher FIO_2 is required, a high-flow mask (e.g., Misty-Ox [Medline]) and a high-flow regulator (that can go up to 30 L/min) are recommended. With all these masks, there is significant deterioration of oxygen delivery as the respiratory rate increases, as when the patient is in respiratory distress. At 30 breaths/min, the FIO_2 delivered by a 15-L oxygen mask can drop from 95% to 60% owing to entrainment of ambient air and dilution of the inspired oxygen concentration. In a study by Wagstaff and Soni,[29] high levels of inspired oxygen concentration were achieved by a 15-L nasal cannula using a Vapotherm system (Equipro) that humidifies and warms the oxygen–air mix and makes it more tolerable to the patient. An alternative is to use a non-rebreather mask in which a reservoir bag with a one-way flap is connected to the mask and fills during the patient's expiration.

Aside from the risk of hypercapnia, there are other risks associated with oxygen therapy. High FIO_2 decreases the amount of inert nitrogen that fills and stabilizes peripheral airways and alveoli while oxygen is being rapidly removed from the alveoli, resulting in atelectasis. Absorption atelectasis causes a decrease in vital capacity and an increase in right-to-left shunt, which leads to worsening of hypoxemia. This is more frequently seen at FIO_2 above 0.7. High FIO_2 can also lead to tracheobronchitis and acute lung injury with capillary leak syndrome.[31] When this happens, it is often difficult to distinguish from worsening of the underlying condition that initially precipitated ARF. In general, FIO_2 of 1.0 can be used for 24 hours and FIO_2 of 0.9 can be used for 72 hours without significant sequelae. FIO_2 of 0.6 or less is usually well tolerated without significant long-term histologic and physiologic changes. If a patient requires very high FIO_2 with the above methods, ventilatory-assist devices should be considered to allow the FIO_2 to be lowered, thereby decreasing the risks of atelectasis and oxygen toxicity. These include noninvasive ventilation using continuous positive airway pressure (CPAP) through nasal or face mask and invasive mechanical ventilation through an endotracheal tube.

Over the past few years, there has been a renewed interest in the use of noninvasive ventilation in the management of ARF. Several pilot studies have shown useful applications of these techniques in avoiding intubation in some patients with ARF. Larger clinical trials are needed to further define the role of noninvasive mechanical ventilation in ARF, especially in those patients with advance directives for no intubation and with potentially reversible processes causing ARF.

Although positive airway pressure can be applied to nonintubated patients, these techniques may lead to gastric distention and vomiting. CPAP is best tolerated at low levels (10 cm H_2O) and for brief periods. Bilevel positive airway pressure allows for the inspiratory pressure to be set at a higher level (e.g., 10 to 20 cm H_2O) than the expiratory pressure (e.g., 0 to 10 cm H_2O). There have been multiple meta-analyses on noninvasive positive pressure ventilation (NPPV), which range from bilevel positive airway pressure machines applied via a full face mask all the way to a conventional ventilator connected to a mask device that covers the whole face. Its success varies according to the purpose and the diagnosis for which it is used. The best survival data and earliest applications were in exacerbations of COPD and acute cardiogenic pulmonary edema. In COPD, the application of NPPV decreased both mortality and length of hospital stay with a number needed to treat of five. Intubation risk was reduced by 28% in a meta-analysis by Keenan and colleagues.[31a] In cardiogenic pulmonary edema, mortality was reduced by 45%.[32] Other trials proved its effectiveness in acute respiratory failure following lung resection, acute asthma, solid organ transplantation, and in immunocompromised patients. NPPV has also been used in weaning patients from mechanical ventilation; the application of NPPV in one study of 443 patients shortened mechanical ventilation by approximately 10.5 days.[33] Other studies, however, have shown increased mortality when NPPV is used in patients requiring vasopressors, lack of improvement of respiratory acidosis, refractory hypoxemia, fatigue, and inability to clear secretions. These clinical parameters should be evaluated 1 hour after initiation of NPPV, when the first arterial blood gas is obtained. Confalonieri developed a chart predicting the success of NPPV that included Acute Physiology and Chronic Health Evaluation II (APACHE II) score, acidosis, level of consciousness, and respiratory rate.[34] As can be imagined, patients with a depressed level of consciousness, a pH less than 7.25, and a respiratory rate greater than 35 are more likely to fail and would probably benefit from urgent intubation without a trial of NPPV.

All studies evaluating NPPV published exclusion criteria that may very well be deemed as contraindications: cardiac or respiratory arrest; hemodynamic instability; the uncooperative patient; and patients with facial trauma, copious secretions, or significant risk of aspiration. Those patients should undergo intubation and conventional mechanical ventilation. Intubation facilitates the delivery of higher tidal volumes and the application of positive end-expiratory pressure needed to avert oxygen toxicity.

Mechanical Ventilation

Mechanical ventilation is a method of supporting intubated patients during illness when spontaneous ventilation is inadequate to sustain life or to achieve a therapeutic target. The clinical objectives are (1) to correct hypoxemia, (2) to correct acute respiratory acidosis, (3) to relieve respiratory distress, (4) to prevent or reverse atelectasis, (5) to rest respiratory muscles or prevent fatigue, (6) to allow sedation and neuromuscular blockade, (7) to decrease systemic or myocardial oxygen consumption, (8) to reduce intracranial pressure through controlled hyperventilation, and (9) to stabilize the chest wall.[35]

In general, mechanical ventilators can be divided into two categories: negative pressure ventilators and positive pressure ventilators. The iron lung is the prototype of negative pressure ventilators that gained popularity during the polio epidemics. Today, newer generations of negative pressure ventilators are still available under different names, such as cuirass, body suit, Porta-Lung, pneumobelt, pneumowrap, pneumosuit, and other more portable devices. They function by creating a negative pressure outside the chest wall, causing chest wall expansion and subsequent inspiration that simulates physiologic breathing. On release of the negative pressure, exhalation is passively accomplished. In the hospital setting, positive pressure ventilators are the mainstay of mechanical ventilation owing to various features and adjunctive modes that allow for more sophisticated delivery of conditioned gas and assistance in ventilation.

Positive pressure inflation of the lung can be achieved with machines that terminate inspiration according to volume, pressure, or time. The latest generation of positive pressure ventilation allows the physician to select among these options and allows for pressure support (a flow-cycled mode of ventilation) and reverse inspiratory to expiratory (I/E) ratio ventilation.

Volume-cycled ventilators deliver preset inspiratory flow to achieve a target volume, regardless of the pressure required. This system guarantees the tidal volume unless the peak pressure during inspiration exceeds the high-pressure limit, in which case the resulting volume is less than the preset volume. High pressure delivered to diseased, noncompliant lungs may predispose to barotrauma. Pressure-cycled ventilators deliver preset positive pressure throughout inspiration; however, the resulting tidal volume is variable depending on the compliance of the lungs. A true time-cycled ventilator does not depend on the patient's lung characteristics or even whether the ventilator is attached to the patient to end inspiration; therefore, it is important to recognize that a complete ventilatory cycle may occur without generating a tidal volume. Pressure support ventilation can be used either as a ventilatory mode or as an adjunctive mode. As a ventilatory mode, the pressure is set to produce a desired level of tidal volume similar to a pressure-cycled system. In an adjunctive mode, the pressure is set just high enough to overcome the tubing and circuit resistance during inspiration such that the level of pressure support does not increase the spontaneous tidal volume of the patient. A pressure support of 5 to 10 cm H_2O is usually adequate for the adjunctive mode.

Volume-cycled ventilators are most commonly used in the intensive care unit. In an assist-control (AC) mode, each patient breath that is recognized by the ventilator is assisted with a preset volume and flow rate in addition to a number of mandatory breaths per minute. In an intermittent mandatory ventilation (IMV) mode, the patient can take spontaneous unassisted breaths between the mandatory breaths. A synchronized IMV (SIMV) mode synchronizes the machine mandatory breaths to the patient's spontaneous breaths to avoid breath stacking. A pressure support system can be used to augment the spontaneous breaths of patients in the SIMV mode while at the same time guaranteeing a minimum number of mandatory breaths.

AC mode allows the patient to rest because each recognized spontaneous breath is assisted. Patients with respiratory muscle fatigue should be allowed to rest on this mode. Patients with sepsis and hypotension benefit from this mode by decreasing respiratory muscle work, which accounts for a significant portion of oxygen consumption during hypoperfusion syndromes. Similarly, in patients with cardiogenic pulmonary edema, decreased work of breathing translates to decreased myocardial oxygen demand. However, in patients with abnormal homeostatic mechanisms, such as hepatic encephalopathy, increased central respiratory drive may result in respiratory alkalosis. The SIMV mode is more homeostatic because the patient can determine the tidal volume needed; however, the work of breathing is higher and proportional to the amount of spontaneous ventilation relative to the assisted ventilation. The SIMV mode is primarily used in patients with severe air flow obstruction who tend to air trap when each breath is a relatively large, positive pressure breath. When the mandatory rate is set beyond the patient's spontaneous rate, or if the patient is completely paralyzed, the two modes are practically indistinguishable and the patient will receive only the mandatory breaths. Newer modes of ventilation include airway pressure release ventilation (APRV) and bilevel modes. The first one allows for CPAP with an intermittent pressure release phase. A P_{high} (high pressure) and P_{low} (low pressure) are set and the patient is allowed spontaneous breathing independent of the ventilator cycle. Rather than continuously distending and deflating the alveoli, the P_{high} maintains inflation during the entire respiratory cycle and only briefly releases to P_{low}, thus aiding in ventilation and CO_2 removal. Oxygenation is improved in this mode through alveolar recruitment by increasing the mean airway pressure (P_{high}) or by increasing the time at P_{high} (T_{high}). Ventilation is improved by changing the pressure gradient between P_{high} and P_{low} or by increasing release frequency. APRV mode may result in lower peak airway pressures and less sedation for the patient but has not been shown to impact mortality.[36]

In addition to ventilator modes, prone positioning has been extensively studied. Most research shows an improvement in oxygenation and PaO_2/FIO_2 ratios. Additionally, Guerin et al. showed significant improvement in 28- and 90-day mortality

when prone positioning was applied early for patients with severe ARDS.[37]

After the mode of ventilation is decided, the tidal volume, respiratory rate, FIO_2, and inspiratory flow rate must be set on the ventilator. The range of tidal volumes used in mechanical ventilation is between 5 and 15 mL/kg of ideal body weight. When low tidal volumes (6 to 8 mL/kg ideal body weight) are used, positive end-expiratory pressure (PEEP) or sighs (generally each sigh volume is 2 to 3 times tidal volume) should be given at set intervals to prevent microatelectasis. As a general rule, with severe airway obstruction or ARDS, 6 mL/kg up to 8 mL/kg tidal volume is reasonable (refer to the ARDSnet.org ventilator chart). Postoperative patients with normal lungs are frequently started on 8 to 12 mL/kg whereas patients with neuromuscular disease receive 10 to 15 mL/kg. It is generally safe to select a tidal volume that generates a peak alveolar pressure of 35 cm H_2O or less (with plateau pressures <30 to 32 cm H_2O). The rate should be chosen in conjunction with the tidal volume to provide minute ventilation that maintains a normal pH. A rate of 12 to 18 breaths/min is usually adequate. Once the patient is stable, the ventilator rate is often adjusted 2 to 4 breaths/min below the total respiratory rate. This prevents excessive work of breathing in the SIMV mode and provides an adequate backup rate in the AC mode.

In emergent situations, the FIO_2 should be set at 0.9 or 1.0 with later adjustments guided by arterial blood gases. The FIO_2 can be titrated down to achieve an SaO_2 of more than 90% (usually a PaO_2 of 60 mm Hg). More than 24 hours with an FIO_2 of 0.9 or greater or prolonged use of an FIO_2 of 0.6 or greater requires the addition of PEEP for prevention of oxygen toxicity. In general, this can be achieved with a PEEP of 5 to 15 cm H_2O. The inspiratory flow rate is usually set by the respiratory therapist at a level of 40 to 55 L/min. It is mandatory for the peak flow setting (inspiratory flow rate) of the ventilator to be greater than the patient's inspiratory flow demand. Otherwise, the patient breathes against the resistance of the ventilator circuitry, which results in the patient "fighting the ventilator." The flow setting should be 3.5 to 4 times the minute ventilation to achieve an I/E ratio of 1:1.2 to 1:1.5. In patients with severe obstructive lung disease, I/E ratios of 1:4 to 1:6 may be necessary.

Complications may arise during the course of mechanical ventilatory support. A deliberate and stepwise approach should be followed in the management process. Patient distress may arise from general discomfort, from inadequate ventilation or from the feeling of dyspnea. If hypoventilation is part of the overall strategy, the patient needs to be sedated. Accidental hypoventilation may result from kinking of the endotracheal tube, mucus plugging, accidental main stem intubation, pneumothorax, ventilator circuit leak, or ventilator disconnection. If the ventilator alarms have been set properly, they are frequently the first indicator of the acute problem, especially in a comatose, sedated, or paralyzed patient. A high-pressure alarm is usually caused by obstruction of the airway or acute change in lung compliance, whereas a low-volume alarm suggests decreased respiratory drive, a leak within the system, or a disconnected ventilator. During a high-pressure alarm distress, the patient should be disconnected from the ventilator and hand ventilated with a bag valve mask at an FIO_2 of 1.0 while a systematic search for the cause is being done. Unequal breath sounds may suggest a pneumothorax or slippage of the endotracheal tube into a main stem bronchus. Acute changes in hemodynamics are more suggestive of the former. Difficulty in hand ventilation should suggest kinking of the tube or mucous plugs; therefore, a suction catheter should be passed for diagnostic and therapeutic purposes. Chest radiography may aid the diagnosis and demonstrate lobar or complete collapse of the lung. If aggressive chest physiotherapy and inhaled mucolytics (e.g., Pulmozyme) are not effective, bronchoscopy may be required. If tension pneumothorax is strongly suspected, placement of a 14-gauge needle (angiocatheter) into the second intercostal space along the midclavicular line can relieve the tension immediately. Once this is done, a chest tube should always be placed whether a tension pneumothorax was present or not since the patient is receiving positive pressure ventilation and the catheter may have punctured the visceral pleura.

When a leak in the circuit is suspected, the ventilator tubing can be changed. If the leak is from the endotracheal tube, it can happen anywhere from the valve of the pillow to the cuff. A three-way stopcock inserted into the valve may correct the problem if the leak comes from the valve, obviating the need to change the endotracheal tube. If it does not stop the leak, the site of the leak may be in the pillow, the pilot line, or the cuff itself and may necessitate replacement of the endotracheal tube over a flexible stylet.

Pneumonia occurs in approximately 30% of patients receiving ventilator support. The risk increases with the duration of ventilator support at a rate of about 1% per day.[3] Pneumonia may be difficult to diagnose in patients with a "white" chest radiograph and may require either empirical therapy with a presumptive diagnosis or the use of bronchoscopy with a sterile brush with greater than or equal to 10^3 CFU/mL on quantitative culture considered a significant finding (or 10^4 on bronchoalveolar lavage or 10^5 on endotracheal aspirate).

Physiologic measurements—such as maximum inspiratory pressure ($PI_{max} = -20$ cm H_2O), vital capacity (VC = 10 mL/kg) and minute ventilation (MV = 15 L/min) are used to determine when a weaning trial should be done. Recently, the ratio of respiratory frequency (f) to tidal volume (V_t) during 1 minute of spontaneous breathing was found to be more accurate.[39] If f/V_t is less than 100 breaths/min per liter, a weaning trial is likely to be successful. The usual method of weaning includes trials of increased spontaneous breathing through a T tube or on pressure support ventilation (PSV, up to 10 cm H_2O). When

patients can breathe spontaneously for more than 30 minutes to 2 hours without a significant change in their hemodynamics, respiratory rate, or minute ventilation, they can usually be successfully extubated.[40]

Extracorporeal Membrane Oxygenation

Extracorporeal membrane oxygenation (ECMO) is a method for providing prolonged cardiopulmonary support to patients with severe acute respiratory failure. There are two types of ECMO: venoarterial (VA), which provides respiratory and hemodynamic support, and venovenous (VV), which provides respiratory support only. The Conventional ventilatory support versus Extracorporeal membrane oxygenation for Severe Acute Respiratory failure (CESAR) trial demonstrated significantly increased survival without disability at 6 months in patients who were randomly assigned to care in an ECMO center in a single United Kingdom center compared to conventional management in non-ECMO centers (63% vs. 47%). This study has several limitations, including the fact that 25% of patients referred for ECMO did not receive this therapy (16 recovered with conventional care and 5 died before transfer). However, several other trials have also demonstrated a survival benefit associated with ECMO for neonates, children, and adults with respiratory failure. Therefore referral to an ECMO center should be considered for adults with severe ARDS who are not improving with conventional management or who may need a bridge to lung transplantation. Guidelines for the use of ECMO are maintained by the Extracorporeal Life Support Organization and available on their website at www.elso.org.[41]

CONCLUSION

Acute respiratory failure implies an inability to maintain adequate oxygenation for tissues or adequate removal of carbon dioxide from tissues. The differential diagnosis should be informed by the radiographic appearance of the chest radiograph and by the patient's history and physical examination. A specific diagnosis should be pursued, which frequently requires ancillary studies such as blood or sputum cultures, bedside spirometry, perfusion lung scan, or a CT angiogram using multidetector scanners. This allows the physician to initiate specific therapy for the underlying cause of acute respiratory failure. These patients often require supportive therapy.

The full reference list for this chapter is available at ExpertConsult.com.

31

Massive Acute Pulmonary Embolism

Narain Moorjani, Susanna Price

Acute pulmonary embolism (PE) represents the sudden obstruction of part or all of the pulmonary arterial vasculature, usually caused by embolization of thrombus from the deep veins within the lower limbs and pelvis. It may also be caused by embolism of air, fat, or amniotic fluid. PE is the third most common cause of cardiovascular death (after coronary artery disease and stroke); more than 600,000 cases are thought to occur in the United States annually.[1] PE has been found in 18% of autopsies and in the majority (70%) of these was considered to be the main or a contributory cause of death.[2] The incidence increases exponentially with age, with the mean age at presentation of 62 years[2,3]; men and women are affected equally.[4]

Although no predisposing factors are identified in approximately 20% of patients (idiopathic or unprovoked PE),[5] the majority have either patient-related or setting-related attributable risk factors (secondary or provoked PE). Patient-related factors include advanced age, previous venous thromboembolism, active cancer, underlying coagulopathy (including Factor V Leiden and prothrombin mutations), smoking, hormone replacement therapy, and oral contraceptives.[6,7] Medical conditions associated with an increased risk of PE include heart failure, stroke, respiratory failure, sepsis, and inflammatory bowel disease.[8] Setting-related risk factors include protracted immobility secondary to major general/orthopedic surgery, major fracture, travel, pregnancy, chemotherapy, or the presence of a central venous line.[9] Commonly, more than one risk factor is present.

Historically, PE was classified according to the anatomic burden of the thrombus in the pulmonary vasculature.[10] Patient outcome is, however, more dependent on the associated hemodynamic compromise, such as the presence of circulatory arrest, hypotension, or right ventricular dysfunction.[5] PE has therefore been reclassified into three different prognostic categories[11,12]:

1. High-risk (massive) PE (20% of cases), which is a life-threatening condition and defined as PE in the presence of:
   a. Arterial hypotension (systolic blood pressure <90 mm Hg or a drop of >40 mm Hg) for more than 15 minutes or requiring inotropic support, which is not caused by a new arrhythmia
   b. Cardiogenic shock (oliguria, lactic acidosis, cool extremities, or altered level of consciousness)
   c. Circulatory collapse in patients with syncope or undergoing cardiopulmonary resuscitation (CPR)
2. Intermediate-risk (submassive) PE (32% of cases), which is defined as PE with a systolic blood pressure greater than 90 mm Hg but echocardiographic evidence of right ventricular (RV) dysfunction or pulmonary hypertension, or the presence of elevated markers of myocardial injury (such as troponin)
3. Low-risk (nonmassive) PE (48% of cases), which is defined as PE with a systolic blood pressure greater than 90 mm Hg and no evidence of RV dysfunction, pulmonary hypertension, or elevated markers of myocardial injury.

Data from the International Cooperative Pulmonary Embolism Registry (ICOPER) demonstrated 90-day mortality for patients with massive PE of 52% compared to 15% for those with submassive and nonmassive PE.[5] Similarly, data from the Management Strategy and Prognosis of Pulmonary Embolism Registry (MAPPET) demonstrated a 65% in-hospital mortality for patients with acute PE requiring CPR compared to 25% for those presenting with cardiogenic shock and 8% for hemodynamically stable patients.[13] The presence of RV dysfunction is associated with a 2-fold increase in 90-day mortality.[14]

PATHOPHYSIOLOGY

Obstruction of flow through the main pulmonary arteries results in increased afterload on the RV. In addition, release of vasoactive mediators, including thromboxane A2 and serotonin, results in pulmonary vasoconstriction and increased pulmonary vascular resistance.[15] The resultant increase in RV wall tension results in displacement of the interventricular septum to the left and impaired left ventricular (LV) filling.[16] If untreated, the RV outflow obstruction also results in reduced preload in the LV, reduced cardiac output, and, eventually, circulatory collapse and shock.[17] Younger patients with otherwise normal underlying cardiac function may tolerate the hemodynamic stress placed by a large PE without developing RV dysfunction or shock. In patients with compromised cardiac function, however, the onset of RV failure and circulatory collapse may be more rapid. In addition, hypoxia may result from the low cardiac output entering the pulmonary circulation, ventilation–perfusion mismatch, and the presence of a right-to-left shunt (through a patent foramen ovale, opened by increased right-sided pressure).[18]

CLINICAL PRESENTATION

The clinical presentation of PE varies widely. Massive PE may present with severe dyspnea at rest, syncope, or even cardiac arrest, whereas nonmassive PE may be asymptomatic or have limited symptoms. Past medical history may include some risk factors for venous thromboembolism. Physical signs include tachycardia, tachypnea, systemic hypotension, and cyanosis. Clinical evidence of RV dysfunction includes distended neck veins, parasternal heave, accentuated pulmonary component of the second heart sound, and a systolic murmur consistent with tricuspid regurgitation. An RV gallop rhythm may also be heard. The presence of a pleural rub, in association with pleuritic chest pain, may be secondary to pleural irritation caused by pulmonary infarction. These clinical features may also be used for risk stratification.[19,20]

DIAGNOSIS AND RISK STRATIFICATION

Clinical features and predisposing risk factors have been incorporated into clinical scoring systems that are used to predict the likelihood of PE and determining subsequent investigations. These include the Wells Score, Simplified Geneva Score, and Pulmonary Embolism Severity Index (PESI; Table 31.1).[19–21] The

TABLE 31.1 Clinical Scoring Systems Used to Determine Risk Following Acute PE

Variable	Points	Variable	Points
Wells Score[19]		Clinical signs	
Predisposing factors		Pain on deep palpation of lower limb and unilateral edema	1
Previous DVT or PE	1.5	Heart rate 75–94 beats/min	1
Recent surgery or immobilization	1.5	Heart rate > 94 beats/min	2
Cancer	1	Clinical probability	Total
Symptoms		PE unlikely	0–2
Hemoptysis	1	PE likely	>2
Clinical signs			
Heart rate >100 beats/min	1.5	**Pulmonary Embolism Severity Index**[21]	
Clinical signs of DVT	3	Age	1 per year
Clinical judgment		Male gender	10
Alternative diagnosis less likely than PE	3	Cancer: active or past history	30
Clinical probability (3 levels)	Total	Heart failure	10
Low	0–1	Chronic lung disease	10
Intermediate	2–6	Heart rate >110 beats/min	20
High	≥7	Systolic blood pressure <100 mm Hg	30
Clinical probability (2 levels)		Respiratory rate >30 beats/min	20
PE unlikely	0–4	Temperature <36°C	20
PE likely	>4	Altered mental status (disorientation, lethargy, stupor, or coma)	60
		Oxygen saturation <90% on room air	20
Simplified Geneva Score[20]		Clinical interpretation (mortality at 30 days)	
Predisposing factors		Class 1: very low mortality risk (0%–1.6%)	<66
Age >65 years	1	Class 2: low mortality risk (1.7%–3.5%)	<86
Previous DVT or PE	1	Class 3: moderate mortality risk (3.2%–7.1%)	<106
Surgery or fracture within 1 month	1	Class 4: high mortality risk (4.0%–11.4%)	<126
Active malignancy	1	Class 5: very high mortality risk (10.0%–24.5%)	>126
Symptoms			
Unilateral lower limb pain	1		
Hemoptysis	1		

DVT, Deep venous thrombosis; *PE,* pulmonary embolism.

most extensively validated and widely used clinical scoring system is the Wells score.[22]

INVESTIGATIONS FOR RISK STRATIFICATION

The chest radiograph (CXR) is usually abnormal in patients with acute PE.[23,24] Although mainly nonspecific, the absence of other features such as atelectasis or pleural effusion can be used to exclude other causes of dyspnea or chest pain. Arterial blood gas (ABG) analysis usually demonstrates hypoxemia (partial pressure of oxygen [PaO_2] <80 mm Hg), with hypocapnia and respiratory alkalosis.[25] In up to 20% of patients, a normal PaO_2 and alveolar-arterial gradient may be found. Alternatively, hypercapnia with respiratory and metabolic acidosis may be seen in patients with massive PE requiring cardiopulmonary resuscitation (CPR). Following assessment of the clinical and hemodynamic status of the patient using a clinical scoring system, the patients are subdivided into different probabilities of PE.

HIGH CLINICAL PROBABILITY

If the patient has a high clinical probability of PE as determined by the clinical scoring systems, then multidetector computed tomography pulmonary angiography (CTPA) is required to determine the presence of thrombus within the pulmonary arterial vasculature.[11] CTPA has become the imaging of choice in patients with suspected PE because of its speed of scanning, widespread availability, and high sensitivity and specificity (>90%).[26] It provides excellent visualization of the pulmonary arterial vasculature, including the main, lobar, and segmental pulmonary arteries along with characterization of extravascular structures (Fig. 31.1).

An alternative imaging modality, such as VQ scintigraphy, may also be required in patients with a contraindication to CTPA, such as those with renal failure or contrast allergy.[27] In hemodynamically unstable patients who cannot be transferred for CTPA, echocardiography may be required.

LOW OR INTERMEDIATE CLINICAL PROBABILITY

If the patient has been classified as having a low or intermediate clinical probability of PE, a D-dimer enzyme-linked immunoabsorbent assay (ELISA) should be performed as the first-line investigation (sensitivity 96% and specificity 39%).[28] Serum D-dimer is a degradation product of cross-linked fibrin and acts as an indirect marker for thrombosis and subsequent fibrinolysis. As the D-dimer ELISA has a high negative predictive value (NPV), its absence effectively rules out acute PE and an alternative diagnosis should be sought.[29] The positive predictive value (PPV) of elevated serum D-dimer levels, however, is low, as although D-dimer is very specific for fibrin, fibrin can be produced in a wide variety of conditions, including aortic dissection, cancer, inflammation, and infection.[30,31] Hence, if positive, the patient should undergo a CTPA.[11]

Once the diagnosis of acute PE has been made, the patients are stratified into low-risk (nonmassive), intermediate-risk (submassive), and high-risk (massive) groups, according to the presence of hypotension, shock and/or RV dysfunction. The clinical status of the patient will differentiate the high-risk (massive) PE from non-high-risk PE patients. Echocardiography can then be used to further delineate non-high-risk PE patients into intermediate-risk PE (with evidence of RV dysfunction) or low-risk PE (with no RV dysfunction) groups.[32] Surrogate markers of RV dysfunction include RV dilatation (RV end-diastolic dimension >30 mm), interventricular septal flattening with paradoxical motion, increased RV/LV ratio (>0.9), RV hypokinesis, pulmonary hypertension (pulmonary artery systolic pressure >30 mm Hg), and increased tricuspid regurgitation jet velocity (>2.6 m/s), which are found in approximately 25% of patients with acute PE (Fig. 31.2).[33,34]

Echocardiography can also be used to exclude other important causes of acute circulatory collapse, including acute myocardial infarction (MI), pericardial tamponade, or type A aortic dissection. Normal RV size and function on echocardiography in a patient

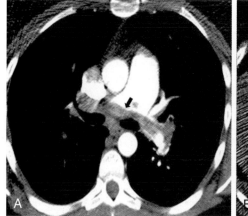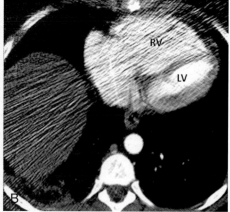

Fig. 31.1 Contrast-enhanced computed tomography pulmonary angiography *(CTPA)* axial images showing (A) a large saddle embolus at the pulmonary artery bifurcation *(arrow)* with extension into both the left and right pulmonary arteries, and (B) evidence of right heart strain shown by enlarged right heart chambers, a right ventricle *(RV)*/left ventricle *(LV)* ratio greater than 1.5, and displacement of the interventricular septum. (Courtesy Dr. Deepa Gopalan, Cambridge, UK.)

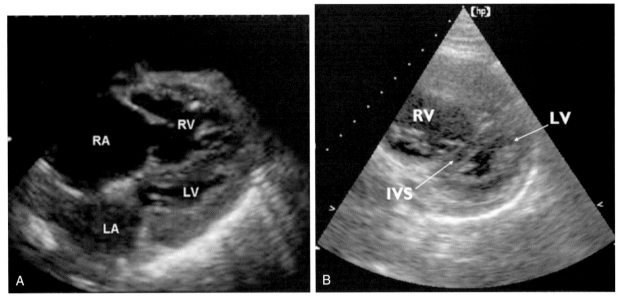

Fig. 31.2 Transthoracic echocardiography images in a patient with massive pulmonary embolism, with (A) subcostal long axis view showing acute right heart dilatation, with the right ventricle *(RV)* larger than the left ventricle *(LV)* and (B) parasternal short axis view showing a small compressed LV, which is D-shaped with a flattened interventricular septum and a dilated RV. *LA,* Left atrium; *RA,* right atrium.

with shock or hypotension virtually rules out acute PE as a cause of hemodynamic instability.[32] The McConnell sign, a distinct echocardiographic feature of acute massive pulmonary embolism, is a regional pattern of RV dysfunction, with akinesia of the mid–free wall and hypercontractility of the apical wall (Video 31.1). Transesophageal echocardiography can provide excellent imaging of the RV and proximal pulmonary vasculature to identify thrombus and can assess RV function and size.[35] In patients with suspected PE with evidence of RV dysfunction, it has a sensitivity of 80% and specificity of 97%.[35] However, it should not be undertaken in hypoxic patients with hemodynamic instability except in special circumstances (i.e., the patient is already intubated and ventilated).

Biomarkers, including serum troponin I or T and brain natriuretic peptide (BNP), may be indirect evidence of RV dysfunction in patients with acute PE.[36] Troponin levels—including troponin I and troponin T rise in PE secondary to increased RV wall tension and end-diastolic pressure—reduced right coronary artery flow, increased RV myocardial oxygen demand, RV myocardial ischemia (even in the presence of normal coronary arteries), and subsequent leakage of the enzymes from the RV myocytes into the bloodstream.[37] They can be used to risk stratify patients with non-high-risk PE into intermediate-risk PE (with elevated troponin levels) or low-risk PE (normal troponin levels).[38] Similarly, plasma B-type natriuretic peptide (BNP) is released from the RV in response to increased pressure and stretch and has been shown to correlate with the presence of RV dysfunction.[39] Elevated levels of both troponin and BNP have been shown to be associated with adverse prognosis and short-term outcomes in patients with acute PE.[40,41] Raised levels of both biomarkers, however, are not specific to PE.

Electrocardiography (ECG) is normal in up to 30% of patients[42] but often demonstrates nonspecific changes, such as sinus tachycardia, atrial fibrillation, or ST/T wave changes.[43,44] Despite having a low sensitivity and specificity, the ECG may demonstrate evidence of right heart strain, such as T-wave inversion in leads V_1 to V_4, P pulmonale, right axis deviation, incomplete or complete right bundle branch block, or the combination of a prominent S wave in lead I, Q wave in lead III, and T-wave inversion in lead III (the classical $S_1Q_3T_3$ pattern, which is present in only 2% to 15% of patients with PE).[45]

As massive PE has a high mortality in the first 6 hours following the onset of symptoms, early diagnosis is paramount in order to instigate timely management. Unfortunately, the diagnosis is frequently first made at autopsy.[46,47]

MANAGEMENT

The primary cause of death in patients with massive PE is low cardiac output. Massive PE should be suspected in patients with major hemodynamic instability accompanied by an elevated central venous pressure, which is not otherwise explained by pericardial tamponade, acute MI, or tension pneumothorax. As the short-term mortality increases depending on the degree of hemodynamic insult caused by obstruction to RV outflow, the choice of initial therapy will also depend on the severity of the hemodynamic insult.

Anticoagulation

Unless there is a strong contraindication, parenteral anticoagulation should be commenced immediately in all patients for whom acute PE is suspected.[12] Options include low-molecular-weight heparin (LMWH), intravenous unfractionated heparin (UFH), or subcutaneous fondaparinux (selective factor Xa inhibitor). Subcutaneous LMWH or fondaparinux are preferred for the majority of patients as they are associated with a lower incidence of thromboembolic events, heparin-induced thrombocytopenia (HIT) and major bleeding (LMWH 1.3% vs. UFH 2.1%), and do not require monitoring.[48,49] Fondaparinux can be given in weight-adjusted doses without monitoring as a once daily subcutaneous injection, as it has a half-life of 15 to 20 hours.[50] UFH is indicated in patients with an increased risk of bleeding or in those for whom thrombolysis is being considered, as its short-acting effects can be directly reversed with protamine.[51] Intravenous UFH should also be used in patients with high-risk (massive) PE, as the effectiveness of LMWH and fondaparinux has not been investigated in this patient population.[48] UFH is also preferred in patients with significant renal impairment (as LMWH and fondaparinux are excreted by the kidney) and in patients with extreme obesity (for whom dosing of LMWH is unpredictable).[11] It is administered intravenously with a bolus of 80 U/kg followed by a continuous infusion of 18 U/kg, which is subsequently adjusted to achieve an activated partial thromboplastin time ratio (aPTTR) between 2.0 and 2.5. The aPTTR is measured 4 to 6 hours following the initial dose, 3 hours after each dose adjustment, and then once daily when the therapeutic aPTTR has been achieved. Anticoagulation with heparin (UFH, LMWH, or fondaparinux) should be continued for at least 5 days.[52] For patients with heparin-induced thrombocytopenia, an alternative non–heparin-based anticoagulant, such as lepirudin, argatroban, or bivalirudin, can be used.[53]

Fibrinolysis

Fibrinolytic drugs (including urokinase, streptokinase, tenecteplase, and recombinant tissue plasminogen activator [rtPA]) actively promote thrombus lysis by hydrolysis of fibrin molecules. They are enzymes that convert circulating inactive plasminogen into its active analogue plasmin. Plasmin is a serine protease enzyme that cleaves fibrin, releasing fibrin degradation products, including D-dimer molecules.[54] These agents are therefore able to induce a more rapid regression of the obstructive thrombotic burden to RV outflow compared to heparin alone.[55,56] The benefits of adding fibrinolytic therapy to heparin, however, must be balanced by the potential side effects, including increased risk of major hemorrhage and transfusion requirements.[57]

Fibrinolytic therapy should ideally be initiated within 48 hours of symptom onset for the greatest benefit but has been shown to have some efficacy up to 14 days.[58,59] Absolute contraindications to thrombolysis include recent major surgery, bleeding, or trauma (within 2 weeks), intracranial hemorrhage, recent stroke (within 2 months), any hemorrhagic stroke, or significant coagulopathy. Relative contraindications include pregnancy, thrombocytopenia, and prolonged cardiopulmonary resuscitation (CPR).[12] Of the 478 patients who received fibrinolysis in the MAPPET registry, just over 40% (n = 193) had more than one relative contraindication.[13] These patients require intensive care monitoring for detection of the complications of acute PE and identification of the hemorrhagic complications of thrombolytic therapy.

The role of thrombolytic therapy for patients with intermediate risk (submassive) PE remains controversial. The effects of thrombolysis in this patient group have been examined in 2 prospective randomized, placebo-controlled trials.[55,60] The MAPPET III trial randomly assigned 256 patients with acute PE and RV dysfunction but without arterial hypotension or shock to heparin plus 100 mg of alteplase (n = 118) or heparin plus placebo (n = 138).[60] The primary endpoint (defined as in-hospital death or clinical deterioration requiring an escalation of treatment, including catecholamine infusion, secondary thrombolysis, endotracheal intubation, CPR, emergency surgical embolectomy, or thrombus fragmentation by catheter) was significantly higher in the placebo group compared to the alteplase group, especially the need for emergency escalation of treatment (24.6% vs. 10.2%, P = .004). There was, however, no mortality difference between the 2 groups (placebo 2.2% vs. alteplase 3.4%, P = .71). There were no episodes of fatal or cerebral bleeding in patients receiving heparin plus alteplase. In the Plasminogen Activator Italian multicenter study 2 (PAIMS 2), 200 patients were randomly allocated intravenous rtPA plus heparin or heparin alone to determine the incidence of pulmonary hypertension following intermediate-risk (submassive) PE.[55] Patients treated with rtPA had a significant reduction in median pulmonary artery systolic pressure as compared to those treated with heparin alone (22 vs. 2 mm Hg; P < .05). At 6 months, 27% of the patients treated with heparin alone developed increased pulmonary artery systolic pressure, suggesting an increased risk of developing long-term chronic thromboembolic pulmonary hypertension.

In a meta-analysis assessing patients with intermediate-risk PE, there was no difference in mortality between those receiving heparin plus thrombolysis compared to heparin alone.[61] The potential benefits of thrombolysis in patients with intermediate risk PE needs to be carefully balanced with the risk of bleeding, especially in patients with absolute and relative contraindications. Even in carefully selected patients without absolute contraindications, the rate of major hemorrhage and hemorrhagic stroke approaches 20% and 3%, respectively.[5] Hence, the clinical benefit of thrombolysis may be present only in a subgroup of patients with intermediate-risk PE, especially in those patients without an elevated risk of bleeding. To further risk-stratify patients in this group, the prospective, international, multicenter, randomized, double-blind Pulmonary Embolism Thrombolysis (PIETHO) trial[62] compared thrombolysis with tenecteplase plus heparin versus placebo plus heparin in 1006 normotensive patients with confirmed PE, RV dysfunction, and elevated troponin levels. The results showed that although death or hemodynamic compromise at day 7 was significantly reduced in the thrombolysis group (2.6% vs. 5.6%, P = .02), thrombolysis was associated with an increased risk of major bleeding in the patients undergoing thrombolysis (extracranial bleeding 6.3% vs. 1.2%, P < .001, and stroke 2.4% vs. 0.2%, P = .003). Current guidelines suggest managing stable patients with intermediate-risk (submassive) PE using therapeutic heparin alone, in a similar manner to low-risk (nonmassive) patients.[12]

In hemodynamically unstable patients (high-risk PE), however, systemic thrombolysis (unless contraindicated) is currently recommended as first-line treatment to decrease the thromboembolic burden on the RV and increase pulmonary perfusion.[51] This is supported by evidence from a prospective randomized controlled trial, in which patients with cardiogenic shock, RV dysfunction, and acute PE were randomized to either streptokinase (1,500,000 IU) followed by intravenous UFH or intravenous UFH alone.[63] The study was stopped early as the 4 patients randomized to streptokinase improved in the first hour after treatment, survived, and at 2-year follow-up were all without pulmonary arterial hypertension, whereas the 4 patients in the heparin-alone group all died within 1 to 3 hours of arrival in the emergency department. These results were confirmed in a meta-analysis of 5 trials with 254 patients that investigated the effectiveness of thrombolysis in patients with high-risk (massive) PE and cardiogenic shock.[57] It showed a significant reduction in recurrent pulmonary embolism or death (9.4% vs. 19.0%; odds ratio, 0.45; 95% confidence interval [CI], 0.22–0.92) with the number needed to treat to prevent one death or recurrent PE being 10. Retrospective data from the ICOPER trial, however, showed that thrombolytic therapy did not significantly reduce 90-day mortality (46.3% vs. 55.1%; hazard ratio, 0.79; 95% CI, 0.44–1.43) in 108 patients with acute PE and cardiogenic shock.[5]

Systemic thrombolysis has been shown to improve hemodynamic parameters in patients with high-risk PE as compared to heparin alone, including a 12% decrease in vascular obstruction, 30% reduction in mean pulmonary arterial pressure, 15% increase in cardiac index, faster improvement in pulmonary blood flow, and improved reduction in the total perfusion defect.[55,64,65] The risk of nonmajor bleeding is significantly increased and major bleeding nonsignificantly increased in patients receiving thrombolysis compared to heparin. Of the 304 patients who received fibrinolysis in the ICOPER registry, 22% had major bleeding complications and 3% had intracranial bleeding.[5,66]

In summary, current guidelines suggest that thrombolytic therapy should be considered for patients with high-risk (massive) PE and an acceptable risk of bleeding complications.[12] Fibrinolysis may be considered for patients with submassive acute PE judged to have clinical evidence of adverse prognosis (new hemodynamic instability, worsening respiratory insufficiency, severe RV dysfunction, or major myocardial necrosis) and low risk of bleeding complications. This, however, needs to be balanced with the increased risk of bleeding. Thrombolytic therapy should be not used in patients with low-risk (nonmassive) PE or stable patients with intermediate-risk (submassive) PE.

Pulmonary Embolectomy

Current indications for surgical embolectomy include patients with massive central PE with contraindications to fibrinolysis or those with persistent hemodynamic compromise or RV dysfunction despite fibrinolytic therapy.[12] In addition, patients with free-floating thrombus within the right heart or with impending paradoxical embolism through a patent foramen ovale should also undergo surgical intervention.[18,67] Before undertaking surgical embolectomy, it is important to radiologically demonstrate a centrally accessible PE, within the main pulmonary trunk, or left or right main pulmonary artery, as patients with the majority of their thrombus burden located peripherally do not benefit from surgery.

Standard surgical technique involves a median sternotomy and institution of cardiopulmonary bypass (CPB), usually with bicaval venous cannulation. This allows careful inspection of the right atrium, interatrial septum, and the RV. In cases in which thrombus is visible in the right atrium on echocardiography, cannulation of the femoral vein and superior vena cava can be used. To minimize myocardial ischemia, the procedure may be performed using normothermic CPB on a beating heart without cross-clamping the aorta. Access to the thrombus is gained via a curved incision in the main pulmonary artery extending into the left pulmonary artery. An additional incision in the right pulmonary artery (between the ascending aorta and superior vena cava) may also be required. Adequate exposure is gained using CPB suction and short episodes of reduced CPB flow. In some patients, cardioplegic arrest with or without systemic hypothermia is required for greater periods of circulatory arrest and better visualization during removal of the thrombus if a patent foramen ovale is present or if intracardiac thrombi are present.[68,69] A combination of curved forceps, Fogarty catheter, suction catheter, and manual compression of the lungs is used to extract the thrombus from the pulmonary arteries. It is important to extract only visible thrombus, which can be achieved up to the level of the segmental pulmonary arteries, and to avoid blind instrumentation of the fragile pulmonary arteries. Intraoperative transesophageal echocardiography can be used to aid thrombus location and extraction.[70] In these patients, protracted weaning of cardiopulmonary bypass may be necessary, especially in patients with RV dysfunction. Bleeding may also be a problem, especially in those who have had preoperative thrombolysis. Heparin is started 6 hours after surgery and continued until warfarin is therapeutic. In patients with persistent RV failure following embolectomy, temporary mechanical support using an RV assist device (RVAD) or extracorporeal membrane oxygenation (ECMO) may also be required.[71]

Compared to medical therapy, surgical embolectomy has been demonstrated to have improved outcomes in patients with massive PE. In a nonrandomized study comparing pulmonary embolectomy versus thrombolysis and best medical therapy, patients in the surgical group had reduced mortality and recurrence of pulmonary embolism.[72] In view of this, some centers have taken a more aggressive approach and extended the indications to also include patients with anatomically extensive PE with RV dysfunction but in the absence of circulatory shock (intermediate-risk PE).[73]

Previously, outcomes following surgical embolectomy were associated with high in-hospital mortality rates.[74] With improved surgical techniques and early intervention, current mortality rates are reported as low as 3.6%.[75] Predictors of early mortality following pulmonary embolectomy include patients with cardiac arrest or undergoing CPR and those with clot extending peripherally into and beyond the subsegmental arteries.[76] Hemodynamically stable patients who undergo surgical intervention have excellent long-term results, with a recent study demonstrating a 3-year survival rate of 83%.[71] The recurrence rate of PE following surgical embolectomy can be as high as 5%.[77]

Surgical embolectomy therefore provides an excellent therapeutic option for patients with high-risk (massive) PE, with comparable early mortality rates and significantly fewer bleeding complications than thrombolysis.[72] Results are worse, however, for those who undergo surgical intervention following CPR or failed thrombolysis.[75]

Catheter-Directed Thrombectomy

Catheter-directed thrombectomy (CdT) is an alternative therapeutic strategy that can be used for the treatment of acute PE. It is usually performed in patients with acute high-risk (massive) PE for whom thrombolysis is contraindicated or has failed and for whom surgical intervention is not available or is contraindicated.[11] CdT is not recommended for patients with low-risk PE or patients with intermediate-risk PE in the absence of hemodynamic instability.[12]

The principal aim of CdT is to achieve rapid debulking of a large central occlusive thrombus to reduce the afterload and strain on the RV, thereby increasing pulmonary and systemic perfusion. The fragmentation process redistributes thrombus into multiple smaller branches further downstream, where the hemodynamic consequence of multiple smaller thrombi in the large volume of the peripheral arterial tree is thought to be less important.[78] Additionally, thrombus fragmentation increases the surface area for exposure to a fibrinolytic agent and intrinsic thrombolytic enzymes to facilitate thrombus dissolution.[79] Using femoral venous access, CdT involves either rheolytic or rotational techniques to disrupt the thrombus in combination with aspiration of the thrombus fragments. Rheolytic techniques use a high-pressured jet system to infuse saline to mechanically disrupt the thrombus.[80] Ultrasound energy can be used to dissociate the fibrin bonds within the thrombus to increase clot permeability and increase the number of receptor sites for fibrinolysis.[81] Rotational techniques involve using a specifically designed thrombectomy catheter, with a covered, high-speed spiral fragmentation tip that rotates at up to 40,000 rpm and also aspirates thrombus fragments.[82]

Complications include distal thrombus embolization, perforation, or dissection of the pulmonary artery, injury to the RV, arrhythmia, pulmonary hemorrhage, pericardial tamponade, and femoral venous injury. To reduce the risk of perforation, only pulmonary artery branches greater than 6 mm should be treated and the procedure should be stopped once the hemodynamic status of the patient improves, irrespective of the angiographic result.[83]

Catheter-directed thrombolysis can be used as an adjunct to CdT,[84] delivering the fibrinolytic agent directly into the PE via a catheter with multiple side holes under fluoroscopic or ultrasound guidance. In combination with CdT, local administration of fibrinolytic agents allows lower doses to be used, as it is delivered directly and the mechanical thrombectomy has increased the surface area of the thrombus available to the drug. The fibrinolytic agent should be injected directly into the thrombus, as any drug injected proximal to the obstructing thrombus will be washed out by the local eddy currents into the nonobstructed pulmonary arteries, thereby reducing its therapeutic efficacy.[85] Results of catheter-directed thrombolysis in patients with acute high-risk (massive) PE were examined in the Pulmonary Embolism Response to Fragmentation, Embolectomy and Catheter Thrombolysis (PERFECT) registry.[86] It assessed 101 patients with acute massive (n = 28) and submassive (n = 73) PE who were treated with catheter-directed mechanical or pharmacomechanical thrombectomy and/or catheter-directed thrombolysis (with rtPA or urokinase). Clinical success—which was defined as hemodynamic stabilization, improvement in pulmonary hypertension and RV strain, and survival to hospital discharge—was achieved in 86% of patients with massive PE and 97% of patients with submassive PE.

ICU MANAGEMENT

The main cause of death in patients with massive PE is cardiogenic shock related to RV dysfunction.[14] Thus, in addition to standard treatment of the critically ill patient, cardiac intensive care management in PE demands consideration of the physiologic role of the RV, knowledge of the mechanisms of RV failure and the pharmacologic and mechanical options available to the intensivist.[87]

The principal roles of the RV are to act as a conduit for blood flow between systemic venous return and the lungs, provide adequate pulmonary flow at an appropriate pressure to allow gas exchange, maintain low filling pressures while avoiding venous congestion and maintaining cardiac output, interact with the pericardium and left heart, and maintain neurohormonal control of the circulation.[88] The RV has important physiologic differences when compared with the LV; these differences become increasingly important when there is an increase in afterload. It has a lower oxygen requirement (lower myocardial mass, preload and afterload), greater extraction reserve, and receives perfusion in both systole and diastole.[89] Thus, as afterload increases, there is a high risk of ischemia with perfusion limited to diastole. The principles of management of RV failure in the context of increased afterload therefore include ensuring optimal preload, maximizing RV contractility, reducing the pulmonary vascular resistance, and achieving adequate aortic root pressure to maintain right coronary artery perfusion.[90]

Optimization of Right Ventricular Preload

Although stroke volume from the RV is highly preload dependent under normal circumstances, in pulmonary hypertension both underfilling and overfilling of the RV may be deleterious.[91] Measured cardiac output may not be an accurate indicator of potential organ damage due to RV failure, as the combination of venous hypertension with only a modest reduction in output may be associated with significant organ dysfunction.[92] Fluid studies in animal models of PE are controversial, with some showing volume loading increasing cardiac index but others demonstrating worsening of shock by induction of RV ischemia and/or reduction in LV filling.[93–95] In the context of massive PE with acute RV failure, a volume challenge may initially increase cardiac output but continued fluid challenges without careful monitoring may result in RV volume overload, venous hypertension, and a progressive fall in cardiac output.[96] This should be suspected if there is a rise in serum lactate, elevation in hepatic enzymes, an abnormal prothrombin time, oliguria, or gastrointestinal dysfunction. Hemodynamic parameters include an increasing V wave on the central venous pressure tracing from increasing tricuspid regurgitation and progressive RV dilatation. In such circumstances, reduction in afterload, removal of volume, and escalation of RV support are indicated, including the use of inotropy and mechanical circulatory support.

Maximizing Right Ventricular Contractility

RV systolic function can be increased with the use of positive inotropic agents or inodilators. A number of studies have been conducted in patients with pulmonary hypertension but no high-quality evidence supports the use of any single vasoactive drug in the context of PE.[97] The most extensively studied inotropic agent is dobutamine.[98] Although low-dose dobutamine (up to 10 μg/kg per minute) improves RV contractility in patients with pulmonary vascular dysfunction, it may, however, demand coadministration of pressor agents. Phosphodiesterase III inhibitors increase RV contractility and also reduce pulmonary vascular resistance but, again, their effects on systemic vascular resistance generally require concomitant administration of pressor agents.[99] The novel agent levosimendan has been shown to reduce pulmonary vascular resistance and increase RV contractility in patients with biventricular dysfunction.[100] Although it has been proposed to improve RV–pulmonary artery coupling in patients with PE, evidence for its use remains limited. The proarrhythmic effects of dopamine significantly limit its use in these patients.

Right Ventricular Afterload

The right ventricle is exquisitely sensitive to increases in afterload. Thus, in addition to the pharmacologic, catheter-based, and surgical techniques described to reduce thrombus burden, manipulation of the pulmonary circulation, modification of ventilatory strategies, maintenance of normocarbia, and avoidance of hypoxia and acidemia may also improve RV function.

Systemic administration of pulmonary vasodilators frequently results in a fall in systemic blood pressure, with the potential to exacerbate RV ischemia and reduce preload. Administration of inhaled pulmonary vasodilators, including nitric oxide, adenosine, prostanoids, phosphodiesterase-5 inhibitors, milrinone, nitroglycerin, and nitroprusside may avoid these systemic effects and act to reduce hypoxic vasoconstriction and improve ventilation-perfusion mismatch.[101] There have been reports of inhaled nitric oxide (iNO) effectively reducing pulmonary vascular resistance and increasing cardiac output in patients with PE, most commonly following surgical embolectomy.[102–104] A recent case series reported rapid and dramatic improvement in hemodynamic parameters and oxygenation in patients with massive PE treated with iNO, suggesting it should be considered as a temporizing agent pending initiation of definitive treatment (thrombolysis, surgery, or catheter-directed thrombectomy) until pulmonary hemodynamics have normalized.[105]

Positive pressure ventilation increases RV afterload and, in adult respiratory distress syndrome, high ventilatory pressures have been associated with increased acute cor pulmonale and increased mortality.[106] This potentially adverse effect has to be balanced against the effects of hypoxia and hypercarbia on the pulmonary circulation, where they act to increase pulmonary vascular resistance and hence RV afterload. Where mechanical ventilation is unavoidable in the context of RV dysfunction, pressures (in particular, positive end-expiratory and plateau pressures) should be limited as far as possible and the inspiratory time should be minimized, especially in patients with restrictive RV physiology.[107]

Coronary Perfusion Pressure

In the context of pulmonary hypertension, when pulmonary vascular resistance exceeds systemic vascular resistance, right coronary artery filling occurs only in diastole. In this scenario, it is essential to maintain aortic diastolic pressure to enable coronary perfusion and avoid ischemia. Although augmentation of aortic root pressure with vasopressors is well established, the beneficial effects must be balanced against potentially detrimental pulmonary vasoconstriction. Sympathomimetic agents include the catecholaminergic vasopressor, norepinephrine, and the noncatecholaminergic vasopressor phenylephrine. The effects on the pulmonary vasculature are complex, relating to dose-dependent α- and β-adrenoreceptor stimulation plus the severity of RV dysfunction.[108] Although arginine vasopressin, acting via the V1 receptor, is a pulmonary vasodilator at low dose, it may cause bradycardia and dose-related myocardial dysfunction at higher doses. There is some evidence, however, that low-dose arginine vasopressin may be of use in cases that are resistant to the usual treatments.[109]

Device Support

A range of devices may be considered to maintain cardiac output in the CICU, including optimization of pacing, Protek-Duo, Impella RP device, ventricular assist devices (VAD) and ECMO. In the critically ill patient with RV dysfunction, atrial arrhythmias are poorly tolerated. Therapeutic options should be to restore and maintain sinus rhythm, optimization of fluid and electrolyte balance, treatment of potential triggers (including sepsis) and institution of pharmacotherapy (amiodarone or digoxin).[110] Ensuring optimal electromechanical activity of the heart can be important but complex and must be individualized to each patient, potentially involving acute temporary pacing (ventricular or atrioventricular),[111] as a restrictive RV that is failing may have a limited stroke volume, requiring a relatively high heart rate to maintain cardiac output. Patients with pulmonary hypertension, however, may have a long duration of systole (indicated by the duration of tricuspid regurgitation on echocardiography), which will limit cardiac filling if the heart rate is excessive. Echocardiography can therefore be used to optimize the heart rate and atrioventricular delay in these patients.

Where cardiogenic shock is present despite all interventions, patients may be considered for advanced mechanical circulatory support. A number of case series have been published using venoarterial extracorporeal membrane oxygenation (VA-ECMO) as a bridge to treatment or recovery in patients with massive PE.[112] Potential advantages over VAD include speed of initiation of therapy, normalization of blood oxygen levels, and bypassing the pulmonary bed, thereby avoiding the potential further elevation of pulmonary pressures.[113] For patients in cardiogenic shock due to massive PE, VA-ECMO can be successful if extracorporeal support is initiated early. Over 48 to 72 hours, emboli will generally either resolve or migrate more distally, allowing patients to be weaned from the mechanical support. VA-ECMO and VAD have also been reported as a successful bridge to recovery in patients who have undergone pulmonary thrombectomy with cardiopulmonary bypass support.[114] Percutaneous right-sided support has also been used in acute RV failure in a range of settings.[115] Although ease of insertion and the ability to also use an oxygenator in the circuit may mean that this will be the preferred mechanical support for massive PE with shock in the future, data are lacking.

Inferior Vena Cava Filter

An inferior vena cava (IVC) filter should be considered in patients with a contraindication to anticoagulation, major bleeding complications during anticoagulation, recurrent embolism while receiving therapeutic anticoagulation, and usually in patients who have required ECMO post-PE.[11,116] They are usually placed in the infrarenal IVC (Fig. 31.3) but can be placed in a suprarenal position if thrombus exists just below the renal veins. The filters can be permanent or retrievable if the patient no longer requires caval interruption.[117] Early complications of IVC filter deployment include device malposition, pneumothorax, hematoma, air embolism, inadvertent carotid artery puncture, and arteriovenous fistula.[118]

The PREPIC trial (Prevention du risque d'embolie pulmonaire par interruption cave), which randomized 400 patients with proximal deep venous thrombosis (DVT) at high risk for PE, demonstrated that placement of an IVC filter significantly reduced the incidence of recurrent PE at 12 days (1.1% vs. 4.8%; $P =$

.03) and at 8 years (6.2% vs. 15.1%; $P = .008$).[119] IVC filters, however, were associated with an increased incidence of recurrent DVT at 2 years (20.8% vs. 11.6%; $P = .02$) and postthrombotic syndrome (40%) and did not improve mortality. As the beneficial effects of implanting an IVC filter in reducing the risk of recurrent PE is accompanied by an increased incidence of recurrent DVT with no effect on overall mortality, the use of an IVC filter in patients with acute PE is not routinely recommended.[12]

LONG-TERM ANTICOAGULATION

The long-term treatment of patients following PE is aimed at preventing extension of the thrombus and recurrent venous thromboembolism.[120] This is achieved with oral anticoagulation using a vitamin K analogue, such as warfarin, aiming for a target international normalized ratio of 2.5 (range, 2.0 to 3.0). The treatment duration is determined by a balance between the risk of recurrence and risk of anticoagulation-related major bleeding. Anticoagulation is recommended for 3 months following a provoked PE, 6 months for an unprovoked PE, and as long as the cancer is active for patients with malignancy.[121] Novel non–vitamin K oral anticoagulant (NOAC) medications—such as dabigatran (factor IIa inhibitor) and rivaroxaban (factor Xa inhibitor)—have been introduced, with the advantage that neither requires dose titration or monitoring.[51] Both have been shown to be noninferior to warfarin with respect to the incidence of recurrent venous thromboembolism or major bleeding.[122,123]

OUTCOMES

Despite the improvement in diagnostic and therapeutic modalities, the contemporary in-hospital mortality rate for patients with PE remains at approximately 7%.[5,124] For patients with high-risk (massive) PE, mortality ranges between 25% and 50%, whereas patients with non-high-risk PE have a lower mortality rate of 3% to 15%. The presence of RV dysfunction and hemodynamic instability are the most significant predictors of a poor early outcome. Long-term predictors of mortality include age and the presence of comorbid conditions, such as congestive heart failure, malignancy, or chronic lung disease. Long-term follow-up of patients following acute PE is required to monitor for the development of chronic thromboembolic pulmonary hypertension.[125]

CONCLUSION

PE is common and potentially lethal, with death usually caused by cardiogenic shock from RV failure. Challenges in diagnosis provided by the often nonspecific symptoms and signs may lead to delay in institution of definitive treatment. Despite the availability of pharmacologic, catheter-based, and surgical interventions, mortality remains high. Strategies to avoid DVT and PE in patients judged to be at risk remain pivotal in reducing PE-associated mortality.

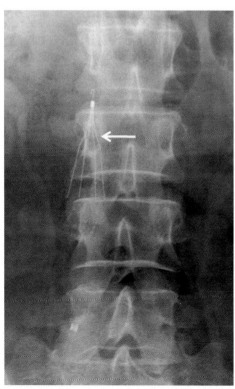

Fig. 31.3 Fluoroscopic image of a temporary caval filter (*arrow*) positioned in the infrarenal vena cava. (Courtesy Dr. Deepa Gopalan, Cambridge, UK.)

The full reference list for this chapter is available at ExpertConsult.com.

32

Pulmonary Hypertension

Demosthenes G. Papamatheakis, William R. Auger

Over the past 2 decades, significant advances have been made in the understanding of the pathophysiology of pulmonary hypertension. In addition, dramatic improvements have occurred in the diagnostic and therapeutic approach of patients afflicted with this disease. The resulting development of new interventions for disease management has fundamentally transformed its natural history and has improved the perception of its various phenotypes. This has enabled a more detailed classification of the various pulmonary hypertension subtypes, leading to a more structured approach to patient care. The purpose of this chapter is to offer the latest information on disease classification, epidemiology, and clinical presentation, and to provide guidance for a systematic approach to both the diagnosis and therapy in patients with pulmonary hypertensive disorders.

DEFINITION OF PULMONARY HYPERTENSION

Pulmonary hypertension (PH) refers to elevated pressures in the pulmonary vascular bed and is defined by a mean pulmonary artery pressure (PAP) greater than or equal to 25 mm Hg confirmed by right heart catheterization.[1] Pulmonary arterial hypertension (PAH), which is an important PH subtype that will be discussed extensively in this chapter, also requires a pulmonary artery occlusion pressure (PAOP) of 15 mm Hg or less and a pulmonary vascular resistance (PVR) greater than 3 Wood units.

The pulmonary circulation extends from the pulmonic valve to the left atrium and consists of the pulmonary outflow track; the right and left main pulmonary arteries; the lobar, segmental, and subsegmental arteries; the pulmonary arterioles; and the capillaries, venules, and larger pulmonary veins. PH may refer to elevated pulmonary artery pressures (precapillary PH), elevated pulmonary venous pressures (postcapillary PH) or, less frequently, a combination of the two. The initial classification of PH included PH without an identifiable cause (primary), and PH with an identifiable cause (secondary). In the last 15 years, however, there has been increasing understanding of the different etiologies of PH, revealing the need for a more nuanced classification scheme. To better demarcate specific categories of the disease, with similar pathophysiologic mechanisms, presentation, and therapies, major changes to the classification of PH were introduced in the 1990s (Box 32.1).[2] Although the general architecture of the classification has been maintained since the introduction of the World Health Organization (WHO) groups in 1998, multiple classification updates have been published by various professional societies, with incremental modifications.[3–5]

CLINICAL PRESENTATION

The symptoms associated with PH are widely nonspecific and are, in large part, related to the severity and stage of the disease. The most common presenting symptoms are dyspnea on exertion

BOX 32.1   Pulmonary Hypertension Classification

Group 1: Pulmonary Arterial Hypertension

1.1 Idiopathic

1.2 Heritable

    1.2.1 BMPR2 mutation

    1.2.2 Other mutations

1.3 Drugs and toxins induced

1.4 Associated with:

    1.4.1 Connective tissue disease

    1.4.2 Congenital heart disease

    1.4.3 Portal hypertension

    1.4.4 Human immunodeficiency virus (HIV) infection

    1.4.5 Schistosomiasis

Group 1′: Pulmonary Veno-Occlusive Disease and/or Pulmonary Capillary Hemangiomatosis

1′.1 Idiopathic

1′.2 Heritable

    1′.2.1 EIF2AK4 mutation

    1′.2.2 Other mutations

1′.3 Drugs, toxins, and radiation induced

1′.4 Associated with

    1′.4.1 Connective tissue disease

    1′.4.2 HIV infection

Group 1″: Persistent Pulmonary Hypertension of the Newborn

Group 2: Pulmonary Hypertension Owing to Left Heart Disease

2.1. Left ventricular systolic dysfunction

2.2 Left ventricular diastolic dysfunction

2.3 Valvular disease

2.4 Congenital/acquired left heart inflow/outflow tract obstruction and congenital cardiomyopathies

2.5 Congenital/acquired pulmonary veins stenosis

Group 3: Pulmonary Hypertension Owing to Lung Diseases and/or Hypoxia

3.1 Chronic obstructive pulmonary disease

3.2 Interstitial lung disease

3.3 Other pulmonary diseases with mixed restrictive and obstructive pattern

3.4 Sleep-disordered breathing

3.5 Alveolar hypoventilation disorders

3.6 Chronic exposure to high altitude

3.7 Developmental lung diseases

Group 4: Chronic Thromboembolic Pulmonary Hypertension and Other Pulmonary Artery Obstructions

4.1 Chronic thromboembolic pulmonary hypertension

4.2 Other pulmonary artery obstructions

    4.2.1 Angiosarcoma

    4.2.2 Other intravascular tumors

    4.2.3 Arteritis

    4.2.4 Congenital pulmonary artery stenoses

    4.2.5 Parasites (hydatidosis)

Group 5: Pulmonary Hypertension With Unclear and/or Multifactorial Mechanisms

5.1 Hematologic disorders: chronic hemolytic anemia, myeloproliferative disorders, splenectomy

5.2 Systemic disorders: sarcoidosis, pulmonary histiocytosis, lymphangioleiomyomatosis

5.3 Metabolic disorders: glycogen storage disease, Gaucher disease, thyroid disorders

5.4 Others: pulmonary tumoral thrombotic microangiopathy, fibrosing mediastinitis, chronic renal failure (with or without dialysis), segmental pulmonary hypertension

Modified from Galie N, Humbert M, Vachiery JL, et al. 2015 ESC/ERS Guidelines for the diagnosis and treatment of pulmonary hypertension: The Joint Task Force for the Diagnosis and Treatment of Pulmonary Hypertension of the European Society of Cardiology (ESC) and the European Respiratory Society (ERS): Endorsed by: Association for European Paediatric and Congenital Cardiology (AEPC), International Society for Heart and Lung Transplantation (ISHLT). *Eur Heart J.* 2016;37:67–119.

and gradual exercise intolerance. Of note, these symptoms tend to be progressive with time, resulting in a steady decline of functional capacity and a worsening in dyspnea. Less common symptoms include easy fatigability, cough, hemoptysis, hoarseness (from compression of the left recurrent laryngeal nerve by an enlarged pulmonary artery), or chest discomfort. In advanced disease, symptoms related to right ventricular (RV) failure start to manifest, including lower extremity edema, abdominal distention, shortness of breath at rest, chest pain, and syncope.

On physical examination, most patients with PH exhibit subtle findings unless they are in RV failure. These include widening of the S2 heart sound and accentuation of its P2 component. In more severe or later-stage disease, possible additional findings include elevated jugular venous pressure, a positive hepatojugular reflux, a fixed split S_2, right-sided S_4 and/or S_3 heart sounds, a murmur associated with tricuspid regurgitation or pulmonic insufficiency, an RV heave, ascites, abdominal distention, hepatomegaly, and/or lower extremity edema. Clubbing is not a common finding in PH, but can be present in cases of comorbid parenchymal lung disease or right-to-left shunt. Cyanosis is also not common unless the above comorbidities are present or in the presence of right-to-left shunting through a patent foramen ovale in cases of severe right atrial pressure elevation.

During the evaluation of the patient with PH, a modified New York Heart Association functional classification is used to stratify symptoms and function of PH patients. In the WHO Functional Classification, patients are categorized into four classes depending on severity of symptoms, as shown in Table 32.1.[6] In addition to functional class (FC), recent guidelines have suggested the use of clinical, laboratory, and other testing data (i.e., presence of syncope, N-terminal pro b-type natriuretic peptide [NT-proBNP] plasma levels, 6-minute walk distance, right heart catheterization hemodynamics) in order to risk-stratify patients to low-, moderate- or high-risk groups, corresponding to a 1-year mortality of less than 5%, 5% to 10%, and greater than 10%, respectively.[2]

TABLE 32.1 World Health Organization (WHO) Functional Classification in Patients With Pulmonary Hypertension

WHO Functional Class	Symptoms (Increased Dyspnea, Fatigue, Chest Pain, or Presyncope)
Class I	No significant symptoms with ordinary physical activity
Class II	Symptoms with ordinary activity; slight limitation of activity
Class III	Symptoms with less than ordinary activity; marked limitation of activity
Class IV	Symptoms with any activity or at rest; unable to perform any physical activity.

Modified from Barst RJ, McGoon M, Torbicki A, et al. Diagnosis and differential assessment of pulmonary arterial hypertension. *J Am Coll Cardiol.* 2004;43:40S–47S.

DIAGNOSIS

One of the biggest challenges in PH management has been delay in diagnosis. Registry data indicate a mean time between symptom onset and diagnosis of PAH (a distinct pulmonary hypertension subgroup) of between 2.3 and 2.8 years.[7,8] Significant efforts have been made to increase awareness of the disease in the medical community and empower physicians to consider it in unexplained dyspnea. This could allow for earlier initiation of the appropriate workup and possible referral to a specialty center with the option to intervene earlier in the disease process. The latter could be beneficial, since it could delay disease progression and the development of right heart failure[9] that, in turn, has been associated with worse prognosis and poorer survival.[10,11] Once PH is suspected, a detailed and thorough history and physical examination can assess for specific risk factors and help identify the possible etiology.

The basis of PH screening is echocardiography and the cornerstone of PH diagnosis is right heart catheterization. However, there are several other studies that play a role in the workup of PH (Fig. 32.1). Echocardiography provides an estimate of the RV systolic pressure (RVSP) based on the tricuspid regurgitant jet velocity and the right atrial (RA) pressure estimate. The tricuspid regurgitant jet velocity can be used to calculate the pressure gradient between the RV and the RA based on the Bernoulli principle (gradient is equal to 4 times the squared regurgitant jet velocity), whereas the RA pressure can, in most cases, be inferred from the size of the inferior vena cava. Although there are no published consensus guidelines on the RVSP value beyond which PH is considered, most echocardiography laboratories use 35 to 40 mm Hg. Moreover, an echocardiogram can give qualitative information regarding the RA (dilatation) and RV (enlargement, hypertrophy, or decreased function) that can indicate right heart dysfunction in the setting of PH.

The recommended diagnostic steps once PH is suspected are to assess for other respiratory abnormalities (pulmonary function tests, polysomnography or overnight oximetry, chest radiograph), an electrocardiogram (ECG) to further evaluate for arrhythmias or other cardiac pathology, ventilation perfusion scintigraphy to rule out chronic thromboembolic pulmonary hypertension, and blood testing for connective tissue diseases (antinuclear antibody, rheumatoid factor), liver disease (liver function tests), and human immunodeficiency virus (HIV) infection. The workup culminates with a right heart catheterization, in which these definitions are used to confirm PH (mean PAP ≥25 mm Hg) and/or PAH (mean PAP ≥25 mm Hg, PAOP ≤15 mm Hg, and PVR >3 Wood units). During the right heart catheterization, a vasodilator or vasoreactivity challenge is performed, which includes the use of a vasodilatory agent (most commonly, inhaled nitric oxide [NO]) to assess acute vasoreactivity. Patients with PAH are considered to have a positive vasoreactivity test if their mean PAP decreases by at least 10 mm Hg and to less than 40 mm Hg.[6] These vasoreactive patients (~5% of the PAH population) tend to have a better prognosis and can be managed with calcium channel antagonists,[12,13] which are not used in nonvasoreactive patients. Interestingly, approximately 50% of these patients will stop being vasoreactive within the first 1 or 2 years of diagnosis and may need additional medical therapy. Fig. 32.1 depicts the diagnostic algorithm for PH.

CLASSIFICATION, PATHOPHYSIOLOGY, AND MANAGEMENT

WHO Group 1

WHO Group 1 PH, or PAH, has a distinct pathophysiology, natural history, and response to treatment. As previously noted, PAH is PH (mean PAP ≥25 mm Hg) with the additional criteria of PVR greater than 3 Wood units and PAOP less than or equal to 15 mm Hg.[1] This is in the absence of other causes of precapillary PH, such as chronic thromboembolic pulmonary hypertension (CTEPH), which can fulfill this definition, but also includes chronic thromboembolic disease. PAH is subcategorized based on etiology, as shown in Box 32.1. Although these etiologic factors seem to be inherently heterogeneous, they result in similar pulmonary vascular pathology, pathobiology, and clinical presentation; thus, they are grouped together.

Epidemiology. The incidence and prevalence of PAH have been derived from several large registries summarized in Table 32.2.[7,14–16] Mean age of onset for PAH has ranged from 36 to 52 years,[14,17] with the younger populations reported from China and the older from Europe and from the United States. All of the above registries show a clear female predominance, ranging from 65% to 80%, although this may be less pronounced in the older populations.

Pathophysiology, Pathobiology, and Pathology. The pathophysiologic basis of PAH is thought to be multidimensional; numerous prior reviews and updates have summarized key findings.[18–22] Although PAH was previously thought to primarily be a disease of excessive pulmonary vasoconstriction, it is now evident that there are additional pathobiologic components playing a role, including endothelial dysfunction, abnormal cell proliferation and apoptosis, shift of cellular metabolism, genetic predisposition, coagulation dysregulation, and inflammation.

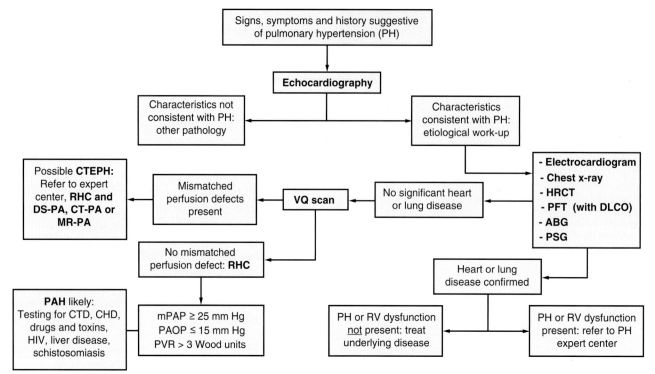

Fig. 32.1 Diagnostic algorithm for suspected pulmonary hypertension. *ABG*, Arterial blood gas; *CHD*, congenital heart disease; *CTD*, connective tissue disease; *CTEPH*, chronic thromboembolic pulmonary hypertension; *CT-PA*, computed tomography pulmonary angiography; *DLCO*, carbon monoxide diffusion capacity; *DS-PA*, digital subtraction pulmonary angiography; *HIV*, human immunodeficiency virus; *HRCT*, high-resolution computed tomography; *mPAP*, mean pulmonary artery pressure; *MR-PA*, magnetic resonance pulmonary angiography; *PAH*, pulmonary arterial hypertension; *PAOP*, pulmonary artery occlusion pressure; *PFT*, pulmonary function testing; *PH*, pulmonary hypertension; *PSG*, polysomnogram; *PVR*, pulmonary vascular resistance; *RHC*, right heart catheterization; *RV*, right ventricle; *VQ*: ventilation perfusion scintigraphy; *x-ray*, radiography. (Modified from Galie N, Humbert M, Vachiery JL, et al. 2015 ESC/ERS Guidelines for the diagnosis and treatment of pulmonary hypertension: The Joint Task Force for the Diagnosis and Treatment of Pulmonary Hypertension of the European Society of Cardiology (ESC) and the European Respiratory Society (ERS): Endorsed by: Association for European Paediatric and Congenital Cardiology (AEPC), International Society for Heart and Lung Transplantation (ISHLT). *Eur Heart J.* 2016;37:67–119.)

TABLE 32.2	Summary of Pulmonary Arterial Hypertension Epidemiology Based on Large Registries		
Registry	**Incidence (Cases Per Million Adult Population)**	**Prevalence (Cases per Million Adult Population)**	**Notes**
Scottish[14]	7.1–7.6	26–52	Retrospective; some data based on disease codes
French[7]	2.4	15	Prospective; hemodynamic and clinical data
REVEAL[15]	2	10.6	Prospective; matched French cohort hemodynamic and clinical data
Spanish[16]	3.2	16	Mostly retrospective, with 2 years of prospective data

Excessive vasoconstriction in PAH has been linked to abnormalities of function or expression of potassium channels located on pulmonary artery smooth muscle cells,[23] impaired production of vasodilators from the endothelium (i.e., NO from endothelial NO synthase),[24,25] and overexpression of vasoconstrictors (i.e., thromboxane A2, endothelin-1, and serotonin).[25–27] Some of these factors, together with vascular effector imbalances (frequently, growth factors—such as platelet-derived growth factor, fibroblast growth factor, and TGFb),[28] impact vascular remodeling by augmenting postapoptotic endothelial cell[29] and pulmonary artery smooth muscle cell proliferation,[29–31] as well as activation of adventitial fibroblasts[32] and metalloproteases.[33] Moreover, these dysregulations can result in an imbalanced prothrombotic microenvironment,[28] causing thrombus formation within the pulmonary circulation, which further exacerbates pulmonary vascular obstruction and lumen narrowing.[34] The role of inflammation in PAH has been confirmed based on pathologic findings of perivascular inflammatory components[35] and is thought to be a significant disease factor, albeit not a well-elucidated one.[36] Finally, it has been hypothesized that, as seen in cancer biology,[37] PAH is characterized by a shift of mitochondrial metabolism from oxidative to glycolytic.[38,39] This is believed to make cells more resistant to apoptosis, hence allowing overproliferation.[37]

Taken together, the above changes result in thickening of the pulmonary artery wall and narrowing of the pulmonary artery lumen, which can eventually be obliterated. These pathologic changes are only present in the arteries (pulmonary veins are not usually affected) and tend to appear in vessels approximately 500 μm in diameter or smaller. Pathologic changes include intimal hyperplasia, medial hypertrophy, and adventitial thickening with perivascular inflammatory infiltrates.[35] End-stage forms of these changes are the previously described complex/plexiform lesions, which can also include in situ thrombotic material.[34,35]

Clinical Presentation and Natural History.
The initial clinical presentation of PAH does not significantly differ from other forms of PH. Registry data reveal that patients may go years with dyspnea on exertion prior to getting the correct diagnosis.[8] Symptoms of right heart failure are more common in PAH than other groups of PH, as the disease severity tends to be higher. Signs and symptoms of underlying disease processes—such as chronic liver disease, HIV/AIDS, congenital heart disease, or connective tissue disease—can also be present. Longer term, PAH has a worse prognosis in general than most other forms of PH and a lower survival rate,[40] mostly owing to disease progression leading to RV dysfunction and failure.

Etiologic categories
Idiopathic. Idiopathic PAH, which is usually diagnosed when other possible causes of PAH have been ruled out, tends to be sporadic in nature. It is the most common form of PAH in the Western world, accounting for approximately 40% to 50% of PAH cases,[7,8,41] and second to congenital heart disease–associated PAH in China (~35% of PAH cases).[17] Idiopathic PAH incidence, as reported by various registries, is estimated to range between 0.9 and 2.6 cases per million adults.[7,14–16] Idiopathic PAH prevalence is estimated to be between 4.6 and 9 cases per million adults.[7,14–16] Although the earlier registries[42] and the ones from China[17] show a younger mean age at diagnosis of idiopathic PAH (approximately 36 years old), most other registries note a mean age of diagnosis between 46 and 65 years old. Female predominance varies depending on the registry but, similar to PAH, ranges from 62% to 83%.[7,14–17,42]

Heritable. Heritable PAH is relatively similar to idiopathic PAH but has a clear association to a genetic defect and accounts for approximately 3% to 4% of PAH cases.[7,8,41] Previously known as familial PAH, heritable PAH has been associated with multiple genetic mutations that are the focus of ongoing research. The most common PAH-associated mutations are encoding for the bone morphogenetic protein receptor type 2 (BMPR2), a member of the tumor growth factor-β (TGF-β) family. This is usually an autosomal dominant trait, which is modulated by factors such as variable expressivity and incomplete penetrance. The latter is estimated to be approximately 27% for both genders (42% in females and 14% in males)[43] and may be affected by female hormones. It is estimated that more than 70% of families with

heritable PAH have one of the more than 300 independent BMPR2 mutations.[44] Moreover, it is thought that up to 26% of sporadic and previously thought to be idiopathic cases of PAH can be attributed to mutations of this gene[45,46] and therefore pose a hereditary risk to other family members. Two other members of the TGF-β cell signaling family have also been associated with heritable PAH (specifically in relation to hereditary hemorrhagic telangiectasia): activin-like kinase-type 1 (ALK1) and endoglin (ENG).[47] In addition, mutations of the bone morphogenetic responsive-gene *SMAD9* (also known as *SMAD8*),[48] the gene encoding for a membrane protein of caveloae caveolin-1,[49] and the gene encoding for the potassium channel KCNK3 have also been implicated in multiple cases of heritable PAH.[50] Interestingly, registry data indicate that patients with heritable PAH tend to develop the disease at a younger age, are more severely ill at diagnosis, and have accelerated disease progression[51] compared to idiopathic PAH, although they both retain a female preponderance (~1.8 : 1)[42] and have similar pathophysiology and pathology.

Drug and toxin related. Expert opinion regarding which drugs and toxins are associated with PAH development has changed over the years. Based on recently published guidelines,[2,4] these substances are categorized based on the level of evidence for association with disease development. A "definite" association is based on large, multicenter epidemiologic studies or an epidemic. A "likely" association is based on multiple case series or a single-center, case-control study. A "possible" association lacks any related studies but features substances that have similar mechanisms of action as the ones in the prior two categories. Finally, an "unlikely" association is based on negative epidemiologic studies that failed to show a link between the substance and the development of PAH. The current drugs and toxins with these defined PAH associations are listed in Table 32.3. Of note, selective serotonin reuptake inhibitors (SSRIs) have been associated with increased risk of primary pulmonary hypertension of the newborn (PPHN) when taken by their mothers during pregnancy.[52] Epidemiologic data are lacking regarding this type of PAH.

Associated. Associated PAH includes PAH in the setting of connective tissue disease, congenital heart disease, HIV infection, portal hypertension, or schistosomiasis (see Box 32.1) and accounts for approximately 50% of all PAH.[7,8,41]

Connective tissue disease–associated PAH (CTD-PAH) has been well described in systemic sclerosis, systemic lupus erythematosus, and mixed connective tissue disease. It can also be seen with rheumatoid arthritis, dermatomyositis, and Sjögrens syndrome.[53,54] It has an estimated prevalence of 2.3 to 10 cases per million adults[7,14,54] and is the most common form of associated PAH in the Western world (15%–30% of all PAH), with systemic sclerosis (particularly the limited cutaneous form) being the most common diagnosis.[7,15,16,54,55] In China, CTD-PAH is the third most frequent form of PAH after congenital heart disease–associated and idiopathic PAH, with systemic lupus erythematosus being the more common diagnosis rather than systemic sclerosis.[17,41,53] Scleroderma-related CTD-PAH has a strong female predominance (~80% females), a mean age of diagnosis greater than 60 years, and a shorter survival time compared to idiopathic

TABLE 32.3	Drugs and Toxins Associated With Pulmonary Arterial Hypertension		
Definite	**Likely**	**Possible**	**Unlikely**
Aminorex	Amphetamines	Cocaine	Oral contraceptives
Fenfluramine	L-Tryptophan	Phenylpropanolamine	Estrogen
Dexfenfluramine	Methamphetamines	St. John's wort	Cigarette smoking
Toxic rapeseed oil	Dasatinib	Amphetamine-like drugs	
Benfluorex		Interferon α and β	
SSRIs[a]		Chemotherapeutic agents[b]	

Modified from Galie N, Humbert M, Vachiery JL, et al. 2015 ESC/ERS Guidelines for the diagnosis and treatment of pulmonary hypertension: The Joint Task Force for the Diagnosis and Treatment of Pulmonary Hypertension of the European Society of Cardiology (ESC) and the European Respiratory Society (ERS): Endorsed by: Association for European Paediatric and Congenital Cardiology (AEPC), International Society for Heart and Lung Transplantation (ISHLT). *Eur Heart J.* 2016;37:67–119.
[a]Increases risk of persistent pulmonary hypertension of the newborn in mothers taking SSRIs during gestation.
[b]Mostly alkylating agents, such as mytomycin C and cyclophosphamide.

PAH[56–58] despite having similar outcome predictors[59] and pathophysiology. The early detection[60] and appropriate management of these patients is very important, as PAH is a leading cause of death in systemic sclerosis.[61]

Congenital heart disease-associated PAH (CHD-PAH) is the second most common form of associated PAH in Europe and the United States (10% to 23% of all PAH) after CTD-PAH[7,15] and the most common form of PAH overall in China (43%).[17] Improvement in childhood CHD management has resulted in a larger number of adult CHD patients with higher disease complexity. A clinical subclassification of this category of associated PAH is now recommended (Box 32.2) to better characterize each individual patient.[2] Depending on their stratification, these patients may have different presentations and prognoses. Eisenmenger syndrome, for example, in which the shunt is now right to left due to high right-sided pressures, can have more dramatic findings and complications (cyanosis, erythrocytosis, hemoptysis, cerebrovascular accidents, brain abscesses, and so on) than other forms. Despite these factors, patients with Eisenmenger syndrome have improved survival compared to untreated idiopathic PAH.[62] Although the reason for this is unclear, RV adaptation since birth and the possible pressure relief from the right-to-left shunt in relation to cardiovascular hemodynamics are mechanisms thought to affect survival.[63] On the other hand, the worst survival in CHD-PAH has been noted in post-CHD repair or PAH patients with small, coincidental defects.[64] Epidemiologic data are not robust, mostly due to their retrospective nature and the lack of uniformity regarding PAH definition or diagnosis in CHD patients. A European survey noted that as many as 28% of CHD adult patients may have pulmonary hypertension,[65] although a more conservative estimate may be closer to 6%.[66] Based on data extrapolated from international registries, CHD-PAH prevalence likely ranges between 1.7 and 12 cases per million adults.[7,14] It is not entirely clear why some patients with CHD will develop PAH compared to others, but the suspected explanation relates to increased blood flow through the pulmonary vascular system. The latter, a direct result from a systemic-to-pulmonary shunt, leads to increased pressures, endothelial dysfunction, vascular remodeling, and eventual pulmonary obstructive arteriopathy as seen in other forms of PAH. The subsequent PVR elevation results in eventual shunt reversal (pulmonary-to-systemic;

BOX 32.2 Congenital Heart Disease–Associated Pulmonary Artery Hypertension Subclassification

1. Eisenmenger Syndrome
This category includes all large intracardiac and extracardiac defects that begin as systemic-to-pulmonary shunts and progress with time to severe elevation of PVR and to reversal (pulmonary-to-systemic) or bidirectional shunting. Cyanosis, secondary erythrocytosis, and multiple organ involvement are usually present.

2. PAH Associated With Prevalent Systemic-to-Pulmonary Shunts
This category includes moderate to large defects, in which PVR is mildly to moderately increased, systemic-to-pulmonary shunting is still prevalent, and cyanosis at rest is not a feature. They are divided into correctable (surgically or with intravascular percutaneous procedure) and noncorrectable.

3. PAH With Small/Coincidental Defects[a]
This category includes PAH with significant PVR elevation in the presence of small cardiac defects (usually ventricular septal defects <1 cm and atrial septal defects <2 cm of effective diameter as assessed by echocardiography), which themselves do not account for the development of the PVR elevation. The clinical picture is very similar to idiopathic PAH and closing the defects is contraindicated.

4. PAH After Defect Correction
This category includes persisting PAH after congenital heart disease repair, either immediately after correction or developing within months to years after correction. This is in the absence of any significant postoperative hemodynamic lesions.

Modified from Galie N, Humbert M, Vachiery JL, et al. 2015 ESC/ERS Guidelines for the diagnosis and treatment of pulmonary hypertension: The Joint Task Force for the Diagnosis and Treatment of Pulmonary Hypertension of the European Society of Cardiology (ESC) and the European Respiratory Society (ERS): Endorsed by: Association for European Paediatric and Congenital Cardiology (AEPC), International Society for Heart and Lung Transplantation (ISHLT). Eur Heart J 2016;37:67-119.
[a]Size applies to adult patients.
PAH, Pulmonary arterial hypertension; *PVR,* pulmonary vascular resistance.

Eisenmenger syndrome) once pulmonary artery pressures start exceeding systemic pressures.[67] The presence of PAH has a documented negative impact on CHD patient outcomes[68] and there should be a high level of suspicion for PAH development and for screening of the disease in this population.[4]

HIV-associated PAH (HIV-PAH) has a relatively low prevalence of approximately 0.45%[69] and does not seem to have changed significantly despite the increased use of highly active antiretroviral therapy (HAART).[70] Nevertheless, the incidence of PAH in patients with HIV may have decreased since the advent of HAART, with some studies suggesting that it may have beneficial effects on pulmonary hemodynamics over time.[71,72] Therefore, the stable prevalence is likely a function of the overall increased survival of HIV-infected patients. Of note, these patients may also present with other comorbidities, such as drug or toxin exposure[73,74] or liver disease, which can also predispose to PH, making determining disease etiology less straightforward. Although the pathogenesis of HIV-PAH is unclear, the resulting pathology is similar to what is seen in idiopathic PAH. There is no evidence that HIV infects pulmonary endothelial cells or that viral proteins are found in the pulmonary vasculature of HIV-PAH patients. Prevailing pathogenetic theories include an indirect role of the virus through inflammatory or tissue growth pathways and/or a possible genetic predisposition being unmasked by the virus.[72]

Approximately 4% to 6% of patients with portal hypertension will develop PAH (portopulmonary hypertension [PoPH]).[75,76] It is mostly related to the presence of portal hypertension regardless of the presence of cirrhosis, the level of hepatic impairment, and the type of liver disease. Although clinically very similar to other forms of PAH, the pathogenesis of PoPH is not well defined. High cardiac output and elevated blood flow through the pulmonary vasculature noted in liver disease and portal hypertension are thought to play a significant role in the development of the disease, with PoPH patients having higher cardiac index (CI) and lower PVR than idiopathic PAH patients.[8,77] Survival of patients with PoPH is similar or even worse than those with idiopathic PAH,[7,8] and the presence of significant PoPH (in contrast to mild PoPH with normal PVR) is a major risk factor for liver transplantation.[78]

Schistosomiasis-associated PAH (Sch-PH) is the most common form of PAH worldwide but is rare in the United States and Europe.[79] This is owing to the very large number of *Schistosoma*-infected individuals found in endemic areas (Sub-Saharan Africa, South America, the Caribbean, the Middle East, and parts of Asia).[80] One of the challenges of Sch-PH is the lack of a widely recognized disease definition, although it is most commonly defined as the presence of PAH in conjunction with active *Schistosoma* infection or prior infection/exposure and evidence of hepatosplenic schistosomiasis, a chronic form of the disease.[81] For those reasons and the variable definitions used for PAH in prior studies,[82,83] the prevalence of Sch-PH is estimated to be between 8% and 25% of patients with chronic hepatosplenic schistosomiasis. The latter represents approximately 10% to 25% of the estimated 20 million people worldwide with chronic schistosomiasis.[79] Sch-PH is now thought to be a reactive arteriopathy in response to parasitic granulomas with pathologic changes similar to idiopathic PAH.

Management. In the last 20 years, the knowledge surrounding PAH management and the available pharmacotherapies have increased significantly. Initial registries showed a 1- and 5-year survival of 68% and 34%, respectively, in incident idiopathic PAH.[84] Almost a decade later, although similar survival can be seen in developing countries,[85] developed countries report survival for all PAH between 79% and 93% for 1 year and 48% and 68% for 5 years.[10,86–90] Although these changes can be partly attributed to increased awareness and recognition of the disease at an earlier stage, inclusion of prevalent and incident cases, analyzing all forms of PAH, and a possibly shifting disease phenotype (i.e., older population),[41] some can also be attributed to the advent of new therapies. The wealth of data derived from multiple registries has also resulted in several prognostic equations or calculators for patient risk stratification[10,84,86,91] that have been validated in subsequent studies.[92–94] Overall, the management of PAH can be divided into general measures, supportive therapies, specific PAH-targeted drug treatments and, eventually, lung transplantation in cases of end-stage disease or atrial septostomy when the latter is not available.[2,95]

General measures are mostly related to recommendations on basic medical interventions as well as physical and daily living activities. These include pregnancy avoidance in female PAH patients, as pregnancy of child-bearing age can result in significant morbidity and mortality,[96,97] psychosocial support, and maintaining some level of physical activity. This can be accomplished in the form of cardiopulmonary rehabilitation, which can be beneficial in PAH patients.[98,99] Other general measures include medication compliance, infection avoidance and prevention, hypoxia avoidance, and genetic counseling. Despite the paucity of evidence regarding their efficacy, these are still recommended for PAH patient management.[2]

Supportive therapies are also based on limited clinical evidence. Anticoagulation is recommended for idiopathic PAH, heritable PAH, and anorexigen-associated PAH based on retrospective data indicating potentially favorable outcomes.[12,100] On the other hand, recent registry data[101,102] are less convincing or even conflicting regarding their efficacy. Diuretics have a clear role in the management of PAH, especially in the setting of decompensated RV failure and volume overload. Although studies are lacking, there is a symptomatic benefit that has been empirically documented. The use of oxygen therapy in hypoxic patients attempts to mitigate hypoxic pulmonary vasoconstriction and comes from studies in chronic obstructive pulmonary disease (COPD).[103] The use of digoxin as a positive inotrope for the dysfunctional RV, and managing anemia and iron deficiency (which are common in patients with PAH) are also therapies that lack long-term evidence.

PAH pharmacotherapy is generally based on inhibiting proliferation and inducing vasodilation, but there seem to be other beneficial effects of these specific medications that have not been clearly defined. Calcium-channel blockers (CCBs) have mostly a vasodilatory effect and were the cornerstone of PAH medical therapy prior to the advent of PAH-specific medications. It is now recognized that they are effective in only a small percentage of patients with idiopathic PAH that are acutely vasoreactive.[12,13] Efficient doses are on the higher end of the spectrum; patients need to be closely monitored for side effects as well as for inadequate response or eventual deterioration, in which case additional PAH-specific therapy should be implemented. In nonvasoreactive patients, CCB treatment is not recommended as there may be side effects without any benefit.[104]

Unlike CCBs, PAH-specific medications work through one of three distinct pathways, including the prostacyclin, endothelin, and NO/cyclic-guanosine monophosphate (cGMP) pathways. These are all thought to work in parallel via pulmonary artery endothelial and smooth muscle cells to regulate vascular contractility and remodeling.

The prostacyclin pathway has both vasodilator and antiproliferative effects[105]; studies show both a decrease in prostacyclin synthase expression[106] and endogenous prostacyclin[25] in PAH. Prostacyclin (prostaglandin I_2) is produced from arachidonic acid within the pulmonary artery (PA) endothelial cells and binds to prostacyclin receptors on the PA smooth muscle cell wall. Through second messengers, it induces cyclic adenosine monophosphate production, which leads to smooth muscle cell relaxation and growth inhibition.[107] Of note, it also acts as an inhibitor of platelet aggregation.[108] Exogenous prostacyclin can have similar effects and is available for therapeutic purposes. Epoprostenol requires continuous intravenous (IV) infusion through a tunneled central venous catheter and has a half-life of 3 to 5 minutes. In unblinded randomized controlled trials in various forms of PAH,[109–111] it improved symptoms, exercise capacity, hemodynamics, and mortality.[110] Treprostinil is an epoprostenol analogue that can be administered subcutaneously and intravenously and has an approximate plasma half-life of 1.5 and 0.5 hours, respectively. The subcutaneous form has been shown to improve symptoms, exercise capacity, and hemodynamics in a randomized controlled trial.[112] Its IV form has similar pharmacokinetics[113] and has been shown to be safe and effective in both shorter-term[114] and longer-term[115] open label, observational studies. One randomized controlled trial on IV treprostinil was stopped early owing to safety reasons and the data are considered unreliable.[116] Treprostinil is also available in inhaled form, which has been shown to improve 6-minute walk distance and quality of life when added to PAH patients on background therapy.[117] The oral form of treprostinil showed a 6-minute walk distance improvement in PAH patients when used as a monotherapy,[118] but this improvement failed to reach statistical significance in patients on background PAH therapy.[119,120] Iloprost, mostly used as an inhaled formulation, has shown improvements in exercise capacity, symptoms, pulmonary vascular resistance, and reduction in clinical events as a PAH monotherapy[121] and improvement in exercise capacity when added on to background PAH therapy.[122] Finally, selexipag is an oral prostacyclin receptor agonist that has been shown to reduce the risk of a composite morbidity and mortality outcome measure in a very large, event-driven randomized controlled trial.[123] Side effects of prostacyclin analogues and prostanoids are similar, including nausea, diarrhea, headaches, extremity and jaw pain, and flushing.

Activation of the endothelin system includes production of endothelin-1 from pre-proendothelin and proendothelin sequentially within the PA endothelial cells. Once released, it can bind with endothelin receptors (ET_A and ET_B) located on the PA smooth muscle cell wall. Although ET_A is thought to cause sustained vasoconstriction and vascular smooth muscle cell proliferation

and ET_B is thought to induce endothelin clearance as well as to increase NO and prostacyclin production from endothelial cells, the end result of their stimulation appears to be pro-proliferative, pro-fibrotic, and pro-inflammatory.[107] Despite the increasing evidence that endothelin and activation of its pathway plays an important role in PAH pathogenesis,[124,125] there are still elements of its pathobiology that have not been elucidated to date. Currently there are three endothelin receptor antagonists (ERAs) available in the United States that block one or both endothelin receptors and therefore have vasodilatory and antiproliferative effects. Ambrisentan selectively antagonizes endothelin receptor A and has shown improvement in exercise capacity, symptoms, hemodynamics, and time to clinical worsening in PAH subgroups in two large randomized controlled trials.[126,127] Bosentan antagonizes both endothelin receptors (A and B) and has shown similar improvements in outcomes in multiple randomized controlled trials.[128–131] Macitentan also antagonizes both endothelin A and B receptors and in a very large, event-driven, randomized clinical trial showed reduction in the composite morbidity and mortality endpoint, as well as increased exercise capacity.[132] Of note, all of these medications have shown efficacy with or without additional PAH therapy and have relatively similar side effect profiles with some variability in the rate of peripheral edema, abnormal liver function tests, and anemia.

The NO/cGMP pathway is based on cGMP-mediated vasodilation and antiproliferation. Intrinsically, endothelial NO synthase (eNOS) produces NO by catalyzing L-arginine oxidation to L-citrulline within the endothelial cell of the PA. NO induces smooth muscle cell relaxation, through soluble guanylate cyclase (sGC) stimulation and cGMP production. Since continuous administration of NO is technically difficult, augmentation of the NO effect can be accomplished by either inhibition of cGMP degradation (phosphodiesterase 5 [PDE5] inhibitors) or induction of cGMP synthesis (sGC stimulation with riociguat). Sildenafil is a selective PDE5 inhibitor that has been shown to improve a combination of exercise capacity, symptoms, hemodynamics, and time to clinical worsening in multiple randomized clinical trials[133–135] as monotherapy or as part of combination PAH therapy. Similar results were noted in a randomized controlled clinical trial with tadalafil[136] and a smaller randomized controlled clinical trial with vardenafil,[137] although the latter is not currently commercially available in the United States. Mild side effects have been reported with PDE5 inhibitors, mostly related to headaches or flushing. Riociguat is an sGC stimulator that increases cGMP and was shown to improve exercise capacity, hemodynamics, FC, and time to clinical worsening in a large randomized clinical trial.[138] Hypotension, syncope, and hemoptysis were its most worrisome side effects; its use in combination with PDE5 inhibitors is contraindicated because of the additive effect of the two drugs on lowering systemic blood pressure.

Treatment with PAH-specific medications is recommended for patients with FC II or worse symptoms. There is now increasing evidence that combination therapy may be better at improving outcomes in patients with PAH when compared with monotherapy.[122,134,136,139] This concept is based on the presence of several parallel pathways at the level of the pulmonary artery smooth muscle cell that can be individually targeted by different medications. Combination therapy can be provided either initially or sequentially and is usually goal oriented. This includes specific treatment targets, such as achieving WHO FC II or I, improvement of 6-minute walk distance to greater than 400 meters, normalization of RV function on echocardiography and of cardiac index on right heart catheterization, and normalization of NT-proBNP plasma levels.[140] If these targets are not met, therapy is generally augmented, whereas improvement in these parameters can be an indicator of better prognosis.[11]

A comprehensive description of these treatment strategies is beyond the scope of this chapter; we encourage consulting the most recent guidelines.[2,95] In addition to using FC as a guide for pharmacotherapy, these guidelines promote patient stratification in low-, moderate-, or high-risk groups based on estimated 1-year mortalities of less than 5%, 5% to 10%, and greater than 10%, respectively (Table 32.4).[2] In summary, initial monotherapy or a combination of oral therapies, including an ERA and a PDE5 inhibitor or a sGC stimulator, are recommended for WHO FC II or low-risk patients. A similar combination or prostacyclin-based treatment with or without an oral agent is usually recommended for FC III or moderate-risk patients. Parenteral prostacyclin-based treatment, with possible additional oral therapies, is recommended for FC IV or high-risk patients. In the case of inadequate clinical response, sequential add-on therapy is recommended, including double or triple combination therapy.[2]

When maximal medical therapy fails or disease continues to progress, lung transplantation is the main therapeutic option.[141] Balloon atrial septostomy can be considered as a bridging therapy to transplant or as a palliative procedure in cases of FC IV patients with syncope and refractory RV failure.[142] Nevertheless, balloon atrial septostomy should be avoided in severe hypoxia or in patients with significant right atrial pressure elevation.

Extracorporeal membrane oxygenation has also been used for bridging to transplant in end-stage lung disease, as well as in cases of severe RV failure and advanced PAH.[143]

Management of the Critically Ill Patient With Pulmonary Arterial Hypertension.

In case of critical illness from severe right heart failure or another underlying disease, patients with PAH may require intensive care unit (ICU) admission. In these instances, treatment is focused on reduction of RV preload and afterload, augmentation of cardiac output, maintenance of systemic blood pressure, and treating any underlying disease process if present.

Evaluation of end-organ function through surrogate markers is recommended in addition to standard vital sign monitoring. In general, signs of poor cardiac output (low mixed or central venous oxygen saturation) and poor tissue (elevated lactate) or kidney (low urine output) perfusion are all poor prognostic signs and indicators of RV failure.

Patients can present with low systemic blood pressure, acute kidney injury, volume overload, worse hypoxia together with worse shortness of breath, lower extremity edema, and/or abdominal distention. Aggressive diuresis to decrease preload to the RV is key in managing these patients, often with intravenous diuretics as decreased gastrointestinal system perfusion can lead to nausea and vomiting or poor absorption of oral medications. In cases of low systemic blood pressure, vasopressor support may be needed to maintain adequate organ and coronary perfusion pressures and avoid cardiovascular collapse. Positive inotropes (dobutamine, dopamine, milrinone, and the like) may also be used to increase cardiac output and help with tissue and kidney perfusion. Afterload reduction of the RV may be achieved with

TABLE 32.4 Pulmonary Arterial Hypertension Patient Risk Stratification and Assessment

Determinants of Prognosis (Estimated 1-Year Mortality)	Low Risk (<5%)	Moderate Risk (5%–10%)	High Risk (>10%)
Clinical signs of right heart failure	Absent	Absent	Present
Progression of symptoms	No	Slow	Rapid
Syncope	No	Occasional	Repeated
WHO functional class	I, II	III	IV
6-minute walk distance	>440 min	165–440 min	<165 min
Cardiopulmonary exercise testing	Peak VO$_2$ >15 mL/min/kg (>65% predicted) VE/VCO$_2$ slope <36	Peak VO$_2$ 11–15 mL/min/kg (35%–65% predicted) VE/VCO$_2$ slope 36–44.9	Peak VO$_2$ <11 mL/min/kg (<35% predicted) VE/VCO$_2$ slope ≥ 45
NT-proBNP plasma levels	BNP <50 ng/L NT-proBNP <300 ng/L	BNP 50–300 ng/L NT-proBNP 300–1400 ng/L	BNP > 300 ng/L NT-proBNP >1400 ng/L
Imaging	RA area <18 cm^2 No pericardial effusion	RA area 18–26 cm^2 No or minimal pericardial effusion	RA area >26 cm^2 Pericardial effusion
Hemodynamics	RAP <8 mm Hg CI ≥2.5 L/min/m^2 SvO$_2$ >65%	RAP 8–14 mm Hg CI 2.0–2.4 L/min/m^2 SvO$_2$ 60%–65%	RAP > 14 mm Hg CI < 2.0 L/min/m^2 SvO$_2$ <60%

Modified from Galie N, Humbert M, Vachiery JL, et al. 2015 ESC/ERS Guidelines for the diagnosis and treatment of pulmonary hypertension: The Joint Task Force for the Diagnosis and Treatment of Pulmonary Hypertension of the European Society of Cardiology (ESC) and the European Respiratory Society (ERS): Endorsed by: Association for European Paediatric and Congenital Cardiology (AEPC), International Society for Heart and Lung Transplantation (ISHLT). *Eur Heart J.* 2016;37:67–119.
Most variables and cut-off values are based on expert opinion.
BNP, β-natriuretic peptide; *CI,* cardiac index; *NT-proBNP,* NT terminal pro-β natriuretic peptide; *RA,* right atrium; *RAP,* right atrial pressure; *SvO$_2$,* mixed venous oxygen saturation; *VE/VCO$_2$,* ventilatory equivalents for carbon dioxide; *VO$_2$,* oxygen consumption; *WHO,* World Health Organization.

the acute use of pulmonary vasodilators (intravenous epoprostenol or treprostinil, inhaled NO, and so on) or up-titration of the dose of already existing therapies.

If the underlying illness is unrelated to PAH, treatment of the disease, while optimizing volume status and avoiding PAH-targeted therapy interruptions, is the recommended approach. Judicious volume replacement, if needed, in patients with PAH and chronic RV dysfunction is important to avoid both diminished RV filling and a detrimental increase in RV preload. This is especially challenging in cases where large amounts of volume replacement are traditionally recommended, such as in sepsis or septic shock. Although elective surgical procedures are usually avoided, the presence of PAH should not exclude patients from life-saving surgery or interventional procedures. Although mortality and the perioperative complication rate may be high[144,145] and there are no data on what type of anesthesia to use during surgery, experts recommend not veering too far from standard operating procedure.

Avoidance of arrhythmias or their prompt treatment is crucial in maintaining normal levels of systemic blood pressure and coronary perfusion. The most common arrhythmias are atrial tachycardias, atrial flutter, and atrial fibrillation. Due to the importance of atrial contraction in a dysfunctional RV, rhythm restoration medically or with electrical cardioversion is most often pursued.[146]

Other treatment measures for the critically ill PAH patient include avoidance of intubation and negative inotropes; oxygen supplementation to maintain normoxia; and the treatment of infections, anemia, or any other condition that may be present. Treatment in specialized centers is also recommended, based on the high mortality (≈40%) reported in this patient population.[147]

WHO Group 1'

Pulmonary veno-occlusive disease (PVOD) and/or pulmonary capillary hemangiomatosis (PCH) have both similarities and differences with PAH, and are therefore considered under a different group (WHO Group 1'). These are relatively uncommon conditions and seem to have significant overlap. Specifically, up to 80% of patients with one disease also have pathologic characteristics of the other; due to other similarities, it has been proposed that PCH may be an angioproliferative process resulting from the effect of PVOD on the postcapillary circulation.[148] The epidemiology of these diseases is not well established, but experts have estimated their incidence at approximately 0.2 cases per million adults.[149] There is increasing recognition of possible associated forms of PVOD/PCH related to toxins and other diseases or risk factors.[150]

Unlike PAH, PVOD/PCH is male predominant and has a worse prognosis.[151] In addition, most of the pulmonary vascular pathology in PAH is within the precapillary circulation, whereas PVOD/PCH has mostly postcapillary vascular pathology with pulmonary venule dilatation, proliferation, and occlusion by fibrous tissue.[148] Although some familial cases of PVOD/PCH have been described, these are usually not related to BMPR2 mutations, as are most cases of PAH. Conversely, biallelic mutations of the eukaryotic translation initiation factor 2 alpha kinase 4 (EIF2AK4)[152] have been described in families with PVOD/PCH.

The clinical presentation of PVOD/PCH is almost identical to PAH and their hemodynamic profile is also relatively similar.[151] Although a lung biopsy is the gold standard for disease confirmation, this is no longer recommended due to increased morbidity in patients with PH. The most helpful diagnostic modality is a high-resolution chest computed tomography (CT), which may show subpleural septal thickening, centrilobular ground-glass nodules, pleural effusions, and mediastinal lymphadenopathy.[151,153] These imaging characteristics together with clinical suspicion (some cases may present with digital clubbing, crackles on lung auscultation, or severe hypoxia compared to PAH), a much lower CO diffusion capacity (DLCO) than expected with PAH, and possible development of pulmonary edema with PAH-specific medications help establish the diagnosis.[151] There are no approved medical therapies for PVOD/PCH; PAH-specific medications may result in harmful pulmonary edema,[150,151] although they may be used in some cases[154] by experienced providers and with close monitoring. Lung transplantation is the only curative option currently available.[154,155]

WHO Group 1"

Pediatric PAH can manifest at any age from infancy to adulthood. Recent registries describe idiopathic, heritable, or CHD-PAH as the most common forms of pediatric PAH,[156] with an estimated incidence and prevalence of idiopathic PAH of 0.5 to 0.7 and 2.1 to 4.4 per million children, respectively,[157,158] or 2.2 and 15.6 of CHD-PAH per million children.[157] PPHN reflects the failure of the pulmonary vasculature to decrease its PVR during birth, which allows for the transition from in utero to neonatal life. This results in sustained elevation of PA pressures and impairment of pulmonary blood flow and oxygenation. The mechanisms related to this are not well described and this type of PH can be associated with multiple neonatal cardiopulmonary diseases.[159] Its prevalence has been estimated at 1.9 per 1000 live births.[160] Although mortality has improved in recent years, it is still as high as 10% and PPHN is linked to a high incidence of neurodevelopmental impairment.[161] Preterm status increases the risk for PPHN[162]; there is controversial evidence regarding maternal use of SSRIs and an increased risk of PPHN.[163]

WHO Group 2

Pulmonary hypertension due to left heart disease (LHD; WHO Group 2 PH) accounts for as many as three-quarters of echocardiographically diagnosed PH cases.[164] Left ventricular (LV) dysfunction (systolic or diastolic) and valvular heart disease are the most common etiologies for this group, although it can also be seen in more uncommon situations (see Box 32.1). The presence of PH in LHD has been associated with worse outcomes and increased symptom severity.[165–167] It tends to have a female predilection similar to PAH, but affects older individuals with systemic hypertension, valvular heart disease, or coronary artery disease.[168]

Definition and Epidemiology. Pulmonary hypertension due to LHD is now defined as mean PAP greater than or equal to 25 mm Hg, a PAOP greater than 15 mm Hg, and a normal or reduced cardiac output.[169] Owing to multiple factors—including variable definitions of PH using different echocardiographic values, the paucity of invasive hemodynamic data, and heterogeneity of the studied populations—the prevalence of PH in LHD is not clear.[170] Although it reportedly ranges between 23% and 83%[171,172] in left heart failure patients, when invasive hemodynamics are used, it is closer to 70%.[173] More specifically, in left heart failure with reduced ejection fraction (HFrEF), echocardiography-based studies note a prevalence between 23% and 48% depending on the population studied (EF threshold used to define reduced EF) and the definition of PH (systolic PAP or RVSP threshold used to define PH).[167,174] Right heart catheter-based studies note a prevalence between 62% and 73%.[165,175] In left heart failure with preserved EF (HFpEF), there is similar variability, with echocardiographic studies noting a prevalence between 36% and 83%[172,176] and right heart catheter-based studies noting a prevalence between 47% and 63%.[173,177] The data on PH prevalence in LHD due to valvular abnormalities have the same issues. Nevertheless, two studies that looked at right heart catheterization data in patients with severe aortic stenosis, using the definition of PH presented earlier, noted a prevalence of 48% to 62%.[178,179]

Pathophysiology and Diagnosis. Development of PH in LHD is mainly related to LV dysfunction resulting in increased filling pressures, transmitted retrograde from the left heart to the pulmonary veins, capillaries, and, eventually, the pulmonary arteries.[180,181] Decreased left atrial compliance and exercise-induced mitral regurgitation may contribute as well.[182] It is not entirely clear how, but it has been suggested that the aforementioned venous congestion may lead to endothelial dysfunction (likely due to NO and endothelin-1 imbalance)[183] which, in turn, can induce pulmonary vasoconstriction and permanent vascular remodeling.[184] The latter may result in further increases of mean PA pressures that appear to be higher than expected for a given PAOP. In theory, this could lead to pulmonary vascular disease with increased RV afterload and subsequent RV failure. Based on these factors, pulmonary hypertension in LHD can either be more "passive" exclusively owing to backwards pressure transmission or more "reactive" owing to additional pulmonary vasoconstriction and remodeling. The latter form of LHD-related PH has also been described as "out of proportion." These terms are nebulous, however, as a clear hemodynamic definition is lacking and are based on the observation that the mean PAP is higher than would be expected for a given PAOP. This can lead to confusion in differentiating between WHO Group 2 PH versus PAH superimposed on LHD, making management decisions harder and placing patients at risk for inappropriate treatment. Practically, PH in LHD could be owing to elevated PAOP and filling pressures without a pulmonary arterial/vascular disease component, a combination of both, or a pulmonary arterial/vascular disease component only, unmasked after diuresis-related PAOP decrease to less than 15 mm Hg. To better elucidate the latter and define its presence, multiple variables have been proposed, including PVR, the transpulmonary pressure gradient (TPG = mean PAP – PAOP) and the diastolic pressure gradient (DPG = diastolic PAP – PAOP). Since an ideal marker of pulmonary arterial/vascular disease should be as independent as possible from changes in PAOP, blood flow, stroke volume, and

pulsatility and should reflect changes in the pulmonary circulation, such as compliance and vessel distensibility,[2,170] DPG seems to be the best candidate. Pulmonary vascular resistance, which is frequently used in practice, is calculated based on flow and pressure, which are interdependent, making it less reliable.[181] TPG, which has previously been used to identify reactive or out-of-proportion pulmonary hypertension in LHD when its value is greater than 12 mm Hg,[169] is also less attractive, as it is affected by increasing PAOP and stroke volume as well as pulsatility.[181] In contrast, the DPG is less affected by PAOP changes[180] for a given stroke volume when compared to systolic PAP or mean PAP.[181] Normal range for DPG has been reported to be between 1 and 3 mm Hg for normal subjects and usually stays below 5 mm Hg in most heart disease patients.[180,181,185]

In order to better differentiate disease processes, recent guidelines[2,170] have moved away from the passive, reactive, and out-of-proportion terminology, adopting instead the term "postcapillary PH" to define LHD-related PH (when mean PAP ≥25 mm Hg and PAOP >15 mm Hg). Moreover, based on the data presented earlier on DPG, a cut-off of less than 7 mm Hg is used to define "isolated postcapillary PH" (DPG <7 mm Hg) versus "combined pre- and postcapillary PH" (DPG ≥7 mm Hg).[170] A PVR of less than 3 Wood units in addition to a DPG of less than 7 mm Hg was subsequently added in the definition of isolated postcapillary PH and conversely greater than 3 Wood units for combined pre- and postcapillary PH.[2,186] This was based on reports of higher mortality when PVR was greater than 3 Wood units in a population with HFrEF and PH,[185] in order to be more consistent with other PH definitions,[2] and to have an additional measure that takes TPG and cardiac output into account.[186] A number of studies since[179,187–189] noted worse prognosis in cases of LHD-associated PH when the DPG was greater than 7 mm Hg, with one notable exception.[190] Despite this controversy in the prognostic value of this measure, its diagnostic value in differentiating between isolated postcapillary and combined pre- and postcapillary PH is still supported. DPG greater than or equal to 7 mm Hg and PVR greater than 3 Wood units, in addition to mean PAP of greater than or equal to 25 mm Hg and PAOP greater than 15 mmHg are thought to best differentiate combined pre- and postcapillary PH in LHD.[186,188]

Although exercise testing and fluid loading have been proposed in order to unmask PH related to LHD in patients with HFpEF, the evidence is still not adequate for specific recommendations. This is due to lack of standardized testing methodology and normative values.

Clinical Presentation. The presentation of PH in LHD is very similar to the presentation of any form of PH, although there may be some signs related to left heart dysfunction. These may include interstitial pulmonary edema, pleural effusions, and crackles on lung auscultation or murmurs owing to mitral or aortic valve disease on cardiovascular examination.

Management. When approaching the patient with WHO Group 2 PH, the initial goal of treatment is to address the underlying disease. In cases of HFrEF, optimizing medical therapy and addressing volume status are key components of management.[191]

Although there is no strong evidence supporting a similar approach to PH in HFpEF patients, it is still usually undertaken. In cases of valvular heart disease, repair or replacement of the diseased valve is also recommended.[191] A second component of LHD-PH management is treatment of any concomitant diseases that can lead to or exacerbate PH, such as COPD or sleep apnea.

Medical treatment of PH-LHD with PAH-specific medications makes sense from a pathobiologic standpoint. As noted earlier, there seems to be a component of endothelial dysfunction[183] that can be targeted by both endothelin receptor and NO pathway-related medications. Moreover, these medications may have additional beneficial effects on myocardial function or remodeling.[170,192] Nevertheless, the results of randomized controlled trials for PAH-specific medical therapy in WHO Group 2 PH have been equivocal.

In HFrEF, all the trials with endothelin antagonists or prostanoids were negative[193] or terminated early owing to side effects[194] or increased mortality.[195] PDE5 inhibitor use in HFrEF has been reported to be safe and well tolerated, with improvement in exercise tolerance (peak VO_2) and hemodynamics (mean PAP, PVR, cardiac output, PAOP).[196–201] A randomized controlled trial looking into the use of riociguat in HFrEF did not meet its primary endpoint of improved walk distance, but noted improvement in hemodynamics and was also well tolerated.[202]

There are fewer data on the use of PAH-specific therapies in HFpEF. Trials with PDE5 inhibitors showed no significant[203] or modest improvements[204] in exercise capacity and hemodynamics. Riociguat in HFpEF did not seem to affect PAP but showed some improvement in exploratory hemodynamic parameters (stroke volume and RV end-diastolic area), was safe, and was well tolerated.[205]

The design of most of these studies could be challenged to some extent, as patient selection was often not based on an invasive hemodynamic diagnosis of PH and some of these patients were not optimized from a volume status perspective prior to treatment initiation. Moreover, most of these studies were not stratifying patients based on the presence of isolated postcapillary PH or combined pre- and postcapillary PH. More recent clinical trials are taking some of these newer definitions into account.

WHO Group 3

Pulmonary hypertension due to lung diseases and/or hypoxia can stem from a diverse group of etiologies (see Box 32.1) and is defined as the presence of PH (mean PAP ≥25 mm Hg) in the setting of one or more of these conditions. The most common lung diseases related to the development of PH are interstitial lung disease (ILD; also referred to as diffuse parenchymal lung disease), COPD, and combined ILD and COPD (commonly referred to as combined pulmonary fibrosis and emphysema [CPFE]).[206] Although sleep breathing disorders (SBD) are also a common cause for WHO Group 3 PH, the disease seems to be milder and easier to manage.[207,208]

Epidemiology. The incidence and prevalence of PH in chronic lung diseases vary widely. This is a function of varying PH etiologies (ILD includes a large number of pathologies), the different tools used to recognize PH and how it was defined for the studies,

and a wide range of underlying disease severity. Based on the current PH definition noted earlier, between 23% and 50% of patients with very severe COPD (mean forced expiratory volume [FEV_1] <30% predicted) have PH.[209–211] Similarly, studies looking at patients with end-stage idiopathic pulmonary fibrosis (IPF) showed a PH prevalence between 31% and 46%, although patients with elevated PAOP were not excluded.[212,213] The prevalence of PH in sleep-related disordered breathing is also relatively high, with similar variability as seen with the other Group 3 PH etiologies.[214,215] Although it reportedly ranges between 17% and 42% in larger studies,[216,217] it is suspected to be closer to 20%. Interestingly, an increased incidence of sleep disordered breathing has been noted in patients with PAH.[218,219]

Pathophysiology. Alveolar hypoxia with subsequent hypoxic pulmonary vasoconstriction and destruction of the pulmonary vascular bed are the most widely accepted mechanisms for the development of PH in chronic lung disease.[220–222] Other mechanisms proposed include respiratory acidosis contributing to pulmonary vasoconstriction and hypoxia-induced polycythemia with increase in blood viscosity, which may result in elevated PA pressures and thrombosis.[222,223] These may lead to endothelial dysfunction and nonreversible pulmonary vascular remodeling, which increases PVR and PAP. Although inflammation has been theorized as a contributing factor, its impact is not clearly defined. Moreover, the relative effect of each of these mechanisms remains to be quantified.[222,224] Similar mechanisms, as well as increased sympathetic activation and dysregulated metabolism, seem to play a role in sleep-related disordered breathing PH.[225]

Clinically, there is accumulating evidence that the development of PH in end-stage lung disease is associated with worse oxygenation, decreased exercise capacity, and shorter survival.[211,226] Whether this is causation or a secondary indicator of worse underlying disease has not been elucidated and the severity of PH does not always correlate with the severity of the underlying lung disease.[209–213,226] Interestingly, from a hemodynamic perspective, patients with COPD-related PH tend to have lower mean PAP, a slower rate of PAP worsening, preserved cardiac output, more diastolic RV dysfunction (vs. systolic RV dysfunction) and are less likely to die from right heart failure compared to PAH.[227,228]

Clinical Presentation and Diagnosis. WHO Group 3 PH patients tend to present with symptoms similar to those of other forms of PH that are also similar to symptoms of their underlying lung disease. They may also present with lower partial pressure of arterial CO_2 and with disproportionately low DLCO.[209,226] The diagnostic algorithm is the same as the one used in pulmonary hypertension in general, including echocardiography and, ultimately, right heart catheterization. In addition to these and the other PH studies, lung imaging (chest radiography and high-resolution CT), pulmonary function testing (spirometry, body plethysmography, and DLCO), and polysomnography are crucial to confirm WHO Group 3 PH.

Management. The basis of WHO Group 3 PH management is treating the underlying hypoxia and chronic lung disease per best current practices.[206] Multiple attempts have been made to assess the efficacy of PAH-specific treatments in these patients. To date, studies with endothelin receptor antagonists[229–231] or with PDE5 inhibitors[232] in diffuse parenchymal lung disease have been negative or showed improvement only in dyspnea and quality-of-life scores. Similarly, in COPD-related PH, trials with these medications have also been negative or lead to conflicting results.[233–235] Inhaled prostanoid therapy is currently being investigated in WHO Group 3 PH, whereas a trial of riociguat in idiopathic interstitial pneumonias was terminated early due to safety concerns.

Owing to the intricacies of distinguishing WHO Group 3 PH from the less common PAH with concomitant lung disease, recent guidelines have attempted to elucidate this. Specifically, if there is "severe" PH with COPD, ILD, or combination of the two (defined as mean PAP ≥35 mm Hg or mean PAP ≥25 mm Hg and a CI <2.0 L/min per m²), there is increased risk of comorbid PAH superimposed on chronic lung disease.[206] In these cases, referral to a center with PH expertise would be beneficial for the patient for more in-depth evaluation of the specific clinical situation and participation in clinical trials or consideration for PAH-specific therapy.

WHO Group 4

Pulmonary hypertension due to chronic thromboembolic disease is categorized as WHO Group 4 pulmonary hypertension. It is defined as mean PAP greater than or equal to 25 mm Hg in the presence of organized pulmonary emboli suggested by persistent perfusion defects on lung perfusion scintigraphy and confirmed radiographically with catheter-based, CT, or magnetic resonance (MR) angiography. In addition to having a different pathophysiologic basis relative to other forms of PAH, CTEPH is the only potentially curable form of pulmonary hypertension with a pulmonary endarterectomy.[236]

Epidemiology. Though experience suggests that CTEPH is under-recognized, it is considered a relatively rare outcome in those patients having survived one or more acute pulmonary embolic events.[237] Several studies have reported incidence rates of CTEPH after acute pulmonary embolism (PE) ranging between 0.57% and 8.8%.[238–243] A recent meta-analysis of 16 studies[244] looking at "all comers" (patients with symptomatic PE; n = 1186), "survivors" (patients with symptomatic PE after 6 month treatment; n = 999), and "survivors without major comorbidities" (no significant cardiopulmonary, oncologic, or rheumatologic disease; n = 1175) reported CTEPH incidence of 0.56%, 3.2%, and 2.8%, respectively. This analysis also revealed that recurrent thromboembolic events and unprovoked PE were associated with a higher risk of developing CTEPH.[244] The prevalence of CTEPH within a 2-year period after acute PE has been reported at 4.8%.[241] Moreover, multiple reports note that a large number of patients with CTEPH do not have a history of PE (25.2%) or deep vein thrombosis (DVT) (43.9%).[245]

Published data provide a better characterization of patients at risk for CTEPH.[245,246] Some of these risk factors include the presence of thrombophilic states, such as antiphospholipid antibody syndromes or lupus anticoagulant[245–247]; elevated levels of factor VIII[248]; factor V Leiden[249]; and von Willebrand factor.[248,249] Other risk factors associated with higher CTEPH incidence include larger perfusion defects or higher levels of pulmonary hypertension at the time of initial PE diagnosis, recurrent PE, splenectomy, ventriculoatrial shunts, infected pacemakers, non-O blood group, thyroid replacement therapy, and history of malignancy.[238,241,246]

Pathophysiology. CTEPH is thought to evolve from a prior episode of acute PE, although the acute event may have been asymptomatic and never diagnosed.[245] Efforts at identifying the pathophysiologic mechanisms of CTEPH have been focused on the transition from an acute thromboembolism to a chronic, endothelialized, endovascular "scar," though the process is incompletely understood. In addition to a possible genetic predisposition for inadequate thrombus dissolution, hypotheses include the concepts of local inflammation, ineffective angiogenesis, and endothelial dysfunction.[250,251]

White blood cell–derived inflammatory infiltrates within the thrombus/vessel-wall complex may result in a chemokine cascade that promotes smooth muscle cell proliferation, fibroblast migration and proliferation, apoptosis inhibition, and endothelin-1 production. Although the specifics are unclear, this may lead to maladaptive vessel-wall remodeling with poor thrombus dissolution and lumen recanalization.[250–253] Moreover, a dysfunctional endothelium may be responsible for ineffective angiogenesis, promoting abnormal thrombus contraction and absorption and resulting in fibroblast proliferation and deregulation of myofibroblast differentiation. These hypotheses, taken together with reports of abnormal fragmentation of fibrinogen variants,[254] provide a plausible mechanism for abnormal thrombus dissolution and maladaptive vessel-wall remodeling, bridging the gap between acute pulmonary embolus and chronic thromboembolic disease.[250,255–257]

Another pathophysiologic feature of CTEPH is the development of a distal pulmonary vasculopathy, which can occur in varying degrees in addition to proximal vessel chronic thrombus. Early observations revealed small-vessel disease with pathologic changes similar to PAH,[258] whereas more recent observations report a more complex distal vasculopathy, associated with bronchial-to-pulmonary venous shunting and collateral blood flow.[259] Whether this downstream vascular pathology is an evolution of chronic thromboembolic disease or is provoked by other factors (i.e., high flow state in the uninvolved vascular bed, genetic predisposition, an infectious process, or other medical condition) remains unclear.[250]

Clinical Presentation and Diagnosis. The most common presenting symptoms of CTEPH are similar to other forms of PH: exertional dyspnea and unexpected exercise intolerance. Other symptoms related to CTEPH can include cough, hemoptysis, palpitations, or atypical chest pain but tend to be relatively uncommon and, in cases of advanced disease, symptoms of RV failure can predominate. Physical examination findings are similar to PAH and can be very subtle or absent altogether. Additional physical findings may be related to prior DVT and venous stasis changes of the extremities, such as varicose veins or skin discoloration. Hypoxia may be present from right-to-left shunt through a patent foramen ovale, significant RV dysfunction, or severe

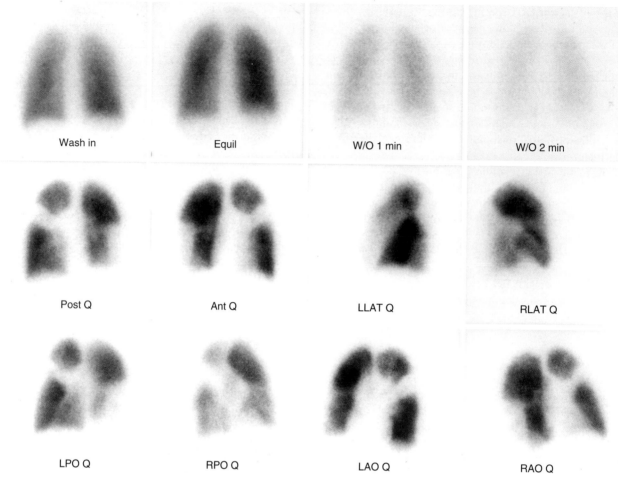

Fig. 32.2 Ventilation perfusion scintigraphy in a case of chronic thromboembolic pulmonary hypertension, demonstrating large perfusion defects (second and third rows) mismatched to the ventilation portion of the scan (first row). *Ant,* Anterior; *Equil,* equilibrium; *LAO,* left anterior oblique; *LLAT,* left lateral; *LPO,* left posterior oblique; *Post,* posterior; *Q,* perfusion; *RAO,* right anterior oblique; *RLAT,* right lateral; *RPO,* right posterior oblique; *W/O,* washout.

ventilation/perfusion ($\dot{V}/\dot{Q}$) mismatch causing cyanosis.[260] Finally, pulmonary flow murmurs or bruits may be heard when auscultating the lungs due to turbulent blood flow through partially obstructed or narrowed vessels.

The initial part of the diagnostic algorithm is identical to other forms of PH. The diverging test in the evaluation of CTEPH is the lung $\dot{V}/\dot{Q}$ scintigraphy scan, which screens for mismatched perfusion defects that might reflect the presence of chronic thromboembolic disease (Fig. 32.2). Despite recent advances in CT imaging of the pulmonary vascular bed, the $\dot{V}/\dot{Q}$ scan remains the recommended standard in screening for CTEPH[261] due to its greater sensitivity.[262,263] Persistent subsegmental or larger perfusion abnormalities in regions of normal ventilation are observed in patients with chronic thromboembolic disease and are distinct from more peripheral, "mottled" perfusion abnormalities sometimes noted in PAH.[264] Although a normal perfusion scan excludes the diagnosis of operable CTEPH, an abnormal perfusion scan is not specific for CTEPH.[265]

Catheter-based, digital subtraction pulmonary angiography (DSA) has been considered the gold standard test for confirming the diagnosis of CTEPH. Angiographic findings may include "pouch" defects, complete obstruction of major vessels, pulmonary artery "webs" or "bands," pulmonary artery wall irregularities, and distinct vessel narrowing, occasionally accompanied by poststenotic dilatation[266] (Fig. 32.3). Other imaging modalities used include CT pulmonary angiography (CTPA) and MR pulmonary angiography (MRA), which can play a pivotal role in the workup of the CTEPH patient.[265]

Defining disease severity from a hemodynamic perspective with right heart catheterization is an essential component of the evaluation. Hemodynamic data can assist with preoperative risk stratification, since higher PVR and severe RV dysfunction increase perioperative mortality.[267–269]

Management. The treatment option providing the greatest opportunity for cure for patients with CTEPH is surgical removal of the thromboembolic material via pulmonary thromboendarterectomy (PTE) surgery (also known as pulmonary endarterectomy, PEA), followed by life-long anticoagulation. Assessment of surgical candidacy necessitates a thorough evaluation at an experienced CTEPH center as to the operability of the chronic thromboembolic lesions. The fundamental elements of the procedure have remained relatively unchanged over the past 2 decades,[268,270] necessitating a median sternotomy, cardiopulmonary

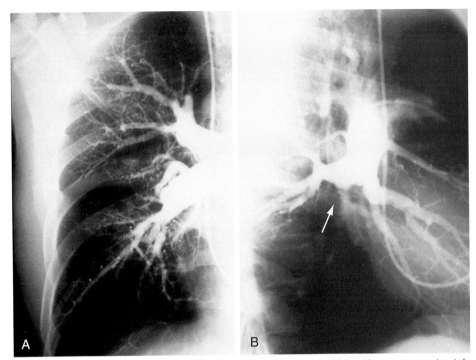

Fig. 32.3 Digital subtraction pulmonary angiography demonstrating multiple pulmonary vascular defects. (A) Posteroanterior view of the right lung showing truncated pulmonary arteries without contrast present in the apex of the right upper lobe and most of the right lower lobe. (B) Lateral view of the same right lung depicting lack of contrast of the entire right lower lobe and abnormal contour of pulmonary arteries with a prominent pouch defect (arrow) where the descending right pulmonary artery terminates abruptly.

bypass, and deep hypothermia (for tissue protection) with circulatory arrest periods in order to provide a bloodless visual field for optimal resection of organized thrombotic material. The favorable short- and long-term outcomes of the surgery with reduction of PA pressures, improvement in RV function and functional status have been consistently reported by multiple centers worldwide.[236,268,270–272] Moreover, as longer-term data have become available, the hemodynamic and resultant functional status improvements are sustained in most patients, along with a favorable impact on long-term survival.[273,274]

Treatment options for CTEPH patients deemed not to be surgical candidates include PH-targeted medical therapy and, in some centers, balloon pulmonary angioplasty. In patients with inoperable CTEPH, sildenafil[275] showed a pulmonary hemodynamic benefit but without significant improvement of the primary endpoint (6-minute walk distance). Similar results were noted in a larger trial with bosentan[276] that included patients with residual pulmonary hypertension following PTE surgery. A recent randomized controlled trial examining the efficacy of riociguat in patients with inoperable CTEPH and persistent pulmonary hypertension following PTE surgery demonstrated a significant improvement in 6-minute walk distance, pulmonary hemodynamics, and WHO FC, as well as a reduction of NT-proBNP levels compared to placebo.[277] These findings were confirmed for up to a year in a subsequent open-label long-term trial.[278]

Another recently emerging treatment option is percutaneous transcatheter balloon pulmonary angioplasty (BPA). Though early reports[279,280] suggested some pulmonary hemodynamic benefit in inoperable patients or poor surgical candidates, a resurgence

of this procedure has documented significant hemodynamic improvements as long as 1 year after BPA.[281–286] The benefits of this procedure in the treatment of CTEPH patients requires further study given ongoing questions regarding appropriate patient selection, long-term outcomes, timing of repeat procedures, and optimal technique to minimize complications.[287]

WHO Group 5

WHO Group 5 PH encompasses many diseases, including a wide range of hematologic, systemic, and metabolic disorders (see Box 32.1). Moreover, the relatively low incidence of these primary pathologies in combination with their significant heterogeneity has resulted in the acquisition of rather superficial knowledge regarding the epidemiology, pathogenesis, or prognosis of associated PH. Mechanisms of PH development range from vascular obliteration and proliferative vasculopathy to extrinsic compression or intrinsic occlusion.[2]

Very little data exist on the use of PAH-specific therapy for Group 5 PH. The large number of diseases, varying pathophysiology, significant overall heterogeneity and relatively low incidence of PH in each subgroup of diseases hinders our ability to design and undertake high-quality clinical trials. In most cases, the underlying disease should be treated and the patients should be referred to tertiary centers with PH expertise. Taken together, there is a clear need for additional research to better understand how these diseases cause PH and, more important, their clinical significance and therapeutic options.

The full reference list for this chapter is available at ExpertConsult.com.

33

Hemodynamically Unstable Presentations of Congenital Heart Disease in Adults

David Gregg IV, Stephanie Gaydos, Rochelle Judd, Elyse Foster

OUTLINE

Recent decades have seen great growth in the number of adults with congenital heart disease (ACHD). Between 1985 and 2000, the number of adults with congenital heart disease has doubled, resulting in approximately 1 million adult survivors in the United States who are increasingly having late complications. This is accompanied by a similar increase in hospitalizations as more adult patients develop late complications of disease.[1] As this population has emerged, adult caregivers are seeing more congenital heart disease in practice but may have little training in providing care for it. The anatomy and nomenclature of congenital heart disease is often intimidating to a cardiologist treating ACHD, but the care in most cases is analogous to that of other adult patients. For example, the care of a young adult with heart failure from a failing systemic right ventricle (RV) is modeled after the deep clinical experience caring for patients with left ventricular (LV) failure. Being aware of congenital anatomy and the complications that are frequently seen in common congenital lesions, however, is important to help focus on the likely diagnosis and optimal treatment plan.

In general, patients with congenital heart disease come to medical attention as adults because they have one or more of the conditions presented in Box 33.1.[2]

Most of these lesions never present as cardiac emergencies. However, unique conditions related to surgical techniques and long-term physiologic burdens do generate potential for emergent presentations in this patient group. These conditions include the history of incisions in the atrium or ventricle affecting the conduction system or forming fibrous scars as the basis for arrhythmias, an anatomic RV functioning as a systemic ventricle for decades, and residual lesions forming substrate for infective endocarditis (Table 33.1). Another example is the fall in systemic vascular resistance in these patients with Eisenmenger syndrome who become pregnant increases the right-to-left shunt and results in arterial desaturation.

Most emergent complications seen in congenital heart disease, however, are similar to the emergency situations seen in adults with acquired rather than congenital heart disease. For example, the diagnosis of ventricular tachycardia in a patient with repaired tetralogy of Fallot is treated in a manner similar to the patient with coronary disease and ventricular tachycardia—unfortunately, with the same uncertain efficacy. What is important to remember is that a patient with repaired tetralogy of Fallot is at risk of developing ventricular tachycardia and to recognize the importance of investigating complaints of palpitations, presyncope, and syncope. Substantial analogies to the care of general cardiac patients exist, but this needs to be combined with knowledge of what complications to expect with what lesion and management needs to be tailored to an ACHD patient's unique anatomy (Table 33.2).

Congenital heart disease can predispose the patient to certain complications that may be responsible for precipitating a cardiac emergency. For example, in a patient with L-transposition of the great vessels and shortness of breath, the RV is acting as the systemic ventricle and is prone to failure. The diagnosis of heart failure is not difficult and treatment is similar to the treatment of congestive heart failure due to other conditions.

BOX 33.1   Complexity of Congenital Heart Disease Lesions in Adults

Simple Lesions That May Escape Early Diagnosis (Native Disease) or Have Had Early Repair

Native Lesions
- Congenital aortic stenosis
- Isolated mitral valve disease
- Isolated patent foramen ovale (PFO) or small atrial septal defect (ASD)
- Isolated small ventricular septal defect (VSD)
- Mild pulmonary stenosis

Repaired Conditions
- Previous ligated or occluded patent ductus arteriosus (PDA)
- Repaired isolated ASD
- Repaired isolated VSD

Moderately Complex Lesions

Asymptomatic in Childhood and Not Repaired
- ASD
- PDA
- Ebstein disease
- Coarctation of the aorta

Underwent Palliative Repair
- Tetralogy of Fallot
- Coarctation of the aorta

Lesions of Great Complexity

Palliated in Childhood
- Single ventricles
- D-transposition of the great vessels with atrial or arterial switch
- Tricuspid atresia with Fontan operation

Not Amenable to a Surgical Procedure
- Severe pulmonary vascular disease (Eisenmenger syndrome)
- Patients with very small pulmonary arteries located where focalization or shunts are not possible

ANATOMIC AND PATHOPHYSIOLOGIC CLASSIFICATION OF CONGENITAL HEART DISEASE

During the formation of the heart and cardiovascular system, there are many opportunities for the development of the lesions of congenital heart disease. The large variety of lesions of congenital heart disease can be confusing. It is helpful for the cardiologist seeing adult patients to think of these lesions in an organized manner. The following classification is helpful in that all congenital heart patients fit into one or more of these categories.

1. *Predominant left-to-right shunt.* Blood that has gone through the lungs and recirculates to the right side of the heart. As a result, the pulmonary blood flow is greater than the systemic blood flow. The shunt can occur at any level (e.g., at the venous level—anomalous pulmonary vein to the superior vena cava; at the atrial level—atrial septal defect [ASD]; at the ventricular level—ventricular septal defect [VSD]; at the arterial level—patent ductus arteriosus [PDA]).

2. *Predominant right-to-left shunt, or "cyanotic disease."* The blood is shunted from the right heart to the systemic circulation, bypassing the lungs. The arterial blood is therefore desaturated. If the amount of desaturated hemoglobin is 5 g/dL or greater, cyanosis can be observed. The systemic blood flow is greater than the pulmonary blood flow. This shunt also can occur at any level of the cardiovascular system (e.g., at the venous level, superior vena cava draining into the left atrium; at the atrial level, tricuspid atresia with an ASD; at the ventricular level, tetralogy of Fallot; at the arterial level, truncus arteriosus).

3. *Stenotic or atretic valves and hypoplastic or atretic ventricles.* The valves can also be incompetent. Either ventricle may be hypoplastic or atretic.

TABLE 33.1   Cardiac Emergencies

	Life Threatening[a]	Not Life Threatening
Arrhythmia	AF with bypass tract Atrial flutter Atrial arrhythmias in Mustard or Fontan procedures CHB with hypotension or CHF and/or ventricular escape Ventricular tachyarrhythmias with symptoms	AF without bypass tract CHB: normal hemodynamics and nodal escape Isolated PVCs Asymptomatic, nonsustained VT Chronic nonischemic chest pain
Ischemia	Ongoing chest pain with ischemic ECG changes	
Ventricular failure	New murmur + fever Compromising pleural effusion or ascites	
Cyanosis	Loss of continuous murmur in patient with BT or central shunt Acute pulmonary infection	Chronic cyanosis
Noncardiac	Hemoptysis Transient ischemic attacks or seizures (new onset)	Gout Biliary colic

[a]Warrants admission to cardiac intensive care unit.

AF, Atrial fibrillation; *BT,* Blalock-Taussig shunt; *CHB,* complete heart block; *CHF,* congestive heart failure; *ECG,* electrocardiogram; *PVCs,* premature ventricular contractions; *VT,* ventricular tachyarrhythmia.

TABLE 33.2 Complications of Congenital Heart Disease

Lesion	Special Considerations
Tetralogy of Fallot	Ventricular tachycardia
	Atrial fibrillation
	Right ventricular dysfunction
	Pulmonary regurgitation (late complication usually associated with moderate to severe regurgitation)
Fontan	Ventricular dysfunction
	Sinus node dysfunction
	Atrial flutter/IART
	Fontan obstruction or leak
	Pulmonary embolus
D-transposition of great arteries	Atrial flutter/IART
	Systemic right ventricular dysfunction
	AV block (uncommon late)
	Baffle systemic AV valve regurgitation
	Sinus node dysfunction with junctional rhythm (usually asymptomatic)
L-transposition of great arteries	Systemic ventricular failure
	AV block
	Systemic AV valve regurgitation
	WPW (2%–4%)
Coarctation	Dissection
	Bicuspid valve with endocarditis, regurgitation, or stenosis
	Early coronary artery disease or heart failure
	Cerebral aneurysm
Left-to-right shunt	Pulmonary hypertension (Eisenmenger syndrome)
	Atrial fibrillation
	Endocarditis (VSD or PDA, rare with ASD)
Right-to-left shunt (cyanotic)	Paradoxical embolus
	Worsening cyanosis
	Brain abscess
	Bleeding diathesis
	Hyperviscosity syndrome with erythrocytosis
	Protein-losing enteropathy
Marfan syndrome	Dissection
	Aortic valve regurgitation
	Mitral valve prolapse

ASD, Atrial septal defect; *AV,* atrioventricular; *IART,* intraatrial reentrant tachycardia; *PDA,* patent ductus arteriosus; *VSD,* ventricular septal defect; *WPW,* Wolff-Parkinson-White syndrome.

4. *Great vessel abnormalities.* Transposition of the great vessels, coarctation of the aorta, PDA, vascular rings, and truncus arteriosus.
5. *Abnormalities of position.* Transposition of the great vessels, L-transposition, dextroposition, and dextrocardia.

Arrhythmias

Arrhythmias are some of the more common emergencies seen in patients with congenital heart disease. There are two types of arrhythmias: bradyarrhythmias (e.g., sick sinus syndrome, sinus arrest, varying degrees of heart block—including complete heart block) and tachyarrhythmias (e.g., atrial fibrillation, atrial flutter, ventricular tachycardia, and fibrillation).

Patients with arrhythmias may complain of palpitations, presyncope, or syncope. With atrial tachyarrhythmias, the patient usually complains of palpitations. Presyncope or syncope occurs with pulse rates of 200 beats/min or more. If the LV is noncompliant with an atrial tachyarrhythmia, especially atrial fibrillation, stroke volume can fall dramatically and the patient may develop syncope. The diagnosis of this type of arrhythmia can be made by electrocardiogram (ECG) if the arrhythmia is persistent. However, even if the patient having syncope or presyncope is in sinus rhythm at the time of the examination, it is most important to consider the possibility that the patient with congenital heart disease, with or without repair, has developed a potentially fatal arrhythmia.

The atrial bradyarrhythmias and tachyarrhythmias encountered in patients with congenital heart disease may result from hemodynamic alterations of the atrium or involve areas of slowed conduction in the areas of scar associated with prior surgery. These may include surgery for ASD repair,[3] both ostium secundum and ostium primum defects, Fontan procedures for tricuspid atresia or single ventricle,[4,5] and the Mustard or Senning procedure for transposition of the great arteries.[6,7]

Lesions affecting the conduction system and causing atrioventricular (AV) block have become less common since surgeons have learned to avoid the conduction system during surgery. However, with any VSD repair, immediate injury or later injury as a result of fibrosis is a possible cause of progressive heart block. With advances in surgical technique and knowledge of the path of the conduction system, heart block after repair of VSD is increasingly rare, with persistent heart block seen in less than 1% of patients.[8]

L-transposition, or corrected transposition of the great vessels, is a lesion in which ventricular inversion has occurred without inversion of the atria or great arteries. In this condition, the anatomic RV is the systemic ventricle and the anatomic LV is the pulmonic ventricle, but the physiologic passage of blood is normal (i.e., the systemic venous return is pumped to the lungs and the pulmonary venous return is ejected into the aorta). The conduction system is also inverted, and the AV node is abnormally located and often dual with elongation of the bundle of His.[9] As a result, these patients have a high rate of AV block, which can occur at all levels of severity—from first to third degree—and which increases in incidence with age at a rate of about 1% to 2% per year.

Atrial Tachyarrhythmias

The diagnosis and treatment of bradyarrhythmias and tachyarrhythmias are the same in patients with congenital heart disease as for those with other lesions. When symptomatic bradycardia and hemodynamic instability (such as hypotension or syncope) are present, a pacemaker is indicated.

Atrial fibrillation, tachycardia, and flutter, when they occur in patients with congenital heart disease, are usually not life threatening.[10,11] These arrhythmias occur in about 20% of patients with ASDs and can recur even after the ASD is repaired, especially when the repair is performed late in life (after the age of 40 years).[3] In some defects, atrial fibrillation or atrial flutter can be very serious and even life threatening. The treatment is similar to that of atrial fibrillation or atrial flutter due to other causes; in patients with hemodynamic instability, immediate cardioversion is indicated. In patients who are hemodynamically stable with noncontracting atria, anticoagulation therapy for 3 weeks before cardioverting is indicated. In such cases, the patient should receive anticoagulation for 3 weeks after cardioversion until mechanical atrial contraction is well established. If the patient is hemodynamically stable, the ventricular response can be slowed with amiodarone, β-blockers, verapamil, or diltiazem. Transesophageal echocardiography (TEE) to rule out evidence of atrial thrombus is preferred if technically feasible, as it reduces the risk of embolization following cardioversion. With atrial tachycardia, 6 mg adenosine given intravenously usually converts the patient to sinus rhythm. If this treatment is unsuccessful, another 6 to 12 mg of adenosine can be given.

Atrial flutter or intraatrial reentrant tachycardia occurs frequently in patients who have undergone a Fontan procedure, with prevalence as high as 50% in adult patients. The presentation is usually subacute but occasionally hemodynamic instability and even sudden death may occur, especially in the setting of 1:1 conduction.[12] The patient should be converted to normal sinus rhythm either pharmacologically or by cardioversion with the caution that antidysrhythmics may exacerbate sinus node dysfunction, AV conduction, or promote 1:1 conduction of an atrial arrhythmia. If atrial flutter recurs, the patient should be referred to an electrophysiologist to map the pathways of flutter, if possible. If this can be done, catheter ablation of the pathway is possible. If atrial flutter or atrial tachycardia recurs incessantly and ablation attempts fail, ablation of the AV node with placement of a dual-chamber pacemaker should be considered. If the patient does not remain in sinus rhythm, then a physiologically responsive pacemaker is the treatment of choice.

Another atrial arrhythmia that can be fatal is atrial tachycardia and subsequent atrial fibrillation in a patient with an antegrade conducting bypass tract. In this condition, the impulse conducts from the atrium to the ventricle over the bypass tract. Especially with sympathetic stimulation or increased conductivity induced by digitalis, the ventricular response can approach 250 to 300 beats/min, and the patient may develop ventricular fibrillation. In patients with a possible AV bypass tract, digoxin should always be avoided. Patients with Ebstein anomaly have 25% incidence of bypass tracts in the posteroseptal location and a bypass tract may be present in 2% to 4% of patients with L-transposition of the great arteries.

In patients with atrial fibrillation and an AV bypass tract (i.e., Wolff-Parkinson-White syndrome), digoxin should always be avoided. In these patients, the ventricular response is controlled with a β-blocker or calcium channel blocker. When present, the AV bypass tract should be ablated.

Ventricular Tachyarrhythmias

Ventricular tachyarrhythmias can occur because of incisions in the RV or LV with fibrous scar forming the substrate for reentrant arrhythmias or, more commonly, with progressive ventricular enlargement with decreased LV or RV function or hypertrophy of the LV or RV.

The development of ventricular tachyarrhythmias late after surgery is not uncommon. This is especially true in patients with tetralogy of Fallot; sudden death later after surgery is seen in about 6% of patients in long-term follow-up.[13] Late sudden death and ventricular arrhythmias in tetralogy of Fallot correlate well with the degree and duration of pulmonary regurgitation, with arrhythmias increasing as continued pulmonary regurgitation results in progressive RV enlargement.[14] As the RV enlarges, there is increased fibrosis, QRS prolongation, and QT dispersion that appears to provide the substrate for ventricular tachycardia.[15,16] Fortunately, it appears that timely pulmonary valve replacement may decrease the incidence of ventricular arrhythmias.[17]

The patient with ventricular arrhythmias may have palpitations, presyncope, or syncope. The diagnosis of ventricular tachycardia can be made on ECG, either on presentation or on an ambulatory ECG. If the arrhythmia is frequent but short lived, an event recorder, which allows continuous ECG monitoring and activation of recording when symptoms occur, may be helpful in making the diagnosis.

Any patient with a history of congenital heart disease presenting with presyncope or syncope must be considered as having a potentially life-threatening arrhythmia. In such patients, if the diagnosis cannot be made on an ECG, electrophysiologic testing should be considered for prognostication and to potentially assist with therapy. Antidysrhythmic therapy has not been shown to be of life-sustaining benefit in congenital heart disease, although it may be important for symptom control. Therefore, the use of an implantable cardioverter-defibrillator (ICD) should be considered in patients considered at high risk for sudden death.

Ischemic Complications

In adult patients with congenital heart disease, ischemic complications related to their congenital defect causing cardiac emergencies are rare. Coronary artery abnormalities in adulthood can generally be categorized as either acquired anomalies resulting from congenital surgical manipulation or as congenital anomalies associated with ectopic origins of the coronary arteries. The potential reasons for the occurrence of myocardial ischemia in adults as related to congenital heart disease are presented in Box 33.2.

The most common anomaly of an ectopic coronary artery origin is anomalous left coronary artery arising from a pulmonary artery (ALCAPA). This condition is nearly always diagnosed in infancy, as it typically causes severe ischemia leading to an extensive anterolateral myocardial infarction (MI). Common presentations include heart failure related to infarction or "angina" manifested by poor feeding or crying at times of exertion (such as feeding). By the age of 1 year, most of these children have been diagnosed or died. Quite rarely, adult patients present with undiagnosed ALCAPA.[19] Presentations include ischemia, sudden death, dilated cardiomyopathy with heart failure, and progressive mitral regurgitation. Extensive collateral flow from a dilated coronary right artery permits survival into adulthood. Prompt repair is indicated.

Cardiologists may also see patients who have undergone surgical correction of ALCAPA in infancy or childhood via a tunnel repair or, occasionally, with simple ligation of the left coronary artery.

BOX 33.2   CHD-Related Etiologies of Myocardial Ischemia

1. Anomalous left coronary artery arising from a pulmonary artery (ALCAPA) with late presentation or with complications resulting after repair in infancy
2. A left coronary artery arising from the right sinus of Valsalva or the right coronary artery arising from the left sinus of Valsalva when these malformations are associated with an interarterial course between the aorta and the pulmonary artery
3. Coronary arteries transposed in the arterial switch operation for transposition of the great vessels, with subsequent compromise
4. Coronary aneurysm, with congenital or inflammatory etiology, such as Kawasaki disease or panarteritis nodosa with associated thrombosis[18]
5. Coronary artery compressed by myocardial muscle bridge
6. Coronary arteriovenous or coronary-cameral fistula
7. Aortic stenosis with myocardial ischemia or pulmonary stenosis with right ventricular ischemia

---

Prior to surgical repair, when the entire coronary circulation is dependent on the right coronary artery and collaterals, patients can develop progressive ischemia with growth, resulting in angina or heart failure. If there are symptoms or signs consistent with myocardial ischemia, the patient should have an assessment of ventricular function by echocardiography or radionuclide scanning and some measure of myocardial viability by positron emission tomography, dobutamine echocardiography, or resting thallium-201 scanning. If ischemic myocardium is found, then revascularization should be performed.

An uncommon condition causing myocardial ischemia is the left coronary artery arising from the right sinus of Valsalva. This lesion may not, and probably usually does not, cause myocardial ischemia in most patients. However, in some patients, sudden and usually transient occlusion of the left coronary artery can occur; the typical setting is in a young adult during or just after exercise. This causes profound ischemia of the LV and is usually manifested by sudden death or syncope and, occasionally, by profound angina, with or without MI. The reason for the sudden ischemic episode is not known. The usual course of such a vessel is obliquely posterior, between the RV outflow tract and the aortic root. This could result in a kinking or compression of the artery during exercise, or possibly in collapse of the orifice of the coronary ostium. However, coronary spasm cannot be ruled out. This type of event may occur after a long history of asymptomatic exercise and with inability to precipitate ischemia with similar exercise after the event.

Less commonly, the right coronary artery arises from the left sinus of Valsalva and causes sudden death, syncope, or inferior MI. This is less often a cause of sudden death because sudden occlusion of the right coronary artery generally leads to inferior MI that is more likely to be hemodynamically tolerated.

Any patient under age 30 years who has presyncope or syncope during exercise or a life-threatening ventricular arrhythmia with an apparently normal heart on ECG should be suspected of having an anomalous origin of the left or right coronary artery from the opposite sinus of Valsalva.[20] Coronary CT or MRI is the recommended imaging modality to define coronary course in this patient group.[21] Definitive identification with invasive catheterization may be required. If such an anomaly is identified, bypass grafting should be considered.

HEART FAILURE IN THE ADULT WITH CONGENITAL HEART DISEASE

The underlying mechanisms for the development of congestive heart failure in the setting of congenital heart disease are similar to those in acquired disease. The causes of congestive heart failure are as follows:

1. Primary pump failure involving either the RV or LV
2. Ventricular hypertrophy and fibrosis leading to diastolic dysfunction
3. Mechanical dysfunction, usually on the basis of valvular disease or failure of a palliative procedure

The onset of heart failure in adults with congenital heart disease is generally gradual; thus, patients usually have chronic or subacute symptoms. Acute presentations are most common in those with sudden valvular incompetence, ischemia (discussed previously), new onset of arrhythmia, or sudden exacerbations of chronic congestive heart failure. Identifying the cause of congestive heart failure in these patients requires an accurate and detailed clinical history and physical examination, a systematic noninvasive evaluation and, frequently, a referral for an invasive hemodynamic evaluation when information remains incomplete.

The clinical history is essential in diagnosing the cause of heart failure in adults with congenital heart disease. Critically important are knowledge of the primary lesion and the presence of associated lesions. One example is coexistence of a bicuspid aortic valve that becomes clinically manifest with stenosis or insufficiency many years following a repair for aortic coarctation. Second, the timing and nature of both palliative procedures and surgical repairs strongly influence late manifestations. Often, a palliative procedure may result in late complications; for example, congenital aortic stenosis treated with surgical valvotomy or balloon valvuloplasty may have recurrent stenosis or progressive aortic regurgitation. Third, the specific procedure performed to achieve the primary repair influences late outcome; for example, a patch placed across the pulmonary annulus (i.e., transannular) to alleviate pulmonary stenosis in teratology of Fallot is associated with progressive pulmonary insufficiency, whereas other procedures, such as RV-to-PA conduit placement, are more likely to be associated with residual stenosis. Finally, the development of acquired disease may influence the natural history of congenital heart disease, such as accelerated atherosclerotic coronary disease in patients with coarctation of the aorta.

The physical examination should be directed toward identifying signs of systemic venous congestion (e.g., elevated jugular venous pressure, leg edema, ascites, pleural effusion) and pulmonary venous congestion (e.g., pulmonary rales). Evidence of ventricular enlargement will be evident on precordial palpation, but the RV and LV may be transposed. Murmurs of valvular stenosis and insufficiency should be carefully noted. Findings of peripheral cyanosis or clubbing in patients with palliated single ventricles may represent the development of venovenous collateral vessels (desaturated systemic venous blood draining directly into the left atrium or pulmonary venous circulation). These collaterals represent a right-to-left intrapulmonary shunt and may cause both hypoxemia and ventricular dysfunction due to chronic volume overload. Hypoxia should also increase suspicion of a pleural effusion or a thromboembolic event in patients with a Fontan circuit, who are more prone to these complications. The absence of a continuous murmur in a patient with a Blalock-Taussig shunt may indicate obstruction or pulmonary vascular disease and explain worsening cyanosis.

The approach to noninvasive diagnosis of heart failure in the adult with congenital heart disease is similar to that for patients with acquired disease, except that knowledge of the anatomy unique to the primary congenital lesion and to surgical repairs is required. Inspection of the ECG for conduction defects and arrhythmias occasionally reveals the cause of heart failure. Echocardiography should be considered early in the presentation of these individuals, with the specific goals as follows:

1. Establishing or confirming the primary and secondary diagnoses
2. Establishing the adequacy of prior surgical repairs, including patch competency and shunt patency
3. Evaluating ventricular systolic and diastolic function
4. Identifying hemodynamically significant valvular dysfunction, either native or prosthetic, and intracardiac shunts

TEE may be superior to transthoracic imaging, especially in evaluation of the atria, interatrial septum, conduits, and prosthetic valves. Although it is a semi-invasive procedure, TEE has been proven safe in critically ill patients once respiratory status is stabilized. Cardiac magnetic resonance imaging (MRI) and computed tomography (CT) may be helpful as well, providing both a cardiac assessment and helping delineate extracardiac pulmonary anatomy. However, both procedures may be impractical in unstable patients.

When the clinical and noninvasive data are inconclusive, cardiac catheterization may be necessary. It is important that the goals of the study be predetermined and that the catheterization be performed by personnel familiar with congenital heart disease. Incomplete information can lead to inappropriate treatment.

Etiologies of Pump Failure

There are several causes of pump failure unique to the population of adults with congenital heart disease. The RV functioning in the systemic circulation is encountered in two groups of patients: those with congenitally corrected transposition of the great arteries (L-transposition) and those with transposition of the great vessels palliated with an interatrial baffle operation (i.e., Mustard or Senning procedures). Although the systemic RV undergoes hypertrophy and is thus able to pump against the increased afterload for many years, late failure is a feature of the natural history of the patient population usually presenting in the fourth or fifth decade of life.[22] The signs and symptoms are those of pulmonary congestion and occasionally low output. It is necessary to exclude obstruction of the pulmonary venous limb of the interatrial baffle, which may also lead to pulmonary venous congestion and may be confused with failure of the systemic ventricle. Likewise, systemic venous congestion may occur in the presence of obstruction to the systemic venous limb of the baffle. These structural lesions may require percutaneous

intervention or surgery. Precipitants such as incessant atrial tachyarrhythmias should be identified, which can lead to ventricular dysfunction.

Another group of patients who are likely to develop "pump" failure are those whose anatomy falls within the broad category of single ventricles. These include hypoplastic left heart syndrome and patients with double-outlet RV, double-inlet LV, tricuspid atresia, and pulmonary atresia with intact ventricular septum. By adulthood, these patients have been treated with a variety of palliative procedures, in most cases to increase pulmonary blood flow, usually through a series of staged surgeries leading to a cavopulmonary connection (i.e., Fontan or Glenn procedure), although adults may infrequently present who have a systemic-pulmonary arterial connection (i.e., Potts or Waterston procedure). Single-ventricle physiology patients who underwent the Fontan procedure have improved survival rates and are presenting with complications in adulthood with increasing frequency, ventricular failure being one fairly inevitable complication. Failure is often multifaceted. The Fontan circulation directly connects systemic venous return to the pulmonary arteries, thereby creating a pumpless, portal-like system. As such, pulmonary venous return is hindered by pulmonary impedance, which creates a state of chronic systemic venous congestion and compromised cardiac preload with chronically low cardiac output.[23] Impairment of any of the components comprising the Fontan system listed here may greatly affect the overall circuit function.

(A) *The venoarterial Fontan connection itself:* At risk of obstruction by thrombus formation, rising systemic venous pressures and increasing coronary sinus pressures causing decreased coronary perfusion pressures
(B) *Pulmonary arteries:* Often prone to recurrent stenosis and related to the underlying congenital defect or thromboembolic obstruction
(C) *Pulmonary capillary network:* Resistance being the primary modulator of cardiac output with resultant compromise from any elevation in pressure
(D) *Pulmonary veins:* May be at risk of obstruction over time owing to an enlarging atrium with septal shift
(E) *Atrioventricular valvar function:* Regurgitation being a main risk factor for late mortality[24]
(F) *Systemic ventricular function*

Other potential causes of late systolic failure seen in ACHD patients include lesions that lead to chronic volume overload of the systemic ventricle. Included in this group are unrepaired shunts—such as ASD, VSD, or a PDA—and congenital causes of aortic and AV valve regurgitation (mitral in the systemic LV and tricuspid in the systemic RV). Congenital defects leading to pressure-overloaded ventricles also contribute to etiologies of systolic heart failure presenting in adulthood, such as residual LV or RV outflow tract obstruction, aortic or pulmonic valve stenosis, or coarctation of the aorta.

Abnormalities of Diastolic Function

Diastolic dysfunction as the cause of RV or LV failure is less common in patients with congenital heart disease than in those with acquired heart disease, but its incidence will increase as congenital patients continue to age. Symptoms of pulmonary congestion may occur in the setting of LV hypertrophy and fibrosis due to long-standing LV outflow tract obstruction, congenital valvular aortic stenosis, or aortic coarctation. Once obstruction is relieved, the hypertrophy regresses, but fibrosis may persist, producing late arrhythmias and even sudden death. A well-recognized consequence of impairment in LV diastolic function that occurs with age is increased left-to-right shunting across an ASD. The increased shunting may contribute to the almost ubiquitous atrial arrhythmias in patients older than 60 years with ASD and ultimately RV failure from volume overload.

RV hypertrophy is most common in the setting of pulmonary valve stenosis. The overwhelming success of surgical and balloon valvuloplasty for this condition in childhood has resulted in normal survival. Patients with repaired tetralogy of Fallot demonstrate LV and RV fibrosis by late gadolinium enhancement on MRI that correlates with ventricular dysfunction, exercise intolerance, and arrhythmia.[25] Similarly increased fibrosis after atrial switch procedures correlates with aging, declining function, and clinical events.[26]

Abnormalities of Valve Function

The sudden development of left-sided valvular regurgitation is most likely to present as acute heart failure. Acute aortic regurgitation associated with congenital heart disease is most likely from destruction of a bicuspid valve owing to endocarditis or from dissection of the aorta in Marfan syndrome. Aortic valve endocarditis may also occur in the setting of discrete fibromuscular subaortic stenosis and may complicate a so-called supracristal (subarterial) VSD. An acute manifestation of the latter is rare. Acute mitral regurgitation may also occur in the setting of endocarditis or as a result of chordal rupture in the presence of mitral valve prolapse. Prosthetic valve dysfunction is discussed later in this chapter.

Failed Palliative Procedures

Systemic-Pulmonary Arterial Shunts.
Systemic-pulmonary shunts (Table 33.3) are employed in cyanotic patients with severely reduced pulmonary arterial blood flow, usually due to outflow obstruction. The three most commonly used shunts were the Waterston procedure, which connects the ascending aorta to the right pulmonary artery; the Potts procedure, which connects the descending aorta to the left pulmonary artery; and the Blalock-Taussig shunt, which connects the subclavian artery directly (classic) or indirectly via a Gore-Tex graft (modified) to the pulmonary artery. The Waterston and Potts procedures are no longer performed because they are associated with a high incidence of congestive heart failure and pulmonary vascular disease. Blalock-Taussig shunts are still routinely performed in infants with complex congenital heart disease, although their creation is nearly always followed by a more extensive palliative or completely reparative surgery that involves take-down of the initial shunt. Therefore, their presence in today's ACHD population is exceedingly rare. If encountered, congestive heart failure, endocarditis, brain abscess, and severe cyanosis due to outgrowing of the shunt or development of pulmonary vascular disease are potential sequelae in these patients. A continuous murmur is a

TABLE 33.3 Palliative Shunts

	Anatomy	Comment
Systemic Arterial–Pulmonary Arterial		
Classic BT	Subclavian artery to PA	Absent ipsilateral radial pulse; continuous murmur
Modified BT	Subclavian to PA conduit	Preserved pulse; continuous murmur
Central shunt	Aorta to PA conduit	Continuous murmur
Waterston	Ascending aorta to RPA	Continuous murmur[a]
Potts	Descending aorta to LPA	Continuous murmur[a]
Systemic Venous–Pulmonary Arterial		
Glenn	Superior vena cava to PA	No murmur; arrhythmias uncommon
Fontan	Total cavopulmonary shunt	No murmur; atrial arrhythmias common
Other		
Rastelli	Right ventricle to PA	Valve degeneration may lead to pulmonary insufficiency murmur.

[a]Continuous murmur may disappear in presence of pulmonary hypertension.
BT, Blalock-Taussig; *LPA*, left pulmonary artery; *PA*, pulmonary artery; *RPA*, right pulmonary artery.

normal finding; its absence indicates obstruction of the shunt. Thus worsening cyanosis and a diminished murmur should prompt urgent catheterization and intervention. Endarteritis may also complicate this type of shunt.

Cavopulmonary Connections.
Cavopulmonary connections (see Table 33.3) consist of a group of palliative procedures commonly performed in patients with tricuspid atresia and other single-ventricle lesions, broadly categorized into the Glenn and Fontan procedures. In the Glenn procedure, the superior vena cava is anastomosed to the right pulmonary artery. However, in older children and adults, the blood supply from the head and neck is rarely adequate for relief of cyanosis. Thus many patients proceed to a total cavopulmonary connection (i.e., Fontan procedure), which is accomplished through a variety of surgical techniques. Supplemental systemic-pulmonary arterial shunts are also used. Pulmonary blood flow is predominantly passive; thus systemic venous pressures are chronically elevated.

The family of Fontan procedures is associated with frequent multiorgan complications, including chylous pleural effusions, liver failure, protein-losing enteropathy, and pulmonary thromboembolic disease. Although they are more likely to present chronically, these complications may occasionally result in an acute decompensation, especially in patients with limited cardiopulmonary reserve, and may be triggered by arrhythmia or a pulmonary thromboembolic event. In addition, increasing pleural effusions compromise respiratory status through atelectasis, exacerbating cyanosis. Ascites from liver failure and hypoalbuminemia may also reduce lung volumes by elevating the diaphragm. Thrombi arising in the deep venous system and right atrium can result in pulmonary emboli, with a rise in pulmonary artery pressures and consequent reduction in pulmonary blood flow. Acutely, TEE and catheterization with angiography may be necessary to exclude conduit obstruction and thromboembolic disease. Acute management may include thoracentesis, paracentesis, and anticoagulation or thrombolytic therapy.

Heart Failure Management Considerations

In general, initial management of the patient in heart failure should be aimed at acute stabilization by reducing preload using diuretics and nitrates, reducing afterload using vasodilators, and providing inotropic support when necessary. However, therapies for heart failure in the patient with congenital disease must be tailored to the individual. For example, in patients with Eisenmenger syndrome or unrepaired tetralogy of Fallot, excessive diuresis can result in a severe fall in cardiac output and afterload reduction with systemic vasodilators may worsen right-to-left shunts. Patients with outflow tract obstruction and secondary hypertrophy are highly dependent on adequate preload and, therefore, are subject to hypotension with diuresis. Thus, the degree of diastolic dysfunction and obstruction necessitates extreme caution with diuresis and avoidance of hypovolemia; slowing of the heart rate is also necessary, when appropriate. Prompt correction of inciting or aggravating conditions, such as arrhythmias and fever, may benefit the patient. For patients in atrial fibrillation or other atrial tachycardia, restoration of sinus rhythm may significantly improve cardiac output. Once the patient is acutely stabilized, further diagnostic procedures can be performed to determine definitive therapy.

Heart failure management for patients with a failing systemic RV requires some special consideration but is generally treated in the same manner as the failing systemic LV. Treatment with inotropic agents may be indicated acutely until adequate afterload reduction can be instituted. The use of β-blocker therapy in the failure of the systemic RV may be of long-term benefit by analogy to LV failure, but only limited studies have been performed in this patient group. The same can be said for angiotensin-converting enzyme inhibitors or angiotensin receptor blockers. There are emerging data demonstrating hemodynamic benefit of cardiac resynchronization therapy in patients with a systemic RV who have evidence of refractory heart failure and ventricular dyssynchrony, though the benefit is smaller than seen with the systemic LV.[27] Patients with intractable cases should be considered for heart transplantation.

The failing single-ventricle patient who has undergone either the Glenn or Fontan palliation requires a thoughtful diagnostic evaluation and therapeutic approach. Similar to patients with a systemic RV, there is a paucity of large, multicenter, longitudinal studies demonstrating benefits with traditional heart failure medications in this patient group.[28] However, these medications continue to be frequently used. There is growing evidence demonstrating benefit of agents such as sildenafil that reduce pulmonary vascular resistance to augment pulmonary blood flow, cardiac filling, and cardiac output in this patient population.[29] Hence, inhaled nitric oxide could be considered in a critical care setting in a patient with Fontan physiology who presents with hypoxia and ventricular dysfunction of uncertain etiology. Fontan conversion to an extracardiac conduit may be considered for refractory atrial tachyarrhythmias thought secondary to atriopulmonary Fontan types. When combined with a Maze procedure, this operation may help control atrial arrhythmias. Catheter ablation has reduced recurrence.[30]

The literature regarding mechanical circulatory support use in ACHD patients who are in heart failure is somewhat limited. In most patients, the principles of utilization are the same as in noncongenital patients, with some exceptions. Ventricular assist device (VAD) placement requires additional consideration in these patients who have already undergone prior—and sometimes multiple—thoracotomies, which increases the surgical complexity of placement. Extracorporeal membrane oxygenation (ECMO) support or intraaortic balloon pump (IABP) use during postoperative care after a repeat cardiac operation in high-risk ACHD patients has been shown in some studies to be associated with significant inpatient mortality.[31] The most challenging patients for VAD placement are adults who have undergone the Fontan procedure. They have severely limited options among existing devices due to their single-ventricle anatomy and the required decision to support either the pulmonic circulation or the systemic circulation. However, few studies have described success with temporary use of such support as a bridge to transplant. There are even fewer studies describing use of Impella devices (Abiomed, Danvers, MA) for such temporary support in acute ventricular dysfunction, and this approach may be seen with increasing frequency until new devices exist for this unique population.[32]

Prosthetic Valve and Prosthetic Material Failure. The presentation of prosthetic valve dysfunction in adults with congenital heart disease is generally similar to that in patients who have had valve replacement for acquired heart disease; however, there are several important differences in patients who had valve replacement during childhood. First, the size of the valve may be an important factor because growth of the patient produces increased requirements for higher stroke volumes. Thus the patient with prosthetic valve mismatch may have diminished exercise tolerance and heart failure. Second, the rate of degeneration of bioprostheses or homografts is faster in young patients; leaflet thickening and tearing may occur as early as 5 years following implantation instead of the expected 10 to 15 years in adult patients.[33] Third, prosthetic valves are more frequently combined with a conduit that can also become obstructed through a process known as pseudointimal thickening.

Other complications of prosthetic valves common in those with acquired and congenital valve disease include endocarditis and thrombosis; the latter is confined primarily to mechanical prostheses. Primary failure is rare in the types of mechanical valves (most frequently, St. Jude bileaflet valves) usually encountered in this population.[34] Prosthetic materials are also used for patch closures of ASDs and VSDs. Operations performed before 1970 were more prone to patch leaks. Although these persistent defects are rarely hemodynamically significant, they represent an important nidus for endocarditis at the site of the jet lesion and are a potential cause of hemolysis.

OTHER CATASTROPHIC EMERGENCIES

Cerebrovascular Disease

Among the neurologic complications of congenital heart disease is subarachnoid hemorrhage as a result of rupture of an aneurysm of the circle of Willis in association with aortic coarctation. Although rupture is more common in those with unrepaired coarctation, patients with repairs remain at risk, especially in the presence of persistent hypertension. Patients with coarctation of the aorta are also at increased risk of thrombotic strokes as a result of long-standing hypertension.

Additional neurologic complications of congenital heart disease include brain abscesses and embolic stroke in the presence of a right-to-left shunt. Brain abscesses may be indicated by new onset of seizures, headache, or unexplained fever. The diagnosis can be made by CT or MRI. In young patients with acute cerebral ischemia, an intracardiac communication responsible for right-to-left shunting should be suspected. Many patients have been shown to have a patent foramen ovale by transthoracic echocardiography or TEE. An ASD may also predispose to a cerebral ischemic stroke.

Thrombotic strokes are rare in patients with cyanotic heart disease and secondary erythrocytosis.[35] Secondary erythrocytosis is a physiologic response to chronic hypoxia in these patients. Prophylactic phlebotomy is not indicated in the absence of symptoms and may, in fact, be harmful. However, the patient with decompensated erythrocytosis (hematocrit >65%), particularly in the context of iron-deficiency anemia, may have moderate to severe hyperviscosity symptoms—including headaches, lethargy, and, less frequently, seizures.[36] Phlebotomy is indicated in these patients only for temporary relief of severe symptoms or preoperatively. Phlebotomy should be limited to removal of one unit of blood at any one time in conjunction with volume replacement with saline. Additionally, these patients benefit from iron replacement in the event of iron-deficiency states, which are common and often overlooked.

Pulmonary Hemorrhage

Pulmonary hemorrhage can occur in patients with Eisenmenger syndrome as a result of pulmonary infarction and pulmonary arteriolar rupture. These life-threatening events may complicate pregnancy and are potentially fatal. However, the differential diagnosis of hemoptysis includes pulmonary edema (which may respond to diuretic therapy) and pulmonary infections.[37] When chest radiography is nondiagnostic, bronchoscopy may be required.

Pulmonary artery hemorrhage may complicate right heart catheterization with a flow-directed, balloon-tipped catheter, especially in the presence of severe pulmonary vascular disease. When it is necessary to perform invasive monitoring, care should be taken not to inflate the balloon in a small pulmonary branch artery but rather to inflate it in a larger branch, then float it out to a smaller branch to obtain the pulmonary capillary wedge pressure.

Control of hemoptysis may be thwarted by the bleeding diathesis that accompanies the polycythemia of cyanotic heart disease. These management issues are beyond the scope of this chapter.

Eisenmenger Syndrome

In Eisenmenger syndrome, irreversible pulmonary vascular disease develops in response to a left-to-right shunt (e.g., VSD, ASD, PDA).[38] There is consequent reversal of shunt flow from right to left and cyanosis. The oxygen saturation is markedly decreased and polycythemia is present. There is ECG and radiographic evidence of RV hypertrophy. These patients have tenuous hemodynamics and are susceptible to severe hypotension in the setting of dehydration or hypovolemia from many causes, including diuretic treatment. Because of fixed pulmonary vascular resistance, there is limited ability to increase cardiac output. Systemic vasodilators are contraindicated because they may result in hypotension and worsening cyanosis with increased right-to-left shunting. Pregnancy is poorly tolerated; a high fetal and maternal mortality is associated with Eisenmenger syndrome.[39] Pulmonary thrombosis, hemorrhage, or both may complicate pregnancy. Endocarditis and arrhythmias are common. As mentioned previously, brain abscess may occur in this setting. Advanced pulmonary vasodilator therapy in this very sick cohort is showing increasing promise as large studies demonstrate greater survival with their use.[40]

CONCLUSION

The numbers of adult patients with congenital heart disease are increasing at a steady rate. These patients require ongoing surveillance for potential residual complications related both to the natural history of their primary lesion and to the palliative and reparative procedures performed. They are not likely to present frequently to emergency departments and cardiac intensive care units; however, appropriate treatment requires an understanding of how the physiology of the particular congenital heart lesion influences clinical presentation and the response to conventional therapies. Awareness of the likely complications to expect with common lesions coupled with a consciousness of the unique anatomy of each individual will improve diagnostic accuracy and help determine the best treatment plan, often based on analogies to general cardiac care.

The full reference list for this chapter is available at ExpertConsult.com.

34

Overdose of Cardiotoxic Drugs

Richard Koch,* Christie Sun, Alicia Minns, Richard F. Clark

Cardiac arrhythmias, myocardial depression, and vasodilation are the major cardiovascular effects observed in poisonings. A large number of therapeutic and nontherapeutic agents can cause toxicity directed toward the cardiovascular system, whether in the setting of an actual overdose or merely a therapeutic misadventure. This chapter addresses some of the most significant and most common cardiovascular toxins. These toxicants are briefly described, including a review of relevant pharmacology, known pathophysiology, clinical manifestations of poisoning, and current management recommendations. In all such cases, consultation with a medical toxicologist or a certified regional poison control center should be considered.

This chapter begins with a review of poisoning due to calcium channel antagonists and β-adrenergic receptor antagonists (β-blockers). These two primary cardiovascular drug classes account for well over half of the life-threatening events and deaths due to cardiovascular agents reported to the American Association of Poison Control Centers each year.[1] Digitalis poisoning is also discussed. Finally, agents that produce cardiotoxicity primarily through sodium channel blockade and those with prominent sympathomimetic toxicity are reviewed.

Not included in this chapter are a number of other cardiotoxic agents that are less commonly encountered or that demonstrate unique mechanisms of toxicity that are beyond the scope of this general discussion. The reader is referred elsewhere for review of these agents, which include clonidine and other antihypertensive agents, antidysrhythmics not noted earlier, cyclosporine,

---

*The views expressed in this article are those of the author and do not necessarily reflect the official policy or position of the Department of the Navy, Department of Defense, or the United States Government.

colchicine, chemotherapeutic agents (doxorubicin; anthracyclines such as daunorubicin and idarubicin), and certain metals (selenium, cobalt, copper, and arsenic).

CALCIUM CHANNEL ANTAGONISTS

Pharmacology

The calcium channel blocking drugs (CCBs) are a heterogeneous class of drugs that block the movement of calcium from extracellular sites through "slow channels" into cells.[2] There are two major categories of these agents: nondihydropyridines, which include phenylalkylamines (e.g., verapamil) and benzothiazapines (e.g., diltiazem); and dihydropyridines (e.g., nifedipine, amlodipine, nicardipine, nimodipine). They are used in a variety of disease states and clinical settings, including coronary vasospasm, supraventricular arrhythmias, hypertension, migraine headache, Raynaud phenomenon, and subarachnoid hemorrhage.[3] In general, CCBs are rapidly absorbed from the gastrointestinal tract and, while the majority undergo extensive first-pass hepatic metabolism yielding low systemic bioavailability, taken in overdose, hepatic enzymes are saturated, reducing the first-pass effect.[4] The volume of distribution of these agents is large, except for nifedipine, and protein binding is high (>90% for all but diltiazem). Additionally, interactions through CYP3A4 or inhibition of P-glycoprotein–mediated drug transport may change clearance or bioavailability.[4–7] Impaired renal function does not affect clearance of CCBs with the exception of a somewhat pharmacologically active metabolite of verapamil that is renally excreted.[8] Terminal half-lives are generally from 3 to 10 hours, but all three classes of CCBs are available in sustained-release preparations, which can result in greatly prolonged half-lives and clinical effects.

Pathophysiology

CCBs can exert profound effects on the cardiovascular system, particularly in overdose. They work by antagonizing L-type or long-acting voltage-gated ion channels in the cardiac pacemaker cells and decreasing phase 2 calcium ion flux in smooth muscle cells of blood vessels. Sinus node depression, impaired atrioventricular (AV) conduction, depressed myocardial contractility, and peripheral vasodilation may result.

Electrophysiologic effects are most prominent with nondihydropyridines and are seen much less often with the dihydropyridines, which work primarily on peripheral vasculature. Sinus node function may be significantly altered by nondihydropyridines in patients with underlying sinus node disease; in excess, these agents may prolong AV nodal conduction sufficient to produce high-grade heart block. The effect of decreased myocardial contractility is most pronounced in overdose or in patients who already have depressed myocardial function from underlying disease or concomitant drugs. Contraction of vascular smooth muscle, particularly arterial, can also be affected by CCBs through inhibition of calcium influx. In overdose, the effect of vasodilation on systemic blood pressure may be profound. However, in some cases, especially those involving the dihydropyridines, vasodilation may be ameliorated by a reflex increase in sympathetic activity, with increased heart rate and cardiac output.

BOX 34.1 **Clinical Features of Calcium Antagonist and β-Blocker Overdose**

Cardiovascular
Hypotension, shock
Dysrhythmias
  Sinus bradycardia
  Second- and third-degree atrioventricular block with nodal or ventricular escape
  Sinus arrest with atrioventricular nodal escape
  Asystole
  Prolonged QRS, ventricular ectopy/tachycardia (propranolol)
Hypertension, tachycardia (pindolol)

Central Nervous System
Lethargy, confusion, coma
Respiratory arrest
Seizures (especially from propranolol)

Gastrointestinal
Nausea, vomiting

Metabolic
Hyperglycemia (verapamil, diltiazem)
Hypoglycemia (β-blockers)
Lactic acidosis

Clinical Manifestations

The most serious consequences of calcium antagonist toxicity result from the pharmacodynamic effects of the specific agent on the cardiovascular system, although unique features of the different agents' specificity profiles may be lost in overdose.[9] Clinical features are summarized in Box 34.1. Bradycardia and conduction defects are among the most frequent electrocardiogram (ECG) findings in overdose of the nondihydropyridines. Additionally, hypotension is present in most significant exposures to any CCB. These features generally develop within 1 to 2 hours of exposure, but the onset of moderate to severe cardiovascular manifestations may be delayed for more than 12 hours when a sustained-release preparation has been ingested.[10]

Patients at particular risk for toxicity from calcium antagonists include those with sinus node dysfunction, AV nodal conduction disease, severe myocardial dysfunction, obstructive valvular disease, hypertrophic cardiomyopathy, hepatic failure (leading to impaired elimination), and concomitant use of β-blockers or digoxin.[11] In addition, verapamil may dangerously accelerate conduction through accessory pathways when administered intravenously to patients with accessory or anomalous AV connections, such as in Wolff-Parkinson-White syndrome.[12] It should not be given to patients with atrial fibrillation and evidence of preexcitation on ECG.

Profound hypotension is the major manifestation of overdose with nifedipine and may produce reflex tachycardia, flushing, and palpitations. Conduction defects are rare unless there is underlying conduction disease, a very large ingestion with loss of receptor specificity, or the presence of coingestants such as β-blockers.[9,11]

Lethargy, confusion, dizziness, and slurred speech are common in CCB poisoning. Coma usually occurs in the setting of cardiovascular collapse with profound hypotension. Seizures are rare. Nausea and vomiting may occur. Metabolic acidosis is common in severely poisoned patients and is likely due to hypoperfusion. Hyperglycemia is also common in overdose with calcium antagonists and is an important diagnostic clue to differentiate poisoning with these medications from others with similar clinical effects. CCBs inhibit calcium-mediated insulin secretion from β-islet cells in the pancreas, impeding the use of carbohydrates, and also increase insulin resistance by unclear mechanisms.[13]

Management

Initial management of poisoning due to calcium antagonists is similar to that for other toxic drug exposures, with initial support of the airway, adequate ventilation, and attention to circulatory status, followed by gastrointestinal decontamination, if appropriate. If accidental or intentional oral overdose has occurred, the administration of activated charcoal orally or through a nasogastric tube is indicated when the patient's airway is not at risk of compromise by potential aspiration. Gastric lavage is not now routinely advocated in the management of overdose patients, except perhaps in recent massive ingestions that present within the first hour. Repeated doses of activated charcoal and the use of whole-bowel irrigation with an iso-osmotic, isotonic lavage solution, such as polyethylene glycol (Go-Lytely) should be considered early in cases involving a slow-release preparation. Recommended rates of whole-bowel irrigation are 2 L/h in adults and 500 mL/h in children via nasogastric tube. Acute changes in the clinical picture can occur rapidly in these ingestions, which should be factored into the decision to decontaminate the patient. Continuous cardiac monitoring should be instituted in anticipation of cardiovascular collapse.

Specific therapy for sinus node depression or AV nodal conduction abnormalities is necessary only when there are signs of hemodynamic compromise or instability. Atropine may be administered but is often ineffective.[14] Temporary cardiac pacing may be considered when severe conduction blocks are present, but because these agents can decrease contractility and peripherally vasodilate, hypotension may persist despite correction of electrical activity and conduction.

Hypotension should be addressed based on the pathophysiology discussed earlier. Treatment should begin with intravenous administration of calcium salts (calcium chloride 10% solution, 10 to 20 mL, or calcium gluconate 10% solution, 30 to 60 mL, followed by either repeat doses or a continuous infusion of 0.2–0.5 mL/kg per hour of calcium chloride or 0.6–1.5 mL/kg per hour of calcium gluconate) though improvement, if observed, may be transient.[15] The optimal dose of calcium is unclear from the available literature, and the danger of hypercalcemia-induced impairment of myocardial contractility and vascular tone must be kept in mind.[16] However, calcium levels have been elevated to as high as 15 to 20 mg/dL in previous case reports without any adverse effects and with an improvement in blood pressure.[17]

Intravenous fluids and vasoconstriction with agents such as norepinephrine, epinephrine, phenylephrine, or dopamine may be successful in correcting hypotension due to peripheral vasodilation. In fact, one study suggests that higher than usual rates of vasopressor administration may be used as the only treatment for hypotension and shock related to CCB toxicity.[18]

Glucagon has had reported successes and failures in cases of calcium antagonist overdose.[19–21] Its use is discussed further in the section on treatment of β-blocker toxicity. As previously noted, calcium antagonists are generally both highly protein bound and extensively distributed in tissue. Therefore enhanced elimination techniques, such as hemodialysis and hemoperfusion, are unlikely to be of benefit; clinical reports have failed to support a role for them in either therapeutic or overdose settings.[22,23]

More recently, use of a hyperinsulinemia/euglycemia therapy (HIT) has gained widespread acceptance as the mainstay of therapy in CCB toxicity. Although there are no controlled studies to support its use, animal studies have demonstrated survival benefit with this treatment[24] as well as many case reports of success with HIT in patients with calcium antagonist poisoning.[25] There is also one human observational study that showed a transient improvement in hemodynamics with HIT in patients that had ingested diltiazem.[26] The proposed mechanisms include exerting a direct inotropic effect on cells without effecting chronotropy, improving calcium pumps in myocardial cells[24,27–29] or reversing insulin resistance, allowing for glucose utilization by the heart. The most recognized insulin dosing regimen is 1 U/kg per hour, along with 0.5 g/kg per hour of glucose using D5, D10, D25, or D50 (the latter two typically require central venous access owing to their vascular irritant effects). In general, serum glucose concentrations should be checked hourly while the patient is on this therapy; however, patients with severe CCB toxicity are typically hyperglycemic and may not even need glucose supplementation. As their toxicity resolves, the glucose levels begin to normalize and glucose supplementation may be added or the insulin infusion may be weaned.

Intravenous fat emulsion (IFE) has been touted as a possible treatment for life-threatening CCB toxicity or for those presenting in cardiac arrest. The majority of studies examining the use of fat emulsion as an antidote dealt specifically with toxicity from local anesthetic agents, such as lidocaine.[30] However, the lipophilicity of CCBs have led many to consider its use during toxicity. The proposed mechanism of action of IFE is that it creates a pharmacologic sink for fat-soluble drugs. Animal studies of CCB toxicity have shown improved survival when treated with fat emulsion; however, there are only a few human case reports of fat emulsion use in CCB toxicity.[31] The dose of fat emulsion is 1.5 mg/kg bolus, which may be repeated several times, followed by an infusion of 0.25 mL/kg per minute over 30 to 60 minutes. In addition to interference with laboratory parameters, there are rare adverse effects, such as hypertriglyceridemia, hypoxemia (with high doses), and hyponatremia.

In severe refractory cases of CCB poisoning, cardiovascular bypass remains a viable option, allowing patients to be supported through the toxic effects of their poisoning as the drug metabolizes.[32,33] Additionally, the successful use of methylene blue has been reported in cases of refractory shock in sepsis and there are case reports of its use in CCB toxicity.[34] The mechanism is thought to be related to nitric oxide scavenging and inhibition of nitric oxide synthase. If patients survive long enough for the medication to be metabolized, they often achieve a complete cardiovascular and neurologic recovery.

β-ADRENERGIC ANTAGONISTS

Pharmacology

Many β-adrenergic antagonists (β-blockers) are available that vary in their pharmacodynamic properties of receptor selectivity, intrinsic sympathomimetic activity, membrane stabilization, bioavailability, lipid solubility, protein binding, elimination route, and half-life. β-Blockers are generally rapidly absorbed from the gastrointestinal tract, with peak plasma concentrations achieved after 1 to 2 hours and with elimination half-lives of 2 to 12 hours for nonsustained-release preparations. Reduced first-pass hepatic extraction and impaired hepatic metabolism in liver disease or in massive overdose may contribute to toxicity by prolonging the half-life of the primary agent or an active metabolite.

Pathophysiology

Poisoning from β-blockers primarily affects the cardiovascular system, disrupting normal coupling of excitation-contraction and impairing ion transport in myocardial and vascular tissue. The mechanism of toxicity from β-blocker poisoning is difficult to fully explain but appears to be related to impaired response to catecholamine stimulation of β-receptors, to disturbances of sodium and calcium ion homeostasis, and to membrane stabilization. Receptor subtype (β1 vs. β2) selectivity may suggest the predominant effect of toxicity due to a given agent; in large overdoses, however, this selectivity is often lost. Membrane stabilizing effects, especially seen in propranolol poisoning—and, to a lesser extent, with acebutolol, betaxolol, carvedilol, and oxprenolol—may result in impaired conduction, prolonged QRS duration, and ventricular ectopy or tachycardia. The lipophilicity of propranolol facilitates central nervous system (CNS) penetration, frequently leading to seizures.

Clinical Manifestations

β-Blocker toxicity is most commonly owing to therapeutic dosing in patients with underlying cardiac disease or to acute overdose. In the setting of acute overdose with a nonsustained-release product, the onset of symptoms can be expected to occur within 6 hours of ingestion.[35]

Generally, poisoning owing to β-blockers shares many clinical features with poisoning owing to CCB (see Box 34.1), but the hallmark of β-blocker poisoning is hypotension, predominantly due to impaired contractility. Sinus node depression and conduction abnormalities are also common. As noted earlier, membrane-stabilizing properties seen most prominently with propranolol may lead to impaired conduction, QRS prolongation, and ventricular arrhythmias.[36,37] Highly β-selective agents (atenolol, nadolol) may produce hypotension with a normal heart rate, but selectivity is frequently lost in large overdose. Overdose of agents with intrinsic sympathomimetic activity, most

notably pindolol, may manifest with hypertension and tachycardia owing to α-stimulation. Sotalol is a unique agent that possesses some class III antidysrhythmic properties and therefore may cause QT prolongation, ventricular tachycardia, and torsades de pointes.[38]

Lethargy and coma may be present in patients with β-blocker poisoning. Seizures are a rare manifestation of β-blocker poisoning, except for propranolol. This appears to be owing to the CNS effects of the drug rather than to hypoperfusion of the CNS.[36,37] Bronchospasm and respiratory depression may occur from overdose with β-blockers but are infrequent. Hypoglycemia may also occur in contradistinction to the hyperglycemia seen in CCB poisoning.[39]

Management

The initial approach to managing a patient with β-blocker overdose is similar to that for CCB overdose.[40] However, β-blockers are receptor antagonists as opposed to CCBs, which block ion channels and movement of calcium into the cell. This may explain why β-blocker poisoning is more responsive than CCB poisoning to therapeutic approaches that either competitively overcome the agent at the blocked receptor (high-dose norepinephrine or epinephrine) or bypass the receptor to achieve a common physiologic endpoint (glucagon).

Glucagon is the mainstay of antidotal therapy for symptomatic β-blocker toxicity. Glucagon is a polypeptide hormone that appears to bypass the β-adrenergic receptor on a cardiac myocyte and increases intracellular levels of cyclic AMP by stimulating a distinct glucagon receptor on the membrane. The resultant promotion of transmembrane calcium flux and intracellular calcium release leads to restoration of chronotropy and inotropy.[41] Although not universally effective, glucagon is of benefit in the majority of β-blocker overdoses.[40] The initial dose of glucagon for symptomatic β-blocker poisoning in the average adult is 3 to 5 mg bolus intravenously. The bolus may be repeated; a continuous infusion of 2 to 5 mg/h or higher may be necessary to maintain conduction and contractility. Nausea and vomiting as well as mild hyperglycemia may occur with these doses; otherwise, the use of glucagon is without significant side effects.

As with CCB toxicity, calcium salts have been reported to be useful in β-blocker toxicity. Calcium infusion can increase blood pressure in hypotensive β-blocker poisonings without any concomitant effect on heart rate.[42] Thus calcium therapy may augment glucagon treatment in these cases. Recommended starting doses are 1 to 3 g of calcium chloride 10% solution (10 to 30 mL) given intravenously. If central line access is not available, calcium gluconate should be used, as calcium chloride can be irritating to peripheral veins. The target of therapy should be a calcium level of 13 to 15 mg/dL.

Similar to CCB poisoning, insulin/euglycemia (HIE) should be considered for severe β-blocker poisoning when patients have not responded to glucagon, calcium, and atropine. A bolus of 1 U/kg is given along with a 0.5 g/kg dose of dextrose. The patient is then started on an infusion of 1 U/kg per hour, which can be increased by 0.5 to 1 U/kg per hour up to 10 U/kg per hour every 10 to 15 minutes when reassessing cardiac function. The patient should be concomitantly started on a dextrose infusion of 0.5 g/kg per hour as these patients are not typically hyperglycemic. When initially started on these infusions, the patient should have blood glucose level monitored every 15 to 30 minutes until stable and then every 1 to 2 hours while therapy is continued. The blood glucose should be targeted to between 100 and 250 mg/dL. Serum electrolytes should be monitored frequently, as hypokalemia may occur. Since there is often a delay in effect from insulin (15 to 60 minutes), a vasopressor will frequently have to be started while insulin takes effect.[40,43]

Some β-blockers, such as propranolol and acebutolol, can also act as membrane-stabilizing drugs and can cause QRS prolongation in overdose. When the QRS duration is widened to greater than 120 ms, treatment with sodium bicarbonate boluses may be required (discussed later). Some animal models and case reports have shown proven benefit with sodium bicarbonate in such circumstances.[44]

Phosphodiesterase inhibitors such as amrinone have not been shown to be of any additional benefit when compared to glucagon for management of β-blocker overdose, but their use might be considered if other therapy is failing.[45,46] These agents may vasodilate and should be discontinued if blood pressure does not immediately respond.

There is no clear advantage to a specific β-adrenergic agonist in the treatment of β-blocker poisoning, although many toxicologists prefer epinephrine and norepinephrine. Isoproterenol was commonly used in the treatment of these poisonings in the past but may not be available at many hospitals. Dose should be titrated to effect with restored perfusion or return of an appropriate heart rate. Successful use of intraaortic balloon pump support in patients in whom other measures were unsuccessful has been reported.[47] Extracorporeal membrane oxygenation (ECMO) is also gaining popularity as a treatment for cardiovascular collapse if other aforementioned treatments have failed. There is currently significant interest in the use of ECMO in poisoning with cardiotoxic drugs such as β-blockers; at this time, however, the data are limited to a small number of case reports.[48,49] ECMO may allow sufficient time for elimination of the toxicant and should be considered when the patient remains profoundly hypotensive despite glucagon, high-dose vasopressors, and HIE.[50]

The use of IFE for β-blocker toxicity is controversial.[51,52] There is theoretical benefit for medications that are significantly lipid soluble (LogD > 2). This has been supported by a small number of case reports but has shown no benefit in others.[52,53] IFE should only be used in the sickest of patients who remain hypotensive or in cardiac arrest despite other therapies.[50,52,53] It must be noted that use of IFE can increase the adverse effects (machine failure, blood clots, fat agglutination in lines) of ECMO and must be considered before starting treatment.[54] The β-blockers that have shown some benefit with IFE include atenolol, carvedilol, nebivolol, and propranolol.

Enhanced elimination measures, such as hemodialysis, are unlikely to be of benefit for most of these medications. Exceptions include those patients with impaired renal function or in the setting of toxicity by a renally excreted agent such as atenolol, acebutolol, nadolol, or sotalol.

DIGOXIN

Pharmacology

Cardiac glycosides, such as digoxin, have been used for centuries in the treatment of a variety of heart diseases. Poisonings, both accidental and intentional, from these agents were once among the most difficult to manage and fatalities were common. With advances in the management of congestive heart failure using newer classes of drugs and the development of digoxin-specific Fab antibody fragments, the incidence of severe digoxin toxicity has declined.

Digoxin is well absorbed after ingestion and, although intravascular concentrations may rise rapidly after oral overdose, tissue distribution may be delayed. The estimated volume of distribution in adults is 7 to 8 L/kg. The kidney excretes over 60% of digoxin unchanged, while digitoxin is metabolized by hepatic enzymes.

Pathophysiology

Cardiac glycosides inhibit the sodium-potassium ATPase pump on cell membranes. As a result, in acute toxic exposures, extracellular and serum potassium concentrations rise along with intracellular sodium and calcium concentrations. Both conduction and contractility are impaired by the drug's effect on cardiac myocytes, but enzyme inhibition occurs throughout the body. There is an increase in automaticity as well as a decrease in depolarization and conduction velocity that are mediated by an increase in vagal tone.

Clinical Manifestations

There are no arrhythmias diagnostic of digoxin toxicity. Several uncommon arrhythmias, such as ventricular bigeminy and bidirectional ventricular tachycardia, are highly suggestive of poisoning by this agent or other cardiac glycosides. The characteristic early cardiac presentation of chronic toxicity is the appearance of premature ventricular contractions in a patient with atrial fibrillation whose ventricular response rate had been previously well controlled. Most patients with chronic, unintentional toxicity will complain first of anorexia and fatigue and will often present with nausea and vomiting. Neurologic symptoms can begin subtly as visual changes—described as blurred vision, decreased visual acuity, or yellow halos—and progress on to confusion, hallucinations, seizures, or coma.[55,56]

Fatalities from digoxin poisoning result most often from cardiovascular collapse. Ventricular dysrhythmias, severe AV block, and depression of myocardial contractility are seen in massive overdose and may be refractory to most conventional therapies. Hyperkalemia can also be significant, especially in acute poisonings, and may contribute to arrhythmias. There was discussion in the past about not treating this hyperkalemia with calcium owing to concern for causing a phenomenon known as "stone heart." However, this concern was not supported in a recent case series.[57]

Management

Before digoxin-specific Fab fragments, the treatment of severe digoxin poisoning consisted of the administration of large doses of atropine and vasopressors, along with the early use of external or transvenous cardiac pacemakers. These therapies are often of little benefit in significant toxicity. The development of digoxin-specific Fab antibody fragments revolutionized the management of these poisonings.

Digoxin-specific Fab fragments (Fab) are ovine-derived immunoglobulin G (IgG) antibodies to digoxin that have had the Fc portion removed by papain digestion to reduce immunogenicity. When administered intravenously to a victim with digoxin toxicity, Fab fragments reverse conduction disturbances, restore contractility, and reestablish sodium-potassium ATPase activity by removing digoxin from receptor sites.[58] Hyperkalemia is also reversed after Fab administration. Signs and symptoms of toxicity should resolve in less than an hour but are often improved within 10 minutes. Patients with severe hypotension or cardiac arrest may not be able to circulate the antibody fragments and may therefore be refractory to treatment.[59]

The dose of Fab fragment recommended to reverse digoxin toxicity is an equimolar dose to that of the ingested cardiac glycoside. A dose of 50 to 100 mg will neutralize 1 mg of digoxin. One vial contains 40 mg; the manufacturer recommends a starting dose of 10 vials when the amount ingested or the level is unknown.[60,61] Tables are available in the Fab package insert or through regional poison control centers to relate the dose of Fab to the measured serum digoxin concentration. Allergic reactions to Fab are extremely rare and skin testing is unnecessary.[58,60] Fab has also been shown to be effective in the treatment of severe cardiac glycoside cardiotoxicity from plants such as oleander containing similar compounds, but larger doses of the Fab may be required.[61,62]

SODIUM CHANNEL BLOCKING AGENTS

Of all categories of cardiotoxic drugs, perhaps the most heterogeneous are those that impair sodium conduction through membrane channels (Box 34.2). These substances are commonly described as having "membrane-stabilizing" effectis on the myocardial cell, altering the electrophysiologic effects on the channel pore or gating system. Substances exhibiting these properties include analgesics, antihistamines, psychotropics, antidepressants, antidysrhythmics, anticonvulsants, and local

---

BOX 34.2 Common Sodium Channel Blocking Drugs

Class Ia antidysrhythmics
Class Ib antidysrhythmics
Class Ic antidysrhythmics
Chloroquine
Quinine
Propoxyphene
Cyclic antidepressants
Phenothiazines
Antihistamines (sedating and nonsedating H, antagonists)
Cocaine
Propranolol
Carbamazepine

---

anesthetics. Many of these medications have unique clinical effects at therapeutic doses but, in overdose, each can produce similar cardiotoxicity. The most common group of sodium channel blocking drugs, and the one to which all others are compared, is the class I antidysrhythmic agents.

Pathophysiology

All sodium channel blocking substances affect conduction of impulses throughout the myocardium by altering the movement of ions through the cell membrane. Sodium, potassium, and calcium ion exchange through channels in the myocardial cell membrane are responsible for the various phases of the action potential. All class I antidysrhythmics block fast sodium channels during various states—open, inactive, or resting. These medications can bind sodium channels, slowing their recovery from open to inactivated state to the resting state. Blockade of these sodium channels decreases the slope of phase 0 of the action potential. This effect leads to a gradual widening of the QRS complex and, in overdose, may eventually culminate in heart block or ventricular dysrhythmias. Class Ic drugs are the most potent sodium channel blockers.[63]

The class I agents can also exert effects on potassium channels during cell repolarization. Blockade of potassium efflux, most commonly displayed by class Ia drugs, leads to prolongation of repolarization and a subsequent increase in QT interval duration.[64] As the duration of repolarization increases, the QT interval lengthens and the opportunity for early afterpolarizations during this relative refractory period increases. Episodes of polymorphic ventricular tachycardia (torsades de pointes) can occur in this situation, especially in the presence of low potassium or magnesium concentrations.[65] Class Ib agents have no effect on potassium channels in the myocardium, leaving the QTc unaffected.[64]

Pharmacology and Clinical Manifestations

Class Ia Antidysrhythmics. Class 1a drugs are potent inhibitors of fast sodium channels, typically in a dose-dependent manner.[63] In addition to sodium channel blockade, which affects the rate of rise of phase 0 on the action potential, depression of slow inward calcium and outward potassium movement may account for reduced action potential plateau and prolonged repolarization. The result is prolongation of the QRS complex as well as the QTc interval, decreased pacemaker automaticity, and a generalized slowing of conduction through the heart.

Quinidine. Quinidine, the prototype of class Ia antidysrhythmics, was released in the United States in the early 1900s. Once widely used for management of arrhythmias, it has now largely fallen out of favor owing to adverse effects. Orally ingested quinidine has good bioavailability, with peak plasma concentrations from 90 minutes to multiple hours depending on the formulation.[66] Quinidine is highly protein bound, with a large volume of distribution throughout the body (3.0 L/kg).[66] Up to 40% of an ingested dose of quinidine may be eliminated by the kidneys with the remainder metabolized to inactive products in the liver.

High therapeutic plasma concentrations of quinidine were found in some individuals who developed both QRS and QT interval prolongation and a sudden loss of consciousness associated with its use was soon described.[66] These symptoms, referred to as "quinidine syncope," were usually associated with polymorphic ventricular tachycardia with an incidence of 2% to 4%.[63] This arrhythmia is often related to a prolonged QT interval, but some studies have determined that quinidine-associated ventricular tachycardia often does not present as torsades de pointes and may not be associated with a prolonged QT interval.[67] Studies have not demonstrated a relationship between quinidine concentrations and the incidence of this arrhythmia.[68,69,70] Hypokalemia, however, is frequently found in patients with quinidine-associated syncope.[65,70]

As quinidine serum concentrations increase, QT interval prolongation is the earliest and most predictable electrocardiographic effect,[71] followed closely by QRS widening. In overdose, QRS widening is almost always present with bundle branch blocks, sinoatrial and AV blocks, sinus arrest, and junctional or ventricular escape rhythms noted at high concentrations.[64,65]

The cause of hypotension from quinidine is multifactorial. Unlike quinidine syncope, quinidine-induced generalized myocardial depression is dose dependent.[65,72] At low doses, especially when administered intravenously, quinidine exerts little negative inotropic effect but is an antagonist of peripheral α_1 receptors, leading to vasodilatation.[65] This effect can result in orthostatic syncope. At toxic concentrations, quinidine causes circulatory collapse owing to a profound negative inotropic effect.[72] In addition to shock, severely poisoned patients can present with recurrent arrhythmias, CNS depression, and renal failure.

The optical isomer of quinidine is quinine; this compound has the capability to produce the same signs and symptoms in overdose.[73,74] Toxic doses of either of these agents can also lead to cinchonism, a condition specific to these compounds named after the tree from which they are derived.[74] This syndrome results in tinnitus, blurred vision, photophobia, confusion, delirium and abdominal pain.[74] Quinine amblyopia may result from large ingestions of these compounds; the visual loss may be complete and sudden. Although vision returns in some patients as toxicity resolves, the loss may be permanent.[75] Coma and seizures can occur with toxic concentrations of these drugs, even in hemodynamically stable individuals.[65] Chloroquine, an antimalarial agent, is structurally related to quinine and quinidine; the cardiotoxicity resulting from chloroquine can be indistinguishable from quinidine.[76]

Quinidine also has antimuscarinic effects and can enhance conduction via the AV node. Furthermore, its potassium channel blockade may cause increased insulin release in the pancreatic islet cells leading to hypoglycemia.[77]

Procainamide. Procainamide is commonly used to treat ventricular or atrial arrhythmias. A therapeutic oral dose of procainamide reaches peak plasma concentration within an hour but massive ingestions can greatly delay absorption and prolong toxicity.[74] Procainamide is metabolized to the compound N-acetylprocainamide (NAPA), which has cardiac activity but does not exhibit the sodium channel blockade of procainamide and, instead, works mainly by prolonging the action potential through blockade of the potassium rectifier current.[78] Like quinidine, both procainamide and NAPA undergo renal elimination and

may accumulate in patients with chronic kidney disease.[79] The therapeutic volume of distribution of procainamide is 2.0 L/kg, with a plasma half-life of 3 to 4 hours, while the volume of distribution of NAPA is 1.25 L/kg with a plasma half-life of 6 to 10 hours.[78] The plasma half-life in overdose may increase significantly.[74]

Cardiotoxicity from procainamide is mechanistically similar to that described from quinidine. Myocardial depression, polymorphic ventricular tachycardia, and other cardiac arrhythmias are all expected at high serum concentrations of procainamide.[74] However, procainamide exerts a less negative inotropic effect and is associated with a lower incidence of ventricular arrhythmias than quinidine.[80,81] Hypotension is mostly seen with intravenous use and usually only during infusions quicker than 20 mg/min.[65] Procainamide overdose can result in severe hypotension and arrhythmias identical to those described with quinidine. Inability to electrically pace the heart of a procainamide-intoxicated patient owing to high pacing thresholds has been described.[82]

Serious toxicity from procainamide includes lethargy, confusion, and depressed mentation along with the cardiotoxicity.[64–66] Other adverse events in acute overdoses include seizures and antimuscarinic effects.[83] Hematologic abnormalities such as agranulocytosis, thrombocytopenia, and hemolytic anemia have been reported with long-term use of procainamide.[84] Procainamide may also produce a lupus-like syndrome.[78] Additionally, since procainamide is structurally similar to amphetamine, patients with procainamide overdose may have a false-positive urine drug screen for amphetamines.[85]

Disopyramide. Disopyramide is a class Ia antidysrhythmic agent that is used mostly in the treatment of patients with hypertrophic cardiomyopathy. Overdose experience with disopyramide is limited in the United States. Peak serum concentrations of disopyramide may be delayed up to several hours in toxic ingestions owing to its antimuscarinic effects on intestinal motility.[65] The protein binding (50%–Th%) and volume of distribution (<1 L/kg) of disopyramide are less than those of quinidine or procainamide; hemodialysis does not seem to affect serum concentrations, at least at therapeutic doses.[86,87] A therapeutic dose of disopyramide has a mean plasma half-life of 6 to 8 hours and is 40% to 60% eliminated by the kidneys.[74] The main hepatic metabolite, mono-N-dealkylated disopyramide, has little cardiac activity but produces more antimuscarinic effects than the parent compound.

Although QT prolongation does not typically occur with therapeutic concentrations of disopyramide, syncopal episodes have been reported.[88] Of all class Ia agents, the negative inotropic effects of disopyramide are most pronounced and hypotension can be seen in poisoning with this agent without concomitant ECG changes.[65,89,90] This may be related to its ability to block myocardial calcium channels.[91] Antagonism of potassium channels in the pancreatic islet cells may cause hyperinsulinemic hypoglycemia as well.[92] Although mild antimuscarinic effects can be noted in poisonings of all class Ia agents, those following disopyramide toxicity are the most clinically significant[65] and can result in sinus tachycardia, blurred vision, altered mental status, seizures, urinary retention, and ileus, at times without accompanying serious cardiotoxicity.[65]

Class Ib Antidysrhythmics. Drugs in this class suppress automaticity similarly to the class Ia agents, but class Ib drugs have rapid on-off binding kinetics for myocardial sodium channels and possess the highest affinity for sodium channels that are in the inactivated state.[74] These compounds typically do not affect the rate of rise of the phase 0 action potential at therapeutic doses. In fact, they can block a small sodium plateau current that reduces the duration of the action potential and shortens the refractory phase. The resultant effects on the ECG include a normal or shortened QT interval and an unchanged QRS duration.[93]

Lidocaine. Lidocaine is the prototype of class Ib antidysrhythmics. Clinically, it is used predominantly as a local anesthetic and to treat ventricular tachycardia. A large first-pass effect is seen with oral dosing of lidocaine and only 30% to 35% of an ingested dose is bioavailable.[94] However, large ingestions have resulted in significant absorption resulting in toxicity.[95] Lidocaine is well absorbed topically through abraded epithelium and from the trachea and bronchi after endotracheal administration.[96] The apparent volume of distribution of lidocaine is 1.3 L/kg, but it is significantly reduced in the presence of congestive heart failure.[97] The liver metabolizes virtually all of a lidocaine dose, with an elimination half-life in therapeutic concentrations of about 2 hours.[74] The most significantly active metabolite is monoethylglycinexylidide (MEGX), which also has a half-life of 2 hours.[98]

For both lidocaine and MEGX, the concern in poisoning is cardiovascular and CNS toxicity. Both compounds are neurotoxic at high concentrations and can cause seizures and apnea.[93] Some individuals experience mild neurologic symptoms at therapeutic plasma concentrations.[93] Since lidocaine rapidly passes through the blood-brain barrier, patients with toxicity usually manifest CNS dysfunction as initial symptoms.[99] Early signs of CNS toxicity from lidocaine include lightheadedness, agitation, confusion, hallucinations, and dysarthria. Some individuals initially complain of tongue or perioral numbness. Progression to seizures or coma can be rapid. Cardiovascular toxicity occurs in massive overdose and typically follows CNS dysfunction. Intrinsic cardiac pacemaker cells are depressed, conduction is delayed, and myocardial contractility is impaired.[100,101] Large intravenous lidocaine doses greater than 1 g have resulted in asystole, complete heart block, and refractory hypotension.[93,100,102]

Phenytoin. Like lidocaine, phenytoin is classified as a class Ib agent and is most commonly used in the management of seizure disorders. Phenytoin absorption from the gastrointestinal tract can be delayed; peak levels after an oral overdose can be delayed up to 24 hours or more.[103] Phenytoin is 90% protein bound: the volume of distribution of the free drug is 0.5 L/kg.[74,103] Signs of toxicity correlate better with free phenytoin levels but most laboratories still assay for both bound and unbound fractions. Phenytoin is metabolized to nontoxic metabolites by the liver. At high concentrations, these enzymes become saturated and the half-life may increase to several days as elimination kinetics change from first order to zero order.[104] Patients with low serum albumin concentrations may be particularly prone to chronic phenytoin toxicity owing to the higher relative fraction of free drug.[74]

Poisoning with phenytoin occurs most often during long-term therapy for epilepsy when a medication inhibiting phenytoin metabolism is added, or when the patient develops a disease state that impairs hepatic mixed function oxidase activity. Acute overdoses occur less frequently, but the resulting clinical presentation is similar.

Phenytoin poisoning primarily causes neurotoxicity manifested as drowsiness, ataxia, dysarthria, and nystagmus. In massive poisonings, coma and seizures can be seen but respiratory depression is infrequent. Cardiac arrhythmias and hypotension are rarely reported with toxic phenytoin ingestions but are often encountered during rapid intravenous infusions.[105] Although phenytoin does have sodium channel blocking effects on myocardial tissue, the diluent of the intravenous solution, propylene glycol, has been implicated as the source of myocardial depression and arrhythmias associated with intravenous infusion.[106] Slowing the rate of infusion can prevent most of these complications.

Mexilitine and moricizine. Overdose experience with other class Ib drugs has been limited. Mexilitine poisoning has caused seizures, ventricular arrhythmias, and impaired myocardial conduction.[107] Other adverse effects of mexilitine are primarily neurologic and comparable to symptoms that occur with lidocaine. Moricizine, which is often classified as a class Ib drug, exhibits both Ib and Ic characteristics. It undergoes extensive and rapid metabolism and is associated with PR and QRS prolongation. Expected effects would include bundle blocks and ventricular arrhythmias.

Class Ic Antidysrhythmics. Class Ic drugs (flecainide, propafenone) bind to sodium channels in the activated state and have the most potent sodium channel blocking effects of all class I antidysrhythmics.[74] Therapeutic concentrations of class Ic agents produce little effect on myocyte repolarization compared with other class I antidysrhythmics.[108] Overdose experience with these drugs is limited but they would be expected to produce similar cardiovascular effects as other class I compounds with no antimuscarinic features.

Flecainide. Flecainide, a derivative of procainamide, is usually used in the treatment of atrial fibrillation or supraventricular tachycardias. Plasma levels peak at 3 hours with minimal first pass effect and no active metabolites.[109] As expected, flecainide toxicity typically causes marked QRS prolongation with minimal QT interval prolongation. In addition to bradycardia, premature ventricular contractions and ventricular fibrillation, flecainide has a negative ionotropic effect similar to quinidine that may worsen congestive heart failure.[110]

Class III Antidysrhythmics. Class III agents (amiodarone, ibutilide, dofetilide) block the rapidly activating component of the delayed rectifier potassium channels.[74] These potassium channels are responsible for phase 3 repolarization in cardiac action potentials without altering conduction velocity during phase 0 or phase 1. Therefore, class III drugs cause an increase in duration of the action potential and an increase in the effective refractory period. On the ECG, this results in prolonged QT intervals. By increasing the refractory period, these drugs are very useful in terminating reentrant arrhythmias.

Amiodarone. Amiodarone is an antidysrhythmic used to terminate reentrant atrial or ventricular arrhythmias and has been a recurrent part the Advanced Cardiac Life Support (ACLS) algorithms.[111] It undergoes hepatic metabolism through cytochrome oxidase systems to produce another pharmacologically active but less potent metabolite, desethylamiodarone.[112] Its half-life is on the order of weeks and a steady state may not be obtained until a month after initiation. The main mechanism of action of amiodarone is prolongation of cardiac myocyte repolarization through blockade of the rapidly activating delayed rectifier potassium channel. However, amiodarone may also block inactivated sodium channels and L-type calcium channels.[113] Expected ECG findings are prolonged QT intervals, ventricular arrhythmias, bradycardia, and conduction block.

Despite its more frequent use today, there are few reported cases of oral amiodarone overdose resulting in significant cardiac toxicity. The low toxicity is likely due to its low and unpredictable oral bioavailability (22% to 86%) and large volume of distribution (>6.0 L/kg).[114] Intravenous overdose of amiodarone has not been reported although hypotension, bronchospasm, and hepatitis from therapeutic doses have been described. Most of the toxic effects reported from amiodarone in the literature are from long-term treatment and appear to be dose related. Chronic use of amiodarone has been associated with pneumonitis, hypothyroidism, thyrotoxicosis, hepatitis, skin discoloration, and corneal damage.[115] Although not well studied, cholestyramine has been suggested as treatment for both acute and chronic amiodarone toxicity for its gastrointestinal binding of unabsorbed amiodarone and blockade of enterohepatic circulation of the drug.[116]

Ibutilide, dofetilide. Both ibutilide and dofetilide are class III antidysrhythmics used for chemical cardioversion of atrial fibrillation or flutter. Both are renally eliminated with half-lives on the order of hours. Due to their effect on the rapidly activating delayed rectifier potassium channels, both drugs can delay action potentials and prolong QT intervals.[74] Ibutilide specifically has a small amount of sodium channel opening effect and can only be administered parenterally, as it undergoes extensive first-pass metabolism. Experiences with overdoses of either drug are limited but expected toxicity would be induction of ventricular arrhythmias. The toxic effect of either drug occurs within 60 minutes of administration and therapeutic use has resulted in torsade de pointes.[113,117] Therefore, a reasonable observational period of 4 to 6 hours is recommended in all patients who received ibutilide or dofetilide.

CYCLIC ANTIDEPRESSANTS

Toxicity from cyclic antidepressants is perhaps the best described of all fast sodium channel blocking compounds. These substances were once responsible for more fatalities than any of the other drugs in this group.[118] After being originally studied for their antihistaminic properties in the 1940s, cyclic antidepressants were introduced into the pharmaceutical market in the United States in the 1960s, rapidly replacing electroshock therapy as a more "humane" treatment for severe depression.

Pharmacology

The first generation of cyclic antidepressant compounds, known as the tertiary amines, includes amitriptyline, imipramine, doxepine, and trimipramine. All are potent inhibitors of myocyte sodium channels. Each undergoes metabolism in the liver. Amitriptyline and imipramine are hepatically converted to the active secondary amines nortriptyline and desipramine, respectively; these compounds were soon marketed as second-generation therapies for depression.[74] The membrane-stabilizing effects of these second-generation agents was soon appreciated as being similar to that of their parent compounds.[74]

Newer antidepressants, categorized as serotonin or norepinephrine reuptake inhibitors (trazodone, fluoxetine, sertraline, bupropion, paroxetine, and others) have demonstrated far less sodium and potassium channel impedance. Although each of these drugs may cause adverse reactions in overdose, their cardiotoxicity appears to be minimal in comparison to the first- and second-generation cyclic drugs. Carbamazepine is an anticonvulsant with structural similarity to the cyclic antidepressants. In overdose, it appears to cause mainly antimuscarinic effects with narrow complex tachycardia, CNS depression, and—rarely—respiratory depression.[76,119] Cyclic antidepressant-like arrhythmias have not been commonly described with carbamazepine.

In therapeutic doses, cyclic antidepressant drugs are rapidly absorbed. Although one might expect delayed gastric emptying as a result of an antimuscarinic effect in large ingestions, clinical signs of cyclic antidepressant toxicity usually appear within 6 hours.[120] Asymptomatic patients without concomitant ingestions should not develop toxicity after 6 hours. Antimuscarinic effects on the central and peripheral nervous systems usually precede cardiotoxicity, but large ingestions of agents with less muscarinic receptor activity, such as imipramine, may present initially with hypotension and arrhythmias. Cardiotoxicity, mental status depression, and seizures resulting from these agents can proceed rapidly, necessitating continuous monitoring.

Cyclic antidepressants are significantly protein bound in circulation and widely distributed in the body (40 L/kg).[74] Hepatic metabolism is the major route of elimination for these compounds with some, such as amitriptyline and imipramine, producing active metabolites. Elimination half-life can be prolonged in overdoses due to enzyme saturation.

Pathophysiology

The pathophysiology of cyclic antidepressant cardiotoxicity results from four main properties: (1) fast sodium channel or membrane-stabilizing effects, (2) muscarinic receptor blockade, (3) α-receptor blockade, and (4) norepinephrine reuptake blockade. Animal data also suggest blockade of delayed rectifier potassium channels as well as the γ-aminobutyric acid (GABA) receptor complex in the brain.[121,122] The cyclic antidepressants also have antihistaminic and serotonin reuptake blockade, but these are unlikely to contribute significantly to cardiac effects.

Cyclic antidepressants block fast sodium channels in a manner similar to quinidine and other class Ia antidysrhythmics, markedly decreasing the slope of phase 0 of the action potential.[74] Prolongation of both the QRS and QT durations has been demonstrated clinically in overdose, but in vitro experiments show that cyclic antidepressants block primarily fast depolarizing sodium currents and actually shorten repolarization.[123,124] QT prolongation resulting from cyclic antidepressant toxicity is mainly attributed to the result of progressive QRS widening with globally impaired myocardial conduction.[124] However, the potential blockade of the delayed rectifier potassium channels may also contribute to QT prolongation.[122] Cardiotoxic effects include ventricular arrhythmias and depressed myocardial contractility.[124]

Cyclic antidepressants block several receptor sites in both the central and peripheral nervous systems, including H_1 and H_2 receptors, dopamine receptors, and muscarinic receptors.[125] This effect on the autonomic nervous system produces a clinical syndrome of dry mouth, blurred vision, sinus tachycardia, altered mental status (ranging from confusion and hallucination to seizures and coma), ileus, urinary retention, and anhidrosis. These signs and symptoms frequently precede the sodium channel blocking effects and are more common with doxepin and amitriptyline than imipramine.[74,125]

Cyclic antidepressants are potent α_1-receptor antagonists. This effect is responsible for the orthostatic hypotension often experienced by patients at the initiation of therapy with these compounds.[74] The resulting vasodilation can be severe in overdose and, combined with the impaired cardiac output from myocardial depression, can lead to refractory hypotension and cardiovascular collapse.[126] α-Receptor blockade of the pupil in patients with cyclic antidepressant toxicity can prevent the anticipated antimuscarinic mydriasis, resulting in an unanticipated miotic pupillary effect.

The hypothesized mechanism of antidepressant action of cyclic antidepressants lies in their ability to block the catecholamine reuptake pump on the presynaptic terminal of neurons.[125] In overdose, this effect can deplete presynaptic catecholamine concentrations, which is thought to contribute to arrhythmias and hypotension.[74]

Hypotension can be present in cyclic antidepressant poisoning without significant arrhythmias. Sinus tachycardia is usually present before the development of ventricular arrhythmias or heart block.[127] Several studies have evaluated the ECG abnormalities predictive of toxicity from these agents. One review found that 33% of patients with QRS intervals greater than 100 ms developed seizures and 14% developed ventricular arrhythmias.[128] There was also a 50% incidence of ventricular arrhythmias in patients with QRS duration exceeding 160 ms.[128] Another study suggested that a rightward terminal vector, best seen in the R wave of lead aVR, may correlate with the degree of cyclic antidepressant toxicity.[129,130] In this study, an R wave in lead aVR greater than 3 mm predicted toxicity. Although the presence of ECG abnormalities can be useful in assessing potential toxicity, none of the findings are 100% sensitive. Absence of these ECG findings is more indicative that cardiac toxicity is not developing.[131]

ANTIPSYCHOTICS (PHENOTHIAZINES, BUTYROPHENONES, AND ATYPICAL AGENTS)

Toxicity from phenothiazine derivative compounds—such as thorazine, thioridazine, and prochlorperazine—may present with effects similar to those of the cyclic antidepressants. Antimuscarinic toxicity is frequently more pronounced in poisonings from these drugs than effects due to their cardiac membrane-stabilizing properties. However, heart block and wide complex tachycardias as well as refractory hypotension are reported in overdoses of these agents.[132,133] Fatalities are rare, even in massive ingestions of these drugs. The most common clinical presentation of phenothiazine overdose is neurotoxicity, manifesting as delirium, agitation, coma, seizures, and other peripheral antimuscarinic effects.

Haloperidol and droperidol are butyrophenone antipsychotic and antiemetic compounds available in the United States. Although these drugs share the potent dopamine receptor blocking properties of the phenothiazines, overdoses of these agents lack the prolonged sedation and antimuscarinic effects most often seen with phenothiazines. Torsades de pointes has been reported with the butyrophenones but usually follows large parenteral dosing.[134] The U.S. Food and Drug Administration issued a box warning in 2001 for droperidol over concerns of QT prolongation and the potential for torsades de pointes. Since then, however, there have been multiple studies that did not detect any significant differences in QT prolongation from droperidol compared to other commonly used medications for sedation.[135,136]

Newer, atypical antipsychotics—such as quetiapine, olanzapine, risperidone, and ziprasidone—seem to have fewer effects on cardiac conduction. Most atypical antipsychotics have inhibitory functions at serotonin receptors in addition to antimuscarinic and dopamine receptor blocking properties. Retrospective data and case reports have demonstrated the ability of some of these drugs to block fast sodium channels and potassium channels, resulting in QRS and QTc prolongation, respectively.[137] In general, these effects are much less common than with the older "typical" antipsychotic agents.

ANTIHISTAMINES

Many H_1-receptor antagonists have been found to exert similar effects on the myocardial action potential as the class Ia antidysrhythmic compounds. Diphenhydramine is the most commonly used medication in this class and has been shown to effectively block fast sodium channels at high concentrations.[138]

In mild to moderate poisonings with these agents, patients most often exhibit a classic antimuscarinic syndrome with sinus tachycardia, dry mouth, and confusion, often marked by hallucinations and psychotic behavior. The toxic syndrome may also include seizures, urinary retention, decreased gastric motility, and coma. Respiratory depression can occur in severe cases, necessitating ventilator support.

In massive poisonings, antihistamines can impair fast sodium channel conduction, resulting in arrhythmias and hypotension similar to that seen with other sodium channel blocking agents.[138–140] Arrhythmias and cardiovascular collapse from these drugs are exacerbated by acidosis and often occur after seizures, which can cause a sudden decline in the serum pH.[138–140]

MANAGEMENT OF SODIUM CHANNEL BLOCKING DRUG TOXICITY

As in the treatment of other cardiotoxic drug overdoses discussed in this chapter, the initial management of poisonings involving sodium channel blocking medications should begin with airway and circulatory support (Box 34.3).[142] Any patient who is not breathing or in whom a patent airway is in question should undergo endotracheal intubation and mechanical ventilation. Combative patients may require sedation and paralysis before an endotracheal tube can be placed. Intravenous line placement, 12-lead ECG, and continuous cardiopulmonary monitoring are also important initial steps in caring for these patients.

Resuscitating the patient poisoned with sodium channel blocking drugs can be challenging. Standard strategies to manage the hypotension resulting from massive ingestions of these agents include intravenous fluid boluses, though hypotension may be refractory, requiring vasopressors. Dopamine is the precursor of norepinephrine and requires uptake into the presynaptic terminals for activation; thus it may be ineffective in treating hypotension caused by agents that block the catecholamine reuptake pump, such as cyclic antidepressants, phenothiazines, and other α_1-receptor–blocking agents.[141] At higher doses, the vasoconstrictive effects of dopamine are antagonized by the α-blocking effects of some of these drugs, potentially leading to unopposed β-receptor stimulation of blood vessels and exacerbating hypotension. For these reasons, vasopressors with more direct α_1-receptor stimulation, such as norepinephrine or phenylephrine, may provide more consistent blood pressure support.

The most helpful adjunct in the management of hypotension due to sodium channel blockade from drug poisoning has proven to be sodium bicarbonate. Sodium bicarbonate has been shown to be effective in raising blood pressure and treating arrhythmias associated with cyclic antidepressants, cocaine, flecainide, quinidine, chloroquine, and diphenhydramine.[143–149]

It is thought to enhance isotropy by accelerating depolarization and increasing intravascular volume and pH. Sodium bicarbonate has been shown in both animal models and human cases of toxicity from these agents to increase blood pressure and improve conduction through the heart. Studies suggest that this is the result of the concomitant effects of both the bicarbonate and sodium components, as they offer a synergistic benefit together when compared to each alone. Thus the beneficial effects are likely secondary to both an increase in blood pH and an increase in extracellular sodium concentration.

Although controlled studies do not exist to support the use of sodium bicarbonate for every drug in this category, its empiric administration to patients with evidence of toxicity from impaired sodium conduction seems prudent. The degree of alkalinization that one must achieve to be of benefit is not well defined. Maintaining serum pH in normal ranges has been sufficient in our practice, but many authors recommend bolus injections of sodium bicarbonate to keep serum pH between 7.45 and 7.50. One common practice is the addition of 50 to 100 mmol sodium bicarbonate (1 to 2 ampules) to 1000 mL of 5% dextrose and water, titrating the infusion to an alkaline pH. This treatment requires frequent analysis of serum pH and sodium, as hypernatremia may result if not monitored closely. Intermittent boluses of sodium bicarbonate, at 1 to 2 mEq/kg, may be more effective. The bolus method is preferred by many toxicologists for the ability to more precisely titrate sodium bicarbonate doses to the effect of a narrowed QRS.

The use of lidocaine has been effective in improving cardiac performance after overdose of membrane-stabilizing drugs[144] and can be administered in cases refractory to sodium bicarbonate. Although it seems counterintuitive to administer another class I antidysrhythmic, the rapid on-off binding of lidocaine may displace other "slower" classes of drugs and reduce the channel blockade.

In some severe cases of sodium channel blocking drug toxicity, ventricular arrhythmias may be refractory to the aforementioned management. Oxygenation should be maintained and resuscitative efforts continued as long as cardiac activity is present. Patients have survived neurologically intact after more than 1 hour of advanced cardiac life support following massive cyclic antidepressant poisoning.[150] Prolonged resuscitation may allow enough drug redistribution from cardiac receptors to restore conduction.

Other therapies to consider in patients with drug-induced cardiotoxicity refractory to standard measures would include intraaortic balloon pump, cardiopulmonary bypass, and IFE therapy. There are also case reports of successful resuscitation of cardiotoxin poisonings using ECMO.[151–153] This treatment has been used intermittently since the late 1990s for patients with cardiogenic shock or cardiac arrest when other treatment modalities have failed. As equipment for ECMO has become easier to utilize, there have been increasing numbers of case reports and animal studies reporting the benefits of its use. The benefit of ECMO is derived from providing both oxygenation and circulatory support without the need for a functional cardiac or pulmonary system. Any poisoning exhibiting severe cardiac dysfunction may be considered for ECMO when all other treatments have failed.[48,49] IFE is another treatment that has been attempted in patients poisoned with cardiotoxic agents that have failed other maximal therapies.[53] A consensus statement of US and international toxicologists based on the best available evidence could give IFE only a neutral recommendation in cardiac arrest and "suggest not using IFE as first-line therapy" in life-threatening toxicity.[52] The panel also suggested that IFE would only have theoretical benefit with lipophilic drugs. IFE and ECMO can lead to significant complications that should be taken into consideration before initiation.[54]

Gut decontamination may prevent absorption after ingestions of any of the agents discussed earlier. If benefit is to be derived from gastric decontamination, it should ideally be initiated within 1 hour of the ingestion. The longer the delay, the more drug escapes into the small intestine, where most absorption occurs. Gastric decontamination using emesis or lavage more than 1 hour after ingestion may be of benefit in drugs that delay gastric emptying, but studies have not shown that gastric decontamination changes clinical outcomes.[154] Syrup of ipecac is no longer recommended as a method of decontamination. Gastric lavage is no longer routinely advocated except for life-threatening poisonings that present within 1 hour of ingestion where no antidote is available.

Activated charcoal has been found to bind most cardiotoxic drugs and may be of benefit in limiting absorption. The timing of activated charcoal administration is also important, but charcoal administration may still be effective in binding drug that has entered the duodenum. It is therefore rational to consider administering a dose of activated charcoal to patients with a history or clinical evidence of ingesting a cardiotoxic substance if no contraindications exist. Unfortunately, there is no strong evidence in most poisonings of improved outcomes when activated charcoal is used in humans. The recommended dose of activated charcoal is 1 g/kg; patients may either drink the aqueous charcoal suspension (which has no taste) or have the dose administered through a nasogastric tube when intubated or uncooperative. Caution should be used when administering activated charcoal to lethargic patients or in those who are unable to protect their airway, as this poses a risk of aspiration. Multiple doses of activated charcoal have been found to be of benefit in poisonings with agents such as theophylline and phenobarbital, but this therapy is not likely to benefit humans poisoned with any of the cardiotoxic agents listed in this chapter. In addition, those drugs that slow gastrointestinal motility may predispose the patient to charcoal bezoar formation when multiple doses are administered.[155]

Extracorporeal removal of drugs using techniques such as hemodialysis or hemoperfusion has proven beneficial in overdoses of compounds such as theophylline, salicylates, and phenobarbital. Most other drugs, including those listed in this chapter, have not been found to be well removed by these modalities.

Several therapeutic considerations should be addressed regarding the antimuscarinic toxicity resulting from agents such as cyclic antidepressants, antihistamines, and phenothiazines. The antimuscarinic signs and symptoms that usually predominate are seldom life threatening; patients typically do well with supportive care measures. Seizures from these agents, in the absence

of severe hypotension or hypoxia, may be related to blockade of muscarinic or other receptors in the brain. They are usually self-limited and easily controlled with benzodiazepines or barbiturates. Sinus tachycardia produced by reduced vagal tone does not require specific treatment. Physostigmine, a short-acting carbamate cholinesterase inhibitor, can reverse CNS toxicity and sinus tachycardia associated with these agents but may exacerbate impaired conduction throughout the heart, rarely resulting in asystole.[156] For this reason, physostigmine is best reserved for patients with altered mental status in whom no cardiac conduction delays are present.

Patients with severe antimuscarinic signs and symptoms may need a urinary catheter if urinary retention occurs. Multiple doses of activated charcoal, as well as food and beverages, should be avoided in those individuals with evidence of impaired gastric motility.

ILLICIT DRUGS

Psychostimulant toxicity is a common cause of emergency department visits. Deaths have been described as a result of the multiorgan effects of these drugs. This is a diverse class of agents that includes cocaine, novel psychoactive agents, and synthetic cannabinoids. The composition of these medications changes rapidly, as some are made illegal and new formulations come to market. In general, the new formulations will have similar clinical effects in toxic concentrations as the three groups described.

Cocaine

Cocaine is an alkaloid derived from the leaves of *Erythroxylon coca* and other trees indigenous to Peru and Bolivia. The alkaloid is dissolved in hydrochloric acid to form a water-soluble salt termed *cocaine hydrochloride* (chemical name, benzoylemethylecgonine). Cocaine hydrochloride is sold as crystals, granules, or white powder. "Crack" (cocaine freebase) is the basic, nonsalt form that is created by the organic esterification of cocaine hydrochloride from a basic solution with ether. When crack is heated, it melts and forms a fat-soluble vapor that can be smoked and rapidly absorbed through the lungs. The name "crack" is derived from the popping sound made by the drug when it is heated. Therapeutically, cocaine is classified as an ester-type local anesthetic and currently limited to use as a mucosal anesthetic.

Pharmacology. Cocaine is well absorbed from the mucous membranes of the nose, lung, and genitourinary and gastrointestinal tracts. Administration can occur through the intravenous, respiratory, intramuscular, and rectal routes. The method and dose of administration determine the onset of action. The "high" from intravenous administration of cocaine peaks within a few minutes after injection. Inhalation of the drug will produce effects within 1 to 3 minutes, but oral ingestion may delay symptoms up to 60 to 90 minutes. The duration of the drug effect depends on the route of administration and varies from 30 to 60 minutes after inhalation to several hours after oral dosing. Plasma concentrations after intranasal use peak within 20 to 30 minutes and gradually decline over the next 60 minutes.[157]

Cocaine is metabolized by nonenzymatic hydrolysis and liver esterases, including plasma cholinesterase. The two major metabolites include benzoylecgonine and ecgonine methyl ester, neither of which crosses the blood-brain barrier. Both compounds are water soluble and are excreted in the urine. Cocaine metabolites may be detected in the urine up to 72 hours after an exposure, although heavy users may have positive urine screens for up to 3 weeks.[158] When a user of cocaine also coingests ethanol, hepatic transesterification will create another pharmacologically active metabolite, cocaethylene. Cocaethylene is not on the routine urine screens for cocaine metabolites.

Pathophysiology. The pharmacologic effects of cocaine in humans include the ability to stabilize membranes and block nerve conduction. The resulting effects on myocardial tissue cause blockade of fast sodium channels leading to widening of the QRS complex with subsequent arrhythmias. The sympathomimetic effects of cocaine are caused by impaired catecholamine reuptake and enhanced catecholamine release at nerve terminals.[157] The increased synaptic concentrations of neurotransmitters stimulate α- and β-receptors throughout the autonomic nervous system, resulting in a cascade of clinical effects. Cocaine may also enhance the release of norepinephrine and dopamine in the CNS.[159] The unique ability of cocaine to inhibit nerve conduction while enhancing vasoconstriction is primarily responsible for its cardiovascular toxicity.[157]

Cocaethylene is also a potent sodium channel blocking agent and appears to prolong the recovery time for the channel compared with cocaine.[160] In animal models, cocaine plus ethanol depressed myocardial contractility more than either agent given alone.[161,162] Once formed, cocaethylene has a longer half-life than cocaine.

The mechanism of cocaine-induced myocardial ischemia is thought to be multifactorial. Cocaine increases myocardial oxygen demand while increasing heart rate and blood pressure. Usually, myocardial oxygen demand results in coronary vasodilatation; however, cocaine taken by some routes can induce coronary vasospasm.[163] Coronary artery thrombus formation has also been implicated as a cause of cocaine-induced myocardial ischemia. Thrombus formation leading to myocardial infarction (MI) has been associated with coronary artery vasospasm.[164] The vasospasm may damage the endothelium and cause release of vasoactive substances, precipitating platelet aggregation. Cocaine may enhance this effect because in vitro studies have demonstrated that cocaine alone may directly stimulate platelet aggregation and platelet thromboxane production.[165] Cocaine activates platelets in whole blood by inducing the release of platelet α-granule contents and by promoting the binding of fibrinogen to the surface of the platelet.[165]

Clinical Manifestations. The clinical effects of cocaine result from diffuse hyperadrenergic stimulation both centrally and peripherally. The peripheral sympathomimetic effects include tremor, mydriasis, urinary retention, and ileus. Adrenergic stimulation of the CNS leads to agitation, hallucinations, seizures, and coma.[166] Patients may experience psychosis, paranoia, and anxiety due to increased dopaminergic transmission.[167]

Cerebrovascular complications from cocaine-induced vasospasm and a hyperadrenergic state include cerebral infarctions, transient ischemic attacks, and subarachnoid and intracranial hemorrhages.[166,167]

Myocardial ischemia and MI are well-documented complications of cocaine use. Ischemia of the myocardium does not require a massive exposure to cocaine and occurs commonly in the young adult with no history of cardiac risk factors. Symptoms of chest pain may be typical, atypical, or absent. A delay of several hours in the onset of chest discomfort may occur after exposure to the drug.[168–170] ECGs from patients with cocaine-associated chest pain may demonstrate a variety of abnormalities, including classic findings of myocardial injury, such as ST segment elevation. However, they may also be normal or have only nonspecific findings. A study of 42 cocaine users with chest pain and normal or nondiagnostic ECGs documented 8 of these patients as having acute MI, defined by total creatinine kinase and myocardial isoenzyme levels.[171] Thus single or even serial ECGs may not be useful in ruling out cocaine-induced ischemia.

Cocaine has been associated with a variety of arrhythmias. Sinus tachycardia is common owing to the sympathomimetic effects. Atrial fibrillation, premature ventricular contractions, ventricular tachycardia, and ventricular fibrillation have all been described.[172] Arrhythmias may occur with or without underlying ischemia. Cocaine can cause sodium channel blockade, widening of the QRS complex, and associated arrhythmias. Toxicity related to sodium channel blockade should be treated with sodium bicarbonate, as previously discussed.

Hypertension is also common with cocaine poisoning. The elevation in blood pressure combined with tachycardia may increase shear forces on the great vessels, resulting in aortic[173] or coronary artery dissection.[174] The intestinal vasculature is susceptible to α-stimulating effects of catecholamines; ischemic colitis has been described in adults[175] as well as in neonates after in utero exposure to cocaine.[176] The uteroplacental vasculature may also respond to cocaine exposure with diminished uterine blood flow after maternal cocaine use.[177]

Extreme hyperthermia is often documented in cocaine overdose. Temperatures are frequently reported in excess of 106°F and are thought to result from a disturbance in thermoregulation due to extensive dopaminergic stimulation combined with excessive musculoskeletal activity and agitation.[178,179] Although cocaine-induced hyperthermia may occur independent of seizure activity, it can be exacerbated by concomitant convulsions.[180] An acute rise in the central body temperature has also occurred after rupture of bags of cocaine ingested by body packers (individuals who conceal illicit drugs in their bodies for smuggling purposes).[181]

Rhabdomyolysis also contributes to the morbidity and mortality of cocaine poisoning. All routes of cocaine exposure have been associated with a rise in serum creatinine phosphokinase level from direct myotoxicity.[181–183] An association has been made between drug-induced hyperthermia and rhabdomyolysis, but observations suggest that cocaine can also induce rhabdomyolysis independently of hyperthermia.[181] Cocaine-induced rhabdomyolysis is associated with myoglobinuric renal failure.[183] Cocaine is not known to be directly toxic to the renal tubules; however, the effects of cocaine on renal blood flow may exacerbate the effects of myoglobinuria.

Novel Psychoactive Substances

Novel psychoactive substances (NPSs) come in many forms and are very popular owing to their wide availability. They can be classified based on their chemical families, which include phenylethylamines, amphetamines, cathinones, piperazines, pipradrols/piperidines, aminoindanes, benzofurans, and tryptamines (Table 34.1).[184] They have varying intoxicating and toxic effects based on their actions on dopamine, serotonin, and norepinephrine. Most of these have no approved uses in the United States but some of the phenylethylamines are used for treatment of narcolepsy, attention deficit disorder, and weight loss. Synthetic cannabinoids are commonly included in the NPSs but will be discussed separately owing to their differing mechanisms. Amphetamines are described as the prototypical agent of this class, as they all have similar mechanisms of action.

Amphetamines have been recognized for their stimulant properties for centuries and continue to be abused by various routes, including intravenous and oral administration. "Ice" is a pure preparation of methamphetamine and is marketed in a solid form, hence its nickname. This preparation is volatile and can be smoked, resulting in rapid absorption and effect. This form of methamphetamine rapidly became one of the leading drugs of abuse in Hawaii and California in the 1980s.[185,186] Illicit laboratories can produce large quantities of methamphetamines because of the ease of availability of most reagents. In recent years, advances and simplification of synthesis techniques have led to many new psychoactive substances being produced and distributed as "legal highs" before legislation could be initiated to make them illegal.[184]

Abuse of amphetamines results in euphoria, with increased self-confidence and well-being. Persistent use with repetitive doses over several days is common. During this "speed run," the user may not sleep or eat owing to the stimulant and anorectic effects of the drug. Chronic use of amphetamines can rapidly lead to tolerance; increasing doses are usually required to maintain euphoria.

Pharmacology. The volume of distribution of amphetamines tends to be large and the half-life ranges from 8 to 30 hours.[187] Elimination is primarily through hepatic transformation, but renal excretion results in significant elimination of certain members of the amphetamine family, such as methamphetamine.[188] Although acidification of the urine may enhance the excretion of some amphetamine derivatives, it may also exacerbate renal toxicity in the presence of rhabdomyolysis and is therefore not recommended.[189]

Pathophysiology. The pharmacologic mechanisms of action of amphetamines are diverse but are thought to rely on indirect effects on catecholamine receptors. These compounds act by entering presynaptic neurons and stimulating the release of endogenous catecholamines, such as norepinephrine and dopamine. Amphetamines also inhibit the reuptake of catecholamines and their breakdown by the monoamine oxidase enzyme system. These effects may last for hours, whereas those of cocaine may resolve within several minutes.[187]

Increased catecholamine release results in stimulation of α- and β-receptors both peripherally and centrally. Dopaminergic and serotonergic receptor stimulation may contribute to the behavioral disturbances and hyperthermic effects that are common with these poisonings.[190] The release of dopamine may be responsible for the pleasurable effects reported with these drugs. Although all members of the amphetamine family may produce a generalized hyperadrenergic state, the pattern of effects with these compounds differs with modification of the parent molecule, resulting in different anorectic, cardiovascular, and hallucinogenic properties.[191]

Clinical Manifestations. Physical findings in amphetamine poisoning are similar to those seen with other sympathomimetic drugs. The cardiovascular toxicity of amphetamines manifests most commonly as tachycardia and hypertension. Arrhythmias are a common cause of death and can include ventricular tachycardia and ventricular fibrillation.[192] Hypertensive emergencies with intracranial hemorrhages and cerebrovascular accidents may be more common with amphetamine and methamphetamine than cocaine abuse.[193] Acute myocardial ischemia, MI, aortic dissection, and dilated cardiomyopathy are also known to occur in the setting of amphetamine use.[194] Diffuse vascular spasm

TABLE 34.1 Novel Psychoactive Substances	
Chemical Name	**Nickname**
Synthetic Cathinones	
4-Methyl-N-ethyl cathinone	4-MEC, Shrimp
α-Pyrrolidinovalerophenone	Alpha PVP, Flakka, Gravel
Benzofurans	
5-(2-Aminopropyl)benzofuran	5-APB, Benzo Fury
6-(2-Aminopropyl)benzofuran	6-APB, Benzo Fury
Piperazines	
3-Chlorophenylpiperazine	mCPP, Legal X
Methoxypiperamide	MeOP, MEXP
Pipradrols/Piperidines	
N-Methyl-3-piperidyl benzilate	JB-336, BZ
(RS)-2-benzhydrylpiperdine	2-DPMP, Ivory Wave
Aminoindanes	
5,6-methylenedioxy-2-aminoindane	MDAI, Woof-Woof, MDog
5-Methoxy-6-methyl-2-aminoindane	MMAI
Tryptamine	
N,N-Dimethyltryptamine	DMT, Fantasia
Phenethylamines/Amphetamines	
3, 4-Methylenedioxymethamphetamine	MDMA, Adam, Ecstasy, XTC
3, 4-Methylenedioxymethamphetamine	MDEA, Eve
3, 4-Methylenedioxyamphetamine	MDA, Love Drug
4-Methyl-2, 5-dimethoxyamphetamine	DOM/STP, Serenity, Tranquility

has also been reported with amphetamine poisoning and may result in death.[195,196]

CNS toxicity is the most common reason for amphetamine-poisoned patients to present to a hospital. Most victims are agitated, anxious, and can become volatile and violent. Tactile and visual hallucinations may contribute to patient agitation, and psychoses similar to paranoid schizophrenia are frequently observed in these patients. Mydriasis and diaphoresis are common. Seizures often complicate amphetamine poisoning.[184,196]

As in acute cocaine intoxication, hyperthermia is well documented in amphetamine poisoning and is associated with increased morbidity and mortality. Hyperthermia may occur independent of seizures and has been associated with rhabdomyolysis, coagulopathy, renal failure, and death.[184,196–198]

Synthetic Cannabinoids

Marijuana has a long history of recreational and medicinal use and is the most widely produced and consumed illicit substance.[199] Synthetic cannabinoids were developed initially in an attempt to provide the therapeutic benefits claimed by botanical cannabis while limiting the psychoactive effects. Around 2004, these synthetic cannabinoids started being produced for use as legal alternatives to marijuana.[199,200] These chemicals were marketed under names such as "K2" or "Spice" and were packaged with statements such as "not for human consumption" or "for aromatherapy use only." Many different compounds have been produced and distributed. It was rapidly recognized by toxicologists that these products had greater effects or potency at smaller doses than standard marijuana. They also seemed to have effects not commonly seen with marijuana use, including tachycardia, arrhythmias, seizures, and delirium.

Pharmacology. The synthetic cannabinoids would be expected to have a large volume of distribution based on their lipophilicity.[200] These compounds are mostly glucuronidated or hydroxylated in the liver and then excreted in the urine. Some of their metabolites are active at cannabinoid receptors, which may increase the length of perceived effects.[199]

Pathophysiology. Synthetic cannabinoids act by stimulating cannabinoid receptors found throughout the body. Two cannabinoid receptors have been identified so far: CB_1 and CB_2. These receptors are G-protein coupled receptors that cause down-regulation of adenylyl cyclase and decrease cellular cyclic adenosine monophosphate (cAMP) levels when activated. This leads to changes in cellular signaling and neurotransmitter release, including acetylcholine, dopamine, norepinephrine, glutamine, and GABA. CB_1 receptors are predominantly in the brain; increased activation leads to modulation of GABA and glutamate neurotransmission. CB_2 is primarily expressed in peripheral tissues of the immune system including the spleen, tonsils, thymus, and gastrointestinal system; activation leads to changes in immunomodulation.[199,200]

Synthetic cannabinoids generally have a much higher potency and affinity for these receptors than delta-9-tetrahydrocannabinol (delta 9-THC) found in marijuana. The changes in GABA and glutamate in the brain are the probable cause leading to the psychosis, seizures, and other central nervous effects often reported with these chemicals, although the exact mechanisms are unclear at this time. The arrhythmias, tachycardia, and hypertension seen with these agents are likely the result of increased release of excitatory neurotransmitters, but this too has not been fully elucidated.[199,200]

Clinical Manifestations. The clinical findings from synthetic cannabinoid overdose are like those seen with the other sympathomimetic drugs. The most commonly reported cardiovascular symptoms are tachycardia, hypertension, chest pain, and arrhythmias. There have been reports of sudden cardiac death after synthetic cannabinoid use. The cause of cardiac death seems to be cardiovascular vasospasm like that described with other sympathomimetic drugs. Acute myocardial ischemia has also been theorized to be caused by increased myocardial oxygen demand resulting from tachycardia and hypertension. A final possible factor for the increased cardiac deaths is the fact that synthetic cannabinoids lead to increased platelet activation that may amplify plaque rupture induced by increased shear forces in the coronary arteries.[200]

In most cases, patients present to medical facilities due to the CNS effects of these agents with psychomotor agitation, psychosis, anxiety, confusion, and changes in memory. Seizures are some of the most severe CNS effects noted from these chemicals but are generally easily controlled with benzodiazepines.[200]

Unlike other sympathomimetic agents, synthetic cannabinoids have not been associated with significant hyperthermia. Other physical signs include dilated pupils, reddened conjunctivae, nausea, vomiting, and shortness of breath. In severe cases, cannabinoids have been associated with ischemic strokes and acute kidney injury requiring hemodialysis.[199,200]

Management. Successful treatment of sympathomimetic poisoning begins with aggressive supportive care. Management of airway, breathing, and circulation are initial priorities. Placement of the patient in a quiet setting may reduce the amount of stimulation and reduce patient agitation; however, the victim must be continuously monitored for potential complications. Vital signs should be obtained frequently and body temperature verified by rectal thermometer if hyperthermia is suspected. Rapid cooling measures should be instituted as soon as hyperthermia is detected; neuromuscular paralysis may be required in severe cases of hyperthermia.

Decontamination of the patient who ingested sympathomimetics or bags containing these drugs begins with the administration of activated charcoal, as described earlier. Whole-bowel irrigation with an isosmotic, isoelectric lavage solution (e.g., Go-Lytely) may enhance the removal of bags from the gastrointestinal tract.[201] Due to the large volume of distribution of these agents, hemodialysis and hemoperfusion are not effective in their removal; however, hemodialysis may be required if acute renal failure develops as a complication of rhabdomyolysis.

Rapid and effective control of hypertension from sympathomimetic poisoning is imperative. The use of β-blockers to control the hypertension associated with sympathomimetics is controversial because these drugs may theoretically potentiate both coronary and peripheral vasoconstriction due to unopposed α-agonist activity.[202,203] Case reports have suggested the use of labetalol as an alternative to nonselective β-blocking agents,[204] but labetalol is a more potent β- than α-antagonist. One study of patients given intranasal cocaine while undergoing angiography demonstrated that labetalol reduced the mean arterial pressure but had no effect on coronary artery vasoconstriction.[205] The current literature supports the use of β-blocking agents in sympathomimetic overdose to control hypertension, with labetalol being the most supported.[206] Vasodilators—such as nitroglycerin, nitroprusside, or phentolamine—can be considered.[207,208]

Cocaine-, NPS-, or cannabinoid-related chest pain must be considered to represent active myocardial ischemia. Therapy should initially include the application of oxygen and the reduction of central sympathomimetic effects with the liberal use of benzodiazepines. Nitroglycerin has been demonstrated to be effective in alleviating cocaine-induced vasoconstriction in diseased and nondiseased coronary arteries.[208] An antiplatelet drug, such as aspirin, may be administered because platelets are activated by cocaine. Heparin may be considered when ischemia is refractory to more conservative management.

Treatment of sympathomimetic-induced arrhythmias begins with the administration of benzodiazepines to sedate the patient and reduce catecholamine release.[209] Wide complex tachycardias from cocaine have been effectively treated with intravenous sodium bicarbonate.[210] Lidocaine may be considered for treatment of arrhythmias secondary to ischemia or refractory to sodium bicarbonate but should be used with caution because it has potentiated cocaine-induced seizures and death in rats.[211]

Benzodiazepines are the mainstay of treatment for the CNS effects of sympathomimetic poisonings. These sedative-hypnotics have been demonstrated to reduce the lethality of both cocaine and amphetamines.[209,212] Butyrophenones have also been effective in reducing the dopaminergic-based delirium associated with amphetamine use.[213] Butyrophenones must be administered cautiously to patients with either cocaine, NPS, or cannabinoid toxicity because most antipsychotic medications may lower seizure thresholds, alter temperature regulation, and cause acute dystonias.

CONCLUSION

Many drugs possess the ability to cause life-threatening cardiotoxicity in overdose. In this chapter, we have outlined some of the most significant and most common agents in this regard, with emphasis on clinical presentation and management. Although primary resuscitative efforts in all disease states should focus on airway and circulation, the varied mechanisms of action of cardiotoxic compounds may require specific therapeutic interventions. Early consultation with a certified regional poison control center or a medical toxicologist may assist in the care of these patients.

The full reference list for this chapter is available at ExpertConsult.com.

PART V

Pharmacologic Agents in the Cardiac Intensive Care Unit

35

Anticoagulation: Antithrombin Therapy

Daniel M. Shivapour, A. Michael Lincoff

OUTLINE

Antithrombotic therapies are a mainstay of contemporary cardiovascular medicine; it is essential for providers in the cardiac intensive care unit (CICU) to have a thorough understanding of these pharmacologic agents. Patients with acute coronary syndromes (ACSs) and those undergoing percutaneous coronary intervention (PCI) account for a substantial proportion of CICU admissions; the thoughtful use of antithrombotic therapies in these settings is required to safely balance the antithrombotic and bleeding risks. The desire to achieve consistent, rapid anticoagulation within a specific therapeutic window has motivated decades of drug development and clinical investigation. The resultant highly evidence-based discipline has improved survival and reduced morbidity, thus forming the basis of contemporary pharmacologic management of coronary artery disease (CAD). While several other categories of medications, such as β-blockers, angiotensin-converting enzyme (ACE) inhibitors and 5-hydroxy-3-methylglutaryl-coenzyme A (HMG coenzyme A) reductase inhibitors (statins) also have robust evidence-supported roles in the long-term treatment of CAD, antithrombotic agents are the only acute therapies that have been convincingly shown to reduce short-term ischemic events associated with ACS and PCI. This chapter offers a broad overview of the coagulation cascade and reviews the clinical evidence supporting the most commonly used anticoagulant therapies, including unfractionated heparin, enoxaparin, fondaparinux, and bivalirudin. Adjunctive pharmacologic management with antiplatelet agents is presented separately in Chapter 36.

HEMOSTASIS AND THE COAGULATION CASCADE

Hemostasis refers to the formation of a platelet-fibrin clot at the site of vascular endothelial injury and involves the activation of platelets as well as the coagulation cascade. Fibrinolysis refers to the dissolution of a platelet-fibrin clot by separate protease reactions. A delicate balance between the carefully regulated systems of coagulation and fibrinolysis is required to keep blood fluid and vessels patent within the circulation; disturbances in either system will cause a tendency toward thrombosis or bleeding.[1] Coagulation, as shown in Fig. 35.1, has often been represented as two independent pathways that converge to a common pathway with thrombin generation as the endpoint of the cascade. This model provides a basic representation of the processes observed in clinical coagulation laboratory testing. The prothrombin time (PT) measures the factors of the extrinsic pathway and activated partial thromboplastin time (aPTT) measures factors of the intrinsic pathway. However, this model is a simplification of a complex physiologic process and has certain inadequacies when applied to the multifaceted in vivo hemostatic processes that involve interactions between cellular-based (e.g., vascular- and platelet-mediated) and soluble coagulation processes. Others have demonstrated that, under normal circumstances, in vivo hemostasis is initiated by tissue factor (TF), a transmembrane glycoprotein that is a member of the class II cytokine receptor superfamily and functions both as the receptor and the essential

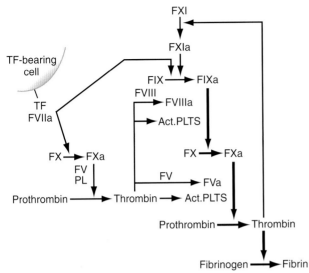

Fig. 35.1 Coagulation cascade. Simplified schematic shows coagulation by activation of factor XII (intrinsic pathway) and factor VII/TF (extrinsic pathway). *Act.,* activated; *F,* factor; *PL,* phospholipids; *PLTS,* platelets; *TF,* tissue factor.

cofactor for factors (F) VII and VIIa.[2,3] Assembly of the TF/FVIIa complex on cellular surfaces leads to the activation of FX and initiates coagulation. TF is constitutively expressed in cells surrounding blood vessels and large organs to form a hemostatic barrier. In addition to its role in hemostasis, the TF/FVIIa complex has been shown to elicit intracellular signaling, resulting in the induction of various genes, thus explaining its role in various biologic functions, such as embryonic development, cell migration, inflammation, apoptosis, and angiogenesis.[4–6]

CELL-BASED MODEL OF COAGULATION

In the cell-based model, coagulation occurs in three overlapping phases: initiation, priming, and propagation.[2] A disruption in vascular endothelium brings plasma into contact with TF-bearing cells; FVII binds to the exposed TF and is rapidly activated by coagulation proteases and by noncoagulation proteases. The FVIIa/TF complex then activates FX and FIX. The activated forms of these two proteins (FIXa and FXa) play very different roles in subsequent coagulation reactions. FXa can activate plasma FV on the TF cell. If FXa diffuses from the protected environment of the cell surface from which it was activated, it can be rapidly inhibited by the TF pathway inhibitor (TFPI) or antithrombin (AT). However, the FXa that remains on the TF cell surface can combine with FVa to produce small amounts of thrombin (the enzyme responsible for clot formation). This thrombin, although not sufficient to cleave fibrinogen throughout a site of injury, nonetheless plays a critical role in amplifying the initial thrombin signal. The initial FVIIa/TF complex is subsequently inhibited by the action of the TFPI in complex with FXa. In contrast to FXa, FIXa is not inhibited by TFPI, and is only slowly inhibited by AT. FIXa moves in the fluid phase from TF-bearing cells to nearby platelets at the injury site.[7]

In the priming (or amplification) phase, low concentrations of thrombin activate platelets adhering to the injury site to release FV from their α-granules. Thrombin cleaves the partially activated FV to yield a fully active form. Thrombin also cleaves FVIII, releasing it from von Willebrand factor. These activated factors bind to platelet surfaces and provide the backbone for thrombin generation that occurs during the propagation phase.[3]

In the propagation phase, the phospholipid surface of activated platelets acts as a cofactor for the activation of the FVIIIa/FIXa complex and the FVa/FXa complex, which accelerates the generation of FXa and thrombin, respectively. The burst of thrombin leads to the bulk cleavage of fibrinogen to fibrin. Soluble fibrin is stabilized by FXIIIa and activated by thrombin to form a fibrin network (i.e., a thrombus).

ARTERIAL THROMBOSIS

Although arterial thrombosis can result from different mechanisms, the most clinically relevant in the context of cardiovascular medicine and PCI are endothelial erosion and plaque rupture. Plaque rupture results in the exposure of thrombogenic substances (e.g., collagen and TF) to the circulation, with the resulting activation of platelets and coagulation cascade that can lead to partial or complete obstruction of the vessel. This sequence of events, coupled with the simultaneous release of vasoactive substances, can result in thrombus formation and vasoconstriction. When this occurs in the coronary circulation, the result is myocardial ischemia and ACS.

ANTITHROMBINS: MECHANISM OF ACTION

Anticoagulant agents specifically target the soluble coagulation cascade proteins required to form fibrin clots. Fig. 35.2 displays the mechanisms of action of the different thrombin inhibitors described here. The heparin derivatives in current clinical use include unfractionated heparin (UFH), low-molecular-weight heparins (LMWHs), and the synthetic pentasaccharide derivative fondaparinux. These are all parenteral agents that must be administered by intravenous (IV) or subcutaneous (SC) injection. They are classified as indirect anticoagulants because they require a plasma cofactor, AT, to exert their anticoagulant activity. By contrast, the direct thrombin inhibitors (DTIs), such as bivalirudin, bind thrombin at its active site and/or its fibrin recognition site (exosite 1), essentially displacing it from fibrin, to provide a direct anticoagulant effect.

UNFRACTIONATED HEPARIN

Pharmacokinetics, Metabolism, and Administration

UFH is a glycosaminoglycan of varying molecular weights that accelerates the action of antithrombin (the enzyme that inactivates thrombin and factor Xa), thereby preventing conversion of fibrinogen to fibrin. It is a natural product that can be isolated from beef lung or porcine intestinal mucosa. It consists of highly sulfated polysaccharide chains with a mean of about 45 saccharide units. Only one-third of the heparin chains possess a unique pentasaccharide sequence that exhibits high affinity for AT; it is this fraction that is responsible for most of the anticoagulant activity of heparin.

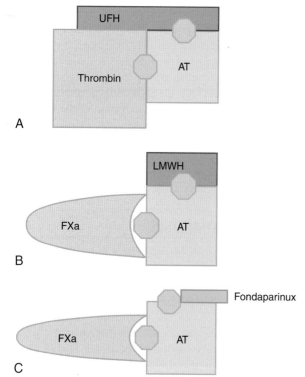

Fig. 35.2 Mechanism of action of heparin derivatives. (A) Unfractionated heparin (UFH) possesses the pentasaccharide unit necessary for its interaction with antithrombin (AT). The UFH/AT complex is able to block the thrombin active site. (B) Low-molecular-weight heparins (LMWHs; short chains) do not bind to exosite 2 of thrombin, in contrast to the longer UFH chains. All LMWH/AT complexes can still bind to factor Xa (FXa). (C) Synthetic pentasaccharides (fondaparinux), similar to LMWHs, bind and activate AT and allow AT to inhibit FXa efficiently. Hirudin and bivalirudin bind to thrombin via the active site and exosite 1, displacing thrombin from fibrin.

UFH must be given parenterally either by continuous IV infusion or by intermittent SC injection. When given SC for treatment of thrombosis, higher doses are needed to overcome the fact that heparin bioavailability after SC injection is only about 30% (however, this is highly variable across individuals).[8] A number of plasma proteins compete with AT for heparin binding, thereby reducing its anticoagulant activity. The levels of these proteins vary among patients. This phenomenon contributes to the variable anticoagulant response to heparin and to the phenomenon of heparin resistance. Heparin is cleared through a combination of a rapid saturable phase and a slower first-order mechanism. Heparin binds to endothelial cells, platelets, and macrophages during the saturable phase. Once the cellular binding sites are saturated, heparin enters the circulation, from where it is cleared more slowly by the kidneys. The complex kinetics of heparin clearance render the anticoagulant response to UFH nonlinear at therapeutic doses, with both the peak activity and duration of effect increasing disproportionately with increasing doses.

Unfractionated heparin can be given in fixed or weight-adjusted doses; nomograms have been developed to aid with initial and maintenance dosing. The doses of UFH recommended for the treatment of ACS are lower than those typically used to

treat venous thromboembolism (VTE) owing to the lower thrombus burden in arterial thromboses. A distinct advantage of UFH is that its anticoagulant effect can be followed (and subsequent dosing titrated) by routine laboratory studies. The test most often used to monitor heparin in the CICU is aPTT. An aPTT ratio between 1.5 and 2.5 (calculated by dividing the reported therapeutic aPTT value by the control value for the reagent) was associated with a reduced risk for recurrent VTE in a large retrospective registry.[9] Based on this study, an aPTT ratio of 1.5 to 2.5 was adopted as the therapeutic range for UFH. Because of different reagents and control values across laboratories, it is important to emphasize that aPTT ratios should be adapted at each institution to the specific reagent used rather than adopting universal/fixed aPTT targets for specific therapeutic indications. Despite these shortcomings, aPTT remains the most commonly used method for UFH monitoring. The aPTT ratio should be measured approximately 4 to 6 hours after the bolus dose of heparin; the continuous IV infusion (maintenance dose) should be adjusted according to the result.

The point-of-care activated clotting time (ACT) can be used to monitor the higher doses of UFH given to patients undergoing PCI or cardiopulmonary bypass surgery as the required level of anticoagulation is beyond the range that can be reliably measured using aPTT assays. Common ACT targets during PCI range from 250 to 300 seconds for UFH monotherapy or 200 to 250 seconds when used concurrently with glycoprotein IIb/IIIa receptor inhibitors or if less intensive anticoagulation is indicated in the setting of increased bleeding risk or other patient-specific factors. Of note, this ideal ACT range has not been examined in the era of routine P2Y$_{12}$ receptor blocker use. At traditional dosing of 50 to 70 U/kg commonly used in PCI, UFH has a dose-dependent half-life of 30 to 60 minutes.

Additional advantages of UFH include its widespread availability, low cost, rapid clearance after the infusion is discontinued, and the ability to reverse its anticoagulant effects with protamine in urgent situations. Potential disadvantages include the higher incidence of heparin-induced thrombocytopenia (HIT) with UFH compared to other heparin preparations, platelet activation, inability to inhibit clot-bound thrombin owing to steric hindrance, circulating inhibitors, and inconsistent pharmacokinetics/pharmacodynamics due to nonspecific binding to multiple other proteins.

Adverse Effects

Bleeding is the major complication of heparin therapy as well as for all other anticoagulants discussed in this chapter. HIT is a condition that can occur following the formation of heparin/platelet factor 4 (PF4) complexes. In HIT, antibodies against a neoepitope on PF4 are produced and bind platelet Fc receptors, resulting in platelet activation. These activated platelets are subsequently removed from the circulation, leading to thrombocytopenia.[10] When HIT is diagnosed, heparin therapy must be immediately discontinued.

Clinical Evidence

UFH was discovered almost 90 years ago and can be thought of as a legacy drug. While its use in the management of patients with non–ST segment elevation-ACS (NSTE-ACS), ST elevation myocardial infarction (STEMI; with or without fibrinolytic agents), and as adjuvant therapy during PCI has been widespread for over 20 years, its supporting evidence base does not meet the standard of nearly every other drug discussed in this chapter. There is no randomized controlled trial establishing its use in PCI; rather, there are only smaller trials examining the relationships between ACT, antithrombotic efficacy, and bleeding.[11–13] Similarly, there are no randomized placebo-controlled trials establishing UFH use in STEMI. The majority of the evidence for its use in ACS was derived from a meta-analysis of six relatively small randomized controlled trials in NSTE-ACS patients that demonstrated a 33% reduction in death or MI among unstable angina patients treated with aspirin plus UFH compared to those treated with aspirin alone.[14]

LOW-MOLECULAR-WEIGHT HEPARINS (ENOXAPARIN)

LMWHs were first introduced in the early 1980s as an alternative to UFH for the prevention of deep vein thrombosis (DVT) in postoperative patients. The LMWH agents are derived from UFH, act via AT, and preferentially inhibit Factor Xa more than thrombin. Three LMWH preparations have been approved by the Food and Drug Administration (FDA) for clinical use in the United States: enoxaparin, dalteparin, and tinzaparin. Enoxaparin is the most rigorously studied of all the LMWH in the setting of ACS, is the agent most commonly used in the United States and, therefore, will be the primary agent discussed in the following section.

Pharmacokinetics, Metabolism, and Administration

Enoxaparin exhibits high bioavailability and much less binding to plasma proteins and endothelial cells than UFH, giving it a more consistent and predictable anticoagulant effect. In addition, LMWH has been reported to have less effect on platelet aggregation than UFH.[15] The LMWHs are most commonly administered SC, although an IV bolus has also been evaluated, most commonly in the STEMI population. Enoxaparin is dosed according to body weight, with 1 mg/kg every 12 hours being the most common dose used in ACS.[16] When given intravenously, enoxaparin has a time to peak effect of 5 to 10 minutes compared with 3 to 5 hours when administered subcutaneously. Enoxaparin's 5- to 7-hour half-life is dose independent; however, dose adjustment is required in patients with renal insufficiency. Other benefits of LMWH include a higher antifactor Xa:IIa ratio, less inhibition by PF4, and an inhibition in the early rise of von Willebrand factor.[17]

Enoxaparin is weakly metabolized in the liver. Renal clearance of active fragments represents about 10% of the administered dose, whereas about 40% of active and inactive fragments combined are excreted renally.

Clinical Evidence

The majority of trials using LMWH in PCI have been in the setting of ACS; the evidence base supporting its use during routine elective PCI is much weaker. Multiple early trials demonstrated

a reduction in death and MI among conservatively managed NSTE-ACS patients (not undergoing routine revascularization) treated with enoxaparin compared with UFH. However, in patients undergoing early invasive management, LMWH was noninferior to UFH for ischemic endpoints but was associated with increased bleeding.[18–21] Select findings from the major clinical trials that provide the evidence base supporting LMWH use in ACS and PCI are summarized in Table 35.1. As with the other agents discussed in this chapter, it is essential to carefully examine the indications, patient populations, and cointerventions in each of these trials as they significantly contribute to the noted differences in results and influence the relative risks and benefits of a given treatment strategy in a particular patient. For example, only one of the landmark NSTE-ACS trials (Superior Yield of the New Strategy of Enoxaparin, Revascularization and Glycoprotein IIb/IIIa Inhibitors [SYNERGY]) utilized contemporary dual antiplatelet therapy (aspirin plus oral $P2Y_{12}$ inhibitors or glycoprotein IIb/IIIa receptor inhibitors [GPIs]).

The relative safety and efficacy of enoxaparin compared to UFH in the setting of PCI was recently examined in a meta-analysis by Silvain and colleagues[22] that included over 30,000 patients and captured a full spectrum of PCI populations (from stable angina patients undergoing elective PCI to primary PCI in STEMI). Enoxaparin was associated with statistically significant reductions in death (risk ratio [RR], 0.66; 95% confidence interval [95% CI], 0.57–0.76; $P < .001$), composite endpoint of death and MI (RR, 0.68; 95% CI, 0.57–0.81; $P < .001$), and major bleeding (RR, 0.80; 95% CI, 0.60–0.85; $P < .001$). Subgroup analyses suggested enoxaparin's mortality benefit was primarily driven by patients with STEMI, although nonstatistically significant trends toward lower mortality were also seen in both elective PCI and NSTE-ACS patient populations. All PCI populations, however, consistently demonstrated statistically significant reductions in bleeding with enoxaparin compared to UFH. Notable limitations of this meta-analysis were that it was not performed with individual patient-level data, approximately one-third of the patients came from nonrandomized studies, and $P2Y_{12}$ usage patterns (e.g., pretreatment protocols) were not well detailed. However, we still believe that the conclusions of the meta-analysis are valid.

In contemporary interventional cardiology practice with routine dual antiplatelet therapy (DAPT) and the increasing utilization of radial artery access for PCI, LMWH use in the United States is still primarily focused on NSTE-ACS patients selected for noninvasive (conservative) management. Large randomized trials incorporating current management techniques would likely be required to definitively establish the role for LMWH as first-line therapy over UFH in primary invasive management. Important practical considerations include the facts that enoxaparin is not reversible with protamine (unlike UFH) and its anticoagulant effect cannot be monitored in the catheterization laboratory with routine lab tests (aPTT or ACT). Special dosing consideration is required when using LMWH in patients with significant renal insufficiency, morbid obesity, and the elderly; if LMWH is used in these patients, anti-Xa levels should be followed carefully and dosing adjusted as required. Heparin-induced thrombocytopenia occurs at lower rates with

TABLE 35.1 Select Major Trials of LMWH by Indication

LMWH	Trial	No. of Patients	Design	Results	Comments
STEMI					
Enoxaparin	STEMI Treated With Primary Angioplasty and Intravenous Lovenox or Unfractionated Heparin (ATOLL), 2011[30]	910	1:1 randomization of prehospital STEMI patients administered 0.5 mg/kg enoxaparin vs. UFH in ambulance	**Composite:** No significant difference in the incidence of composite endpoint events at 30 days (death, complication of MI, procedure failure, or major bleeding; 28% vs. 34%, $P = .06$).	The main secondary endpoint (composite of death, recurrent ACS, or urgent revascularization) was significantly reduced in the enoxaparin treatment group (7% vs. 11%; $P = .015$).
Enoxaparin	Facilitated Intervention with Enhanced Reperfusion Speed to Stop Events (FINESSE), 2010[31]	2452	STEMI patients randomized to either enoxaparin vs. UFH in primary PCI or facilitated PCI with GPI + half-dose reteplase	**Composite:** Significantly reduced death, MI, urgent revascularization, or refractory ischemia at 30 days in the enoxaparin treatment arm (5.3% vs. 8%; $P = .0005$) as well as all-cause mortality through 90 days (3.8% vs. 5.6%; $P = .046$).	Facilitated PCI performed in 33% of patients in the trial. Nonintracranial major/minor bleeding was not significantly different between the treatment groups.
Early Invasive Management of NSTE-ACS					
Enoxaparin	A to Z Trial, 2004[20,32]	3987	NSTE-ACS patients randomized to receive either enoxaparin or UFH in combination with ASA and tirofiban	**Composite:** No significant difference in the incidence of composite endpoint events (death, MI, or refractory ischemia) at 7 days (8.4% vs. 9.4% for UFH, $P = .048$). **Major Bleeding:** The incidence of major bleeding complications was higher with enoxaparin (0.9% vs. 0.4%, $P = .05$).	NSTEMI criteria met in 74% of patients, and an early invasive strategy was pursued in 55% of study patients. In a prespecified subgroup analysis, there was no difference in outcome for the patients treated with an early invasive strategy, whereas there was a significant reduction in the primary endpoint for patients treated with a noninvasive (conservative) strategy.
Enoxaparin	Superior Yield of the New Strategy of Enoxaparin, Revascularization and Glycoprotein IIb/IIIa Inhibitors (SYNERGY), 2004[21,33]	10,027	NSTE-ACS patients planned for an early invasive strategy randomized to enoxaparin or UFH in combination with ASA plus $P2Y_{12}$ or GPI	**Composite:** No significant difference in the incidence of composite endpoint events (death or nonfatal MI) at 30 days (14.0% vs. 14.5% for UFH). **Major Bleeding:** The incidence of in-hospital major bleeding complications was higher with enoxaparin (9.1% vs. 7.6%, $P = .008$).	There remained no difference in composite endpoint rates at 6 and 12 months. UFH may be preferable to enoxaparin owing to the increased bleeding risk highlighted by this trial in the population of NSTE-ACS patients with high bleeding risk undergoing an early invasive strategy pretreated with contemporary DAPT.
Conservatively Managed NSTE-ACS (Noninvasive)					
Enoxaparin	Efficacy and Safety of Subcutaneous Enoxaparin in Non–Q-Wave Coronary Events (ESSENCE), 1997[19,34]	3,171	NSTE-ACS patients treated with ASA randomized to enoxaparin vs. UFH therapy for a minimum of 48 hours to a maximum of 8 days	**Composite:** Enoxaparin had a lower rate of composite endpoint events (death, MI, or recurrent angina) at 30 days (19.8% vs. 23.3% for UFH, $P = .016$). **Major Bleeding:** There was no difference between the groups in the 30-day incidence of major bleeding complications (6.5% vs. 7.0%). **Repeat Revascularization:** The need for repeat revascularization procedures at 30 days was significantly less in the patients assigned to enoxaparin (27.1% vs. 32.2%, $P = .001$).	Revascularization was not intended in this trial. A one year follow-up analysis found that the benefits were maintained for both the composite endpoint (32% vs. 36% for UFH, $P = .022$) and the need for repeat revascularization (36% vs. 41%, $P = .002$).

TABLE 35.1   Select Major Trials of LMWH by Indication—cont'd

LMWH	Trial	No. of Patients	Design	Results	Comments
Enoxaparin	Thrombolysis in Myocardial Infarction (TIMI)-11B, 1999[18]	3910	NSTE-ACS patients treated with ASA randomized to enoxaparin vs. UFH therapy for a minimum of 3 days. This trial also included an outpatient phase (followed to day 43)	**Composite:** Enoxaparin had a lower rate of composite endpoint events (death, MI, or urgent revascularization) at 9 days (12.4% vs. 14.5% for UFH, $P = .048$). **Major Bleeding:** No difference between the groups in the predischarge incidence of major bleeding complications (1.5% vs. 1.0%).	Revascularization was not intended in this trial. The benefit of enoxaparin was limited to the patient population with elevated troponin.
Elective PCI					
Enoxaparin	Safety and Efficacy of Enoxaparin in Percutaneous Coronary Intervention Patients (STEEPLE), 2006[35]	3528	Patients randomized to 0.5 or 0.75 mg/kg enoxaparin vs. UFH (targeted to ACT and stratified by provisional GPI use)	**Composite:** The 0.5 mg/kg enoxaparin dose reduced composite bleeding events by 31% at 48 hours (5.9% vs. 8.5%; $P = .01$), while the 0.75 mg/kg dose was no different than UFH. Also, target anticoagulation levels were achieved in significantly more patients in both enoxaparin groups (0.5 mg/kg dose, 79%; 0.75 mg/kg dose, 92%) than patients who received UFH (20%, $P < .001$).	No significant differences in ischemic outcomes were found; however, this trial was not powered to provide a definitive comparison of efficacy in the prevention of ischemic events.
Reviparin	Reduction of Restenosis After PTCA, Early Administration of Reviparin in a Double-Blind, Unfractionated Heparin and Placebo-Controlled Evaluation (REDUCE), 1996[36]	612	Single-lesion CAD patients treated with PTCA randomized to fixed-dose LMWH vs. UFH. Patients also received low-dose SQ reviparin or placebo injections for 28 days following PCI	**Composite:** No difference between the groups at 30 days for the composite endpoint of death, MI, need for reintervention or bypass surgery (33.3% vs. 32%; $P = .707$). **Major Bleeding:** No difference between the groups within the 35 days following PTCA for major bleeding complications.	No significant differences between the groups in the incidence of angiographic restenosis over 30 weeks; however, a secondary endpoint (requirement of bailout intervention) was reduced in the reviparin group (2.0% vs. 6.9%; $P = .003$).

ACT, Activated clotting time; *ASA,* aspirin; *CAD,* coronary artery disease; *GPI,* glycoprotein IIb/IIIa receptor inhibitors; *LMWH,* low-molecular-weight heparins; *MI,* myocardial infarction; *NSTE-ACS,* non–ST elevation acute coronary syndrome; *NSTEMI,* non–ST elevation myocardial infarction; *PCI,* percutaneous coronary intervention; *PTCA,* percutaneous transluminal coronary angioplasty; *STEMI,* ST elevation myocardial infarction; *SQ,* subcutaneous; *UFH,* unfractionated heparin.

LMWH than with UFH; however, platelet counts should still be monitored routinely after treatment.

SYNTHETIC PENTASACCHARIDES (FONDAPARINUX)

Fondaparinux is a synthetic analog of the heparin pentasaccharide sequence that causes an AT-mediated, selective inhibition of FXa. It exerts its effect exclusively on FXa with no action on thrombin (its molecular structure is too short to bridge AT to thrombin).[23]

Pharmacokinetics, Metabolism, and Administration

Fondaparinux shares many of the pharmacodynamic and pharmacokinetic advantages of the LMWHs relative to UFH.

The specific anti-Xa activity of fondaparinux is approximately seven-fold higher than that of LMWHs. HIT is unlikely to occur with fondaparinux because it does not bind to platelets or PF4 and therefore does not induce the formation of heparin/PF4 complexes that serve as the antigenic target for the antibodies that cause HIT. However, fondaparinux also fails to interact with protamine sulfate; therefore, as with the LMWHs, the effect of fondaparinux is not reliably reversed with protamine. Fondaparinux has little or no effect on routine coagulation tests, such as aPTT or ACT, rendering these tests unsuitable for monitoring its clinical effects. If monitoring is required, the anticoagulant effect of fondaparinux can be measured with dedicated anti-Xa assays.

Fondaparinux can be administered subcutaneously with a time to peak effect of approximately 2.5 hours and a half-life of approximately 20 hours in patients with normal renal function, allowing for a predictable anticoagulant effect with once-daily dosing. Fondaparinux exhibits linear pharmacokinetics when given in doses ranging from 2 to 8 mg.[24] A daily 2.5-mg SC dose is used in patients with ACS and for thromboprophylaxis in medical and surgical patients. A dose of 7.5 mg is used for treatment of VTE. As a synthetic molecule, fondaparinux has no antigenic properties. The drug is excreted unchanged in the urine. Consequently, dose adjustments are necessary in patients with renal insufficiency; fondaparinux should not be used in patients with severe renal failure.

Clinical Evidence

The foundation for fondaprinux use in ACS comes from two large randomized clinical trials that included patients treated with PCI. The Comparison of Fondaparinux and Enoxaparin in Acute Coronary Syndromes (OASIS-5) trial, in which approximately 40% of patients underwent PCI, demonstrated that NSTE-ACS patients treated with fondaparinux had noninferior rates of the composite endpoint (death, MI, or refractory ischemia) at 9 and 30 days. When compared with enoxaparin, with or without adjunctive GPI use, the fondaparinux treatment group had significantly lower rates of major bleeding (2.4% vs. 5.1%, $P < .00001$). At 6 months, fondaparinux produced a significant reduction in all major endpoints; however, in the subset of patients who underwent PCI, there was no difference in the primary endpoint at any time point.[25]

The findings of the subsequent Organization for the Assessment of Strategies for Ischemic Syndromes (OASIS-6) trial, which examined fondaparinux versus UFH in a higher-risk STEMI population, were largely similar. As in OASIS-5, adjunctive GPI administration was permitted, with adjustment of fondaparinux and UFH dosing in these patients. Overall, the fondaparinux treatment arm had significantly lower rates of the primary composite endpoint (9.7% vs. 11.2%; 95% CI, 0.77–0.96; $P = .008$) at 9 days, with benefits persisting out to 6 months. As was seen in OASIS-5, in the 29% of patients who underwent primary PCI, fondaparinux was not superior to UFH.[26] Of particular importance, in both the OASIS-5 and OASIS-6 trials, fondaparinux was associated with increased catheter-related thrombus formation ($P < .001$) as well as higher overall rates of coronary complications (e.g., abrupt vessel closure, no reflow, perforation; $P = .04$) during PCI.

These findings led to the Fondaparinux with Unfractionated Heparin During Revascularization in Acute Coronary Syndromes (FUTURA/OASIS-8) trial that evaluated the addition of low-dose versus standard-dose UFH to fondaparinux during PCI. In a population of NSTE-ACS patients, there was no difference in the primary composite endpoint (major bleeding, minor bleeding, or access site complications) or in the prespecified secondary endpoints (composite bleeding at 48 hours, death, MI, or target vessel revascularization within 30 days) between the low-dose and standard-dose UFH groups. Catheter thrombosis occurred less often than in the prior OASIS-5 and OASIS-6 trials; however, it was not significantly different between the low- and standard-dose UFH dosing populations.[27]

Therefore, similar to LMWH, the use of fondaparinux in contemporary practice is typically reserved for patients with a high risk of bleeding selected for a conservative management strategy, as it has not been shown to confer added benefit over UFH or LMWH in patients undergoing PCI. Because of the unique concerns with catheter thrombosis, fondaparinux is not recommended for use as the sole anticoagulant agent during PCI. It is important that patients treated with fondaparinux who go on to have PCI do so with the addition of other parenteral antithrombotic therapy, such as UFH or bivalirudin.

DIRECT THROMBIN INHIBITORS (BIVALIRUDIN)

DTIs are derivatives of hirudin, a polypeptide first isolated from the salivary glands of the medicinal leech, *Hirudo medicinalis*.[28] Hirudin and its derivative, bivalirudin, are bivalent molecules that are capable of binding the active site and fibrin-binding site of thrombin. By contrast, argatroban is a univalent DTI that binds only the active site. Rather than catalyzing the production of endogenous thrombin inhibitors, DTIs bind directly to thrombin and inhibit its interaction with substrate, thereby preventing fibrin formation, thrombin-mediated activation of the coagulation cascade and thrombin-induced platelet aggregation. Although indirect thrombin inhibitors, such as heparin and LMWH, lead to the inactivation of only circulating thrombin, DTIs are capable of inactivating clot-bound heparin as well. It is important to note that, in comparison to heparin derivatives, HIT has not been reported in patients receiving bivalirudin and, in fact, the DTIs are the primary parenteral treatment for patients with HIT.

Bivalirudin is a synthetic 20-amino acid DTI. It is the most widely used DTI in the United States, has the largest evidence base supporting its clinical use, and is the only DTI approved by the FDA for use in ACS and PCI. The following section is therefore limited to this agent.

Pharmacokinetics, Metabolism, and Administration

Bivalirudin is a parenteral agent that is most frequently administered as a weight-based bolus (usually 0.75 mg/kg) followed by an infusion (usually 1.75 mg/kg per hour) through the completion of PCI. Bivalirudin has a half-life of approximately 25 minutes and a response that is linearly proportional to its dosing, with coagulation parameters returning to baseline approximately 1 to 2 hours after its discontinuation in patients with normal renal function. Elimination of bivalirudin is through a combination of renal excretion and proteolytic cleavage, both by endogenous proteases and thrombin itself. Special dosing of bivalirudin infusions is required in patients with renal insufficiency based on the severity of renal impairment; its use should be avoided in patients with end-stage renal disease. Special caution should also be exercised with its use in patients at extremes of weight and in the elderly.

Bivalirudin has several intrinsic advantages over UFH and LMWH in the setting of PCI: it does not require a cofactor (such as AT), it has no known natural inhibitors (such as PF4), it has a more predictable bioavailability, and it does not directly activate platelets. Unlike UFH, bivalirudin does not require periprocedural monitoring with ACT levels after it is administered.

Clinical Evidence

Multiple randomized clinical trials over a 20-year period have examined bivalirudin in nearly all PCI settings (STEMI, NSTE-ACS, and elective PCI), comparing it to various anticoagulation regimens (most notably UFH and UFH and routine GPI). Select findings from the major clinical trials that provide the foundational evidence supporting bivalirudin use in PCI are summarized by indication in Table 35.2. In early trials, bivalirudin monotherapy was demonstrated to consistently reduce the incidence of major bleeding by approximately 40% compared to UFH and GPI without an increase in ischemic events.

Bivalirudin monotherapy had largely replaced the use of UFH and routine GPI in patients undergoing PCI. However, several concurrent advances in contemporary PCI—such as radial artery access; newer, thinner drug-eluting stent designs with second-generation antiproliferative drugs; and routine use of improved third-generation oral $P2Y_{12}$ inhibitors—have led to the reevaluation of bivalirudin against UFH-only regimens. In several of these recent trials—including Novel Approaches in Preventing and Limiting Events III Trial (NAPLES-III), Minimizing Adverse Haemorrhagic Events by Transradial Access Site and Systemic Implementation of AngioX (MATRIX), and How Effective are Antithrombotic Therapies in Primary Percutaneous Coronary

TABLE 35.2 Select Major Trials of Bivalirudin by Indication

Trial	No. of Patients	Design	Results	Comments
STEMI				
Harmonizing Outcomes with Revascularization and Stents in Acute Myocardial Infarction (HORIZONS-AMI), 2008[37]	3602	STEMI patients randomized to UFH + GPI vs. bivalirudin during PCI (with provisional GPI allowed if clinically needed)	**Composite:** No significant difference in the composite primary endpoint at 30 days (death, MI, urgent target vessel revascularization, or stroke). **Major Bleeding:** Bivalirudin alone reduced major bleeding complications compared to UFH + GPI (4.9% vs. 8.3%; $P < .001$).	Provisional GPI was used in 7.2% of patients in the bivalirudin group with large thrombus burden. Bivalirudin reduced cardiovascular death (1.8% vs. 2.9%; $P = .03$) and all-cause mortality (2.1% vs. 3.1%; $P = .047$) at 30 days; however, bivalirudin was associated with an increased risk of acute stent thrombosis within 24 hours of PCI (1.3% vs. 0.4%; $P < .001$).
European Ambulance Acute Coronary Syndrome Angiography (EUROMAX), 2013[38]	2218	STEMI patients randomized to UFH + provisional GPI vs. bivalirudin during PCI and continued for at least 4 hours post-procedure (with provisional GPI allowed if clinically needed)	**Composite:** No significant difference in the composite primary endpoint at 30 days (death, MI, urgent target vessel revascularization, or stroke). **Major Bleeding:** Bivalirudin alone reduced major bleeding complications (2.6% vs. 6.0%; $P < .001$) compared to UFH + GPI.	Representative of contemporary PCI practice, with all patients receiving DAPT (including 40% with third-generation agents prasugrel or ticagrelor) and over 45% of patients with radial artery access. Bivalirudin was again associated with an increased risk of acute stent thrombosis (1.6% vs. 0.5%; $P = .02$) despite prolonged infusion after PCI. There was also a trend toward higher rates of reinfarction at 30 days, although the study was not adequately powered to assess this.
Unfractionated Heparin vs. Bivalirudin in Primary Percutaneous Coronary Intervention (HEAT-PPCI), 2014[39]	1829	STEMI patients randomized to UFH vs. bivalirudin during PCI (with provisional GPI allowed in both arms if clinically needed)	**Composite:** UFH demonstrated significantly lower rates of the composite primary endpoint at 28 days (death, MI, urgent target vessel revascularization, or stroke) compared to bivalirudin (5.7% vs. 8.7%; $P = .01$). **Major Bleeding:** No significant difference in the rates of major bleeding complications.	Representative of contemporary PCI practice, with over 90% of patients receiving DAPT (including third-generation agents prasugrel or ticagrelor) and over 75% of patients with radial artery access. Rates of "bailout" GPI use were not significantly different between the groups (13% in the bivalirudin group; 15% in the UFH group). Again noted was a greater risk of reinfarction with bivalirudin, driven by increased acute stent thrombosis (3.4% vs. 0.9%; $P = .001$).

Continued

TABLE 35.2   Select Major Trials of Bivalirudin by Indication—cont'd

Trial	No. of Patients	Design	Results	Comments
Bivalirudin in Acute Myocardial Infarction vs, Heparin and GPI Plus Heparin Trial (BRIGHT), 2015[40]	2194	STEMI patients randomized to UFH vs. UFH + GPI vs. bivalirudin with a post-PCI infusion	**Composite:** Bivalirudin reduced the rates of the primary composite endpoint at 30 days (all-cause death, MI, ischemia-driven target vessel revascularization, stroke, or bleeding) compared to both UFH and UFH + GPI (8.8% vs. 13.2% vs. 17.0%, respectively; $P < .001$). **Major Bleeding:** Bivalirudin reduced major bleeding compared to UFH alone or UFH + GPI (4.1% vs. 7.5% vs. 12.3%, respectively; $P < .001$).	No differences in stent thrombosis within 24 hours, at 30 days, or at 1 year.
Minimizing Adverse Hemorrhagic Events by Transradial Access Site and Systemic Implementation of Angiox (MATRIX), 2015[41]	7213	ACS patients (48% STEMI, 52% NSTE-ACS) randomized to bivalirudin vs. UFH. Patients in the bivalirudin group were subsequently randomly assigned to either receive or not receive a post-PCI bivalirudin infusion	**Composite:** No significant difference in the composite primary endpoint (death, MI, or stroke). Post-PCI continuation of bivalirudin infusion did not significantly decrease the rate of urgent target-vessel revascularization, definite stent thrombosis, or net adverse clinical events compared with bivalirudin infusion during the PCI procedure only. **Major Bleeding:** No significant difference in the rates of reduced major bleeding complications.	While this large contemporary study should have been the definitive trial comparing bivalirudin to UFH, there was marked imbalance in the rates of GPI use between the heparin and bivalirudin arms, making this an impure comparison of bivalirudin to true heparin monotherapy (as it is currently used in contemporary PCI). Additionally, this study did not correct for multiple testing of secondary endpoints; therefore, differences for these endpoints with borderline P values must be interpreted with caution.

Early Invasive Management of NSTE-ACS

Trial	No. of Patients	Design	Results	Comments
Bivalirudin Angioplasty Study, 1995[42,43]	4098	Unstable angina or postinfarct angina patients undergoing PTCA randomized to high-dose UFH alone or bivalirudin	**Composite:** No significant difference in the composite primary endpoint (in-hospital death, MI, abrupt vessel closure, or rapid clinical deterioration of cardiac origin). However, a reanalysis of the trial dataset subsequently published in 2001 reported that bivalirudin significantly reduced composite primary endpoint events at 7 days ($P = .039$) and 90 days ($P = .012$), with a trend toward reduced events at 180 days. **Major Bleeding:** Patients treated with bivalirudin had lower incidence of bleeding (3.8% vs. 9.8%; $P < .001$).	No coronary stenting was performed in this trial, significantly limiting its generalizability to contemporary practice. There was no routine GPI use in this trial.
Acute Catheterization and Urgent Intervention Triage Strategy (ACUITY), 2006[44,45]	13,819	NSTE-ACS patients randomized to bivalirudin alone vs. bivalirudin + GPI vs. heparin (UFH or LMWH) + GPI	**Composite:** No differences in the primary composite endpoint at 30 days (death, MI, unplanned revascularization). **Major Bleeding:** Bivalirudin alone reduced major bleeding compared to heparin + GPI or bivalirudin + GPI (3.1% vs. 5.7% vs. 5.3%, respectively; $P < .001$).	In the subsequent substudy of 7789 patients who underwent PCI, there were no differences in the primary ischemic endpoint, again finding less bleeding in the bivalirudin-alone treatment arm (driven predominantly by fewer access site and retroperitoneal hemorrhages).

TABLE 35.2 Select Major Trials of Bivalirudin by Indication—cont'd

Trial	No. of Patients	Design	Results	Comments
Intracoronary Stenting and Antithrombotic Regimen: Rapid Early Action for Coronary Treatment (ISAR-REACT) 3, 2008[46]	4570	Stable angina and NSTE-ACS patients undergoing PCI treated with 600 mg clopidogrel randomized to bivalirudin vs. very high-dose UFH monotherapy	**Composite:** No significant difference in the composite primary endpoint (death, MI, urgent target vessel revascularization). **Major Bleeding:** Bivalirudin reduced major bleeding complications compared to very-high-dose UFH (3.1% vs. 4.6%; $P = .008$).	The UFH dose used in this trial (140 U/kg) was much higher than is used in contemporary interventional practice (50–70 U/kg). There was no routine GPI use in this trial.
Intracoronary Stenting and Anti-thrombotic Regimen: Rapid Early Action for Coronary Treatment (ISAR-REACT) 4, 2011[47]	1721	NSTE-ACS patients randomized to bivalirudin alone vs. UFH + GPI	**Composite:** No significant difference in the composite primary endpoint (death, MI, urgent target vessel revascularization). **Major Bleeding:** Bivalirudin reduced major bleeding complications compared to UFH + GPI (2.6% vs. 4.6%; $P = .02$).	
Elective PCI				
Randomized Evaluation in PCI Linking Angiomax to Reduced Clinical Events (REPLACE)-2, 2003[48]	6010	Patients undergoing elective PCI (or urgent PCI without MI) randomized to UFH + GPI vs. bivalirudin with provisional GPI allowed	**Composite:** No difference in the primary composite endpoint at 30 days (death, MI, urgent repeat revascularization, or in-hospital major bleeding). **Major Bleeding:** Bivalirudin significantly reduced in-hospital major bleeding rates (2.4% vs. 4.1%; $P < .001$).	All patients received aspirin and 85% received an oral P2Y$_{12}$ inhibitor. Provisional GPI was used in 7.2% of patients in the bivalirudin group.
Novel Approaches for Preventing or Limiting Events (NAPLES) III, 2015[49]	837	Consecutive cardiac biomarker-negative patients at increased bleeding risk undergoing elective PCI were randomized to UFH vs. bivalirudin alone	**Composite:** No difference in the primary composite endpoint of in-hospital major bleeding.	Limited generalizability to contemporary practice as this was a relatively small, single-center study of patients undergoing elective PCI with 100% femoral access used.

ASA, Aspirin; *DAPT,* dual antiplatelet therapy; *GPI,* glycoprotein IIb/IIIa receptor inhibitors; *LMWH,* low-molecular-weight heparins; *MI,* myocardial infarction; *NSTE-ACS,* non–ST elevation acute coronary syndrome; *PCI,* percutaneous coronary intervention; *PTCA,* percutaneous transluminal coronary angioplasty; *UFH,* unfractionated heparin.

Intervention (HEAT-PPCI)—bivalirudin was not found to significantly reduce bleeding and, in one trial in a contemporary STEMI population (HEAT-PPCI), UFH alone was demonstrated to reduce ischemic events compared to bivalirudin. Another such trial (BivaliRudin in Acute Myocardial Infarction vs. Glycoprotein IIb/IIIa and Heparin: a Randomised Controlled Trial [BRIGHT]), again in a contemporary STEMI population, found ischemic events and major bleeding reduced by bivalirudin compared to UFH.

The relative safety and efficacy of bivalirudin compared to UFH in the setting of PCI was recently examined in a meta-analysis by Cavender and colleagues that included 16 trials with nearly 34,000 patients and captured a full spectrum of PCI populations (from stable angina patients undergoing elective PCI to primary PCI in STEMI), stratified according to the use of GPI.[29] In their analyses, ischemic complications were slightly more frequent among patients receiving bivalirudin-based regimens compared to UFH-based regimens (RR, 1.09; 95% CI, 1.01–1.17), regardless of the clinical indication for PCI or the GPI strategy used. The impact of bivalirudin on bleeding events, however, was significantly impacted by the GPI strategy utilized. No significant bleeding differences were found in comparisons of bivalirudin monotherapy with UFH monotherapy; however, it is noteworthy that the one large trial comparing bivalirudin to UFH monotherapy that observed increased bleeding with UFH monotherapy used much higher UFH doses (140 U/kg) than are conventionally used in contemporary PCI. Another important limitation of this meta-analysis is that it predated the MATRIX trial that demonstrated both a bleeding and mortality advantage of bivalirudin over UFH in ACS patients (albeit in the setting of a marked imbalance in GPI usage between the bivalirudin and UFH arms, thus making it an impure comparison of bivalirudin to UFH monotherapy). Therefore, in the contemporary PCI era, in which GPIs are not routinely used, the role of bivalirudin over standard dose (70 to 100 U/kg) UFH monotherapy with third-generation DAPT is less clear.

CONCLUSION

AT therapy in the CICU setting for the treatment of cardiovascular disease has rapidly evolved and has become a highly evidence-based discipline guided by decades of rigorous investigation. While considerable attention has been given to the technological advances in PCI itself, the majority of benefit with regard to improving survival and reducing morbidity in the treatment CAD can be attributed to the significant advances in the adjunctive pharmacotherapy used. This chapter has provided a broad overview of each of the categories of anticoagulant agents used in the CICU for patients following ACS and/or PCI. A fundamental goal of therapy is to achieve a robust antithrombotic effect using a combination of antiplatelet and antithrombotic medications while at the same time limiting the associated risks of bleeding. A thorough understanding of the antithrombotic pharmacology reviewed in this chapter is required to select patient-tailored medication regimens for the various clinical circumstances encountered in the CICU setting. While there are multiple anticoagulants with a significant foundation of clinical evidence supporting their use, unfractionated heparin has remained a durable choice and has many properties that favor its use (widespread availability, low cost, short duration, easy point-of-care monitoring, and rapid reversal with protamine). While several new antithrombotic agents are currently under investigation, the "holy grail" for new antithrombotic therapies remains to achieve a predictable, uniform response that offers improved efficacy without unacceptably increasing bleeding complications.

Acknowledgment

The authors acknowledge the contributions of Drs. Michael Nguyen, Yuri Pride, and C. Michael Gibson, who were the authors of this chapter in the previous edition.

The full reference list for this chapter is available at ExpertConsult.com.

36

Antiplatelet Therapy

Ryan E. Wilson, Khaled M. Ziada

Over the last 3 decades, clinical management and outcomes of patients presenting with acute coronary syndromes (ACSs) have improved dramatically. Better understanding of the role of the platelet in the pathophysiology of the ACS has been the fundamental pillar for that progress. The development and availability of effective pharmacologic agents and the advance of coronary revascularization procedures have been the tools by which scientific advances were translated into reductions in morbidity and mortality of patients across the spectrum of ACS, from those with ST elevation myocardial infarction (STEMI) or those with non-ST segment elevation ACS (NSTE-ACS).

PLATELET AND ACUTE CORONARY SYNDROMES

Plaque rupture and luminal thrombus formation are the sentinel events that convert the atherosclerotic disease process from a slowly progressive condition causing insidious luminal obstruction to an acute coronary event marked by rapid deterioration of clinical condition and possible death. Plaque rupture is a term that describes the development of a gap in the fibrous cap, exposing its collagen and the underlying lipid-rich core to flowing blood.[1] This event results in activation of the circulating platelets, which, in turn, initiates a sequence of events involving the activated platelet: adhesion, aggregation, and secretion (Fig. 36.1).

Platelet activation occurs via multiple stimuli, including adenosine diphosphate (ADP) and thromboxane (TX) A_2, but collagen and thrombin are the two most potent platelet activators. Once collagen is available for binding, platelet adhesion and activation depend on two major collagen receptors located on the platelet membrane, the integrin glycoprotein (GP) Ia/IIa ($\alpha 2\beta 1$) and GP VI. Both receptors generate activation signals that enhance platelet thrombus formation. Thrombin is also a potent stimulus for platelet activation by binding and cleaving platelet protease–activated receptors (PAR), PAR_1, and PAR_4. This process forms a tethered-ligand that acts to initiate transmembrane signaling, also leading to platelet activation.[2–4]

Once activated, platelet adhesion occurs when platelet GP Ib-IX-V binds to tissue von Willebrand factor (vWF).[5] At least one other receptor that participates in platelet adhesion includes the platelet receptor Ia/IIa, which binds to collagen fibrils.[6] Platelet aggregation soon follows and is primarily mediated by the GP IIb/IIIa complex ($\alpha IIb\beta 3$). GP IIb/IIIa adhesion proteins are found on platelets and megakaryocytes. They are the most abundant glycoprotein found on the platelet surface, with approximately 80,000 copies. The GP IIb/IIIa complex requires platelet activation,

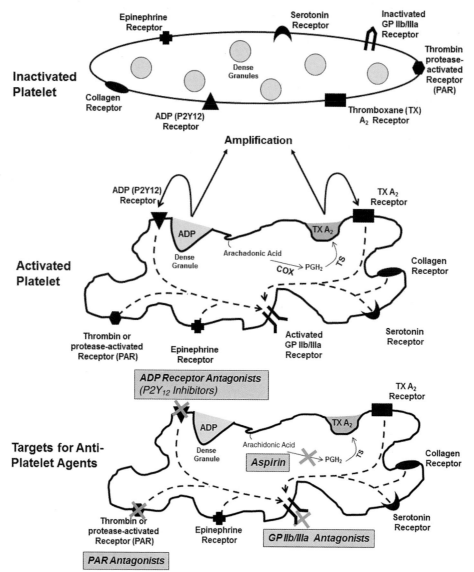

Fig. 36.1 In the inactive state, the platelet is rich with membrane receptors and contains dense granules (*top*). When the membrane receptors are stimulated, the platelet is activated (*middle*), leading to conformational changes and a cascade of events, which result in deformational change and activation of the final common pathway of platelet activation: the glycoprotein (GP) IIb/IIIa receptor complex. Activation of that receptor leads to binding of fibrinogen, aggregation of platelets, and formation of a platelet-rich thrombus. *Bottom,* Sites of action of the most commonly used platelet inhibitors in clinical practice: aspirin inhibits the cyclooxygenase enzyme and reduces formation of thromboxane A2, thienopyridines inhibit the P2Y$_{12}$ receptor, vorapaxar inhibits the protease-activated receptors, and GP IIb/IIIa inhibitors inhibit the activated GP Ib/IIIa receptor.

which causes a conformational change in the receptor, thereby becoming a high-affinity fibrinogen binding receptor. Fibrinogen bridges activated platelets, forming a platelet plug. The cytosolic portion of the GP IIb/IIIa complex stimulates actin rearrangement, resulting in platelet spreading, aggregation, and clot retraction. Hence, GP IIb/IIIa receptor antagonists are powerful antiplatelet drugs.[2–4]

Activated platelets secrete substances from their granules that stimulate further activation and aggregation. These mediators include, but are not limited to, ADP, TXA$_2$, fibrinogen, fibronectin, and thrombospondin. There are at least two receptors that bind

ADP: P2Y$_{12}$ and P2Y$_{12}$. Commercially available agents that block the P2Y$_{12}$ receptor include clopidogrel, prasugrel, ticagrelor, and cangrelor. Thromboxane A$_2$ is an arachidonic acid metabolite and a strong platelet stimulator. The production of TXA$_2$ depends on the cyclooxygenase pathway, which is irreversibly inhibited by aspirin (see Fig. 36.1).[2–4] The aforementioned steps of adhesion, aggregation, and secretion are presented in a stepwise fashion for simplicity, but in reality, these processes occur simultaneously. By better understanding the molecular mechanisms, targets for future and more effective antiplatelet agents can be defined (see Fig. 36.1).

NON–ST SEGMENT ELEVATION ACUTE CORONARY SYNDROME

Platelet activation is central to the process of coronary thrombus formation, the sentinel pathophysiologic step in ACS. Therefore, antiplatelet therapy is the cornerstone of treatment in NSTE-ACS. Numerous clinical trials have established that appropriate antiplatelet therapy in NSTE-ACS reduces mortality and other ischemic events. When antiplatelet therapy is used in the cardiac intensive care unit (CICU), it is imperative that physicians ensure that their patients are receiving these agents at the appropriate dosages and while cautiously observing for side effects, namely, bleeding complications.

The field of antiplatelet therapy for NSTE-ACS has evolved and changed rapidly over the last few decades. While aspirin was the only available agent for many years, the 1990s were dominated by the development and use of intravenous GP IIb/IIIa inhibitors. These agents demonstrated the value of effective and rapid platelet inhibition, but were associated with increased bleeding complications. In the late 1990s and early 2000s, $P2Y_{12}$ inhibitors were developed. Their value of GP IIb/IIIa inhibitors took some time to clarify, but soon they were supplanting intravenous agents because of ease of use, reduced cost, and less concern about bleeding. Newer $P2Y_{12}$ inhibitors demonstrated higher efficacy and further improvement in outcomes, but again at the cost of excess bleeding. The newer thrombin receptor antagonists appeared to have lower bleeding complications in the early trials but subsequently were found to have the same features: enhanced efficacy with increased risk of bleeding. The most recent addition to the antiplatelet armamentarium is the intravenous $P2Y_{12}$ inhibitor, cangrelor, which provides immediate inhibition and can be followed by an oral agent that inhibits the same receptor.

Acetylsalicylic Acid (ASA or Aspirin)

The importance of effective and early use of aspirin in ACS was established decades ago. Fortunately, the awareness of this fact among the public and health care professionals encountering these patients is very high. In many instances, patients reach for aspirin as they are calling emergency medical services for the acute onset of chest pain. The dispatchers receiving the calls instruct patients to use aspirin if they have it available and first responders immediately provide it upon arrival to the scene. For those who did not receive it, almost all patients with chest pain are given aspirin in the emergency department.

When aspirin is given acutely as a tablet it should be chewed in order to achieve rapid platelet inhibition within approximately 20 minutes. Aspirin blocks the production of TXA_2 by irreversibly acetylating a serine residue on cyclooxygenase 1. This prevents the conversion of arachidonic acid to prostaglandin H_2, a precursor of TXA_2. TXA_2 causes vasoconstriction and platelet aggregation.[7] Unless there is a well-documented severe allergic reaction, all patients with ACS should be treated with 162 mg to 325 mg of nonenteric coated aspirin promptly after presentation.[8] The American College of Cardiology (ACC)/American Heart Association (AHA) guidelines for treatment of NSTE-ACS give aspirin a class IA recommendation for its immediate and indefinite use

in this patient population.[8,9] Regardless of whether the patient will require percutaneous or surgical revascularization, the first dose should be followed by indefinite daily ASA: 81 mg/day in patients treated concomitantly with ticagrelor and 75 to 325 mg/day in all others.[8]

The benefit of aspirin in unstable angina has been demonstrated in several trials. In the Veterans Administration Cooperative Trial, 1266 men with unstable angina were randomized to either aspirin or placebo. The incidence of death or acute myocardial infarction (MI) was reduced by 51% in the aspirin group (5.0% vs. 10.1%, $P = .0005$). Examined individually, both nonfatal MI and death were dramatically reduced by more than 50% in the aspirin group, although the reduction in death did not quite reach the level of statistical significance (3.4% vs. 6.9%, $P = .005$ for acute MI and 1.6% vs. 3.3%, $P = .054$).[10] Further confirmation of the benefit of aspirin in reducing death and nonfatal MI was demonstrated in other trials.[11]

Despite the extensive body of literature describing the benefits of aspirin, more conclusive data about the appropriate dosing have not been available until the last few years. As little as 30 mg/day of aspirin chronically can completely inhibit serum TXB_2 production[12]; many studies suggest equal benefit with doses of less than 150 mg daily compared to higher doses when taken long term.[13] While only 30 mg/day of aspirin are needed to inactivate TXA_2 production, the rapidity of platelet inactivation should also be considered in the context of ACS. In a small study involving 18 healthy volunteers, chewing 162 mg and 324 mg, but not 81 mg of aspirin resulted in maximal inhibition of TXA_2 within 15 minutes.[14]

Many large, blinded, controlled trials in addition to several meta-analyses of placebo-controlled trials have evaluated the optimal aspirin dose in treating patients with nearly every clinical manifestation of atherosclerosis, including stroke, transient ischemic attack (TIA), percutaneous coronary and peripheral interventions, carotid endarterectomy, and MI. In all of these trials, there is no relationship between increasing aspirin dosage and improved clinical efficacy.[13] However, increasing aspirin doses significantly increases the risk of bleeding. An analysis of 31 trials including 192,036 patients examined the association between aspirin dose and bleeding complications. Data were divided into several categories, including major bleeding, minor bleeding, gastrointestinal, stroke, fatal/life threatening, and total bleeding episodes. In all categories, aspirin doses higher than 100 mg/day were associated with significantly more events.[15]

The Clopidogrel and Aspirin Optimal Dose Usage to Reduce Recurrent Events–Seventh Organization to Assess Strategies in Ischemic Syndromes (CURRENT-OASIS) 7 trial enrolled 17,263 patients with ACS who underwent early percutaneous coronary intervention (PCI) in a 2 × 2 randomized factorial design: 600 mg versus 300 mg loading dose of clopidogrel and high-dose (300 to 325 mg) versus low-dose (75 to 100 mg) of daily aspirin. The primary outcome was cardiovascular death, MI, or stroke at 30 days. There was no significant difference in the primary outcome between the high-dose and low-dose aspirin groups (4.1% vs. 4.2%; $P = .76$).[16] Major bleeding was also not different in the high-dose and low-dose aspirin groups (1.5% vs. 1.3%, $P = .2$), but high-dose aspirin recipients reported more minor bleeding events

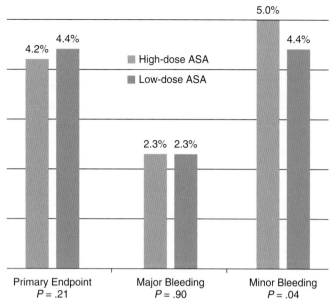

Fig. 36.2 Efficacy and safety of various aspirin doses in acute coronary syndrome (ACS) patients. In the Clopidogrel Optimal Loading Dose Usage to Reduce Recurrent Events/Optimal Antiplatelet Strategy for Interventions (CURRENT/OASIS 7) trial conducted on ACS patients treated with percutaneous coronary intervention, there was no difference in the composite primary endpoint (cardiovascular death, myocardial infarction, or stroke at 30 days) between those receiving high-dose (300–325 mg) or low-dose (75–100 mg) of aspirin. While there was no difference in major bleeding events, the high dose was associated with a significant increase in minor bleeding events.[16] *ASA,* Acetylsalicylic acid.

(Fig. 36.2). Very similar conclusions could be drawn from The Treatment with ADP Receptor Inhibitors: Longitudinal Assessment of Treatment Patterns and Events after Acute Coronary Syndrome (TRANSLATE-ACS) study, in which 10,123 patients with MI who underwent PCI were discharged on dual antiplatelet therapy, including either 325 or 81 mg of aspirin. At 6 months, there were no statistically significant differences between the 2 groups in the rate of major adverse cardiovascular events (death, MI, stroke, or unplanned revascularization) with an adjusted hazard ratio (HR) of 0.99 (95% confidence interval [CI], 0.85–1.17). However, bleeding complications were significantly more frequent with high-dose aspirin (24.2% vs. 19.5%; adjusted odds ratio [OR], 1.19; 95% CI, 1.05–1.34). The increased bleeding events were mostly in minor bleeding events not requiring hospitalization.[17]

Adenosine Diphosphate Receptor Antagonists

The oral ADP receptor antagonists include ticlopidine, clopidogrel, prasugrel, and ticagrelor. Ticlopidine is rarely used due to its unfavorable side effect profile of nausea, vomiting, diarrhea, neutropenia, and—rarely—thrombotic thrombocytopenic purpura along with a longer time to onset of platelet inhibition than clopidogrel; thus, it will not be discussed.

Clopidogrel. The introduction of clopidogrel to the field of ACS management has had a dramatic effect on the algorithms

of therapy used all over the world. Moreover, it introduced the concept of dual antiplatelet therapy (DAPT) and the class of $P2Y_{12}$ inhibitors, which remain the mainstay of therapy today.

The daily dose of clopidogrel is 75 mg. In circumstances when rapid platelet inhibition is desired, such as ACS, a loading dose of clopidogrel 300 or 600 mg for NSTE-ACS or 600 mg for STEMI can be given. The loading doses demonstrate additional antiplatelet aggregation properties when compared to aspirin alone and are considered as class I recommendations by the respective ACC/AHA guidelines.[8,18,19]

When added to aspirin in patients with NSTE-ACS, clopidogrel offers additional reduction in vascular events and death, as established in the Clopidogrel in Unstable Angina to Prevent Recurrent Events (CURE) study.[20] The study randomized 12,562 patients presenting with NSTE-ACS to receive aspirin plus clopidogrel versus aspirin plus placebo. The study was designed to examine two primary outcomes: the first was a composite of cardiovascular death, MI, or stroke and the second comprised the first primary outcome plus refractory ischemia. At 9 months, patients receiving aspirin plus clopidogrel had a statistically significant reduction in both primary outcomes (9.3% vs. 11.4%, $P < .001$ and 16.5% vs. 18.8%, $P < .001$; Fig. 36.3).[20]

Several observations solidified the role of clopidogrel in management of this patient population. The benefit appeared within 24 hours of presentation and was seen irrespective of baseline risk stratification.[21] Additionally, the continuation of clopidogrel after hospitalization in this group of patients further reduced subsequent ischemic vascular events (cardiovascular death, MI, or stroke). The reduction in vascular events was independent of concomitant use of antiplatelet and antithrombotic medication, antihypertensives, lipid-lowering therapy, or coronary intervention.[22] However, a statistically significant increase in bleeding complications was seen in patients on DAPT (major bleeding 3.7% vs. 2.7% and minor bleeding 5.1% vs. 3.4%, $P \leq .001$ for both).[20]

With most patients with NSTE-ACS being referred to coronary angiography and revascularization early in the course of their admission to the CICU, it is important to clearly define the value of clopidogrel therapy in patients undergoing PCI. The PCI CURE substudy examined whether treatment with clopidogrel plus aspirin prior to PCI reduced postprocedure ischemic complications. Patients were pretreated with aspirin and either clopidogrel or placebo. After stenting, over 80% of patients were started on open-label clopidogrel agent for 4 weeks and then resumed taking placebo or clopidogrel for an additional 8 months. In the clopidogrel arm, the primary outcome of death, MI, or urgent target vessel revascularization within 30 days was significantly reduced compared to those receiving aspirin alone (4.5% vs. 6.4%, $P = .03$). In patients receiving clopidogrel for at least 8 months, there were fewer events of cardiovascular death, MI, or revascularization from any cause ($P = .03$) (see Fig. 36.3).[23]

The loading dose of clopidogrel given early in the course of NSTE-ACS therapy has changed over time as well. The 600-mg dose has been found to inhibit platelets more rapidly and effectively than the 300-mg dose.[24–26] Clinically, this may translate into fewer short-term ischemic events after PCI. Cuisset et al. demonstrated that patients who received the 600-mg loading

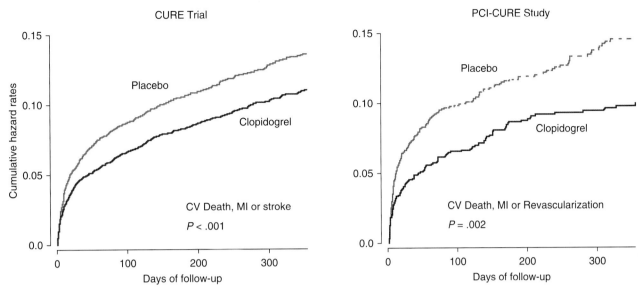

Fig. 36.3 Role of clopidogrel in treatment of acute coronary syndrome patients. In the Clopidogrel in Unstable Angina to Prevent Recurrent Events (CURE) trial, clopidogrel therapy (compared to placebo) was associated with a significant reduction in major ischemic complications in the first 30 days (*left*).[20] Outcomes of the majority of CURE patients who underwent percutaneous coronary intervention (PCI) were reported in PCI-CURE. Continuation of clopidogrel therapy resulted in further reduction in the composite endpoint of major ischemic complications in this prespecified analysis. The mean duration of clopidogrel therapy in this group was 9 months (*right*).[23] *CV,* Cardiovascular; *MI,* myocardial infarction.

dose of clopidogrel prior to PCI for an NSTE-ACS had fewer subsequent ischemic events (defined as cardiovascular death, acute or subacute stent thrombosis, recurrent ACS, and stroke) within 1 month when compared to those receiving a 300-mg loading dose (5% vs. 12%; *P* = .02).[25] These findings were subsequently confirmed in the Antiplatelet Therapy for Reduction of Myocardial Damage During Angioplasty 2 (ARMYDA-2) trial, in which the higher loading dose resulted in a reduced incidence and size of periprocedural MI.[27]

The AHA/ACC guidelines for management of NSTE-ACS give clopidogrel a class IB indication in patients who cannot take aspirin. With an early invasive strategy, a preprocedural loading and maintenance dose of clopidogrel or ticagrelor should be given (class IB). If an ischemia-guided strategy is taken and no intervention is performed, clopidogrel or ticagrelor is recommended for up to 12 months (class IB), although ticagrelor is preferred. If intervention is performed, the patient should receive clopidogrel, prasugrel, or ticagrelor for at least 12 months (class IB).[8,18,19] Ticagrelor is preferred over clopidogrel in early invasive and initial ischemia-guided strategies (class IIa).[8]

Prasugrel. The second ADP receptor antagonist to gain U.S. Food and Drug Administration (FDA) approval was prasugrel. Like clopidogrel, prasugrel is a thienopyridine prodrug that must be converted into its active metabolite in order to irreversibly bind to the P2Y$_{12}$ receptor. The loading dose of prasugrel (60 mg) appears more potent than 600 mg of clopidogrel. Similarly, the maintenance dose of prasugrel (10 mg) maintains a higher degree of platelet inhibition than a daily dose of 150 mg of clopidogrel.[28]

The largest clinical investigation to date to examine prasugrel was the Trial to Assess Improvement in Therapeutic Outcomes by Optimizing Platelet Inhibition with Prasugrel–Thrombolysis in Myocardial Infarction (TRITON–TIMI) 38.[29] In that study, 13,608 patients with moderate-to-high-risk ACS scheduled for PCI were randomized to receive prasugrel (a 60-mg loading dose and a 10-mg daily maintenance dose) or clopidogrel (a 300-mg loading dose and a 75-mg daily maintenance dose) for 6 to 15 months. All patients received aspirin in addition to the thienopyridine agent. The primary efficacy endpoint was a combined endpoint of cardiovascular death, nonfatal MI, or nonfatal stroke, while the key safety endpoint was major bleeding. There was a statistically significant 19% reduction in the primary endpoint (cardiovascular death, nonfatal MI, or stroke) in the prasugrel group (Table 36.1). The use of prasugrel was also associated with significant reduction in other ischemic complications, such as MI, urgent target-vessel revascularization, and stent thrombosis.[29]

However, prasugrel therapy was associated with increased bleeding complications. Major bleeding not related to coronary artery bypass graft (CABG) was more frequent with prasugrel compared to clopidogrel therapy (2.4% vs. 1.8%, HR, 1.32; 95% CI, 1.03–1.68; *P* = .03). Even more concerning, a similar statistically significant increase was noted in fatal bleeding (0.4% vs. 0.1%; *P* = .002).[29] Efforts were then made to identify subgroups of patients in whom the harm caused by increased bleeding complications supersedes the benefit of reduced ischemic events. Patients who had a previous stroke or TIA had net harm from prasugrel (HR, 1.54; 95% CI, 1.02–2.32; *P* = .04), patients greater than or equal to 75 years of age or weighing less than 60 kg had no net benefit from prasugrel (HR, 0.99; 95% CI, 0.81–1.21;

TABLE 36.1 **Pivotal Randomized Trials Comparing Efficacy and Safety of Newer P2Y$_{12}$ Inhibitors to Clopidogrel**

	TRITON TRIAL[29,a]				PLATO TRIAL[32,b]			
	Prasugrel	Clopidogrel	HR (95% CI)	P Value	Ticagrelor	Clopidogrel	HR (95% CI)	P value
Efficacy Endpoints								
Composite primary endpoint[c] (CV death, MI, or stroke)	9.9%	12.1%	0.81 (0.73–0.90)	<.001	9.8%	11.7%	0.84 (0.77–0.92)	<.001
All-cause mortality	3.0%	3.2%	0.95 (0.78–1.16)	.64	4.5%	5.9%	0.78 (0.69–0.89)	<.001
Stent thrombosis (definite or probable)	1.1%	2.4%	0.48 (0.36–0.64)	<.001	2.2%	2.9%	0.75 (0.59–0.95)	.02
Safety Endpoints[d]								
Non-CABG major bleeding (TIMI criteria)	2.4%	1.8%	1.32 (1.03–1.68)	.03	2.8%	2.2%	1.25 (1.03–1.53)	.03
CABG-related major bleeding (TIMI criteria)	13.4%	3.2%	4.73 (1.9–11.82)	<.001	5.3%	5.8%	0.94 (0.82–1.07)	.32
Intracranial bleeding	0.3%	0.3%	1.12 (0.58–2.15)	.74	0.3%	0.2%	1.87 (0.98–3.58)	.06
Major or minor bleeding (TIMI criteria)	5.0%	3.8%	1.31 (1.11–1.56)	.002	11.4%	10.9%	1.05 (0.96–1.15)	.33

CABG, Coronary artery bypass graft; *CI*, confidence interval; *CV*, cardiovascular; *HR*, hazard ratio; *MI*, myocardial infarction; *PCI*, percutaneous coronary intervention; *TIMI*, Thrombolysis in Myocardial Infarction.
[a]More than 13,000 patients with ACS undergoing PCI, randomized in a 1:1 blinded fashion.
[b]More than 18,000 patients with ACS, randomized in a 1:1 blinded fashion.
[c]At 15 months of follow-up for TRITON but only at 12 months for PLATO.
[d]Selected bleeding endpoints reported in both trials using TIMI criteria to facilitate comparison and perspective.

$P = .92$ and 1.03; 95% CI, 0.69–1.53; $P = .89$, respectively). Accordingly, prasugrel is contraindicated in patients with previous history of stroke or TIA (class III) and not recommended for those age 75 years or older or who weigh 60 kg or less (FDA black box warning).[29]

It is important to note that the TRITON trial examined the role of prasugrel as an adjunct to an early invasive strategy and thus was given at the time of PCI. It was unclear if the reduction in ischemic events noted in TRITON can be replicated in patients treated medically or using a selective ischemia-guided strategy. For that purpose, The Targeted Platelet Inhibition to Clarify the Optimal Strategy to Medically Manage Acute Coronary Syndromes (TRILOGY ACS) study was conducted, a randomized, double-blind trial of approximately 10,300 patients with high-risk NSTE-ACS who were intended to undergo medical therapy. Patients were randomized to clopidogrel versus prasugrel, with aspirin as background antiplatelet therapy in both arms. More than 72% of patients were younger than 75 years and received prasugrel 10 mg/day, but those older than 75 years or who weighed less than 60 kg were treated with 5 mg daily. At 17 months, the reduction of the primary endpoint (cardiovascular death, MI, or stroke) in the prasugrel arm was not statistically significant (13.9% vs. 16.0%; HR 0.91; 95% CI, 0.79–1.05; $P = .21$). The trial concluded that among patients with NSTE-ACS treated medically, prasugrel did not significantly reduce the frequency of adverse ischemic events compared with clopidogrel with similar risks of bleeding.[30]

Ticagrelor. Ticagrelor is an ADP P2Y$_{12}$ receptor inhibitor. Unlike clopidogrel and prasugrel, ticagrelor is a reversible, direct-acting agent. Ticagrelor is a more potent platelet inhibitor with a more rapid onset of action than clopidogrel.

The role of ticagrelor in contemporary therapy of ACS was established in the Study of Platelet Inhibition and Patient Outcomes (PLATO) trial, a multicenter, double-blind, randomized trial that compared ticagrelor to clopidogrel therapy with background aspirin. The study compared ticagrelor (180 mg loading dose, 90 mg twice daily thereafter) and clopidogrel (300 to 600 mg loading dose, 75 mg daily thereafter) for the prevention of cardiovascular events in 18,624 patients admitted with ACS, with or without ST segment elevation. The composite primary endpoint (cardiovascular death, MI, or stroke at 12 months) occurred in 9.8% of patients receiving ticagrelor compared to 11.7% in the clopidogrel group (HR, 0.84; 95% CI, 0.77–0.92; $P < .001$) (see Table 36.1). It is important to note that cardiovascular death and all-cause death were reduced in the ticagrelor group (4.0% vs. 5.1%, $P = .001$ and 4.5% vs. 5.9%, $P < .001$, respectively). No significant difference in the rates of major bleeding was found between the ticagrelor and clopidogrel groups (11.6% and 11.2%, respectively; $P = .43$). However, ticagrelor was associated with a higher rate of major bleeding not related to CABG (4.5% vs. 3.8%; $P = .03$).[31] There was also a treatment difference noted by region and North Americans appeared to have less of a benefit from ticagrelor than Europeans. This was later attributed to a higher dose of aspirin therapy in the North American patients.[32]

These findings led to the recommendation to give a daily maintenance dose of 81 mg of aspirin when ticagrelor is being coadministered.[8,18] In light of the PLATO trial, ticagrelor was given a class IIA recommendation in the 2014 NSTE-ACS

American guidelines[8] and a class IA recommendation in the European guidelines and in the subsequent ACC/AHA update on DAPT.[19,33]

Dyspnea was more common in the ticagrelor group than the clopidogrel group (13.8% vs. 7.8%), but this only led to discontinuation of the drug in 0.9% of patients compared to 0.1% in the clopidogrel group.[31] The dyspnea is thought to be an adenosine-mediated effect that was mild and short lived. Most patients had resolution of symptoms if they continued on therapy. Bradycardia was slightly more common in the ticagrelor group (4.4% vs. 4%), but there was no statistical difference in pacemaker insertion, syncope, or heart block between the two groups.

Cangrelor. Cangrelor is a rapid-acting, reversible, nonthienopyridine adenosine triphosphate (ATP) analogue that is administered intravenously (IV) to block the ADP receptor $P2Y_{12}$.[34] There were three large-scale trials to study the efficacy and safety of cangrelor in the setting of ACS: Cangrelor versus Standard Therapy to Achieve Optimal Management of Platelet Inhibition (CHAMPION) PCI, CHAMPION PLATFORM, and CHAMPION PHOENIX.

CHAMPION PCI was conducted on more than 8000 ACS patients undergoing PCI to compare two antiplatelet strategies: cangrelor (30 μg/kg IV bolus given before PCI and followed by an infusion of 4 μg/kg per minute for 2 to 4 hours) and clopidogrel 600 mg orally prior to PCI. The primary endpoint (a composite of death, MI, or ischemia-driven revascularization at 48 hours) was not significantly different between cangrelor and clopidogrel arms (7.5% vs. 7.1%; OR, 1.05; 95% CI, 0.88–1.24; $P = .59$). There was no difference in major bleeding according to the Thrombolysis in Myocardial Infarction (TIMI) or Global Use of Strategies to Open Occluded Coronary Arteries (GUSTO) criteria.[34]

CHAMPION PLATFORM was a double-blind, placebo-controlled study that randomized 5362 patients undergoing PCI to either cangrelor or placebo at the time of PCI, followed by clopidogrel 600 mg. The primary endpoint was similar and enrollment was stopped when an interim analysis concluded that the trial would be unlikely to show superiority (primary endpoint occurred in 7.0% of the cangrelor patients and 8.0% of the placebo patients, $P = .17$). There was, however, a statistically significant decrease in two prespecified secondary endpoints with cangrelor versus placebo: stent thrombosis (0.2% vs. 0.6%; OR, 0.31; 95% CI, 0.11–0.85; $P = .02$) and all-cause death (0.2% vs. 0.7%; OR, 0.33; 95% CI, 0.13–0.83; $P = .02$).[35]

The latest CHAMPION PHOENIX trial included 11,145 patients undergoing urgent or elective PCI. They received IV cangrelor or a loading dose of 600 mg or 300 mg of clopidogrel. The primary endpoint was the composite of death, MI, ischemia-driven revascularization, or stent thrombosis at 48 hours, which occurred in 4.7% of the cangrelor group and 5.9% in the clopidogrel group (adjusted OR, 0.78; 95% CI, 0.66–0.93; $P = .005$). The key secondary endpoint was stent thrombosis at 48 hours, which occurred in 0.8% of the cangrelor group and 1.4% in the clopidogrel group (OR, 0.62; 95% CI, 0.43–0.9; $P = .01$). The primary safety endpoint of severe bleeding at 48 hours

occurred in 0.16% of the cangrelor group and 0.11% of the clopidogrel group (OR, 1.5; 95% CI, 0.53–4.22; $P = .44$). These findings led to the conclusion that cangrelor significantly reduced the rate of ischemic events, including stent thrombosis, during urgent or elective PCI, with no significant increase in severe bleeding.[36]

A pooled analysis of patient-level data from the three CHAMPION trials compared cangrelor with clopidogrel or placebo to assess its effects on thrombotic complications during and after PCI.[37] The use of cangrelor reduced the odds of death, MI, and ischemia-driven revascularization at 48 hours (3.6% for cangrelor vs. 4.4% for the control group, $P = .0014$). Stent thrombosis was decreased from 0.8% in the control group to 0.5% in the cangrelor group ($P = .0008$). There was no difference in the primary safety outcome of GUSTO severe or life-threatening bleeding (0.2% in both groups), but cangrelor did cause and increase in GUSTO mild bleeding (16.8% vs. 13%, $P < .0001$). Currently, there are no ACC/AHA guideline recommendations for the use of cangrelor in any setting.

Vorapaxar

Vorapaxar is an oral protease-activated receptor-1 (PAR-1) antagonist that inhibits thrombin-induced platelet activation. Thrombin activates platelets through two PARs, PAR-1 and PAR-4, and stimulates a more rapid platelet activation response. Preclinical models showed that selective PAR-1 inhibition resulted in potent reduction in thrombin-induced platelet aggregation and preserved primary hemostatic function.[38]

The Thrombin Receptor Antagonist for Clinical Event Reduction in Acute Coronary Syndrome (TRACER) trial was a multinational, double-blind, randomized trial that compared vorapaxar (loading dose of 40 mg and daily maintenance dose of 2.5 mg) with placebo in 12,944 patients who had NSTE-ACS. The primary endpoint (composite of cardiovascular death, MI, stroke, recurrent ischemia with rehospitalization, or urgent coronary revascularization) was reduced with vorapaxar, but the reduction did not reach statistical significance. However, a composite of cardiovascular death, MI, or stroke was significantly reduced with vorapaxar (14.7% vs. 16.4%; HR, 0.89; 95% CI, 0.81–0.98; $P = .02$). The trial was terminated early after a safety review showed that rates of moderate to severe bleeding and intracranial hemorrhage were significantly increased with use of vorapaxar.[38] Given the failure to meet the primary endpoint and the increased bleeding complications, there are no indications for vorapaxar in treatment of ACS.

Glycoprotein IIb/IIIa Receptor Antagonists

Platelet aggregation depends on the GP IIb/IIIa receptor located on the surface of platelets. Often called the final common pathway, the GP IIb/IIIa receptor on the activated platelet undergoes a conformational change that allows binding of fibrinogen and vWF, which, in turn, cross-links with GP IIb/IIIa receptors on other activated platelets, promoting platelet aggregation.

The GP IIb/IIIa receptor antagonists were initially approved as adjunctive pharmacologic agents that reduce the ischemic complications of PCI, particularly in patients at high risk of abrupt closure in the prestent era. The significant success of these agents in reducing abrupt closure and periprocedural myonecrosis established the importance of aggressive platelet inhibition in reducing ischemic complications. It was only natural that these agents be tested in other clinical situations in which the activated platelets play a fundamental role, namely, ACS. It is also important to note that most of the evidence demonstrating the efficacy of IIb/IIIa inhibitors in reducing ischemic complications was accumulated prior to the routine use of clopidogrel and prior to approval of newer and more potent ticagrelor and prasugrel. The intravenous IIb/IIIa receptor antagonists available for use in the United States include abciximab, eptifibatide, and tirofiban.

Abciximab. Abciximab was the prototype of all intravenous GP IIb/IIIa receptor antagonists. It is a chimeric human-murine monoclonal antibody that irreversibly binds to the GP IIb/IIIa receptor. Abciximab also cross-reacts with the $\alpha_v\beta_3$ (vitronectin) receptor.[39] It has a plasma half-life of approximately 30 minutes and is cleared through the reticuloendothelial system but, once bound to the platelet, it remains nearly irreversibly bound and maintains some GP IIb/IIIa blockade for the lifespan of the platelet, 10 to 14 days. The dose of abciximab approved for use in conjunction with other antithrombotics in the setting of PCI is a bolus of 0.25 mg/kg 10 to 60 minutes prior to intervention, followed by an infusion of 0.125 µg/kg per minute (10 µg/min maximum) for 12 hours. During the abciximab infusion, platelet levels should be monitored; the infusion should be discontinued if the level falls below 100×10^9 cells/L.

Numerous landmark trials have established the value of abciximab as an adjunct to heparin for anticoagulation during PCI. Those trials included both stable and unstable patients.[40–43] In an early randomized trial of more than 1200 ACS patients, abciximab was administered 18 to 24 hours prior to PCI and continued for 1 hour afterwards in the treatment group. The primary endpoint (death, MI, or urgent intervention within 30 days) was significantly reduced in the abciximab group (11.3% vs. 15.9%, $P = .012$).[44] Interestingly, the benefit of intense antiplatelet therapy was observed within 24 hours, even before revascularization was attempted (Fig. 36.4). Further analysis demonstrated the benefit of intense and early platelet inhibition by abciximab was mostly limited to patients presenting with elevated serum troponin levels (see Fig. 36.4).[45]

In contrast to the aforementioned studies, GUSTO IV-ACS evaluated the efficacy of abciximab therapy in ACS patients not undergoing early revascularization. In this context, abciximab use (bolus and 24- to 48-hour infusion) was not associated with any reduction in death or MI at 30 days. In fact, at 48 hours, a higher mortality rate was seen in patients receiving abciximab.[46] The reason for this excess mortality is unclear. One possibility is that the antiplatelet effects of abciximab become unpredictable and tend to diminish with time; subtherapeutic dosing or insufficient platelet inhibition by IIb/IIIa inhibitors may actually be deleterious in patients with higher levels of inflammation.[47]

Eptifibatide. Eptifibatide is a cyclic heptapeptide competitive inhibitor of platelet GP IIb/IIIa. Eptifibatide binding to the IIb/IIIa receptor is reversible and the drug's efficacy is dependent

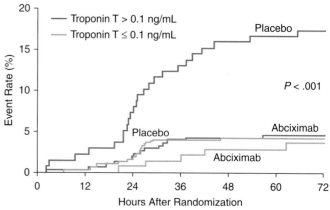

Fig. 36.4 Benefit of IIb/IIIa inhibitors in high-risk acute coronary syndrome (ACS) patients. In the c7E3 Fab Antiplatelet Therapy in Unstable Refractory Angina (CAPTURE) trial, high-risk ACS patients received abciximab for 18 to 24 hours before percutaneous coronary intervention (PCI) and for 1 hour after the procedure. Major adverse cardiac events at 30 days were significantly reduced in the abciximab arm. The reduction in events was significantly more apparent in those with troponin elevation on presentation *(red line graph)*. The reduction in events with abciximab in the troponin negative patients *(blue line graph)* was not statistically significant. Importantly, differences between abciximab and placebo were noticed within the first 24 hours—that is, before PCI—indicating that the reduction in ischemic events was driven by the intense platelet inhibition.[44]

on maintaining a high serum concentration that allows a steady state of IIb/IIIa receptor blockade. In ACS patients, eptifibatide is given as an IV bolus of 180 µg/kg followed by a continuous infusion of 2 µg/kg per minute. In patients with a creatinine clearance less than 50 ml/minute, the continuous infusion is given at 1 µg/kg per minute. High levels of platelet inhibition occur within 1 hour, with platelet function normalizing 4 to 8 hours after discontinuation. It is primarily secreted in the urine.

The benefit of eptifibatide in patients with acute coronary syndrome was established in the Inhibition of Platelet Glycoprotein IIb/IIIa with Eptifibatide in Patients with Acute Coronary Syndrome (PURSUIT) trial. This randomized, placebo-controlled trial included 10,948 NSTE-ACS patients. Most patients received aspirin and heparin, and were then randomized to receive placebo or eptifibatide (IV bolus of 180 µg/kg followed by an infusion at 1.3 or 2 µg/kg per minute). The duration of therapy extended to 72 hours (or 96 hours if PCI occurred later in the hospitalization) or until the patient left the hospital. The primary endpoint was a composite of death and nonfatal MI at 30 days. In the eptifibatide group, there was a 1.5% absolute reduction in the incidence of the primary endpoint (14.2 vs. 15.7%; $P = .04$), with this effect occurring in most major subgroups.[48,49] Further investigation of the PURSUIT cohort revealed that eptifibatide reduced the rates of death and MI in patients before and after PCI, in stented and nonstented patients and in those who did not undergo PCI, although the reduction in primary events appeared greater in patients who had an early PCI.[50]

The Early Glycoprotein IIb/IIIa Inhibition in Patients With Non–ST Segment Elevation Acute Coronary Syndrome

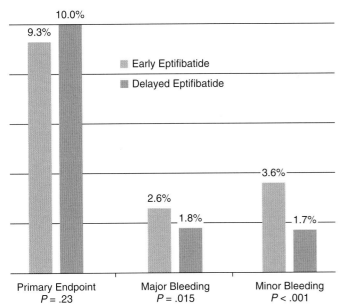

Fig. 36.5 Contemporary use of IIb/IIIa Inhibitors in ACS patients. In the Early Glycoprotein IIb/IIIa Inhibition in Non–ST Segment Elevation Acute Coronary Syndrome (EARLY ACS) trial, high-risk ACS patients were randomized to early routine use of eptifibatide at the time of admission or delayed provisional use at the time of percutaneous coronary intervention. Clopidogrel was used in 75% of all patients. The primary composite endpoint (death, myocardial infarction, recurrent ischemia requiring urgent revascularization, or thrombotic bailout at 96 hours) was not different between the two groups, but bleeding complications were more frequent with the early routine use of eptifibatide.

(EARLY-ACS) trial is an important experiment examining the role of eptifibatide and IIb/IIIa inhibitors in contemporary management of ACS in which $P2Y_{12}$ inhibitor use is widespread. Patients were randomly assigned to either early, pre-PCI double-bolus eptifibatide or delayed, provisional eptifibatide at the time of PCI. Upstream preprocedure clopidogrel was administered in 75% of the population. Upstream eptifibatide therapy did not result in a significant reduction in the primary efficacy endpoint (a composite of death, MI, recurrent ischemia requiring urgent revascularization, or the occurrence of a thrombotic complication during PCI at 96 hours). However, the risk of major bleeding in the early eptifibatide group was 2.6% compared to 1.8% (P = .02) in the delayed provisional group (Fig. 36.5).[51] Thus the use of GP IIb/IIIa receptor antagonists has significantly shifted from an upstream drug to an adjunctive medication given at the time of PCI, usually in a bailout fashion.

Tirofiban. Similar to eptifibatide, tirofiban is a small-molecule, reversible antagonist of the platelet GP IIb/IIIa receptor. Tirofiban is cleared renally and platelet function returns to normal 4 to 8 hours after discontinuation.

The initial randomized trials attempting to establish a role for tirofiban in management of ACS were unsuccessful in achieving that goal because benefits in reducing ischemic complications did not reach statistical significance for the prespecified endpoint.[42,52] In a subsequent randomized trial, Platelet Receptor

Inhibition in Ischemic Syndrome Management in Patients Limited by Unstable Signs and Symptoms (PRISM-PLUS),[53] 1915 NSTE-ACS patients were randomized to receive tirofiban, heparin, or tirofiban plus heparin for a mean of 71.3 ± 20 hours. The primary composite endpoint included death, MI, or refractory ischemia. Angiography and revascularization were typically performed after 48 hours. The frequency of the composite endpoint at 7 days was lower among patients receiving tirofiban plus heparin than those receiving heparin alone (12.9% vs. 17.9%; risk ratio [RR], 0.68; P = .004). The significantly improved outcomes in the tirofiban plus heparin arm were preserved at 30 days (18.5% vs. 22.3%; P = .03) and at 6 months (27.7% vs. 32.1%; P = .02). It is important to note that the third arm of randomization in the study (those receiving tirofiban without heparin) was stopped prematurely due to an excess mortality at 7 days (4.6% compared to 1.1% for patients treated with heparin alone).

The 2014 ACC/AHA guidelines for management of patients with NSTE-ACS who undergo an early invasive strategy state that GP IIb/IIIa inhibitors may be considered as part of the initial antiplatelet therapy in patients treated with DAPT with intermediate/high-risk features (class IIb). The preferred options are eptifibatide or tirofiban. Both require renal dose adjustments for creatinine clearance less than or equal to 50 mL/min and less than or equal to 30 mL/min, respectively. In patients with NSTE-ACS and high-risk features (e.g., elevated troponin) not adequately pretreated with clopidogrel or ticagrelor, it is useful to administer a GP IIb/IIIa inhibitor (abciximab, double-bolus eptifibatide, or high-dose bolus tirofiban) at the time of PCI (class IA). Abciximab should be used only if there is no appreciable delay in angiography and PCI is likely to be performed. In patients referred for CABG, short-acting intravenous GP IIb/IIIa inhibitors (eptifibatide or tirofiban) should be discontinued at least 2 to 4 hours before surgery and abciximab at least 12 hours before to limit blood loss and the need for transfusion (class IB).[8]

ST SEGMENT ELEVATION MYOCARDIAL INFARCTION

The paramount importance of early reperfusion in acute STEMI has been well established.[54] The preferred mechanism by which such reperfusion is achieved has shifted over the years from thrombolytic therapy to primary PCI.[1,55] In either case, patients presenting with acute STEMI usually arrive at the CICU with therapy already administered, either in the ambulance, the emergency department, and/or in the catheterization laboratory.

While the purpose of antiplatelet therapy in and of itself is not to achieve initial reperfusion in patients with STEMI, antiplatelet agents can play a significant role as adjunctive therapies to improve the outcome of reperfusion therapy.

While effective in dissolving arterial thrombi, fibrinolytic agents can activate thrombin and promote platelet aggregation, potentially leading to rethrombosis. This procoagulant activity has been demonstrated in several studies. Fibrinopeptide A levels, when used as a measure of thrombin activity, significantly increased after the infusion of both streptokinase (SK) and tissue plasminogen activator (tPA) in patients presenting with acute STEMI.[56] The increased thrombin is thought to be due to upstream activation of coagulation factors, as prothrombin levels are also elevated in patients receiving tPA.[57] More direct evidence of platelet activation with thrombolysis is demonstrated by assessing TX biosynthesis in patients receiving SK after presenting with a STEMI. Major enzymatic metabolites of TXA_2, urinary 2,3-dinor-TXB_2 and plasma 11-dehydro-TXB_2 were markedly increased in patients receiving SK therapy. Platelets are the main source of TXA_2, suggesting marked platelet activation after the infusion.[58] Thus, the addition of effective antiplatelet therapy is important in preserving the patency of the infarct-related artery that is prone to platelet-mediated reocclusion.

Similarly, there is ample evidence for the benefits of antiplatelet agents in the setting of primary PCI. The benefits of antiplatelet therapy are manifested by improved flow, reduced embolization, reduced infarct size, and/or improved clinical outcomes.

Aspirin

The benefit of aspirin in the treatment of STEMI was clearly demonstrated in the second International Study of Infarct Survival (ISIS-2) trial, in which more than 17,000 patients were randomized to receive an intravenous SK, 1 month of 160 mg aspirin, both, or neither within 24 hours of a suspected acute MI. Vascular death was significantly reduced in patients receiving aspirin compared to placebo (9.4% vs. 11.8%, $p < .0001$). The reduction in mortality in those receiving aspirin was very similar to patients receiving SK compared to placebo infusion (9.2% vs. 12%, $P < .0001$; Fig. 36.6). However, the greatest reduction in mortality occurred when aspirin and SK were used in combination.[59]

When comparing 162 mg aspirin with 325 mg aspirin, both doses seem equally effective in lowering mortality in patients with an STEMI. However, recent data suggest that the 162-mg dose is associated with fewer episodes of bleeding. This was noted in a study in which acute mortality and bleeding risk was evaluated in fibrinolytic-treated STEMI patients. Data were obtained from a combined analysis of GUSTO I and GUSTO III trials.[60] After adjustment for other variables, aspirin dose (162 mg vs. 325 mg) was not associated with a difference in 24-hour, 7-day, or 30-day mortality rates. There was also no difference in MI between the two groups. However, the 325-mg dose was associated with a significant increase in moderate/severe bleeding using the GUSTO prediction model (OR, 1.14; 95% CI, 1.05–1.24; $P = .003$).[60]

Aspirin therapy is also proven to prevent reocclusion and recurrent ischemia after thrombolysis. In a meta-analysis of 32 studies that included angiographic assessment after receiving thrombolytic therapy (heparin plus SK or heparin plus tPA), patients receiving aspirin had a significantly lower rate of reocclusion (11% vs. 25%; $P < .001$).[61]

The ACC/AHA 2013 guidelines for the management of STEMI recommend aspirin, 162 to 325 mg, be given prior to primary PCI, preferably nonenteric coated and in chewable form for faster onset of action, in STEMI patients (class IB). After PCI, aspirin should be continued indefinitely at a dose of 81 to 325 mg (class IA) but 81 mg is the preferred maintenance dose (class IIA).[18]

ADP Receptor Antagonists

Clopidogrel. Clopidogrel is considered a reasonable alternative to aspirin in patients with STEMI who are unable to tolerate

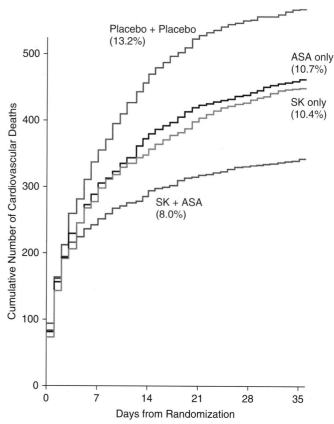

Fig. 36.6 Impact of aspirin on mortality in ST elevation myocardial infarction patients. In the Second International Study of Infarct Survival (ISIS-2) trial, patients with suspected acute myocardial infarction were randomized in a 2 × 2 factorial design to receive acetylsalicylic acid (ASA) versus placebo and streptokinase (SK) versus placebo. A 23% relative reduction in mortality was achieved with ASA therapy alone, which was almost identical to that of thrombolytic therapy. Patients with best outcomes in this trial were those randomized to both ASA and streptokinase. (From Randomized trial of intravenous streptokinase, oral aspirin, both, or neither among 17,187 cases of suspected acute myocardial infarction: ISIS-2. ISIS-2 [Second International Study of Infarct Survival] Collaborative Group. *Lancet.* 1988;2:349–360.)

aspirin.[1] More important and more commonly, these agents are used in addition to aspirin for the demonstrable reduction in adverse ischemic outcomes in STEMI patients. The benefits can be seen in the early phase as adjuvants to the reperfusion strategy (primary PCI or thrombolytic therapy) and also as long-term maintenance therapy for secondary prevention.

Two trials have evaluated the role of clopidogrel in addition to aspirin compared with aspirin alone in medically treated STEMI patients: Clopidogrel as Adjunctive Reperfusion Therapy—Thrombolysis in Myocardial Infarction 28 (CLARITY-TIMI 28) and Clopidogrel and Metoprolol in Myocardial Infarction (COMMIT). In CLARITY-TIMI 28, 3491 patients younger than 75 years, with a recent (≤12 hours) STEMI received a loading dose of clopidogrel 300 mg followed by 75 mg daily or matching placebo after receiving fibrinolytic therapy. All patients received aspirin; heparin was given when fibrin-specific thrombolytic agents were used. The composite endpoint included an occluded infarct-related artery on angiography, death, or recurrent MI before angiography. In patients treated with clopidogrel and aspirin, the infarct-related artery was more likely to be patent (88.3% vs. 81.6% in the aspirin only group, P < .001). Addition of clopidogrel also resulted in a 30% reduction in recurrent MI (from 3.6 to 2.5%; P = .08). Similar trends were seen at 30 days.[62]

The COMMIT study included greater than 45,000 patients with an acute MI (87% with ST segment elevation and 6% with left bundle branch block) not undergoing PCI, who received clopidogrel 75 mg daily (n = 22,961) or placebo (n = 22,891) in addition to aspirin 162 mg daily until discharge or for up to 28 days (mean therapy of 14.9 days). No loading dose of clopidogrel was given and approximately half of the patients received fibrinolytic therapy before or shortly after enrollment. Mortality was significantly reduced in all patients receiving clopidogrel compared to placebo (1726 events in the clopidogrel group vs. 1845 in the placebo group, corresponding to a significant 7% relative risk reduction). Those receiving clopidogrel also had a significant 14% relative reduction in the risk of reinfarction and a nonsignificant 14% relative reduction in the risk of stroke. Furthermore, when specifically examining those receiving fibrinolytic therapy, there was a significant 11% relative reduction in the risk of adverse events in the fibrinolytic group that received clopidogrel compared to placebo.[63]

The widespread use of stents eventually led to the very early administration of DAPT in STEMI patients. Direct evidence of the benefit of clopidogrel in the treatment of STEMI patients emerged from a prespecified analysis of the CLARITY-TIMI 28 trial that examined the effect of clopidogrel pretreatment of STEMI patients undergoing PCI.[64] In PCI-CLARITY, 1863 patients undergoing PCI received aspirin and either clopidogrel 300 mg loading dose, then 75 mg once daily, or placebo initiated with fibrinolysis and given until coronary angiography was performed (2–8 days after initiation of the study drug). Open-label clopidogrel with the 300 mg loading dose was recommended for those undergoing coronary stenting. The primary endpoint was the composite of cardiovascular death, recurrent MI, or stroke from PCI to 30 days after randomization. Pretreatment with clopidogrel significantly reduced the incidence of the composite primary endpoint (3.6% vs. 6.2%; P = .008). Pretreatment with clopidogrel also reduced the incidence of MI or stroke prior to PCI (4.0% vs. 6.2%; P = .03) and there was a highly significant reduction in cardiovascular death, MI, or stroke from randomization through 30 days (7.5% vs. 12.0%; P = .001).

Patients with prior MI, ischemic stroke, or peripheral vascular disease were found to have further reduction in recurrent events when clopidogrel was administered in addition to aspirin. This was demonstrated in a subgroup of 9478 patients from the Clopidogrel for High Atherothrombotic Risk and Ischemic Stabilization, Management, and Avoidance (CHARISMA) trial. With a median follow-up of 27.6 months, the rate of cardiovascular death, MI, or stroke was significantly reduced when clopidogrel was added to aspirin compared to placebo plus aspirin: 7.3% versus 8.8% (HR, 0.83; 95% CI, 0.72–0.96; P =.01). Hospitalizations for ischemia were also significantly reduced (11.4% vs. 13.2%; HR 0.86; 95% CI, 0.76–0.96; P = .008).[65]

In patients less than 75 years of age who receive fibrinolytic therapy, it is reasonable to administer an oral loading dose of clopidogrel 300 mg (class IA). Patients older than 75 years may proceed without a loading dose of clopidogrel. Long-term maintenance therapy (e.g., 1 year) of clopidogrel 75 mg daily is indicated in STEMI patients irrespective of whether they underwent reperfusion therapy.[1,66] DAPT should be continued for at least 12 months after drug-eluting stent (DES) implantation (class IC).[18]

Prasugrel. In TRITON TIMI-38, patients presenting with STEMI represented 3534 of 13,608 (25.9%) patients in the study. As previously discussed, the study as a whole achieved its primary efficacy endpoint: a statistically significant reduction in the composite of cardiovascular death, nonfatal MI, or stroke. In the STEMI subgroup, the results were similar, with a significant reduction in the primary endpoint in the prasugrel arm (HR, 0.79; 95% CI, 0.65–0.97; P = .02).[29]

Prasugrel has not been studied concomitantly with fibrinolytic therapy and therefore does not currently have a role in that setting.

Ticagrelor. In the PLATO trial, 37.5% of the ticagrelor-treated patients and 38% of the clopidogrel-treated patients presented with a STEMI. In STEMI patients, there was a 1.9% absolute risk reduction (16.3% relative risk reduction) of the composite endpoint of death from vascular causes, MI, or stroke at 12 months with ticagrelor. Among patients who received a stent during the study, the rate of definite stent thrombosis was lower in the ticagrelor group than in the clopidogrel group (1.3% vs. 1.9%; P = .009).[31]

The more rapid onset of action of ticagrelor compared to clopidogrel appeared to offer some potential benefit to STEMI patients if administered early. A double-blind, randomized trial including more than 1800 STEMI patients undergoing primary PCI compared the potential benefit of prehospital administration (180-mg loading dose in the ambulance) to administration of the same loading dose after arrival in the catheterization laboratory and immediately prior to the procedure. Although there was no significant difference in either the primary efficacy (ST segment resolution or infarct-related artery patency) or safety endpoint (bleeding complications), there was a clinically relevant advantage to prehospital administration of ticagrelor loading, namely, a statistically significant reduction in definite stent thrombosis within the first 24 hours and more significantly at 30 days.[67]

The 2013 ACC/AHA guidelines for the management of STEMI recommend a loading dose of a P2Y$_{12}$ receptor inhibitor as early as possible at the time of primary PCI. The options include clopidogrel 600 mg, prasugrel 60 mg, or ticagrelor 180 mg (class IB). After coronary stenting, DAPT should be continued for at least 1 year as follows: clopidogrel 75 mg daily, prasugrel 10 mg daily, or ticagrelor 90 mg twice daily (class IB). Clopidogrel, prasugrel, or ticagrelor can be continued beyond 1 year after DES placement (class IIb).[18]

The 2016 ACC/AHA guideline update for the duration of DAPT therapy gives a class IIa recommendation to use ticagrelor in preference to clopidogrel after an NSTE-ACS or STEMI. They give the same class IIa recommendation to use prasugrel in preference to clopidogrel in patients with no prior history of stroke or TIA and no high-risk bleeding features.[19] There is still a class I recommendation to continue DAPT therapy for 12 months after an NSTE-ACS or STEMI, but it is considered reasonable to discontinue DAPT after 6 months in patients treated with a DES who are at high risk for bleeding complications or who develop significant overt bleeding (class IIb).[19]

The European Society of Cardiology (ESC) 2012 guidelines for the management of STEMI make the same recommendations for loading patients with clopidogrel, prasugrel, or ticagrelor. They give a class I recommendation for prasugrel and ticagrelor over clopidogrel in patients treated with PCI. There is also a class I recommendation to continue DAPT therapy for 12 months after a STEMI with a "strict minimum" of 1 month after treatment with a bare metal stent and 6 months after treatment with a DES (class IIb).[68]

Ticagrelor has not been studied with fibrinolytic therapy and therefore should be avoided in that setting.

Cangrelor

The CHAMPION PHOENIX trial had 962 (17.6%) STEMI patients in the cangrelor group and 1030 (18.8%) in the clopidogrel group. There were 27 (2.8%) events in the cangrelor group and 38 (3.7%) in the clopidogrel group (OR, 0.75; 95% CI, 0.46–1.25; P = NS). The events included death from any cause, MI, ischemia-driven revascularization, or stent thrombosis within 48 hours.[36]

There are currently no guideline recommendations for the use of cangrelor in the setting of STEMI; however, it may be a reasonable option for a patient who is unable to swallow a pill or who would require rapid antiplatelet therapy and has not received any DAPT at the time of primary PCI.

Vorapaxar. Vorapaxar has not been studied in the setting of STEMI and therefore is not recommended in that clinical setting.

Glycoprotein IIb/IIIa Inhibitors and Primary Percutaneous Coronary Intervention. The use of GP IIb/IIIa inhibitors in patients undergoing nonemergent PCI has been well studied in numerous randomized trials.[41,42,44,69] Several lessons were learned from those trials that were employed in the subsequent utilization of those agents during primary PCI. With increasing baseline risk, the advantage of these agents in reducing ischemic complications becomes more robust.[44,70,71] Additionally, the increased bleeding complications noted in earlier GP IIb/IIIa inhibitor trials were controlled by weight adjusted heparin dosing and early removal of femoral access sheaths.

Abciximab is the most studied GP IIb/IIIa inhibitor in patients receiving primary PCI. Despite some reduction in ischemic complications when abciximab is used in conjunction with primary PCI, there has been no large-scale randomized controlled trial to demonstrate evidence of reduced mortality in the STEMI population using this approach.

Numerous clinical trials have attempted to demonstrate a role for abciximab in reducing ischemic complications.[72–76] In these trials, patients undergoing primary PCI were randomized to abciximab or placebo with a composite clinical endpoint of death, reinfarction, and target lesion revascularization. In all trials, there was a significant reduction in 30-day ischemic events in patients receiving abciximab after PCI. None of these trials were individually powered to detect a mortality benefit.

In the Intracoronary Stenting and Antithrombotic Regimen-2 (ISAR-2) trial, the composite endpoint was reached in 5.0% of the abciximab group and 10.5% of the control group (P = .038). There was no statistically significant difference in the composite endpoint at 1 year.[72] In the Abciximab before Direct Angioplasty and Stenting in Myocardial Infarction Regarding Acute and Long-Term Follow-up (ADMIRAL) trial, the composite endpoint was reached in 6.0% of the patients in the abciximab group versus 14.6% in the placebo group (P = .01). At 6 months, the corresponding figures were 7.4% and 15.9% (P = .02).[73] The reduction in the primary endpoint with abciximab was similar in the Abciximab and Carbostent Evaluation (ACE) trial (4.5% and 10.5%, respectively; P = .023). Additionally, the composite of 6-month death and reinfarction was lower in the abciximab group than in the placebo group (5.5% and 13.5%, respectively; P = .006).[74] In the Controlled Abciximab and Device Investigation to Lower Late Angioplasty Complications (CADILLAC) trial, a large randomized trial examining the role of abciximab with primary PCI, either balloon angioplasty alone or stenting, abciximab was associated with a reduction in urgent target vessel revascularization. However, there was no reduction in reinfarction, stroke, or death.[76]

Despite the lack of a 30-day mortality benefit in any of these individual trials, the meta-analysis of De Luca et al., which included randomized comparisons of abciximab versus placebo in both primary and facilitated PCI, demonstrated a statistically significant reduction in 30-day (2.4% vs. 3.4%; P = .047) and 6-month (4.4% vs. 6.2%; P = .01) mortality with abciximab.[77] The benefit of abciximab was offset by a significant increase in the risk of bleeding when abciximab therapy was combined with fibrinolysis. However, the risk of bleeding was not increased when abciximab was used with primary PCI without thrombolytic therapy, resulting in a statistically significant reduction in adverse ischemic events that was not offset by the bleeding complications.

Two more recent clinical trials better define the role of abciximab in contemporary primary PCI: Facilitated Intervention with Enhanced Reperfusion Speed to Stop Events (FINESSE) and Intracoronary Abciximab Infusion and Aspiration Thrombectomy in Patients Undergoing Percutaneous Coronary Intervention for Anterior ST-Segment Elevation Myocardial Infarction (INFUSE-AMI). FINESSE was a large prospective controlled clinical trial that randomized 2452 STEMI patients to one of three treatment arms: primary PCI with abciximab administered in the catheterization laboratory, facilitated PCI with abciximab administered prior to arrival in the catheterization laboratory, and facilitated PCI with abciximab and half-dose reteplase administered prior to arrival in the catheterization laboratory.[78] The primary endpoint of the trial was a composite of all-cause mortality, readmission for heart failure, ventricular fibrillation, or cardiogenic shock. The patency rate of the infarct-related artery was significantly higher in combined facilitated PCI. However, at 90 days, there was no difference between the treatment arms (10.7%, 10.5%, and 9.8%, respectively, P = NS). The rate of TIMI major bleeding was highest in the facilitated PCI group (4.8%), with a trend toward increased intracranial hemorrhage. This study cast doubt on the role of GP IIb/IIIa inhibitors as effective adjunctive therapy in primary PCI and further confirmed the increased risk of bleeding associated with the combination of GP IIb/IIIa inhibitors and fibrinolytic therapy. INFUSE-AMI was a smaller but randomized and controlled trial assessing two strategies to reduce distal embolization and improve outcomes in 452 anterior STEMI patients. The first therapy was aspiration thrombectomy and the second was an intracoronary bolus of abciximab 0.25 mg/kg administered in the infarct-related artery, using a local drug delivery catheter. The primary endpoint was infarct size (percentage of total left ventricular mass) at 30 days as assessed by cardiac magnetic resonance imaging. While aspiration thrombectomy had no impact on the primary endpoint, patients receiving abciximab had a significant reduction in infarct size (median 15.1% vs. 17.9%; $P = .03$).[79] The study was not powered to detect differences in clinical outcomes.

Fewer data exist on small molecule GP IIb/IIIa inhibitors in the setting of primary PCI. There is, however, evidence of noninferiority of both eptifibatide and tirofiban in comparison to abciximab regarding efficacy and safety endpoints.[80,81]

In the ACC/AHA 2013 guidelines, there are no class I recommendations for GP IIb/IIIa inhibitors in STEMI and primary PCI. The use of any of the three approved GP IIb/IIIa inhibitors in conjunction with heparin at the time of primary PCI is considered reasonable and given a class IIa recommendation. Two additional applications of GP IIb/IIIa inhibitors are given class IIb recommendation: intracoronary injection of abciximab during primary PCI or GP IIb/IIIa inhibitor administration prior to arrival in the catheterization laboratory for those set to undergo primary PCI.[82]

Glycoprotein IIb/IIIa Inhibitors and Thrombolytic Therapy.

A significant body of literature addresses the role of GP IIb/IIIa inhibitors when used as adjuvants to thrombolytic therapy, with most studies evaluating abciximab.[83–87] There was no evidence that GP IIb/IIIa inhibitors in conjunction with fibrinolysis resulted in any reduction in mortality. These findings were confirmed in a large meta-analysis demonstrating the lack of efficacy and the increased risk of bleeding complications with the combination therapies.[77]

Eptifibatide has also been studied in combination therapy with thrombolytic agents in patients with an acute STEMI. Similar to the abciximab trials, death at 30 days was similar among patients receiving thrombolytic therapy alone and the combination of eptifibatide and tPA.[88]

The term "facilitated PCI" was previously used to describe a strategy of pharmacologic antithrombotic therapy combined with primary PCI, with the hope of capturing the benefit of early onset of therapy administered through simple IV access and the effectiveness of revascularization offered by delayed PCI. The pharmacologic intervention was usually in the form of full- or half-dose of a thrombolytic agent and/or a GP IIb/IIIa receptor antagonist. Patients were immediately transferred for planned PCI within 90 to 120 minutes. However, these approaches have failed to provide any improvement in outcomes and, in fact, had more adverse outcomes.[18,82,89,90] Hence, current guidelines do not recommend the use of these approaches in STEMI patients.

ANTIPLATELET THERAPY AND BLEEDING COMPLICATIONS

The development of modern interventional techniques and potent antiplatelet agents has led to significant reduction in ischemic complications in patients with ACS. However, potent antiplatelet therapies are, by design, associated with a risk of bleeding, particularly in the context of interventional and surgical procedures. Similarly, the risk of bleeding is augmented by the combination of potent antiplatelet agents with fibrinolytics and/or anticoagulant therapy. It is the balance between the reduction in ischemic complications and the incidence and severity of bleeding complications that determines the value and clinical utility of a specific antiplatelet agent. ACS patients in the CICU who are typically treated with one or more of these agents should be monitored diligently for signs and symptoms of bleeding.

The literature on bleeding complications related to antiplatelet agents is quite extensive. However, the lack of uniform methodology in assessing and reporting bleeding complications has hindered efforts to compare efficacy and safety of each of the agents when combined with antithrombotic drugs and/or interventional procedures.

Aspirin

It has been well established that aspirin increases the risk of gastrointestinal hemorrhage; however, this appears to occur with chronic and not acute therapy. In a meta-analysis of 66,000 patients on chronic aspirin therapy, gastrointestinal hemorrhage occurred in 2.47% of patients taking aspirin compared with 1.42% on placebo (OR, 1.68; 95% CI, 1.51–1.88); the number needed to harm was 106 based on an average of 28 months of therapy.[91] It is important to note, however, as demonstrated in the ISIS-2 trial, when used alone in patients with acute MI, aspirin was not associated with an increase in intracerebral hemorrhage or bleeding requiring transfusion.[58] Nonetheless, it should be emphasized that acute MI patients are rarely treated with aspirin alone. As previously discussed in this chapter, numerous investigations have demonstrated an increased risk of bleeding with larger doses of aspirin with no clear reduction in ischemic events.[13,15,16]

Clopidogrel

Not surprisingly, the combination of aspirin and clopidogrel has been found to increase the likelihood of bleeding. In the CURE trial, major bleeding occurred more frequently in patients receiving clopidogrel compared to placebo (3.7% vs. 2.7%; RR, 1.38; $P = .001$). There were no increased episodes of life-threatening bleeding requiring surgical intervention or hemorrhagic stroke. The most common cause of bleeding was gastrointestinal hemorrhage and bleeding at arterial puncture sites.[20]

The heightened risk of bleeding becomes a significant issue when patients are transferred for surgical revascularization soon after admission with the diagnosis of ACS. In the United States, such transfers usually occur within 1 or a few days and the effect of clopidogrel administered at the time of admission cannot be reversed. Clopidogrel has been found to increase the risk of bleeding in patients undergoing CABG if taken within 5 days of surgery. This was initially demonstrated in the CURE trial, in which 910 patients who stopped taking clopidogrel at least 5 days prior to bypass surgery had no increase in bleeding complications (4.4% in patients taking clopidogrel and 5.3% for those taking placebo). However, if clopidogrel was stopped less than 5 days prior to surgery, the likelihood for bleeding was higher during and after CABG (9.6% for clopidogrel vs. 6.3% for placebo; RR, 1.53; $P = .06$). Therefore the ACC/AHA guidelines recommend that CABG surgery be postponed, if possible, for at least 5 days after administration of clopidogrel and for at least 24 hours prior to urgent on-pump CABG, if possible (class IB).[8] On clinical grounds, this is not always feasible and many patients still undergo bypass surgery within this 5-day period.[92] It is therefore imperative that there is full communication, understanding, and preparation among the medical and surgical teams caring for such patients in the operating room and the postoperative ICU.

Prasugrel

In the TRITON-TIMI 38 trial, prasugrel was associated with more bleeding complications than clopidogrel (see Table 36.1). Major bleeding occurred in 2.4% of patients treated with prasugrel and 1.8% treated with clopidogrel (HR, 1.32; 95% CI, 1.03–1.68; $P = .03$). Life-threatening bleeding occurred in 1.9% versus 0.9% in the clopidogrel group ($P = .01$). Fatal bleeding occurred in 0.4% versus 0.1% ($P = .002$). These data follow the trend of more potent antiplatelet therapy causing more bleeding events. Accordingly, prasugrel therapy should be withheld for 7 days prior to CABG or other surgeries (class IC).[18]

Intracranial hemorrhage occurred more frequently with prasugrel. The increased risk was noted in older patients, those with low body mass index, and those with a history of stroke or TIA.[29] The FDA approval of the drug was accompanied by a black box warning not to use it in such populations.[8]

Ticagrelor

The PLATO trial showed similar rates of bleeding between ticagrelor and clopidogrel (11.6% and 11.2%, respectively; $P = .43$), but ticagrelor was associated with a higher rate of major bleeding not related to CABG (4.5% vs. 3.8%, $P = .03$).[31] There was also no significant difference in the rates of major bleeding according to the Thrombolysis in Myocardial Infarction (TIMI) criteria (7.9% with ticagrelor and 7.7% with clopidogrel, $P = .57$) or fatal or life-threatening bleeding (5.8% in both groups, $P = .70$; see Table 36.1). The absence of a significant difference in major bleeding was consistent among all subgroups without significant heterogeneity except with regard to the body mass index ($P = .05$ for interaction).[31] Ticagrelor should be discontinued 5 days prior to a planned CABG and at least 24 hours before urgent on-pump CABG, if possible (class IB).[8]

Glycoprotein IIb/IIIa Receptor Antagonists

GP IIb/IIIa inhibitors have also demonstrated an increased risk of bleeding, although the incidence and severity of such bleeding complications varies from one study to another. In the Evaluation in PTCA to Improve Long-Term Outcome with Abciximab GP IIb/IIIa Blockade (EPILOG) trial, the increased incidence of minor TIMI bleeding with abciximab was eliminated with weight-adjusted heparin dosing and early removal of arterial sheathes.[42] With those lessons learned, there was no difference in major or minor bleeding complications between ACS patients receiving abciximab or placebo in the Intracoronary Stenting and Antithrombotic Regimen: Rapid Early Action for Coronary Treatment 2 (ISAR-REACT 2) trial.[71] In the meta-analysis by De Luca et al., abciximab in acute STEMI was not associated with an increased risk of bleeding unless combined with thrombolytic therapy.[77] Like abciximab, the incidence of bleeding with eptifibatide varied depending on the study. In the Platelet Glycoprotein IIb/IIIa in Unstable Angina: Receptor Suppression Using Integrilin Therapy (PURSUIT) trial, patients receiving eptifibatide had an increased incidence of bleeding and required more blood transfusions.[75]

Certain patient populations—including women, elderly, and those with acute renal insufficiency—have an increased risk for bleeding with GP IIb/IIIa inhibitor therapy. Observations from the Can Rapid Stratification of Unstable Angina Patients Suppress Adverse Outcomes with Early Implementation of the American College of Cardiology/American Heart Association Guidelines (CRUSADE) registry demonstrated that women treated with GP IIb/IIIa inhibitors had higher rates of major bleeding compared to men (15.7% vs. 7.3%, $P < .0001$). Furthermore, when compared to men, women more frequently received excessive dosing of GP IIb/IIIa inhibitors (46.4% vs. 17.2%, $P < .0001$; adjusted OR, 3.81, 95% CI, 3.39–4.27). This excessive dosing caused more bleeding in both women and men; however, the rate of bleeding attributable to dosing was much higher in women (25.0% vs. 4.4%).[93]

Elderly patients are also at a higher risk for bleeding. Octogenarians were traditionally excluded from clinical trials assessing the efficacy of GP IIb/IIIa inhibitors but are often prescribed one of these agents in the context of high-risk ACS and/or high-risk PCI. In a retrospective analysis of 459 patients who received GP IIb/IIIa inhibitors, the risk of bleeding was increased, with vascular access and gastrointestinal tract representing the most common sites. Events were not always related to prior history of peptic ulcer disease and/or peripheral vascular disease in this patient population.[94]

Patients with renal insufficiency are also known to be at an increased risk of bleeding complications and in-hospital mortality when undergoing PCI. This bleeding risk is increased further with GP IIb/IIIa inhibitors. In 4158 patients undergoing PCI, use of abciximab showed a trend toward major bleeding in patients with renal insufficiency (OR, 1.18; $P = .06$).[95] In a smaller retrospective analysis, ACS patients with renal insufficiency who received *any* GP IIb/IIIa inhibitor had an increased risk of major bleeding ($P < .001$).[96]

The bleeding complications associated with CABG and GP IIb/IIIa inhibitor use have not been widely studied. One study examining abciximab administration prior to urgent CABG surgery demonstrated the increased need for platelet transfusions, which nearly reached statistical significance ($P = .059$). There was no increase in major blood loss or transfusions, but surgical exploration for bleeding was significantly more frequent in those who received abciximab (12% vs. 3%).[97] Short-acting GP IIb/IIIa receptor antagonists (eptifibatide and tirofiban) should be discontinued 2 to 4 hours prior to urgent CABG and abciximab should be discontinued 12 hours prior to CABG.[98]

CONCLUSIONS AND FUTURE DIRECTIONS

Acute arterial thrombosis is one of the world's primary causes of mortality today; antiplatelet agents remain the cornerstone of therapy to treat and prevent these events. Over the last 50 years, through hundreds of trials and involving over a half-million patients, the benefits of antiplatelet therapies have been identified and the risks highlighted. However, despite such extensive investigation, questions remain about mechanisms, routes of administration, dosing, combined use, and failure of therapy to prevent subsequent events. As great as past advances have been

in the application of platelet inhibitors to clinical practice, it appears that we have just begun to scratch the surface. We continue to push the envelope of higher potency with acceptable bleeding risks and have developed more rapid-acting agents for use in ACS. Agents targeting platelet receptors for novel agonists such as serotonin, collagen, and TXA_2 are in clinical testing. At the same time, our knowledge of the biology and physiology of platelets continues to expand; with it will come new agents that target as yet unidentified platelet-centered processes that contribute to atherothrombotic disease.

The full reference list for this chapter is available at ExpertConsult.com.

37

Inotropic and Vasoactive Agents

Andreia Biolo, Michael M. Givertz, Wilson S. Colucci

OUTLINE

Inotropic and vasoactive agents often play an important role in the management of hemodynamic instabilty in the intensive care setting. This chapter discusses the relevant pharmacology and clinical indications for the parenteral inotropic, vasodilator, and vasoconstrictor agents most frequently used in the cardiac intensive care unit (CICU).

These agents are used to correct or stabilize hemodynamic function; therefore in many cases their proper selection and dosing requires hemodynamic information based on a pulmonary artery catheter, an intraarterial pressure monitor, and electro-cardiographic monitoring (Table 37.1). However, the use of a pulmonary artery catheter did not show benefit either in acute decompensated heart failure patients in the Evaluation Study of Congestive Heart Failure and Pulmonary Artery Catheterization Effectiveness (ESCAPE) trial[1] or in a meta-analysis of 13 randomized trials including more than 5000 critically ill patients.[2] This lack of benefit may result from the absence of effective strategies to use in combination with pulmonary artery catheter information. These studies also demonstrated no increased mortality or hospitalization associated with pulmonary artery catheter use. Based on the available information, there is no indication for **routine** use of a pulmonary artery catheter in patients hospitalized for decompensated heart failure. Nevertheless, a pulmonary artery cathether may provide valuable information and help to guide therapy in specific conditions (e.g., patients who have respiratory distress, clinical evidence of impaired perfusion, or worsening renal function in whom the presence of congestion is unclear, and patients with no response to empiric adjustment of therapies

who may need consideration for mechanical circulatory support or transplantation).[3]

SYMPATHOMIMETIC AGENTS

Dopamine

Dopamine is the immediate precursor of epinephrine and norepinephrine. It has both cardiac and vascular sites of action, depending, in part, on the dose used[4,5] (Table 37.2). At low doses (1 to 3 µg/kg per minute), dopamine directly activates dopaminergic receptors in the kidney and splanchnic arteries, thereby causing vasodilation of these beds. The resultant increase in renal blood flow leads to increased urine output and sodium excretion. At moderate doses (3 to 8 µg/kg per minute), dopamine is a weak partial agonist of myocardial β_1-receptors and causes the release of norepinephrine from sympathetic nerve terminals in the myocardium and vasculature. The direct stimulation of myocardial β-adrenergic receptors exerts positive chronotropic and inotropic effects. The increased release of norepinephrine from nerve terminals (a tyramine-like effect) also contributes to myocardial stimulation but in addition may exert a mild vasoconstrictor effect due to stimulation of vascular α-adrenergic receptors. At high doses of dopamine (5 to 20 µg/kg per minute), the effect of peripheral α-adrenergic stimulation predominates, resulting in vasoconstriction in all vascular beds and leading to increases in mean arterial pressure and systemic vascular resistance. At high doses, the vasoconstrictor effect overshadows the dopaminergic vasodilator effects so that renal blood flow decreases

TABLE 37.1 Comparative Hemodynamic Effects of Commonly Used Positive Inotropic Agents

	+ dP/dt	PCWP	SVR	CO
Dobutamine	↑↑	↓	↓	↑
Dopamine (low dose)	↔	↔	↓	↔↑
Dopamine (high dose)	↑↑	↑	↑↑	↑↔↓
PDE III inhibitors	↑	↓↓	↓↓	↑↑
Levosimendan	↑	↓↓	↓↓	↑

CO, Cardiac output; *PDE,* phosphodiesterase; *PCWP,* pulmonary capillary wedge pressure; *SVR,* systemic vascular resistance.

TABLE 37.2 Receptor Activities of Several Sympathomimetic Agents

	MYOCARDIAL	VASCULAR		
	β_1/β_2	α_1	β_2	Dopaminergic
Dobutamine	+++	++	++	0
Dopamine (low dose)	0	0	0	+++
Dopamine (high dose)	+++	+++	0	+++
Isoproterenol	+++	0	+++	0
Norepinephrine	+++	+++	+	0

0, No activity; *+,* low activity; *++,* moderate activity; *+++,* high activity.

and urine output may decline. However, in patients with acute decompensated heart failure, the dose required for improving systemic and renal hemodynamics may be higher (on the order of 4 to 6 µg/kg per minute) than the usual "low-dose" range, leading to the suggestion that severe heart failure may impair the renal effects of dopamine.[6]

Given its varying actions, there are several potential uses for dopamine in the CICU. In patients with decompensated heart failure, dopamine may be used at low infusion rates to improve renal function by increasing renal blood flow.[7,8] However, the effects of low-dose dopamine (2 µg/kg per minute) in patients with acute heart failure and impaired renal function were recently investigated in the Renal Optimization Strategies Evaluation (ROSE) trial, and no impact on diuresis or renal function was observed.[9] Low-dose dopamine is frequently combined with one or more other inotropic (e.g., dobutamine) or vasodilator (e.g., nitroprusside) agents.[10]

In patients with severe compromise of the arterial pressure or frank cardiogenic shock, higher doses of dopamine are used to increase systemic vascular resistance. At these higher doses, the increased left ventricular afterload is partially offset by the positive inotropic action. In addition, when it is necessary to use vasoconstrictor doses of dopamine to manage systemic hypotension in the setting of myocardial failure, it is often useful to add dobutamine to augment the level of positive inotropic support beyond that provided by dopamine alone. When used alone at vasoconstrictor doses in patients with left ventricular failure, dopamine may increase both left and right heart filling pressures[11] (Fig. 37.1 and Table 37.3). This effect reflects increased left and right ventricular afterload and increased peripheral venoconstriction, the latter causing increased return of venous blood to the heart. To counteract these actions,

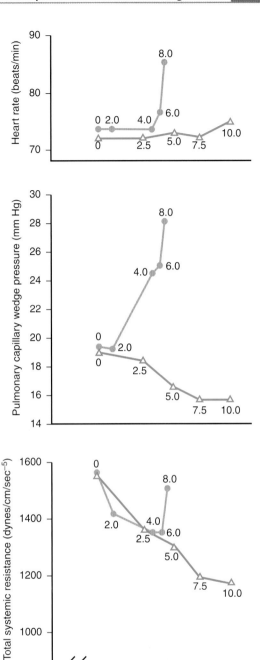

Fig. 37.1 Comparative effects of dopamine (pink) and dobutamine (blue) on heart rate, pulmonary capillary wedge pressure, and total systemic resistance in patients with moderate to severe heart failure. Each agent was titrated over the doses shown. These data illustrate that dopamine, when given alone at vasoconstrictor doses to patients with severe heart failure, increases left heart filling pressures. (Modified from Leier CV. Regional blood flow responses to vasodilators and inotropes in congestive heart failure. *Am J Cardiol.* 1988;62:86E.)

high-dose dopamine is sometimes combined with vasodilators (e.g., nitroglycerin).[12]

The inotropic responses to dopamine may be attenuated due to desensitization of the β-adrenergic pathway and depletion of myocardial catecholamine stores, both of which are common in

TABLE 37.3 **Intravenous Drug Selection in Patients With Elevated Left Heart Filling Pressures and a Reduced Cardiac Output**

Systemic Vascular Resistance	High	Normal	Low
Initial agents	Nitroprusside Nitroglycerin	Nitroprusside Milrinone Dobutamine/ nitroprusside	Dobutamine

patients with chronic severe myocardial failure.[13,14] Although generally well tolerated at low doses, higher infusion rates of dopamine may result in unwanted sinus tachycardia and/or arrhythmias (supraventricular and ventricular). Other adverse effects of dopamine include digital gangrene in patients with underlying peripheral vascular disease, tissue necrosis at sites of infiltration, and nausea at high doses. Local infiltration may be counteracted by the local injection of the α-adrenergic antagonist phentolamine.

Dobutamine

Dobutamine is a direct-acting synthetic sympathomimetic amine that stimulates β_1-, β_2-, and α-adrenergic receptors (Table 37.2). Clinically, it is available as a racemic mixture in which the (+) enantiomer is both a β_1- and β_2-adrenergic receptor agonist and an α-adrenergic receptor competitive antagonist, and the (−) enantiomer is a potent β_1-adrenergic receptor agonist and an α-adrenergic receptor partial agonist.[15,16] The net effect of this pharmacologic profile is that dobutamine causes a relatively selective stimulation of β_1-adrenergic receptors; accordingly, dobutamine's primary cardiovascular effect is to increase cardiac output by increasing myocardial contractility. This positive inotropic effect is associated with relatively little increase in heart rate. The drug causes modest decreases in left ventricular filling pressure and systemic vascular resistance due to a combination of direct vascular effects and the withdrawal of sympathetic tone[17] (Table 37.3). Dobutamine also directly improves left ventricular relaxation (positive lusitropic effect) via stimulation of myocardial β-adrenergic receptors.[18] Dobutamine has no effect on dopaminergic receptors and therefore no direct renal vasodilator effect. However, renal blood flow often increases with dobutamine in proportion to the increase in cardiac output.

Dobutamine is a valuable agent for the initial management of patients with acute or chronic systolic heart failure characterized by a low cardiac output.[19] It is often initiated at an infusion rate of 2.5 µg/kg per minute (without a loading dose) and titrated upwards by 2.5 µg/kg per minute every 15 to 30 minutes until the hemodynamic goal is reached or a dose-limiting event occurs, such as unacceptable tachycardia or arrhythmias. Maximum effects are usually achieved at a dose of 15 µg/kg per minute, although higher infusion rates may occasionally be used. In patients with more severe decompensation, and presumably greater β-adrenergic receptor down-regulation, dobutamine can be started at 5 µg/kg per minute. If the maximally tolerated infusion rate of dobutamine does not result in a sufficient increase in cardiac index, a second drug (e.g., milrinone) may be added.[10,20] In patients with elevated systemic vascular resistance and/or left heart filling pressures, the coadministration of a vasodilator such as nitroprusside or nitroglycerin may be required. In patients who remain hypotensive on dobutamine, consideration should be given to the addition of a pressor dose of dopamine and/or the use of mechanical support.

Other clinical situations in which dobutamine is effective include cardiogenic shock complicating acute myocardial infarction (MI), low cardiac output following cardiopulmonary bypass, and as a bridge to cardiac transplantation.[21] There is some evidence that intermittent infusion of dobutamine can result in sustained improvement in hemodyamics and functional status for days to weeks after the infusion is stopped.[22–24] However, there are limited clinical data to suggest that the intermittent use of dobutamine either has no effect on outcomes[25] or may increase mortality.[26]

Dobutamine may increase heart rate, thereby limiting the dose that can be infused. However, in some patients with very depressed cardiac output, the improvement in hemodynamic function may cause a withdrawal of sympathetic tone such that heart rate falls. Hypotension is uncommon, but can occur in patients who are hypovolemic. Arrhythmias, including supraventricular and ventricular tachycardia, may limit the dose. Likewise, myocardial ischemia secondary to increased myocardial oxygen consumption may occur. Some patients with chronic severe heart failure may be tolerant to dobutamine or tolerance to dobutamine may develop after several days of a continuous infusion.[27] In this situation, the addition or substitution of a phosphodiesterase inhibitor may be helpful. Hypersensitivity myocarditis has also been reported with chronic infusions of dobutamine and should be suspected if a patient develops worsening hemodynamics in association with fever or peripheral eosinophilia.

Isoproterenol

A synthetic sympathomimetic structurally related to epinephrine, isoproterenol is a nonselective β-adrenergic receptor agonist with little or no effect on α-receptors (Table 37.2). Its cardiovascular effects include increased myocardial contractility, heart rate, and atrioventricular conduction due to stimulation of myocardial β_1- and β_2-adrenergic receptors, and vasodilation of skeletal muscle and pulmonary vasculature due to stimulation of vascular β_2-adrenergic receptors. Isoproterenol increases cardiac output and lowers both systemic and pulmonary vascular resistance.

Owing to its propensity to increase heart rate, isoproterenol has relatively limited applications in the CICU. However, isoproterenol may be useful in the management of torsades de pointes that is refractory to magnesium,[28] inotropic and chronotropic support immediately following cardiac transplant,[29] and treatment of pulmonary hypertension secondary to acute pulmonary embolism.[30] Isoproterenol is usually administered as a continuous infusion at 0.5 to 5 µg/min. The dose of isoproterenol may be limited by tachycardia, increased myocardial oxygen consumption leading to ischemia, and by atrial or ventricular arrhythmias.

Epinephrine

Like isoproterenol, epinephrine stimulates β_1- and β_2-adrenergic receptors in the myocardium, thereby causing marked positive chronotropic and inotropic responses. Unlike isoproterenol, it also has potent agonist effects at vascular α-adrenergic receptors causing increased arterial and venous constriction. Because of this latter effect, epinephrine (like high-dose dopamine and norepinephrine) plays little role in the acute management of heart failure, except when complicated by severe hypotension. Epinephrine may be useful for the treatment of low cardiac output, with or without bradycardia, immediately following cardiopulmonary bypass or cardiac transplantation.[31] Continuous infusions may be started at a low dose (0.5 to 1 µg/min), and titrated upwards to 10 µg/min, as needed. The use of epinephrine may be limited by tachycardia, arrhythmias, increased myocardial oxygen consumption leading to ischemia, and oliguria from renal vasoconstriction.

In the setting of cardiac arrest, standard-dose epinephrine may be used as per the Advanced Cardiac Life Support (ACLS) protocol (1 mg intravenous push or via endotracheal tube every 3–5 minutes) to manage asystole, ventricular fibrillation, pulseless ventricular tachycardia, or electromechanical dissociation.[32] In this scenario, high-dose epinephrine (0.1 to 0.2 mg/kg) is not recommended for routine use, except for special circumstances, such as for β-blocker or calcium channel blocker overdose. Epinephrine may also be infused at 2 to 10 µg/min to manage symptomatic bradycardia that is unresponsive to atropine while awaiting placement of an external or temporary transvenous pacemaker.

Norepinephrine

The myocardial and peripheral vascular effects of this endogenous catecholamine are similar to those of epinephrine except that norepinephrine causes little stimulation of vascular β_2-adrenergic receptors and therefore causes more intense vasoconstriction (see Table 37.2). Norepinephrine may be used to provide temporary circulatory support in the setting of hypotension (e.g., following cardiac surgery or with cardiogenic shock complicating acute MI or pulmonary embolism). Norepinephrine is infused at doses of 2 to 10 µg/min. As with epinephrine, the use of norepinephrine in the CICU may be limited by arrhythmias, myocardial ischemia, renal impairment, or tissue necrosis at the site of local infiltration.

PHOSPHODIESTERASE INHIBITORS

The breakdown of adenosine 3',5'-cyclic monophosphate (cyclic AMP [cAMP]) is mediated by a membrane-bound enzyme, phosphodiesterase (PDE). In myocardium and vascular smooth muscle, the predominant isoform of this enzyme, termed type III, is inhibited by the type-III selective PDE III inhibitors amrinone and milrinone, leading to an increase in intracellular cAMP concentrations. In the myocardium, intracellular cAMP increases both contractility and the rate of relaxation (positive lusitropic effect). PDE III inhibitors are also potent vasodilators in the systemic and pulmonary vasculature.[33–35]

In patients with decompensated heart failure, type III PDE inhibitors increase cardiac output by increasing stroke volume. Balanced arterial and venous dilation causes decreases in right atrial, pulmonary artery, pulmonary capillary wedge, and mean arterial pressures. Because PDE inhibitors exert both positive inotropic and vasodilator actions, their net hemodynamic effects differ from those of dobutamine and nitroprusside. Thus, for a comparable increase in cardiac output, the PDE inhibitor milrinone decreases systemic vascular resistance and left ventricular filling pressure to a greater extent than dobutamine[36] (Fig. 37.2; also see Table 37.3). Conversely, for a comparable decrease in arterial blood pressure, milrinone increases cardiac output to a greater extent than nitroprusside[37] (Table 37.4).

PDE inhibitors are used for the treatment of heart failure characterized by low cardiac output, high filling pressures, and elevated or normal systemic vascular resistance. They may also be useful in the management of low cardiac output following cardiopulmonary bypass and as a bridge to cardiac transplant,[38] especially in patients tolerant of dobutamine. The positive inotropic effects of these drugs add to those of digoxin and may be synergistic with those of sympathomimetics such as dobutamine[39,40] (Fig. 37.3). When excess β-blocking agents have been

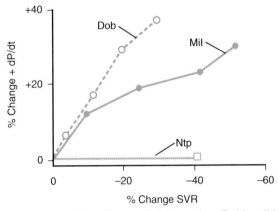

Fig. 37.2 The relative effects of dobutamine (Dob), milrinone (Mil), and nitroprusside (Ntp) on left ventricular contractility, as reflected by peak + dP/dt, and systemic vascular resistance (SVR) in patients with severe heart failure. (From Colucci WS, Wright RF, et al. Positive inotropic and vasodilator actions of milrinone in patients with severe congestive heart failure. Dose-response relationships and comparison to nitroprusside. *J Clin Invest.* 1985;75:643.)

TABLE 37.4	Comparative Hemodynamic Effects of Intravenous Vasodilators		
	PCWP	**SVR**	**CO**
Nitroprusside	↓↓	↓↓	↑
Nitroglycerin	↓↓	↔↓	↑↔↓
PDE III inhibitors	↓↓	↓↓	↑↑
Hydralazine	↓	↓↓	↔↑
ACE inhibitor	↓↓	↓↓	↑
Nesiritide	↓↓	↓↓	↑

ACE, Angiotensin-converting enzyme; *CO*, cardiac output; *PCWP*, pulmonary capillary wedge pressure; *PDE*, phosphodiesterase; *SVR*, systemic vascular resistance.

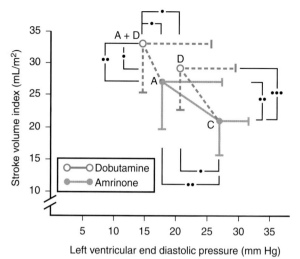

Fig. 37.3 Hemodynamic effects of dobutamine (D), amrinone (A) and the combination (A + D) in patients with moderate to severe heart failure. The additive effect of the two agents may exceed the effect of either agent alone. (Modified from Gage J, Rutman H, Lucido D, LeJemtel TH. Additive effects of dobutamine and amrinone on myocardial contractility and ventricular performance in patients with severe heart failure. *Circulation.* 1986;74:367.)

given, PDE inhibitors may be more effective than β-adrenergic stimulation for increasing cardiac output.

Inamrinone

Inamrinone (formerly amrinone) is administered as an intravenous bolus of 0.5 to 0.75 mg/kg over 2 to 3 minutes, followed by a continuous infusion at 5 to 10 µg/kg/min titrated to hemodynamic goals. The major dose-limiting effects of inamrinone are tachycardia, atrial or ventricular arrhythmias, and hypotension. The latter effect is most likely to occur in patients who are hypovolemic. Thrombocytopenia, which is seldom severe, occurs in 5% to 10% of patients. This effect is dose dependent, occurring with higher doses and/or more prolonged infusions, and appears to be owing to decreased platelet survival.[41] Other adverse effects include liver function abnormalities, fever, and nausea.

Milrinone

In patients with heart failure, milrinone is administered as a 25 to 50 µg/kg intravenous bolus over 10 minutes followed by a constant infusion at 0.25 to 0.75 µg/kg/min. If a lower dose (i.e., 25 µg/kg) is used to initiate therapy and the response is not adequate, a second bolus of 25 µg/kg may be given before increasing the infusion rate. However, milrinone is frequently started without a bolus in order to avoid an excessive lowering of blood pressure. The dose is then titrated to the lowest dose at which the desired hemodynamic effect is obtained. With this approach, up-titration should occur at intervals of no less than 2 to 4 hours. The dose of milrinone tolerated may be limited by tachycardia or arrhythmias. In addition, relatively volume-depleted patients may not tolerate its vasodilator effects and will experience hypotension that may necessitate stopping the drug. Thrombocytopenia is rarely seen with milrinone. Milrinone has

a half-life of 30 to 60 minutes in patients with heart failure. It can be used alone or in combination with other agents (e.g., dobutamine or nitroprusside).

The routine use of milrinone was assessed in the OPTIME CHF trial, a study of 949 patients admitted to the hospital with an exacerbation of heart failure. Under these circumstances, a 48-hour infusion did not reduce the subsequent need for hospitalization and was associated with an increased risk of arrhythmias and sustained hypotension.[42] It is important to note that patients requiring inotropic support (with shock or severe hypotension) were excluded from this trial. Thus, milrinone, like dobutamine, should be reserved for the short-term management of patients with symptomatic hemodynamic compromise that is not responsive to diuretics and vasodilators. In addition, the administration of milrinone for several weeks to months may be of value in the maintenance of adequate hemodynamics in end-stage patients awaiting transplantation or mechanical support.

CALCIUM-SENSITIZING AGENTS

Positive inotropic agents, such as dobutamine and milrinone, act by increasing myocyte calcium influx; therefore, they may be associated with increased arrhythmias. An alternative approach that may avoid such complications is to enhance myocardial response to a given concentration of calcium with a class of molecules referred to as "calcium sensitizers."[43] Several calcium sensitizers have been reported; most have additional effects, such as phosphodiesterase inhibition, which may contribute significantly to their clinical profile.

Levosimendan

Levosimendan, the most widely studied calcium sensitizer,[44] increases myocardial contractility by increasing myofilament sensitivity to calcium. Levosimendan is also a potent vasodilator owing to activation of adenosine triphosphate-dependent potassium channels in vascular smooth muscle cells leading to decreases in both preload and afterload. In patients with severe heart failure, levosimendan administration increases cardiac output and reduces pulmonary capillary wedge pressures and systemic vascular resistance (see Table 37.1).[45,46]

The hemodynamic effects are dose dependent at doses ranging from 0.05 to 0.6 µg/kg/min, with a higher incidence of side effects (headache, nausea, and hypotension) with doses above 0.2 µg/kg per minute.[47] Levosimendan is completely metabolized prior to excretion. Approximately 5% of a dose is converted to a highly active metabolite OR-1896 (that exhibits hemodynamic effects similar to those of levosimendan) with an elimination half-life of 75 to 80 hours (compared to 1 hour for levosimendan itself). Because of the long half-life of this active metabolite, these effects last for up to 7 to 9 days after discontinuation of a 24-hour infusion of levosimendan.[45]

Several clinical trials have evaluated the efficacy of levosimendan in patients with heart failure, both compared to placebo[48,49] or dobutamine.[50,51] It is approved for clinical use in several European and South American countries. The data from these trials suggest symptomatic benefit with levosimendan in the short term in acutely decompensated subjects but with more frequent hypotension and arrhythmias. Therefore, both the efficacy and safety of levosimendan are still uncertain in this scenario. Levosimendan has been studied and may be useful in other situations, such as the perioperative and postoperative setting, ischemic heart disease, and cardiogenic as well as septic shock.[44]

OTHER PARENTERAL INOTROPES

Digoxin

Although digoxin can be given intravenously, it is seldom used as a positive inotropic agent in the acute management of heart failure. Digoxin is often useful for the control of a rapid ventricular rate in patients with or without heart failure complicated by atrial fibrillation or atrial flutter.

VASODILATORS

For many patients with decompensated heart failure characterized by low cardiac output, high filling pressures and elevated systemic vascular resistance, a parenteral vasodilator is the initial agent of choice, either alone or in combination with an inotropic agent (see Table 37.1).

Nitroprusside

Nitroprusside is a sodium salt of ferricyanide and nitric acid. Its reduction by intracellular glutathione leads to the local production of nitric oxide, which mediates the drug's potent vasodilator effect.[52] The onset of action is rapid, in 1 to 2 minutes, making it an ideal agent for use in urgent situations that require rapid dose titration and a predictable hemodynamic effect. Nitroprusside is both an arterial and venous dilator; therefore, it reduces both filling pressures and vascular resistance (systemic and pulmonary). Stroke volume and cardiac output increase; pulmonary artery, pulmonary capillary wedge, and right atrial pressures decrease (Fig. 37.4). In patients with heart failure, heart rate is generally unchanged or may fall due to reflex sympathetic withdrawal.[53]

There are several indications for the use of nitroprusside in the CICU.[54] The most common indication is acute decompensated heart failure manifested by low cardiac output, elevated filling pressures, high systemic vascular resistance, and a systolic blood pressure adequate to maintain vital organ perfusion, usually 90 mm Hg or greater. This hemodynamic picture is often seen with acute MI, acute mitral or aortic regurgitation, and fulminant myocarditis. In acute MI, nitroprusside may be particularly useful if the infarction is complicated by significant hypertension, mitral regurgitation secondary to papillary muscle rupture, or rupture of the ventricular septum.[55] Acute valvular regurgitation secondary to endocarditis, aortic dissection, or ruptured chordae is another situation in which nitroprusside may be used effectively, often as a bridge to more definitive therapy (e.g., valve replacement or repair).[56] Nitroprusside is often used in patients with chronic heart failure due to dilated cardiomyopathy, both to manage acute decompensation and to determine whether pulmonary hypertension is reversible during the evaluation for cardiac transplantation.[57,58] Nitroprusside is often the parenteral agent of choice for treating hypertensive

emergencies.[59] A recent study showed increased cardiac output with nitroprusside administration in patients with severe aortic stenosis and left ventricular dysfunction presenting with severe heart failure, suggesting that it may be useful in this context as a bridge to aortic valve replacement or oral vasodilators.[60]

The infusion of nitroprusside should be guided by close hemodynamic monitoring, ideally with a pulmonary artery catheter and arterial line. Nitroprusside may be started at a rate of 10 to 20 µg/min and increased by 20 µg/min every 5 to 15 minutes until the hemodynamic goal is achieved (e.g., a systemic vascular resistance of 1000 to 1200 dynes/sec/cm^5 and a pulmonary capillary wedge pressure of 16–18 mm Hg) while maintaining an adequate systolic blood pressure (generally ≥80 mm Hg). Doses of 300 µg/min or higher are seldom required and increase the risk of toxicity.

Nitroprusside is a potent vasodilator and its use may be limited by hypotension. In patients with underlying coronary artery disease, drug-induced hypotension accompanied by reflex tachycardia may worsen myocardial ischemia. In patients with decompensated heart failure, hemodynamic deterioration may occur following the withdrawal of nitroprusside, apparently due to a transient "rebound" increase in systemic vascular tone.[61] Other adverse effects of nitroprusside are due to the accumulation of its metabolites, cyanide and thiocyanate.[62] The accumulation of cyanide results in lactic acidosis and methemoglobinemia and may manifest itself as nausea, restlessness, and dysphoria. Cyanide toxicity is most likely to occur in patients with liver dysfunction or following prolonged infusions but may occur even in patients with normal hepatic function who have received the drug for only a few hours. If cyanide toxicity is suspected, serum levels should be drawn and the infusion stopped. In severe cases, treatment with sodium nitrate, sodium thiosulfate, or vitamin B$_{12}$ may be necessary. Cyanide is converted in the liver to thiocyanate, which is cleared by the kidney. The half-life of elimination of thiocyanate is 3 to 7 days. Thiocyanate toxicity generally occurs gradually and is manifested by nausea, confusion, weakness, tremor, hyperreflexia, and, rarely, coma. Thiocyanate toxicity is more likely to occur in patients with renal insufficiency and with prolonged infusions or high rates of infusion. If mild, it can be managed by cessation of the drug; in severe cases, hemodialysis may be necessary.

Nitroglycerin

When administered parenterally, nitroglycerin has an immediate onset of action and a plasma half-life of 1 to 4 minutes. It is cleared by vascular endothelium, hydrolyzed in the blood, and metabolized in the liver. At lower infusion rates, its main cardiovascular effect is venodilation, with a resultant fall in ventricular volumes and filling pressures. At higher infusion rates, nitroglycerin also causes arterial dilation, resulting in decreases in both pulmonary and systemic vascular resistances[53] (see Table 37.4).

Nitroglycerin plays several important roles in the CICU.[54] In the setting of cardiogenic pulmonary edema, especially when due to myocardial ischemia or MI, nitroglycerin provides immediate symptomatic relief and improves both hemodynamics and oxygen saturation.[63] By causing direct coronary vasodilation, nitroglycerin also has the theoretical advantage of improving myocardial

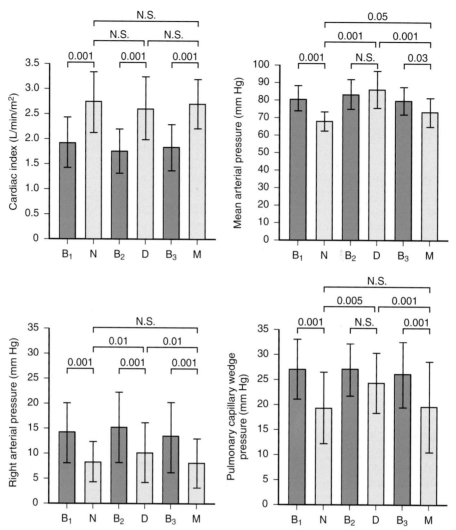

Fig. 37.4 Shown are the comparative effects of nitroprusside (N), dobutamine (D), and milrinone (M) on cardiac index, mean arterial pressure, right atrial pressure, and pulmonary capillary wedge pressure in patients with severe heart failure. The agents were administered in doses that caused comparable increases in cardiac index. Under these conditions, nitroprusside and milrinone significantly reduced mean arterial pressure, but dobutamine had no effect. All three agents reduced right atrial pressure, although the effect of dobutamine was less pronounced. Both nitroprusside and milrinone significantly reduced pulmonary capillary wedge pressure; this effect was significantly more pronounced than the effect of dobutamine. (Modified from Monrad ES, Baim DS, Smith HS, et al. Milrinone, dobutamine, and nitroprusside: comparative effects on hemodynamics and myocardial energetics in patients with severe congestive heart failure. *Circulation.* 1986;73:III168.)

perfusion and limiting infarct size.[64] Intravenous nitroglycerin is often useful in the management of patients with new-onset heart failure or acute decompensation of chronic heart failure, particularly in patients who are refractory to diuretic therapy and continue to manifest elevated right- and left-sided filling pressures, in patients with disproportionate right-sided failure, and in patients in whom nitroprusside is not tolerated.

Intravenous nitroglycerin is usually started at a low infusion rate of 20 to 30 μg/min, and increased by 10 to 20 μg/min every 5 to 10 minutes until the desired response is observed or a dose of 400 μg/min is reached. In patients with decompensated heart failure, upward titration should be guided by filling pressures

and systemic vascular resistance. While awaiting intravenous access, nitroglycerin can be administered by the sublingual, buccal, or transdermal route.

Use of nitroglycerin may be limited by hypotension, which may require discontinuation of the drug and/or supportive care with intravenous fluids and leg elevation. Other common side effects related to vasodilation include headache, flushing, and diaphoresis. Some patients with heart failure will not respond to the acute administration of nitroglycerin.[65] This resistance is usually seen in patients with significant right-sided failure and peripheral edema and often resolves following diuresis.[66] In addition, patients may develop pharmacologic tolerance to nitroglycerin. Strategies to prevent the development of such tolerance include avoidance of excessive dosing, limiting fluid retention, and the use of intermittent dosing.[67,68]

Nesiritide

Nesiritide (recombinant human brain natriuretic peptide [BNP 1-32]) is identical to and mimics the actions of the endogenous BNP molecule. Clinical studies with intravenous infusion of nesiritide in patients with decompensated heart failure have shown that it exerts potent dose-related vasodilation that is rapid in onset and sustained for the duration of drug infusion.[69] Balanced arterial and venous vasodilation is reflected by decreases in systemic vascular resistance, systemic arterial pressure, pulmonary capillary wedge pressure, and right atrial pressure. Vasodilation occurs without a change in heart rate and is associated with increases in stroke volume and cardiac output.

Administration of nesiritide in the short-term treatment of acute decompensated heart failure resulted in a dose-dependent reduction in pulmonary capillary wedge pressure and improved clinical status compared to placebo.[70] When compared to standard vasoactive agents, nesiritide produced a similar improvement in clinical status and dyspnea. In another randomized trial, nesiritide reduced pulmonary capillary wedge pressure significantly more than nitroglycerin but with a similar improvement in dyspnea and clinical status.[69] However, the largest randomized controlled trial, Acute Study of Clinical Effectiveness of Nesiritide in Decompensated Heart Failure (ASCEND-HF), found that nesiritide only slightly reduced dyspnea, had no effect on death or rehospitalization rates, and significantly increased episodes of hypotension.[71] Similar results were obtained in the smaller Reevaluation of Systemic Early Neuromuscular Blockade (ROSE trial), in which low-dose nesiritide (0.005 µg/kg/min without bolus for 72 hours) had no significant effect on 72-hour cumulative urine volume or symptoms compared to placebo in patients with acute heart failure.[9] When compared to dobutamine, nesiritide appears to be less likely to cause ventricular arrhythmias and may be associated with clinical benefit (reduced 6-month mortality and a trend toward lower heart failure readmission).[72,73]

Nesiritide is given as an initial intravenous bolus of 2 µg/kg, followed by a continuous infusion of 0.01 µg/kg per minute. The dose is increased (usually by 0.005 µg/kg per minute, preceded by a bolus of 1 µg/kg) if there is no therapeutic response, after 3 to 24 hours, up to a maximum of 0.03 µg/kg/min. The main adverse effect is dose-related hypotension. If this occurs, the infusion should be discontinued and restarted when the blood pressure has stabilized, at a 30% lower dose without a repeat bolus.

There has been concern about the possible effects of nesiritide on survival and renal function. Randomized trials and meta-analyses have yielded conflicting results on 30-day mortality and worsening renal function among patients treated with nesiritide.[74-76] However, the largest study (ASCEND-HF) did not confirm those findings.[71]

In summary, nesiritide seems to increase rates of hypotension, does not alter rates of death or rehospitalization at 30 days, and shows a borderline significant trend toward reducing dyspnea, with no significant impact on renal function. Its use is reserved for carefully selected patients with severe acute decompensated heart failure who remain dyspneic despite adequate therapy and who are not hypotensive or in cardiogenic shock.

Hydralazine

Hydralazine is a potent direct-acting arteriolar smooth muscle dilator that causes both pulmonary and systemic vasodilation. While nitroprusside and nitroglycerin are generally preferred as parenteral vasodilators in the acute management of heart failure, there are specific situations in which hydralazine given intravenously may be a useful or necessary alternative. In particular, hydralazine may be useful in patients who have become toxic with nitroprusside or continue to have an elevated systemic vascular resistance despite the use of a maximally tolerated dose of nitroprusside or nitroglycerin. In addition, hydralazine may be safely administered to pregnant patients with heart failure[77] or severe hypertension.[78,79]

When used parenterally, hydralazine should be started at a low dose (5 mg given as an intravenous bolus every 4 to 6 hours), and increased gradually up to 25 to 30 mg, as tolerated. The onset of action is rapid and the magnitude of the hemodynamic effects may be unpredictable. Blood pressure should therefore be monitored with an intraarterial line. Nausea may be a limiting side effect in the acute setting.

Enalaprilat

Enalapril, a commonly used oral angiotensin-converting enzyme (ACE) inhibitor, is cleaved by plasma and tissue esterases to form enalaprilat, the active form of the drug. When given parenterally, enalaprilat acts as a balanced vasodilator, resulting in decreased right and left heart filling pressures.[80] Enalaprilat is given as an intravenous bolus (0.625 to 1.25 mg every 6 hours). Although the onset of action is rapid (minutes), the duration of effect is prolonged (several hours). The major adverse effect is hypotension, which is more commonly seen in patients who are volume depleted.

Enalaprilat may be of value in the treatment of acute decompensation in patients with chronic heart failure.[81] However, owing to the somewhat unpredictable magnitude of the response and its prolonged duration of action, enalaprilat is not a first-line agent for the treatment of patients with MI or new-onset heart failure.

The full reference list for this chapter is available at ExpertConsult.com.

38

Intensive Diuresis and Ultrafiltration

Marlies Ostermann, Claudio Ronco

Fluid overload has been recognized as a serious complication of cardiac disease. It is associated with an increased risk of respiratory failure, prolonged need for mechanical ventilation, the development of acute kidney injury (AKI), a longer stay in the hospital, and increased mortality rate.[1–5] Patients with chronic kidney disease (CKD) and heart disease are particularly at risk.

Congestive heart failure (CHF) is a common reason for hospitalization. Furthermore, 25% of patients with CHF are readmitted within 30 days.[2] The treatment options are limited and include diuretics and ultrafiltration, together with correction of any precipitating factors. Management can be challenging, especially in patients with hemodynamic instability. The aim of this chapter is to review the role of commonly used diuretics and ultrafiltration strategies and to outline remaining gaps in knowledge.

DIURETICS

Types of Diuretics and Physiologic Efficacy

Diuretics can be classified in terms of their site of action and behavior along the nephron (Table 38.1). With the exception of spironolactone and mannitol, diuretics are protein bound. They act from within the tubular lumen. Loop diuretics are transported from the plasma into the proximal tubular cells via organic anion transporters. From there, they are secreted into the luminal space. The quantity that enters the tubule depends on the intrinsic secretory capacity of the proximal tubule as well as the presence of other substances that also depend on cellular uptake via organic anion transporters, such as urea nitrogen and certain drugs. Loop diuretics selectively block the $Na^+/K^+/Cl^{2-}$ cotransporter in the luminal membrane of the ascending loop of Henle and generate greater water loss than sodium loss, resulting in the production of hypotonic urine.

Patients with an estimated glomerular filtration rate (GFR) of approximately 15 mL/min/1.73 m^2 secrete only 10% to 20% of the amount of loop diuretic secreted by patients with a normal GFR receiving the same dose. As a result, higher doses are needed to elicit a similar diuretic response. In addition, in patients with a reduced GFR, the filtered load of extracellular fluid and sodium is lower, which limits the maximum achievable response to any further diuretic.

Other factors that influence drug availability in the tubular lumen and diuretic response include the actual dose administered, absolute bioavailability (for orally administered drugs), renal blood flow, and the presence of competing drugs and metabolites.

INDICATIONS FOR INTENSIVE DIURESIS

Decompensated Congestive Heart Failure

Volume overload and abnormal fluid distribution are defining features in decompensated CHF and the main reason for hospital admission and readmission. Loop diuretics are administered in up to 90% of patients hospitalized for CHF. A Cochrane review

TABLE 38.1	Characteristics of Commonly Used Diuretics in Fluid Overload			
Type of Diuretic	Site of Action	Physiologic Effect	Most Common Indications Related to Fluid Accumulation	Most Important Side Effects
Loop diuretics (furosemide, bumetanide)	Thick ascending limb of loop of Henle	Blockade of $Na^+/K^+/Cl^-$ cotransport system leads to inhibition of Na^+ reabsorption	AKI CKD CHF Chronic liver disease	Otoxicity Hyperuricemia Electrolyte disorders Drug hypersensitivity
Thiazides (bendrofluazide, hydrochlorothiazide) Metolazone	Distal tubule; metolazone also acts on the loop of Henle	Blockade of Na^+/Cl^- transport system leads to inhibition of Na^+ reabsorption	CKD	Hyperglycemia Drug hypersensitivity Cholestatic jaundice Hepatitis Agranulocytosis
Aldosterone antagonists (spironolactone)	Aldosterone receptors in the distal tubule	Blockade of Na^+ retaining action of aldosterone	Chronic liver disease CHF	Gynecomastia Gastrointestinal side effects Drug hypersensitivity Agranulocytosis
Osmotic agents (mannitol)	Active in whole nephron following glomerular filtration	Reduced passive reabsorption of water	Cerebral edema	Skin necrosis (in case of extravasation) Renal failure Seizures
Potassium-sparing diuretics (amiloride, triamterene)	Late portion of the distal tubule and cortical collecting duct	Inhibition of K^+ secretion	To minimize K^+ loss during treatment with loop diuretics or thiazides	Hyperkalemia
ANP/BNP (nesiritide)	Afferent and efferent glomerular arterioles	Increase in GFR by dilation of afferent glomerular arteries and constriction of efferent arteries	Acute heart failure	Renal failure Skin necrosis (in case of extravasation)

AKI, Acute kidney injury; *ANP*, atrial natriuretic peptide; *BNP*, B-type natriuretic peptide; *CHF*, congestive heart failure; *CKD*, chronic kidney disease; *GFR*, glomerular filtration rate.

concluded that, based on 14 controlled studies ($n = 525$ patients), there was evidence that conventional diuretics in CHF reduced the risk of worsening heart failure and death when compared to placebo.[6] Diuretic use was also associated with a 28% to 33% increase in exercise tolerance compared to other drugs. However, it was noted that diuretic prescriptions were not standardized and most studies were small with a follow-up period of only 4 to 24 weeks. In addition, diuretics have well-known side effects (see Table 38.1). Although they may induce a decrease in ventricular filling and fall in cardiac output, this is usually not clinically important unless patients are overdiuresed. The margin of safety of aggressive diuresis is determined by the amount of extravascular edema and the Starling curve of the individual patient. Patients with predominantly diastolic dysfunction are at greater risk of overdiuresis than patients with severe systolic dysfunction.

Acute Decompensated Heart Failure

The management of fluid overload in acute decompensated heart failure is a clinical challenge due to the lack of consistent data from randomized controlled trials and the resulting lack of formal evidence-based treatment guidelines.[7] For decades, intravenous loop diuretics formed the mainstay of therapy to reduce congestion and decrease ventricular filling pressures. However, many patients with acute heart failure are not substantially volume overloaded despite the presence of pulmonary or peripheral

edema.[8,9] In this case, removing too much volume may reduce the necessary preload and may actually be harmful.

There are other potential risks with administering loop diuretics in this situation, including the risk of neurohormonal activation, hypovolemia and systemic vasoconstriction, electrolyte disturbances, and deterioration of renal function. For these reasons, aggressive diuresis should be avoided unless there is clear evidence of intravascular fluid overload.

Chronic Kidney Disease

There are complex interactions between cardiac and renal function and a large proportion of patients with CHF also suffer from CKD.[10,11] In advanced CKD, urine output may be reduced and patients often (but not always) develop progressive sodium and water retention. Loop diuretics are the preferred diuretics. Thiazides (with the exception of metolazone) cease to be effective when the estimated GFR falls to below 30 mL/min/1.73 m². Metolazone remains active in patients with a low GFR. As renal function deteriorates further and patients respond less well, renal replacement therapy (RRT) may be the only option to remove fluid.

Chronic Liver Disease

Chronic liver congestion and ascites are common features in patients with advanced CHF. For large-volume ascites, there are two therapeutic strategies: paracentesis and administration of diuretics at increasing doses until an adequate amount of ascitic fluid has been removed. Randomized trials comparing both approaches support paracentesis as the method of choice.[12] Although there is no difference with respect to long-term mortality, large-volume paracentesis is faster, more effective, and associated with fewer adverse events than diuretic therapy. However, regardless of the strategy used, diuretics should be included in the maintenance therapy to prevent or delay recurrence of ascites.

DIURETIC RESISTANCE AND MEDICAL MANAGEMENT OF REFRACTORY EDEMA

Diuretic resistance is a major problem as heart failure progresses and renal function deteriorates. Affected patients remain symptomatic and often need escalating doses of diuretics or combination therapies[13,14] (Table 38.2). The significance of diuretic resistance is substantiated by data from large national registries showing that approximately 40% of hospitalized heart failure patients are discharged with unresolved congestion.[15,16] Furthermore, their risk of dying is increased and they have a 3-fold increase in rehospitalization.

Combination of Diuretics

The combination of alternative classes of diuretics creates a state of "sequential nephron blockade" in which multiple sites of sodium reabsorption are inhibited.[13] Combinations of diuretics also reduce the risk of side effects from a single drug given at high dose.

Thiazides and metolazone are often combined with loop diuretics. They inhibit sodium reabsorption in the distal convoluted tubule and thus can counteract compensatory distal tubular hypertrophy induced by loop diuretics. Although the

combination can be effective in maintaining an acceptable fluid balance, there are few data to suggest any mortality or morbidity benefit.

The Safety and Efficacy of the Combination of Loop With Thiazide-type Diuretics in Patients with Decompensated Heart Failure (CLOROTIC) study is an ongoing randomized placebo-controlled trial that aims to explore whether the addition of hydrochlorothiazide to a furosemide regimen is a safe and effective strategy to improve diuretic resistance and symptoms resulting from heart failure.[17]

The Randomized Aldactone Evaluation (RALES) trial showed that in patients with CHF, spironolactone (25 to 50 mg daily) in combination with an angiotensin-converting enzyme inhibitor and a loop diuretic with or without digoxin was associated with a significantly reduced mortality at 24 months and significant reduction in hospitalization for heart failure.[18]

Intravenous Bolus Versus Continuous Infusion Therapy

There is some evidence that loop diuretics given as a continuous infusion are more effective than intermittent boluses, but the data are not consistent. In a randomized crossover study comparing bumetanide boluses with a continuous infusion in volunteers with CKD (mean estimated GFR 17 mL/min/1.73 m^2), a greater net sodium excretion was observed during continuous infusion than with regular bolus administration despite comparable total 14-hour drug excretion.[19]

A randomized controlled trial comparing furosemide infusion versus bolus administration in 59 critically ill patients with fluid overload showed that patients in the bolus group needed a significantly higher total dose of furosemide to achieve target diuresis.[20] Mean urine output per dose of furosemide was significantly higher in the infusion group, but there was no difference in hospital mortality, number of patients requiring ventilatory support, change in serum creatinine, or change in estimated GFR. The Diuretic Optimization Strategies Evaluation (DOSE) trial found no benefit of continuous-infusion furosemide compared to the same dose given intermittently in patient symptoms or change in renal function.[20a] However, the median furosemide infusion dose was only 6.7 mg/h. Superior diuresis has been found when a loading dose followed by higher infusion doses are used.[20b] Based on these data, it appears that diuresis is easier to achieve with a continuous infusion of high-dose (20 to 40 mg/h) furosemide and the risk of toxicity appears to be reduced compared to high-dose intermittent bolus therapy.[20c]

Combination With Albumin

Severe hypoalbuminemia can contribute to diuretic resistance.[14] There are several potential explanations. First, albumin is considered to be necessary to deliver furosemide via renal blood flow to the proximal tubules, where it is secreted into the tubular lumen. In the case of hypoalbuminemia, the amount of diuretic delivered to the tubule is reduced. Second, hypoalbuminemia reduces the intravascular volume available for removal. Third, in patients with significant proteinuria, diuretics bind to albumin in the tubular fluid so that less active drug is available to interact with the tubular receptor.

TABLE 38.2   Mechanisms of Diuretic Resistance and Management Strategies

Mechanisms of Diuretic Resistance	Therapeutic Strategies
Variable enteral absorption due to gut edema	Change from oral to intravenous administration
Worsening CKD	Increased doses of diuretics
Acute deterioration of renal function (owing to nephrotoxic exposure)	Discontinuation of nephrotoxins
Hypoalbuminemia	Correction of hypoalbuminemia
Severe proteinuria (binding of active diuretic within the tubular lumen)	Treatment of the underlying renal disease
Loop diuretic–induced compensatory distal tubular hypertrophy	Combination diuretic therapy
Co-administration of drugs that enhance fluid retention (fludrocortisone, minoxidil)	Discontinuation of competing drugs
Co-administration of drugs with high [Na$^+$] (saline, piperacillin)	Discontinuation of competing drugs
Reduced cardiac output	Inotropic support
Intraabdominal hypertension	Measures to reduce intraabdominal pressure

CKD, Chronic kidney disease.

The role of albumin supplementation to overcome these problems remains unclear. In a study including patients with cirrhosis and ascites, the administration of premixed loop diuretic and albumin (40 mg of furosemide and 25 g of albumin premixed versus 40 mg of furosemide) did not enhance the natriuretic response.[21] In contrast, a randomized controlled crossover study in 24 patients with CKD and hypoalbuminemia showed significant differences in urine output between treatment with furosemide alone and furosemide and albumin.[22] However, at 24 hours, there were no longer any significant differences.

ULTRAFILTRATION

Rationale for Mechanical Fluid Removal

Ultrafiltration (UF) involves the removal of an iso-osmotic solution of plasma water and electrolytes from whole blood across a semipermeable membrane. During UF, the circulating blood volume is maintained by recruitment of interstitial fluid into the intravascular space (plasma refilling). The plasma refilling rate varies among patients and is dependent on the serum oncotic pressure and capillary permeability. Ideally, UF and plasma refilling should occur at a similar rate to prevent hemodynamic instability. When the rate of removal of plasma water exceeds the refilling capacity, hypotension develops. The ultrafiltrate is isotonic and consists of water and nonprotein-bound small and middle molecular weight solutes, in contrast to diuretic-induced urine, which is hypotonic.

Options for Ultrafiltration

Techniques to remove fluid mechanically include isolated UF and RRT with hemodialysis, hemofiltration, or peritoneal dialysis[23] (Table 38.3). UF involves the removal of an iso-osmotic solution of plasma water and electrolytes, whereas RRT also provides clearance of metabolic and uremic solutes. Both techniques can be applied intermittently and continuously. Fluid removal is better tolerated when conducted with lower UF rates over longer periods.

Benefits of Ultrafiltration

Compared with diuretic therapy, fluid removal by extracorporeal techniques is fully controllable and adjustable. It is a strategy to reset fluid status to euvolemia (Fig. 38.1). In addition, the fluid removed with extracorporeal techniques is isotonic, whereas urine produced following diuretic administration is usually hypotonic. In patients with acute decompensated heart failure, the average urinary sodium concentration after furosemide administration is 60 mmol/L, leaving behind 80 mmol of excess sodium for every liter of urine output.[24] This, combined with neurohormonal activation, may explain why the initial weight loss after diuretics is rapidly negated.[25] By restoring euvolemia and removing sodium, UF may be successful at restoring diuretic responsiveness. Finally, in patients with fluid overload and absent kidney function, mechanical fluid removal is the only option.

Peritoneal dialysis is an alternative mode of fluid removal.[26,27] With peritoneal dialysis, water and solutes are removed via the peritoneal membrane driven by an osmotic gradient between the dialysate solution in the peritoneal cavity and the capillary blood. The fluid removed is isotonic to plasma fluid. Peritoneal dialysis allows individualized fluid removal and solute clearance, as determined by the patient's needs. Compared to intermittent hemodialysis, it is associated with less hemodynamic instability and myocardial stress.[26]

Several observational studies have confirmed the role of peritoneal dialysis for patients with CHF, in particular for those with associated CKD and refractory heart failure.[26,27] Other studies

---

TABLE 38.3 Options for Mechanical Fluid Removal

Modality	Blood Flow Rate (mL/min)	Fluid Removal Rate (mL/h)	Advantages	Disadvantages
SCUF	50–100	0–300	Slower and more sustained fluid removal	Immobilization
Intermittent UF	250–400	0–2000	Shorter procedure than continuous UF Anticoagulation not essential	Higher risk of hemodynamic instability
CRRT	50–100	0–300	Provision of UF and solute clearance Slower and more sustained fluid removal Less hemodynamic instability during fluid removal Adjustment of fluid removal to patient's needs at any time Requires some form of anticoagulation	Immobilization
IRRT	250–400	0–2000	Provision of UF and solute clearance Anticoagulation not essential	Higher risk of hemodynamic instability with fluid removal Fluctuating fluid balance Metabolic fluctuations
Peritoneal dialysis	Not applicable	0–500	UF and solute clearance No need for venous access Reduced risk of hemodynamic instability No need for anticoagulation	Need for peritoneal catheter Contraindicated in patients immediately after abdominal surgery Special expertise required

CRRT, Continuous renal replacement therapy; *IRRT,* intermittent renal replacement therapy; *SCUF,* slow continuous ultrafiltration; *UF,* ultrafiltration.
Modified from Rosner MH, Ostermann M, Murugan R, et al. Indications and management of mechanical fluid removal in critical illness. *Br J Anaesth.* 2014;113(5):764–71.

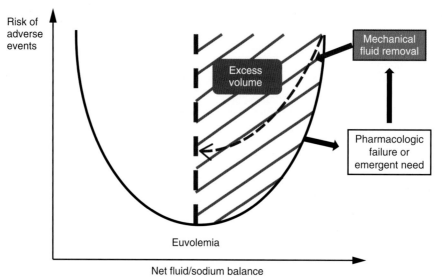

Fig. 38.1 Management of fluid overload during critical illness.

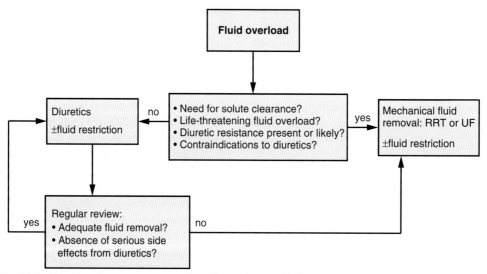

Fig. 38.2 Algorithm for management of cardiac patients with fluid overload. *RRT,* Renal replacement therapy; *UF,* ultrafiltration.

have demonstrated a slower decline in renal function with peritoneal dialysis compared to intermittent hemodialysis.[28,29] However, randomized controlled studies directly comparing peritoneal dialysis and diuretic therapy in CHF are lacking.

Indications for Mechanical Fluid Removal

The indications for mechanical fluid removal depend predominantly on the impact that fluid overload has on the patient, the apparent and expected trajectories, the likelihood of successful fluid removal with pharmacologic measures, and the risk of serious side effects from diuretics (Fig. 38.2).

The Acute Disease Quality Initiative (ADQI) expert group[23] suggested the following indications for mechanical fluid removal:

- Fluid overload after pharmacologic failure, that is, patients with fluid overload who have not responded adequately to diuretics
- Presence of serious adverse effects of diuretics, that is, patients with fluid overload who need to discontinue diuretics

- High chance of diuretic failure, that is, patients with fluid overload and significantly impaired renal function in whom treatment with diuretics is unlikely to be effective in a timely manner and in whom the risk of prolonged and progressive fluid overload is high
- Combined fluid overload and solute accumulation, that is, patients who need both fluid removal and solute clearance

In cases of localized fluid accumulation in a confined compartment, such as isolated pleural effusions or large-volume ascites, UF is less likely to be effective and fluid removal by direct drainage should be considered.

CLINICAL STUDIES

Several clinical trials have been conducted using continuous or intermittent UF in patients with CHF with mixed results[30-41] (Table 38.4). In the Ultrafiltration versus Intravenous Diuretics for Patients Hospitalized for Acute Decompensated Heart Failure

TABLE 38.4 Recent Randomized Controlled Trials on the Use of Mechanical Fluid Removal in Patients With Congestive Heart Failure

Study	Patients	Treatment Groups	Ultrafiltration Protocol	Main Results
RAPID-CHF, Bart et al., 2005[31]	40 patients with CHF and FO	Early single 8-hour UF vs. standard care	Fluid removal rate at discretion of clinical team	Significantly greater fluid removal with UF No significant difference in renal function
UNLOAD, Costanzo et al., 2007[32]	200 patients with CHF and FO	Single session of UF within first 24 hours of admission vs. IV diuretics	Duration and rate at discretion of clinical team	Significantly greater fluid removal with UF Lower hospitalization rate at 90 days in UF group No significant difference in renal function
UNLOAD substudy, Rogers et al., 2008[35]	19 patients with CHF, FO, and EF <40%	As per UNLOAD protocol	As per UNLOAD protocol	No difference in total fluid removal No significant difference in change of GFR
ULTRADISCO, Giglioli et al., 2011[38]	30 patients with decompensated HF	Slow, continuous UF vs. furosemide infusion	Duration and UF rate as guided by hemodynamic monitoring using pressure recording analytical method	Significantly greater weight loss with UF Improvement in cardiac index and stroke volume in UF group No significant difference in renal function
Hanna et al., 2012[39]	36 patients with advanced HF	UF vs. conventional diuretic Rx	Fixed UF rate at 400 mL/h for first 6 hours and 200 mL/h thereafter	Faster and greater fluid removal in UF group Shorter hospital stay in UF group No change in hospital readmission rate No significant difference in renal function
CARESS-HF, Bart et al., 2012[33]	188 patients with decompensated HF and worsened renal function	UF vs. stepped diuretic algorithm	Fixed UF rate at 200 mL/h Use of vasoactive drugs was prohibited (except as rescue Rx)	No difference in weight loss between groups No difference in 60-day hospitalization More adverse events in UF group Significant rise in serum creatinine in UF group
CUORE, Marenzi et al., 2014[36]	56 patients with CHF	UF as first-line treatment versus standard medical Rx	Duration and rate of UF at discretion of clinical team	No difference in weight reduction at discharge Lower 1-year rehospitalization rate in UF group No significant difference in renal function
AVOID-HF, Constanzo et al., 2016[37]	224 patients with HF (terminated early)	UF vs. intravenous loop diuretics	Adjustable UF rate	Greater fluid removal and total fluid loss in UF group Lower 30-day hospitalization rate in UF group Significantly more adverse events in UF group

CHF, Congestive heart failure; *EF*, ejection fraction; *FO*, fluid overload; *GFR*, glomerular filtration rate; *HF*, heart failure; *Rx*, therapy; *UF*, ultrafiltration.

(UNLOAD) trial and the Relief for Acutely Fluid-Overloaded Patients With Decompensated Congestive Heart Failure (RAPID-CHF) trial, UF was associated with significantly greater fluid removal than diuretic therapy[31,32] (see Table 38.4). In contrast, in the Cardiorenal Rescue Study in Decompensated Heart Failure (CARRESS-HF) trial, weight loss was similar in the UF and medical management groups.[33] However, patients included in this study had worse baseline renal function and received a more intensive diuretic regimen compared to the previous studies.

The reported effects of mechanical fluid removal on renal function also vary.[33,35,36] Some studies have demonstrated improved renal function that could be explained by better cardiac performance and relief of renal congestion. In contrast, a substudy of the UNLOAD trial showed no difference in the change in GFR of both groups (3.4 and 3.6 mL/min, respectively)[35] and the CARRESS-HF trial was terminated early due to a higher incidence of renal dysfunction in the UF group.[33] These discrepancies in reported renal effects may be attributable to differences in the rate of fluid removal and potential imbalance between UF rate and vascular refill capability together with variations in the medical management of heart failure. More recently, attempts have been made to correct for this variability. In the Continuous Ultrafiltration for Congestive Heart Failure (CUORE) study,

patients with severe acutely decompensated heart failure were randomized to standard medical therapy versus UF.[36] In patients randomized to UF, hematocrit was continuously monitored and the rate of fluid removal was adjusted accordingly. There was no significant difference in serum creatinine levels between both groups.

Finally, the large-scale Aquapheresis Versus Intravenous Diuretics and Hospitalization for Heart Failure (AVOID-HF) trial compared UF and medical treatment in acute heart failure and used adjustable, rather than fixed, treatment regimens in both arms.[37] The study was terminated early after enrollment of 224 patients. At 30 days, the UF group had fewer heart failure and cardiovascular events. There was no difference in renal function between both groups from 24 hours after initiation of treatment to 90 days after randomization. However, significantly more UF patients experienced an adverse effect or a serious adverse event, including bleeding and infections. Ultimately, a decision was made to terminate the trial due to safety concerns and slower-than-projected enrollment.

Despite differences in patient selection, study design, and UF protocol, existing studies confirmed that treatment with UF relieves signs and symptoms of congestion and can improve quality of life. Some studies also demonstrated decreased length of stay in the hospital and reduced 90-day readmission rate, but a mortality benefit with UF has not been established. In addition, some studies clearly demonstrated that UF can have serious adverse effects if applied without adjustment to the characteristics of the individual patient and that patients undergoing mechanical UF need to be monitored closely.

ONGOING LIMITATIONS

Providing optimal care to patients with acute decompensated CHF is challenging, especially owing to limited therapies available and important gaps in knowledge. A major limitation relates to the correct assessment of fluid status, which even experienced clinicians find difficult.[42] Clinical signs—such as central venous pressure, skin turgor, and peripheral edema—are often used as surrogate markers, but they lack sensitivity and specificity. It has been clearly shown that patients with CHF without any symptoms and no clinically recognized volume overload were, in fact, hypervolemic.[43]

The optimal diuretic regimen for patients with CHF is not known. Similarly, the optimal practice of applying UF remains uncertain, including patient selection, timing, mode of UF, rate of UF, method of monitoring, and duration of treatment. Further studies are urgently required to fill these gaps in knowledge.

Techniques are available to monitor the effects of fluid removal, including online-hematocrit recording, relative blood volume monitoring, bioimpedance spectroscopy, and biomarkers. Online monitoring of hematocrit in the withdrawal line detects changes in hematocrit as a result of an imbalance between fluid removal and vascular refill. These devices can be programmed so that fluid removal is terminated if the increase in hematocrit exceeds the threshold set by the treating clinician and resumed when the hematocrit falls below the prespecified limit. Despite improved technologies, none of the available monitoring devices have been sufficiently evaluated to know if they reliably predict the adequacy of fluid removal and prevent the development of hypotension.

USE OF ULTRAFILTRATION IN CLINICAL PRACTICE

Current European and North American practice guidelines suggest that UF should be offered only under experienced supervision.[44,45] In this case, the UF prescription should include the method (UF or RRT, intermittent vs. continuous, with or without diuretics), target fluid balance, and endpoints detailing when to stop fluid removal.[23] The UF rate should not exceed 250 mL/h and should be adjusted regularly. If solute clearance is required and RRT is necessary, the dose needs to be specified.

During UF, the target fluid removal rate should be adjusted regularly as guided by the patient's effective circulating volume and capability to refill the vasculature from the extravascular compartments to avoid hemodynamic instability.

Diuretics may be added to extracorporeal fluid removal, especially when using intermittent UF techniques and sufficient renal function is maintained. This combination ensures some control of fluid balance while the extracorporeal therapy is not operative.

FUTURE OF EXTRACORPOREAL FLUID REMOVAL

The future of UF may encompass the process of simplification and miniaturization of the dedicated technology. The principles of extracorporeal fluid removal provide an opportunity to consider the possibility of miniaturizing the devices designed for isolated UF and attaching them directly to the patient's body. The same processes involved in reducing the size and complexity of the UF machines for ambulatory patients (wearable UF systems) can be applied to the critically ill patient. Simplification will make extracorporeal UF a routine treatment avoiding complicated procedures or large-bore catheters. Miniaturization will provide the necessary mobility so that routine clinical care, including prone positioning and procedures, can continue while UF takes place.

The question is whether extracorporeal fluid removal therapy should remain a rescue therapy in case of diuretic failure or whether it should be considered as a routine treatment option to prevent fluid accumulation in patients who require high-volume fluid administration. It is well known that fluid overload, even in small proportions, can be dangerous and is associated with poor outcomes.[1,4,46] The elective use of a small dedicated device for extracorporeal fluid removal may represent an interesting option for the future, especially if the complications related to the procedure are reduced to a minimum.

CONCLUSIONS

In CHF patients with severe fluid overload, diuretics remain first-line treatment.[47] Ultrafiltration is a promising modality for fluid removal, especially in situations in which pharmacologic treatment has failed, is unsafe, or unlikely to be effective. However, the benefits are limited to short-term improvement of symptoms and reduced risk of hospitalization. So far, there are no data showing that long-term survival improves or health care costs can be reduced.

The decision between UF alone versus RRT depends on the clinical needs of the individual patient. The proposed algorithm by the ADQI group suggests to consider UF if diuretic therapy has failed or is unsafe or additional solute clearance is required[23] (see Fig. 38.1). Current European and North American practice guidelines suggest that UF should be offered only under experienced supervision.[44,45] If applied, a customized and individualized UF prescription is essential to avoid complications, including intravascular hypovolemia and hemodynamic instability. More research is urgently required to determine the optimal strategy of managing patients with decompensated CHF.

The full reference list for this chapter is available at ExpertConsult.com.

39

Antidysrhythmic Electrophysiology and Pharmacotherapy

Pamela K. Mason, Rohit Malhotra

OUTLINE

The management of critically ill patients is often complicated by cardiac arrhythmias. Patients with acute cardiac ischemia, heart failure, respiratory failure, or renal failure are at risk for different arrhythmias, including atrial fibrillation, supraventricular tachycardia, ventricular tachycardia, and ventricular fibrillation. This includes patients both with and without a history of cardiac arrhythmias. Over the last several decades, procedural methods of managing cardiac arrhythmias have provided patients with more options. From pacemakers to implantable cardioverter-defibrillators to catheter ablation, advances have improved patients' longevity and quality of life. Procedural options to manage cardiac arrhythmias are often impractical in the cardiac intensive care unit (CICU) setting, however. Thus antidysrhythmic agents continue to be the mainstay for arrhythmia management in the CICU.

While antidysrhythmic medications are valuable tools, they have the potential for side effects and drug interactions. Some of these side effects can be life threatening. Of utmost concern is that many antidysrhythmic drugs have potential proarrhythmic

effects.[1-3] Another important consideration is that antidysrhythmic medications are incompletely effective for many conditions. A complete understanding of the indications, use, and monitoring required for each medication is important for managing patients effectively and safely. The purpose of this chapter is to review the basic electrophysiology of arrhythmias and the pharmacology of the antidysrhythmic drugs that are commonly used in the CICU.

CARDIAC ACTION POTENTIAL

The action potentials of individual cardiac cells determine the overall electrical activity of the heart. Different cardiac cells have differently shaped action potentials. Of particular import, the sinoatrial (SA) node, atrioventricular (AV) node, and His-Purkinje system all have slightly different normal action potentials.[4,5] Various ion channels are implicated in the different phases of each action potential. Activity at these ion channels is the basis for antidysrhythmic pharmacology. Antidysrhythmic drugs alter the shape of the action potentials of various cells. This imparts both the antidysrhythmic therapeutic effects and proarrhythmic side effects. While a detailed description of cellular electrophysiology is beyond the scope this chapter, a basic understanding of the fundamentals of ion channels and action potential production is helpful for a better understanding of antidysrhythmic drugs. These features determine how the different antidysrhythmic medications are classified, which arrhythmias each agent most effectively treats, and the monitoring required to avoid dangerous proarrhythmia.

The inherent pacemaker of the heart is the sinus node, which is located in the high right atrium. This tissue has slow response with delayed upstroke during depolarization. The AV node has a similarly shaped action potential. Both the sinus node and the AV node are rich with autonomic innervation, both sympathetic and parasympathetic. However, the His-Purkinje action potential represents fast response tissue with rapid depolarization of the cardiac cell and has little in the way of autonomic innervation.

Sinoatrial Node and Atrioventricular Node Action Potential

The SA node is located in the anterolateral portion of the right atrium, at the junction of the superior vena cava and the right atrium, near the crista terminalis and the right atrial appendage. This structure is heavily innervated and has a highly protected vascular supply. Cardiac action potentials are broadly composed of four phases. In general, the cell membrane is at resting equilibrium at −90 mV at phase 4. Depolarization occurs during phase 0, and repolarization occurs over phases 1, 2, and 3. However, the SA node action potential differs from ventricular action potentials in that phases 1 and 2 are not present (Fig. 39.1).

Depolarization of the sinus node initiates with the slow leak of sodium across the cell membrane via the inward sodium channels (I_f) that generate what is termed "funny" current. Once the cell charge rises from −60 mV to −50 mV, the latter portion of phase 4 commences, with activation of transient inward calcium channels (I_{CaT}). Influx of calcium leads to activation of the L-type (long-acting) calcium channels (I_{CaL}). Once the cell depolarizes to −30 mV, phase 0 initiates. Phase 0 is characterized by prolonged and more rapid influx of calcium via L-type calcium channels with deactivation of the I_f and I_{CaT} channels. These L-type calcium channels influx calcium slowly relative to phase 0 in other portions of the cardiac conduction system. Subsequently, potassium channels open and begin repolarization. As these potassium channels open, the cell membrane potential reaches a peak of about 10 mV and the cell begins to repolarize. These potassium channels cause the cell to hyperpolarize, causing the L-type calcium channels to close. The efflux of potassium and the closure of the calcium channels brings the cell back to its resting potential. The sodium-potassium adenosine triphosphatase (Na^+/K^+-ATPase) is a membrane pump that helps to regulate the ion concentrations and maintain the resting membrane potential. The AV node action potential is very similar to the action potential of the SA node.[6]

Both the SA node and the AV node receive sympathetic and parasympathetic innervation. Activation of the parasympathetic nervous system increases vagal tone and can precipitate bradycardia in the SA node via activation of acetylcholine receptors and increased cyclic guanosine monophosphate (cGMP) production. In the AV node, parasympathetic activation can lead to prolongation of the PR interval and transient heart block. Conversely, activation of the sympathetic nervous system leads to tachycardia and can lead to more rapid AV nodal conduction.[7]

His-Purkinje Action Potential

While the SA node action potential has only three phases (4, 3, and 0), the His-Purkinje and ventricular action potentials have phases 1 and 2 (Fig. 39.2). The cell rests at phase 4, predominantly through efflux of potassium through open potassium channels. Phase 0 occurs when sodium channels open, leading to rapid influx of sodium that shifts the cell membrane charge from −90 mV to +10 mV. As sodium channels open, the potassium channels close, leading to more rapid depolarization. At peak depolarization, inward potassium channels open, leading to a slight decline in depolarization. Calcium efflux channels via long-acting L-type calcium channels then lead to slow repolarization through phase 2. During phase 3 of the action potential, potassium efflux begins and the calcium channels close. As potassium effluxes, the membrane potential returns to baseline (phase 4). During these phases (0 through 3 and the early portions of phase 4), the cell membrane cannot be depolarized, preventing multiple wavefronts of depolarization. Antidysrhythmic medications impact these channels, but owing to the duplication of channels in SA, AV, and His-Purkinje cells, the medications can impact different portions of the conduction system.

CLASSIFICATION OF ANTIDYSRHYTHMIC MEDICATIONS

Two systems are used to classify antidysrhythmic medications. The most commonly used system remains the Vaughan Williams

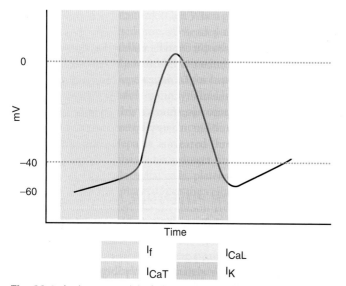

Fig. 39.1 Action potential of sinoatrial and atrioventricular nodal cells. I_{CaL}, Inward long-acting calcium channels; I_{CaT}, transient inward calcium channels; I_f, inward sodium channels; I_K, inward potassium channels.

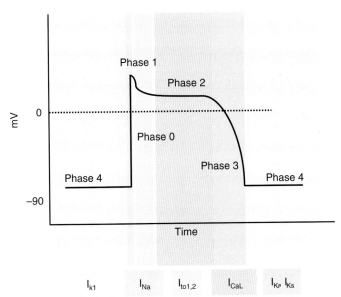

Fig. 39.2 Action potential of His-Purkinje cells. I_{CaL}, Inward long-acting calcium channels; I_K, inward potassium channels; I_{Kr}, rapidly activating delayed rectifier potassium current; I_{Ks}, slowly activating delayed rectifier potassium current; I_{Na}, inward sodium channels; $I_{to1,2}$, transient outward potassium current 1 and 2.

classification system[8–10] (Table 39.1). This system was introduced several decades ago and has undergone some modification. The Vaughan Williams system attempts to classify the different drugs based upon mechanism of action. This system has always had weaknesses in that many drugs have multiple ion channel effects or do not work through the ion channels at all. It also does not account for different potencies within the classes or other effects on cardiac physiology. Because of this, a new system was proposed, called the Sicilian Gambit[11] (Table 39.2). This is a much more complex system, but one that attempts to link more directly each medication to the relevant arrhythmias at the cellular level (Table 39.3). While this system has never really supplanted the Vaughan Williams system for classifying these drugs, it is presented here because it does provide a more detailed framework for the understanding of how many of the individual drugs work.

Class I Antidysrhythmic Medications

The Vaughan Williams class I drugs are sodium channel blockers. They are classified into IA, IB, and IC drugs based upon their potency and effects on conduction velocity. Class IA drugs decrease conduction and increase refractoriness. Class IB drugs decrease refractoriness, while class IC drugs decrease conduction (Fig. 39.3). The class IC drugs are the most potent with the slowest binding and dissociation, class IA drugs are the least potent with the fastest binding and dissociation, and class IB drugs are moderate in potency.[12]

All class I drugs, particularly the class IC drugs, demonstrate "use dependence."[13] Since IC drugs have very slow binding and dissociation, faster heart rates lead to an increasing number of blocked receptors. This can lead to a dramatic reduction in conduction velocity. On the surface electrocardiogram (ECG), this manifests as prolongation of the QRS complex. This can be

TABLE 39.1 Modified Vaughan Williams Classification of Antidysrhythmic Medications

	Drug Effects
Class I: Na$^+$ Channel Blockers	
IA	Moderate slowing of conduction
Quinidine	with prolonged refractoriness
Procainamide	
Disopyramide	
IB	Slight slowing of conduction
Lidocaine	with minimal decrease in
Mexiletene	refractoriness
IC	Marked slowing of conduction
Flecainide	with slight prolongation of
Propafenone	refractoriness
Class II: β-Blockers	β-Adrenergic receptor
Metoprolol	antagonism
Atenolol	
Class III: K$^+$ Channel Blockers	Prolongation of refractoriness
Amiodarone	
Dronedarone	
Sotalol	
Ibutilide	
Dofetilide	
Class IV: Ca^{2+} Channel Blockers	Block calcium entry
Verapamil	
Diltiazem	
Class V: Other	
Adenosine	
Digoxin	

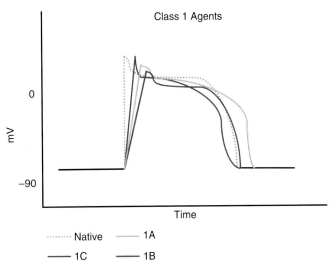

Fig. 39.3 Effects of class I antidysrhythmic drugs on the action potential of His-Purkinje cells.

seen when the drug is being administered in a patient who is tachycardic. QRS complex widening can also be seen as a manifestation of class IA and IC drug toxicity.

It should be noted that the class IC drugs have limited utility in the CICU setting. Several important studies involving IC drugs, the Cardiac Arrhythmia Suppression Trial (CAST) and CAST II

TABLE 39.2 The Modified Sicilian Gambit

Mechanism	Arrhythmia	Desired Effect	Example Drugs
Automaticity			
Enhanced	Inappropriate sinus tachycardia	Decrease phase 4 depolarization	β-Blockers
	Idiopathic ventricular tachycardia (some)	Decrease phase 4 depolarization	Na$^+$ channel blockers
	Atrial tachycardia	Decrease phase 4 depolarization	Muscarinic receptor agonists
	Accelerated idioventricular rhythms	Decrease phase 4 depolarization	Ca^{2+} or Na$^+$ channel blockers
Triggered Activity			
EAD	Torsade de pointes	Shorten action potential	β-Blockers
		EAD suppression	Ca^{2+} channel blockers
			Mg^{2+}
			β-Blockers
DAD	Digoxin-induced arrhythmias	Block calcium entry	Ca^{2+} channel blockers
	Right ventricular outflow tract tachycardia	Block calcium entry	Ca^{2+} channel blockers
		DAD suppression	β-Blockers
Na$^+$ Channel–Dependent Reentry			
Long excitable gap	Typical atrial flutter	Depress conduction and excitability	Class IA and class IC Na$^+$ channel blockers
	Atrioventricular reciprocating tachycardia	Depress conduction and excitability	Class IA and class IC Na$^+$ channel blockers
	Monomorphic ventricular tachycardia	Depress conduction and excitability	Na$^+$ channel blockers
Short excitable gap	Atypical atrial flutter	Prolong refractory period	K$^+$ channel blockers
	Atrial fibrillation	Prolong refractory period	K$^+$ channel blockers
	AV reciprocating tachycardia	Prolong refractory period	Amiodarone and sotalol
	Polymorphic and uniform ventricular tachycardia	Prolong refractory period	Class IA Na$^+$ channel blockers
	Bundle branch reentry	Prolong refractory period	Class IA Na$^+$ channel blockers and amiodarone
Na$^+$ Channel–Dependent Reentry			
	Atrioventricular nodal reentrant tachycardia	Depress conduction and excitability	Ca^{2+} channel blockers
	Atrioventricular reciprocating tachycardia	Depress conduction and excitability	Ca^{2+} channel blockers
	Verapamil-sensitive ventricular tachycardia	Depress conduction and excitability	Ca^{2+} channel blockers

DAD, Delayed afterdepolarization; *EAD,* early afterdepolarization.

TABLE 39.3 Actions of Antiarrhythmic Drugs Used in Critical Care

Drug	CHANNELS					RECEPTORS					PUMPS	CLINICAL EFFECTS			ECG INTERVAL EFFECT		
	Na$^+$ Fast	Na$^+$ Medium	Na$^+$ Slow	Ca^{2+}	Ca^{2+}	γ α	β	M2	A1		Na$^+$/K$^-$- ATPase	LV Function	Sinus Rate	Extracardiac	PR	QRS	QT
Lidocaine	Low											$\rightarrow$	$\rightarrow$	Med			$\downarrow$
Procainamide		ASB			Med							$\downarrow$	$\rightarrow$	High	$\uparrow$	$\uparrow$	$\uparrow$
Verapamil	Low			High		Med						$\downarrow$	$\downarrow$	Low	$\uparrow$		
Diltiazem				Med								$\downarrow$	$\downarrow$	Low	$\uparrow$		
Sotalol					High		High					$\downarrow$	$\downarrow$	Low	$\uparrow$		$\uparrow$
Amiodarone	Low			Low	High	Med	Med					$\rightarrow$	$\downarrow$	High	$\uparrow$		$\uparrow$
Propanolol	Low						High					$\downarrow$	$\downarrow$	Low	$\uparrow$		
Adenosine									Agonist			?	$\downarrow$	Low	$\uparrow$		
Digoxin								Agonist			High	$\uparrow$	$\downarrow$	High	$\uparrow$		$\downarrow$

Potency of blockade: *Low,* low potency; *Med,* medium potency; *High,* high potency.
ASB, Activated state blocker.

trials showed little efficacy in preventing arrhythmias in addition to causing excess mortality.[1,3] These medications are not safe to be used in patients with structural heart disease. Further, they are only available in oral form and some are renally cleared, making these drugs unsuitable for most critically ill cardiac patients.

In contrast, several of the IA and IB drugs are used extensively in the CICU setting. The availability of intravenous (IV) formulations and their relative safety in patients with coronary artery disease and heart failure make procainamide (IA) and lidocaine (IB) two of the important antidysrhythmics for cardiac patients.

These will be discussed in more detail in the Antidysrhythmics of Clinical Relevance section.

Class II Antidysrhythmic Medications

The class II antidysrhythmic medications are also known as β-blockers. They inhibit the β-adrenergic receptor and thus largely create their effects at the SA and AV nodes. They also contain mild sodium channel blocking effects. In cardiac patients, the benefits of β-blockers cannot be overstated. They increase survival in patients with multiple cardiac conditions, including coronary artery disease and heart failure. They decrease sudden cardiac death events for patients with implantable defibrillators. The likely mechanism of class II drugs in preventing tachyarrhythmia is by suppressing sympathetic activity.[14] Increased sympathetic tone can lead to an increase in triggered activity caused by afterdepolarizations; β-blockers may suppress this. Different β-blockers can assist with management of acute arrhythmias as well. Some arrhythmias, including supraventricular tachycardia, can be terminated and suppressed with β-blockers. The ventricular response to some arrhythmias, including atrial fibrillation and atrial flutter, can be reduced by slowing conduction via the AV node.

Class III Antidysrhythmic Medications

The class III antidysrhythmic medications demonstrate potassium channel blocking properties. They prolong the plateau phase of the action potential, which slows repolarization and extends the action potential duration (Fig. 39.4). This increases the refractory period and causes prolongation of the QT interval on the surface ECG.

Class III drugs demonstrate "reverse use dependence,"[13] meaning that they have greater activity at slower heart rates. Thus the potential for QT interval prolongation is magnified at lower heart rates.[15] QT prolongation is the most important proarrhythmic risk of this class of medications. Prolongation of the QT interval increases the risk of "R on T" phenomena, which can cause torsades de pointes, a potentially lethal arrhythmia. The degree of QT interval prolongation and thus the risk of torsades de pointes caused by the different class III medications

varies widely. Dofetilide can cause such significant QT prolongation that inpatient loading of this medication is recommended. In contrast, amiodarone rarely causes any QT prolongation and only rarely has proarrhythmic effects.[16] Amiodarone is one of the most important antidysrhythmic medications in the CICU setting; it is detailed in the Antidysrhythmic Medications of Clinical Relevance section.

Class IV Antidysrhythmic Medications

The class IV antidysrhythmic drugs block the slow calcium channels. This class includes only the nondihydropyridine calcium channel blockers, which are the only calcium channel blockers that have electrophysiologic effects. Their most significant sites of action are in the SA and AV nodes. These medications slow spontaneous phase 4 depolarization. This can lead to both bradycardic effects at the SA node and delayed conduction through the AV node.[17] Thus these medications can be very useful to slow the rapid ventricular response from arrhythmias, such as atrial fibrillation or flutter, or suppress supraventricular tachycardia similarly to β-blockers. Unlike β-blockers, however, they do not directly suppress adrenergic input.

Calcium channel blockers can also affect phase 2 of the action potential of ventricular myocytes. Thus, calcium channel blockers inhibit early afterdepolarizations that are an important cause of arrhythmias in conditions that cause prolongation of the action potential.[18] They are particularly useful for suppressing left ventricular (LV) fascicular tachycardias.

It is important to note that calcium channel blockers are negatively inotropic. Thus they are to be avoided, if possible, in patients with heart failure.[19] While the mechanisms of action of calcium channel blockers and β-blockers are different, many of their resultant effects are similar. In general, β-blockers are better first-line therapy in most situations.

Atypical Antidysrhythmic Medications

One of the many weaknesses of the Vaughan Williams classification system is that there are several medications that are unclassified. These medications are often grouped together with an unofficial "class V" designation. Digoxin, which has multiple electrophysiologic effects, is included in this group. It is one of the oldest antidysrhythmic drugs and has fallen out of favor for all conditions except as a second line agent for rate control of atrial fibrillation. Adenosine, which is used for acute termination of arrhythmias, is also included in this class. These are both important in the critical care setting and are discussed in the Antidysrhythmic Medications of Clinical Relevance section.

PHARMACOKINETICS OF ANTIDYSRHYTHMIC DRUGS

The pharmacokinetics of the various antidysrhythmic medications are complicated and an extensive discussion of these principles is outside the scope of this chapter. It is, however, important to remember that a drug's absorption, distribution, metabolism, elimination and half-life affect the dosing, frequency, and potential side effects.[20] Many of these factors are altered in patients when they are critically ill, making management of antidysrhythmic

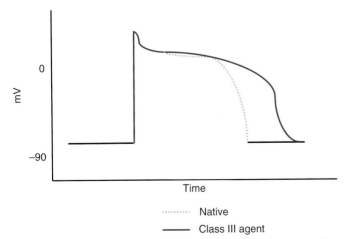

Fig. 39.4 Effects of class III antidysrhythmic drugs on the action potential of His-Purkinje cells.

TABLE 39.4	Pharmacokinetics of Antidysrhythmic Drugs Used in Critical Care						
Drug	Bioavailability (F)	Vd (L/kg)	Protein Binding (%)	Elimination Half-Life (h)	Therapeutic Range (μg/mL)	Biotransformation and Excretion	Metabolites
Procainamide	75–95	1.5–2.5	15–25	2–4	4–10 (17–42.5 μmol/L)	Liver: acetylation Kidney: 60% unchanged	N–Acetylprocainamide (class III effects)
Lidocaine	NA	1–2	1–2	65–75	0.3–2	1.5–5 (5.7–21.3 μmol/L)	Monoethylglycylxylidine, glycine xylidine (inactive)
Ibutilide	NA	11	40	6		Liver: omega oxidation	
Amiodarone	20–50	Large	> 96	≥60 d	0.5–3.0	Liver: deethylation	Desethylamiodarone (class III effects)
Verapamil	15–30	4–5	90	3–7	0.1–0.15	Liver: high first-pass extraction	Norverapamil (Ca²⁺ channel blocker effects)
Diltiazem	50	5	70–80	3–4.5	120–200 ng/mL	Liver	
Digoxin	60–80	7.5	20–30	40	0.5–2.0 ng/mL	Kidney: >90% unchanged	

medications different in this setting than in stable patients. The basic pharmacokinetics of antidysrhythmic drugs are presented in Table 39.4.

The bioavailability of a drug is the amount of an orally administered drug that reaches the circulation unchanged. The two major factors that affect bioavailability are gut uptake and first-pass clearance through the liver. Gut uptake is affected by drug dissolution, gastric pH, bacterial flora, and transporter proteins, such as P-glycoprotein. During first-pass clearance, hepatocytes metabolize and excrete certain drugs into bile. Both of these processes can be altered in critically ill patients.

In the critical care setting, many medications are given in an intravenous form; therefore, the principles of drug absorption do not apply. Some of the antidysrhythmic drugs, such as lidocaine, are so heavily metabolized during the first pass that oral forms are not even available.[21] It is important to remember these concepts in cases in which oral formulations are used or during patient recovery when they are converted from intravenous (IV) to oral medications.

Certain tissues, including most of the central organs, receive the best perfusion and are termed the central compartment. Skin and muscle compose the peripheral compartment and adipose tissue is considered the deep compartment. The penetration of different drugs into these areas is variable and affects the volume of distribution of the drug. The volume of distribution for a drug is the theoretical volume through which a drug is distributed and correlates with drug dose and the plasma level. The volume of distribution can be affected by the actual plasma volume or perfusion of the various compartments. It can also be affected by binding to proteins. For example, α_1-glycoprotein is an important binder of many antidysrhythmic drugs and its concentration increases in patients with shock or trauma.

These principles are very important for several of the commonly used antidysrhythmic drugs in the CICU. The most important drug with slow penetration into the deep compartment is amiodarone. Amiodarone has a large volume of distribution; thus its onset of action is delayed. It also has a long elimination half-life. Amiodarone is often given as a load in order to reach effective plasma concentrations more quickly. In contrast,

lidocaine toxicity becomes more common in patients with heart failure since the volume of distribution may be decreased dramatically. Most of the antidysrhythmic medications are metabolized hepatically via the cytochrome P450 system. Metabolites of some drugs may be as or more potent than the parent drug or have completely different actions. Amiodarone is metabolized to desethylamiodarone, which possesses clinically relevant class II antidysrhythmic and vasodilator properties. Procainamide, which is a class IA agent, is converted to N-acetylprocainamide (NAPA), which has class III effects. The administration of multiple drugs that are metabolized via the cytochrome P450 system can alter elimination of one or more of the drugs.

ANTIDYSRHYTHMIC MEDICATIONS OF CLINICAL RELEVANCE IN THE CRITICAL CARE SETTING

Many antidysrhythmic drugs are of little use within the critical care setting. Table 39.5 lists the dosing and administration of the antidysrhythmic medications most commonly used in the CICU.

Class IA

Procainamide is the only class IA agent that is commonly used in the CICU. It is a pharmacologically complicated medication that it is metabolized via acetylation from a sodium channel blocker to NAPA that has potassium channel blocking properties. Procainamide therefore decreases conduction velocity and prolongs the His-Purkinje action potential and thus the effective refractory period.[22] It can also suppress automaticity in the SA and AV nodes and triggered activity in normal Purkinje fibers.[23,24] Procainamide can prolong the QT interval. There is genetic variation in acetylation of the parent drug whereby some patients have rapid acetylation and others have slow acetylation. This is important for drug monitoring.

Indications. Procainamide has two major indications. Historically, it has been utilized as first-line therapy for management

TABLE 39.5 Usual Dosing of Antidysrhythmic Drugs Used in Critical Care

	INTRAVENOUS		ORAL (MG)		Peak Plasma Concentration (Oral Dosing in Hours)
Drug	Loading	Maintenance	Loading	Maintenance	
Procainamide	6–15 mg/kg at 0.2–0.5 mg/kg/min	2–6 mg/min	500–1000	350–1000 q3–q6h	1
Lidocaine	1–3 mg/kg over 15–45 min	1 mg/kg/h			
Propanolol	1–3 mg at 1 mg/min			10–200 q6–8h	4
Ibutilide	1–2 mg				
Amiodarone	5 mg/kg over 10–30 min	720–1000 mg q24h	For VT: 1200–1600 qd for 1–2 wk then 600–800 qd for 2–4 wk For SVT: 600–800 qd for 2 wk	For VT: 200–400 qd For SVT: 200 qd	
Verapamil	10 mg over 1–2 min			80 mg q12h up to 320 mg/d	1–2
Adenosine	6–12 mg				
Digoxin	1 mg over 24 h in divided doses	0.125–0.25 mg q24h	1 mg over 24 h in divided doses	0.125–0.25 mg q24h	1–3

SVT, Supraventricular tachycardia; *VT,* ventricular tachycardia.

of stable ventricular tachycardia.[25,26] Although amiodarone is increasingly administered for that indication, procainamide is still commonly used.[27,28] Procainamide also remains the treatment of choice for treating pre-excited atrial fibrillation in the setting of Wolff-Parkinson-White syndrome.[29]

Electrocardiographic Effects. The effects of procainamide on the surface ECG are a reflection of the sodium channel blocking properties of the parent drug and the potassium channel blocking properties of the NAPA metabolite. Patients demonstrate use-dependent widening of the QRS at faster heart rates. QRS widening also occurs with high plasma concentrations. The PR interval and QT intervals can lengthen.[30] Widening of the QRS interval by greater than 25% suggests levels in which toxicity may occur and may be useful to monitor therapy.[31]

Side Effects. Procainamide has a wide variety of side effects that can be dangerous for patients and require vigilant monitoring. In addition to the proarrhythmic effects related to QT prolongation that can lead to torsade de pointes, procainamide has other clinically important cardiac effects. Procainamide can be negatively inotropic and, especially in the intravenous form, can cause hypotension. These are limiting side effects in the CICU, where patients often have LV dysfunction and hypotension. Noncardiac effects, such as pancytopenia and agranulocytosis, can be life threatening. The timing of these reactions can be unpredictable, and can occur months after the medication is started. Systemic lupus can occur with prolonged use. Headaches, gastrointestinal effects, and mental disturbances can also occur.

Administration. Procainamide is used almost exclusively in the IV form in the CICU. Oral forms can be compounded but, in addition to being rarely used in the inpatient setting, they are not recommended for long-term outpatient use owing to their side effects and inferior efficacy to other drugs for most arrhythmias. As the IV administration is generally given for acute

arrhythmias, it is often initiated as a loading dose. There are several different protocols commonly used. A gram of procainamide can be administered over 20 to 30 minutes. This is often used to convert preexcited atrial fibrillation. Procainamide can also be given as 6 to 15 mg/kg at 0.2 to 0.5 mg/kg per minute. Care should be taken to reduce the dose in the setting of renal or cardiac impairment. Care should also be taken in monitoring for ECG changes and hypotension. Following the loading dose, maintenance should be administered at 1 mg/kg per hour. The metabolism of this drug is widely variable, including the acetylation to NAPA; thus, levels of both procainamide and NAPA should be monitored with prolonged usage. The procainamide level should be less than 12 μg/mL. The sum of both procainamide and NAPA should be less than 30 μg/mL.

Class IB

Lidocaine is the only medication in this class that is useful in the CICU. Historically, lidocaine was commonly used for ventricular arrhythmias.[32] However, it has fallen out of favor compared to other antidysrhythmics, particularly amiodarone.[33,34] Lidocaine exerts most of its actions on the Purkinje fibers and has little effect on the SA or AV nodes.[35] Lidocaine is a sodium channel blocker that decreases conduction velocity. Compared to other sodium channel blockers, it shortens the action potential and decreases automaticity by decreasing the slow or phase 4 diastolic depolarization.[36] It can be helpful in both reentrant and automatic arrhythmia suppression.

Indications. Lidocaine has become a secondary agent in the CICU that is most commonly used for both stable VT and unstable ventricular arrhythmias that are refractory to β-blockers and amiodarone.[37] Other antidysrhythmic agents are superior in these circumstances. One special consideration is that since lidocaine is not a QT-prolonging medication, if a patient has severe QT prolongation and torsade de pointes, it would be preferred over other antidysrhythmic medications that may cause additional QT prolongation. That being said, rapid pacing, isoproterenol, and magnesium infusions are superior treatments in this situation.[38]

In the past, lidocaine was thought to be of benefit in patients with myocardial infarctions for primary and secondary prevention of ventricular arrhythmias. This was based on small, nonrandomized data that focused on prevention of ventricular arrhythmias and not mortality. There have been subsequent studies that demonstrated no mortality benefit from lidocaine, particularly as prophylactic therapy.[39–41] Therefore prophylactic lidocaine in the setting of acute myocardial infarction is not recommended.

Electrocardiographic Effects. There are generally no changes seen on the ECG in patients receiving therapeutic doses of lidocaine.[42] As it shortens the action potential, the QRS prolongation that can be seen with procainamide is not seen with lidocaine. Lidocaine has no class III properties and the QT interval is not affected.

Side Effects. The most common toxicities of lidocaine are central nervous system (CNS) effects, particularly mental status changes.[43] In most cases, these are mild and resolve with cessation or dose reduction. Elderly patients and those with congestive heart failure are at higher risk of CNS toxicity.[44] In addition, since lidocaine is mostly cleared hepatically, liver failure predisposes to toxicity. Tremors are the first CNS symptom with early toxicity; seizures occur at extremely high plasma concentrations. Bradyarrhythmias, hypotension, and decreased inotropy can occur but only at very high plasma levels.

Administration. There are several important factors that affect dosing and administration of lidocaine. First, the first-pass clearance of lidocaine is so high that it is administered only in IV form. Second, it has a very short half-life of less than 3 hours. The metabolites have only weak antidysrhythmic properties. Third, it is highly bound to α-acid glycoproteins, which are increased in heart failure patients. Finally, the reduced volume of distribution in heart failure leads to higher concentrations of the drug.

In general, a loading dose of 1 to 3 mg/kg is administered over several minutes followed by maintenance infusions of 1 to 4 mg/min. For acute arrhythmia treatment, patients can be bolused several times if needed until the steady state is reached by the maintenance infusion, which can take 3 to 4 hours.[45] Dosing needs to be decreased in patients with hepatic dysfunction or heart failure. Therapeutic levels of lidocaine are between 1.5 to 5 μg/mL. Monitoring for CNS side effects should also be done to assess for toxicity.

Class IC

This class of antidysrhythmic medications is no longer used in the critical care setting. The Cardiac Arrhythmia Suppression Trial (CAST) and CAST II were critical in establishing that these medications can increase arrhythmic deaths in patients after myocardial infarction.[1,3] Flecainide and propafenone are the only two medications in this class left on the market. Encainide and moricizine are no longer available, partially due to their proarrhythmic side effects. Flecainide and propafenone are used in the outpatient setting, predominantly for atrial arrhythmias. The fact that they cannot be used in patients with structural heart disease or significant renal dysfunction and that they are available only in oral formulations make them of little value in the CICU.

Class II

β-Blockers are critical to the management of many cardiac conditions, including arrhythmias. Unlike most antidysrhythmic medications, β-blockers have been shown to reduce mortality in a variety of situations, including heart failure, acute myocardial infarction, and coronary artery disease.[46–49] They also decrease the rate of shocks for patients with implantable cardioverter-defibrillators and prevent degeneration of ventricular tachycardia to ventricular fibrillation.

β-Blockers may bind to β_1 receptors, β_2 receptors, or both. Some β-blockers also block α1 receptors. β_1 Receptors are found in the cardiovascular system. β_2 Receptors are noncardiac and lead to β-blocker side effects, such as pulmonary bronchospasm. α_1 Receptor antagonism causes additional arteriolar vasodilation; drugs with α_1 receptor blockade tend to be used more commonly for hypertension or heart failure than arrhythmias (Table 39.6).

While all β-blockers have class effects, there are slight differences in the various drugs. For example, pindolol has less of a bradycardic effect than many of the other β-blockers due to its intrinsic sympathomimetic action. As many of the beneficial cardiovascular effects seem to be observed with the β-blockers that cause the most bradycardic effects, pindolol is rarely used by cardiologists. There are also differences in the indications for the various drugs based upon clinical trial data. Carvedilol, bisoprolol, and the long-acting form of metoprolol, all oral medications, are indicated for long-term treatment of patients with heart failure in the setting of LV dysfunction.

The myriad benefits of β-blocker therapy are, for the most part, a result of blocking the effects of adrenergic stimulation.[50] Adrenergic stimulation can cause a variety of negative electrophysiologic findings, including increased automaticity, triggered activity, reentrant excitation, and delayed afterdepolarizations.

TABLE 39.6 Dosing and Metabolism of Commonly Used β-Blockers

Drug	β1 Selective	IV Dosage	Half-Life	Elimination	Other Properties
Atenolol	Yes	5 mg q 10 min up to 10 mg	6–9 h	Renal	None
Esmolol	Yes	500 μg/kg loading; 50–300 μg/kg/min maintenance	9 min	Blood esterase	None
Labetalol	No	20 mg IV push; 2 mg/min infusion up to 300 mg	3–4 h	Hepatic	α-Blockade
Metoprolol	Yes	5 mg q 2–5 min up to 15 mg	3–4 h	Hepatic	None
Propanolol	No	1 mg/min up to 5 mg	3–4 h	Hepatic	Membrane stabilization

Indications. β-Blockers are used to treat multiple arrhythmias. They can be used to suppress some forms of supraventricular tachycardia, including AV nodal reentrant tachycardia. They slow the ventricular response for atrial fibrillation and atrial flutter. As β-blockers exert most of their influence on the SA and AV nodes, they generally do not convert these rhythms. They decrease ventricular arrhythmias in patients with acute myocardial infarction. Adrenergically mediated ventricular arrhythmias respond well to β-blockers, including right ventricular outflow tract tachycardia. β-Blockers reduce the risk of sudden cardiac death in patients with congenital long QT syndrome.

Electrocardiographic Effects. In patients in sinus rhythm, β-blockers commonly slow the sinus rate and produce bradycardia. In high doses or in patients with native conduction system disease, PR prolongation can be seen as well. β-Blockers do not cause QT prolongation or QRS widening.

Side Effects. Compared to other antidysrhythmic medications, β-blockers are well tolerated. From a cardiovascular standpoint, all β-blockers can cause bradycardia and hypotension, although the degree of risk for each drug is dependent on which adrenergic receptors it binds. Since the use of any β-blocker to control a tachyarrhythmia can be limited by hypotension, blood pressure needs to be monitored closely. β-Blockers improve survival for patients with heart failure and LV dysfunction and should be considered first-line therapy in this setting.[51]

The most common non-cardiac side effect of β-blockers is exacerbation of bronchospasm in patients with asthma or chronic obstructive pulmonary disease.[52] β-Blockers with β_2 selectivity are most likely to cause bronchospasm, but even drugs with predominantly β_1 selectivity should be used cautiously in susceptible patients. Other uncommon noncardiac side effects include a blunted response to hypoglycemia, fatigue, and depression.[53,54]

Administration. There are a number of different β-blockers with different receptor selectivity, half-lives, and modes of elimination. While β-blockers have class effects, these differences should inform drug selection for individual patients. For example, atenolol is not a good β-blocker for patients with severe renal impairment, as it is predominantly renally cleared. In addition, some β-blockers are available only in oral or intravenous forms. Table 39.6 outlines the IV β-blockers that are most commonly used in the CICU for treatment of arrhythmias.

Class III

The weaknesses of the Vaughn Williams classification system of antidysrhythmic drugs are apparent when reviewing the class III drugs. Nominally, these medications have potassium channel blocking properties. However, many of these drugs have other properties as well. In particular, amiodarone also has sodium channel blocking properties, calcium channel blocking properties, and β-blocker properties; thus amiodarone does not behave in ways that a pure class III drug would be expected to. There are a number of class III drugs, but amiodarone remains one of the most important antidysrhythmic medications for patients in the

CICU and will be discussed in detail. Ibutilide is an IV drug used only for the acute conversion of atrial arrhythmias. Historically, sotalol was available only in oral form in the United States but, more recently, an IV form has been approved that may be of use in critically ill patients. Although it is not yet widely available, it does seem to be effective for termination of atrial fibrillation.[55]

Amiodarone. Amiodarone is one of the most effective antidysrhythmic medications for both atrial and ventricular arrhythmias across a range of different mechanisms, including automatic and reentrant. It is available in both oral and IV forms; the oral form has high bioavailability. It has little proarrhythmic effects and, despite being a class III drug, does not cause significant QT prolongation in most settings.[56–58] These features make it a very useful drug for treatment of arrhythmias, particularly in critically ill patients. Despite these favorable characteristics, it has the potential for multiple side effects, some of which can be serious and life threatening. These side effects are often, although not always, found during long-term oral therapy. Thus amiodarone is a first-line medication, especially for life-threatening ventricular arrhythmias.

Amiodarone is classified as a class III medication due to its ability to block IK_r and IK_s, leading to action potential prolongation and increased refractory periods in atrial and ventricular tissues.[59] However, it also a significant blocker of sodium and calcium channels and demonstrates the effects of these classes. It is a weak β-blocker and α_1 blocker, which can result in bradycardia and hypotension. It also decreases peripheral conversion of T4 to T3 and impairs T3 binding to myocytes, causing cellular hypothyroidism.[60] The magnitude of the various effects is different in the oral versus IV forms, with the oral form demonstrating decreased automaticity, increased action potential duration, and prolongation of the QT interval.[61]

Indications. With its multiple class effects and limited proarrhythmic effects, amiodarone is a versatile antidysrhythmic drug. It is efficacious in converting and suppressing atrial fibrillation as well as in the acute treatment of ventricular arrhythmias. Amiodarone is part of the advanced cardiac life support (ACLS) guidelines for management of ventricular fibrillation and pulseless ventricular tachycardia.[26] However, it is approved by the U.S. Food and Drug Administration (FDA) only for the treatment of ventricular arrhythmias. Nevertheless, amiodarone has been studied for multiple conditions over the last several decades and guidelines statements for the treatment of atrial fibrillation and ventricular tachycardia include amiodarone as a treatment option. It is important to note that amiodarone, unlike other antidysrhythmic drugs, is both a vasodilator and is not a negative inotrope. Thus it can be used safely in patients with coronary artery disease and LV dysfunction.[62–64]

The use of amiodarone for the long-term suppression of ventricular arrhythmias has been controversial in the past.[65–70] A review of the available literature would suggest that oral amiodarone is unlikely to be of benefit in long-term primary or secondary prevention of sudden death. However, in the acute setting, IV amiodarone is the mainstay for treatment of lethal ventricular arrhythmias in most situations.

Amiodarone is clearly superior to other antidysrhythmic medications for the treatment of atrial fibrillation.[71,72] For critically ill patients, the rapid ventricular response associated with atrial fibrillation can complicate other conditions. Restoration of sinus rhythm can improve hemodynamics in some patients with heart failure, renal failure, or sepsis. Amiodarone has been shown to decrease postoperative atrial fibrillation in cardiac surgery patients.[73]

Electrocardiographic effects. Due to its multiple cellular mechanisms of action, amiodarone causes a variety of ECG findings. Sinus bradycardia and PR prolongation are common. Furthermore, mild QRS widening can be seen. QTc prolongation can also be seen but is usually mild and rarely proarrhythmic. While administration of most class III medications requires inpatient monitoring of the QT interval, amiodarone can be started as an outpatient. Amiodarone demonstrates reverse use dependence; as a result, the QT prolongation is generally seen more prominently at slower heart rates.

Side effects. The side effects of amiodarone occur mostly in the setting of long-term oral administration. Patients can have bradycardia, hepatic dysfunction, hypothyroidism, hyperthyroidism, ophthalmologic changes, CNS effects, neuropathy, skin discoloration, and, most concerning, pulmonary fibrosis. Patients on amiodarone have to be monitored for the development of these side effects in the outpatient setting. Table 39.7 lists the most common drug interactions with amiodarone.

In the inpatient setting, the most significant concerns are the potential for the development of hypotension, bradycardia, or proarrhythmia during the administration of intravenous amiodarone. The risk of acute pulmonary lung toxicity is quite low. However, the risks may be higher in critically ill patients and, if it does occur, early recognition is of paramount importance so that the medication can be stopped and corticosteroids can be administered.

Administration. For acute management of arrhythmias, a 150-mg IV loading dose is given over 10 minutes. After this, an IV infusion of 1 mg/min is given for 6 hours followed by an infusion of 0.5 mg/min, which provides a total of just over 1 g of amiodarone in 24 hours. A maintenance infusion of 0.5 mg/min or intermittent intravenous loading doses can be continued for patients who cannot take oral medications. The intravenous form can reach steady state quickly.

The oral form of amiodarone is very lipophilic and thus has a very large volume of distribution. Thus, oral administration does not start to have an effect for several days and the half-life of oral amiodarone is extremely long. To achieve steady state, a patient must have upwards of 10 g to thoroughly saturate the peripheral and deep compartments.

There is no renal metabolism of amiodarone, which is another advantage in critically ill patients who may have acute renal failure. It is entirely metabolized via the liver and the gut. The liver metabolite desethylamiodarone is active and has a very long half-life. There should be adjustment of the dose for patients with liver dysfunction; liver function tests should be monitored closely.

Ibutilide. Ibutilide blocks Ik$_r$, leading to an increase in action potential duration and atrial and ventricular refractoriness. It is available only in IV form.

Indications. Ibutilide is indicated only for the acute conversion of atrial fibrillation and atrial flutter to sinus rhythm.[29,74] It is more likely to be effective for atrial flutter than atrial fibrillation and is more likely to be effective for shorter episodes of atrial arrhythmias. The success rate for conversion of atrial fibrillation is only approximately 30%. Electrical cardioversion is certainly more effective but requires sedation. Ibutilide can also be used to facilitate electrical cardioversion in patients who have atrial fibrillation refractory to prior electrical cardioversions.[75]

Electrocardiographic effects. Ibutilide can be a very potent QT prolonging agent, with resultant risks of torsade de pointes. It does not cause significant bradycardia or alter other ECG intervals.

Side effects. One of the advantages of ibutilide is that it has few side effects beyond the QT prolongation. The infusion does not cause hypotension. The risk of torsade de pointes is not insignificant at 3.6% to 8.3%; very close monitoring is warranted with administration of this medication.[76,77]

Administration. Ibutilide should be administered in a very controlled setting. Patients need to be on continuous telemetry monitoring. An external defibrillator must be immediately

TABLE 39.7	**Drug Interactions With Amiodarone**		
Drug	**Result**	**Risks**	**Mechanism of Interaction**
Apixaban	Increases apixaban levels	Increased risk of bleeding	Inhibits CYP3A4 P-glycoprotein
Cyclosporine	Increases cyclosporine levels	Increased risk of CNS and GI side effects, hypertension	Inhibits CYP3A4 P-glycoprotein
Dabigatran	Increases dabigatran levels	Increased risk of bleeding	P-glycoprotein
Digoxin	Increases digoxin levels	Increased risk of arrhythmia, CNS, and GI side effects	P-glycoprotein
Rivaroxaban	Increases rivaroxaban levels	Increased risk of bleeding	Inhibits CYP3A4 P-glycoprotein
Simvastatin	Increases statin levels	Increased risk of liver toxicity and rhabdomyolysis	Inhibits CYP3A4
Warfarin	Increases INR	Increased risk of bleeding	Inhibits CYP2CP Inhibits CYP1A2

CNS, Central nervous system; *GI,* gastrointestinal; *INR,* international normalized ratio.

available. Potassium and magnesium levels should be optimized. The usual dosing is 1 mg infused over 10 minutes. The infusion should be stopped in the event of either marked QT prolongation or conversion to sinus rhythm. A second dose can be given after 10 minutes if neither of the above endpoints occurs. The drug is hepatically metabolized and renally excreted, with the half-life ranging from 2 to 12 hours. Continuous telemetry must be monitored for at least 4 hours after the infusion. Longer monitoring is warranted in patients with hepatic dysfunction.

Class IV

Only the nonhydropyridine calcium channel blockers, verapamil and diltiazem, have electrophysiologic effects and fall within this class. These medications slow phase 4 conduction and decrease conduction velocities in the SA and AV nodes. They also have antiadrenergic properties. Thus, overall, they behave similarly to β-blockers. They are very effective at slowing the ventricular response in atrial fibrillation or atrial flutter. Verapamil and diltiazem can shorten the plateau phase of the ventricular action potential and thus decrease early afterdepolarizations, which may help reduce torsade de pointes in certain circumstances.

Indications. The major use of the calcium channel blockers is for the treatment of atrial arrhythmias.[78] Both IV diltiazem and verapamil are effective in decreasing the ventricular response of atrial fibrillation and atrial flutter. They can also suppress forms of supraventricular tachycardia, particularly AV nodal tachycardia. As with other AV nodal blockers, they should not be used in patients with Wolff-Parkinson-White syndrome.

There are specific forms of ventricular tachycardia that are particularly sensitive to calcium channel blockers. Right ventricular outflow tract tachycardia and familial catecholaminergic polymorphic ventricular tachycardia can be treated with calcium channel blockers as well as β-blockers.

Electrocardiographic Effects. For patients in sinus rhythm, calcium channel blockers slow the sinus rate and can lead to bradycardia. They can also cause PR prolongation. Like β-blockers, they do not change the QRS or QT duration.

Side Effects. Both diltiazem and verapamil can cause hypotension, particularly in the IV forms. They both can cause flushing due to the vasodilator effects. They should be used with caution in conjunction with other drugs that have similar electrophysiologic effects, particularly β-blockers and digoxin. It should be noted that verapamil has several very important drug interactions. It cannot be used with dofetilide, as verapamil affects the renal clearance of that drug and can lead to severe QT prolongation. It also can interact with amiodarone and cause profound bradycardia. Calcium channel blockers have not been shown to be beneficial for patients with coronary artery disease or heart failure. Thus, when rate control medications are needed, β-blockers are preferable to calcium channel blockers in the CICU.

Administration. In the critical care setting, verapamil and diltiazem are often given in the IV form, as they both undergo significant first-pass elimination. Verapamil can be loaded at 5 to 20 mg over several minutes. A maintenance infusion at 0.005 mg/kg per minute is given when patients are unable to take oral medications. Diltiazem can be loaded with a 20-mg bolus. Repeated boluses can be given as well as maintenance infusions.

Atypical Antidysrhythmics (Class V)

Digoxin. Digoxin is a cardiac glycoside and one of the oldest antidysrhythmic medications available. It has many electrophysiologic effects; the most important ones are autonomic, increasing parasympathetic and decreasing sympathetic activity.[79] It also decreases automaticity in the SA node and increases refractoriness of the AV node.

Indications. The only remaining indication for digoxin is as a second-line agent for rate control of atrial fibrillation or atrial flutter. As digoxin exerts most of its influence autonomically, its effectiveness in the critical care setting when patients are under stress is reduced. It should never be used as sole therapy for rate control but rather as an additional medication when β-blockers and calcium channel blockers are not completely effective. Digoxin does not cause hypotension, which can make it useful as an additional medication when increasing the dose of β-blockers or calcium channel blockers is limited by hypotension. Digoxin was used in the past for heart failure due to its ability to improve contractility via inhibition of Na^+/K^+-ATPase, increasing intracellular calcium. It has now fallen out of favor owing to the clinical data demonstrating little beneficial effect with increases in mortality.[80]

Electrocardiographic effects. At nontoxic doses, digoxin does not exert obvious effects on the sinus rate, PR interval, QRS duration, or QT interval. Patients treated with digoxin often develop downsloping of the ST segment, which is known as "digoxin effect." At toxic doses, patients can have a variety of arrhythmias, including AV block, atrial tachycardias, junctional tachycardias, and bidirectional ventricular tachycardia.

Side effects. At therapeutic levels, digoxin does not have many side effects. However, clearance is substantially affected by renal function and patients can become toxic easily, with changes in renal function, which is common in acutely ill patients. Elderly patients are particularly prone to toxicity. Low serum potassium levels increase the risks of toxicity as digoxin competes with potassium for the binding site on Na^+/K^+-ATPase. At toxic levels, digoxin causes a wide variety of noncardiac side effects, including nausea, vomiting, headaches, and visual disturbances.

Digoxin toxicity can cause a variety of arrhythmias. Classically, patients will develop automatic rhythms (atrial tachycardia or junctional tachycardia) with high-grade AV block. Bidirectional ventricular tachycardia is less common but is considered pathognomonic for digoxin toxicity.

Digoxin has a variety of drug interactions. One of the most important is the interaction with amiodarone. Patients who are receiving amiodarone to convert atrial fibrillation to sinus rhythm may also be receiving medications for rate control. Digoxin is a substrate for the P-glycoprotein system, of which amiodarone is a potent inhibitor. Administration of digoxin and amiodarone together can increase digoxin levels dramatically by increasing bioavailability and decreasing clearance.

Treatment of digoxin toxicity is urgent. The medication should be stopped and electrolyte levels corrected, though pseudohyperkalemia may develop due to potassium displacement from the myocytes. The only exception to this is the administration of calcium, which should be avoided as it can precipitate arrhythmias due to the Na^+/K^+-ATPase blockade. In urgent settings, the digoxin immune FAB antibody can be administered.[81] Owing to protein binding, digoxin is not removed by dialysis.

Administration. Digoxin dosing must take into consideration that it is principally excreted via the kidney. Thus, renal insufficiency places patients at increased risk for digoxin toxicity through reductions in both volume of distribution and clearance, requiring doses to be lowered. Regular monitoring of digoxin levels is important for preventing toxicity. In general, serum digoxin concentrations should be less than 2.0 ng/mL. For patients with heart failure, they should be less than 1.0 ng/mL.

If rapid effects are needed, digoxin can be loaded IV. Up to 1 mg can be infused in divided doses over 24 hours. Patients with renal insufficiency should receive reduced loading doses depending on the severity of the renal dysfunction. Due to the relatively long distribution time, the recommended dosing strategy is 50% of the total loading dose followed by 25% for the subsequent two doses, spaced 6 hours apart. Oral maintenance doses should be 0.125 mg or 0.25 mg daily, depending upon the renal function. However, for patients who are unable to take oral medications, IV digoxin can be given but at reduced doses, as the oral form has only 60% to 80% bioavailability.

Adenosine. Adenosine is an endogenous nucleoside found in most tissues of the body. It affects potassium and calcium channels via α_1 and α_2 receptors, in addition to G proteins. The half-life is only seconds, and the primary activity is the outward potassium current (I_{KAdo}) found in atrial tissue.[82] It inhibits the I_f channel, which decreases sodium influx in the SA and AV nodes, resulting in a negative chronotropic effect. Adenosine has indirect antiadrenergic effects, which may be important to its antidysrhythmic properties. It slows automaticity and conduction in the SA and AV nodes.

Indications. The primary indication of adenosine is for the termination of supraventricular tachycardias that depend on the AV node for a reentrant circuit. This would include AV nodal reentrant tachycardia and AV reentrant tachycardia. Adenosine should be used in caution in patients with AV reentrant tachycardia in the setting of known Wolff-Parkinson-White syndrome, as it can induce atrial fibrillation, which can be life threatening in rapid conduction down the accessory pathway.

Adenosine can terminate some atrial tachycardias due to its effects in atrial tissue. It is thought that about 10% of atrial tachycardias may be adenosine responsive. Right ventricular outflow tract tachycardia may be adenosine responsive as well.[83]

Adenosine can also be used for diagnostic purposes when the diagnosis of atrial flutter or atrial fibrillation is unclear. For these rhythms, the AV node blocks and the absence of QRS complexes allow for evaluation of the underlying atrial waveforms, particularly the presence or absence of flutter waves. Adenosine is sometimes used to attempt to differentiate ventricular tachycardia from supraventricular tachycardia with aberrancy. This is generally not recommended, as it can be misleading and unsafe in the setting of ventricular tachycardia in which expert ECG interpretation should provide the diagnosis.

Electrocardiographic effects. Adenosine causes transient AV block. This leads to termination of AV nodal–dependent reentrant arrhythmias or slowing of the ventricular response in atrial fibrillation or atrial flutter.

Side effects. The extremely short half-life of adenosine makes the possibility of side effects very limited.[84] From a noncardiac standpoint, adenosine can cause facial flushing and chest pain as a result of the vasodilator effects. It can also cause bronchospasm in patients who are prone to reactive airways. The shortening of the refractory period in the atrium and ventricle puts patients at risk for premature contractions. There is approximately a 10% chance of inducing atrial fibrillation with adenosine administration.[85]

Administration. Adenosine needs to be given as a rapid IV bolus in order to be effective. This is due to the extremely rapid red blood cell metabolism of the drug. Preferably, it should be given via a central venous IV. Doses of 6 to 12 mg can be given as a rapid IV push followed by a saline flush. If no evidence of AV nodal blockade is seen, another larger bolus, up to 18 mg, can be given. The half-life is so short that repeat doses can be given within 30 seconds. Caution should be used in heart transplant patients, in whom the drug is more likely to cause prolonged block.

CONCLUSION

Antidysrhythmic medications are the mainstay of arrhythmia management for patients in the CICU setting. While these drugs are vital for arrhythmia treatment, they have a variety of side effects and drug interactions and are often incompletely effective. Until new drugs are developed, we must continue to rely on these currently available medications. An understanding of mechanisms of of action, metabolism, and possible side effects of currently available antidysrhythmic medications will allow clinicians to provide patients with targeted therapy to minimize toxicity and maximize therapeutic benefit.

The full reference list for this chapter is available at ExpertConsult.com.

40

Analgesics, Tranquilizers, and Sedatives

Bryan Simmons, Alexander Kuo

OUTLINE

Analgesics, tranquilizers, and sedatives are among the most commonly prescribed medications in the intensive care unit (ICU) and are frequently used for the management of pain, agitation, and delirium. These medications are not benign; as the patient population becomes older with more comorbidities, the management of these drugs can profoundly impact patient outcomes in the cardiac ICU (CICU). Thus it is important for the cardiac intensivist to be familiar with not only these medications but also with the management of pain, agitation, and delirium in an ICU setting. Very few studies have specifically evaluated the management of pain, agitation, and delirium in the CICU patient population. Instead, clinical decision making is based upon extrapolation of data from surgical and medical ICU patients.

This chapter reviews the general concepts in assessing and treating pain, agitation, and delirium in the ICU. The most commonly used and validated assessment tools for pain, agitation, and delirium are presented. Finally, the most common analgesics and sedatives available for use in the critical care setting are described, with special attention paid to those drugs of greatest usefulness in the CICU. Mechanisms of action, pharmacodynamics, pharmacokinetics, and clinical uses of these agents are addressed.

PAIN MANAGEMENT

The International Association for the Study of Pain (IASP) defines pain as "an unpleasant sensory and emotional experience associated with actual or potential tissue damage, or described in terms of such damage."[1] Pain is very common in the ICU, with roughly 50% of medical and surgical ICU patients experiencing moderate to severe pain during their ICU course.[2] Undesirable short-term consequences of pain include catecholamine-induced vasoconstriction, increased oxygen consumption, and a neurohormonal response leading to impaired healing and catabolism.[3,4] Poorly treated acute pain can lead to long-term consequences, such as posttraumatic stress disorder and chronic pain.[5] Thus adequate pain control is a vital aspect in the care of the CICU patient.

Routine assessment of pain has been associated with improved outcomes in critical care patients, including decreased duration of both the ICU stay and mechanical ventilation.[6] The gold standard of pain assessment remains self-reported pain. Reporting and quantifying of pain can be aided with tools such as the visual analog scale (VAS), a continuous graphic line anchored by endpoints labeled *no pain* and *extreme pain*.[7] Patients quantify their pain by pointing to a location on this line. With intubated patients unable to self-report pain, psychometric pain assessment tools can be employed. The two most validated methods are the Behavioral Pain Scale (BPS) and the Critical-Care Pain Observation Scale (CPOT). BPS is a 12-point scale based upon three items: compliance with mechanical ventilation, movement of the upper extremities, and facial expressions.[8] Originally validated in postoperative cardiac surgery patients, CPOT is an 8-point system based upon four items: facial expressions, body movements, muscle tension, and compliance with the ventilator.[9] It is important to emphasize that vital signs (tachycardia, hypertension) alone offer a poor assessment of pain in the ICU patient population.

For the treatment of pain in critical care patients, a few general concepts should be kept in mind. First, pain should be anticipated with certain activities, such as bedside procedures, and should be treated preemptively. Second, pain is a common cause of agitation and delirium in ICU patients. Thus, pain should be suspected, evaluated, and treated prior to administration of sedatives in delirious and agitated patients, a practice known as an *analgesia first approach*. Finally, while the mainstay of pain management in the ICU remains opioid analgesics, a multimodal approach to analgesia has the potential to reduce opioid requirements and their side effects.

Opioids

Receptor Physiology. Opioid receptors are found throughout the peripheral and central nervous system as well as pituitary, adrenal, and immune cells.[10] In the central nervous system, there are three main types of opioid receptors: mu (μ), delta (δ), and kappa (κ), each with subtypes resulting from posttranslational modifications. Ultimately, binding of an agonist to the opioid receptor results in hyperpolarization of the neuron and decreased action potential propagation. The highest density of receptors is in the substantia gelatinosa of the cerebral cortex and spinal cord, periaqueductal gray areas, thalamus, and hippocampus.[11] Of these areas, laminae II through V of the substantia gelatinosa and the periaqueductal gray areas appear to have the highest concentration of μ-receptors and have the greatest impact on analgesia.

Morphine. Morphine is the prototypic opiate agent. It has traditionally been used as the primary analgesic in the management of acute myocardial ischemia and for sedation in patients with underlying myocardial disease.[12] Morphine has an onset time of action of 5 to 10 minutes and has a terminal elimination half-life ($t_{1/2\beta}$) between 2 and 4.5 hours.[13,14] Morphine is unique compared with other commonly used opioid agents in that it has relatively low lipid solubility (Table 40.1). This results in lower penetration across the blood-brain barrier and significantly slower time to peak effect (20 to 30 minutes).

Morphine is metabolized by both the liver and the kidneys. Although the liver is responsible for the majority of its metabolism, 40% is metabolized by the kidneys.[15] Owing to the high hepatic extraction ratio, morphine clearance can be significantly reduced in patients with shock or reduced hepatic blood flow.[16] Morphine-3-glucuronide is the major metabolite, but it possesses much less opiate activity and has significant neuroexcitatory properties.[17] In contrast, morphine-6-glucuronide accounts for roughly 10% of morphine metabolism and is more potent than its parent compound.[18] In patients with renal failure, the accumulation of this metabolite can result in excess or prolonged respiratory depression. Thus morphine should be used with caution in patients with shock, renal failure, hepatic failure, or multiorgan dysfunction.

Morphine has distinct hemodynamic properties that make it advantageous in certain cardiac patients. Perhaps the most important of these is morphine's ability to decrease venous and arterial tone.[19,20] It appears that the increase in venous capacitance produced by morphine is relatively greater than the decrease in arterial resistance.[21] This effect on venous capacitance is dose related; large doses may result in hypotension.[22] In some cardiac patients, this modest decrease in preload is desirable. In the dosages commonly used in the critical care setting, morphine has no direct effect on the inotropic state of the heart.[23] However, morphine-induced histamine release resulting from rapid or large doses of morphine can induce a transient positive inotropic and chronotropic state. Overall, the net chronotropic effect of morphine is to slow the heart rate under normal conditions. The exact mechanism by which morphine achieves this action is not certain, but it is thought to involve both a stimulation of the central vagal nucleus and a direct depressive effect on the sinoatrial node.

Many of morphine's side effects are dose related and can be minimized by reducing the doses administered to patients. The most dangerous side effect of morphine is respiratory depression. All opiate agonists share the property of depressing ventilation; this is primarily accomplished by decreasing the central ventilatory response to carbon dioxide.[13] This respiratory suppression may

TABLE 40.1 Physicochemical and Pharmacokinetic Data of Commonly Used Opioid Agonists

	Morphine	Hydromorphone	Fentanyl	Remifentanil
pKa	8	8.9	8.4	7.1
Percent unionized at pH 7.4	23		<10	67
Octanol/H_2O partition coefficient	1.4	1.28	813	17.9
Percent bound to plasma protein	20–40	8–19	84	80
$t_{1/2\pi}$ (min)	1–2.5		1–2	0.5–1.5
$t_{1/2\alpha}$ (min)	10–20		10–30	5–8
$t_{1/2\beta}$ (hr)	2–4	2–3	2–4	0.7–1.2
V_{dcc} (L/kg)	0.1–0.4	0.03–0.43	0.5–1.0	0.06–0.08
V_{dss} (L/kg)	3–5	3–4	3–5	0.2–0.3
Clearance (L/min/kg)	15–30		10–20	30–40
Hepatic extraction ratio	0.8–1	0.5	0.8–1	NA

$t_{1/2\pi}$, first distribution half-life; $t_{1/2\alpha}$, second distribution half-life; $t_{1/2\beta}$, elimination half-life; V_{dcc}, volume of distribution at central compartment; V_{dss}, volume of distribution at steady state.

Modified from Bailey PL, Egan TD, Stanley TH. Narcotic intravenous anesthetics. In: Miller RD, ed. *Anesthesia*, 5th ed. New York: Churchill Livingstone; 2000:312.

lead to progressive hypercapnia, carbon dioxide narcosis, and obtundation with apnea. High-risk patients—such as those with morbid obesity, obstructive sleep apnea, or advanced age—should receive additional monitoring for signs of excessive sedation and respiratory compromise when receiving opioids.

The central nervous system side effects of morphine and all opiates include drowsiness, lethargy, and potentially excessive sedation. All opioids may cause or exacerbate delirium in the elderly population and other at-risk patients. In addition to the direct central respiratory depression described previously, excessive sedation with morphine can worsen respiratory compromise by causing upper airway obstruction and obstructive apnea. Euphoria with morphine has been noted but is less common than with other opioids. Dysphoria can also occur. As in respiratory depression, the central depressant effects are dose related and progressive.

The other organ systems most commonly affected by morphine (or any opioid) are the gastrointestinal (GI) and genitourinary (GU) systems. Morphine has many GI effects, including nausea, emesis, constipation, generalized slowing of the GI tract, and spasm of the sphincter of Oddi. Morphine has been reported to cause urinary retention by increasing urethral sphincter and detrusor tone.[24] Hyponatremia secondary to the syndrome of inappropriate secretion of antidiuretic hormone is occasionally seen with the administration of large doses of morphine.[25]

Morphine may cause the release of histamine, although true allergic reactions to morphine are quite rare.[26] The release of histamine is from mast cells rather than basophils; the mechanism is nonimmunologic but not thoroughly understood.[27] The release of histamine can lead to a flushing sensation, intense pruritus, hypotension, and tachycardia. When histamine-related hypotension occurs, treatment includes discontinuing morphine, ruling out other causes of anaphylactic or anaphylactoid type of reactions, administering intravenous fluids for hypotension, and administering histamine type 1 and type 2 blocking agents.[13]

The main reason to administer intravenous morphine in the CICU is to produce analgesia and sedation, especially in the setting of acute myocardial ischemia or acute cardiogenic pulmonary edema. The acute venodilatory effects of intravenous morphine, combined with its analgesic and sedative properties, make it useful in cardiac patients. In contrast to fentanyl, morphine—with its long clinical duration and low lipid solubility—is best suited to administration by intermittent boluses rather than continuous infusion. Morphine may best be avoided in the hemodynamically unstable patient because it is more likely to induce hypotension than other opiates and in patients with multiorgan dysfunction owing to the risk of an excessively prolonged effect.

Hydromorphone. Hydromorphone is a semisynthetic opioid that was introduced into clinical practice in 1926.[17] Structurally very similar to morphine, hydromorphone is a hydrogenated ketone derivative of morphine; however, it is roughly 8 times more potent. Following intravenous administration, the onset of action is roughly 5 minutes, with maximal effect achieved at 20 minutes. Although it is still very water soluble, it is more fat soluble than morphine, resulting in a slightly faster onset of action and peak effect when compared to morphine. The analgesic effect of parenterally administered hydromorphone lasts roughly 3 to 4 hours in the absence of liver and renal failure. Hydromorphone is metabolized primarily in the liver to hydromorphone-3-glucuronide (H3G) and dihydroisomorphine glucuronide. Like morphine-3-glucuronide, H3G has neuroexcitatory properties. However, unlike morphine, hydromorphone does not have active metabolites, making it safer to use in patients with renal dysfunction.

The cardiovascular and hemodynamic effects of hydromorphone are not as well studied as morphine and fentanyl. However, it has proven to be hemodynamically well tolerated and is a common alternative to morphine for pain control in the ICU. Given its long duration of action and lack of metabolites, hydromorphone is suited for both intermittent bolus and continuous infusion. Unlike morphine, hydromorphone is not associated with histamine release and may have a lower frequency of nausea. The side effect profile is otherwise very similar to that of morphine, including respiratory depression, impairment of mental status, constipation, or general slowing of the GI tract.

Fentanyl. Fentanyl and remifentanil are members of the phenylpiperidine class of opiate agents.[13] In terms of analgesic properties, fentanyl is approximately 80 times more potent than morphine because of its greater affinity for the μ-opiate receptor.[15] For many years, fentanyl has been used extensively for procedural sedation and in the operating room owing to its high potency, rapid onset, and short initial duration of action. Owing to these properties, it is now commonly used as an analgesic and sedative in the critical care setting.

Although fentanyl has similar elimination kinetics to morphine, fentanyl is approximately 40 times more lipid soluble than morphine, leading to significant differences in clinical effects.[13,15] Its high lipid solubility allows rapid entry across the blood–brain barrier, resulting in a rapid onset and peak effect within minutes of intravenous administration. This also allows rapid redistribution away from the brain to inactive organ groups, such as muscle and adipose tissue. The redistribution is responsible for fentanyl's short clinical duration of action in bolus form. This rapid onset and brief clinical effect make it useful for procedural analgesia in the ICU. These pharmacokinetic properties also make fentanyl more suitable for continuous infusion than morphine. In addition, the dose can be easily titrated.

After prolonged infusions, fentanyl's duration of action becomes significantly prolonged. The actual $t_{1/2\beta}$ of fentanyl is similar to morphine at 2 to 4.5 hours.[15] As the total cumulative dose of fentanyl increases, the inactive tissues become saturated and the duration of fentanyl's clinical effects becomes progressively longer as the drug clearance then depends upon the much longer $t_{1/2\beta}$. This concept is known as *context-sensitive half-time*, in which the half-time of the drug's clinical effects depend upon the context of total duration of infusion. Fentanyl is metabolized primarily by the liver and to a lesser degree by the kidney without active metabolites of clinical significance.

When used in analgesic doses, fentanyl has minimal direct hemodynamic effects and no direct inotropic effects.[28,29] However, fentanyl can cause hypotension through dose-dependent bradycardia thought to reflect direct stimulation of the central vagal nucleus by fentanyl.[30] Fentanyl can cause hypotension indirectly by decreasing central sympathetic outflow.[31] This effect is supported by the observation that patients with high basal levels of sympathetic tone, especially when they are hypervolemic, are more likely to become hypotensive when given fentanyl.[13] It is important to note that the combination of synthetic opioids and benzodiazepines, especially midazolam, can cause significant decreases in blood pressure.[32]

The side effect and toxicity profile of fentanyl are similar to morphine, with several exceptions. The pharmacokinetic properties of fentanyl can result in rapid apnea and oversedation if not used with caution; therefore this drug should be used only in a monitored setting. Fentanyl does not release histamine from mast cells in humans.[33] It has been rarely reported to cause true anaphylactic reactions.[13]

Few studies have formally addressed the role of fentanyl in the CICU. In comparison to morphine, fentanyl does not have the same vasodilatory effects that may be beneficial in the setting of myocardial ischemia or acute cardiogenic pulmonary edema. However, fentanyl's rapid kinetics, neutral hemodynamic profile, and lack of active metabolites make it useful for procedural analgesia and a better choice in patients with organ dysfunction or hemodynamic instability.

Remifentanil. Remifentanil is chemically related to fentanyl and possesses similar pharmacodynamic properties with a rapid onset of action but is slightly more potent than fentanyl. Remifentanil is unique in that its metabolism is independent of organ function. Instead, remifentanil is metabolized by nonspecific plasma esterases located primarily within erythrocytes.[34] The primary metabolite is a carboxylic acid derivative with no opiate activity that is eventually excreted in the urine. The widespread metabolism of remifentanil results in a rapid clearance with a $t_{1/2\beta}$ of 9 minutes. In addition, the context-sensitive half-time remains short, even following prolonged infusions.[35] For example, following infusion of remifentanil for over 8 hours, the context-sensitive half-time remains roughly 3 minutes. In comparison, a 3-hour infusion of fentanyl has a context-sensitive half-time of 180 minutes.[36] Thus the effects of remifentanil will subside very quickly, even after a prolonged infusion.

Remifentanil has vagotonic and sympatholytic effects, leading to bradycardia and hypotension, particularly with bolus administration.[34] The use of remifentanil infusions in cardiac surgical patients provides better control of the hemodynamic response to painful stimuli but results in a greater requirement for vasopressor support and a longer time to extubation attributed to a problematic transition to a stable pain regimen in the periextubation period.[37,38] Like all opioids, other side effects of remifentanil include apnea, respiratory depression, and muscle rigidity, all of which can occur quickly with bolus administration. Nausea, vomiting, and pruritus are also common side effects. Remifentanil is not known to cause histamine release and rarely causes allergic reactions. As with all opioids, the side effects are reversible with opioid antagonists.

Opioid Antagonists

The effects of opioids are rapidly reversed with the use of an opioid antagonist. The most commonly used is naloxone, which can achieve full reversal with 0.4 to 2 mg administered intravenously, intranasally or intramuscularly. However, the elimination half-life of naloxone, approximately 1 hour, is shorter than commonly used opioids. Thus redosing or a continuous infusion of naloxone and close monitoring may be required to prevent recurrence of respiratory depression. Caution must be used when administering opioid reversal, as it can precipitate acute opiate withdrawal, extreme pain, and a dangerous increase in sympathetic tone, especially in patients on chronic or high-dose opioids. In nonemergent situations, it is prudent to titrate small divided doses of 0.02 to 0.04 mg for a more controlled opioid reversal.

Opioid-induced constipation can be safely treated in the ICU with enteral naloxone or a selective peripheral μ-opioid antagonist, such as enteral naloxegol, alvimopan, or subcutaneous methylnaltrexone.[39] Enteral naloxone has low risk of analgesia reversal due to its poor systemic bioavailability resulting from its high first-pass hepatic metabolism, although patients on high doses of opioids are still at risk.[40,41] Typical dosing of enteral naloxone is 0.4 to 4 mg repeated 3 to 4 times daily.

Ketamine. Ketamine is a phencyclidine derivative that primarily acts as a noncompetitive antagonist to N-methyl-D-aspartate (NMDA) receptors but also has activity at other receptors, including opiate receptors. It was initially developed as a "dissociative anesthetic" owing to its psychomimetic effects and combined properties of analgesia, amnesia, and hypnosis. Owing to emergence delirium and dysphoria, it is no longer commonly used as a primary anesthetic. Because of its unique properties, however, it is finding increasing popularity as an adjunct for pain and sedation.

Ketamine is water soluble at the pH of intravenous preparations but becomes highly lipid soluble in the bloodstream, resulting in a rapid onset of effect within 1 minute of intravenous administration. Like fentanyl, ketamine has a rapid initial redistribution half-life ($t_{1/2\alpha}$) of 7 minutes and a longer $t_{1/2\beta}$ of 2 to 4 hours. Metabolism is predominantly hepatic via the cytochrome P450 system, in which ketamine is converted into its active metabolite, norketamine. It is then hydroxylated and conjugated to more water-soluble metabolites that are excreted in the urine. Due to its high hepatic extraction ratio and active metabolites, ketamine's effects can be prolonged in patients with hepatic or renal failure or when concomitant drugs cause inhibition of the P450 enzyme system. Clinically, ketamine's rapid redistribution to inactive tissues accounts for its short duration of clinical action in bolus form, approximately 10 minutes. With increasing total cumulative doses, peripheral tissue becomes saturated and the clinical effect becomes significantly prolonged.[42,43]

In subanesthetic doses, ketamine provides opiate-sparing analgesic effects. Unlike opiates, ketamine may preserve airway reflexes and is less likely to depress respiratory drive. Ketamine does not cause slowing of the GI tract. Ketamine can also cause increased salivation and relaxation of bronchial smooth muscle tone. Hemodynamically, ketamine is a sympathomimetic, resulting in increased heart rate, blood pressure, and cardiac output in healthy patients but may also be a direct cardiac depressant. In one randomized controlled study of critically ill patients, ketamine used in emergent tracheal intubation did not cause hemodynamic instability compared to etomidate.[43] This unique sympathomimetic property may be desirable in some CICU patients and best avoided in others depending upon their cardiovascular pathology.

Ketamine causes disassociate anesthesia in high doses and a psychomimetic effect and analgesia at lower doses. Common side effects at sedative and analgesic doses are vivid dreams, hallucinations, and dysphoria. Side effects are generally dose dependent. Ketamine has both proconvulsant and anticonvulsant properties, with anticonvulsant effects generally predominating.[44]

Clinically, adjunctive pain dosing for nonintubated patients is 0.1 to 0.5 mg/kg per hour. Owing to ketamine's unique combination of sedative and analgesic effects with preservation of respiratory reflexes and a stable hemodynamic profile, it is also an effective procedural analgesic when used in divided doses of less than 1 mg/kg. For this use, it is often combined with midazolam to ameliorate its potentially unpleasant psychomimetic effects. Caution must still be used because ketamine may have a synergistic sedative effect with other agents. Nevertheless, because of these beneficial properties compared to opiates, ketamine is finding increasing use in the critical care population as an analgesic adjuvant and an analgosedative.

Other Nonopioid Analgesics

The use of nonopioid analgesics is recommended in the ICU population to decrease the amounts of opiates administered and their associated side effects.[45] Commonly used nonopioid analgesics in the ICU include nonsteroidal antiinflammatory agents (NSAIDs), acetaminophen, and neuropathic pain medications, such as gabapentin and carbamazepine.

NSAIDs produce analgesia primarily by decreasing tissue inflammation in the periphery by inhibiting cyclooxygenase (COX), an enzyme responsible for the formation of prostaglandin. Prostaglandins are important mediators of tissue inflammation, nociceptive signal initiation, and peripheral sensitization. Two main isoforms of COX exist: the constitutively expressed COX-1 is responsible for platelet aggregation and maintaining gastric mucosal protection; the inducible COX-2 enzyme mediates inflammation, fever, and pain.[48] Selective COX-2 inhibitors, such as celecoxib, do not affect platelet aggregation or gastric mucosal protection. However, they may be associated with an increase in cardiovascular thrombotic events, including myocardial infarction (MI).[46] NSAIDs have also been associated with an increased risk of heart failure in patients with preexisting heart failure.[47] Other side effects include platelet inhibition (nonselective COX inhibitors) and renovascular vasoconstriction that may increase the risk of renal injury. Avoiding NSAIDs is recommended in patients at risk of heart failure, MI, or renal failure. All NSAIDs are metabolized by the liver and excreted by the kidneys.

Although the mechanism is not fully understood, acetaminophen also seems to be a COX inhibitor. However, it acts primarily within the central nervous system, with very little peripheral antiinflammatory activity. It is nonetheless an effective analgesic and antipyretic. Acetaminophen undergoes hepatic metabolism to N-acetyl-p-benzoquinone imine, which in sufficient doses can cause hepatic failure. If used within recommended doses, acetaminophen is well tolerated in CICU patients.

Many CICU patients may suffer from neuropathic pain that is commonly the result of diabetic neuropathy. In such patients, gabapentin or carbamazepine may be beneficial as an adjunct to opioids. Gabapentin is an anticonvulsant that inhibits voltage-gated calcium channels; it is shown to be a useful adjunct in treatment of peripheral neuropathies. Side effects are generally well tolerated and include dizziness, mild sedation, and nausea. Carbamazepine is also an anticonvulsant that acts as a sodium channel blocker. It has been shown to be effective in neuropathic pain conditions, particularly trigeminal neuralgia. However, it does have significant side effects, including cardiac dysrhythmias, heart failure, dizziness, nausea, and somnolence.

AGITATION AND SEDATION MANAGEMENT

Agitation and anxiety are common among CICU patients and can impede recovery.[48] Poorly controlled agitation can lead to undesirable stress and resulting complications. Appropriate pharmacologic management of agitation allows for patients to safely tolerate routine care and procedures in the ICU.[49] The evidence is clear that oversedation of ICU patients results in negative outcomes.[50-52] Periodic assessment of agitation and sedation is a prerequisite for their appropriate management.

Several assessment tools have been developed to monitor the depth of sedation in critically ill patients. The most widely used and validated methods are the Sedation-Agitation Scale (SAS) and the Richmond Agitation-Sedation Scale (RASS).[45] The SAS was originally developed in a study evaluating haloperidol use for sedation in agitated, critically ill patients.[53] It was subsequently validated in a variety of ICU settings, including cardiac patients.[54-57] The SAS is a 7-point numerical scale that describes the level of sedation on a continuum from unarousable (1) to dangerously agitated (7), with calm and cooperative patients given a 4. Similarly, the RASS is a 10-point scale that describes the level of agitation or sedation on a continuum ranging from −5 to +4 (Table 40.2).[58] There are four levels of agitation (+4 combative to +1 restless), one level corresponding to calm and cooperative (0 calm) and five levels of sedation (−1 drowsy to −5 unarousable). The RASS has also been validated in multiple settings, including cardiac surgical and CICU patients.[55,58-60] Both the SAS and RASS have proven to have great interrater reliability and correlate with the processed electroencephalogram (EEG) bispectral index values of sedation.[55]

There are a few concepts central to management of agitation and administration of sedatives in an ICU setting. First, underlying identifiable and treatable causes such as hypoglycemia, hypoxia, pain, underlying psychiatric disorders, or delirium should be addressed and treated before resorting to sedative medications. This frequently results in the administration of analgesics prior to other sedatives (*analgesic-first approach*). In fact, one study demonstrated that completely avoiding

TABLE 40.2 Richmond Agitation-Sedation Scale (RASS)

Score	Description	
+4	Combative	Violent, immediate danger to self or others
+3	Very agitated	Removes catheters, tubes, and more or is aggressive toward others
+2	Agitated	Nonpurposeful movement; ventilator dyssynchrony
+1	Restless	Anxious, but not aggressive
0	Alert and calm	
−1	Drowsy	Sustained (>10 seconds) awakening with eye contact to voice
−2	Light sedation	Briefly (<10 seconds) awakens with eye contact to voice
−3	Moderate sedation	Movement without eye contact to voice
−4	Deep sedation	No response to voice, movement to physical stimuli
−5	Unarousable	No response to verbal or physical stimuli

Modified from Sessler CN, Gosnell MS, Grap MJ, et al. The Richmond Agitation-Sedation Scale: validity and reliability in adult intensive care unit patients. *Am J Respir Crit Care Med* 2002;166:1338–1344.

TABLE 40.3 Physicochemical Characterization of Three Benzodiazepines

	Diazepam	Lorazepam	Midazolam
Molecular weight	284.7	321.2	362
pKa	3.3 (20°C)	11.5 (20°C)	6.2 (20°C)
Water soluble	No[a]	Almost insoluble	Yes[a]
Lipid soluble	Yes,[a] highly lipophilic	Yes, relatively less lipophilic	Yes,[a] highly lipophilic

Modified from Sasajima M. Analgesic effect of morphine-3-glucuronide. *Keio Ogaka.* 1970;47:421.
[a]pH dependent: pH >4 = lipid soluble, pH <4 = water soluble.

sedatives while controlling pain with morphine and delirium with haloperidol resulted in an increased number of mechanical ventilation-free days.[61]

Numerous studies have demonstrated that prolonged and deep sedation leads to worse outcomes, including an increased duration of mechanical ventilation and ICU length of stay.[50,51] For mechanically ventilated and sedated patients, this has led to the practice of daily awakening trials in which sedation is held to allow patients to "wake up" for a period of time.[52] Awakening trials have been shown to decrease the amount of sedatives administered as well as the length of ICU stay and the duration of mechanical ventilation. It was subsequently shown that when daily awakening trials are performed in conjunction with spontaneous breathing trials (SBTs), there is not only a reduction in duration of mechanical ventilation and ICU stay but also a reduction in hospital length of stay and 12-month mortality.[62] It is now generally accepted that maintaining lighter levels of sedation (RASS 0 to −1), when possible, is ideal for most ICU patients. In doing so, there is no additional benefit of daily sedation interruption.[63] While maintaining lighter levels of sedation may be associated with an increased stress response, this has not translated to an increased risk of adverse physiologic consequences, such as myocardial ischemia.[64,65] Nonetheless, many CICU patients are at high risk for such events; thus the appropriate level of sedation should be considered for each patient individually.

Finally, the choice of sedative remains controversial. When compared to a nonbenzodiazepine, there is evidence to suggest that benzodiazepine-based sedation is associated with an increased ICU length of stay, possibly an increased duration of mechanical ventilation, and an increased incidence of delirium.[66–69] However, there does not seem to be any mortality benefit of

a benzodiazepine versus nonbenzodiazepine regimen.[66,67,69–70] Dexmedetomidine may offer benefit over other medications in patients with delirium. A few trials have shown a reduction in delirium when a dexmedetomidine-based sedation regimen is used when compared to a benzodiazepine-base regimen.[66,67] These results suggest that either benzodiazepines are deliriogenic or dexmedetomidine is effective in preventing or treating delirium.

Benzodiazepines

Historically, benzodiazepines were the most commonly used sedative agents in the ICU, having been in use for several decades. The benzodiazepines are small, lipid-soluble molecules that act as agonists at the benzodiazepine (BNZ) receptor.[71] The BNZ receptor is part of the larger γ-aminobutyric acid (GABA) receptor complex in which other drugs, such as barbiturates, also act.[72] GABA is one of the primary inhibitory neurotransmitters of the human central nervous system. Activation of the GABA receptor complex causes a net influx of chloride ions into the cell, resulting in hyperpolarization and resistance to excitation.[73] There are two main GABA receptors in the central nervous system: the GABAa complex and the GABAb complex. The benzodiazepines have their main activity at the GABAa complex.[14] The binding of a benzodiazepine to its receptor results in a conformation change of the GABAa receptor complex that facilitates binding of the neurotransmitter GABA.[71] Benzodiazepine receptors are found in greatest concentration in the olfactory bulb, cerebral cortex, cerebellum, hippocampus, substantia nigra, and inferior colliculus.[71]

In the United States, the three benzodiazepines most commonly used in the CICU are diazepam, lorazepam, and midazolam. Although these agents work similarly at the receptor level, they are quite different with respect to their pharmacology and physical properties (Table 40.3). Midazolam is roughly three times more potent than diazepam, whereas lorazepam is five times more potent than diazepam.[71] In general, all three compounds are highly lipid soluble but lorazepam is less so than diazepam or midazolam.[74] The onset of peak clinical activity is similar for all three on the order of a few minutes; the slightly slower onset of lorazepam is related to its lower lipid solubility. However, the $t_{1/2\beta}$ is quite different among these three drugs. Midazolam has a relatively short half-life of 2 to 3 hours, lorazepam has an intermediate half-life of 10 to 20 hours, and diazepam has a long half-life of 20 to 50 hours.[71]

The benzodiazepines are metabolized in the liver where the parent compounds undergo extensive biotransformation. Diazepam undergoes biotransformation to a number of products, two of which (oxazepam and desmethyldiazepam) are potent and long-acting BNZ receptor agonists. These metabolites result in the prolonged sedative effect seen with diazepam.[14] Lorazepam is also highly metabolized, but its metabolites are rapidly excreted by the kidneys and none have significant clinical activity.[75] Midazolam is biotransformed to compounds known as hydroxymidazolams, but controversy exists regarding whether these compounds have any benzodiazepine activity.[76] Several studies in elderly patients and the critically ill have shown prolongation of midazolam's $t_{1/2\beta}$ and its sedative effect.[77,78] This is caused by several factors, including increased volume of distribution and extensive fatty tissue uptake after prolonged infusion. One study investigating the effect of prolonged midazolam infusions in critically ill patients found that the mean time from administration to awakening in patients with renal failure was approximately 44 hours (control, 13 hours). The time to awakening in two patients with renal and hepatic failure was greater than 120 hours.[79] Although these same factors could affect lorazepam, its lower lipid solubility and inactive metabolites appear to make it less likely to cause prolonged sedation.[14]

With respect to hemodynamics, the benzodiazepines have a reputation for safety in patients with cardiac disease, especially coronary artery disease.[80,81] When administered alone, the benzodiazepines cause a mild decrease in arterial blood pressure that is related to a decrease in systemic vascular resistance, with other cardiac indices only minimally affected.[71] Notably, midazolam has more of a blood pressure–lowering effect than the other intravenous benzodiazepines.[82] The combination of benzodiazepines and opioids is synergistic in lowering blood pressure resulting from reduced central sympathetic tone.[83,84] Although the majority of these data are from the cardiac anesthesia literature, in which much higher doses are used, hypotension is still a concern in CICU patients, even when the doses are significantly lower.

Benzodiazepines have several uses in the CICU. Midazolam, lorazepam, and diazepam are all equally efficacious as anxiolytics and induce anterograde amnesia. All three are also effective as sedatives for mechanically ventilated patients but benzodiazepines do not have intrinsic analgesic properties. If painful procedures are anticipated, benzodiazepines should be used in conjunction with an opioid or other analgesics. All the benzodiazepines are effective when used for the acute termination of seizures. It is believed that lorazepam may be the drug of choice in the termination of status epilepticus because its longer half-life allows treatment with another longer-acting anticonvulsant to be begun before seizures can recur.[85,86] Benzodiazepines are also useful for the treatment of acute alcohol withdrawal and may be useful in the treatment of acute cocaine intoxication.[14]

Overall, benzodiazepines are very safe sedative agents, with high therapeutic indices and minimal hemodynamic effects.[14] The main side effects of benzodiazepines in the CICU population are excessive sedation and respiratory depression. Excessive sedation is a dose-related phenomenon that may lead to an inability to protect or maintain a patent airway in the nonintubated patient.

Benzodiazepines also cause central respiratory depression but to a much lesser degree than opiates. Benzodiazepines flatten the ventilatory response curve to hypercarbia but, unlike opioids, they do not shift the curve to the right.[71,87] Apnea can occur with benzodiazepines but it is usually related to the administration of large doses or upper airway obstruction from sedation. The combination of an opioid and benzodiazepine has a synergistic central respiratory depressive effect and results in a much higher risk of respiratory compromise.[71]

The sedative and respiratory side effects of benzodiazepines can be reversed by the BNZ receptor antagonist flumazenil,[88] but it must be used with caution. It has a relatively short elimination half-life compared with the longer-acting benzodiazepines; therefore, recurrent sedation may occur after the flumazenil effect has terminated.[71] Additionally, seizures and acute withdrawal symptoms have been reported in patients with chronic benzodiazepine tolerance treated with flumazenil.[89] Of note, flumazenil is not as effective at reversing the amnestic effects of the benzodiazepines as it is at reversing other side effects.[90]

Diazepam and lorazepam are water insoluble and therefore require vehicles for intravenous injection. Diazepam injection is prepared with propylene glycol, alcohol, and benzyl alcohol as vehicles; lorazepam is prepared with polyethylene glycol and benzyl alcohol vehicles.[71] These solvents are known to cause phlebitis with peripheral intravenous injection.[71] Midazolam has pH-dependent water solubility without the need for these additional intravenous carrier agents. Propylene glycol toxicity has been reported with high-dose intravenous diazepam administration and may also occur with lorazepam.

Recently, multiple studies have shown that prolonged administration of benzodiazepines to critically ill patients may increase the risk for the development of delirium.[91] Furthermore, plasma concentrations of benzodiazepines or other sedatives did not correlate well with sedation scores, suggesting that the effects of the drug are influenced by other factors, especially age. These reports should decrease enthusiasm for the use of benzodiazepines in critically ill elderly patients.

Propofol

Introduced into clinical practice in 1977, propofol is an alkylphenol that is water insoluble, necessitating a lipid carrier for intravenous administration. Propofol is a rapid-acting, highly lipid-soluble central nervous system depressant with hypnotic and amnestic properties. These properties are mediated primarily through the β-subunit of the GABAa receptor.[92] At low doses, propofol potentiates the effect of GABA on the GABAa receptor; at higher doses, propofol directly activates GABAa receptors.[93]

Propofol pharmacokinetics display a rapid $t_{1/2\alpha}$ of 2 to 8 minutes and a slower $t_{1/2\beta}$ of 1 to 3 hours.[94] Although propofol is lipophilic, a protracted period of sedation following discontinuation of prolonged infusions does not occur with propofol as it does with fentanyl and midazolam. A study using propofol for sedation in mechanically ventilated CICU patients demonstrated a rapid time to extubation and full recovery (1 and 2 hours, respectively) in patients receiving infusions of propofol.[95] This rather unique ability is related to its extremely high clearance, which is greater than liver blood flow.[94] Therefore, although propofol has high hepatic clearance, it appears that other routes of elimination exist to explain its short clinical duration of action. Respiratory elimination may be partially responsible for this phenomenon.[96]

Much of the data regarding the cardiovascular and hemodynamic effects of propofol have been generated in the setting of general anesthesia or sedation for surgery. The most prominent effect of propofol on hemodynamics is a decrease in arterial blood pressure.[97,98] This hypotension appears to be related to both peripheral vasodilation and possibly a negative inotropic effect.[71] Propofol infusions appear to decrease both myocardial blood flow and myocardial oxygen demand by roughly equal magnitudes.[71] Conflicting chronotropic responses have been reported in patients receiving propofol, including increases, decreases, or no change in heart rate.[99–101]

Propofol is a highly potent drug with a narrow therapeutic range. The most serious side effects are arterial hypotension and central apnea. If propofol is used in nonintubated patients, it can rapidly lead to apnea or airway obstruction. Other side effects of propofol include dystonic or choreiform movements not associated with abnormal EEG activity.[102] Pain at the injection site and phlebitis are well-known side effects that can be prevented by avoiding administration into small hand veins.[103] Because propofol is dissolved and administered in a lipid carrier, hypertriglyceridemia can occur with prolonged infusions or high doses, especially in the ICU setting. Rarely, this has been associated with acute pancreatitis.[104]

Propofol infusion syndrome (PRIS) is one of the most serious side effects of propofol. It is associated with metabolic acidosis, refractory heart failure, progressive and refractory bradycardia, fever, lipemia, increased creatine phosphokinase, myoglobinemia and myoglobinuria.[105] The maximum recommended dose from the manufacturer is 4 mg/kg per hour for adults; all reported cases of PRIS received doses higher than this recommended dose.[106] All practitioners are encouraged to adhere to the maximum limits suggested and to be watchful for signs of PRIS.

The two most common indications for propofol in the CICU have been sedation for elective electrical cardioversion and for mechanical ventilation.[107] A study comparing propofol, methohexital, and midazolam as sedatives for the elective electrical cardioversion of patients with supraventricular arrhythmias demonstrated that all three agents were efficacious but the time to awaken was more rapid in the propofol and methohexital groups.[108] Although hemodynamics were well maintained in this group of stable patients, it is prudent to avoid the use of propofol in the setting of cardioversion for hemodynamic instability because of propofol's known cardiovascular depressive effects.

There have been no randomized controlled studies specifically investigating the safety or efficacy of propofol for sedation in the CICU patient. There are, however, several studies addressing its use in the medical-surgical ICU and in the postoperative cardiac surgery patient.[109–118] The experience from these studies suggests that when propofol is used in sedative doses ranging between 5 and 50 μg/kg per minute (0.3 and 3 mg/kg per minute), there is excellent patient tolerance and minimal side effects.

In a study directly comparing propofol and midazolam for short-term sedation of mechanically ventilated patients after coronary artery bypass graft (CABG) surgery, there was no difference in the number of hypotensive episodes during the maintenance phase of the study, although there was a significantly higher number of hypotensive episodes in the propofol group during propofol loading.[118] Despite the mild to moderate degree of hypotension that accompanies the use of this agent, ICU patients sedated with propofol appear to have no compromise in oxygen delivery.[114] Furthermore, patients treated with propofol were found to have a parallel and equal decrease in myocardial oxygen supply and demand, implying that this agent is safe in the setting of coronary artery disease.[99]

Although propofol does not have analgesic properties, ICU patients sedated with propofol were noted to have a lower supplemental narcotic requirement than patients sedated with midazolam.[112,118] Several studies comparing propofol to midazolam in patients sedated for prolonged periods showed a significantly shorter time to awakening and time to extubation in patients sedated with propofol.[95,108] This experience has not been universal; in two studies comparing propofol with midazolam in postoperative CABG patients, there was no significant difference in time to extubation.[115,118] It is notable that, in these studies, the duration of sedation was relatively short.

Propofol infusions are widely used and a good option for mechanically ventilated patients. There is little published experience specifically in the CICU patient population. Experience in the medical-surgical and postoperative CABG patient population, however, suggests that this therapy is safe and efficacious. Propofol's main advantage over other sedative agents is rapid awakening after prolonged infusions and improved minute-to-minute control of sedation.[107] The available literature supports the use of sedative doses of propofol in the CICU only for mechanical ventilation.

Dexmedetomidine

Dexmedetomidine is the active dextro-isomer of medetomidine and is a highly selective α_2-adrenergic receptor agonist. It exhibits a high ratio of specificity for the α_2- versus α_1-receptor and has eight times the potency as clonidine at the α_2-receptor. It is therefore considered a full agonist at the α_2-receptor.[119] As an α_2-adrenergic agonist, dexmedetomidine exhibits sedative, anxiolytic and analgesic properties.[120] Dexmedetomidine has a unique sleep-like quality of sedation and has the benefit of minimal respiratory depression when used alone.

Dexmedetomidine works at α_2-receptors both peripherally and centrally; however, the sedative and anxiolytic effects of the drug are mediated through stimulation of central α_2-receptors. Activation of these receptors attenuates central nervous system excitation, especially in the locus coeruleus.[121] Stimulation of central α_2-receptors also leads to a decrease in sympathetic outflow and augmentation of cardiac vagal activity.[122] In addition, α_2-receptors modulate pain pathways within the spinal cord. Activation of the α_{2c}-receptor subtype produces an analgesic effect by accentuating the action of opioids.[123] Finally, dexmedetomidine's interaction with α_2-receptors located on blood vessels and sympathetic terminals mediates vasoconstriction and inhibits norepinephrine release, respectively.[122]

Dexmedetomidine has an onset of action of approximately 15 minutes, with peak concentrations reached within 1 hour following continuous infusion. It exhibits a rapid distribution phase with a $t_{1/2\alpha}$ of approximately 6 minutes and a $t_{1/2\beta}$ of approximately 2 hours. The drug is highly protein bound and has a large volume of distribution.[124] Dexmedetomidine is highly metabolized by the liver, undergoing glucuronidation and cytochrome P450-mediated metabolism. Therefore, patients with severe hepatic insufficiency may require lower doses.[124] The metabolites of dexmedetomidine are excreted renally.[125]

The recommended dose of dexmedetomidine is 1 μg/kg loading infusion over 10 minutes, followed by a continuous intravenous infusion of 0.2 to 1.4 μg/kg per hour.[121] The bolus of dexmedetomidine may result in a transient increase in blood pressure and a reflex decrease in heart rate, especially in younger patients.[126] This response is likely related to direct vasoconstriction of peripheral vessels.[124] Alternatively, patients may experience profound hypotension and bradycardia with the bolus dose.[127] Most intensivists simply start a continuous infusion of dexmedetomidine between 0.2 and 0.7 μg/kg per hour since omitting the bolus dose may avoid the undesirable hemodynamic effects.[128] During a continuous infusion of dexmedetomidine (0.2–0.7 μg/kg per hour), patients typically experience a slight decrease in blood pressure, heart rate, and cardiac output.[122] This effect is mediated by sympatholysis, as indicated by the fact that patients taking β-blockers do not experience heart rate slowing.[122]

Other side effects of dexmedetomidine include significant bradycardia; sinus arrest may occur in patients with high vagal tone or during rapid administration. Dexmedetomidine should be avoided in patients with advanced heart block and ventricular dysfunction.[129] Doses of the drug should be reduced in patients with hepatic impairment because the drug is highly metabolized by the liver. Its metabolites are excreted in the urine but have not been studied, so cautious dosing in renal failure is prudent. Mild respiratory depression is seen with bolus dosing of dexmedetomidine due to sedation.[122] Finally, prolonged use of dexmedetomidine may be associated with withdrawal phenomena upon discontinuation, including nausea, vomiting, and hypertension.

Dexmedetomidine is approved for use by the US Food and Drug Administration as a sedative for less than 24 hours duration. Studies in ICU patients have shown that compared with propofol, dexmedetomidine produces similar levels of sedation and time to extubation with less opioid requirements.[121] One study by Herr et al.[130] examined dexmedetomidine versus propofol-based sedation regimens in post-CABG patients. The results showed that dexmedetomidine provided safe and effective postoperative sedation in this patient population while reducing the need for analgesics, β-blockers, antiemetics, epinephrine, and diuretics. Since dexmedetomidine provides sedation without decreasing respiratory drive, it can be used as a sedative during weaning from mechanical ventilation and throughout the extubation period. This can be useful in anxious patients who might otherwise require large doses of propofol or benzodiazepines to tolerate the endotracheal tube during SBT. In addition, dexmedetomidine may be beneficial in patients who have a high tolerance to opioids. Finally, when compared to benzodiazepines, dexmedetomidine may be associated with decreased duration or incidence of delirium.[66,67] One study, in a cardiovascular surgical ICU setting, demonstrated that a dexmedetomidine-based sedation regimen decreased the duration of delirium with a trend toward a decreased incidence of delirium.[131] Recent studies have suggested that dexmedetomidine has a treatment or prophylactic effect against delirium in ICU patients, but further work is required to confirm these results.[132,133]

DELIRIUM MANAGEMENT

Delirium is a disturbance in attention, awareness, and cognition that develops over a short period of time and tends to fluctuate over the course of the day.[134] Subtypes include hyperactive and hypoactive delirium. Hyperactive delirium is characterized by restlessness, occasional combativeness, and frequent attempts at removing monitors, catheters, and endotracheal tubes. In contrast, hypoactive delirium is illustrated by apathy, decreased responsiveness, and withdrawal.[135] While the underlying pathophysiology of delirium remains unclear, there are multiple risk factors, including advanced age, underlying dementia, alcohol use, higher severity of illness, coma, and administration of sedative medications.[136] For many years, delirium was underdiagnosed and underappreciated in the ICU.[137] However, it is now recognized as a common problem in both ventilated and nonventilated patients and has been associated with an increase in adverse outcomes, including length of ICU stay, length of hospital stay, duration of mechanical ventilation, and mortality.[138–141] Given the increasing age and acuity of ICU patients along with the adverse effect of delirium on outcomes, there is growing interest in the prevention and treatment of delirium.

Emphasis is placed upon the early detection and prevention of delirium, since there is a 10% increase in mortality for each additional day of delirium.[139] There are multiple delirium screening tools in clinical practice; the two most validated are the Confusion Assessment Method for the ICU (CAM-ICU) and the Intensive Care Delirium Screening Checklist (ICDSC).[142,143] The CAM-ICU is a four-step process designed for providers without formal psychiatric training that screens patients for the cardinal features of delirium: acute onset or fluctuating course, inattention, disorganized thinking, and altered consciousness. Patients that screen positive are diagnosed with delirium. The CAM-ICU was originally validated in medical and coronary ICU patients but has since been validated in multiple other ICU settings. The ICDSC is a checklist of eight items corresponding to the *Diagnostic and Statistical Manual of Mental Disorders, 4th edition* (DSM-IV) diagnostic criteria for delirium.[143] Like the CAM-ICU, the ICDSC has been validated across multiple ICU settings. Screening tools should be utilized on a regular basis, preferably at least every nursing shift, particularly for high-risk patients. Without the use of validated screening tools, delirium will be correctly identified in only 35% and 28% of patients by nursing staff and physicians, respectively.[144]

Nonpharmacologic prevention of ICU delirium involves limiting predisposing clinical factors, reorientation activities, and early mobilization. Clinical factors that may predispose patients to delirium include hypoxia, infection, dehydration, pain, poor nutrition, sensory impairment, and sleep disturbances.[145] Verbal reminders of the year, day, and time as well as visual cues such as a calendar or clock are helpful in reorienting delirious patients. Maintaining exposure to daylight may also be helpful. Early mobilization is one particularly effective nonpharmacologic intervention that decreases the duration of delirium.[146] Early physical and occupational therapy in intubated patients shortens the duration of delirium by 2 days.

Pharmacologic management of delirium is limited. Although antipsychotics are commonly used in the management of delirium, there are limited data to suggest that they are effective. Most studies evaluating prophylactic use of haloperidol or atypical antipsychotics have shown no benefit in the prevention of delirium.[147] The same is true with regard to treating established delirium with antipsychotics. However, a small randomized controlled trial demonstrated a decrease duration of delirium with quetiapine administration.[148] The prophylactic use of dexmedetomidine has shown some promise in reducing delirium. One randomized trial in cardiac surgical patients demonstrated a reduction in the duration and a trend toward a decreased incidence of delirium in patients receiving dexmedetomidine.[131] In patients requiring sedation for mechanical ventilation, dexmedetomidine is preferred over benzodiazepines for reducing delirium.[66,149] In a recent randomized trial in patients with agitated delirium preventing them from being extubated, the addition of dexmedetomidine decreased the time to extubation and accelerated the resolution of delirium.[133]

Haloperidol

Haloperidol is one of the most commonly used members of the butyrophenone class of neuroleptic major tranquilizers.[150] It has a moderately rapid rate of onset, with a $t_{1/2\alpha}$ of 3 to 19 minutes and a $t_{1/2\beta}$ of 10 to 19 hours.[14] Respiratory depression and hypotension rarely occur.[14] Initially developed as an oral neuroleptic agent, haloperidol has gained favor as an intravenous agent for the management of delirium in critically ill medical patients.[109] The intravenous route of administration seems to decrease the incidence of extrapyramidal side effects compared with the oral route.[151] Intermittent intravenous bolus administration is recommended to treat acute delirium.[14] Standard doses range from 2 to 10 mg administered every 10 to 15 minutes until the desired effect is obtained. If around-the-clock dosing is needed, the patient may be started on a divided intravenous dose based on the loading dose or on a continuous infusion.

Although widely used, haloperidol has serious side effects that may be especially concerning for CICU patients. A prolonged QT interval, torsades de pointes, ventricular arrhythmias, and cardiac arrest have been reported in patients treated with intravenous haloperidol.[152–161] Daily electrocardiograms are warranted to follow the QT interval in all patients receiving haloperidol. In addition to the cardiovascular effects, haloperidol may cause extrapyramidal effects, such as akathisia and oropharyngeal dysfunction.[154,155] Neuroleptic malignant syndrome and dystonic reactions may also occur.[53,156] Despite

these side effects, haloperidol has a long history of clinical use and has been shown to be a safe and efficacious treatment of agitation and delirium in patients with an intraaortic balloon pump.[157]

Olanzapine

Olanzapine is a second-generation antipsychotic agent that belongs to the thiobenzodiazepine class. It is a selective monoaminergic antagonist with a high affinity for multiple receptors, including serotonin 5HT2/2C and 5HT6, dopamine D1-4, histamine H1 and adrenergic α_1 receptors. It is available in oral and intramuscular forms but is more commonly given orally in the ICU. The oral form of olanzapine is well absorbed with good bioavailability. It reaches peak concentrations in approximately 6 hours and its $t_{1/2\beta}$ is approximately 21 to 54 hours. The drug undergoes direct glucuronidation and cytochrome P450-mediated oxidation. Renal dysfunction does not appear to impact pharmacokinetics.[158] If patients can take medications by mouth, it is a good alternative to haloperidol for the treatment of ICU delirium and, in fact, may be better tolerated with fewer side effects. In one study of olanzapine versus haloperidol, the patients taking olanzapine had no extrapyramidal side effects.[154] The drug is typically administered orally in doses that range from 2.5 to 10 mg daily.

Side effects of olanzapine include orthostatic hypotension that is likely the result of α_1-receptor antagonism. QT prolongation has been reported with atypical antipsychotics such as olanzapine but is less common than with haloperidol.[159] Olanzapine is not approved for the treatment of patients with dementia-related psychosis and should be avoided in this patient population.[157] Other side effects include hyperglycemia, neuroleptic malignant syndrome, and hyperlipidemia.

Quetiapine

Quetiapine is another orally administered second generation atypical neuroleptic agent with similar properties and pharmacologic effects to olanzapine. It is a benzisoxazole derivative like other drugs in this class such as risperidone. It is also a selective monoaminergic antagonist with activity at many receptors including serotonin, dopamine, histamine, and α_1-adrenergic and α_2-adrenergic receptors. Oral bioavailability is high; the drug undergoes extensive hepatic metabolism and elimination, with a half-life of 6 hours. Clearance is not significantly altered by renal dysfunction. Like other atypical neuroleptics, quetiapine has a lower incidence of extrapyramidal side effects compared with haloperidol. Due to its prominent anticholinergic effects, quetiapine is more associated with sedation that may be beneficial in the treatment of nighttime agitation associated with delirium.[160] Typical dosing starts at 25 mg nightly and can be titrated to effect or given in divided doses throughout the day to a maximum daily dose of 200 mg.

Side effects of quetiapine are similar to other drugs in this class and include orthostatic hypotension, QT prolongation, hyperglycemia, neuroleptic malignant syndrome, and hyperlipidemia. Notably, neutropenia and agranulocytosis have also been reported; thus, patient blood counts should be monitored while receiving this drug. Quetiapine is also not approved for the treatment of patients with dementia-related psychosis and should be avoided in this patient population. Few studies have directly compared the use of quetiapine to other neuroleptics in the ICU patient population with delirium but, when additional sedating properties are needed, it is an effective alternative or adjunct to other medications for the treatment of agitated delirium.[148,161]

Acknowledgment

We acknowledge the contributions of Kristina R. Sullivan, William B. Cammarano, and Jeanine P. Wiener-Kronish, who were the authors of this chapter in the previous edition.

The full reference list for this chapter is available at ExpertConsult.com.

41

Pharmacologic Interactions

Shoshana Zevin

Concomitant administration of several drugs is common in the treatment of cardiovascular diseases. Often, combinations of drugs are necessary and result in improved outcomes. With a large number of medications, however, there is also an increased concern about drug interactions. Although the number of potential interactions is great, many are inconsequential. Conversely, drug interactions can have significant adverse effects or even be lethal.[1,2]

Many drug interactions can be prevented by recognizing the drugs and the patients at risk. Situations with a high likelihood for clinically significant adverse drug interactions include the following[1-3]:

1. A large number of drugs. The risk is significantly higher when more than 10 drugs are concurrently administered.
2. Drugs with a steep dose response relation when even small changes in the drug level lead to profound changes in its action

3. Drugs with a narrow therapeutic index
4. Concomitant administration of drugs known as liver enzyme inducers or inhibitors (e.g., rifampin and cimetidine)
5. Elderly patients
6. Critically ill patients

It is important to be aware of the possibility of drug interactions in the cardiac intensive care unit (CICU) because many of these patients receive high-risk drugs, are elderly, and may have circulatory failure or be critically ill. It is also important to inquire about the use of herbal supplements and medicines, as many of these products can interact with drugs and cause adverse events. Drug interactions may mimic worsening or progression of the underlying disease with manifestations such as arrhythmia or congestive heart failure (CHF).

Mechanisms of interactions may be pharmacokinetic, affecting drug absorption, bioavailability, metabolism, or renal excretion, or pharmacodynamic, occurring at the sites of action in the heart, such as sinoatrial (SA) and atrioventricular (AV) nodes, the intraventricular conduction system, and the smooth muscle.[3]

This chapter discusses interactions of drugs commonly used in the CICU, with emphasis on interactions with other cardiovascular drugs.

VASODILATORS

Nitrates

The chief interactions of nitrates are pharmacodynamic. Nitrates (e.g., nitroglycerin, isosorbide dinitrate, isosorbide mononitrate) are widely used both in patients with angina and in those with CHF. A limitation in nitrate therapy is the development of tolerance, which is time dependent.[4] Many theories are proposed to explain this phenomenon,[5–7] including nitrate resistance,[8] pseudotolerance (i.e., activation of counterregulatory responses, such as secretion of catecholamines, angiotensin II, and endothelin),[9] and "true" tolerance resulting from impaired bioconversion to nitric oxide (NO)[10,11] and increased generation of superoxide.[7,12]

There are several reports of agents that limit or reverse nitrate tolerance when coadministered with nitroglycerin or isosorbide dinitrate. These include N-acetylcysteine, angiotensin-converting enzyme (ACE) inhibitors,[13,14] angiotensin receptor blockers (ARBs),[15] carvedilol,[16] hydralazine,[12] ascorbic acid,[17] folic acid,[18] and L-arginine.[19] However, there are not enough data to make definite recommendations on drug combinations to prevent nitrate tolerance.

The combination of nitrates with hydralazine has long been known to be beneficial in CHF and is still used in patients who are intolerant of ACE inhibitors and in African-American patients who have reduced capacity for endogenous production of nitric oxide.[20] These drugs may interact at the site of smooth muscle, involving inhibition of pyridoxal-dependent enzymes by hydralazine and resulting in an increased availability of sulfhydryl groups and prevention of nitrate tolerance by decreasing superoxide production and scavenging of reactive oxygen species.[12,21]

A clinically significant interaction occurs between nitrates and phosphodiesterase type 5 (PDE5) inhibitors, such as sildenafil and tadalafil, commonly used to treat erectile dysfunction. Inhibition of PDE5 results in increased cyclic guanosine monophosphate (cGMP) levels, which are generated from endogenously derived NO. Nitrates exert their effect via biotransformation to NO and generation of cGMP. Coadministration of nitrates and PDE5 inhibitors causes significant reduction of blood pressure via a synergistic increase in cGMP levels, resulting in symptomatic hypotension and even death.[22–24] PDE5 inhibitors are contraindicated for patients treated with nitrates. Conversely, nitrates should not be started within 24 hours of using sildenafil and 48 hours of using tadalafil.[25]

Another pharmacodynamic interaction occurs when nitrates are used with β-blockers, calcium channel blockers, or both as part of an intensive antianginal regimen, resulting in hypotension with reduced coronary flow. The result may be worsening of angina.[26]

ANGIOTENSIN-CONVERTING ENZYME INHIBITORS AND ANGIOTENSIN RECEPTOR BLOCKERS

ACE inhibitors (Table 41.1) are widely used for the treatment of CHF and hypertension and to prevent remodeling after myocardial infarction (MI).

Interactions involving ACE inhibitors are primarily pharmacodynamic and are based on their mechanism of action. The principal mechanism of action is lowering of angiotensin II levels, resulting in vasodilation and suppression of aldosterone release. ACE inhibitors also inhibit the degradation of bradykinin and increase prostaglandin synthesis, both of which may contribute to vasodilation.

The main interaction of concern is between ACE inhibitors and potassium supplements or potassium-sparing diuretics. These combinations can result in rapid development of hyperkalemia, especially in the presence of diminished renal function.

TABLE 41.1 Drug Interactions With Angiotensin-Converting Enzyme Inhibitors (ACEI)

Interacting Drug	Effect	Mechanism	Comments
Potassium supplements or potassium-sparing diuretics	Hyperkalemia	Inhibition of aldosterone release	Avoid combinations, monitor potassium levels
Angiotensin receptor blockers	Hyperkalemia	Dual inhibition of RAS	Monitor potassium levels, blood pressure, and renal function
	Hypotension Renal failure		
Diuretics	Hypotension	Inhibition of angiotensin II–mediated response to hypovolemia	Reduce dose or temporarily discontinue the diuretic before starting ACEI
	Renal failure		
NSAIDs	Inhibition of hypotensive effect of ACEI	Inhibition of kinin-mediated prostaglandin synthesis	Monitor blood pressure
Lithium	Lithium toxicity	Reduction of Na concentration in the proximal tubules by ACEI, causing increased lithium reabsorption	Reduce lithium dose by 50%, monitor lithium blood levels
Sulfonylurea	Hypoglycemia	Increased sensitivity to insulin	Monitor blood glucose

NSAIDs, nonsteroidal antiinflammatory drugs; RAS, renin-angiotensin system.

There is a beneficial effect in the synergism between ACE inhibitors and diuretics (e.g., thiazides and furosemide) in the treatment of hypertension and CHF. In a sodium-depleted patient or one with high renin levels, however, the combination can result in hypotension and worsening of renal failure. In such patients, the physician should start with a lower-than-normal dose of ACE inhibitor, temporarily lower the dose of diuretic, or discontinue the diuretic before administration of an ACE inhibitor. There is no evidence of a significant pharmacokinetic interaction between ACE inhibitors and diuretics. A synergistic effect on blood pressure reduction was also observed between various ACE inhibitors and calcium antagonists without pharmacokinetic interactions.[27] No significant interactions have been found between ACE inhibitors and β-blockers or digoxin.[27,28]

Among the interactions of ACE inhibitors with noncardiovascular drugs, the most notable is with nonsteroidal antiinflammatory drugs (NSAIDs) because of their opposing effects on prostaglandin synthesis. The result is an attenuation of the antihypertensive effects of ACE inhibitors, predisposition to renal failure, or both.[29,30] There are conflicting reports on the interactions between ACE inhibitors and low-dose aspirin.[31,32] However, a retrospective analysis did not demonstrate an adverse effect of aspirin on the survival of patients with left ventricular (LV) systolic dysfunction treated with ACE inhibitors.[33]

There are reports of lithium toxicity when patients on chronic lithium therapy were started on ACE inhibitors. Because renal excretion of lithium is dependent on glomerular filtration and on sodium concentration in the proximal tubule, the possible mechanism of interaction may be the reduction of both by ACE inhibitors, especially in volume-depleted patients.[27,28]

A life-threatening anaphylactoid reaction has been described in a patient treated with ACE inhibitors while on hemodialysis with a polyacrylonitrile membrane (AN69). The possible mechanism of this interaction is activation of the kinin-kallikrein system by the surface of the AN69 membrane, resulting in an increased production of bradykinin, the breakdown of which is inhibited by ACE inhibitors.[27] No adverse reactions were reported with other dialysis membranes.

ACE inhibitors increase insulin sensitivity; there have been several reports of hypoglycemia when captopril or enalapril was given to patients receiving glibenclamide, although others did not observe this effect.[34–36] It seems prudent to monitor for possible hypoglycemia when ACE inhibitors are given to patients who are already receiving oral antihypoglycemic agents.

ARBs have low potential for interaction with other drugs. Among ARBs, only losartan and irbesartan undergo significant metabolism by cytochrome P-450 enzymes (CYP2C9 and CYP3A4). Rifampin significantly reduces the area under the drug concentration in blood plasma versus time curve (AUC) as well as the half-life of losartan and its active metabolite; an increased dose of losartan may be indicated during concomitant administration with rifampin.[37] However, no clinically significant interactions have been found between losartan and erythromycin, digoxin, or warfarin and between irbesartan and digoxin, nifedipine, or hydrochlorothiazide.[38] There was a report of a significant interaction between valsartan and lithium resulting in lithium toxicity.[39]

Attenuation of the hypertensive effect of ARBs may result from concomitant administration of NSAIDs via mechanisms similar to the interaction with ACE inhibitors.[38]

Combination of ACE inhibitors and ARBs provides a dual and more effective blockade of the renin-angiotensin system (RAS). However, the combination therapy is associated with a significantly increased risk of adverse events, such as hyperkalemia, kidney damage, and hypotension, particularly in patients with diabetic nephropathy.[40,41] There are conflicting data on the use of dual RAS blockade with β-blockers in patients with CHF. The Valsartan Heart Failure Trial (Val-HeFT) suggested an increased mortality in patients treated with triple therapy compared with an ACE inhibitor and β-blocker alone, while the Candesartan in Heart failure—Assessment of Mortality and Morbidity (CHARM) and Valsartan in Acute Myocardial Infarction (VALIANT) trials did not find any increase in mortality in patients on triple therapy.[42–44] The meta-analysis of more than 68,000 patients from 33 randomized controlled trials of combination therapy with an ACE inhibitor and an ARB found an 18% decrease in hospitalizations for CHF but did not find any mortality benefit with combination therapy compared with monotherapy, while the risk of adverse events was very high (41% to 68%).[41] Thus combination therapy should be avoided in the majority of the patients.

Sacubitril/Valsartan

Recently, a fixed-dose combination of the neprilysin inhibitor sacubitril and the ARB valsartan was approved for patients with CHF. Reduced LV function after the combination was shown to reduce the risk of cardiovascular death and hospitalizations due to CHF exacerbation.[45] Drug interactions are similar to those occurring with ARBs—that is, increased risk of hyperkalemia with potassium-sparing diuretics or potassium supplements, particularly in patients with chronic kidney disease, diabetes, or hypoaldosteronism. Worsening of renal failure can occur with concomitant use of NSAIDs; lithium toxicity has also been described.

INOTROPIC DRUGS

Dopamine and Dobutamine

Vasoactive amines are used in the CICU to treat CHF and shock. Both drugs are metabolized in the liver: dopamine by catechol-O-methyltransferase and monoamine oxidase; dobutamine by catechol-O-methyltransferase. Dopamine is inactivated in alkaline pH and, therefore, should not be administered in the same infusion as bicarbonate.[46]

Although there are not many reports in the literature about drug interactions involving vasoactive amines, such interactions could be expected in patients treated with monoamine oxidase inhibitors, requiring lowering the dose of dopamine. The dose of vasoactive amines should be adjusted in patients treated with tricyclic antidepressants because of the possibility of an increased pressor effect.

Changes in blood pressure and in blood flow to the liver will affect the metabolism of high-extraction drugs, such as lidocaine and lipophilic β-blockers (e.g., propranolol, metoprolol). As a result, doses of inotropic drugs that increase cardiac output will also increase liver blood flow and accelerate the clearance of lidocaine, requiring an increased dose of lidocaine. Conversely, when dopamine is used in high doses, resulting predominantly in α-activation and vasoconstriction, liver blood flow decreases and lidocaine clearance would be expected to do the same.

Low-dose dopamine prevents norepinephrine-induced decreases in renal plasma flow in healthy volunteers.[47] However, it is not clear whether the same effect is found in critical care patients. A multicenter study of low-dose dopamine use in critical care patients did not find any improvement in renal outcomes and there were more adverse effects in patients on dopamine.[48,49]

There is a report of interaction between dobutamine and low-dose carvedilol resulting in severe hypotension.[50] The proposed mechanism is a fall in systemic vascular resistance due to excessive β_2 receptor activation caused by a selective β_1 receptor blockade by low-dose carvedilol. This interaction may be expected with other selective β_1 blockers.

Digoxin

Digoxin is a drug with a narrow therapeutic range and is subject to many drug interactions, both pharmacokinetic and pharmacodynamic (Table 41.2).

Interactions Affecting Absorption and Bioavailability. Digoxin tablets are absorbed slowly; therefore agents that increase gastrointestinal motility (e.g., metoclopramide) may decrease its absorption, whereas agents that slow gastrointestinal transit (e.g., propantheline, other anticholinergic agents) may increase its absorption.[51] Elixir preparations are usually not subject to these interactions because their absorption is more rapid.

Treatment with high-dose chemotherapeutic agents resulting in intestinal mucosal injury can reduce digoxin absorption from tablets by as much as 50% but does not significantly affect absorption from elixir.[52]

In about 10% of patients, digoxin that is not absorbed in the upper gastrointestinal tract or that is excreted in the bile is reductively metabolized by the anaerobic bacterium *Eubacterium lentum*, which is part of the normal flora of the colon. Such metabolism can account for about 40% of digoxin elimination. These patients may be recognized by the characteristic of needing higher-than-usual doses of digoxin to achieve therapeutic levels. In this group of patients, treatment with broad-spectrum antibiotics (e.g., erythromycin, tetracycline) can result in significantly increased bioavailability and digoxin toxicity.[53]

Cholesterol-binding resins (e.g., cholestyramine, colestipol) bind digoxin in the gut and may reduce its absorption by 20% to 30%. This effect can be avoided by giving digoxin at least 1 hour before the resins.[54] Sucralfate has been reported to decrease the absorption of digoxin.[55] No significant interaction has been found between digoxin and antacids.[56]

Intestinal P-glycoprotein (P-gp) plays an important role in the bioavailability of digoxin.[57] Rifampin increases P-gp content in the intestine and decreases digoxin bioavailability, resulting in significantly lower digoxin AUC after oral administration.[58] On the other hand, drugs that inhibit intestinal P-gp increase digoxin bioavailability and AUC. Dipyridamole was shown to increase digoxin bioavailability in vitro and in vivo; however, the effect on AUC was slight and clinically insignificant.[59] Carvedilol significantly decreased oral clearance of digoxin in children, resulting in digoxin toxicity in some cases.[60] However,

TABLE 41.2 Drug Interactions With Digoxin

Interacting Drug	Serum Digoxin Levels	Mechanism	Comments
Cholestyramine, colestipol	D	Decreased absorption	Wait 1 h after digoxin administration
Metoclopramide	D	Decreased absorption due to increased GI motility	Monitor digoxin levels; substitute elixir for tablets
Erythromycin	I (only in small percentage of patients)	Increased bioavailability due to decreased gut metabolism	Monitor digoxin levels, adjust dose
Anticancer drugs	D	Decreased absorption due to mucosal injury	Monitor digoxin levels; substitute elixir for tablets
Sucralfate	D	Decreased absorption	Do not administer within 1 h of digoxin
Amiodarone	I	Decreased clearance (P-gp inhibition)	Decrease digoxin dose, monitor levels
Dronedarone	I	Decreased clearance (P-gp inhibition)	Decrease digoxin dose, monitor levels
Cyclosporine	I	Decreased clearance of digoxin (P-gp inhibition)	Monitor digoxin levels, decrease dose
Diuretics	I	Decreased renal clearance in hypovolemia; increased toxicity due to hypokalemia/ hypomagnesemia	Monitor serum potassium and magnesium levels; monitor digoxin levels
Itraconazole	I	Decreased clearance (P-gp inhibition)	Decrease digoxin dose, monitor levels
Propafenone	I	Decreased renal clearance	Monitor digoxin levels, adjust dose
Quinine, quinidine	I	Decreased renal clearance (P-gp inhibition)	Decrease digoxin dose, monitor blood levels
Spironolactone	I	Decreased renal clearance (P-gp inhibition)	Monitor levels
Ticagrelor	I	Decreased renal clearance (P-gp inhibition)	Monitor levels
Verapamil	I	Decreased renal excretion (P-gp inhibition)	Decrease digoxin dose, monitor levels
Rifampin	D	Increased bioavailability (intestinal P-gp induction)	Monitor levels

D, Decrease; *GI*, gastrointestinal; *I*, increase; *P-gp*, P glycoprotein.

in adults, carvedilol caused only a modest increase in digoxin bioavailability and AUC.[61]

St. John's wort (*Hypericum perforatum*) is an herbal medicine frequently used for treatment of depression. *H. perforatum* induces intestinal P-gp, resulting in a 1.4-fold increased expression of duodenal P-gp in humans.[62] Coadministration of St. John's wort and digoxin caused a 25% decrease in AUC and a 33% reduction in trough and C_{max} concentrations of digoxin.[63]

Interactions Affecting Elimination. Digoxin is eliminated primarily by renal excretion via the ATP-dependent efflux pump, P-gp.[57,64-66] Basic drugs—among them, amiodarone, dronedarone, clarithromycin, itraconazole, quinine, quinidine, verapamil, spironolactone, cyclosporine A, propafenone, and ritonavir—decrease the renal clearance of digoxin by inhibiting P-gp in the kidney.[67-72] Carvedilol causes significant increases in digoxin AUC and C_{max} in men but not in women.[73] The explanation may be that men have a higher P-gp activity compared with women and, thus, are more sensitive to the effects of inhibiting drugs.

Because the combination of digoxin with drugs that inhibit its elimination results in increased toxicity, the physician should reduce the digoxin dose by 50% when starting another drug, such as quinidine or amiodarone. Because of the long half-life of digoxin, even after dose reduction there is still a potential for toxicity during the first week after adding another drug to the regimen. Patients must be monitored closely during this period.

Pharmacodynamic Interactions. Digitalis effect and toxicity are enhanced in the presence of hypokalemia and hypomagnesemia. Toxicity may be present even when digoxin blood levels are within the therapeutic range. Because digoxin is often used with diuretics, which can cause electrolyte abnormalities, it is important to monitor and correct deficiencies even though potassium and magnesium blood levels do not always accurately reflect body stores.[74] Concomitant administration of digoxin and sympathomimetic or vagolytic drugs may mask digitalis toxicity because of opposing effects on cardiac conduction. This effect is used therapeutically when digoxin is administered at the beginning of quinidine therapy to prevent rapid AV node conduction as a result of the vagolytic effect of quinidine.

Coadministration of digoxin with sympatholytic drugs (e.g., β-blockers) or calcium antagonists (e.g., verapamil, diltiazem) may result in additive AV block or bradyarrhythmia.

ANTIDYSRHYTHMIC DRUGS

Drug interactions with antidysrhythmic drugs are presented in Table 41.3. A detailed review was published by Trujillo and Nolan.[75]

Class 1A

Quinidine. Quinidine is a drug with many adverse side effects and interacts with many other drugs.

Pharmacokinetic interactions. Quinidine is primarily metabolized in the liver with only about 20% excreted in the urine. It is subject to interactions with drugs that either induce or inhibit liver

enzymes. Among the enzyme inducers, phenobarbital, phenytoin, and rifampin accelerate the metabolism of quinidine, resulting in decreased blood levels. Therefore, when any of these drugs is added, the quinidine dose should be increased, and when these drugs are stopped, the quinidine dose should be decreased. The dose adjustment may be as great as threefold.[76]

There have been conflicting reports about the effect of nifedipine on quinidine blood levels.[77] However, quinidine pharmacokinetics do not appear to be significantly changed by nifedipine or felodipine.[77] Cimetidine, verapamil, and amiodarone inhibit quinidine metabolism and necessitate downward dose adjustment.[78-80]

Even though renal excretion accounts for only 20% of quinidine clearance, clearance is influenced by urine pH; alkalinization of urine (e.g., with intensive antacid therapy) may result in a moderate increase in quinidine levels.[81]

Pharmacodynamic interactions. The combination of quinidine with other class 1A drugs (e.g., disopyramide, procainamide) or with class 3 drugs (e.g., amiodarone, sotalol) can result in QT prolongation and increased risk of torsades de pointes.[82,83]

Moxifloxacin, a methoxyquinolone antibiotic, prolongs QT interval, and must be used with caution with class 1A or class 3 drugs.[84] Hypokalemia, hypomagnesemia, or both—common with diuretic treatment—can increase QT prolongation and the risk of torsades de pointes from quinidine or other drugs.[85]

A proarrhythmic effect of combining amiloride and quinidine has been described, probably resulting from a synergistic increase in sodium channel blockade.[86]

Quinidine has also been reported to potentiate the anticoagulant effects of warfarin by direct inhibition of clotting factor synthesis in the liver. It inhibits neuromuscular transmission and prolongs the duration of anesthesia when used with curare or succinylcholine.[87]

Procainamide. Procainamide is both metabolized and excreted renally; its active metabolite, *N*-acetyl procainamide (NAPA), is cleared primarily by renal excretion. The major mechanism is tubular secretion with little reabsorption; therefore, urine pH changes do not cause significant changes in blood procainamide concentration. Conversely, other basic drugs that are secreted by renal tubules (e.g., cimetidine, ranitidine, trimethoprim) significantly inhibit procainamide secretion.[88,89] Levofloxacin, but not ciprofloxacin, significantly inhibits renal clearance of procainamide and NAPA.[90]

Additive effects of combined treatment with other class 1A or class 3 drugs, or other drugs that cause QT prolongation, are the same as for quinidine.

Disopyramide. Disopyramide is metabolized by liver enzymes. Enzyme inducers (e.g., rifampin, phenytoin, barbiturates) enhance the metabolism of disopyramide and may cause subtherapeutic blood levels.[91] Enzyme inhibitors such as cimetidine are expected to decrease disopyramide clearance and to increase blood levels. Macrolide antibiotics—including erythromycin, clarithromycin, and azithromycin—inhibit P450 enzymes and there are reports of disopyramide toxicity during concomitant administration.[92-94]

TABLE 41.3 Drug Interactions With Antidysrhythmic Drugs

Drug	Interacting Drug	Effect	Mechanism	Comments
Quinidine (Q)	Rifampin Phenytoin Phenobarbital	Decrease in Q levels	Induction of Q metabolism	Increase Q dose, monitor Q levels
	Cimetidine Amiodarone Verapamil	Increase in Q levels	Inhibition of Q metabolism	Decrease Q dose, monitor Q levels
	Antacids	Increase in Q levels	Alkalinization of urine, reduced Q tubular secretion	Monitor Q levels, change can be minor
	Procainamide	Proarrhythmic effect	Additive Q-T prolongation	Use combination with caution; monitor Q-T and potassium levels
	Disopyramide Amiodarone Sotalol	Torsades de pointes		
	Succinylcholine	Prolonged neuromuscular blockade	Inhibition of neuromuscular transmission (muscarinic receptors)	
Procainamide (P)	Cimetidine Trimethoprim Levofloxacin	Increased P levels	Reduced tubular secretion of P	Reduce P dose, monitor P levels
Disopyramide (Di)	Rifampin	Decreased Di levels	Acceleration of Di metabolism	Increase Di dose or avoid combination (increased anticholinergic effects with Di metabolite)
	Phenytoin Macrolides	Increased Di levels	P-450 inhibition	Decrease Di dose or avoid combination
Lidocaine (L)	Cimetidine Amiodarone Fluvoxamine	Increased L levels	Inhibition of L metabolism	Reduce L infusion rate
	Phenobarbital	Decreased L levels	Acceleration of L metabolism	Increase L dose
	β-Blockers	Increased L levels	Decrease in L clearance due to reduction in hepatic blood flow	Reduce L infusion rate
Mexiletine (M)	Quinidine Rifampin	Increased M levels	Inhibition of M metabolism	Reduce M dose or avoid combination
	Phenytoin	Decreased M levels	Acceleration of M metabolism	Increase M dose
Flecainide (F)	Cimetidine Amiodarone Quinine	Increased F levels	Inhibition of F metabolism	Decrease F dose
	Antacids	Increased F levels	Alkalinization of urine, decrease in tubular secretion	Minor effect
Encainide (E)	Quinidine	Increased E levels; diminished efficacy due to reduced formation of active metabolite	Inhibition of E metabolism	Avoid combination
	Cimetidine	Increased E levels; enhanced activity due to inhibition of active metabolite clearance	Inhibition of E metabolism	Avoid combination
Propafenone (Pr)	Quinidine	Increased Pr levels and β-blockade	Inhibition of Pr metabolism	Decrease Pr dose or avoid combination
Amiodarone (A)	Digoxin Flecainide Lidocaine Procainamide Quinidine Simvastatin Cyclosporine	Increased levels of the interacting drugs	Inhibition of the drug's metabolism by A	Monitor serum A levels, adjust dosages

Continued

TABLE 41.3   Drug Interactions With Antidysrhythmic Drugs—cont'd

Drug	Interacting Drug	Effect	Mechanism	Comments
	Phenytoin Warfarin			
	Class 1A and 1C drugs	Proarrhythmic effect, torsades de pointes	Additive Q-T prolongation	Avoid combination or monitor Q-T.
	β-Blockers Ca channel blockers	Hypotension, bradycardia, AV	Additive depression of conduction	Monitor blood pressure and pulse rate; avoid combination in conduction disorders and heart failure
Adenosine (Ad)	Theophylline (T)	Antagonizes Ad effect	Competition for Ad receptors	Ad ineffective for patients on T
	Dipyridamole	Increased Ad levels and effect	Inhibition of Ad reuptake	Decrease Ad dose by 50%–75%

Class 1B

Lidocaine. Lidocaine is extensively metabolized by the liver, with a high extraction ratio; therefore, its clearance is dependent on hepatic blood flow. Lidocaine is usually administered as a bolus followed by continuous intravenous infusion. The distribution of a bolus to the tissues is slowed in patients with severe CHF and shock and may result in high blood levels and toxicity.[95] To avoid this, a bolus dose of lidocaine in these situations should be given slowly.

Drugs that decrease hepatic blood flow (e.g., β-blockers) decrease lidocaine clearance, whereas drugs that increase hepatic blood flow (e.g., dopamine and dobutamine) can be expected to increase clearance.[96]

Lidocaine clearance changes with liver enzyme inducers and inhibitors; it decreases with cimetidine and increases with phenobarbital.[97] Amiodarone has been reported to reduce lidocaine clearance, resulting in high lidocaine plasma levels and seizures.[98] Fluvoxamine, a CYP1A2 inhibitor, significantly reduced lidocaine clearance.[99] An interaction with mexiletine resulting in increased plasma lidocaine levels and toxicity has been reported.[100] The purported mechanism is displacement of lidocaine from tissue binding sites. It is recommended that the rate of lidocaine infusion be adjusted by 25% to 50% in the presence of potential drug interactions.

Increased cardiotoxicity resulting in SA block has been reported with concomitant use of lidocaine and quinidine or procainamide.[81,101]

Mexiletine. Mexiletine is extensively metabolized by the liver, mainly by cytochrome P-450 isozyme 2D6—the activity of which is genetically determined—and, in part, by isozyme 1A2. Mexiletine metabolism is inhibited by quinidine.[102] Fluvoxamine, a CYP1A2 inhibitor, causes significant increases in mexiletine AUC.[103] The enzyme inducers rifampin and phenytoin have been shown to enhance its metabolism.[104]

Class 1C

Flecainide. Flecainide is eliminated by renal excretion and hepatic metabolism. Changes in urine pH are expected to affect its clearance; alkalinization of urine will result in higher plasma concentrations. Cimetidine, quinine, and amiodarone have been reported to inhibit the clearance and increase plasma concentrations of flecainide.[105,106]

Encainide. Encainide is extensively metabolized by the liver with significant first-pass effect and its metabolism is genetically determined. Its metabolites are active and are responsible for the majority of its pharmacologic activity.[107] Quinidine inhibits encainide metabolism, resulting in diminished pharmacologic activity.[108] Cimetidine inhibits the metabolism of the active metabolites of encainide even more than it inhibits encainide metabolism, resulting in enhanced pharmacologic activity.[109]

Propafenone. Propafenone is metabolized by cytochrome P-450 isozyme 2D6; thus its metabolism is subject to genetic polymorphism of 2D6. About 10% of whites are poor metabolizers of this drug. When propafenone is administered to extensive metabolizers, quinidine, a potent inhibitor of 2D6 enzyme, inhibits its clearance, resulting in higher blood levels and a significant increase in pharmacologic effect.[110,111] Conversely, rifampin, a P-450 inducer, increases propafenone clearance.[112] Propafenone has been reported to inhibit the metabolism of theophylline.[113]

Class 3

Amiodarone. Amiodarone has a number of significant pharmacokinetic and pharmacodynamic drug interactions.

Pharmacokinetic interactions. Amiodarone is an inhibitor of certain cytochrome P-450 enzymes. Amiodarone potentiates the effect of warfarin and causes enhanced anticoagulation.[114,115] Because the half-life of amiodarone is very long, this effect may take up several weeks to reach maximum intensity. Conversely, after amiodarone is discontinued, its effect on warfarin metabolism can persist for several months. Amiodarone also elevates the blood levels of digoxin, quinidine, procainamide, flecainide, lidocaine, metoprolol, simvastatin, cyclosporine, and phenytoin.[98,116-119] It is recommended that dosages of warfarin and digoxin be decreased by half when amiodarone is added.[75]

Pharmacodynamic interactions. The combination of amiodarone with class 1A or class 1C drugs can result in enhanced antidysrhythmic efficacy. However, when combined with class 1A drugs, such as quinidine, amiodarone can result in marked QT prolongation and an increased risk of torsades de pointes.[74] Another pharmacodynamic interaction with calcium antagonists or β-blockers may result in SA node depression with excessive bradycardia or sinus arrest.[120] This effect may persist for weeks after discontinuing amiodarone. However, the combination of amiodarone and β-blockers is usually safe and may be beneficial in some post-MI patients.[121]

Dronedarone. Dronedarone is a derivative of amiodarone, lacking the iodine moiety. Dronedarone and its active metabolite, N-desbutyldronedarone (NDBD), were shown to inhibit CYP3A4 and CYP3A5 in a time- and concentration-dependent manner.[122] It was found to increase plasma levels and toxicity of CYP3A4 substrates tacrolimus[123] and sirolimus.[124] A 50% to 75% reduction of sirolimus dose is suggested prior to initiating dronedarone.

Unlike amiodarone, dronedarone causes only a mild inhibition of CYP2C9 and, thus, does not cause a significant increase of warfarin levels or international normalized ratio (INR) prolongation.[125]

Dronedarone also inhibits P-glycoprotein.[126] Concomitant administration of dronedarone and digoxin may result in significantly increased digoxin levels and increased cardiovascular mortality in patients on combination therapy compared with patients on digoxin alone.[127]

Sotalol. The administration of aluminum and magnesium hydroxide decreases sotalol absorption.[128] Separation of the drugs by 2 hours avoids the interaction. Sotalol is excreted primarily unchanged by the kidneys. The same pharmacodynamic effects for the combination with class 1A drugs would be expected for sotalol as with amiodarone. Hypokalemia can aggravate the risk of torsades de pointes with this combination.[129] Torsades de pointes has been reported after the combination of sotalol and terfenadine.[130] The combination of sotalol with other β-blockers may produce bradycardia, AV block, or exacerbation of CHF.[131]

Class 4

Adenosine. Adenosine is used for acute treatment of supraventricular tachycardia. Dipyridamole inhibits adenosine reuptake, causing increased blood concentrations. Patients on dipyridamole should receive one-fourth the standard dose of adenosine. Theophylline competes with adenosine for the same receptors and, thus, inhibits its action.[132]

Calcium Channel Blockers. The most commonly used calcium channel blockers (e.g., verapamil, diltiazem, nifedipine; Table 41.4) are extensively metabolized by the liver; therefore, their metabolism is dependent on hepatic blood flow. Because of their extensive hepatic metabolism, they undergo significant first-pass metabolism in the liver, with a low level of bioavailability.[133] Verapamil and diltiazem also inhibit some P-450 enzymes, thus affecting the metabolism of other drugs.

Pharmacokinetic interactions. Cytochrome P-450 enzyme inducers (e.g., rifampin, phenytoin, phenobarbital) decrease the bioavailability and increase the clearance of verapamil and diltiazem. St. John's wort also significantly decreases verapamil bioavailability through induction of first-pass metabolism in the gut.[134] Conversely, the enzyme inhibitor cimetidine increases the bioavailability and decreases the clearance of calcium antagonists.[135–137] Macrolide antibiotics clarithromycin and telithromycin also inhibit CYP3A4; their combination with

verapamil may result in significant verapamil toxicity.[138,139] Felodipine metabolism is inhibited by itraconazole and erythromycin, resulting in significant increases in plasma concentrations and AUC.[68,140]

Grapefruit juice, which inhibits some P-450 enzymes, has been found to increase the bioavailability of some dihydropyridine calcium antagonists. The most significant interaction was with felodipine and nitrendipine, whereas nifedipine bioavailability was not significantly affected.[141] Verapamil increases digoxin concentration by inhibiting its renal excretion through P-gp.[142] Diltiazem has been reported to increase digoxin concentration, but this effect is not always present, and digoxin levels are affected to a lesser degree than with verapamil.[135] Nifedipine does not have a significant effect on digoxin concentration.[143]

Verapamil and diltiazem are inhibitors of CYP3A4 and thus are expected to inhibit the clearance of drugs metabolized by this enzyme. Verapamil and diltiazem significantly increase peak plasma levels and AUC of simvastatin and atorvastatin,[144–146] and there are reports of rhabdomyolysis with these combinations.[147,148] Verapamil and diltiazem have been reported to increase cyclosporine plasma levels, necessitating a reduction of cyclosporine doses.[149,150] The same interaction was observed between diltiazem and sirolimus[151] and diltiazem and tacrolimus.[152,153] Verapamil has also been reported to increase blood levels of prazosin. This pharmacokinetic interaction, along with a possible pharmacodynamic interaction, may result in hypotension.[154] Verapamil inhibits theophylline metabolism.[155] Verapamil and diltiazem significantly decrease the metabolism of midazolam, potentially causing excessive sedation. They also inhibit the metabolism of the anticonvulsants carbamazepine and phenytoin.[156,157]

Because verapamil is highly bound to plasma proteins, its displacement can result in transient toxicity. Complete AV block has been precipitated by ceftriaxone and clindamycin, which are also highly bound drugs, in a patient receiving verapamil.[158]

Pharmacodynamic interactions. Many calcium antagonists depress cardiac contractility and conduction; thus, they can cause sinus bradycardia or arrest, AV block, asystole, hypotension, and CHF.[159] There is a greater risk of these events when calcium channel blockers are coadministered with other drugs that can have similar effects on the heart, such as β-blockers. Verapamil and diltiazem have the greatest effect on conduction and contractility and, therefore, the most reported interactions with β-blockers; nifedipine has also been implicated in such interactions, however.[135,159–162] The combination of calcium antagonists and β-blockers can be desirable and necessary to control angina or the ventricular response in atrial fibrillation, but patients should be closely monitored. The probability of adverse interactions is increased in the elderly and when the patient has underlying CHF or conduction disorders. Intravenous verapamil should be avoided in patients treated with β-blockers because asystole has been reported as a complication of such therapy.[162] Development of CHF is also a risk when administering verapamil with other negative inotropic agents, such as disopyramide. Hypotension with verapamil and quinidine has been described, possibly as a result of additive α-adrenergic blocking effects.[163] An interaction between verapamil and clonidine that

TABLE 41.4 **Drug Interactions With Calcium Channel Blockers**

Drug	Interacting Drug	Effect	Mechanism	Comment
Verapamil Diltiazem	β-Blockers	Bradycardia, sinus arrest, heart block, heart failure	Additive effect on myocardial contractility and conduction	Avoid combination in elderly patients and in those with heart failure or conduction abnormalities
	Cimetidine	Increased bioavailability	Inhibition of metabolism	Decrease dose of Ca blockers
Felodipine Nitrendipine	Grapefruit juice	Increased bioavailability	Inhibition of metabolism	Monitor blood pressure and side effects
Verapamil (V) Diltiazem (D)	Rifampin	Decreased levels	P-450 induction; decreased bioavailability and increased clearance	Increase V and D doses
Verapamil (V)	Clarithromycin	Increased V levels	Inhibition of metabolism	Decrease V dose
Verapamil	Digoxin (D)	Increased D levels, heart block, asystole in D toxicity	Inhibition of P-gp, additive depression of conduction	Decrease D dose, monitor serum levels, avoid Ca blockers in digitalis toxicity
Verapamil	Prazosin (Pz)	Increased Pz levels, excessive hypotension	Inhibition of metabolism, additive α-blockade	Monitor blood pressure
Verapamil Diltiazem	Simvastatin (S) Atorvastatin (A)	Increased S and A levels Increased risk of myotoxicity	CYP3A4 inhibition	Avoid high S and A doses; use another statin
Verapamil	Theophylline (T)	Increased T levels	Inhibition of T metabolism	Decrease T dose, monitor T levels
	Quinidine	Hypotension (after verapamil IV)	Additive α-blockade	Use verapamil IV cautiously
	Clonidine	Complete AV block, hypotension	Additive myocardial depression	Use combination cautiously
	Halothane	Excessive bradycardia	Additive myocardial depression	Avoid combination if possible
Verapamil Diltiazem	Cyclosporine (Cy)	Increased Cy levels	Inhibition of Cy metabolism	Decrease Cy dose, monitor serum levels
Verapamil	Phenytoin (Ph)	Increased Ph and C levels	Inhibition of Ph and C metabolism	Decrease anticonvulsant dose, monitor levels
	Midazolam (Md)	Increased Md levels and effect	Inhibition of Md metabolism	Reduce Md dose
	Disopyramide	Heart failure	Additive negative inotropic effect	Avoid combination
Diltiazem	Sirolimus (Sir) Tacrolimus (Tac)	Increased Sir and Tac levels	Inhibition of metabolism	Decrease dose, monitor levels
Nifedipine	Magnesium sulfate	Neuromuscular blockade	Additive effect on depletion of intracellular calcium	
	Quinidine (Q)	Decreased Q levels	Increased clearance of Q(?); effect found in men with left ventricular failure	Monitor Q levels

results in severe hypotension and atrioventricular block has been reported.[164]

Verapamil is contraindicated in patients with digitalis toxicity because of additive depression of the SA and AV nodes.[165] An interaction between nifedipine and intravenous magnesium sulfate was reported in a woman with preeclampsia, resulting in neuromuscular blockade in the presence of normal magnesium levels. The possible mechanism is depletion of intracellular calcium by the additive actions of the calcium antagonist and magnesium.[166]

Interactions between calcium channel blockers and anesthetic agents have been described, notably a pronounced bradycardia when halothane was given to a patient on verapamil.[135]

Calcium can negate some of the effects of calcium antagonists and has been used to treat their overdose or adverse effects. Calcium reverses the negative inotropic effect and partly reverses AV conduction depression caused by calcium channel blockers but does not reverse sinus node depression or vasodilation.[159,167]

β-Blockers. β-Blockers (Table 41.5) can be divided into two groups based on their disposition: the lipophilic drugs (e.g., propranolol, metoprolol, timolol) and the more hydrophilic drugs (e.g., atenolol, nadolol, pindolol). The lipophilic drugs are extensively metabolized by the liver and are subject to a significant first-pass metabolism. The hydrophilic drugs have little first-pass metabolism, although absorption is less complete. The hydrophilic β-blockers are mostly excreted unchanged by the kidneys.

Pharmacokinetic interactions. Absorption of all β-blockers is reduced by concomitant administration of antacids or cholesterol-binding resins. For the drugs with high first-pass metabolism (e.g., propranolol, metoprolol), rifampin, phenytoin, and phenobarbital decrease bioavailability and increase clearance, resulting in low blood concentrations. Cimetidine has the opposite effect.[168–171]

Hydralazine has an effect on propranolol and metoprolol disposition whereby it increases the bioavailability of these

TABLE 41.5 Drug Interactions With β-Blockers

Drug	Interacting Drug	Effect	Mechanism	Comments
All β-blockers	Antacids	Decreased concentrations	Reduced absorption	Separate dosing by 1 hour
	Verapamil	Bradycardia, AV block, sinus arrest, hypotension, heart failure	Additive effect on myocardial contractility and conduction	Avoid combination in elderly and in patients with heart failure or conduction disturbance
	Diltiazem			
	Amiodarone			
	Epinephrine (adrenalin)	Severe hypertension	Unopposed effect on α receptors	Avoid epinephrine with patients on β-blockers
Propranolol (Pp)	Rifampin	Reduced bioavailability	Accelerated metabolism	Increase the doses of Pp and Me
Metoprolol (Me)	Phenytoin			
	Phenobarbital			
	Cimetidine	Increased bioavailability	Inhibition of metabolism	Decrease the dose
	Hydralazine	Increased bioavailability and clearance; usually, increase in Pr levels	Increased hepatic blood flow, accelerated metabolism, and saturation of first-pass metabolism	Adjust Pr dose to achieve β-blockade
Metoprolol (Me)	Quinidine	Increased levels	Inhibition of metabolic clearance	Decrease the dose of Me
Carvedilol	Digoxin (D)	Increased D and Cy levels	Inhibition of P-gp	Decrease D and Cy dose, monitor levels
	Cyclosporine (Cy)			

AV, Atrioventricular.

β-blockers by increasing hepatic blood flow, saturating the metabolizing enzymes. By the same token, by increasing hepatic blood flow, hydralazine increases propranolol clearance, but the increase in bioavailability exceeds the increase in clearance. Therefore, the net result is an increase in propranolol blood levels.[172] Metoprolol is metabolized by the cytochrome P-450 isozyme 2D6; its metabolism is genetically determined. Quinidine inhibits metoprolol clearance in extensive metabolizers.[173] There is some evidence that desethylamiodarone, a metabolite of amiodarone, can increase metoprolol serum concentration by inhibiting CYP2D6.[174] β-Blockers themselves, by decreasing hepatic blood flow, reduce clearance of other extensively hepatically metabolized drugs, such as lidocaine. Carvedilol and propranolol significantly inhibit P-gp, which can lead to an increase in serum concentrations of drugs such as digoxin and cyclosporine.[73,175] Doses of both drugs should be adjusted if combined with carvedilol.

Pharmacodynamic interactions. Because the major effects of β-blockers are depression of cardiac contractility and conduction, their combination with drugs exerting similar effects may result in excessive bradycardia, sinus arrest, AV block, CHF, and hypotension. Especially implicated is a combination of β-blockers with verapamil, but adverse effects with diltiazem and nifedipine have also been reported, especially in patients with CHF or underlying conduction disorders.[161,162] The combination of β-blockers and disopyramide, which also has a significant negative inotropic effect, may precipitate CHF.

The interaction between β-blockers and epinephrine can be very serious. Nonselective β-blockers, and selective ones in high doses, also block β_2 receptors, which mediate arterial vasodilation. Administration of epinephrine to a patient receiving nonselective β-blockers can result in unopposed action on α receptors and cause a serious increase in blood pressure that could be catastrophic.[176]

Chronic treatment with β-blockers has also been shown to increase the sensitivity to pressor effects of norepinephrine and angiotensin about twofold; the mechanism is unclear.[177]

ANTITHROMBOTIC AND ANTICOAGULANT DRUGS

Aspirin

Aspirin is a mainstay of antithrombotic therapy in patients with ischemic heart disease. Most aspirin interactions are pharmacodynamic. The most significant interaction is with warfarin, resulting in excessive bleeding by producing additive effects through their different effects on hemostasis. This additive effect is diminished when both drugs are used in low doses.[178]

Concomitant use of low-dose aspirin and NSAIDs may increase gastrointestinal bleeding; the use of aspirin with selective cyclo-oxygenase (COX)-2 inhibitors may abolish their gastroprotective effect.[179] In addition, NSAIDs—in particular, ibuprofen—may interfere with the antithrombotic effects of low-dose aspirin, especially when the ibuprofen dose is given before aspirin or with chronic use.[180,181] However, short-term use of over-the-counter ibuprofen does not appear to result in a clinically meaningful loss of cardioprotection.[182]

Ticagrelor

Unlike thienopyridines, ticagrelor is an active drug and does not require bioactivation. It is a substrate of both CYP3A4 and P-gp.[209] When ticagrelor is administered with potent CYP3A4 inhibitors, such as ketoconazole, a 2.4-fold increase in ticagrelor C_{max} was observed.[209] Conversely, discontinuation of phenytoin, a potent CYP3A4 inducer, resulted in improved platelet inhibition with ticagrelor.[211] Rifampin, another CYP3A4 inducer, decreased ticagrelor C_{max} by 73% and increased its clearance by 110%.

Morphine administration in healthy volunteers caused a reduction in ticagrelor AUC by 23%, but there was no effect on platelet aggregation.[212]

Ticagrelor was found to cause an increase in simvastatin C_{max} two- to threefold; thus, administration of ticagrelor with simvastatin doses higher than 40 mg is not recommended. In contrast, the effect on atorvastatin levels was only a 23% increase.[213]

Inhibition of P-gp by ticagrelor resulted in increased levels of digoxin; thus, monitoring of digoxin levels when initiating or discontinuing ticagrelor is recommended.[213]

Warfarin

Warfarin (Tables 41.6 and 41.7) is subject to many drug interactions, both pharmacokinetic and pharmacodynamic. As many as 80 interactions have been described; most of these have been known for many years. The consequences of warfarin interactions can be catastrophic (e.g., fatal bleeding or thrombosis). Most consequences can be avoided by checking the concomitant medications and adjusting the warfarin dose accordingly, especially when starting or discontinuing another drug. Warfarin metabolism is stereoselective. The more potent S isomer is metabolized by CYP2C9, whereas the less potent R isomer is metabolized by CYP1A2 and CYP3A4. CYP2C9 is subject to genetic polymorphism, and *2 and *3 alleles are associated with poor warfarin metabolism.[214] CYP2C9 polymorphism contributes to the variability in warfarin dosage as well as in drug-drug interactions.[215]

Pharmacokinetic Interactions

Enhancing the anticoagulant effect. Drugs that enhance the anticoagulant effect of warfarin (see Table 41.6) do so by inhibiting warfarin metabolism. Among drugs that inhibit warfarin metabolism are anti-infectives (metronidazole, macrolides, trimethoprim-sulfamethoxazole, fluoroquinolones, azole antifungals), cardiovascular drugs (amiodarone, diltiazem, propafenone), lipid-lowering drugs (fenofibrate, gemfibrozil, lovastatin), antidepressants (selective serotonin inhibitors, such as fluvoxamine and sertraline), gastrointestinal drugs (cimetidine, ranitidine, omeprazole) and other drugs such as allopurinol, anabolic steroids, and tamoxifen.[216,217] The time course of the interactions is difficult to predict because it depends on the half-lives of the interacting drug and warfarin and the vitamin K–dependent clotting factors II, VII, IX, and X. For most drugs, the interactions start within 2 to 3 days after administration and reach their maximal effect in 1 to 2 weeks.

Inhibiting the anticoagulant effect. Drugs such as cholestyramine and colestipol inhibit the anticoagulant effect of warfarin by decreasing its absorption (see Table 41.7). Most of the drugs that antagonize the anticoagulant response do so by accelerating warfarin metabolism. Among these drugs are rifampin, phenytoin, barbiturates, and carbamazepine.[216,217] Nafcillin and dicloxacillin also accelerate warfarin metabolism; high doses of warfarin may be required to achieve therapeutic prothrombin time prolongation in the presence of these drugs.[218]

TABLE 41.6 Drug Interactions With Warfarin: Increased Anticoagulation

Interacting Drug	Mechanism	Comment
Allopurinol	Inhibition of warfarin metabolism	Reduce warfarin dose, monitor PT
Amiodarone		
Propafenone		
Diltiazem		
Cimetidine		
Ranitidine		
Omeprazole		
Quinolones		
Macrolides		
Co-trimoxazole		
Metronidazole		
Azole antifungals		
Lovastatin		
Gemfibrozil		
Fenofibrate		
Fluvoxamine		
Sertraline		
Phenylbutazone		
Sulfinpyrazone		
Broad-spectrum antibiotics	Reduction in vitamin K availability	Primarily in malnourished patients
Acetaminophen	Inhibition of vitamin K–dependent carboxylase	Variable effect
Quinidine	Inhibition of clotting-factor synthesis	Adjust warfarin dose, monitor PT
NSAIDs	Depression of platelet function	Avoid combination; monitor PT
Clopidogrel		
SSRIs		
Cefamandole		
Moxalactam		

NSAIDs, Nonsteroidal antiinflammatory drugs; *PT,* prothrombin time; *SSRIs,* selective serotonin reuptake inhibitors.

TABLE 41.7 Drug Interactions With Warfarin: Decreased Anticoagulation

Interacting Drug	Mechanism	Comments
Barbiturates	Accelerated metabolism of warfarin	Increase warfarin dose, monitor PT
Carbamazepine		
Griseofulvin		
Phenytoin		
Nafcillin		
Rifampin		
Cholestyramine	Decreased absorption of warfarin	Allow at least 1 hour after warfarin administration
Colestipol		
Vitamin K	Antagonizes warfarin action	Avoid combination

PT, Prothrombin time.

Pharmacodynamic Interactions. Warfarin acts by inhibiting the synthesis of vitamin K–dependent clotting factors. Most of the vitamin K is obtained from food, with a small amount synthesized by intestinal bacteria. Treatment with antibiotics may reduce the amount of vitamin K produced by intestinal flora and thus cause an enhanced sensitivity to warfarin. However, the degree of INR change following this interaction is highly variable.[216] Acetaminophen has been reported to potentiate the effect of warfarin inhibiting vitamin K–dependent carboxylase. There is a significant interindividual variation in the magnitude of this effect.[219] Drugs that depress the synthesis of clotting factors (e.g., quinidine, salicylate in high doses) also enhance the anticoagulant effect of warfarin.[220]

The most significant interactions are those resulting from the additive effects of other drugs affecting hemostasis by a different mechanism, resulting in an increased risk of bleeding. Such drugs include aspirin; NSAIDs; clopidogrel; some third-generation cephalosporins that inhibit platelet function; and heparin, which affects other clotting factors.[221,222] Selective serotonin reuptake inhibitors may inhibit platelet aggregation by depleting platelet serotonin levels and thereby cause an increased risk of bleeding with warfarin.[223] Drugs that injure gastrointestinal mucosa—such as NSAIDs and, to lesser degree, COX-2 inhibitors—also increase the risk of gastrointestinal hemorrhage.[221,224]

Some herbal preparations—such as garlic, ginger, ginseng, ginkgo biloba, and the Chinese herb danshen—have been shown to have antiplatelet activity and may increase the risk of bleeding when used concomitantly with warfarin.[225]

Drugs that antagonize the effects of warfarin are vitamin K analogues, foods, and enteral formulas containing high amounts of vitamin K. Oral contraceptives inhibit the anticoagulant effect by increasing the synthesis of clotting factors VII and X.

Heparin and Low-Molecular-Weight Heparins

The significant interactions of heparin and low-molecular-weight heparins are with other drugs that affect hemostasis, such as aspirin, NSAIDs, and warfarin. Concomitant use of glycoprotein IIb/IIIa antagonists, particularly in elderly patients, is also associated with an increased risk of major bleeding.[235] There have been reports of interactions with intravenous nitroglycerin, in which the anticoagulant effect of heparin is reduced and therefore higher heparin doses are required, but subsequent studies have not supported this observation.[236–238]

THIENOPYRIDINES

Ticlopidine

Ticlopidine has a different antithrombotic action than aspirin—inhibition of adenosine diphosphate (ADP)–dependent platelet aggregation. It is cleared primarily through hepatic metabolism. Ticlopidine has been shown to inhibit some P-450 enzymes. It reduces theophylline clearance.[183,184] Contrary to expectations, ticlopidine was reported to significantly decrease plasma cyclosporine levels. The mechanism responsible for this action is unknown.[185]

Clopidogrel

Clopidogrel has largely replaced ticlopidine because of a lower incidence of neutropenia. Clopidogrel is a prodrug and is metabolized to an active drug by CYP2C19, which significantly contributes to the first oxidative step, and by CYP3A4, which is involved in the second oxidative step.[186] Carriers of the loss of function allele of CYP2C19 have 30% lower levels of active metabolite and a 25% reduction in platelet inhibition ex vivo.[187] Proton pump inhibitors (PPIs) are commonly used in patients who are on dual antiplatelet therapy (DAPT) to prevent gastrointestinal bleeding. PPIs are both substrates and inhibitors of CYP2C19, with omeprazole having the strongest effect and, in decreasing order, esomeprazole and lansoprazole. Reduced levels of clopidogrel active metabolite and higher platelet–reactivity index ex vivo were found in subjects treated with clopidogrel and PPIs,[188,189] prompting a U.S. Food and Drug Administration warning about concomitant treatment in 2009. However, the clinical significance of this interaction is not clear. Clinical outcomes studies have been inconsistent, with observational studies reporting increased risks of recurrent MI in patients treated with clopidogrel and PPIs,[190,191] whereas a post hoc analysis of randomized trials and a retrospective cohort study did not identify such risks.[191,192] Observational data suggested an increased risk of acute coronary events not only with omeprazole but also with pantoprazole and esomeprazole.[193]

Given the potentially increased risk of gastrointestinal bleeding on DAPT, the American College of Cardiology/American College of Gastroenterology/American Heart Association (ACCF/ACG/AHA) issued a consensus document on the concomitant use of PPIs and thienopyridines in 2010.[194] The document states that clinical decisions must balance overall risks and benefits of cardiovascular and gastrointestinal complications. A review of published studies on this issue found that 74% did find an increased clinical risk with clopidogrel and PPIs.[195]

Fluoxetine, a CYP2C19 and CYP3A4 inhibitor, decreased clopidogrel AUC and C_{max} by 20.6% and 25.3%, respectively, in healthy volunteers. Similar effects were observed with ketoconazole.[196]

Concerns have been raised about a potential interaction causing decreased efficacy of clopidogrel with some statins that inhibit CYP3A4, such as atorvastatin and simvastatin. Indeed, there are several reports of a reduced antiplatelet effect of clopidogrel with atorvastatin in vitro.[197,198] However, other studies have not found this effect[199] and no adverse effect on cardiovascular outcomes has been found when clopidogrel was administered with CYP3A4-inhibiting statins compared with statins with no effect on CYP3A4.[200–203]

Clopidogrel strongly inhibits CYP2C8. In healthy volunteers, a maintenance dose of clopidogrel increased the AUC of repaglinide (a CYP2C8 substrate) fourfold.[204] Thus, clopidogrel should not be prescribed with repaglinide because of the risk of hypoglycemia.

Morphine delays the antiplatelet activity of clopidogrel in patients with ST elevation MI, probably by delaying gastric emptying and intestinal absorption.[205,206]

The addition of clopidogrel to aspirin has a synergistic effect on platelet inhibition and in some patients has been shown to overcome ex vivo aspirin resistance assessed by aggregometry, flow cytometry, and platelet resistance index.[201]

Prasugrel

Prasugrel, like clopidogrel, is a prodrug that requires CYP3A4 for its activation. However, there are few clinically significant interactions with prasugrel. Grapefruit juice reduced the C_{max} and AUC of the primary active metabolite of prasugrel, but the effect on antiplatelet activity was negligible.[207] Ritonavir, an antiretroviral drug and a potent CYP3A4 inhibitor, was shown to reduce the bioactivation of prasugrel.[208] Other CYP3A4 inhibitors, such as ketoconazole and PPIs, have been shown to reduce the rate of generation of prasugrel active metabolite but not its overall exposure. There was no effect of administration of these drugs on peak inhibitory platelet activity (IPA) after loading dose of prasugrel or on IPA on maintenance dose.[209,210]

DIRECT ORAL ANTICOAGULANTS (DOACS)

DOACs are oral inhibitors of factor IIa (dabigatran) and of factor Xa (rivaroxaban and apixaban). They have far fewer drug interactions than warfarin and are approved for use in nonvalvular atrial fibrillation and in the prevention and treatment of venous thromboembolism. Combination of these drugs with antiplatelet agents or with other anticoagulants can result in an increased risk for bleeding.

Dabigatran

Dabigatran is a prodrug and is absorbed via P-gp. Thus its bioavailability, plasma concentration, and AUC are increased by concomitant therapy with potent inhibitors of P-gp (such as amiodarone, dronedarone, clarithromycin, ketoconazole, and verapamil) and decreased with potent P-gp inducers (such as rifampin, carbamazepine, and phenytoin).[226,227] The increase in dabigatran plasma levels was limited when dabigatran was administered 2 hours prior to verapamil administration.[228] The clinical significance of the interactions is not clear and no dose adjustments are recommended for concomitant use with amiodarone and clarithromycin in patients with normal renal function. However, concomitant therapy with P-gp inhibitors should be avoided in patients with moderate to severe renal failure and in patients over 80 years. Coadministration with P-gp inducers is not recommended.[229]

In the Randomized Evaluation of Long-Term Anticoagulation Therapy (RE-LY) study, 38.4% of the patients received concomitant antiplatelet therapy at some point. Concomitant use of either aspirin or clopidogrel increased the risk of major bleeding compared with dabigatran alone (hazard ratio [HR], 1.6) whereas the use of DAPT increased the risk even more (HR, 2.3). The absolute risk of bleeding was highest with the 150 mg twice-daily dose of dabigatran.[230]

Rivaroxaban and Apixaban

Both drugs are metabolized by CYP3A4 and are substrates for P-gp. Combination therapy with drugs that are either inhibitors of both CYP3A4 and P-gp (i.e., ketoconazole, clarithromycin)

or inducers of CYP3A4 and P-gp (rifampin, carbamazepine, phenytoin) should be avoided.[229,231]

Aspirin did not alter the pharmacokinetics and the anti-Xa activity of rivaroxaban.[232] However, concomitant use of aspirin and rivaroxaban in the Rivaroxaban Once Daily Oral Direct Factor Xa Inhibition Compared with Vitamin K Antagonism for Prevention of Stroke and Embolism Trial in Atrial Fibrillation (ROCKET AF) was associated with an increased risk of major bleeding (HR, 1.32) and death (HR, 1.27).[233] In patients with acute coronary syndromes, the addition of apixaban to antiplatelet therapy increased the risk of major bleeding compared with placebo: HR of 6.6 for aspirin monotherapy and HR of 2.58 for DAPT.[234]

LIPID-LOWERING DRUGS

Drug interactions with lipid-lowering drugs are displayed in Table 41.8. The significant interactions with hydroxymethylglutaryl-coenzyme A reductase inhibitors (e.g., lovastatin, simvastatin, pravastatin, fluvastatin, atorvastatin, rosuvastatin) are pharmacokinetic, leading to high statin concentrations in the peripheral blood and muscle tissue, and pharmacodynamic, leading to additive or synergistic muscle toxicity.

Concomitant use of simvastatin, lovastatin, and atorvastatin with CYP3A4 inhibitors (such as erythromycin, clarithromycin, fluconazole, verapamil, diltiazem, and amiodarone) results in a significantly increased AUC of statins and, particularly when high doses of statins are used, in myotoxicity and rhabdomyolysis.[239,240] CYP3A4 inhibitors have no appreciable effect on plasma levels of pravastatin and rosuvastatin, which are not metabolized by CYP3A4.[240] Cytochrome P-450 inducers, such as rifampin and carbamazepine, can significantly reduce the AUC of simvastatin and atorvastatin.

The uptake of statins into the liver is mediated by organic anion transporter OATP1B1. This mechanism is particularly significant for hydrophilic statins, such as pravastatin and rosuvastatin. Inhibitors of OATP1B1 include cyclosporine, clarithromycin, and protease inhibitors ritonavir, saquinavir, and indinavir. Coadministration of these drugs with statins results in an increased AUC of statins and an increased risk of rhabdomyolysis.[240]

Concomitant use of statins and fibrates results in increased risk of myopathy and rhabdomyolysis because of their additive risk. The risk of interaction with gemfibrozil is the greatest because, in addition to the pharmacodynamic interaction, gemfibrozil also inhibits CYP2C8, which metabolizes the active form of simvastatin and lovastatin, and OATP1B1.[240] Gemfibrozil also increases plasma levels of other CYP2C8 substrates, particularly the glucose-lowering drugs repaglinide, rosiglitazone, and pioglitazone.[240]

Clofibrate and gemfibrozil increase the anticoagulant effect of warfarin by inhibiting its hepatic metabolism.

Cholesterol-binding resins (e.g., cholestyramine, colestipol) bind to acidic drugs, such as digoxin, warfarin, thiazide diuretics, thyroid hormones, and sulfonylureas in the gut, thereby interfering with their absorption.[241] Cholestyramine also decreases the bioavailability of ezetimibe.[240] Probucol can prolong the QT

TABLE 41.8 Drug Interactions With Lipid-Lowering Drugs

Drug	Interacting Drug	Effect	Comments
Simvastatin Lovastatin Atorvastatin	Macrolides Fluconazole Amiodarone Diltiazem Verapamil	Rhabdomyolysis via increased statin levels (CYP3A4 inhibition)	Avoid combination if possible; otherwise, monitor CPK
Simvastatin Lovastatin	Gemfibrozil	Rhabdomyolysis via increased statin levels (CYP2C8 and OATP1B1 inhibition)	Avoid combination if possible; otherwise, monitor CPK
HMG-CoA reductase inhibitors	Cyclosporine	Rhabdomyolysis via increased statin plasma levels (OATP1B1 inhibition)	Avoid combination if possible; otherwise, monitor CPK; decrease dose when combined with cyclosporine
	Clarithromycin Ritonavir Saquinavir Indinavir		
HMG-CoA reductase inhibitors	Fibrates	Rhabdomyolysis	Avoid combination if possible; otherwise, monitor CPK
Clofibrate Gemfibrozil	Warfarin	Increased anticoagulation (inhibition of warfarin metabolism)	Monitor PT, adjust warfarin dose
Probucol	Class 1A antidysrhythmic	Additive Q–T prolongation; risk of torsades de pointes	Avoid combination
Cholestyramine Colestipol	Digoxin Ezetimibe Thiazide diuretics Warfarin Sulfonylurea Thyroid hormones	Binding in the gut and decreased absorption of the interacting drugs	Separate administration of bile acid sequestrants by 2–3 hours

CPK, Creatine phosphokinase; *PT*, prothrombin time.

interval and thus create an additive risk for torsades de pointes when administered with class 1A or class 3 drugs.[242]

DIURETICS

Most of the drug interactions with diuretics are pharmacodynamic. There is a synergistic effect when a loop diuretic is administered with a thiazide; this combination is used in refractory edematous states (e.g., severe CHF) in which loop diuretic efficacy is limited because of enhanced sodium reabsorption in the distal tubules. Because this combination may result in massive fluid and electrolyte loss, the thiazide should be started at low doses.[243] Care should be exercised when an ACE inhibitor is added to a diuretic because the inhibition of angiotensin II response may result in profound hypotension and renal failure. Reduction in the diuretic dose or temporary withdrawal of the diuretic is prudent before starting an ACE inhibitor.[27,28] NSAIDs and COX-2 selective inhibitors raise blood pressure and significantly increase the incidence of CHF. Thus, they can be expected to diminish

the response to loop and thiazide diuretics.[244,245] There are reports of indomethacin inhibiting the antihypertensive actions of the diuretics, although other NSAIDs, specifically diclofenac and sulindac, did not have this effect.[246]

Diuretics reduce the renal excretion of lithium because sodium depletion causes enhanced tubular reabsorption of lithium. Lithium doses should therefore be reduced by 25% when adding diuretics and plasma levels should be monitored. There is a risk of additive ototoxicity when loop diuretics are used with aminoglycosides, especially with high doses of the diuretic and in patients with renal failure.

Concomitant use of potassium-sparing diuretics with ACE inhibitors or angiotensin receptor blockers can result in severe hyperkalemia, particularly in patients with spironolactone doses higher than 25 mg/day, the elderly, and patients with impaired renal function and diabetes mellitus.[247]

The full reference list for this chapter is available at ExpertConsult.com.

PART VI

Advanced Diagnostic and Therapeutic Techniques: Indications and Technical Considerations

42

Central Venous Access Procedures

Thomas M. Przybysz, Alan C. Heffner

PERIPHERAL INTRAVENOUS CANNULATION

Patients in the cardiac intensive care unit (CICU) require reliable intravenous access.[1-3] Dependable peripheral vein cannulation technique is an essential tool to establish intravenous access in critically ill patients.

Equipment

Equipment for peripheral venous access includes the following: (1) 16-, 18-, and 20-gauge intravenous (IV) catheter over needle units with backup supplies, (2) alcohol swabs, (3) tourniquet, (4) TB or 3-mL syringe with 1% lidocaine, (5) 25-gauge needle, (6) short connector IV tubing flushed with sterile crystalloid, and (7) Steri-Drape and tape to secure the access.

Technique

Although any vein may be utilized for emergency access, distal upper extremity veins and superficial jugular veins are prime peripheral cannulation targets. Note that highly mobile sites may limit reliability following insertion. For example, cannulation at the antecubital fossa requires the arm to maintain a straight position. When present, Y-shaped venous confluences are preferred targets. The dorsal hand, wrist, and forearm are common access sites. Use of a proximal tourniquet or blood pressure cuff accentuates the venous targets. Avoid tying the tourniquet in a tight knot. Focused manual pressure may be applied to distend a superficial jugular vein. Actively pumping the fist hastens venous engorgement at upper extremity sites.

Steps for inserting a peripheral intravenous line are shown in Fig. 42.1. Always wear clean gloves. When targeting a venous Y-confluence, aim for the branch point. Local anesthesia may be infiltrated prior to cannulation but is not required. Apply traction with the nondominant hand to anchor the vein and keep the skin taut. Advance the catheter-over-needle assembly through the skin and into the vein while monitoring for a blood flash at the needle hub. The initial flash represents needle-tip penetration. Advance 1 to 2 mm to ensure that the entire needle tip is within the vessel before advancing the catheter into the vein. Maintain the needle in position and release the tourniquet. Next, remove the needle and discard it. Connect the intravenous

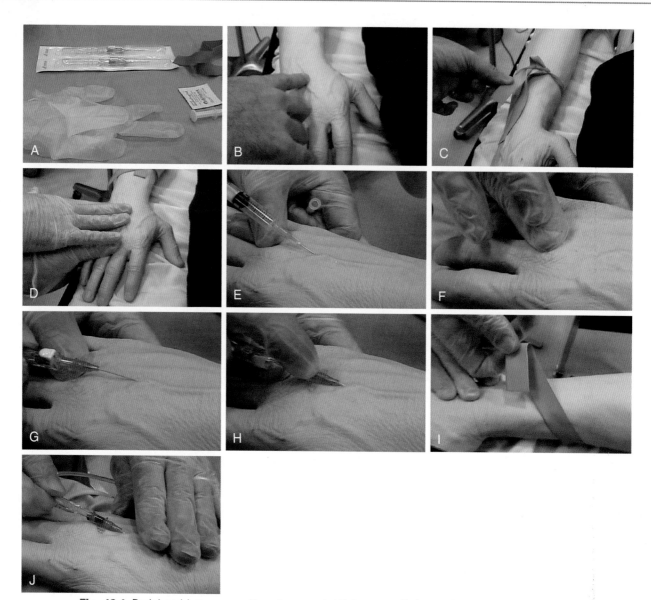

Fig. 42.1 Peripheral intravenous line placement. (A) Lay out all the equipment in an organized way. (B) Look for a good vein, ideally one shaped like an inverted Y. (C) Make sure that the tourniquet can be undone with one hand. (D) Try to get the vein to stand out. (E) Apply alcohol wipe and administer lidocaine. (F) Pull the skin taut and keep it taut. (G) Approach at a shallow angle to get the needle and catheter tip in. (H) Without letting go of the taut skin, advance the catheter. (I) Undo the tourniquet. (J) Hold down above the catheter.

connector tubing and secure the catheter. Monitor for subcutaneous infiltration while gently flushing the catheter with sterile crystalloid.

Clinical Pearls

- Prepare all equipment, including backup supplies, prior to the first venipuncture attempt.
- Long intravenous tubing represents the greatest resistance to flow. For rapid large-volume resuscitation, a 16-gauge catheter is equally efficient to larger catheters.
- Y-shaped venous confluences are easily anchored and represent high-yield targets for peripheral venous cannulation.

- Advancing 1 to 2 mm after the initial blood flash ensures that the needle tip is within the vein. Failure to advance the needle following initial blood flash is a common mistake.
- Adequately secure the IV access immediately after insertion.

Complications

Known complications of peripheral venous access are phlebitis, infection, and extravasation. Adequate skin preparation, limited punctures, and diligent site monitoring are recommended to reduce complications. Poorly functioning access sites should be removed immediately once alternative access is obtained.

CENTRAL VENOUS ACCESS GENERAL PRINCIPLES AND PREPARATION

Central venous access is indicated in CICU patients who require reliable intravenous access, vasopressor administration, hemodynamic monitoring, temporary transvenous pacing, and hemodialysis access.[4] Contraindications to central access are relative, depending on alternative vascular access options and the urgency of the situation. Anatomic distortion, local infection, and existing hardware justify avoiding specific sites when possible. Coagulopathy is not a contraindication to central access placement, but the procedural risk and patient benefits should be carefully weighed.[4–6]

Central access is often required emergently and obtaining consent may not be practical. In nonemergent circumstances, consent should be obtained prior to cannulation and should highlight the benefits and risks of the procedure. Infection, bleeding, arterial injury, venous thrombosis, and pneumothorax are all important risks to discuss.[7,8] After consent is obtained, dedicate several minutes to optimal site selection and preparation.

Most nonemergent central venous catheters in the CICU are placed in the internal jugular or subclavian vein. If ultrasound is available, the site should be investigated prior to skin preparation and draping. Abnormal vascular anatomy or visible clots may prohibit a preferred site. The Trendelenburg position is recommended for subclavian and jugular access if the patient can safely tolerate repositioning. A patient in severe respiratory distress may require intubation prior to obtaining central access. The neutral body position is ideal for most central lines with a few modifications. Patients may need to have breast tissue or an abdominal pannus retracted by an assistant or secured with tape to access a site.

Once the site is selected and the patient is positioned, the skin should be cleaned. Chlorhexidine-based solutions reduce central line–associated blood stream infection (CLABSI) compared with povidone iodine-alcohol solutions.[9–11] Full sterile precautions consisting of hat, face mask, eye shield, sterile gown, sterile gloves, and large sterile drape should be used for all central access procedures.[12] A table large enough to accommodate the central line kit should be ergonomically positioned within the provider's arm reach. Supplies should not be placed on the sterile drape as patients can unexpectedly move during the procedure. The insertion site should be anesthetized with 1% lidocaine. Ultrasound guidance is recommended for access procedures when available. It may be used to confirm appropriate anatomy and landmarks prior to instrumentation or provide dynamic real-time imaging to track needle penetration.

SELDINGER TECHNIQUE

The modified Seldinger guidewire technique is standard for central venous and arterial access procedures. Initial vessel puncture is obtained with a large-bore, 18-gauge introducer needle or catheter-over-needle assembly. Needle trajectory and depth should be monitored closely throughout the procedure. Continuous negative pressure is applied to the aspirating syringe during needle advancement and withdrawal. Initial blood flash may be first recognized during needle withdrawal. The ability to continuously aspirate while maintaining strict control of the needle requires practice. Novice providers should be closely supervised. Venous puncture confirmation is important for central venous access procedures to avoid inadvertent arterial cannulation. Blood color, pulsatility, and ultrasound visualization may be misleading in certain circumstances.[13] A 30-cm length of intravenous or pressure tubing can be used to gauge or transduce pressure prior to vessel dilation.[14] The pressure tubing may be connected directly to the introducer needle or angiocath inserted over the needle or via guidewire.

The guidewire is next advanced through the introducer needle to approximately 20 cm. The needle must remain stationary before the wire is inserted. Bracing the hand against the patient to steady the needle and avoid accidental needle movement is a common technique. The guidewire should pass easily with minimal resistance. If resistance is encountered, remove the wire, reconfirm blood aspiration, or reposition the needle trajectory or guidewire J-tip orientation prior to readvancing the guidewire. With the wire stabilized at 20 cm, the needle is removed and a small stab incision at the guidewire exit site is completed with a No. 11 scalpel. While stabilizing the guidewire, the tissue tract dilator is advanced over the guidewire through the skin and connective tissue to reach the vessel. Care must be taken to avoid advancing the wire and dilator together, as this can bend the wire and damage the vessel. The wire should always slide easily within the dilator during proper technique. Next, the dilator is removed while keeping the wire stationary and maintaining hemostasis at the site with firm pressure. The vascular catheter is then advanced into position over the guidewire using the same technique. Finally, the guidewire is removed, the catheter lumens are flushed, and the catheter is secured to the skin at the appropriate depth (usually 15 to 20 cm depending on access site and patient size).

Clinical Pearls

- Arrange all supplies on a bedside table prior to starting the procedure.
- Place the guidewire on the field in close proximity and brace the needle during syringe removal and guidewire insertion to avoid losing the target vessel during these steps.
- Stabilizing the guidewire while advancing the dilator helps prevent guidewire kinking and vessel injury.
- Hold the dilator close to the skin while advancing in small increments.
- Novice operators focus heavily on procedural mechanics and may not identify patient deterioration during the procedure. Bedside assistance or supervision is highly recommended.

INTERNAL JUGULAR VEIN

Relevant Anatomy

The internal jugular vein originates at the jugular foramen and descends to join the subclavian vein. In the mid to lower neck, it lies lateral and then anterolateral to the carotid artery. At the level of the thyroid cartilage, the vein lies deep to the sternocleidomastoid muscle. The vessel emerges from behind the muscle into the triangle created by the sternal and clavicular insertions of the sternocleidomastoid muscle, just above the clavicle. Right-sided jugular cannulation is preferred owing to the direct path to the superior vena cava and to avoid risk to the left-sided thoracic duct.

Landmark Technique

Steps for internal jugular central venous line placement are shown in Fig. 42.2. Turn the patient's head 15 to 30 degrees to gain exposure to the access site. Turning the neck farther will compress and flatten the vessel. It is useful to mark the surface landmarks before starting the procedure. The apex of the sternocleidomastoid triangle or medial border of the posterior sternocleidomastoid muscle is a common needle insertion point. The carotid artery can be palpated medial to this point. A 22-gauge finder needle is inserted 30 degrees to the skin and aimed toward the ipsilateral nipple. After the internal jugular vein is located, the finder needle is kept in place, and the larger 18-gauge introducer needle mounted on a 5-mL slip tip syringe is inserted adjacent to the needle finder and along the same trajectory. Typical jugular vein depth is less than 2 cm from the skin surface but needle trajectory and patient variation may require deeper needle insertion. Following needle puncture, insert the catheter using the Seldinger technique as described earlier.

Ultrasound-Guided Technique

Ultrasound-guided central line placement aids in identifying anatomic variations and is associated with improved success and reduced complications.[15,16] Real-time dynamic ultrasound allows the provider to visualize the needle tip during insertion. It is important to recognize that the needle shaft and tip have a similar appearance. Vigilantly monitor needle insertion depth during the procedure.

Clinical Pearls

- The sternocleidomastoid triangle and carotid artery pulsation are important surface landmarks.
- Insert the needle at the apex of sternocleidomastoid triangle to maximize distance from the lung and avoid pneumothorax.
- Orient the ultrasound screen to minimize head turning during the procedure.
- An angiocatheter and pressure tubing allow accurate confirmation of venous access and can prevent inadvertent arterial dilation or catheter placement, which are associated with arterial occlusion and stroke.

Complications

It is important to know how to manage pitfalls and complications associated with internal jugular cannulation. The most critical complications arise from carotid artery puncture or cannulation. Recognized puncture of the artery with immediate needle withdrawal and application of firm but nonocclusive pressure is usually uncomplicated. Major bleeding can lead to neck hematoma and airway compromise. Arterial cannulation can result in cerebrovascular insufficiency, vessel thrombosis, or pseudoaneurysm formation. If this occurs, leave the catheter

in place and consult a vascular surgeon for assistance with removal. Advancing the guidewire too deeply can induce dysrhythmias that are usually relieved by withdrawing the guidewire.

SUBCLAVIAN VENOUS CANNULATION

Subclavian venous access is a common and often preferred access site based on the low risk of mechanical and infectious complications.[17] Site-specific contraindications include clavicle distortion or indwelling local hardware (i.e., pacemakers or implantable cardioverter-defibrillators) and severe coagulopathy that may promote bleeding at this noncompressible site.

Technique

Steps for subclavian central venous line placement are shown in Fig. 42.3. The left subclavian vein is the preferred site owing to low incidence of catheter malposition and direct insertion trajectory for emergency transvenous pacemaker or pulmonary artery catheter placement. Consider prioritizing cannulation ipsilateral to severe unilateral lung disease or an indwelling chest drain to minimize patient decompensation in the event of a procedure-related pneumothorax.

Set up for the central line as described earlier with proper position and full sterile equipment. Consider having an assistant apply gentle caudal traction to the ipsilateral arm.[18] Ultrasound guidance for subclavian cannulation is not standard but is described.[19] Inject 1% lidocaine at the injection site for anesthesia. The introducer needle is inserted 2 cm lateral and inferior to the midclavicular point. Aim for the suprasternal notch and pass beneath the clavicle. Intentionally contacting the clavicle to "walk" the needle down the clavicle helps to maintain the needle in a plane parallel to the floor to reduce the risk of pneumothorax.[20] Following vessel puncture, insert the catheter via the Seldinger technique as described earlier.

Complications

Pneumothorax and subclavian arterial puncture are common concerns with the subclavian access approach but the rate of mechanical complication remains low.

Clinical Pearls

- To avoid pneumothorax, the needle should be maintained parallel to the floor during insertion.
- The subclavian vein is the preferred venous access site to reduce mechanical and infectious complications.

FEMORAL VENOUS CANNULATION

Femoral venous catheters are generally avoided in favor of internal jugular or subclavian venous access but still have a role in certain scenarios, such as emergency situations and for hemodialysis access when the right internal jugular vein is not an option.[21] The femoral site has historically been associated with an increased risk of infection, but more recent literature suggests only minor increased risk.[22,23] Venous thrombosis is more common compared with jugular and subclavian vein access.[24]

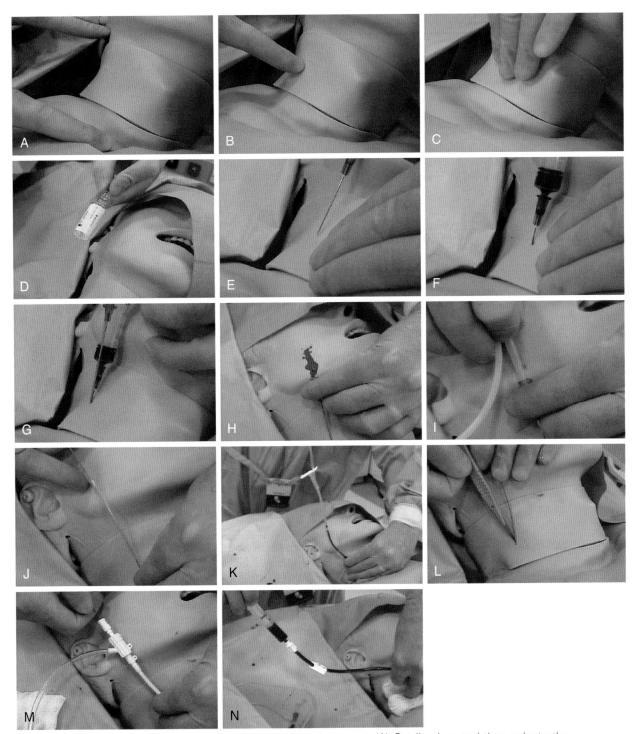

Fig. 42.2 Internal jugular central venous line placement. (A) Get lined up and then palpate the sternal notch (lower finger) and mastoid process (upper finger) to identify the sternocleidomastoid muscle. (B) Without any imaging guidance, go in at about the halfway point. (C) Palpate the carotid artery but do not press down on it to avoid compressing and flattening the internal jugular vein, making it hard to hit. (D) Use local anesthetic judiciously. (E) It is crucial to be close to the carotid artery but aiming away from it (at the ipsilateral nipple). If this is performed under ultrasound guidance, the carotid artery and internal jugular vein are adjacent to each other. (F) Proceed until dark venous blood is observed, usually 1 to 2 cm deep. (G) Once the finder is in, place the needle directly on top of the finder to exactly reproduce the approach angle. (H) If the blood is bright and squirts out in pulsatile fashion, the attempt has missed and hit the artery. (I) Assuming that did not happen, advance the wire, keeping an eye out for ectopy. (J) Once the wire is in, again check that it is in the right place. Slide the 18-gauge catheter down the wire, pull the wire out, and connect the catheter to the extension tubing. (K) Hold the tubing up, make sure that the blood goes up to central venous pressure height and not to arterial height (it would climb all the way to the top and squirt out). This is a quick and effective way of ensuring the correct location. Proceed with the standard Seldinger technique. (L) Nick, dilate, flush, sew, and dress. (M) If a cordis is being placed, the dilator and cordis should be placed as a unit. (N) Aspirate and flush, without leaving anything open to air, which could lead to an air embolus.

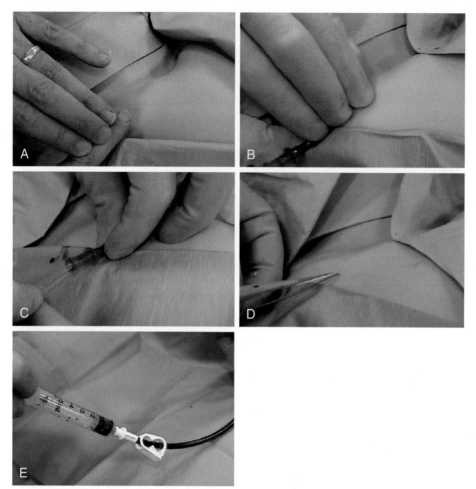

Fig. 42.3 Subclavian central venous line placement. (A) The needle should target the sternal notch, but always angle away from the lungs. If the needle needs to be depressed, press down on top with three fingers so that the whole needle goes down flat as a single unit rather than just pointing the tip down. (B) The needle is in the clavicle and the upper fingers are pressing the needle down as a unit so that it goes down but is still inclined away from the lung. (C) Once the needle is in, the subclavian area has a distinct advantage over the internal jugular vein area, as the needle is held between the clavicle and the first rib and is better secured. (D) Wire, nick, dilate, and flush. Do not go too medially to avoid getting stuck between the first rib and the clavicle. (E) Aspirate, flush, sew, and dress.

Steps for inserting a femoral central venous line are shown in Fig. 42.4. The ipsilateral leg should be slightly abducted and externally rotated for access site exposure. The anatomic structures can be recalled by the mnemonic NAVEL (nerve, artery, vein, empty space, lymphatics-oriented lateral to medial). Use of ultrasound is recommended if available. The introducer needle is inserted 1 to 2 cm below the inguinal crease with the aim of puncturing the femoral vein as it emerges beneath the inguinal ligament. Vessel puncture and instrumentation above the inguinal ligament risks procedure-related hemorrhage that may be concealed in the retroperitoneum and is not easily compressible. The needle is advanced at a 20- to 30-degree angle to the skin toward the arterial pulsation. Preparation and Seldinger technique have been described earlier.

Complications

Retroperitoneal hemorrhage can occur from posterior vessel injury without any evidence of superficial bleeding or hematoma formation and may go unrecognized.

Clinical Pearls

- It is ergonomically easier for right-handed operators to target the right femoral vein.
- Avoidance of this site or modified technique with a straight guidewire may be required in patients with indwelling inferior vena cava filters.
- Any clinical consideration of a retroperitoneal hemorrhage must be ruled out immediately with a CT scan.

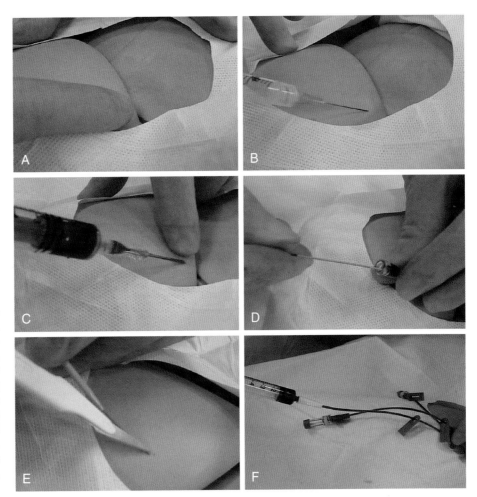

Fig. 42.4 Femoral central venous line placement. (A) The mnemonic NAVEL is very useful for reviewing the anatomic landmarks (nerve, artery, vein, empty space, lymphatics). (B) Apply local anesthesia generously. (C) Using the hollow needle, advance until dark venous blood is observed. (D) Hold the needle steady, wire it up, and proceed using the standard Seldinger technique. (E) Nick the skin, dilate, and pass the line. (F) Aspirate, flush, sew in place, and apply dressing.

RADIAL ARTERIAL CANNULATION

Continuous invasive arterial access is indicated for close blood pressure monitoring and for reliable serial blood gas sampling. The radial artery is the most commonly selected site.[25–29] This site is contraindicated following radial artery harvest as a bypass conduit and in cases of preexisting arterial insufficiency to the hand.

Equipment

Equipment for radial arterial line placement includes the following: (1) antiseptic skin preparation, (2) a wrist board to hold the position once completed, (3) tape, (4) 1% lidocaine in a small syringe with a 25-gauge needle, (5) 20-gauge vascular cannula—a prefabricated arterial catheter-over-needle assembly with attached guidewire and sheath is common, with peripheral intravenous cannulas being an alternative option, and (6) transducer and pressure tubing.

Technique

Steps for inserting a radial arterial line are shown in Fig. 42.5. First, as with all procedures, explain the procedure and obtain consent. Consider real-time ultrasound guidance, which may be associated with greater first-pass success.[30] Set up all equipment prior to starting the procedure. Sitting in a comfortable position at the bedside is recommended over standing and bending over the target. Extend the target site wrist 20 degrees to flatten the thenar eminence and gain exposure to the site. Extending the wrist over a towel roll may help. Tape the hand to maintain this position. Apply chlorhexidine-based antiseptic skin preparation solution and allow it to dry followed by infiltration of local anesthetic at the intended puncture site. Target the distal vessel just proximal to the flexor crease. This allows a more proximal artery target in case of vasospasm or hematoma following a failed first attempt.

Puncture the skin and slowly advance the needle or catheter-over-needle assembly at a 15- to 30-degree angle along the long axis of the target vessel. The vessel lies less than 0.5 cm deep in most situations, which is more superficial than commonly recognized. Once inserted beyond the anticipated target depth, slowly withdraw the needle under close guidance while monitoring for blood flash. Some operators prefer a through-and-through technique in which the needle is intentionally inserted through and beyond the artery, with flash monitored during needle withdrawal. Once punctured, pressurized arterial blood should flow from the catheter or up the attached sheath. A flexible, straight guidewire is advanced over the wire to maintain access to the vessel. A 20-gauge catheter is then advanced in place over the guidewire and the needle and guidewire are removed.

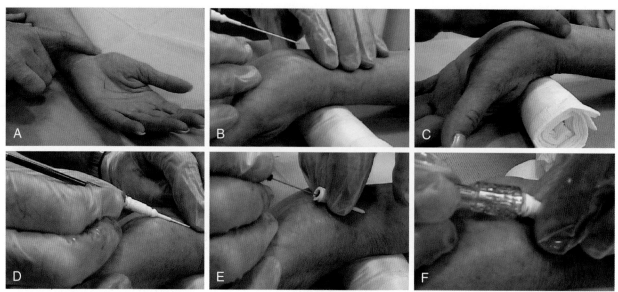

Fig. 42.5 Radial arterial line placement. (A) To approach the radial artery, one needs to go over the thenar eminence. (B) Extending the wrist allows a straight shot to the radial artery. (C) Approach at a shallow angle to get the needle in, then slide up a little more to get the catheter in as well. (D) Make sure that the blood keeps flowing as you advance. (E) Slide the catheter in, then hold down above the line so that the blood does not squirt out. (F) It is recommended to use a Luer-Lok to avoid disconnecting the line.

Following confirmation of arterial blood withdrawal, connect the pressure tubing to the catheter. Check the arterial tracing to ensure an appropriate waveform. Secure the catheter and wrist position with an arm board. If the first attempt fails, apply pressure to maintain hemostasis and reinsert at the same site or just proximal.

Clinical Pearls

- Prepare all equipment and orient yourself in a comfortable position prior to attempting insertion.
- Apply chlorhexidine skin preparation and ensure sterile insertion technique as in central venous access procedures.
- Approach the artery via a shallow 15- to 30-degree angle.
- Recognize the superficial position of the target vessel.
- The wire should pass easily and smoothly without resistance.
- Remove the catheter and consider vascular surgery consultation for signs of distal extremity ischemia.

Complications

Distal arterial ischemia is the most feared complication, but is uncommon. Despite tradition, the Allen test is not a good screening test for arterial collateralization of the hand. The arterial catheter should be removed for evidence of distal ischemia. Other important complications include infection, dissection, vasospasm, arterial aneurysm, and vascular sclerosis.

FEMORAL ARTERIAL CANNULATION

Indications and Contraindications

Femoral arterial access[31–33] is indicated for close blood pressure monitoring and arterial access for frequent blood sampling. The femoral site is often selected for patients in shock or with absent or diminished radial pulses. This site is contraindicated in patients with recent femoral or iliac artery surgery, infection at the site, and severe aortoiliac disease, as monitoring will be inaccurate.

Equipment

The equipment for femoral arterial line placement includes the following: (1) antiseptic skin preparation and sterile barrier equipment, (2) 1% lidocaine in a small syringe with a 25-gauge needle, (3) 18- or 16-gauge single-lumen cannula—often contained in prefabricated arterial or venous access kits, and (4) transducer and pressure tubing.

Technique

Steps for inserting a femoral arterial line are shown in Fig. 42.6. If the operator is right-handed, the right femoral artery is easier to approach. Prep and drape in sterile fashion and have an assistant nearby. Apply local anesthetic. The ipsilateral leg should be slightly abducted and externally rotated for access site exposure. The lateral to medial anatomic landmarks can be recalled by using the mnemonic NAVEL. The needle is inserted 1 to 2 cm below the inguinal crease in anticipation of puncturing the femoral artery as it emerges beneath the inguinal ligament. Needle puncture above the inguinal ligament risks procedure-related hemorrhage that may be concealed in the retroperitoneum and is not easily compressible. The needle is inserted at a 20- to 30-degree angle to the skin toward the arterial pulsation. Ultrasound guidance should be used if available. Following arterial puncture, the arterial cannula is inserted via the Seldinger technique as described earlier, with the exception that guidewire-assisted insertion of the thin-walled arterial cannula does not require a tissue tract dilator or skin incision.

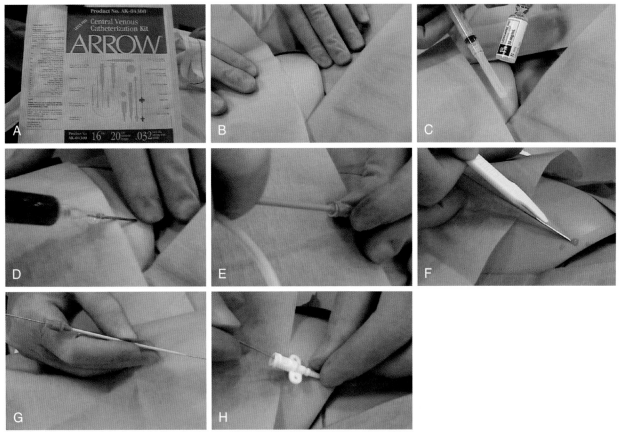

Fig. 42.6 Femoral arterial line placement. (A) Shown is a good kit for a femoral arterial line. The needle is soft-tipped so that it does not erode and cause retroperitoneal bleeding. (B) Palpate the femoral pulse and remember the mnemonic NAVEL for anatomic structures going lateral-to-medial (nerve, artery, vein, empty space, lymphatics). (C) Apply local anesthetic generously. (D) Using the big hollow needle, advance until bright blood is observed. (E) Once the needle is in, proceed with the Seldinger technique, making sure that the wire goes in easily. (F) A small nick is enough for the 16-gauge catheter to go in easily. (G) Dilate with caution to avoid a major bleed. (H) Slide the catheter up, check the location again, connect the tubing, sew in place, and apply dressing.

Clinical Pearls

- Optimize patient and provider positioning prior to starting the procedure.
- The femoral artery is smaller than most central venous access targets. Pre-position the guidewire for rapid insertion through the needle to avoid losing access to the vessel.
- Any clinical consideration of a retroperitoneal hemorrhage must be ruled out immediately with a computed tomographic scan.

Complications

Vascular complications—including hemorrhage, arterial thrombosis with malperfusion, pseudoaneurysm, dissection, and arteriovenous fistula—are rare but well recognized. Appropriate technique and monitoring following placement are important. Occult bleeding deep to the vessel and in the retroperitoneum may occur with puncture superior to the inguinal ligament. The absence of superficial hematoma formation does not exclude the presence of a retroperitoneal hemorrhage. Arterial cannulas are associated with catheter-associated bloodstream infection and deserve vigilant sterile technique and maintenance.[34]

The full reference list for this chapter is available at ExpertConsult.com.

43

Temporary Cardiac Pacing

Ali A. Sovari, Paria Zarghamravanbakhsh, Michael Shehata

Temporary cardiac pacing delivers electrical cardiac stimulation to treat a cardiac bradyarrhythmia until the underlying problem resolves or a permanent pacing solution is provided. Temporary cardiac pacing is most commonly used for symptomatic bradycardia and is occasionally used to determine whether a patient requires permanent pacing. The important factors that determine whether a patient requires a temporary or permanent pacemaker include the patient's rhythm, hemodynamic tolerance of the rhythm, and/or symptoms related to the dysrhythmia. There are several methods for temporary pacing of the heart (transcutaneous, transvenous, transesophageal, transthoracic, and epicardial). Among these methods, transvenous and transcutaneous cardiac pacing are the most commonly used procedures.

BRADYARRHYTHMIAS

Bradyarrhythmias can be classified into five groups: sinus bradycardia, sinus pause, junctional rhythm, sinoatrial (SA) exit block, and idioventricular rhythm (Table 43.1). Junctional and idioventricular rhythms commonly occur in the setting of complete heart block. Atrioventricular (AV) conduction blocks may also result in bradycardia and require pacemaker implantation. Like the classification of SA exit blocks, AV blocks are defined in three groups. First-degree AV block refers to a conduction delay in the AV node appearing as a prolonged PR interval on the surface electrocardiogram (ECG). This is, in fact, an AV delay and not a true conduction block. Second-degree AV block is divided into types 1 and 2. In type 1 AV block, the conduction through the AV node slows with each beat and appears on the ECG as beat-to-beat progressive PR prolongation followed by a P wave with no associated QRS complex. The following conducted P wave shows the shortest PR interval in a typical Wenckebach phenomenon. In type 2 second-degree AV block, AV node conduction block happens abruptly with no prior PR prolongation. If this happens with more than one P wave consecutively,

it is called high-degree AV block. In third-degree AV block or complete heart block, there is no AV conduction; therefore, atrial and ventricular rhythms and rates are dissociated from each other. Complete heart block, type 2 second-degree AV block, and high-degree AV block are commonly indications for pacemaker implantation (Table 43.2).

Signs and Symptoms of Bradyarrhythmias

The decision for pacemaker implantation depends on the hemodynamic consequences of bradycardia, such as hypotension along with associated signs and symptoms related to bradycardia, including:

- Dizziness
- Lightheadedness
- Weakness
- Dyspnea on exertion
- Fatigue
- Shortness of breath
- Confusion
- Syncope
- Cyanosis
- Hypotension

PERMANENT VERSUS TEMPORARY CARDIAC PACING

All indications for permanent cardiac pacing are considered indications for temporary cardiac pacing (see Table 43.2). Whether a patient requires permanent or temporary cardiac pacing is partly based on the potential reversibility of the bradycardia. When the cause of bradycardia is reversible or is unknown at the time of initial diagnosis, a temporary pacemaker is preferred over a permanent device.

Although the presence of bradycardia generally is a prerequisite for pacemaker implantation, relative bradycardia is a possible

TABLE 43.1	**Different Types of Bradyarrhythmias**	
Bradyarrhythmias	**Definition**	**ECG Changes**
Sinus bradycardia	• Rate: <60 beats/min • Rhythm: regular • P waves: normal in morphology and duration • PR interval: between 0.12 and 0.20 sec	
Sinus pause	• Sinus node fails to generate an impulse • No P wave or its associated QRS and T wave • Lasting from 2.0 sec to several minutes	
Junctional rhythm	• AV node becomes the principal pacemaker • Rate: 40–60 beats/min	
Idioventricular rhythm	• Ventricle becomes the principal pacemaker • Wide QRS complexes (more than 120 msec) • Rate: lower, between 20 to 40 beats/min	
Sinoatrial Exit Block[a]		
Second-degree type 1 SA block	• Shortening of the PP interval until a P-QRS-T complex is dropped • Takes progressively longer for each SA node impulse to exit the node until an impulse fails to exit the node	
Second-degree type 2 SA block	• Impulse generated in the SA node occasionally fails to propagate into the atria, which appears as a dropped P-QRS-T complex • PP interval surrounding the dropped complexes is two times (or a multiple) the baseline PP interval	
Third-degree SA exit block	• None of the generated impulses exits the SA node • Pause or junctional rhythm	

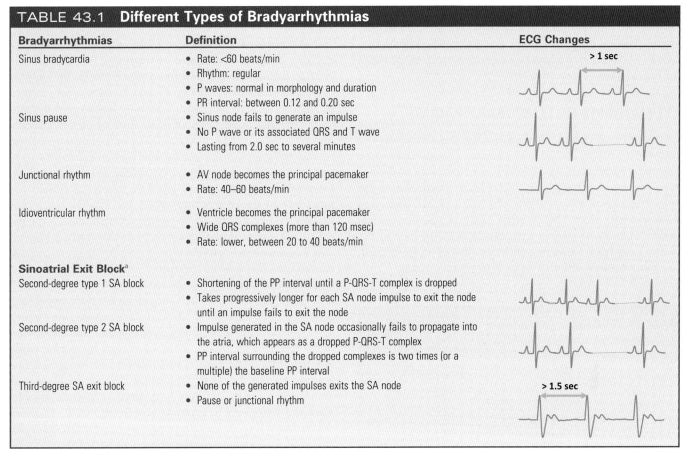

[a]First-degree SA block, which is a delay between generation of impulse in SA node and its exit from the node, is not detectable on surface ECG.
AV, Atrioventricular; *SA,* sinoatrial.

TABLE 43.2	**Indications and Contraindications for Permanent and Temporary Cardiac Pacing Based on Causes**	
	Indications	**Contraindications**
Permanent cardiac pacing	• Any symptomatic bradycardia • Sinus node dysfunction • Acquired Mobitz II or third degree atrioventricular block in adults • Hypersensitive carotid sinus syndrome and severe neurocardiogenic syncope • After cardiac transplantation • Pacing to prevent ventricular tachycardia • Patients with congenital heart disease	• Local infection at implantation site • Active systemic infection with bacteremia • Severe bleeding tendencies (relative contraindication) • Active anticoagulation therapy (relative contraindication)
Temporary cardiac pacing	• Reversible injury to the sinus node or other parts of the conduction system after cardiac surgery (e.g., injuries, postcoronary bypass) • Chest and cardiac trauma associated with temporary sinus node or AV node dysfunction • Metabolic and/or electrolyte imbalance (e.g., hyperkalemia) • Drug-induced bradyarrhythmia (e.g., digitalis toxicity) • Infectious diseases (e.g., Lyme disease or bacterial endocarditis)	• Asymptomatic patient with stable rhythm (e.g., a first-degree AV block or a Mobitz 1 or stable escape rhythm)

AV, Atrioventricular.

exception. Relative bradycardia implies that the rate is too slow for the patient's medical condition but is not technically bradycardia (<60 beats/min). For example, following cardiac transplant, a higher than normal heart rate is often required to maximize hemodynamic performance of the transplanted, denervated heart.

Another example of relative bradycardia is chronotropic incompetence, the inability to increase the heart rate during exertion or periods of increased demand. Chronotropic incompetence includes the inability or a delay to achieve maximum heart rate, heart rate instability during exercise, and inadequate heart rate recovery following exercise. Although these patients have normal sinus rhythm at rest, the heart rate does not increase appropriately during demand or exertion. Such patients may require a pacemaker to adequately meet hemodynamic demands during exertion.

TYPES/FORMS OF TEMPORARY PACING

Of the different types of temporary pacing, transcutaneous and transvenous pacing are the most commonly used (Table 43.3). Epicardial pacemakers are commonly used following cardiothoracic surgery in which the pacemaker leads are attached to the epicardium of the atrium and/or ventricle and then connected to an external pacer. The expected length of time for pacing, desired stability of pacing, cost, and level of urgency in the patient's condition are among the factors that affect the decision to choose between different types of temporary pacing.

TABLE 43.3 **Advantages and Disadvantages of Different Types of Temporary Pacing**		
	Advantages	**Disadvantages**
Transcutaneous pacing	• Method of choice in case of emergencies (asystole or cardiac symptoms)	• Least reliability • Least convenient • Skin tingling, burning • Musculoskeletal contractions
Transvenous pacing	• Enhanced patient comfort • Greater reliability • The ability to pace the atrium • Stability of pacing system	• Requires central venous access • Complications that result from obtaining venous access (venous thrombosis, inadvertent arterial puncture)
Temporary permanent transvenous pacing	• Higher stability • Provides data by interrogation	• Expensive

Transcutaneous Pacing

Transcutaneous pacing is the fastest method to initiate temporary cardiac pacing. It is indicated as treatment for symptomatic bradyarrhythmias and is part of advanced cardiac life support in patients with bradycardia or asystole. Transcutaneous cardiac pacing may be associated with a burning sensation of the skin and/or skeletal muscle contractions. Because of this, patients who are conscious and hemodynamically stable should be sedated.

Transcutaneous cardiac pacing equipment consists of a pacing unit, pads (cardiac electrodes), and a cardiac monitor (Fig. 43.1). In nonemergency situations, the first step is to explain the procedure to the patient and obtain the baseline heart rate, rhythm, and vital signs. Before electrode application, wipe the patient's skin with alcohol and shave body hair carefully to avoid skin abrasions, which can elevate the pacing threshold and increase discomfort. The anterior electrode has negative polarity and should be placed either over the cardiac apex or at the position of lead V_3. The posterior electrode, which has positive polarity, should be placed inferior to the scapula or between the right or left scapula and the spine. After skin preparation and application of the pads, the pacemaker is turned on and the pacing mode selected. If the patient is in cardiac arrest with bradycardia or asystole, pacing should be initiated at the maximum current output to ensure that capture is achieved as soon as possible. Then, the current can be gradually reduced to 5 to 10 mA above the threshold for capture. The presence of a wide QRS complex after each pacing stimulus suggests but does not confirm capture. Cardiac capture should be confirmed by assessing the pulse, blood pressure, and clinical status of the patient. In healthy individuals, the pacing threshold is usually less than 80 mA. The pacing threshold can be increased in some conditions, such as obesity, myocardial ischemia, metabolic derangements, pneumothorax, and by poor skin-to-electrode contact.

Transvenous Pacing

Transvenous pacing requires central venous access. This method has several advantages over the transcutaneous method, such as enhanced patient comfort and stability of pacing wires but it

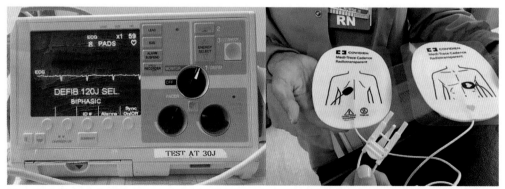

Fig. 43.1 External defibrillator and transcutaneous pacing system. Three knobs on the pacing system allow setting the device for pacing, choosing the rate, and then choosing the output to have appropriate cardiac capture. Two external pads are attached to the appropriate part of the chest and back of the patient, as shown on the pads.

cannot be initiated as rapidly as transcutaneous pacing. In emergency situations, transcutaneous pacing is the initial method of choice and can be followed by transvenous pacing to pace for a longer period of the time, allowing evaluation of the requirements for permanent pacing.

The requirements for transvenous pacing are a central venous access kit, a pacing lead, a temporary external transvenous pacing generator (single-chamber or dual-chamber) and external defibrillator, along with the following:

- Sterile gown, gloves, cap, and face shield
- Drapes or towels for skin preparation
- Lidocaine, sterile gauze, syringes, scalpel, saline flush, catheter, dilator, needle, wire, suture, needle driver
- Fluoroscopy is commonly used for intracardiac lead placement. If fluoroscopy is not available, ECG guidance or echocardiography may be used instead.

The first step in transvenous pacing is obtaining venous access (Video 43.1). Before obtaining venous access, the subcutaneous tissue and area around the course of the needle should be anesthetized with lidocaine 1% or 2%, with or without epinephrine. If the pacer wire is going to be inserted under fluoroscopic guidance, the most common access site is the right femoral vein. When the pacer is to be inserted without fluoroscopic guidance (usually by ECG guidance at the bedside), a balloon flotation catheter is used, and the most common sites of venous access are the internal jugular and subclavian veins.

The following steps are taken to insert a temporary pacer at the bedside using ECG guidance, with insertion of a temporary pacer under fluoroscopic guidance being more straightforward (see Video 43.1). After obtaining venous access and placing a transvenous sheath, the balloon-tipped catheter is inserted through the sheath into the vein and is advanced 20 cm (the catheter has markers for each 10 cm). It is then inflated to be advanced with blood flow. The distal electrodes of the catheter are connected to the V_1 lead of the ECG device to record a unipolar ECG. This allows sensing of atrial and ventricular ECGs as the lead enters these chambers. Alternatively, the lead can be paced at maximum output during the insertion, and detection of atrial or ventricular capture will guide the operator as to chamber location. The catheter is advanced through the vein until it reaches the right atrium (RA). When the catheter enters the RA, atrial waves are recorded that confirm the catheter position in the RA; or, if the lead is paced at maximum output, then atrial position of the lead is confirmed by atrial capture on a surface ECG or monitor. Advancing further, when the catheter passes the tricuspid valve and enters the right ventricle (RV) and the catheter is in contact with the RV endocardium, the ventricular signal is very large (usually >4 mV) and produces ST segment elevation as an indication of an injury current. From the morphology of the paced QRS on the surface ECG, one can determine the catheter position within the RV. For example, if the catheter is in the apex, the morphology of the captured paced beat is negative in inferior leads (II, III, aVF). If the lead is in the high septum or RV outflow tract, then the captured paced morphology is positive in the inferior leads. In an emergency, the highest output should be tried first; output should then be gradually reduced until the capture is lost and the pacing threshold

is determined. If the situation is not an emergency, the rate is set 10 to 20 beats/min above the intrinsic heart rate and the output is initially set low and then gradually increased until capture occurs. The output should be set to a value at least three times higher than the threshold to ensure a safe margin for any change that occurs in the capture threshold. The ideal capture threshold is less than 1 mA.

The lead and sheath are secured to the skin with suture and a transparent dressing applied. The patient is reevaluated daily, including checking for infection, threshold testing, and evaluation of the paced surface ECG.

Permanent Temporary Pacemaker

The permanent temporary pacemaker (PTPM) is a permanent pacing system with an active fixation lead that is used for temporary purposes but with the lead externalized through the skin to a standard pacemaker pulse generator. PTPM is indicated when temporary pacing should be used for a longer period of time or when more stability is required. Patients with temporary transvenous systems are usually restricted to bed rest and are monitored in intensive care units (ICUs). Patients with PTPM, however, have a more stable and reliable pacing system and may, therefore, be monitored and treated outside of the ICU.

With this method, the lead usually is implanted via either the internal jugular or subclavian vein under fluoroscopic guidance (Fig. 43.2). A peel-away sheath is used to obtain venous access. Fluoroscopy is required for insertion of the active fixation lead and the lead is then inserted through the sheath and advanced to the RV under fluoroscopic guidance. The ideal position is usually in the mid to apical portion of the RV septum. The septal position of the lead can be determined using a left anterior oblique fluoroscopic view. The tip-screw mechanism is then activated to fix the lead in the appropriate position. After measuring sensing, impedance, and pacing threshold and finding a position with satisfactory measurements, the peel-away sheath is removed, the lead suture sleeve is advanced to the puncture site, and the lead is sutured over the sleeve to the skin. The lead is then connected to a standard pacemaker pulse generator. This pacemaker can be taped to the neck or upper chest depending on the access site.

The main advantage of this method is the stability of the pacing lead. In addition, the device can be interrogated and gives more information about the percentage of paced beats and the patient's underlying rhythm than a standard temporary transvenous pacemaker. One recent application of the PTPM is following transcatheter aortic valve replacement (TAVR) in which patients may develop transient complete heart block soon after the procedure. The PTPM can provide a safe and stable method of pacing for these patients until further evaluation determines their need for a permanent pacemaker. Another group of patients who benefit from this method of pacing are those pacer-dependent patients with pacemaker infections in whom the infected permanent system is removed. It may take days to weeks for their infection to be adequately treated before they can safely receive another permanent pacing device. During this treatment period, PTPM can be a valuable tool for safe and stable temporary pacing.

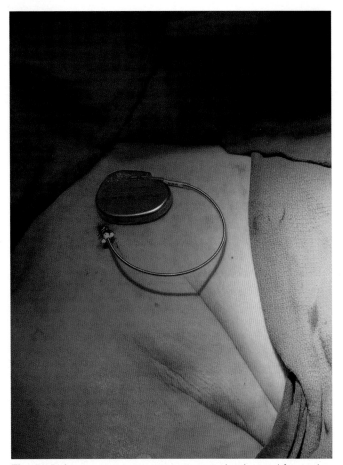

Fig. 43.2 A permanent temporary pacemaker is used for pacing for longer than the usual indications and when more stability is required. The active fixation lead is inserted into the right ventricle under fluoroscopic guidance. The sleeve is sutured to the skin, and the pulse generator is connected to the lead and is covered by a dressing.

CONCLUSIONS

Temporary cardiac pacing is used for treatments of bradycardia. Hemodynamics can often be stabilized using temporary cardiac pacing until further investigation of the etiology of bradycardia is performed, transient causes of bradycardia resolve, or a contraindication for permanent pacing is identified. Transvenous, transcutaneous, epicardial, and permanent-temporary pacemakers are the most common methods of temporary cardiac pacing. Each of these methods provides certain advantages. Familiarity with different types of temporary pacing and the indications and contraindications of each method is very important in the CICU, allowing selection of the most appropriate method for each individual patient's condition.

Pericardiocentesis

Ali S. Sovari

Pericardiocentesis was first described in 1840 and has since became the primary method for diagnosing the etiology of a pericardial effusion and treating pericardial tamponade. Initially, the procedure was performed blindly through a subxiphoid approach. Later, fluoroscopy and electrocardiography (ECG) were used to guide the procedure. Since 1979, echocardiography has been used for direct visualization of cardiac structures and adjacent vital organs during the procedure.

The accumulation of pericardial fluid is usually owing to inflammation or infection of the pericardium and adjacent structures. Alternatively, pericardial fluid egress can be compromised by infiltration of the pericardium with malignant cells with resultant accumulation of fluid in the pericardial space. *Hemopericardium* can result spontaneously from coagulation abnormalities or as a result of surgical complications, trauma, dissection of an aortic aneurysm, or myocardial rupture. *Chylopericardium* is a pericardial effusion composed of chyle—a milky white and opaque fluid, with a triglyceride level greater than 500 mg/dL and a cholesterol/triglyceride ratio less than 1. The primary form is rare; secondary chylopericardium may be owing to radiation, subclavian vein thrombosis, infections (e.g., tuberculosis), mediastinal tumors, following cardiac and aortopulmonary surgeries, or from any process that damages the thoracic duct. Although the cholesterol content is high, chylopericardium should not be confused with cholesterol pericarditis, in which the fluid is clear and contains cholesterol crystals, foam cells, macrophages, and giant cells. *Pneumopericardium* is rare, occurring in the setting of chest trauma, following medical interventions (e.g., catheter ablation of arrhythmias), fistula formation, and a variety of gas-forming infections. Table 44.1 summarizes the most important causes of pericardial effusion. Approximately 20 to 30 mL of fluid accumulation in the pericardial space is required for detection by different imaging modalities. An increase in the size of the cardiac silhouette on chest radiograph is typically seen when at least 250 mL of fluid has accumulated in the pericardial space. The rate of fluid accumulation is the critical factor in determining the hemodynamic effects and associated clinical signs and symptoms. A slow accumulation of a large amount of pericardial fluid may have no significant hemodynamic effect, whereas with an acute pericardial effusion, even a small volume can result in tamponade physiology.

CLINICAL PRESENTATION

Chest pain is a common presenting symptom when the cause of pericardial effusion is acute, subacute, or chronic pericarditis. Shortness of breath commonly occurs when the hemodynamic effect of a pericardial effusion is significant. Fever, cough, hoarseness, and hiccups can also be present depending on the causes of the pericardial effusion and its effect on adjacent structures, such as the bronchial tree and phrenic nerve.

On physical examination, patients with pericardial tamponade usually appear anxious and uncomfortable. Depending on the hemodynamic effects of the pericardial effusion, signs such as tachycardia, tachypnea, jugular venous distention, pulsus paradoxus, elevated central venous pressure, and diminished pulse pressure may be present. A pericardial friction rub may be detected with a small effusion in the setting of pericarditis. If pericardial fluid compresses the adjacent lung, dullness to percussion, egophony, and bronchial breath sounds at the angle of the left scapula may be elicited (Ewart sign). Massive cardiomegaly with a left pleural effusion can produce a similar finding, with dullness in the left axillary area. In a retrospective analysis of patients with pericardial effusion, cardiac tamponade was most strongly associated with the following five features on bedside examination: symptoms of dyspnea, tachycardia, pulsus paradoxus of greater than 10 mm of mercury, elevated jugular venous pressure, and cardiomegaly on chest radiograph.[1]

DIAGNOSTIC TESTS

The chest radiograph may show an enlarged cardiac silhouette. Lungs are usually clear unless the patient is in heart failure or has significant lung disease. The absence of vascular congestion

TABLE 44.1   Causes of Pericardial Effusion

Categories	Examples	Categories	Examples
Idiopathic infections	• Bacteria (e.g., staphylococci, streptococci, pneumococci, *Haemophilus influenzae*, *Mycoplasma* species, *Neisseria* species, *Borrelia burgdorferi*, *Chlamydia* species, *Legionella* species, *Salmonella* species, *Mycobacterium tuberculosis*, *Mycobacterium avium*). • Viral (e.g., coxsackievirus, adenovirus, Epstein-Barr virus, echovirus, cytomegalovirus, infectious mononucleosis, parvovirus B19, influenza, mumps, varicella, hepatitis B, HIV) • Fungal (e.g., histoplasmosis, aspergillosis, blastomycosis, coccidioidomycosis, *Candida* species, *Nocardia* species) • Rickettsial organisms • Parasitic (toxoplasmosis, amebiasis)	Autoimmune diseases	• Systemic lupus erythematosus • Rheumatoid arthritis • Scleroderma • Polyarteritis nodosa • Temporal arteritis • Mixed connective tissue disorder • Inflammatory bowel diseases • Sarcoidosis • Behçet disease • Myasthenia gravis
Neoplasm	• Metastatic (e.g., lung or breast carcinoma, lymphoma, leukemia, melanoma) • Primary (e.g., rhabdomyosarcoma, lipoma, teratoma, fibroma, fibrosarcoma, angioma, angiosarcoma, mesothelioma)	Trauma	• Blunt • Penetrating • Iatrogenic (e.g., perforation caused by catheter insertion or pacemaker implantation, status postcardiopulmonary resuscitation)
Myocardial infarction	• Rupture of ventricular aneurysm	Others	• Hypothyroidism • Amyloidosis and autoimmune diseases • Chylopericardium • Uremia • Radiation • Pneumopericardium • Postcardiothoracic surgery • Idiopathic thrombocytopenic purpura • Postpericardiotomy syndrome • Dissecting aortic aneurysm
Drugs	• Procainamide • Hydralazine • Warfarin • Heparin • Thrombolytics • Methysergide • Isoniazid • Cyclosporine		

in the lung fields of patients with pericardial effusion and tamponade is an important radiographic clue.

On ECG, signs of acute pericarditis in the form of diffuse ST segment elevation and PR segment depression may be seen. The ECG hallmark of pericardial effusion is low-voltage QRS complexes, reflecting the electrical insulation of the pericardial fluid. Low voltage is defined as a QRS amplitude less than 0.5 mV in the limb leads and less than 1 mV in the precordial leads. However, low QRS voltage is neither a sensitive nor specific sign for pericardial effusion; therefore, it should not be used to confirm a suspected diagnosis of pericardial effusion or to rule it out. Electrical alternans, the beat-to-beat variation of the amplitude of QRS voltage, is another ECG finding suggestive of a large pericardial effusion or cardiac tamponade. With large pericardial effusions and no clinical tamponade, the heart has some freedom of movement; therefore, small variations in the QRS amplitude can be seen in many cases. However, significant alternans in the P wave, QRS complex, and T wave, or total electrical alternans, is a specific finding for cardiac tamponade.

Routine laboratory studies prior to pericardiocentesis should include complete blood count, prothrombin time/international normalized ratio (INR), activated partial thromboplastin time, and a basic metabolic panel. Cardiac enzymes, thyroid-stimulating hormone, autoantibodies, and viral or rickettsial serologic tests

are indicated depending on the clinical information and differential diagnosis.

Routine tests on pericardial fluid often include cell count with differential, lactate dehydrogenase (LDH), protein, glucose, Gram stain, and routine bacterial cultures. Smears for acid-fast bacilli; adenosine deaminase; mycobacterial, fungal, and viral cultures; and cytology are indicated depending on the degree of suspicion for specific infectious or malignant etiologies. In contrast to pleural effusions or ascites, there are few data regarding the chemical and cell-count parameters of pericardial effusions to aid diagnosis. Most pericardial effusions are exudates but no biochemical or cell-count parameter is useful for differentiating among the individual causes or among various groups of pericardial disorders.[2]

Echocardiography is the best method of making the diagnosis of pericardial effusion. It can detect a pericardial effusion as small as 30 mL. Small nonloculated pericardial effusions usually present in the posterior pericardial space with the patient in the supine position. As the amount of fluid increases, it starts to accumulate anteriorly and laterally. Large effusions are usually circumferential, allowing free motion of the heart within the fluid (swinging of the heart). Important echocardiographic findings may include swinging of the heart within the effusion, right atrial (RA) collapse, early right ventricular (RV) collapse, reciprocal changes in right and left ventricular volume, and respiratory variation in ventricular filling and ejection.

INDICATIONS FOR PERICARDIOCENTESIS

The key factors in making the decision to perform pericardiocentesis include the patient's symptoms, the amount of pericardial fluid and its hemodynamic effects, and the need for diagnostic tests on the pericardial fluid. In asymptomatic patients, pericardiocentesis is rarely indicated. In addition, if the amount of pericardial fluid is small, it may be very difficult to access and drain. Occasionally, pericardial fluid drainage is required for diagnostic purposes even if the patient is asymptomatic from the effusion.

The indications for pericardiocentesis are as follows:
- Pericardial tamponade or large pericardial effusions
- Symptomatic pericardial effusions
- Suspicion of purulent pericarditis
- Effusions of unclear etiology
- Pericardial effusions that compress other organs (e.g., trachea, lung)

THE PERICARDIOCENTESIS PROCEDURE[3]
(Video 44.1)

- Elective or urgent pericardiocentesis should be performed by experienced individuals; otherwise, the surgical approach should be pursued.
- An echocardiogram should be obtained prior to the pericardiocentesis procedure to confirm that the effusion is at least of moderate size and is not loculated.
- The procedure should be performed in an environment equipped with two-dimensional echocardiography and/or fluoroscopy. Echocardiographically guided pericardiocentesis can be performed at the bedside with no exposure to radiation from fluoroscopy.
- If the clinical situation permits, any clotting abnormality should be corrected.
- An ECG should be obtained before the procedure and ECG monitoring should be continued during the procedure. If the pericardiocentesis needle touches the myocardium, the current of injury causes ST segment elevation on the ECG monitor.
- The pericardiocentesis tray and associated equipment should include:
  - An 18- to 20-gauge cardiac needle or long central venous catheter with needle introducer
  - A three-way stopcock
  - Syringes (10, 20, and 60 mL)
  - Antiseptic chlorhexidine and alcohol or povidone-iodine solution
  - ECG monitor
  - Specimen collection tubes for fluid analysis and cultures; fluid receptacle (1 L vacuum bottle)
  - Pressure tubing and transducer (for pericardial pressure measurement, if needed)
  - Small-gauge needle for local anesthesia and 1% to 2% lidocaine
  - Sterile gloves, mask, gown, dressing materials (sterile transparent plastic drape), and gauze
  - Surgical blade (No. 11)
  - Sterile isotonic sodium chloride solution (for flushing catheter)
  - Emergency medications (e.g., atropine, lidocaine, epinephrine)
  - Defibrillator with monitor
- Position the patient at a 30- to 45-degree, head-up angle to permit pericardial fluid to pool on the inferior surface of the heart. Palpate the subxyphoid process, about a finger-width below the edge of the rib. This location avoids difficulty in advancing the catheter through fibrous tissue closer to the lower part of the sternum itself.
- Prepare the site in a sterile manner and drape, covering everything but a small area around the subxyphoid process. After infiltration of the skin and subcutaneous tissues with lidocaine, make a small incision (approximately 5 mm) to decrease the resistance during needle insertion. Separate the subcutaneous tissue with forceps.
- Connect the needle with a three-way stopcock. Ensure that the syringe with 1% lidocaine is connected to the three-way stopcock on the opposite side of the needle connection. Connect the pressure tubing and transducer on the side port of the three-way stopcock. If ECG monitoring will be used, attach a sterile alligator clip connected to an ECG recorder to the metal part of the needle.
- Insert the pericardial needle. Advance the needle through the skin, first perpendicularly to the chest and then angled lower to a plane nearly parallel with the floor, moving under the subxyphoid process toward the left shoulder. More lidocaine can be given gently through the pericardial needle as it is advanced. If the patient is obese, a longer needle and some force may be required to tip the syringe under the subxyphoid process toward the heart.
- Advance the needle into the pericardial space. Passage of the needle through the skin causes the needle to become occluded by subcutaneous tissue. Flush any tissue that may have accumulated during passage before entering the pericardium, a tough fibrous membrane. Use caution when advancing the needle through the diaphragm, as excessive forward pressure may result in a sudden jump through the pericardium into a cardiac chamber.
- Confirm the intrapericardial position with hemodynamics or echo contrast imaging. As the needle advances, colored fluid or blood in the syringe signals likely entry into the pericardium (note that chronic effusions are often clear yellow, occasionally serosanguineous, or, less commonly, dark brown. Acute effusions resulting from trauma, cancer, myocardial rupture, or aortic dissection are frankly bloody). Pericardial pressure can be seen on turning the stopcock and should be nearly the same as RA pressure in tamponade. If the pressure shows an RV pressure waveform, the needle has gone too far and should be pulled back into the pericardial space. Echocardiographic guidance is also confirmatory of correct positioning. After entering the pericardial space, an injection of 5 to 10 mL of agitated saline through the needle appears

as microbubble contrast and confirms the intrapericardial needle position. If the needle tip is in the RV, the bubbles will be seen in the RV cavity and will be dispersed rapidly by RV ejection.

- When the needle tip is inside the pericardial space, a soft floppy-tip guidewire is passed through the needle. This guidewire should be advanced posteriorly around the heart. This wire position is important to ensure that the needle has not punctured the heart and the wire is not inserted into the RV, in which case the wire will go up the RV outflow tract and will induce frequent premature ventricular contractions or ventricular tachycardia.

- The needle is exchanged over a guidewire for a multiple side-hole pericardial drainage catheter. Pericardial and RA pressures are measured again, the effusion is aspirated, and pressures are measured once more after the pericardial space is empty. If the catheter will not drain or the exact position of the catheter is uncertain, a small amount of radiographic or echo contrast medium may be injected to assess the problem. Contrast medium pools in the dependent portion of the pericardial space, but rapidly washes out of a vascular space if a cardiac chamber has been entered inadvertently. Bloody pericardial fluid may be owing to chronic disease or from acute trauma during the procedure. Chronic bloody effusions have a lower hematocrit value than blood and will not clot rapidly when placed in a red-top tube.

- Obtain serial echocardiograms before and after removal of the pericardial drainage catheter to confirm the absence of fluid reaccumulation. In the absence of significant fluid reaccumulation, the pericardial drain can usually be removed after 24 to 48 hours. Should fluid recur, consider a surgical pericardial window.

COMPLICATIONS

Potential complications of pericardiocentesis include ventricular puncture, cardiac arrest, pneumothorax, liver laceration, laceration of a coronary artery or vein, pericardial tamponade, bleeding, and ventricular and atrial arrhythmias. With the advent of echocardiographic guidance, the morbidity and mortality rates of pericardiocentesis have been significantly reduced. Blind pericardiocentesis, which has a significantly greater complication rate than echocardiographically or fluoroscopically guided procedures, should be undertaken only in emergency situations in patients with significant hemodynamic instability. A very high mortality has been observed in patients undergoing pericardiocentesis when presenting with pulmonary arterial hypertension complicated by pericardial effusion.[4] It is important to be aware of contraindications for pericardiocentesis and avoid the procedure in those situations. Other contraindications to pericardiocentesis include myocardial rupture, aortic dissection, skin infection at the access site, and severe bleeding disorders.

The full reference list for this chapter is available at ExpertConsult.com.

45

Invasive Hemodynamic Monitoring

Joshua D. Mitchell, David L. Brown

Hemodynamics is derived hydrodynamics, the physics of the motion and action of water. The dimensions of hemodynamics include flow, pressure, static resistance, dynamic impedance, reflectance and compliance, branching effects, viscosity, fluid friction, turbulence, and other physical characteristics.[1]

The goals of hemodynamic assessment and manipulation in the critically ill patient are to ensure adequate organ blood flow, oxygen supply,[2] and ultimately to improve survival. Noninvasive parameters to measure organ perfusion include systolic and diastolic blood pressure, body temperature, heart rate, urine output, and respiratory frequency.[3] Although these established clinical signs of organ perfusion should be routinely used for monitoring, they may have limited value as accurate indicators of cardiovascular function.[4] Important pathophysiology may remain obscured if judged solely on clinical signs[2]; further invasive, quantitative measurements may be needed for optimal diagnosis and treatment. The development of bedside intravascular catheterization procedures allowed, for the first time, meaningful application of hemodynamic monitoring in the care of selected critically ill patients.[5]

SYSTEMIC ARTERIAL BLOOD PRESSURE

The continuous measurement of arterial pressure is essential in hemodynamic monitoring. Arterial pressure is the input pressure for organ perfusion.[6] It is usually monitored noninvasively with a sphygmomanometer. In the cardiac intensive care unit (CICU), however, a more invasive technique with insertion of an indwelling arterial catheter into either the arm (brachial or radial sites) or groin (femoral arterial site) is often used to provide more precise monitoring. The advantages of arterial catheterization over noninvasive techniques are continuous monitoring of arterial pressure and its waveform and providing a site for repetitive blood sampling.[6]

Arterial pressure is a function of both vasomotor tone and cardiac output (CO). Local metabolic demands determine local vasomotor tone that, in turn, determines blood flow distribution.[6] Perfusion pressure and local vascular resistance determine organ perfusion of all capillary beds. Flow is proportional to local metabolic demand if there is no hemodynamic instability to cause increased sympathetic tone.[6] CO primarily determines

465

arterial pressure in the setting of varying degrees of local blood flow, and because it is proportional to local metabolic demand, there is no normal value in an unstable, metabolically active patient.[6] The literature currently suggests maintaining previously nonhypertensive patients at a mean arterial blood pressure (MAP) of 65 mm Hg,[6,7] consistent with the initial MAP target recommended by the Surviving Sepsis Guidelines.[8] In a clinical trial that examined the effects of resuscitative efforts with fluid and vasopressors in circulatory shock patients to varying MAP targets ranging from 60 to 90 mm Hg, no increased organ blood flow could be determined above a MAP of 65 mm Hg.[9] However, there is evidence in the septic shock literature that a MAP of 75 to 85 mm Hg may reduce the development of acute kidney injury in patients with chronic arterial hypertension.[10] As a result, it has been suggested to consider more individualized targets for older patients with hypertension or atherosclerosis and in patients with septic shock.[8]

Box 45.1 displays indications for arterial catheterization. The transducers used for blood pressure measurement are connected to the circulation via fluid-filled tubing. The accuracy of the system is optimized when the catheters and tubing are stiff, the total length of tubing is not excessive, the number of stopcocks is limited and residual air bubbles are eliminated.[2] The "zeroing" of the transducer at the appropriate level in relation to the patient (i.e., mid-thorax) must be correct to prevent errors caused by hydrostatic pressure of the fluid column.[2,11] In most cases, the choice of location for insertion of the catheter is the radial artery because femoral artery cannulation is more often associated with displacement during patient movement and hemorrhage that is more difficult to control.[1] Although arterial catheterization is an invasive procedure with inherent risks (temporary vascular

---

BOX 45.1 **Arterial Catheterization**

Probable Indications for Arterial Catheterization

- Guide to management of potent vasodilator drug infusions to prevent systemic hypotension
- Guide to management of potent vasopressor drug infusions to maintain a target mean arterial pressure
- As a port for the rapid and repetitive sampling of arterial blood in patients in whom multiple arterial blood samples are indicated
- As a monitor of cardiovascular deterioration in patients at risk for cardiovascular instability

Useful Applications of Arterial Pressure Monitoring in the Diagnosis of Cardiovascular Insufficiency

- Differentiating cardiac tamponade (pulsus paradoxus) from respiration-induced swings in systolic arterial pressure; tamponade reduces the pulse pressure but keeps diastolic pressure constant. Respiration reduces systolic and diastolic pressure equally, such that pulse pressure is constant.
- Differentiating hypovolemia from cardiac dysfunction as the cause of hemodynamic instability. Systolic arterial pressure decreases more following a positive pressure breath as compared with an apneic baseline during hypovolemia. Systolic arterial pressure increases more during positive pressure inspiration when LV contractility is reduced.

Modified from Polanco PM, Pinsky MR. Practical issues of hemodynamic monitoring at the bedside. *Surg Clin North Am.* 2006;86(6):1431–1456.

---

occlusion 20% and hematoma 14%), most complications are not severe, with permanent ischemic damage, sepsis, and pseudoaneurysm occurring in less than 1% of cases.[12]

RIGHT HEART AND PULMONARY ARTERY CATHETERIZATION: HISTORICAL PERSPECTIVE

Right heart catheterization permits additional measurements of CO, right heart, and pulmonary pressures that make it possible to calculate other derived hemodynamic parameters, such as cardiac work indices and systemic and pulmonary vascular resistance.[2] These fundamental hemodynamic variables help further describe the disordered physiologic state with sufficient precision to enhance management decisions and aid in the care of critically ill patients.[13,14]

The first known cardiac catheterizations were conducted by Hale in 1711 using brass pipes to enter the right ventricle (RV) and left ventricle (LV) of the heart of a horse through the internal jugular vein and carotid artery.[15] Werner Forssmann later performed the first human cardiac catheterization in 1929 when he successfully placed a catheter into his own right atrium (RA) after practicing with cadavers. Subsequent investigations conducted by Dickinson Richards and André Cournand on right heart physiology would earn them the Nobel Prize in Medicine in 1956, along with Forssmann.[11] Lewis Dexter was the first to measure pulmonary capillary wedge pressure (PCWP) and oxygen saturation after introducing a stiff catheter under fluoroscopic guidance to the distal pulmonary artery (PA) in 1947. Subsequent work from his laboratory noted PCWP to be a reliable estimate of left atrial (LA) pressure.[16]

The physiologic and anatomic data obtained over the years led to the development of important concepts, such as pressure manometry and CO measurement. Initially, right heart catheterization was exclusively performed in the cardiac catheterization laboratory primarily to diagnose congenital and valvular heart lesions.[17] However, the increasing numbers of admissions to CICUs for hemodynamic instability from ischemic heart disease prompted an expanded role for invasive hemodynamic monitoring. The 1960s ushered in the establishment of coronary care units (CCUs) to manage cardiac arrhythmias in the setting of acute myocardial infarction (MI).[1,18] It was noted that profound hemodynamic changes might be the primary factor in arrhythmic deaths.[1] However, practical limitations in transporting critically ill patients to a cardiac catheterization suite and the increased risk of induction of cardiac arrhythmias limited the application of invasive hemodynamic monitoring.[1]

In 1970, motivated by a lack of understanding of the hemodynamic perturbations in patients admitted with ischemia or infarction, Swan developed a balloon-tipped, flow-guided catheter that for the first time established a reliable and safe way to perform bedside catheterization in specialized cardiac care units.[19] The initial study by Swan et al.[19] involved 100 patients in whom successful bedside hemodynamic monitoring was performed. They concluded that it was possible to safely catheterize the PA at the bedside without fluoroscopy in a high proportion of patients. The information gained proved to be important in understanding the abnormal pathophysiology of various acute cardiac conditions and thereby altered management in these patients.[5]

The widespread use of PA catheters would follow this landmark report. The relative ease of hemodynamic monitoring transformed the care of cardiac pump failure in the CCU. It allowed the recognition of hemodynamic subsets in MI, the diagnosis of right ventricular MI, provided additional prognostic insight, and allowed for the selection and monitoring of vasoactive and inotropic therapies.[20]

The PA catheter allows for determination of various fundamental hemodynamic parameters, including measurement of CO by thermodilution (TD), RA, RV, PA, and pulmonary capillary wedge pressures; and sampling of blood from the PA, RV, and RA. Pulmonary vascular and systemic resistance, as well as RV and LV stroke work, can then be derived. Further developments included continuous measurement of PA blood oxygen saturation[21] and near-continuous or instantaneous cardiac output.[22]

PULMONARY ARTERY CATHETER

The catheter most commonly used is a 7.5 Fr thermodilution catheter. It is a triple-lumen radiopaque catheter, 110 cm long and made of polyvinylchloride. The outside is marked with black rings every 10 cm from the tip that allow determination without fluoroscopy of the appropriate catheter length at which to inflate the distal balloon. The distal lumen terminates at the tip of the catheter, whereas the RA lumen terminates 30 cm proximal to the tip. There is a venous infusion lumen 1 cm proximal to the RA lumen. A thermistor bead located 3 to 5 cm from the tip is connected to an external thermistor connector by a wire. The external thermistor is, in turn, linked to a computer that allows for determination of CO by the thermodilution (TD) method.[14,19,20] A latex balloon with a maximum inflating capacity of 1.0 to 1.5 mL is positioned at the tip. Upon inflation, the balloon engulfs the catheter tip, cushioning the transmitted force, limiting irritation and injury of endocardial surfaces and reducing the frequency of arrhythmias.[19] The inflated balloon facilitates flow-directed advancement of the catheter through the right heart into the PA. Once inflated in a distal branch of the PA, the balloon occludes the vessel and allows for measurement of PCWP through the catheter tip. Most catheters are heparin coated to reduce thrombogenicity. In addition, electrodes implanted in some catheters allow for pacing and electrocardiographic recording. The inclusion of fiberoptics in other catheters allows continuous measurement of oxygen saturation in the PA. The catheter can serve multiple functions, including measurement of CO by TD, PA temperature, intracardiac pressures (RA, RV, PA, PCW) and PA occluded pressure. Blood sampling can be done through the active lumens of the catheter.

Equipment and Signal Calibration

Properly functioning electronic monitoring equipment is essential. The fluid-filled PA catheter is connected via semirigid pressure tubing to pressure transducers. These transducers consist of a fluid-filled dome, a diaphragm, and a strain gauge Wheatstone bridge arrangement.[14] An electric current directly proportional to the fluid motion is amplified and transmitted to the oscilloscope equipment for display. Other factors that influence accurate reproduction of a biologic signal include frequency response, natural frequency, damping, and catheter whip artifact.

The system must have a frequency response of flat to 15 to 20 Hz to be adequate for human studies. Pressure waveforms are not reliable in patients with excessively rapid heart rates of greater than 180 beats/min. The length of the pressure tubing determines the natural frequency of fluid-filled systems. Excessively long tubing will drop the natural frequency to below physiologic range, causing an overamplification of signal, resulting in falsely elevated pressure readings. The recommended length of pressure tubing is 3 to 4 feet.[14] Damping is the opposite effect, with a loss of physiologic signal that most commonly results from air trapped in the circuit. Because air, unlike fluid, is compressible, less motion is transmitted to the diaphragm per unit of pressure. Damping of the PA pressure signal may make it difficult to discern from the PCWP tracing. Catheter whip artifact results from motion imparted to the catheter with each cardiac contraction. High-frequency filters can eliminate this artifact.[14]

Accurately measuring pressure signals requires proper calibration of the monitoring system. With a patient supine, the pressure transducer is aligned with the fourth intercostal space midway between the front and back of the chest.[14] This site serves as the standard zero reference point. The calibration of the monitor involves the introduction of a known pressure signal. This can be done either internally or externally. Zero reference and calibration should be checked each day of hemodynamic monitoring.[14] Box 45.2 lists the required equipment for PAC insertion. Prepackaged kits with these materials are available.

Catheter Insertion

Catheter equipment should be inspected and calibrated. All lumens should be flushed with normal saline and should be free of air. Potential insertion sites include the internal jugular, subclavian, and femoral veins (Table 45.1). Although the site of insertion is at the discretion of the operator, the right internal

---

BOX 45.2   Equipment Required for Swan-Ganz Catheter Insertion

Appropriate Swan-Ganz catheter
Dilator-sheath-side arm assembly
Three-way stopcocks
Pressure tubing
Transducers
18-gauge, thin-walled Cook needle
Sterile gowns, drapes, gloves
1% lidocaine
Heparinized saline
J-tipped guidewire
Towel clips, syringes, suture material
Electrocardiography and pressure-monitoring equipment
Intravenous line
Atropine
Defibrillator unit
21-gauge Micropuncture Access Set (Cook Medical; optional)
Ultrasound (optional)

TABLE 45.1	Comparison of Venous Access Routes	
Vein	**Advantages**	**Disadvantages**
Internal jugular	Rapidly accessible Does not interfere with CPR Provides a straight route to the heart Less restrictive to patient movement	Air embolism, carotid artery puncture, and tracheal injury may occur. Pneumothorax (more common in the left than the right internal jugular vein). Thoracic duct injury (left internal jugular vein only).
Subclavian	Rapidly accessible Allows free neck and arm movement Easier to keep sterile	Air embolism, more frequent pneumothorax and hemothorax; subclavian artery puncture; injury to nerve bundle may occur.
Femoral	Rapidly accessible Does not interfere with CPR	Sepsis, in situ thrombosis, and pulmonary embolism may occur. Usually requires fluoroscopy.

CPR, Cardiopulmonary resuscitation.

jugular vein is preferable because of the straight course to the superior vena cava. Meticulous preparation of the chosen site with aseptic technique is crucial. The operator and any assistants should be in sterile gown, gloves, face masks, and caps. Any other personnel in the room should wear masks and caps.

The patient should be properly prepped, draped, and placed in the Trendelenburg position. The site is then accessed percutaneously through a modified Seldinger technique. After local anesthesia, an 18-gauge, 7.6-cm Cook needle with attached syringe is inserted bevel up at approximately 45 degrees between the heads of the sternocleidomastoid muscles toward the ipsilateral nipple while palpating the ipsilateral carotid artery. After free-flowing venous blood is obtained, the syringe is disconnected from the needle and a 40-cm-long J-tipped guidewire is inserted into the needle and passed gently into the vein. The guidewire should pass without any resistance and should never be advanced if any resistance is encountered. The needle is then removed and the skin puncture is enlarged with a scalpel blade. The dilator sheath system is then advanced over the guidewire into the vein with a gentle rotating movement. Once the sheath is properly positioned, the wire and dilator should be removed and the sheath sutured in place. Ultrasound-guided insertion of the needle and a micropuncture system are commonly used to further reduce complications.[23,24]

Prior to insertion, the PAC should be inspected for bends and kinks and the balloon tested with air inflation underwater to evaluate for leaks. The catheter should then be connected with pressure tubing to calibrated pressure transducers. Finally, a plastic sleeve is placed over the catheter to preserve the sterile length of the catheter outside of the body for future manipulation.

The catheter is then inserted and advanced approximately 10 cm before the balloon is inflated with 1 to 1.5 mL of air. In most patients, the catheter will reach the RA 10 to 15 cm from the internal jugular or subclavian vein. Once in the RA, the catheter should be quickly advanced under continuous pressure and electrocardiographic monitoring across the tricuspid valve, through the RV, PA, and into the PCWP position. The catheter should reach the PA approximately 50 to 55 cm from the internal jugular vein. One should suspect catheter coiling if significantly greater lengths are required. Fig. 45.1 illustrates typical pressure waveforms.

After achieving the wedge position, deflation of the balloon should allow the deflated catheter to recoil into the proximal PA. The balloon should be slowly inflated while PA pressure is continuously monitored. With inflation, the catheter should then float to a wedge position. The goal is occlusion of a distal vessel impeding blood flow to that area. PCWP tracings without inflation of the distal balloon indicates distal migration of the catheter. With the balloon deflated, the catheter should be repositioned by slow withdrawal 1 to 2 cm at a time. Inability to secure a proper PCWP tracing can be due to patient movement, mechanical ventilation, positive end-expiratory pressure (PEEP) and eccentric balloon inflation.[14] Catheter position should be checked routinely by overpenetrated chest radiographs.[14] To minimize the risk of endothelial damage to the PA, PA rupture, or pulmonary infarction, time in the wedge position should be kept to a maximum of about 8 to 15 seconds.[14] End-expiration diastolic pulmonary pressures should approximate mean wedge pressure in the absence of increased pulmonary arteriolar resistance, such as with pulmonary hypertension or pulmonary embolus.[14]

The pressure recorded through a wedged end-hole catheter is that of the next active vascular system which, in most circumstances, is the LA or LV at end diastole. This assumes that the vascular system distal to the catheter tip provides a direct connection to the LA without any anatomic or functional interruption. The ideal placement of the catheter is the lower lung zone. In zone 3, the most dependent portion, both PA and venous pressures exceed alveolar pressure, thereby maintaining an open vascular system from the catheter tip to the LA.[14] In the upper lung, or zone 1, alveolar pressure exceeds PA and venous pressures, keeping the capillaries closed, disrupting the system and preventing accurate measurement of LA pressures. The arterial pressures in the central lung, or zone 2, should exceed alveolar pressure, but low pulmonary venous pressure may prevent retrograde transmission of pressures from the LA. Fortunately, most of the lung in the supine position is in zone 3 and flow-guided catheters will usually enter this zone. A lateral chest radiograph can confirm position of the catheter tip below the LA.

PULMONARY ARTERY OCCLUSION AND WEDGE PRESSURE

Pulmonary capillary wedge pressure is a phase-delayed, amplitude-damped version of LA pressure. During diastole with a nonstenotic mitral valve, the pulmonary venous system, LA, and LV is a continuous circuit and the PCWP is then reflective of the LV

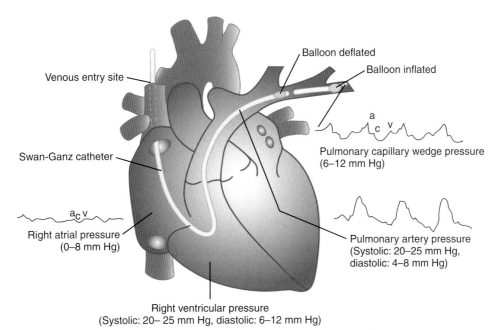

Fig. 45.1 Normal hemodynamic pressures. (Modified from Swan HC. The pulmonary artery catheter. *Dis Mon.* 1991;37:518.)

diastolic pressure.[20] The level of PCWP is important for two reasons. First, it provides the measure of hydrostatic pressure that is responsible for forcing fluid out of the pulmonary vascular space. In addition, the capillary pressure is directly related to diastolic fiber stretch according to Starling's principle, which states that the strength of contraction is proportional to myocardial fiber length/LV volume.[20] When applied to construct a cardiac function curve, it is often called LV filling pressure or preload.

The pulmonary artery occluded pressure (PAOP) is obtained after inflating the distal balloon of the PAC in a large branch of the PA (about 10 mm in size). A static column of fluid is created between the site of occlusion and where the venous flow resumes as other venous branches connect downstream.[7] As downstream pulmonary flow decreases, the PA pressure decreases to a minimal value reflecting that pressure.[6] The compliance of the vasculature relative to the catheter causes a slight dampening of the pressure signal. Therefore, PAOPs are lower than PA diastolic pressure with dampened waveforms.[6] The PCWP is obtained when a catheter tip engages a small PA vessel (<2 mm) as opposed to an occlusion pressure obtained from balloon inflation in a medium to large vessel. The anatomic territory affected by the wedge is smaller than that affected by the occlusion pressure, thereby subjecting each to varying forces that generate a pressure. The term "occluded pressure" was historically preferred to "wedge pressure," but currently they are used interchangeably.[1]

The natural oscillation in intrathoracic pressure associated with respiration directly affects intraluminal pulmonary vascular pressure. During spontaneous breathing, the highest pulmonary pressures occur at end-expiration. This is the opposite of mechanical positive pressure ventilation, in which the lowest pulmonary pressures occur at end-expiration.[6] To minimize this artifact, recorded pressures should be made at end-expiration. Even at end-expiration, PAOP measures can still be overestimated if pleural pressures are elevated at end-expiration. Factors such as hyperinflation, air trapping, and PEEP in relation to lung and chest wall compliance increase pleural pressure to varying degrees.[6]

CARDIAC OUTPUT AND MIXED VENOUS OXYGEN CONSUMPTION

Though CO can be measured by several techniques, the two most commonly used are the indicator thermodilution technique and the Fick oxygen technique. Both are based on the theoretical principle devised by Adolf Fick in 1870, which states that the total uptake or release of any substance by an organ is the product of blood flow to the organ and the arteriovenous (AV) concentration difference of the substance.[25] The clinical marker most commonly used is oxygen; the difference between arterial and venous oxygen content is the uptake of oxygen as it flows through the lungs.[25]

Indicator Dilution Method

Stewart was the first to use the indicator dilution method to determine CO in 1897.[26] There have been a number of indicators used in the past but the most commonly used today is the "cold" indicator in the TD method. This technique measures the change in the temperature of blood caused by introduction of a known quantity of cold upstream from a point of temperature measurement.[25] Typically cold saline is injected into the RA. This results in cooling of the blood that is measured downstream by a thermistor to produce a TD curve. The area under the curve represents the integral of the instantaneous mixing temperature at the sensing point[25] (Fig. 45.2). CO is automatically computed from these measurements using a small microprocessor. Accurate calculation of CO by TD assumes that the injectate mixes

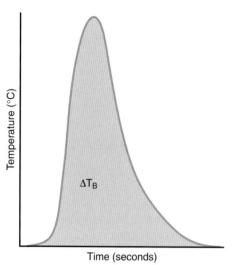

Fig. 45.2 Sample thermodilution curve shows the change in instantaneous mixed temperature at the sensing point (thermistor) versus time. (Modified from Ehlers KC, Mylrea KC, Waterston CK, et al. Cardiac output measurements: a review of current techniques and research. *Ann Biomed Eng.* 1986;14:219–239.)

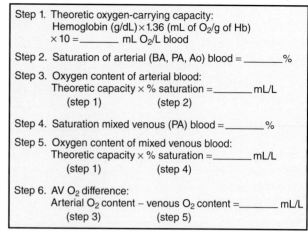

Fig. 45.3 Calculation of oxygen content and arteriovenous (AV) oxygen difference when using the reflectance oximetry method. *Ao*, Aorta; *BA*, brachial artery; *PA*, pulmonary artery. (Modified from Baim DS, ed. *Grossman's Cardiac Catheterization, Angiography, and Intervention.* 7th ed. Philadelphia: Lippincott Williams & Wilkins; 2006:154.)

completely with the blood and its concentration can be measured correctly. Though Felger described the TD method in 1954, it gained wide clinical use only after Swan and Ganz developed a multi-lumen PAC with a distal thermistor.[25]

The validity of results depends on the precision of the technique. The injection technique should be smooth and rapid to avoid dispersion of the injectate. Multiple measures should be taken and averaged to avoid ventilatory cycle-specific patterns.[6] The presence of significant tricuspid regurgitation can introduce error into the calculation and overestimate the CO. In a patient with a left-to-right intracardiac shunt, measurement of the RV CO would not reflect LV function. CO measurements via the TD method show good correlation with the Fick method for CO in the range of 3 to 6 L/min.[27,28] In the case of low-flow states, loss of indicator may occur because of warming of the blood by the walls of cardiac chambers. Grondelle and colleagues noted that TD measurement overestimated CO consistently in patients with CO less than 3.5 L/min (with the greatest discrepancy in patients with CO <2.5 L/min).[27,29]

A modification of the standard TD method now allows for continuous CO monitoring. The PA catheter was modified, with placement of a blood-warming filament on the catheter at the region of the catheter injectate port. The catheter filament delivers heat to the flowing blood with a random on/off sequence that is continuously repeated with approximate total heating time of about 50%. CO is derived from the reconstructed washout curve using an equation analogous to the Stewart-Hamilton equation used for solution-based flow measurements.[22] This advance simplifies the assessment of CO at the bedside by eliminating the need for accurate repeated injection of solution but is not available on all PA catheters.

Fick Method

With the Fick method of CO measurement, pulmonary blood flow is determined by measuring the AV difference of oxygen across the lungs and the rate of uptake by blood across the lungs. If there are no intracardiac shunts, pulmonary and systemic blood flow should be equal and the CO equals oxygen consumption divided by AV oxygen difference.[11]

$$CO\ (vol/time) = \frac{O_2\ consumption\ (mass/time)}{[arterial - venous\ O_2\ content]\ (mass/vol)}$$

The oxygen consumption can be either directly measured or calculated. Direct measurement is performed with exhaled breath analysis using a spirometer, such as the metabolic rate meter (MRM) or the Deltatrac II (Datax-Ohmeda).[11] In a steady state, oxygen consumption can be determined by having the patient breathe pure oxygen from the spirometer with a carbon dioxide absorber and measuring oxygen uptake directly by the net gas flux.[25] Normal oxygen consumption in a resting individual is approximately 250 mL O_2/min. Calculation of the $\dot{V}/O_2$ can be done with rearranging the Fick equation: $\dot{V}/O_2$ (mL O_2/min) = CO × (CaO$_2$ – CvO$_2$), where CaO$_2$ is the arterial oxygen content and CVO$_2$ is the mixed venous blood content. Normal CaO$_2$ and CVO$_2$ are 20 mL O_2/dL and 15 mL O_2/dL, respectively.

Oxygen consumption can also be estimated using a nomogram based on age, sex, height, and weight. The AV difference is calculated by obtaining blood from a peripheral artery and the pulmonary artery for a mixed venous sample. The oxygen saturation is then multiplied by theoretical oxygen-carrying capacity to yield the oxygen content of the sample (Fig. 45.3).

Mixed venous oxygen saturation (SvO$_2$) reflects the relationship between oxygen consumption ($\dot{V}/O_2$) and oxygen delivery (DO$_2$).

$$SvO_2 = oxygen\ delivered\ (SaO_2 \times Hb \times CO)$$
$$- oxygen\ consumed\ (\dot{V}/O_2)$$

It should be measured from blood drawn from the distal tip of the PA catheter to allow for adequate mixing of superior vena cava, inferior vena cava, and coronary sinus samples. The normal range of SvO$_2$ is 60% to 80%. If the SvO$_2$ is normal, one can assume that tissue perfusion is adequate, whereas high or low values reflect an imbalance between oxygen supply and demand. A low SvO_2 reflects either decreased oxygen delivery (i.e., decreased Hb, SaO_2, or cardiac output) or increased oxygen demand. Conversely, high SvO_2 reflects increased oxygen delivery or decreased oxygen demand, such as in the case of sepsis or, more generally, the systemic inflammatory response syndrome (SIRS).

Pulmonary and Systemic Vascular Resistance. The pulmonary vascular resistance (PVR) and systemic vascular resistance (SVR) are computed values using measurements from the PA catheter.

$$PVR\ (dyne \times sec/cm^5) = 80 \times \frac{Mean\ PAP - PAOP}{CO}$$

$$SVR\ (dyne \times sec/cm^5) = 80 \times \frac{MAP - RA}{CO}$$

Normal PVR is less than 250 dyne $\times$ sec/cm^5. If pulmonary hypertension is associated with increased PVR, causes are primarily within the lung, such as pulmonary embolism, pulmonary fibrosis, essential pulmonary hypertension, or pulmonary veno-occlusive disease. Normal PVR in the setting of pulmonary hypertension is more indicative of elevation of LV filling pressures. Normal SVR ranges from 800 to 1200 dyne $\times$ sec/cm^5. Low SVR indicates a vasoplegic state, while increased SVR indicates vasoconstriction.

COMPLICATIONS OF PULMONARY ARTERY CATHETERIZATION

As with any invasive procedure, complications are an inherent risk of PA catheterization. Multiple observational and randomized studies have investigated the incidence and significance of adverse events related to PA catheter use. Complications have been associated with catheter insertion (pneumothorax, arrhythmia, atrioventricular block) and those associated with the catheter once in place (pulmonary infarction, local thrombosis, pulmonary artery rupture, catheter-related infection).

Arrhythmias and Atrioventricular Block

Although ventricular and atrial ectopy are not uncommon, sustained ventricular arrhythmias are rare. Ventricular tachycardia has been reported in 12% to 68% of patients undergoing PA catheterization.[30,31] Most episodes resolve with catheter movement and seldom require treatment. PA catheter-related arrhythmia does not appear to influence patient outcome.[31]

In patients with preexisting left bundle branch block (LBBB), the insertion of a PA catheter may be associated with the development of concomitant right bundle branch block (RBBB), thereby resulting in complete heart block. However, Sprung and coworkers studied 293 patients undergoing 307 PAC insertions and found a 3% incidence of new RBBB.[32] They found no difference between the incidence of complete heart block in patients with preexisting LBBB and development of RBBB and those with no underlying conduction disease. Though prophylactic pacemaker placement is not indicated, the use of PA catheters that provide for ventricular pacing is advisable in patients with preexisting LBBB.

Pulmonary Vascular Damage

Pulmonary infarctions appear to range in incidence from 7%[33] in earlier studies to 1.3% in later studies.[34,35] These may occur as a result of either damage to the pulmonary endothelium, emboli originating from the catheter shaft, or prolonged placement of the catheter in the distal PA. Infarct can be avoided by minimizing the time the catheter is in the distal PA and by preventing migration of the tip into the distal pulmonary vessel.[1] These small, segmental infarcts usually resolve within 48 hours and, though undesirable, appear to be of limited clinical significance. Chest radiographs should be obtained daily to monitor position of the catheter tip.

PA rupture, though rare, is the most serious complication of PA catheter use, occurring in up to 0.2% of patients undergoing PAC insertion.[34,36–38] In a retrospective review of more than 32,000 patients with PA catheters in a single institution over 17 years, Kearney and Shabot reported 10 patients with PA rupture (0.031%) with 70% mortality.[37] All 10 patients were over the age of 60 years and five had baseline pulmonary hypertension. All 10 patients developed hemoptysis. Risk factors for PA rupture include advanced age, pulmonary hypertension, and cardiopulmonary bypass surgery.[1,37,39] Inflation of the balloon in a peripheral diseased pulmonary vessel may produce enough force to cause rupture; however, even a deflated catheter tip in the wedge position can cause arterial erosions.[1] The clinician must be careful to limit the length of time the catheter is in a peripheral artery, inflate the balloon only when the catheter position is known, and to confirm a safe "parking spot" for the deflated catheter in the main PA or proximally in the right or left branches of the PA.[1] A PA catheter that allows for surveillance of appropriate position by monitoring RV pressure via a middle lumen located 10 cm from the distal tip is available.[40] Recording a ventricular pressure tracing from this lumen may help ensure that the catheter is in the appropriate position.

Infection

Strict sterile technique is of paramount importance with any invasive procedure. The incidence of catheter-related infection ranges from 0.5% to 2%.[34,41] A recent randomized control study on PA catheter use in 433 patients found catheter-related infection to be the most common adverse outcome with an incidence of 1.9%.[42] Mermel and colleagues prospectively examined 297 PAC cases for infection and found a 22% incidence of local infection of the introducer sheath with only a 0.7% incidence of bacteremia.[43] The patient's skin was noted to be the single most common source of infection. Most investigators agree that the risk of catheter-related sepsis increases when a catheter is left in place more than 72 hours.[34,41,43]

Thrombosis

A thin fibrin coating will usually envelop PA catheters within 24 hours of insertion.[1] In an autopsy series of 32 patients, thrombosis was identified in 53% and fibrin deposition was identified in 66% of patients along the entire length of the PA catheter.[44] The incidence of thrombosis was significantly higher in cases in which the catheter was left in place more than 36 hours. There appears to be no difference in the incidence of pulmonary emboli in those with and without thrombi.[45] Though these thrombi can possibly embolize or become infected, the incidence and clinical significance appears to be low.

PA catheter use in the CICU and its complication profile is similar to the procedure performed at other locations; however, there are some important caveats. For instance, the use of anticoagulation, such as antiplatelet and antithrombin therapy, in the setting of acute coronary syndromes increases the propensity for bleeding and hematoma formation. In addition, the majority of CICU patients are already at increased risk for morbidity and mortality owing to their underlying conditions. The overall morbidity of PAC use should not exceed 2% to 5%. Swan estimated the added mortality risk in the CICU environment to be less than 0.25%.[1]

INDICATIONS FOR PULMONARY ARTERY CATHETERIZATION

Hemodynamic data derived from PA catheterization may aid in diagnosis as well as guide management. Despite the widespread use of PA catheters, the effect on patient outcome remains controversial. The accepted indications for PA catheterization have been based largely on expert opinion.[46] The decision to place a PA catheter should be based on a clinical question regarding a patient's hemodynamic status that cannot be answered with noninvasive assessment. The use of hemodynamic data to differentiate various cardiopulmonary disorders is presented in Table 45.2. There needs to be an intent to act on the information gathered by invasive hemodynamic monitoring to justify PA catheter placement. Examples of how hemodynamic data can influence choice of therapy are presented in Table 45.3. In general,

TABLE 45.2	**How Hemodynamic Profiles Differentiate Cardiopulmonary Disorders**	
Disorder	**Hemodynamic Profile**	**Comments**
Acute ischemic RV dysfunction	Increased RA, decreased SV, decreased CO, decreased AP, RA greater than or equal to PCWP	Steep y descent RV diastolic dip and plateau (square root sign) Volume loading may unmask hemodynamic changes
Acute mitral regurgitation	Increased PCWP, prominent v waves, sometimes reflecting onto the PA tracing as well	V waves may not always differentiate mitral regurgitation from ventricular septal rupture
Acute ventricular septal rupture	Oxygen step-up from RA to RV and PA	RV forward output exceeds LV forward output Early recirculation on the thermodilution curve
Shock		
Ventriculopenic	Increased RA, decreased SV, decreased CO, decreased AP, increased SVR	
Hypovolemic	Decreased or low-normal PCWP, decreased SV, decreased CO, decreased AP, increased SVR	Orthostatic tachycardia
Early septic	Increased PA, increased PVR, increased CO, decreased AP, decreased SVR	SVR is elevated and cardiac output is lowered in later stages
Noncardiac pulmonary edema	Normal PCWP	Normal heart size
Acute massive pulmonary embolism	Decreased SV, decreased CO, decreased AP, increased PA, increased PVR, normal PCWP	PCWP normal despite elevated pulmonary artery systolic and diastolic pressures
Chronic precapillary pulmonary hypertension	Increased RA, increased RV systolic pressure, increased PA, increased PVR, normal PCWP	Left-sided pressures often normal PA and RV systolic pressures may reach systemic levels
Acute cardiac tamponade	Increased RA, increased PCWP, RA equal to PCWP, decreased SV, decreased CO, decreased AP	Paradoxical pulse Blunted y descent Prominent x descent on RA tracing
Constrictive pericarditis	Increased RA, increased PCWP, dip and plateau in RV pressure, M- or W-shaped jugular venous pressure with preserved x and steep y descent	Paradoxical pulse rare Positive Kussmaul sign common May simulate ischemic RV dysfunction or restrictive cardiomyopathy
Restrictive cardiomyopathy	Findings are similar to those described for constrictive pericarditis, but PCWP may be higher than RA; difference between PCWP and RA may be exaggerated by exercise	Simulates constrictive pericarditis; however, PA systolic pressure is usually >50 mm Hg and diastolic plateau is less than one-third peak RV systolic pressure. Thus, other tests are often needed for differentiation from constrictive pericarditis
Tricuspid regurgitation	Increased RA, increased RV end-diastolic pressure	Blunted x descent, prominent v wave, steep y descent Ventricularization of RA pressure

AP, Mean arterial pressure; *CO,* cardiac output; *LV,* left ventricular pressure; *PA,* mean pulmonary artery pressure; *PCWP,* pulmonary capillary wedge pressure; *PVR,* pulmonary vascular resistance; *RA,* mean right atrial pressure; *RV,* right ventricular pressure; *SV,* stroke volume; *SVR,* systemic vascular resistance.

TABLE 45.3   Using Hemodynamic Data to Choose Therapy

Clinical Diagnosis	Hemodynamic Data	Suggested Therapy
Acute pulmonary edema	Increased PCWP, decreased CO	Diuretics, vasodilators Hemofiltration/dialysis if edema is associated with oliguria or anuria Intraaortic balloon counterpulsation support in special circumstances
Low-Output or Shock Syndromes		
Absolute or relative hypovolemia	Decreased PCWP	Volume expansion
Ischemic right ventricular dysfunction	Increased RA, normal PCWP, normal PA	Volume expansion with or without inotropic agents
Early sepsis	Increased CO, decreased SVR, decreased AP	Volume loading Vasopressors/inotropic drugs Specific treatment for causative organism
Ventriculopenia	Increased PCWP, increased PA, decreased CO, decreased AP	Reduce preload with diuretics and/or vasodilators Inotropic agents and intraaortic balloon counterpulsation in special circumstances
Pulmonary embolism	Increased RA, decreased CO, decreased AP, increased PA, normal PCWP	Thrombolytic or anticoagulant therapy after scintigraphic or angiographic confirmation
Cardiac tamponade	Increased RA, RA equals PCWP, paradoxical pulse	Echocardiographic confirmation, if time permits Pericardiocentesis

AP, Mean arterial pressure; *CO,* cardiac output; *PA,* mean pulmonary artery pressure; *PCWP,* pulmonary capillary wedge pressure; *RA,* mean right atrial pressure; *SVR,* systemic vascular resistance.

patients requiring invasive monitoring include those with circulatory collapse, cardiogenic shock, and severe heart failure. RV infarct, ventricular septal rupture, and cardiac tamponade are currently more appropriately diagnosed with echocardiography.

Clinical Applications

Pulmonary Edema. At times, determination of the etiology of pulmonary edema through radiographic and clinical means may be difficult.[47] Often these patients are critically ill, have severe blood gas abnormalities, and have radiographic evidence of generalized interstitial and alveolar infiltrates. In noncardiogenic pulmonary edema, the PCWP would be normal to low. This distinction is critical for the appropriate choice of therapy (i.e., diuretics, vasodilators, and/or inotropes in cardiogenic pulmonary edema versus supportive care in the case of adult respiratory distress syndrome).

For many forms of shock, an empiric trial of volume expansion may be indicated. PA catheterization is considered in patients when these initial strategies may be contraindicated, have failed, or when there are coexisting features of cardiac and noncardiac etiologies making therapeutic decisions difficult. Following the diagnosis, PA catheterization may be helpful in effectively titrating doses of diuretics, vasodilators, inotropes, or vasopressors.

Pericardial Tamponade. Pericardial tamponade is a clinical diagnosis characterized by distant heart sounds, pulsus paradoxus, and hypotension that is best confirmed by echocardiography. When echocardiography is unavailable or technically suboptimal, PAC can provide evidence for the diagnosis. The low ventricular volume during systole creates a dominant *x* descent on the RA tracing. The *y* descent is attenuated or absent. During inspiration, the mean RA pressure declines, allowing one to distinguish tamponade from constriction and RV infarction,[13] which display paradoxical increases in RA pressure with inspiration due to

reduced ventricular filling from a poorly compliant pericardium or myocardium (Fig. 45.4). Early diastolic filling is also blunted in tamponade, further differentiating it from constriction.[48] Therapeutic intervention should never be delayed in unstable patients to await PA catheterization.

Acute Decompensated Heart Failure. Invasive hemodynamic measurements may be useful for effectively treating some episodes of severe acute decompensated heart failure by allowing more precise adjustments of therapy, including diuretics, vasopressors, vasodilators, and inotropes[49] based on real-time assessment of hemodynamics. Stevenson and colleagues outlined a concept of "tailored therapy" for advanced heart failure in 152 patients awaiting heart transplant that included use of nitroprusside, furosemide, and oral vasodilators with targets for PCWP and SVR.[50] They demonstrated a correlation between mortality and failure to improve PCWP during therapy.

Acute Myocardial Infarction. It has never been the practice to routinely use PA catheters in the setting of uncomplicated acute MI. A prospective study by Gore et al. analyzed PA catheter use in acute MI over the 1970s and 1980s in hospitals in Worchester, Massachusetts.[51] More than 96% of the instances of PA catheterization were in the setting of congestive heart failure, hypotension, and cardiogenic shock. A retrospective analysis of two large randomized acute coronary syndrome trials looking at PA catheter use found an overall rate of 2.8%. Those undergoing PAC insertion were more likely to have ST elevation MI and Killip class III or class IV.[52] As per previous American College of Cardiology/American Heart Association (ACC/AHA) guidelines, indications for PAC are related to specific complications of MI, including (1) hypotension, low CO, and cardiogenic shock owing to LV failure; (2) acute mechanical complications (mitral regurgitation [MR] from papillary muscle rupture/ischemia,

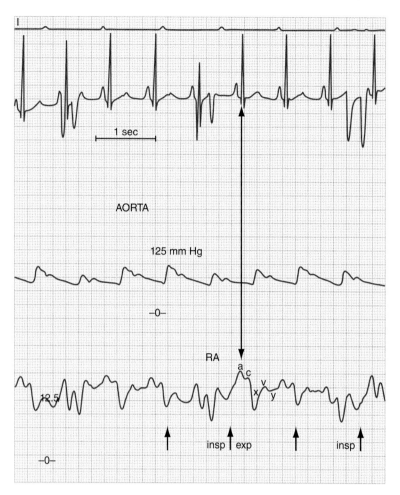

Fig. 45.4 Right atrial (RA) and aortic pressure tracings from a patient with pericardial tamponade. Aortic pressure declines by 20 mm Hg during inspiration (pulsus paradoxus). RA pressure declines normally during inspiration. A dominant *x* descent can be seen. (Modified from Sharkey SW. Beyond the wedge: clinical physiology and the Swan-Ganz catheter. *Am J Med.* 1987;83:118.)

ventricular septal defect [VSD], or ventricular free wall rupture); (3) complicated RV infarction; and (4) heart failure or pulmonary edema refractory to usual management.[46]

Shock/Low Cardiac Output. Diminished CO is frequently multifactorial but most often due to decreased contractility because of infarct or ischemia. Mechanical causes, such as MR and VSD, though less frequent, are not uncommon causes of low CO states.[20] Assessing filling pressures and hemodynamic criteria with a PA catheter can help differentiate cardiogenic shock from other etiologies and can guide therapy. Patients that exhibit progressive hemodynamic deterioration with cardiac indices less than 1.8 L/min/m^2, elevated PA pressure, and PCWP above 25 mm Hg may require mechanical ventilation, afterload reduction, heart rate control, various vasoactive medications, or ventricular assist devices. CO measurements can be followed to assess the response to therapy.[1] An analysis of the Should We Emergently Revascularize Occluded Coronaries for Cardiogenic Shock (SHOCK) registry of patients with acute MI complicated by cardiogenic shock found overall use of PA catheters in 66% of patients. However, there was a significant decrease in use from the early to late 1990s.[53] Though no data prove a survival benefit in cardiogenic shock associated with the use of PA catheters, most studies have been limited by selection bias that precludes clear conclusions.[51,54]

Mitral Regurgitation Due to Papillary Muscle Rupture. Though acute MR can be accurately diagnosed by echocardiography, severe MR associated with papillary muscle rupture is an indication for prompt right and left heart catheterization and cardiac surgery evaluation for possible valve replacement. The retrograde ejection of blood into a normal-sized, noncompliant LA causes a giant *v* wave on the wedge pressure tracing. The giant *v* wave is transmitted to the PA tracing, yielding a bifid PA waveform composed of a pulmonary systolic wave and *v* wave[13] (Fig. 45.5). Inflation of the balloon obliterates the systolic wave as the catheter is wedged but the *v* wave remains. Careful attention needs to be paid to avoid mistaking the PCWP and PA tracing in these patients. The systolic wave in the PA tracing occurs earlier in the QRS cycle than does the *v* wave. Prominent *v* waves are not specific to acute MR but can also be seen with acute VSD or any situation in which a noncompliant LA experiences abruptly increased retrograde blood flow. Bedside PA catheterization may help guide vasodilator therapy in acute MR.

Ventricular Septal Defect. Echocardiography is highly sensitive and specific for the diagnosis of VSD and can provide quantitative measures regarding the magnitude of the shunt, pulmonary artery pressures, and RV function.[46] Though not typically required, PA catheterization can be helpful if echocardiography is unavailable or suboptimal in evaluating the magnitude of the shunt. Clinical

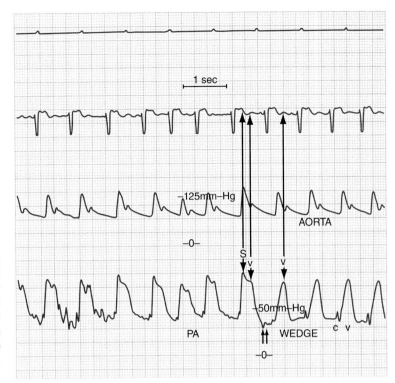

Fig. 45.5 Arterial, pulmonary artery (PA), and wedge pressure waveforms in a patient with acute mitral regurgitation. A prominent v wave is present in pulmonary artery and wedge tracings. The bifid PA waveform reflects the systolic (S) and v wave. The *double arrow* denotes inflation of the balloon and wedging, which obliterates the S wave. (Modified from Sharkey SW. Beyond the wedge: clinical physiology and the Swan-Ganz catheter. *Am J Med.* 1987;83:115.)

differentiation between acute MR and VSD can be difficult. Rupture of the septum causes acute volume overload from LV into the RV with increased pulmonary to systemic blood flow ratio greater than 2:1.[13] The diagnosis is confirmed with the presence of a step-up in oxygen saturation of greater than 10% between the RA and PA.[11]

Right Ventricular Infarction. RV infarction complicates acute inferior wall MI in up to 30% of cases.[13] The characteristic hemodynamic profile of acute RV dysfunction includes RA pressure disproportionately increased relative to PCWP, a steep y descent, and an RV pressure tracing that may show a diastolic dip and plateau referred to as the square root sign[14] (Fig. 45.6). Though a prominent x and y descent are typical, the y descent may exceed the x descent because of the presence of a dilated noncompliant RV that is confined by the pericardium.[13] During inspiration, the RA pressure may increase, called the Kussmaul sign.[13] Tricuspid insufficiency due to papillary muscle dysfunction and RV dilation may complicate RV infarction.[13] Volume loading may be necessary to unmask these hemodynamic abnormalities in up to 50% of patients.[14]

Constrictive Pericarditis. As in tamponade, constrictive pericarditis produces diastolic pressure equalization with elevated right- and left-sided filling pressures. However, unlike tamponade, constriction produces an early diastolic dip followed by a pressure plateau in both RV and LV pressure tracings.[14] The RA tracing displays the characteristic M or W shape with a preserved x descent and a prominent early y descent (Fig. 45.7).

Restrictive Cardiomyopathy. The hemodynamic profiles of restrictive cardiomyopathy and constrictive pericarditis mirror each other as both display the characteristic M- or W-shaped RA pressure tracing and diastolic dip and plateau pattern in the RV and LV. Criteria exist to help differentiate the two. Classically, in restrictive cardiomyopathy, the left ventricular end diastolic pressure (LVEDP) tends to be higher than the right ventricular end diastolic pressure (RVEDP) and the RVEDP is usually less than one-third the RV systolic pressure.[14] The RV systolic pressure is generally also less than 50 mm Hg in constriction. If all three of these criteria are concordant, then the probability of accurate classification is 90%, but 25% of patients may not be able to be classified.[55] Constriction is also marked by increased ventricular interdependence, with increased RV filling in inspiration associated with decreased LV filling. A measure of the ratio of RV to LV systolic area during inspiration and expiration has been found to have 100% predictive accuracy.[56]

Controversies

The PAC became a widely used monitoring device in critically ill patients after its introduction in 1971, but its initial use was based only on assumed benefit and the desire to understand the hemodynamic profiles of various disease states. Retrospective analyses from the 1980s[51,54] studying PAC use in acute MI found no difference in mortality after adjusting for severity of illness. In 1996, a retrospective observational study of more than 5500 cardiac and noncardiac critically ill patients concluded that, after adjustment for treatment selection bias, use of a PAC was actually associated with increased mortality and length of stay.[57] An accompanying editorial proposed a moratorium on PAC use.[58] This prompted a response by multiple organizations, including the ACC and AHA, who issued a consensus statement stating that, despite attempts to account for selection bias by the authors, flaws in the data existed. Patients with lack of response

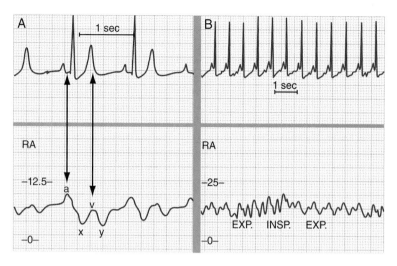

Fig. 45.6 (A) Right atrial (RA) pressure waveform in a patient with right ventricular infarction. Note the steep *x* and *y* descents. (B) The inspiratory increase of RA pressure in right ventricular infarction is known as the Kussmaul sign. (Adapted from Sharkey SW. Beyond the wedge: clinical physiology and the Swan-Ganz catheter. *Am J Med.* 1987;83:116.)

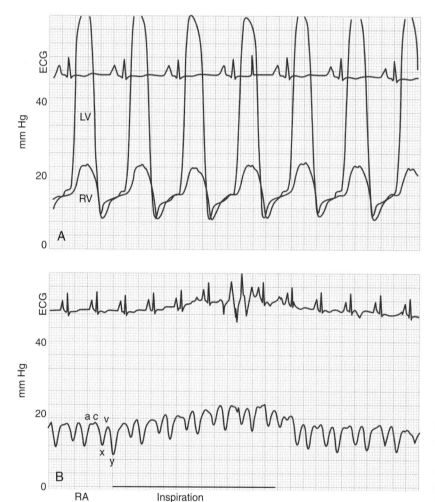

Fig. 45.7 (A) Simultaneous right ventricular (RV) and left ventricular (LV) tracings show equalization of end-diastolic pressures along with the "square root sign" (i.e., early diastolic dip and late diastolic plateau). (B) Kussmaul sign—the inspiratory increase in right atrial pressure.

to initial therapy were more likely to undergo PAC placement. In addition, patients with PACs in place were more likely to enter the study with multiorgan failure, respiratory failure, and congestive heart failure—all factors associated with higher mortality. These criticisms did not discount the possibility that PAC use may be associated with detrimental outcomes but instead highlighted the need for further trials, randomized if possible.

However, the statement also cautioned that even data from randomized trials may not resolve the issue because of the difficulty in controlling for the effects of therapies administered and enrolling the large numbers of patients necessary for a definitive study.[46]

In 2005, two large multicenter randomized trials were published examining the effectiveness of PA catheterization in the management of critically ill patients. The first reported on more than 1000 critically ill patients enrolled between 2001 and 2004. Patients were randomized to PAC insertion or no PAC use. The authors found no statistical difference in hospital mortality between the groups (68% vs. 66%; adjusted hazard ratio, 1.09; 95% confidence interval, 0.94–1.27; $P = .39$).[59] It also found that the less than 10% complication rate did not directly lead to an increase in mortality. Later that year, the second trial was published. Patients admitted with severe symptomatic and recurrent heart failure from 2000 to 2003 were randomized to PA catheterization or no PAC insertion. The authors found that therapy in both groups led to substantial reduction in symptoms, jugular venous pressure, and edema. The use of a PAC did not significantly affect the primary endpoint of 6-month mortality.[42] Therefore basing the decision to administer vasodilator and diuretic therapy on PAC data plus clinical judgment was not superior to decisions based on clinical judgment alone.[42] The authors did note that there was a trend toward better outcomes using PAC-guided therapy in centers with large numbers of patients. Ultimately, the data from both trials found PAC use to be safe and did not substantiate previous retrospective reports of excessive mortality associated with PAC use.

Safe and effective PAC use should be predicated on careful catheter placement, attention to measurement techniques, and thoughtful interpretation of the data. Iberti and colleagues published a multicenter evaluation of physician knowledge of PAC use in 1990.[60] The authors used a 31-question multiple-choice examination of 496 physicians to assess physician understanding of PAC use. They found a mean test score of 67% correct. Mean scores varied independently by training and with the frequency of PAC use in clinical practice.

Every physician who performs hemodynamic monitoring should understand the indication for the procedure, should be technically competent with insertion techniques, and have the ability to interpret data obtained.[61]

Acknowledgment

We acknowledge the contributions of Dr. Robin Matthews and the late Dr. H.J.C. Swan, who were authors of this chapter in previous editions.

The full reference list for this chapter is available at ExpertConsult.com.

46

Temporary Mechanical Circulatory Support Devices

Mark Gdowski, Jonathan D. Wolfe, David L. Brown

OUTLINE

Clinicians practicing in the cardiac intensive care unit (CICU) are challenged with increasingly complex patients who often require hemodynamic support to improve end-organ perfusion and reduce mortality. The high mortality associated with cardiogenic shock has been the stimulus for technological advances that provide life-sustaining hemodynamic support when maximum pharmacologic therapy is ineffective. Numerous devices to augment cardiac output (CO) have been developed that can be placed surgically or percutaneously (Fig. 46.1). Each approach has device-specific characteristics (Table 46.1), advantages and disadvantages, different effects on hemodynamics (Table 46.2), and different complication profiles (Table 46.3). This chapter will explore four categories of devices, provide practical guidance on device management, and examine the evidence behind indications for the use of each.

INTRAAORTIC BALLOON PUMP

The intraaortic balloon pump (IABP) is one of the most frequently placed mechanical circulatory support devices. The device is used in managing cardiogenic shock, intractable angina, myocardial ischemia, during high-risk percutaneous coronary intervention (PCI), in cardiac surgery, and for patients with refractory heart failure or arrhythmias awaiting definitive therapy.[1] It relies on the concept of diastolic augmentation and afterload reduction to improve the function of ischemic and/or failing myocardium. The concept was originally proposed by Moulopoulos et al. in 1962 and validated by demonstration of an improvement in hemodynamic parameters in experimental animal models.[2] The first report of human use by Kantrowitz appeared 6 years later.[3] Although most commonly placed in the patient in the catheterization laboratory, the IABP can be placed at the bedside by experienced operators. Practitioners in the CICU need to be familiar with the fundamental principles of IABP counterpulsation therapy to effectively manage patients. Characteristics of the IABP are summarized in Table 46.1.

Physiologic Principles

The primary goal of IABP counterpulsation is to increase myocardial oxygen supply while decreasing oxygen demand.

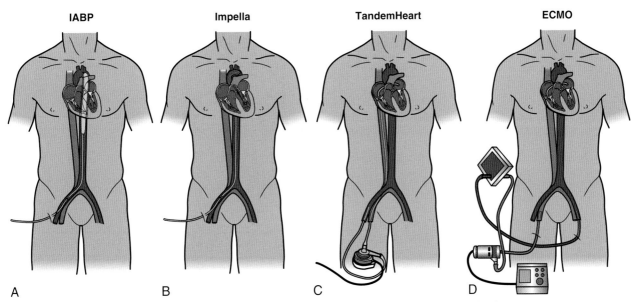

Fig. 46.1 Comparison of the most commonly used temporary mechanical circulatory support devices. (From Scheidt S, Wilner G, Mueller H, et al. Intraaortic balloon counterpulsation in cardiogenic shock. *N Engl J. Med.* 1973;288:979).

TABLE 46.1 Characteristics of Temporary Mechanical Circulatory Support Devices

Device Characteristics	IABP	Impella	TandemHeart	VA ECMO
Pump mechanism	Pneumatic	Axial flow	Centrifugal	Centrifugal
Cannula size	8 Fr	13–23 Fr	21 Fr inflow, 15–17 Fr outflow	18–21 Fr inflow, 15–17 Fr outflow
Insertion	Percutaneous	Percutaneous or surgical cutdown	Percutaneous	Percutaneous and surgical
Maximum implant duration	7–10 days	7–21 days (model dependent)	14–21 days	21–28 days
Delivered flow	0.5–1 L/min	1.5–5 L/min (model dependent)	4 L/min	3–6 L/min

IABP, Intraaortic balloon pump; *VA ECMO,* venoarterial extracorporeal membrane oxygenation.
From Combes A, Brodie D, Chen Y, et al. The ICM research agenda on extracorporeal life support. *Intensive Care Med.* 2017;43:1306–1318.

TABLE 46.2 Effect of Temporary Mechanical Circulatory Support Devices on Hemodynamics

Hemodynamic Parameter	IABP	Impella	TandemHeart	VA ECMO
MAP	Increase	Increase	Increase	Increase
Afterload	Reduced	Neutral	Increased	Increased
Coronary perfusion	Slightly Increased	Unknown	Unknown	Unknown
LV stroke volume	Slightly Increased	Reduced	Reduced	Reduced
LV preload	Slightly Reduced	Slightly Reduced	Reduced	Reduced
LVEDP	Slightly Reduced	Reduced	Reduced	Increased
Peripheral tissue perfusion	Neutral	Improved	Improved	Improved

IABP, Intraaortic balloon pump; *LV,* left ventricular; *LVEDP,* left ventricular end-diastolic pressure; *MAP,* mean arterial pressure; *VA ECMO,* venoarterial extracorporeal membrane oxygenation.
Modified from Werdan K, Gielen S, Ebelet H, et al. Mechanical circulatory support in cardiogenic shock. *Eur Heart J.* 2014;35:156–167; and Combes A, Brodie D, Chen Y, et al. The ICM research agenda on extracorporeal life support. *Intensive Care Med.* 2017;43:1306–1318.

During diastole, the balloon inflates, resulting in a volume of blood being displaced toward the proximal aorta. During systole, the balloon rapidly deflates, creating a vacuum effect resulting in a decrease in left ventricular (LV) afterload. To optimize these two hemodynamic effects, the IABP must inflate and deflate in synchrony with the cardiac cycle. The single most important determinant of effective counterpulsation is the timing of the IABP relative to the cardiac cycle.[4] Once proper timing has been established, IABP counterpulsation improves myocardial oxygen delivery via an increase in coronary perfusion pressure, reduces cardiac work by decreasing systolic blood pressure and afterload, and improves forward blood flow in patients with impaired cardiac contractile function.[5] Modern IABPs now use a closed-loop control system to automatically optimize pump timing.[6–10]

Several factors influence the hemodynamic effect of an IABP: the volume of the balloon, its position in the aorta, the underlying

TABLE 46.3 **Complications of Temporary Mechanical Circulatory Support Devices**				
Complication	IABP	Impella	TandemHeart	VA ECMO
Limb ischemia	+	++	+++	+++
Hemolysis	+	++	++	++
Hemorrhage	+	++	+++	+++

IABP, Intraaortic balloon pump; *VA ECMO,* venoarterial extracorporeal membrane oxygenation.
From Combes A, Brodie D, Chen Y, et al. The ICM research agenda on extracorporeal life support. *Intensive Care Med.* 2017;43:1306–1318.

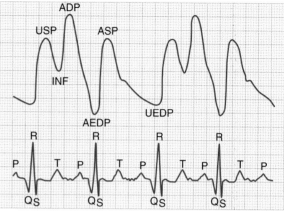

Fig. 46.2 Optimal timing of an intraaortic balloon pump (IABP). Arterial pressure tracing from a patient with an IABP. The balloon was set at 2:1 to evaluate timing. Inflation (INF) was timed to the dicrotic notch to follow aortic valve closure. There is augmentation of diastolic pressure (ADP) and reduction of the end-diastolic pressure with augmented beats (AEDP) compared with the unaugmented end-diastolic pressure (UEDP). The augmented systolic pressure (ASP) is often lower than the unaugmented systolic pressure (USP) as well. (Modified from Hollenberg S, Saltzberg M, Soble J, Parrillo J. Heart failure and cardiomyopathy. In: Crawford MH, Dimarco JP, Paulus WJ, eds. *Cardiology.* London: Mosby; 2001.)

heart rate and rhythm, the compliance of the aorta, and systemic vascular resistance.[11] An increase in arterial elastance (a property that is affected by compliance) is associated with a greater degree of hemodynamic improvement from an IABP.[12] Despite the presence of multiple factors that can cause variability in the effects of an IABP, a majority of patients exhibit a specific hemodynamic response (see Table 46.2), including a decrease in systolic pressure, an increase in diastolic pressure (which may subsequently enhance coronary blood flow to a territory perfused by an artery with a critical stenosis), a reduction in heart rate, a decrease in the mean pulmonary capillary wedge pressure (PCWP), and an increase in CO.[13] The reduction in aortic pressure caused by the rapid deflation of the balloon decreases LV afterload and diminishes myocardial workload.[5] Two indices that are measured during IABP counterpulsation are the tension-time index (TTI), which is the time integral of LV pressures during systole, and the diastolic pressure-time index (DPTI), which is the time integral of the proximal aortic pressures during diastole. Proper balloon inflation augments diastolic pressure (i.e., increases DPTI), whereas rapid balloon deflation decreases LV afterload (i.e., decreases TTI). The endocardial viability ratio (DPTI:TTI), which reflects the relationship between myocardial oxygen supply and demand, will increase with optimal IABP counterpulsation.[5,14]

Monitoring of IABP Counterpulsation

The appropriate timing of balloon counterpulsation to the mechanical events of the cardiac cycle must be monitored to ensure that the patient is deriving maximal hemodynamic benefit (Fig. 46.2). To maximize diastolic augmentation, the balloon should inflate at end systole, immediately after closure of the aortic valve. Balloon inflation augments coronary perfusion pressure, thereby providing greater myocardial oxygen delivery. Mean diastolic pressure (MDP) correlates well with coronary perfusion and, hence, oxygen delivery.[5] Smith and colleagues confirmed that maximal coronary perfusion occurs when balloon inflation coincides with end systole.[8,15] The timing of balloon deflation, which decreases LV oxygen consumption, should occur at end diastole. Deflation before the LV ejection of blood creates a vacuum effect in the proximal aorta that, in turn, reduces afterload and peak systolic pressure.

The triggering of balloon counterpulsation requires a predictable, reproducible, and reliable trigger event. The most commonly used trigger is the electrocardiographic (ECG) waveform. Inflation of the balloon begins at end systole, which correlates with the

middle of the T wave, while deflation of the balloon begins at end diastole and correlates with the R wave. IABP systems recognize other potential triggers, such as arterial pressure waveforms (most often used during cardiopulmonary resuscitation [CPR]) and ventricular or atrioventricular pacer spikes. A suboptimal hemodynamic effect results when IABP counterpulsation is not appropriately timed to the mechanical events of the cardiac cycle.[16] Loss of the optimal hemodynamic effect occurs when balloon IABP counterpulsation is not appropriately timed to the mechanical events of the cardiac cycle. Mahaffey and colleagues have described four different scenarios involving faulty coupling of balloon IABP counterpulsation with the cardiac cycle[16] (Fig. 46.3).

During early inflation, the balloon inflates before closure of the aortic valve. Pressure augmentation is thus superimposed upon the systolic aortic pressure tracing, leading to a decrease in LV emptying (a decrease in stroke volume), a decrease in cardiac output, an increase in LV afterload, and an overall increase in myocardial oxygen consumption. In this scenario, there is loss of the distinct systolic peak of the central aortic pressure waveform and loss of the dicrotic notch (see Fig. 46.3A). To correct early inflation, the timing interval should be slowly increased until the onset of inflation occurs at the dicrotic notch.

During late inflation, the dicrotic notch on the aortic pressure waveform is clearly visualized. The balloon inflates well beyond closure of the aortic valve. In this scenario, diastolic augmentation of the central aortic pressure is decreased, whereas LV afterload is minimally affected. The classic morphologic finding on the central aortic pressure tracing is the presence of a distinct dicrotic notch, with the augmented diastolic pressure wave occurring well afterward (see Fig. 46.3B). To correct late inflation of the

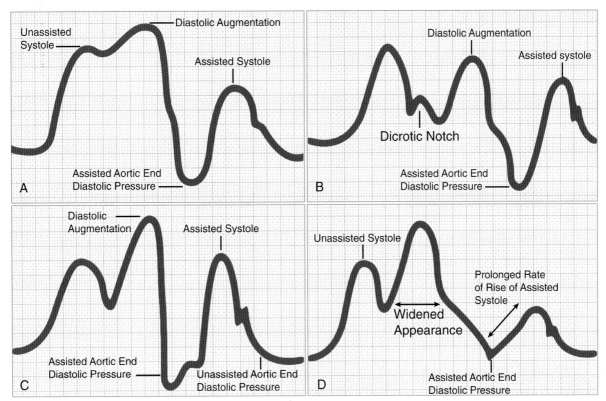

Fig. 46.3 Incorrect timing in intraaortic balloon counterpulsation. (A) Early inflation: loss of dicrotic notch and distinct systolic peak of the aortic pressure waveform. (B) Late inflation: dicrotic notch is clearly visualized with the augmented diastolic pressure curve occurring well afterward. (C) Early deflation: peaked augmented diastolic wave along with a U-shaped wave preceding the onset of systole. (D) Late deflation: loss of a distinct valley representing the end-diastolic pressure before the central aortic systolic waveform. (From Krishna M, Zacharowski K. Principles of intra-aortic balloon pump counterpulsation. Continuing education in anaesthesia. *Crit Care Pain.* 2009;9(1):24–28. Reproduced with permission from Datascope.)

IABP, the timing interval should be gradually decreased until the onset of inflation coincides with the dicrotic notch on the arterial pressure waveform.

During early deflation, the balloon deflates prematurely; consequently, the benefits of diastolic augmentation are lost. Analysis of the arterial pressure tracing reveals the presence of a peaked diastolic augmentation wave along with a U-shaped wave preceding the onset of systole (Fig. 46.3C). To correct early deflation, the timing interval should be increased until the augmented diastolic wave becomes appropriate.

During late deflation, the balloon is deflated after the onset of systole and the opening of the aortic valve. The resultant hemodynamic profile is like the one observed with early inflation: afterload is increased, leading to increased LV work and myocardial oxygen consumption along with reduced stroke volume and CO. Analysis of the arterial pressure tracing usually reveals the loss of a distinct valley representing the end-diastolic pressure before the central aortic systolic wave (see Fig. 46.3D). To correct late deflation, the timing interval should be decreased gradually until the balloon deflates before the onset of systole.

Contraindications to IABP Counterpulsation

When IABP therapy is being considered, the risks and benefits of this modality must be individually assessed for each patient. Absolute contraindications include significant aortic regurgitation, suspected aortic dissection, clinically significant abdominal or thoracic aortic aneurysm, distal aortic occlusion or severe stenosis, and chronic end-stage heart disease with no anticipation of recovery. Relative contraindications include severe peripheral arterial disease (PAD), contraindications to anticoagulation, uncontrolled sepsis, and sustained tachyarrhythmias (heart rate >160 beats/min).[17]

IABP counterpulsation in a patient with aortic regurgitation can potentially lead to further cardiac decompensation. During balloon inflation, an increased regurgitant volume may be generated across the incompetent aortic valve, resulting in increased LV volumes. Data from animal studies have demonstrated increased regurgitant flow but also enhanced LV stroke volumes, despite the increased diastolic volumes.[18] Therefore, although patients with severe aortic valvular insufficiency should be excluded from IABP therapy, patients with lesser degrees of aortic regurgitation can be considered but with close monitoring during the initial phase of therapy. Patients with vascular abnormalities—such as distal aortic stenosis, aortic dissection, or aortic aneurysm—have a significantly increased risk of catastrophic vascular complications. The presence of PAD or iliofemoral grafts increases the risk of complications associated with balloon insertion and removal. Sustained tachyarrhythmias with heart rates exceeding 160 beats/

BOX 46.1   Insertion and Removal of the Intraaortic Balloon Pump

The following steps are involved during insertion of an intraaortic balloon pump:

1. An initial physical examination focusing on peripheral vasculature should be conducted, including palpation and demarcation of the femoral, popliteal, dorsalis pedis, and posterior tibial pulses and auscultation for femoral and abdominal bruits.
2. The side with the better arterial pulsations should be selected for insertion.
3. The inguinal region should be inspected for landmarks and the femoral artery should be identified.
4. The inguinal region should be prepared and draped in a sterile fashion.
5. Following administration of a local anesthetic agent, a skin incision is made 2 to 3 cm below the inguinal ligament.
6. Using a modified Seldinger technique, the femoral artery is cannulated with a needle and a J-tipped guidewire is then advanced through the needle after brisk flow of arterial blood is confirmed.
7. The guidewire should be advanced to the level of the descending aorta under fluoroscopic guidance.
8. A dilator is inserted and removed until an arterial sheath can be safely placed.
9. The intraaortic balloon is passed over the guidewire to a position just distal to the origin of the left subclavian artery.
10. The guidewire is subsequently removed and the catheter lumen is aspirated to remove any residual air or thrombus.
11. The intraaortic balloon is connected to the drive system console and counterpulsation can subsequently begin.
12. The hemodynamic tracing should be inspected for proper timing.
13. A chest radiograph should be obtained to document correct positioning.
14. The intraaortic balloon catheter and femoral sheath should be secured with sutures.

BOX 46.2   Insertion and Removal of the Intraaortic Balloon Pump

1. Anticoagulation should be stopped; confirm that the activated clotting time is less than 180 seconds or the activated partial thromboplastin time is less than 40 seconds.
2. Conscious patients should receive a low-dose narcotic and/or analgesic agent.
3. The securing sutures are cut.
4. The drive system console is turned off.
5. The intraaortic balloon is completely deflated by aspiration with a 20-mL syringe attached to the balloon inflation port.
6. The sheath and intraaortic balloon catheter are pulled as one unit.
7. Blood is allowed to flow from the arterial access site for a few seconds to remove any thrombi.
8. Manual pressure is applied above the puncture site for 30 minutes or longer if hemostasis is not obtained. A mechanical compression device can also be used to help apply pressure to promote hemostasis.
9. Distal arterial pulsations are palpated.
10. The patient should remain recumbent for a minimum of 6 hours to prevent any subsequent hemorrhage or vascular complications at the arterial access site.

---

min hamper the ability of the balloon to accurately track the mechanical events of the cardiac cycle and provide hemodynamic support.

Insertion, Removal, and Complications

The most commonly used approach for percutaneous placement is cannulation of the femoral artery. Once it is concluded that the patient no longer requires circulatory support, the removal of the IABP is also a straightforward process. Mahaffey and colleagues have devised a simple stepwise approach to device insertion and removal (Boxes 46.1 and 46.2).[16]

A thorough vascular examination should precede the insertion of the IABP. This examination should include palpation of all lower extremity pulses along with auscultation of the lower half of the abdomen and of the femoral arteries. The femoral artery with the best palpable pulsation should be selected to minimize vascular complications.[1] The balloon (7.5 Fr) is inserted percutaneously over a guidewire using a sheath (8–9 Fr) although a sheathless approach has been used. The downsizing of IABP catheters (from early single-lumen balloons) has significantly reduced the incidence of ischemic peripheral vascular complications, especially in patients with small or atherosclerotic arteries. In patients with severe peripheral atherosclerosis or distal abdominal aortic aneurysms, the IABP can be inserted through the axillary, subclavian, or brachial arteries.

Following insertion of the device (see Box 46.1), fluoroscopy can be used to confirm that the device has been placed in the descending thoracic aorta distal to the origin of the left subclavian artery. IABP counterpulsation can begin thereafter, with augmentation using one inflation for each cardiac cycle (1:1 ratio) being ideal for optimal hemodynamic support. However, adjusting counterpulsation timing is best done with the console set at 1:2 pumping so that the pressure tracings with and without counterpulsation can be compared. Daily chest radiographs and continuous monitoring of hemodynamic parameters ensures stable placement and appropriate timing of the device.

No conclusive data support the requirement for intravenous anticoagulation in the setting of IABP use. A trial of 153 patients found no difference in vascular complications in patients undergoing IABP therapy with and without continuous heparin anticoagulation.[19] Industry guidelines do not require continuous anticoagulation therapy, especially when the device is set at a 1:1 assist ratio. Currently, it is reasonable to use intravenous heparin with the goal of maintaining an activated partial thromboplastin time (aPTT) of 60 to 75 seconds in a patient without contraindications to anticoagulation and when IABP counterpulsation therapy is planned for longer than 24 hours or at lower assist ratios.[1]

Although no conclusive data exist in the literature, some authorities recommend gradual weaning of the balloon pump before it is finally removed. In patients in whom the IABP was placed to treat hemodynamic instability, a gradual reduction in the assist ratio from 1:1 to 1:2 and then to 1:3 over several hours is frequently employed. If hemodynamic stability is demonstrated at lesser assist ratios, the device can be safely removed (see Box 46.2).

Complications arising from IABP counterpulsation therapy can be categorized into vascular and nonvascular events. In two studies of nearly 40,000 patients, death due directly to an IABP or IABP placement was less than 0.05%. Major complications—including major limb ischemia, severe bleeding, balloon leak, and death related directly to device insertion or to device failure—occurred in 2.6% of patients (see Table 46.3).[20]

The true incidence of complications associated with placement of an IABP is difficult to ascertain. Studies citing complication rates differ in the indications for IABP counterpulsation therapy, insertion technique (surgical or percutaneous), duration of use, and the specific definitions of complications.[20–24] The most commonly reported complications are bleeding and arterial trauma.[1]

Vascular complications remain the most common serious complications to occur in patients with an IABP. The most common types of vascular complications include limb ischemia, vascular laceration necessitating surgical repair, and major hemorrhage.[25–27] Arterial obstruction and limb ischemia can occur when the IABP is inadvertently placed into either the superficial or profunda femoral artery instead of the common femoral artery, as these arteries are usually too small to accommodate the IABP without compromising blood flow to the leg. Prompt removal of the device and contralateral insertion (with avoidance of an excessively low needle puncture) is recommended. Arterial dissection can occur with improper advancement of a guidewire with subsequent insertion of the IABP into a false lumen. Less common vascular complications include spinal cord or visceral organ ischemia, cholesterol embolization, cerebrovascular accidents, sepsis, and balloon rupture. Balloon rupture is uncommon and usually owing to the balloon inflating against calcified plaque in the aorta. Because the helium gas used to inflate the balloon is insoluble in blood, helium embolization can cause prolonged ischemia or stroke. These patients can be treated with hyperbaric oxygen to maintain tissue viability. Numerous analyses have been attempted to identify clinical variables that predispose to a higher rate of complications. The presence of PAD (including a history of limb claudication, femoral arterial bruit, or absent pulsations) has been the most consistent clinical predictor of complications.[28–30] These complications are more common in women (related to the size of the vessels) and patients with a history of diabetes mellitus and hypertension who are more likely to have PAD.

Clinical Efficacy and Indications

IABP counterpulsation therapy improves the hemodynamic and metabolic derangements that result from circulatory collapse.[17] Historically, this modality has been mainly used in the setting of acute ischemic syndromes associated with hemodynamic decompensation. In the decades since its introduction, more data have accumulated supporting the use of IABP therapy in a variety of clinical scenarios.

Unstable Angina. Data are sparse regarding the use of IABP counterpulsation in patients with unstable angina. These data date back several decades; the use of IABP counterpulsation in this patient population is based on observational studies and clinical experience. Gold and colleagues studied 11 patients experiencing persistent angina despite aggressive medical therapy

after an acute myocardial infarction (MI); nine of these patients exhibited symptomatic improvement following placement of an IABP.[31] Fuchs and colleagues examined seven patients who had proximal left anterior descending coronary arterial stenoses exceeding 90% along with unstable angina.[32] The use of IABP counterpulsation before intervention improved symptoms and enhanced coronary blood flow as assessed with a Doppler flow wire.[32] The 2014 American College of Cardiology/American Heart Association (ACC/AHA) practice guidelines for the management of patients with non-ST elevation acute coronary syndromes state that it may be reasonable to consider IABP counterpulsation therapy in patients with unstable angina that is continuing or recurring despite intensive medical therapy.[33]

Acute Myocardial Infarction. Routine use of IABP counterpulsation in patients with acute MI, including ST segment elevation myocardial infarction (STEMI), is not indicated, though there may be patients who benefit from its use. Primary PCI in patients with STEMI has reduced mortality but it is widely recognized that some patients develop reperfusion injury or fail to achieve reperfusion at the cellular level owing to microvascular embolization that limits myocardial salvage even if the occluded coronary artery has been successfully recanalized by PCI.[34–36]

In the pre-PCI era, Ohman and colleagues conducted a trial of 182 patients with acute MI who were randomized to prophylactic IABP counterpulsation therapy for 48 hours or standard medical therapy.[37] Patients randomized to IABP experienced less recurrent ischemia and a significantly lower rate of reocclusion of the infarct-related artery (8% vs. 21%; $P < .03$) at follow-up angiography 5 days later. The composite endpoint of death, stroke, reinfarction, need for emergent revascularization, or recurrent ischemia was significantly lower in patients randomized to IABP (24% vs. 13%; $P < .04$).

The Primary Angioplasty in Myocardial Infarction-II (PAMI-2) trial randomized 437 patients who underwent primary percutaneous transluminal coronary angioplasty (PTCA) to 36 to 48 hours of IABP following primary or standard care. Prophylactic IABP counterpulsation after primary PTCA showed no benefit over standard therapy in decreasing all-cause mortality or adverse cardiovascular events, including infarct-related artery reocclusion.[38]

A registry of 1490 acute MI patients treated by primary PTCA was analyzed by Brodie and colleagues.[39] In this observational study, 105 patients had an IABP placed before PCI, whereas 108 patients had an IABP inserted following the completion of PCI. Although the patients with an IABP placed before PCI exhibited a higher prevalence of cardiogenic shock and multivessel coronary artery disease, they experienced substantially higher procedural success rates and fewer adverse events (e.g., dysrhythmias and shock) during the PCI. In this observational study, the initiation of IABP counterpulsation therapy before PCI was an independent predictor of lower periprocedural complications.

The Counterpulsation to Reduce Infarct Size Pre-PCI Acute Myocardial Infarction (CRISP AMI) trial randomized 337 patients with anterior STEMI without cardiogenic shock to routine IABP counterpulsation before primary PCI or primary PCI alone to determine if its use reduced infarct size, assessed by cardiac magnetic resonance imaging.[40] Patients randomized to IABP showed no reduction in infarct size at 3 to 5 days compared to those who received no IABP. All-cause mortality at 6 months (2% vs. 5%; P = .12) and the composite endpoint of death, new or worsening heart failure and shock favored IABP use (5% vs. 12%; P = .03). More important, a substudy of patients with large MIs (defined by summed ST deviation ≥15 mm) and persistent ischemia (ST resolution after PCI >50%) showed a significant mortality reduction with IABP placement (0 vs. 5 deaths; P = .046).[41]

A meta-analysis of IABP use in acute MI patients in the absence of cardiogenic shock showed no mortality benefit.[42] Thus the routine use of IABP counterpulsation in patients with acute MI, including STEMI, is not indicated.

Cardiogenic Shock. Cardiogenic shock occurs in 5% to 10% of patients with acute MI and is associated with high mortality rates even in patients who undergo early revascularization with PCI or coronary artery bypass graft surgery (CABG).[43] The 30-day mortality rate for the 0.8% of Global Utilization of Streptokinase and Tissue Plasminogen Activator for Occluded Coronary Arteries (GUSTO I) trial patients with cardiogenic shock treated with thrombolytic therapy was 58%.[44] In the interventional era, the mortality rate of cardiogenic shock remains as high as 50%.[45,46]

Early use of IABP in acute MI complicated by cardiogenic shock was based predominantly on small retrospective studies performed in the thrombolytic era that suggested improved outcomes.[47,48] A meta-analysis of IABP use in patients with acute MI suggested a reduction in in-hospital mortality in patients with cardiogenic shock.[49] The Intraaortic Balloon Pump in Cardiogenic Shock (IABP-SHOCK) trial randomized 45 patients with cardiogenic shock complicating acute MI treated with PCI to IABP or standard therapy. Mechanical support was associated only with modest reductions of the Acute Physiology and Chronic Health Evaluation (APACHE) II score as a marker of severity of disease, improvement in cardiac index, reduction of inflammatory state, or reduction of brain natriuretic peptide (BNP) biomarker status compared with medical therapy alone.[50]

The Intraaortic Balloon Pump in Cardiogenic Shock II (IABP-SHOCK II) trial was one of the first large, multicenter randomized trials to compare IABP counterpulsation and standard medical therapy alone in patients with acute MI complicated by cardiogenic shock and treated with early revascularization.[51] A total of 600 patients were randomized to IABP or no standard care. All patients underwent early revascularization (by PCI or CABG) and received optimal medical therapy. At 30 days, 119 patients in the IABP group and 123 patients in the control group died (39.7% vs. 41.3%; P = .69). There were no significant differences in secondary endpoints, including length of stay in the intensive care unit, duration of catecholamine therapy, and renal function. There was no difference in 1-year mortality (52% vs. 51%; P = .91) between the groups.[52] Despite being the largest randomized trial performed in patients with cardiogenic shock, there were many limitations. The trial anticipated a 30-day mortality of 56% in the control group, but it was significantly lower than anticipated and thus was underpowered to address the primary

hypothesis. Despite evidence suggesting that IABP placement before primary PCI results in reduced mortality compared with insertion after primary PCI, 86% of patients in the IABP-SHOCK II trial had the IABP inserted following PCI.[53] Also, there was a large crossover from the control group to the IABP group and use of LV assist devices in the control group.

Based on clinical trials, routine use of IABP in acute MI patients with cardiogenic shock is not indicated. The 2013 ACC/AHA practice guidelines for the management of STEMI currently give the use of IABP counterpulsation a class IIa indication for acute MI patients in cardiogenic shock who do not stabilize with pharmacologic therapy.

High-Risk Percutaneous Coronary Intervention. An IABP is often used for mechanical circulatory support in patients undergoing high-risk PCI. These patients often have a higher risk of procedural morbidity and mortality due to severe LV dysfunction, multivessel coronary artery disease, or uncontrolled angina. In this subset of patients, placement of an IABP before the intervention may be beneficial from the enhancement of coronary perfusion pressure and stabilization of hemodynamic parameters. The IABP may also allow them to better tolerate procedural complications, such as coronary artery dissection or the development of no-reflow.

Small retrospective studies of elective IABP counterpulsation support before high-risk PCI have found favorable outcomes with no major adverse events within 72 hours of the intervention.[54,55] Briguori and colleagues described 133 consecutive patients who underwent high-risk PCI.[56] The patients were divided into those with an elective preprocedural placement of an IABP and those with provisional (i.e., standby) usage of an IABP. Among patients with a low LV ejection fraction (LVEF), the rate of major adverse cardiac events (acute MI, shock, stroke, emergent CABG, or death) was 17% in the standby IABP group versus 0% in the group that received a preprocedural IABP (P = .001).

The Balloon Pump-Assisted Coronary Intervention Study (BCIS-1) was one of the first randomized controlled trials to examine the use of elective IABP in high-risk PCI patients.[57] A total of 301 patients scheduled to undergo high-risk single-vessel or multivessel PCI were randomized to PCI with or without an IABP. There was no significant difference in major adverse cardiovascular events, including MI or stroke, in the elective IABP group compared with the control group (15.2% vs. 16.0%; P = .85). There were no differences in major secondary endpoints between the two groups except for major procedural complications, including ventricular tachycardia/fibrillation, cardiopulmonary arrest, and prolonged hypotension, all of which were less common in the IABP group. All-cause mortality at 51 months was significantly lower in the elective IABP group compared to the control group (42 patients vs. 58 patients; P = .039).[58] The 2011 ACC/AHA/Society of Cardiovascular Angiography and Intervention (SCAI) practice guidelines currently assign the use of elective IABP as an adjunct to PCI in a carefully selected subgroup of patients with a class IIb indication.

Cardiac Surgery. The literature regarding the use of IABP counterpulsation in cardiac surgery is conflicting. Low cardiac output syndrome occurs in approximately 5% to 10% of patients following open-heart surgery and is associated with increased mortality. Some studies suggest that placement of prophylactic IABP before CABG in patients with certain high-risk features—including critical coronary arterial anatomy (including left main disease), severe LV dysfunction, or unstable angina—may be beneficial.[59–61]

In a small prospective study, Christenson and colleagues randomized 60 consecutive high-risk patients who were to undergo CABG to either conservative management or to preoperative IABP commencing 2, 12, or 24 hours before surgery.[60] Most of these patients had LV dysfunction, unstable angina, and/or left main stenosis. Although no mortality benefit was observed, patients who were randomized to preoperative IABP of any duration had significantly higher cardiac output, a shorter duration of mechanical ventilation, and a reduced length of hospitalization.

In 141 hemodynamically stable, high-risk patients who underwent CABG, 38 (27%) of whom underwent prophylactic IABP before surgery, after risk-adjustment, prophylactic IABP was associated with a reduction in postoperative low cardiac output syndrome (adjusted odds ratio [OR] 0.07; $P = .006$) and postoperative MI (adjusted OR, 0.04; $P = .04$) as well as a shorter length of hospital stay (10.4 days vs. 12.2 days; $P < .0001$).[62] A meta-analysis performed by Field and colleagues of five randomized clinical trials of prophylactic IABP before CABG or standard care concluded that preoperative IABP counterpulsation may be beneficial in specific high-risk patient groups.[63] Future clinical trials are needed to assess its true effectiveness.

Other. IABP counterpulsation can also be used in a variety of other clinical situations. In patients with severe end-stage cardiomyopathy with refractory heart failure who are awaiting cardiac transplantation or LV assist device (LVAD) placement, IABP counterpulsation can be used as a bridging modality. There have been several case series and studies that have reported successful bridging with IABP counterpulsation in patients with cardiogenic shock who require cardiac transplantation or an LVAD.[64,65] IABP counterpulsation in this setting decreases aortic systolic pressure and impedance; thus, it can promote systolic unloading of the LV, leading to an increased stroke volume. The use of IABP counterpulsation has also been shown to improve right ventricular (RV) failure, as unloading the LV can increase performance of the RV and improve outcomes in carefully selected patients.[66]

Incessant ventricular tachyarrhythmias are occasionally treated with IABP counterpulsation to unload the LV or to improve perfusion to ischemic myocardium. Several anecdotal reports have described cessation of ventricular tachycardia and fibrillation following the initiation of IABP counterpulsation therapy.[17]

Conclusion

IABP counterpulsation is one of the most frequently used mechanical circulatory support devices in the CICU setting owing to its ease of use, safety, and availability. Based on the dual physiologic concept of diastolic augmentation and systolic afterload reduction, it can be an important strategy to improve the function of an ischemic and failing heart in selected patients.

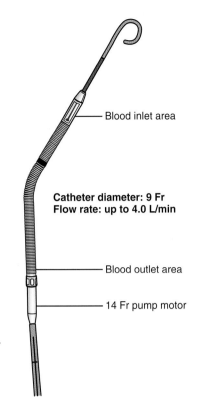

Catheter diameter: 9 Fr
Flow rate: up to 4.0 L/min

Blood inlet area

Blood outlet area

14 Fr pump motor

Fig. 46.4 Components of the Impella CP device. (Courtesy of Abiomed, Inc.)

Although routine use is clearly not indicated in a variety of clinical settings based on randomized clinical trials, IABP counterpulsation may still be beneficial in selected subgroups of patients. Future randomized clinical trials are required to help understand which patients may benefit from IABP counterpulsation.

LEFT VENTRICLE TO AORTA SUPPORT DEVICES

Catheter-mounted, temporary ventricular pumps were described as early as 1975 and were first used in humans in the 1990s.[67] The concept evolved into the Impella (Abiomed, Inc.) LV to aorta support devices. The Impella is a miniature axial flow pump attached to a catheter (Fig. 46.4). Most commonly, devices are inserted percutaneously or surgically to position the pump across the aortic valve with the inflow in the LV and the outflow into the aorta (Fig. 46.5). The first device was approved by the US Food and Drug Administration (FDA) in 2008 for partial circulatory support during cardiac procedures not requiring cardiopulmonary bypass.[68] Subsequent FDA-approved indications have expanded as alterations have been made to the device, resulting in a family of devices that are used for cardiac support during high-risk percutaneous procedures, LV support in cardiogenic shock and, most recently, for circulatory assistance in the setting of RV failure.

Current device models include the Impella 2.5, Impella CP, Impella 5.0, and Impella RP (Video 46.1). All devices except the Impella RP provide LV circulatory support. The recently approved Impella RP provides RV circulatory support.[69–71] This section will focus on the LV Impella devices.

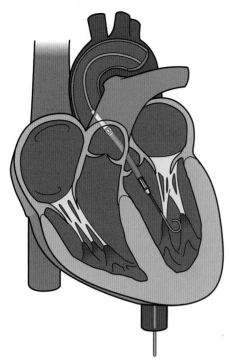

Fig. 46.5 Illustration of an Impella device positioned across the aortic valve. (From Thiele H, Smalling RW, Schuler GC. Percutaneous left ventricular assist devices in acute myocardial infarction complicated by cardiogenic shock. *Eur Heart J.* 2007;28:2057–2063.)

Physiology and Monitoring

The Impella devices contain a miniature pump with a rotating impeller based on the principle of the Archimedes Screw.[72] The pump is mounted on a flexible catheter and inserted percutaneously or surgically through the arterial system and advanced to position the distal end of the pump in the LV apex with the proximal end in the ascending aorta. Blood is aspirated out of the LV and ejected into the aorta. The devices are most commonly inserted through the femoral artery but alternative access sites, such as the subclavian and axillary arteries, have been described (see Table 46.1).[73–75] Unlike the IABP, the Impella systems do not require timing or a trigger based on the ECG or arterial pressure. By unloading the LV, the pump reduces myocardial oxygen consumption, improves mean arterial pressure, and reduces PCWP (see Table 46.2).[76] Adequate RV function is necessary to maintain LV preload in cases of biventricular failure or unstable ventricular arrhythmias.[77]

The 12 Fr Impella 2.5, 14 Fr Impella CP, and 21 Fr Impella 5.0 provide a maximum flow rate of 2.5, 3 to 4, and 5 L/min, respectively.[68,78] The Impella 2.5 and Impella CP are inserted percutaneously (see Video 46.1). The Impella 5.0 requires surgical cutdown due to the large cannula size. The pumps consist of inflow and outflow areas, a motor, and a pump pressure monitor. Heparin and glucose are continuously infused into the motor housing to prevent backflow of blood. The pump is attached to a flexible 9 Fr catheter that houses the motor power leads and lumens for pressure measurement and heparin infusions. The catheter's most proximal end contains a hub for attachment of a console cable and side arms for attachment of pressure measurement tubing.

Impella devices are used with an automatic controller that can be run off a built-in rechargeable battery or from an electric power cord. The controller features a display that users interact with to determine pump positioning and the quality of pumping function. The degree of support for patients can be set by changing the revolutions per minute (RPM) in set levels designated as P1 to P9 on the controller.[79] The flow of heparin and saline into the motor is regulated by the "purge cassette" and can be monitored on the controller display.[80]

In addition to the use of radiography and echocardiography, appropriate Impella placement may be verified by the pressure waveform generated from the pressure sensor at the distal end of the pump. The placement signal is used to verify whether the Impella pump is correctly positioned in the LV or the aorta by evaluating the pressure differential on a pulsatile waveform. Appropriate placement can also be assessed on the display using the motor current waveform, which is a measure of the energy intake of the Impella pump. The energy used by the Impella varies with motor speed and the pressure difference between the inflow and outflow areas of the pump. When the Impella is positioned correctly with the inlet area in the LV and the output in the ascending aorta, the motor current should be pulsatile because of the pressure difference between the two areas. When the intake and output are on the same side of the aortic valve, the motor current will be dampened owing to the lack of a pressure differential.[80]

The Impella 2.5 and CP devices have been approved for up to 4 days and the Impella 5.0 is approved for up to 6 days. Although much longer use has been reported, the requirement for hemodynamic support beyond these timelines should result in consideration of a more durable form of cardiac support.[81] Once weaning is desired, the pump power can be slowly reduced over time to reduce the level of cardiac support. If the patient's hemodynamics remain stable, the device can be pulled proximally into the aorta. If continued hemodynamic stability is observed, the device can then be removed entirely.

Contraindications and Complications

Appropriate evaluation prior to insertion of an Impella device is crucial in determining potential contraindications or patient-specific risk factors for complications. Careful physical examination and imaging technology are necessary to assess the patient's vasculature and select an appropriate arterial access site. Traditional angiography, magnetic resonance angiography, or computed tomography angiography are often used for this purpose. Echocardiography is important to assess for LV thrombus, mechanical aortic valves, severe aortic stenosis, or aortic regurgitation. Insertion of a pulmonary artery catheter should also be considered to provide continuous hemodynamic monitoring of cardiac output, central venous pressures, and mixed venous oxygen saturation (SvO_2).

Contraindications to the use of Impella devices include mechanical aortic valves or LV thrombus. The device should not be placed in patients with severe PAD owing to the risk of embolism during insertion. A minimum vessel diameter of 7 mm is required for the Impella 5.0 owing to the cannula size. Preexisting septal defects are considered a relative contraindication as, theoretically, the device could worsen right-to-left shunting. Severe aortic stenosis and regurgitation are considered relative indications, although Impella use in critical aortic stenosis has been reported.[82] Anticoagulation is necessary to prevent thrombus formation on the pump housing and catheter. Therefore the device should not be inserted in patients who cannot tolerate anticoagulation. Obesity, scar tissue related to previous vascular procedures, and tortuous vasculature may increase the risk of complications.

The most common complications include limb ischemia, vascular injury, and bleeding (see Table 46.3).[83] Vascular complications include hematoma or pseudoaneurysm formation, arteriovenous fistula creation, and retroperitoneal hemorrhage. Hemolysis is reported in up to 10% of patients with Impella devices due to the sheer stress of the rotating impeller on red blood cells. Repositioning the device may reduce the degree of hemolysis. Patients with persistent hemolysis associated with acute kidney injury should have the device removed.[84]

Clinical Efficacy and Indications

Numerous case reports, case series, and observational studies of various Impella devices have been reported for a wide range of indications. Many demonstrate improved hemodynamics and outcomes. Unfortunately, few randomized controlled trials are available. Most available data address Impella use in patients with cardiogenic shock and prophylactic use in patients undergoing PCI.

Cardiogenic Shock. Several observational studies have evaluated the role of Impella in the setting of cardiogenic shock. Three studies evaluated the use of the Impella 2.5 in the setting of acute MI complicated by cardiogenic shock and demonstrated improved hemodynamics.[83,85,86] Two studies evaluated the Impella 5.0 in refractory cardiogenic shock and also demonstrated improved hemodynamics.[87,88] Most studies report mortality but, as these are observational studies, none report mortality compared to a control population.

One retrospective cohort study compared the Impella 2.5 to IABP counterpulsation in patients with cardiogenic shock following cardiac arrest or in patients with risk factors for cardiogenic shock after angiography. Mortality between the two groups was similar, with equal rates of vascular complications. There was a trend toward a higher rate of bleeding with the Impella device.[89]

Only one randomized controlled trial evaluated the utility of an Impella device in cardiogenic shock. In the Efficacy Study of LV Assist Device to Treat Patients With Cardiogenic Shock (ISAR-SHOCK), 26 patients with cardiogenic shock after acute MI were randomized to Impella 2.5 versus IABP. The primary outcome was the change of cardiac index from baseline to 30 minutes after implantation. Mortality at 30 days was considered a secondary outcome. The trial demonstrated that the cardiac index was significantly higher in the Impella arm versus the IABP arm (Impella ΔCI: 0.49 ± 0.46 L/min/m^2; IABP ΔCI: 0.11 ± 0.31 L/min/m^2; $P = .02$). There was no difference in mortality between the two groups.[90]

High-Risk PCI. Numerous observational studies in over 1000 patients have demonstrated the safety and efficacy of the Impella device in the setting of high-risk PCI.[91–96] Some of the studies were funded by the manufacturers of Impella devices, introducing a risk of bias. Studies are limited to the Impella 2.5; data regarding the use of the Impella CP or Impella 5.0 in this setting are lacking. A retrospective cohort study comparing outcomes of patients undergoing high-risk PCI with periprocedural support from Impella 2.5 ($n = 13$) versus IABP ($n = 62$) showed similar efficacy and a similar incidence of bleeding complications between the two groups.[97]

Only one randomized controlled trial exists that evaluates the utility of Impella in patients undergoing high-risk PCI. In the Prospective, Multicenter, Randomized Controlled Trial of Impella 2.5 Versus Intra-aortic Balloon Pump in Patients Undergoing High-Risk Percutaneous Coronary Intervention (PROTECT II), patients with symptomatic, complex three-vessel coronary artery disease or unprotected left main coronary artery disease and severely depressed LV function undergoing nonemergent high-risk PCI were randomized to Impella 2.5 (n = 225) versus IABP (n = 223). The primary endpoint was adverse events during and after the PCI procedure at discharge or at 30-day follow-up, whichever was longer. Components of the primary outcome included all-cause mortality, MI, stroke or transient ischemic attack, repeat revascularization procedure, need for cardiac or vascular operation, acute renal insufficiency, severe intraprocedural hypotension requiring therapy, CPR, ventricular tachycardia requiring cardioversion, aortic insufficiency, or angiographic failure of PCI. The study demonstrated that, relative to IABP, Impella provided superior cardiac power output. However, there was no difference in the primary outcome between the two groups at 30 days. At 90 days, there was a statistically nonsignificant trend toward improved outcomes with Impella. PROTECT II was terminated early owing to futility.[98]

Conclusion

Impella use is increasing in frequency and is an intriguing option for patients with cardiogenic shock or as prophylaxis during high-risk PCI. Compared to the IABP, Impella devices consistently demonstrate improved hemodynamics (see Table 46.2). However, Impella use has not translated into improved outcomes and is associated with a high rate of complications. Current evidence is largely limited to the Impella 2.5 and Impella 5.0 devices; whether the percutaneous design and enhanced cardiac support provided by the Impella CP will translate into improved outcomes is unknown. Further randomized clinical trials evaluating the use of Impella are necessary.

LEFT ATRIUM TO AORTA SUPPORT DEVICES

The TandemHeart percutaneous ventricular assist device (Cardiac Assist, Inc.) is the only commercially available left atrium to aorta assist device. This percutaneous device pumps blood extracorporeally from the left atrial via a transseptally inserted cannula to the ileofemoral arterial system, thereby bypassing the LV (see Table 46.1). This device entered the market in 2005 and is FDA approved to provide extracorporeal circulatory support for up to 6 hours.[68,79]

Physiology and Monitoring

The TandemHeart has four components: a transseptal cannula, a centrifugal pump, a femoral arterial cannula, and a control console. A 21 Fr cannula is inserted into the right femoral vein, advanced to the right atrium, and finally into the left atrium via a transseptal puncture (Fig. 46.6A).[72,99] The fenestrated cannula aspirates blood from the left atrium via a large end hole and 14 smaller side holes (Fig. 46.6B).[79] Blood flows to a 15 to 19 Fr arterial perfusion cannula inserted into the common femoral artery. The flow of blood is propelled by an extracorporeal centrifugal pump containing a spinning impeller. The pump has both a motor chamber and a blood chamber that are separated by a polymer membrane. An electromagnetic motor rotates the impeller between 3000 and 7500 RPM. The size of the arterial cannula determines the maximum flow rate. The 15 Fr arterial cannula can support flow rate up to 3.5 L/min, whereas the 19 Fr arterial cannula can achieve flow up to 5 L/min.[79] Heparinized saline flows continuously into the lower chamber of the pump, providing lubrication, cooling, and preventing thrombus formation. An external controller controls the pump and contains a 60-minute backup battery in case of power failure.

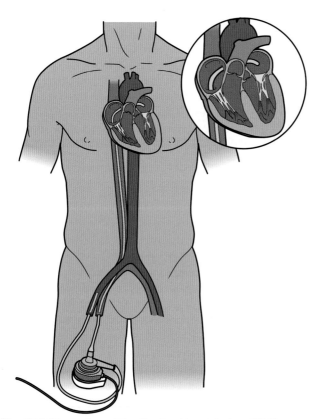

Fig. 46.6 Illustration of the TandemHeart device. (A) Placement of the TandemHeart demonstrating an arterial catheter and a transseptal venous catheter connected to the centrifugal pump. (B) Close-up of the transseptally inserted fenestrated venous catheter. (From Thiele H, Smalling RW, Schuler GC. Percutaneous left ventricular assist devices in acute myocardial infarction complicated by cardiogenic shock. *Eur Heart J.* 2007;28:2057–2063.)

An FDA-approved oxygenator can be added to the circuit to provide oxygenation in addition to circulatory support.

The hemodynamic effects of the TandemHeart are superior to the IABP (see Table 46.2). Similar to the Impella device and unlike the IABP, the TandemHeart does not require a trigger or timing based on the cardiac cycle. As the TandemHeart device works in parallel with the LV, any intrinsic CO from the LV is additive to the support of the device. By virtue of unloading the LV, the TandemHeart results in increased CO, increased mean atrial pressure, decreased PCWP, and decreased central venous pressure.[100] Both the LV and RV have decreased filling pressures, resulting in reduced ventricular workload and oxygen demand, and an increase in cardiac power index.[101,102] However, due to an increase in afterload and a decrease in preload, ventricular contraction may decrease. As a result, the LV often provides only a minimal contribution to CO, resulting in relatively nonpulsatile arterial pressure tracing.

The amount of cardiac support provided by TandemHeart can be increased or decreased by changing the RPM on the centrifugal pump. Although only FDA approved for 6 hours, in practice, devices are often used for a week or more.[103] Weaning is facilitated by monitoring hemodynamic stability while slowly reducing the RPM on the centrifugal pump. If hemodynamic stability is confirmed, the pump can be turned off and removed.

Contraindications and Complications

Initial evaluation is similar to other percutaneous support devices. Imaging modalities and physical examination are necessary to evaluate the patient's vasculature. Expertise with transseptal puncture technique is required and is often a barrier to the use of TandemHeart given that proficiency with this technique is not universal among interventional cardiologists. Upon insertion of the transseptal cannula, appropriate placement must be verified using a combination of echocardiography, pressure transduction, and blood gas analysis from the distal port.

Contraindications for the use of TandemHeart include severe PAD, which may preclude the placement of the arterial cannula, contraindications to anticoagulation, and left atrial thrombus. Adequate RV function or support is necessary to maintain appropriate left atrial pressure for optimal device function.[77] There is limited experience using the TandemHeart in the setting of ventricular septal defects or severe aortic regurgitation.[104,105] Obesity, scar tissue related to previous vascular access procedures, and tortuous vasculature may increase the risk of complications.

Complications include arterial dissection, groin hematoma, limb ischemia, hemolysis, and thromboembolism (see Table 46.3).[106] Complications unique to the transseptal puncture technique, such as cardiac tamponade, may be increased in anticoagulated patients. Additionally, dislodgement of the left atrial cannula back into the right atrium will cause severe right-to-left shunting and associated hypoxemia. The cannula may also migrate into a pulmonary vein, which may cause device malfunction.

Clinical Efficacy and Indications

There are currently no randomized control trials evaluating the TandemHeart device. The TandemHeart to Reduce Infarct Size

(TRIS) trial that intended to randomize patients with STEMI to either TandemHeart or usual care prior to PCI was withdrawn before enrollment. Current evidence is limited to case series or observational comparisons with other types of percutaneously inserted cardiac support devices.

Cardiogenic Shock. In one of the earliest trials describing its use, 18 patients with acute MI complicated by cardiogenic shock were treated with TandemHeart. Patients were noted to have improved hemodynamics, including increased cardiac index and mean arterial pressure with decreased PCWP and central venous pressure. Mortality was 44%.[99] In a much larger study of 117 patients with cardiogenic shock despite vasopressors and/or IABP, support with TandemHeart was used for a mean of 5.7 days. TandemHeart resulted in improved cardiac index and decreased lactate. Mortality at 30 days was 40.2%. Complications were numerous and included bleeding around the arterial cannula in 29% of patients, vascular complications in 5% of patients, and limb ischemia in 3.4% of patients.[106]

Two studies compared outcomes between TandemHeart and the IABP in patients with cardiogenic shock. A 2005 study of patients with cardiogenic shock after MI compared outcomes between patients treated with an IABP ($n = 20$) and TandemHeart ($n = 21$). Compared with the IABP, TandemHeart demonstrated improved hemodynamics, including improved cardiac power index. However, mortality at 30 days was similar between the two groups (45% vs. 43%). Furthermore, TandemHeart was associated with more complications, including severe bleeding (IABP, $n = 8$ vs. TandemHeart, $n = 19$) and limb ischemia (IABP, $n = 0$ vs. TandemHeart, $n = 7$).[101] A 2006 randomized control trial of 42 patients across 12 centers compared patients with cardiogenic shock randomized to IABP ($n = 14$) or TandemHeart ($n = 19$). Patients treated with TandemHeart had improved hemodynamics compared to those treated with an IABP. However, survival was not different between the two groups at 30 days; TandemHeart use was associated with more adverse events than the IABP.[102]

High-Risk Percutaneous Coronary Intervention. A 2016 single-center observational study of 74 patients treated with TandemHeart for elective, urgent, emergent, and emergent salvage cases suggested that TandemHeart is a viable option for high-risk PCI. Up to 13% of patients had ischemic limb injury associated with the arterial catheter and 31% of patients had major bleeding.[107]

Two trials compare TandemHeart with Impella devices for high-risk PCI. In a 2013 single-center observational study, 68 patients underwent high-risk PCI with TandemHeart support ($n = 32$) or Impella 2.5 ($n = 36$). There was no difference in mortality or major vascular complications at 30 days between the two groups.[108] A 2016 meta-analysis reviewed 8 studies of 205 combined patients that utilized TandemHeart and 12 studies of 1345 patients that utilized Impella 2.5 for support during high-risk PCI. Mortality at 30 days was 8% for the TandemHeart group and 3.5% for the Impella group. Bleeding rates were 3.6% with the TandemHeart group and 7.1% with the Impella group.[109]

Conclusion

The TandemHeart device provides impressive hemodynamic support and remains an option for patients with cardiogenic shock or high-risk PCI. However, its insertion requires experience with transseptal puncture, which is a major barrier, and the device is used infrequently at many centers as a result. Additionally, rates of complications, including bleeding and limb ischemia, warrant careful considering of the use of this device if other options are available, particularly in emergency settings.

EXTRACORPOREAL MEMBRANE OXYGENATION

Cardiopulmonary bypass was used as early as the 1950s during cardiac surgery.[110,111] Modifications of cardiopulmonary bypass led to the development of extracorporeal membrane oxygenation (ECMO) that was first used successfully in humans for treatment of respiratory failure in 1972.[112] Early devices were fraught with complications, limiting their utility. ECMO technology has advanced dramatically in the past several decades. Subsequent improvements have reduced complications and allowed for expanded use of these devices for a variety of indications.[79] The two basic configurations of ECMO are venovenous (VV) ECMO and venoarterial (VA) ECMO. VV ECMO can be used to oxygenate blood and remove carbon dioxide in patients with respiratory failure. VA ECMO provides both hemodynamic and respiratory support. This section will focus on VA ECMO used to provide temporary cardiac support.

PHYSIOLOGIC PRINCIPLES OF ECMO

The ECMO circuit consists of a blood pump, membrane oxygenator, conduit tubing, and a heat exchanger (see Table 46.1).[113] In VA ECMO, a drainage catheter is inserted into the venous circulation, which drains blood through an oxygenator and returns it to the arterial system using a pump (Fig. 46.7). VA ECMO is a supportive therapy with the goals of improving oxygen delivery and carbon dioxide removal while resting the heart and lungs to facilitate recovery. When recovery is not possible, VA ECMO may be used as a bridge to definitive therapy with a permanent ventricular assist device or cardiac transplant. Minimizing complications in this setting is crucial.[114]

The VA ECMO circuit can be set up in different ways. Although other vessels may be used, most commonly the femoral artery and vein are cannulated. Regardless of the setup, the drainage cannula is positioned in the vena cava or right atrium and the return cannula is positioned to deliver blood retrograde to the aorta. Blood flowing anterograde from the LV will meet resistance from blood flowing retrograde from the ECMO circuit. This nonphysiologic configuration has differing effects on the RV and LV. For the RV, drainage of blood from the venous system results in decreased preload, reduced RV output, and reduced pulmonary blood flow. For the LV, blood delivered retrograde into the arterial system results in increased mean arterial pressure and, consequently, increased afterload (see Table 46.2).[114] The

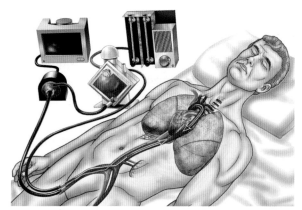

Fig. 46.7 Illustration of a patient with femoral venoarterial (VA) extracorporeal membrane oxygenation (ECMO). Deoxygenated venous blood from the femoral vein is infused through the ECMO circuit, and oxygenated blood is returned retrograde to the femoral artery *(red arrow)*. Poorly oxygenated blood flowing anterograde from the left ventricle *(purple arrow)* will meet with resistance from the blood returned retrograde from the ECMO circuit. (From Abrams D, Combes A, Brodie D. Extracorporeal membrane oxygenation in cardiopulmonary disease in adults. *J Am Coll Cardiol.* 2014;63(25):2769–2778.)

resultant increase in afterload often leads to reductions in LV stroke volume. The degree of reduction depends on residual LV function and the integrity of the aortic and mitral valves. Increasing hemodynamic support by increasing flow through the VA ECMO circuit further increases afterload. Concomitant increases in LV end-diastolic pressure may cause LV dilation, decreased coronary blood flow, and reduced subendocardial perfusion. The amount of support can be titrated by changing the flow rate on the blood pump. Rates as high as 10 L/min can be accommodated with large-bore cannula.[79] However, ECMO generally provides between 3 and 6 L/min of support.[115] High flow also increases left atrial pressure and may precipitate pulmonary edema. Increases in afterload may be further exacerbated by the vasoconstrictive effects of vasopressor medications. Systemic hypertension is common; weaning of vasopressors and the addition of antihypertensive medications may be necessary to prevent complications.

Oxygenation and removal of carbon dioxide is facilitated by an oxygenator that uses a semipermeable membrane as an artificial lung to separate gas from blood. In VA ECMO, deoxygenated blood is pulled from the venous system and oxygenated blood is returned to the arterial system. Oxygenation is determined by the amount of blood flow through the ECMO circuit, gas flow through the oxygenator, and the contribution from the patient's own pulmonary function. The rate of carbon dioxide removal is regulated by the flow of blood through the ECMO circuit and gas flow through the oxygenator, known as the sweep gas flow rate. Adjustments may be made guided by arterial blood gas analysis.[116,117]

Monitoring of ECMO

Once cannulation has occurred and patients are connected to the ECMO circuit, flow through the circuit is slowly uptitrated to achieve appropriate respiratory and hemodynamic targets. Frequent adjustments may be necessary to achieve adequate arterial oxyhemoglobin saturation, mean arterial pressure, and venous oxygen saturation. Light sedation may be necessary to maintain patient comfort.

Anticoagulation is essential during ECMO and is typically achieved with intravenous unfractionated heparin. Anticoagulation with the direct thrombin inhibitors argatroban and bivalirudin has been reported and is used in the case of heparin-induced thrombocytopenia.[118] Anticoagulation is usually titrated based on activated clotting time (ACT). There is no universally agreed upon anticoagulation protocol; target ACT varies between institutions.[117] Alternatives to the ACT have been proposed and include titration based on aPTT, anti-factor Xa levels, and thromboelastography.[119]

The artificial material in the ECMO circuit results in activation of the coagulation, fibrinolytic, and complement pathways, which can result in both bleeding and thrombotic complications. As a result, platelets are continuously consumed.[120] Current practice is to maintain platelet levels over 50,000/mL; some centers maintain levels over 100,000/mL. Hemolysis, hemorrhage, and decreased bone marrow production due to critical illness may result in a decreased hemoglobin concentration. Hemoglobin levels have historically been kept at or near normal levels because adequate oxygen delivery depends not only on adequate blood flow but also on hemoglobin concentration. Accordingly, hemoglobin is often maintained between 12 and 14 mg/dL.[121] Recent reports using newly improved ECMO circuits suggest that ECMO may be safely performed with a hemoglobin below 8 mg/dL. However, these data have not yet been incorporated into widespread practice.[115,122] Owing to the requirement for aggressive transfusion parameters, patients frequently receive dozens of blood product tranfusions.[123]

For ventilated patients, ventilator settings should be minimized once adequate oxygenation and carbon dioxide removal is facilitated with the ECMO circuit. This allows avoidance of ventilator-associated lung injury and oxygen toxicity. An ultraprotective lung strategy with target plateau pressures less than 20 cm H_2O and FiO_2 less than 0.5 is often used to improve outcomes.[124] Reduction in ventilator settings decreases intrathoracic pressure, which may facilitate venous return and CO. Early tracheostomy may be beneficial.

While near maximum flow rates are typically used for patients on VV ECMO, the flow rates used with patients on VA ECMO must be high enough to facilitate hemodynamic and oxygenation goals but low enough to allow for sufficient preload to maintain intrinsic CO. LV output must be monitored frequently owing to the risk of LV distention. Aggressive diuresis may be necessary. Ultrafiltration can also be added to the ECMO circuit to facilitate volume removal. LV output is assessed using the pulsatility on an arterial line waveform in combination with echocardiography. If LV output cannot be maintained, ionotropes, an IABP, or Impella devices may be inserted to improve forward flow.[125–127] If cardiac output remains low despite these interventions, LV decompression may be necessary. Techniques include transatrial balloon septostomy or surgical insertion of an LV or right upper pulmonary vein drainage catheter.[120]

Contraindications to the Use of ECMO

General criteria for initiating VA ECMO include severe cardiac failure that is potentially reversible and unresponsive to standard therapy. ECMO should not be considered for patients who have preexisting conditions that are incompatible with recovery, such as severe neurologic injury and advanced malignancy.

Insertion, Removal, and Complications

Insertion. ECMO requires a multidisciplinary team, including a surgeon, anesthesiologist, perfusionist, cardiologist, pulmonologist, and intensivist. Once it has been decided that ECMO will be initiated, the patient is anticoagulated and the cannula are inserted. If ECMO is initiated after cardiac surgery, the cannulas may be connected centrally to the same outlets used for cardiopulmonary bypass. If peripheral cannulation is desired, the cannulas are inserted percutaneously using the Seldinger technique. The size of the cannulas chosen is determined based on the expected amount of circulatory support required for the patient based on residual LV function. Often, the largest possible cannula is used. For adults, inflow cannulas are available between 18 and 21 Fr and outflow cannulas are between 15 and 22 Fr.[115] In VA ECMO, a venous cannula is typically placed in the femoral vein and advanced to the venocaval junction. The arterial cannula is typically placed in the common femoral artery. Given the large cannula sizes used in ECMO, ischemia to the limb ipsilateral to the arterial cannula is common. To compensate, a distal arterial cannula may be inserted into the posterior tibial artery to provide flow to perfuse the lower limb.[128]

If the femoral vessels are unsuitable for cannulation owing to severe PAD or prior arterial bypass, other arteries may be utilized. The right carotid, right subclavian, and axillary arteries have been used.[129] Cannulation of the right carotid carries the risk of cerebral infarction and should be used cautiously. The subclavian artery has the advantage of potentially allowing patient ambulation.

Removal. The duration of ECMO support is typically 5 to 10 days, with a maximum implant time of 3 to 4 weeks.[115] Once patients have recovered sufficiently to warrant consideration of weaning, weaning may be initiated as a series of trials. To facilitate a trial, the support provided by the ECMO circuit is decreased incrementally while monitoring hemodynamic and respiratory stability. There is no universally accepted protocol for weaning. As VA ECMO also provides for gas exchange, the pump flow cannot be decreased without ensuring that respiratory support is adequate. Also, completely turning off the pump increases the risk of thrombus formation in the ECMO circuit, but short periods of reducing flow to 1 L/min can be performed. Since assessment of LV function may be compromised when the VA ECMO circuit is providing full support, cardiac monitoring during the weaning process with transthoracic or transesophageal echocardiography has been proposed.[130] If weaning is successful and the decision is made to discontinue ECMO entirely, the cannulas are removed and the venous and arterial access sites are compressed manually for at least 30 minutes to achieve hemostasis.

Complications. Advances in ECMO technology aimed at reducing complications include low-resistance gas exchange membranes, highly durable centrifugal pumps, heparin-coated tubing, and improved cannulas.[120] Major complications include bleeding, thromboembolism, neurologic injury, and cannulation-related injury (see Table 46.3). Bleeding is the most common complication, occurring in 27% to 50% of patients, and may be severe enough to require intervention.[119,123,131] Both anticoagulation and platelet dysfunction contribute to bleeding. Cannulation-related injury includes hemorrhage, dissection, distal ischemia, and compartment syndrome. Major bleeding from surgical wounds should prompt exploration. Modern heparin-coated ECMO circuits allow for anticoagulation to be held. Discontinuation of anticoagulation for up to 20 days has been reported without complication.[132]

Thrombus may develop within the ECMO circuit or the patient's vasculature with an incidence of 8% to 16%.[119,123] Routine inspection of all tubing and connectors for signs of clot formation is necessary. Changes in the pressure gradient across the oxygenator may reflect thrombus formation. Large clots necessitate immediate circuit exchange. If anticoagulation must be held or if there is heightened concern for thrombus development, circuits primed with anticoagulant may be kept at the bedside for urgent exchange. Intracardiac thrombosis may also develop if there is stasis owing to poor LV function.

Neurologic injury occurs in up to 50% of patients with cardiac failure or those for whom ECMO is administered during cardiopulmonary resuscitation.[133] Coma, encephalopathy, anoxic brain injury, stroke, brain death, and myoclonus have all been observed. Cerebral hypoxia is of particular concern for patients with femoral artery cannulation. Oxygenated blood returning from the circuit to the aorta will preferentially perfuse the abdominal viscera instead of the brain, heart, and upper extremities. To detect this complication, arterial oxyhemoglobin saturation should be monitored in the upper extremities.

Other complications include pulmonary edema and pulmonary hemorrhage due to elevated LV end-diastolic and left atrial pressures that may warrant LV or left atrial venting. Infection related to cannulation may result in prolonging the duration of ECMO or increased length of hospital stays.[134] Heparin-induced thrombocytopenia may also develop and should prompt changing the anticoagulant to a direct thrombin inhibitor. Hemolysis, thrombocytopenia, acquired von Willebrand's syndrome, disseminated intravascular coagulation, acute kidney injury, and air emboli have all been reported.[120,135]

Clinical Efficacy and Indications

ECMO has numerous indications in adult populations. While randomized controlled trials exist demonstrating the utility of ECMO in respiratory failure and acute respiratory distress syndrome, there are no such trials for cardiac support or following cardiopulmonary arrest.[136] In practice, ECMO is often used as a salvage therapy or a temporary bridge to definitive therapy with ventricular assist devices or cardiac transplant.[115] As a result, conducting a controlled trial for cardiac failure is challenging owing to the lack of an ethically defensible control group. The available evidence supporting the use of VA ECMO in cardiogenic shock and cardiopulmonary arrest is presented next.

Cardiogenic Shock. Studies have demonstrated the utility of ECMO for patients with cardiogenic shock from acute MI, acute decompensated heart failure, myocarditis, stress-induced cardiomyopathy, and postcardiotomy shock.[115,137–139] Miniaturized VA ECMO devices have even been shown to facilitate interhospital transfer for patients with cardiogenic shock.[140]

A 2008 observational study of 81 patients with refractory cardiogenic shock due to medical causes ($n = 55$), postcardiotomy ($n = 16$), or following cardiac transplantation ($n = 10$) and treated with VA ECMO found a 42% patient survival to discharge. More than half of patients had at least one major ECMO-related complication. Long-term quality of life for ECMO survivors was worse than age-matched controls but better than patients on dialysis, after acute respiratory distress syndrome, or with advanced heart failure.[141]

A 2010 study compared 30-day outcomes between STEMI patients with cardiogenic shock refractory to IABP and ionotropic agents in two different time periods. One group ($n = 115$) received usual care, but ECMO therapy was available to the other group ($n = 219$) and used in 46 patients. Mortality at 30 days was lower in the group with ECMO availability (41% vs. 30%; $P < .04$).[142]

A 2017 meta-analysis of 24 studies and 1926 patients placed on ECMO for refractory cardiogenic shock after cardiac surgery showed a survival to discharge rate of 31%.[143] A 2016 study of 4227 Taiwanese patients placed on ECMO for cardiogenic, postcardiotomy, traumatic or septic shock showed an average 30-day mortality of 60% and 1-year mortality of 77%. In patients with cardiogenic shock, mortality at 30 days was 66% and 77% at 1 year.[144]

The Extracorporeal Life Support Organization has maintained an international registry of patients receiving ECMO support since 1989. Their most recent report of 78,397 adults and children showed that survival for patients on ECMO was higher when it was used for respiratory support than for cardiac failure or following CPR. However, cardiogenic shock was the most common indication for VA ECMO. Among 9025 adult patients with cardiogenic shock, survival to discharge was 41%.[145]

Cardiac Arrest. VA ECMO support has emerged as an intriguing option for patients with refractory cardiopulmonary arrest and has been the subject of numerous trials.[146–153] In one of the largest trials comparing patients with refractory cardiac arrest treated with conventional CPR ($n = 321$) to those treated with VA ECMO support ($n = 85$), the primary outcome was survival to discharge with minimal neurologic impairment. Among propensity-matched patients, patients treated with ECMO showed improved 6-month survival (OR, 0.48; $P = .003$).[154]

In a meta-analysis of 20 studies, including 833 patients for whom VA ECMO was initiated for refractory out-of-hospital cardiac arrest, overall survival to discharge was 22%. Thirteen percent of patients were considered to have a good neurologic outcome.[155] In a 2016 meta-analysis of nine studies of ECMO used in patients with refractory cardiopulmonary arrest, ECMO was associated with an absolute increase of 30 days survival of 13% compared with patients in whom ECMO was not used (95% CI, 6% to 20%; $P < .001$; number needed to treat [NNT], 7.7) and a higher rate of favorable neurologic outcome at 30 days (absolute risk difference, 14%; 95% CI, 7% to 20%; $P < .0001$; NNT, 7.1).[121]

According to the Extracorporeal Life Support Organization registry, VA ECMO has been used for 2885 adult patients with refractory cardiopulmonary arrest since 1989. Overall survival to discharge was 29%.[145]

Conclusions

VA ECMO is becoming a commonly used method of temporary cardiac support. It has advantages of providing full cardiac and respiratory support as well as utility in biventricular failure. Considerable expertise is required for proper maintenance of ECMO circuits and complications are common and may be severe. However, ECMO remains an exciting and unique option for otherwise viable patients as salvage therapy for cardiogenic shock and cardiopulmonary arrest refractory to conventional resuscitation methods.

█ S U M M A R Y

Numerous devices are available to provide temporary mechanical cardiac support for a variety of indications. Selection of a device should be based on individual patient characteristics in addition to a thorough understanding of device concepts, advantages, and disadvantages. While each device can augment CO and provide hemodynamic support, evidence suggests that improving hemodynamics alone may not translate into improved survival. Therefore, while mechanical support devices may be life saving for an individual patient, continued improvement in technology and high-quality evidence are necessary before routine use should be considered.

The full reference list for this chapter is available at ExpertConsult.com.

47

Ventricular Assist Device Therapy in Advanced Heart Failure

Ulrich Jorde, Daniel B. Sims, Dmitri Belov

OUTLINE

The development of reliable left ventricular assist devices (LVADs) has revolutionized heart failure (HF) management. In the cardiac intensive care unit (CICU) context, LVADs are encountered in three situations: first, selection of the appropriate heart failure patients for mechanical circulatory support (MCS) and preoperative evaluation; second, management of these patients perioperatively; and third, treatment of complications and prevention of adverse events. This chapter addresses these issues.

TECHNOLOGY OF LEFT VENTRICULAR ASSIST DEVICES

The initial LVADs were volume displacement pumps known as pulsatile-flow devices. They filled during device diastole and ejected during device systole. As a result, all patients would have a pulse and a measurable systolic and diastolic blood pressure. The HeartMate XVE (Thoratec Corp.) and the Novacor pump, both implantable durable LVADs, could support the systemic circulation. However, both pumps had multiple moving parts, including bearings, valves, and pusher plates that were subject to failure. In addition, the pulsatile pumps were bulky, noisy, and their implantation required a major operation.

A paradigm shift in the field of assisted circulation occurred with the introduction of durable, implantable continuous-flow devices. The rationale for continuous flow was the observation that the initial pulsatile flow in the aorta is progressively dampened, transforming into continuous nonpulsatile flow at the level of the capillary (Fig. 47.1). Continuous-flow LVADs have only a single moving part and propel blood forward in a steady, continuous fashion with an axial or centrifugal rotor or an impeller. With this simplified design, the risk of mechanical failure has been greatly reduced. Continuous-flow pumps are also smaller, lighter, and operate in virtual silence.

Currently, the HeartMate II (St. Jude Medical) and the HeartWare HVAD (HeartWare) are the only US Food and Drug Administration (FDA)–approved continuous-flow LVADs. The HeartMate II is capable of providing up to 10 L/min of support and is surgically inserted into a preperitoneal pocket (Fig. 47.2A). Blood is pulled out of the LV into the LV inflow cannula, accelerated by a rotor, and then ejected into the outflow graft, which is anastomosed to the ascending aorta. A percutaneous driveline exits in the upper abdomen and connects the device with a portable controller and two batteries for mobile operation, or to a power base unit (PBU) and a wall outlet when a patient is stationary for several hours (e.g., while sleeping). The device provides a constant flow of blood with one back-up speed used in case of a sudden drop of preload. The actual flow is calculated based on the power consumed and is not measured. The typical operating speed range is 8600 to 9600 rpm. Despite antithrombotic coating with titanium microbeads, anticoagulation with a target international normalized ratio (INR) of 2.0 to 3.0 and aspirin are recommended.

In distinction to the axial-flow HeartMate II, the HVAD is a miniaturized centrifugal pump (Fig. 47.2B). The smaller size of this device allows implantation into the pericardial space and, often, a shorter operation. The housing contains an impeller suspended by magnets and the device is capable of providing 10 L/min of flow. The usual operating speed range is 2400 to 2800 rpm.[1]

The Jarvik 2000 (Jarvik Heart, Inc.) is an axial-flow LVAD positioned directly inside the LV and can be implanted through a lateral thoracotomy (Fig. 47.2C). The outflow graft can be anastomosed with the descending aorta, eliminating the need for a more traumatic median sternotomy. Also, the unique feature of this LVAD is that the driveline can be tunneled to a retroauricular area to decrease the risk of infections and allow for submersion in water (i.e., swimming). The Jarvik 2000 is currently in clinical trials in the United States.

It is important to appreciate that the presence of a continuous-flow device does not necessarily eliminate the presence of a palpable pulse on physical examination. This has an important consequence when measuring a patient's blood pressure. In the

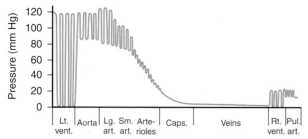

Fig. 47.1 Pressure and pulsatility distribution in the systemic circulation. *Caps.,* Capillaries; *Lg. art.,* large artery; *Lt. vent.,* left ventricle; *Pulm. art.,* pulmonary artery; *Rt. vent.,* right ventricle; *Sm. art.,* small artery.

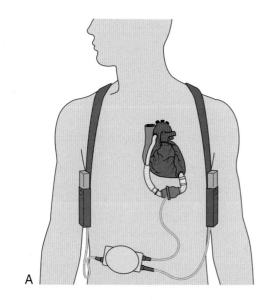

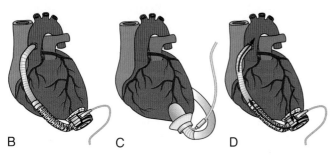

Fig. 47.2 Axial (A, C) and centrifugal (B, D) left ventricular assist devices. (A) St. Jude HeartMate II. (B) HeartWare HVAD. (C) Jarvik 2000. (D) St. Jude HeartMate 3.

absence of a palpable pulse, mean arterial pressure (MAP) is measured via Doppler. The blood pressure cuff is inflated above where the Doppler tones are heard, and then the return of sounds auscultated via Doppler is taken as the MAP. MAP measured by Doppler overestimates pressure in the presence of palpable pulse and should not be reported.[2] Instead, auscultation of the Korotkoff sounds should be performed.

Specific adverse effects related to continuous-flow physiology have emerged. First, nonpulsatile blood flow can lead to gastrointestinal bleeding often owing to arteriovenous malformations

(AVMs). Second, the aortic valve may no longer open, leading to aortic valve fusion and the development of aortic insufficiency. Third, nonpulsatile flow could potentially predispose to pump thrombosis.[3]

The HeartMate 3 (St. Jude Medical) is a new intrapericardial centrifugal pump with a fully magnetically levitated impeller designed to overcome the shortcomings of older-generation pumps (Fig. 47.2D). A distinctive feature of the HeartMate 3 is an artificial pulsatility created by changing the impeller rotation speed at fixed time intervals (30 times/min). Clinical outcomes with the HeartMate 3 were recently compared with the HeartMate II pump in the MOMENTUM 3 trial.[4] There were no significant differences between the groups in the rates of death or disabling stroke; however, a striking difference was observed in suspected or confirmed pump thrombosis (0% vs. 10.1% at 6 months; $P <$ .001) and rate of reoperation for pump malfunction (0.7% vs. 7.7%, $P =$ .002) favoring the newer HeartMate 3.[4] It is anticipated that because of these important advantages, the HeartMate 3 has the potential to advance the field of MCS.

BRIDGE TO TRANSPLANTATION

Bridge to transplantation (BTT) refers to the implantation of a durable LVAD in a patient with end-stage HF with the intent of improving the hemodynamics and clinical course until a donor heart is available. Because the demand for donor hearts is always higher than the supply, it is impossible to allocate a donor heart for everyone who needs it in a timely fashion. LVADs are a readily available cardiac replacement while the patient is waiting for a donor heart. As the donor shortage has worsened, the proportion of transplant recipients who required bridging with a durable LVAD increased from 26% in 2004 to more than 50% in 2014.[5] In their 2001 landmark study, Frazier et al. summarized the multicenter experience with the pulsatile HeartMate VE LVAD on 280 heart transplant candidates.[6] The outcomes were compared with a retrospectively matched cohort of 48 patients. This trial resulted in an impressive improvement of survival from 29% to 67% in the LVAD group at 180 days (Fig. 47.3A). These data indicated that continued management of these mostly desperately ill patients who were failing medical therapy (including an intraaortic balloon pump) without any LVAD support carries a grave prognosis. The outcome is even more impressive considering that the mean waiting time for a donor heart in the control group was only 4 days.

Miller et al. evaluated outcomes of 133 patients listed for heart transplantation and bridged with the continuous-flow HeartMate II device.[7] The primary outcome was defined as "recovered, transplanted or alive on device by 180 days." Of the patients, 75% achieved the primary outcome, 19% died while on support, and 4% became ineligible for a transplantation due to irreversible medical complications during LVAD support. Investigators of the ADVANCE trial[1] selected the same primary outcome and time point as in Miller et al. and compared the HeartWare HVAD with a cohort from The Interagency Registry for Mechanically Assisted Circulatory Support (INTERMACS) database who received almost exclusively axial-flow devices. An impressive 90.7% of patients receiving an HVAD achieved the

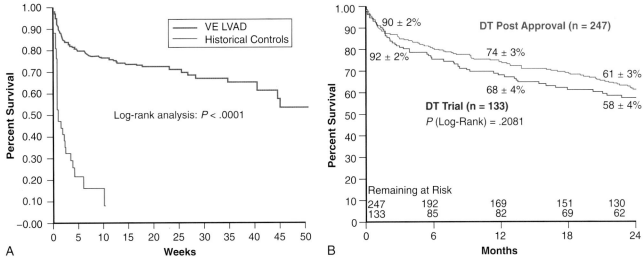

Fig. 47.3 Improvement of probability of survival in advanced heart failure patients treated with a left ventricular assist device. (A) Frazier et al.[6] compared outcomes of patients listed for transplantation and bridged with a HeartMate XVE versus historical cohorts. (B) Jorde et al.[14] demonstrated a trend toward better survival in the HeartMate II DT post-FDA approval group compared to the initial clinical trial,[13] with an absolute difference of 74% vs. 68% at 1 year and 61% vs. 58% at 2 years. *DT,* Destination therapy; *LVAS,* left ventricular assist system. (A, From Frazier OH, et al. Multicenter clinical evaluation of the HeartMate vented electric left ventricular assist system in patients awaiting heart transplantation. *J Thorac Cardiovasc Surg.* 2001;122[6]:1186–1195. B, From Jorde UP, et al. Results of the destination therapy post-Food and Drug Administration approval study with a continuous flow left ventricular assist device: a prospective study using the INTERMACS registry [Interagency Registry for Mechanically Assisted Circulatory Support]. *J Am Coll Cardiol.* 2014;63[17]:1751–1757.)

primary endpoint. The patients in the control arm, who almost exclusively received a HeartMate II pump, had a similar success rate of 90.1%.

These early studies in a BTT population have proven that prompt implantation of an LVAD is the only meaningful chance for survival available to the sickest patients. These studies also demonstrated a substantial reversibility of organ damage: that is, implantation of LVADs was followed by a significant improvement in biochemical markers of kidney and liver injury.[8] Poor durability remained a significant impediment in early LVAD trials.[6,9] More recent LVAD models have improved durability and a reduced rate of adverse events. The more favorable adverse effects profile was achieved, at least in part, by miniaturization of LVADs with less dissection and surgical trauma required during the implantation.

DESTINATION THERAPY

Destination therapy (DT) refers to the implantation of an LVAD in a patient with end-stage HF who is not a candidate for heart transplant or who is unwilling to undergo a transplant. The most recent INTERMACS report[10] indicated that the number of LVADs implanted for BTT (45.7%) was almost equal to the number of LVADs implanted for DT. However, some experts suggest that LVADs still remain underutilized and expect increased use of LVADs for DT.[11] It is important to highlight that heart transplantation currently remains the "gold standard" for management of end-stage HF. As a result, patients who receive a DT

LVAD are older and have more comorbidities—important facts to consider when interpreting DT trial results.

In the landmark Randomized Evaluation of Mechanical Assistance for the Treatment of Congestive Heart Failure (REMATCH) trial, patients with end-stage HF were randomly assigned to undergo HeartMate I implantation or continued medical management.[12] The principal finding of REMATCH was a significantly better survival of patients randomized to the HeartMate I LVAD compared to medically managed patients. Estimates of survival at 1 and 2 years were 52% and 23% in the device group and 25% and 8% in the medical therapy group, respectively. Analysis of mortality revealed that sepsis and LVAD failure were the leading causes of death.[12] Of note, all device failure events occurred during the second year as durability was lacking owing to the multiple moving parts in the pulsatile-flow pump.

In 2009, Slaughter et al.[13] published outcomes of the first randomized trial comparing two LVADs for DT. The patients were assigned to receive either a pulsatile-flow HeartMate I or a continuous-flow HeartMate II. The primary study endpoint, "survival free from disabling stroke and reoperation to repair or replace the LVAD at two years" was achieved by 46% and 11% of patients in HeartMate II and HeartMate I groups, respectively. The survival in the HeartMate II group was better than the survival in the HeartMate I group (58% vs. 24%). Also, the HeartMate II LVAD had a lower hazard of adverse events compared to the HeartMate I LVAD: pump replacement hazard ratio (HR), 0.12 (95% confidence interval [CI], 0.06 to 0.26); right heart failure HR, 0.30 (95% CI, 0.16 to 0.57), sepsis HR, 0.35 (95% CI,

0.21 to 0.57), and cardiac arrhythmias HR, 0.53 (95% CI, 0.33 to 0.83).[13]

More recently, Jorde et al.[14] presented an analysis of a postapproval "real-world" HeartMate II experience in 247 patients. Several interesting observations were made. First, survival at 12 and 24 months improved to 74% and 61%, respectively; the best survival was achieved in less sick patients (Fig. 47.3B). Second, the risk of some serious adverse events over a 2-year period was even less than in the HeartMate II trial: bleeding 12% (vs. 30%), right heart failure 18% (vs. 23%), sepsis 19% (vs. 41%) and any arrhythmia 37% (vs. 56% in Slaughter et al).[13,14] Impressively, with increased familiarity with and management of the pump, the survival rate and adverse-event profile improved outside of the clinical trial setting.

In addition to the quantity of life, emphasis should be placed on the quality of life (QOL) post-LVAD and its equal importance to longevity. In this context, two important issues are worth considering. First, QOL does improve post-LVAD implantation. For example, in the HeartMate II DT trial, 80% of patients on a continuous-flow LVAD were in New York Heart Association (NYHA) class I or II 24 months postimplantation with a remarkable improvement of their scores on The Minnesota Living with Heart Failure and The Kansas City Cardiomyopathy Questionnaires.[13] Finally, the improvement in exercise capacity, which is one of the components in QOL assessment, is often less than predicted due to limitations related to a suboptimal increase in cardiac output (CO) during exercise and associated comorbidities.[15,16]

BRIDGE TO RECOVERY

A different approach for management of HF consists of a combination of MCS with aggressive medical therapy to promote LV recovery. If LV function normalizes, the device could potentially be explanted. Initial enthusiasm with "bridge to recovery" (BTR) dropped off after the realization that only a small proportion (1% to 2%) of patients in large datasets could be weaned from MCS.[17] However, when patients were initially classified as BTR at time of implant, they did have higher rates of recovery compared to BTT or DT (11.2% vs. 1.2%). Younger age, nonischemic etiology, and short duration of HF were variables associated with a greater likelihood of recovery. Recently, enthusiasm for a BTR strategy has been renewed by promising short-term results from the Remission from Stage D Heart Failure (RESTAGE-HF) study.[18]

PATIENT SELECTION AND EVALUATION

If a patient is found to be a suitable candidate for an LVAD, particular attention should be paid to the patient's candidacy for heart transplantation and the timing of implantation. Because most of the indications for MCS evolved from historical indications for heart transplantation, a common clinical dilemma is whether to proceed with an LVAD implant or wait for cardiac transplantation. If the patient is a candidate for heart transplantation and if a prolonged wait time for a donor heart is anticipated, it might be reasonable to proceed with a durable LVAD if no contraindications

exist to ensure hemodynamic and clinical stability while on the waiting list. In addition, patients on LVADs are less likely to become deconditioned and lose muscle mass than those on chronic inotropic therapy.[19] Conversely, in a stabilized patient with a favorable blood type and projected short wait time for a donor heart, the best decision might be to wait for a primary transplant without a bridging LVAD. It is important to note that in the United Network of Organ Sharing (UNOS) registry, overall posttransplant survival of patients requiring bridging with an LVAD is the same as patients who are transplanted without having received an LVAD first, with the only exception being patients with increased transplant urgency status due to device infection who possibly have decreased survival.[20]

For the purpose of prognostication and rapid assessment of patients with severe symptomatic HF, a staging system was developed known as the INTERMACS profiles.[21] INTERMACS profile I ("crash and burn") includes the sickest patients with cardiogenic shock who are hemodynamically unstable despite inotropes and/or counterpulsation. Death is imminent without escalation of support for these patients. A temporary MCS might be a good option in some of these patients while assessing potential reversibility of LV and end-organ damage. If the LV damage is beyond recoverable (or is unlikely to recover without durable LVAD) and the need for assisted circulation persists, evaluation for a durable LVAD should be performed.

Currently, the majority (66%) of patients evaluated for LVAD are INTERMACS profile II ("sliding") and INTERMACS profile III ("stable on inotropes"); the benefit of LVAD is well proven in these patients.[10] Long-term therapy with inotropes is associated with poor survival and it is reasonable to proceed with an evaluation for durable LVAD as soon as the patient is declared inotrope dependent. An important observation can be made comparing 1-year survival of INTERMACS II and III patients with the sickest INTERMACS I profile. When an LVAD is implanted for INTERMACS profile I patients, survival to hospital discharge is only 70.4%. When an LVAD is implanted for INTERMACS profile II or III patients, survival to discharge is improved at 93.5% and 95.8%, respectively.[22] As a result of this observation, fewer LVADs are now implanted for INTERMACS profile I (only 14.3% in 2014). An appropriate strategy for these very sick patients has evolved to include temporary MCS to allow for reversal of end-organ damage and achievement of clinical stability prior to proceeding with a durable LVAD.

One-fifth of LVADs are implanted into patients not receiving inotropes or temporary MCS (INTERMACS profiles IV to VII).[10] The recent Risk Assessment and Comparative Effectiveness of Left Ventricular Assist Device and Medical Management in Ambulatory Heart Failure Patients (ROADMAP) trial addressed suitability of these patients for MCS.[23] In this observational trial, outcomes of 200 advanced HF noninotrope-dependent patients with NYHA classes IIIB/IV symptoms were evaluated. In a nonrandomized fashion, patients with 6-minute walk distance less than 300 m and at least one hospitalization for HF in the last year could elect to have an LVAD implanted or elect to continue with optimal medical therapy. While LVAD patients experienced more frequent adverse outcomes (mainly bleeding), NYHA class and health-related QOL were still better with an LVAD[23] compared to medically managed

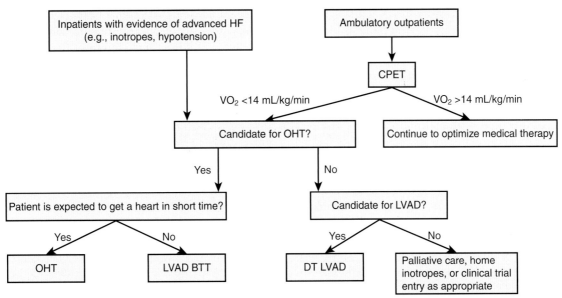

Fig. 47.4 A simplified algorithm of patient selection for left ventricular assist device (LVAD) support. Currently, only patients who are not candidates for OHT should be considered for DT LVAD. *BTT,* Bridge to transplantation; *CPET,* cardiopulmonary exercise test; *DT,* destination therapy; *LVAD,* left ventricular assist device; *OHT,* orthotopic heart transplantation.

patients. Findings from the ROADMAP study could yield two interpretations: (1) noninotrope-dependent patients who are severely functionally limited may be appropriate for LVAD therapy and (2) the identical 1-year mortality rates argue for a watchful waiting approach. A proposed algorithm for LVAD evaluation is presented in Fig. 47.4.

Absolute contraindications for LVAD implantation are any irreversible end-stage organ damage that can limit survival after LVAD surgery. This includes cirrhosis, permanent hemodialysis, dementia or severe stroke, severe COPD, and malignancy with life expectancy less than 2 years.[24] In the CICU setting, important additions to this list include terminal multiorgan failure, ongoing bacteremia, incessant ventricular tachycardia, significant coagulation abnormalities, high bleeding risk, contraindications to anticoagulation with warfarin, severe RV dysfunction, and pregnancy. All contemporary LVADs require the patient's or caregiver's ability to comprehend and act upon controller alarms, change batteries, and clean the driveline exit site. Patients and caregivers who are unable to take care of the device due to a medical or psychosocial issue cannot be considered for a durable LVAD. The decision about advanced cardiac therapies in patients with a history of cancer should be made in conjunction with an oncologist. Typically, even patients with recently treated cancer may be candidates for DT if their estimated life expectancy is more than 2 years.[24]

A number of conditions represent obstacles to achieving optimal life expectancy and QOL. These important relative contraindications for LVAD include severe peripheral vascular disease, poorly controlled diabetes with complications, severe malnutrition, frailty, and lack of a supportive caregiver. Chronic kidney dysfunction traditionally belongs to this group; however, the numeric value for a low glomerular filtration rate (GFR) or an elevated creatinine to set as a contraindication is a subject of ongoing debate. Previous studies demonstrated that renal

function usually improves post-LVAD in the majority of patients; however, it starts to decline again after 1 year of support.[25] We consider presence of a primary renal disease with creatinine 2.5 mg/dL or greater despite optimization of hemodynamics with inotropes and/or temporary MCS as a relative contraindication for DT LVAD. However, in exceptional cases, an option of LVAD bridging followed by a combined heart-kidney transplantation may be considered.

Although transplantation remains the gold standard for management of end-stage HF patients, some important advantages of LVADs over heart transplantation exist. Individuals with pulmonary vascular resistance greater than 5 Wood units can be supported by an LVAD in the absence of concomitant RV failure.[11,26] Several publications indicate that so-called "fixed" pulmonary hypertension (pulmonary hypertension that does not improve despite medical therapy) does, in fact, improve post-LVAD implantation.[26,27] Second, obesity with a body mass index greater than 35 kg/m² is only a relative contraindication for MCS. In addition, improvement of hemodynamics and clinical state with an LVAD may allow a morbidly obese patient to undergo bariatric surgery and thus lose weight to become a heart transplant candidate. Third, on rare occasions in patients who would be unable to tolerate immunosuppressive therapy owing to drug interactions or are otherwise unwilling to undergo a transplant for personal reasons, DT LVAD offers better survival than optimal medical therapy.[14]

Because of the complexity of the decisions in advanced HF patients, LVAD centers have specialized protocols and teams dedicated to selecting appropriate candidates for MCS. A standard minimal workup should include evaluation by a heart failure specialist, social worker, psychiatrist, palliative care team, and a cardiothoracic surgeon. We found that palliative care consultants are particularly helpful coordinating decision making; such consultation is now mandated by the Center for Medicare Services for DT implants. Because all contemporary FDA-approved LVADs require antithrombotic therapy, a history of bleeding diathesis must be investigated and documented. Individuals with a prior unprovoked deep venous thrombosis or pulmonary embolism should have a full hypercoagulable workup performed and be evaluated by a hematologist. Infectious diseases, nephrology, and hepatology consultants should see the patients as appropriate. For hospitalized decompensated patients, placement of a pulmonary artery catheter is required for optimization of right-sided pressures prior to the surgery (right atrial pressure below 15 mm Hg is a reasonable goal). For patients with a history of coronary artery bypass graft surgery, a chest computed tomographic (CT) scan is indicated to map bypass grafts and prevent trauma to them during the surgery.

Cardiac anatomy and the presence of concomitant structural heart disease, including intracardiac thrombi, should be evaluated with an echocardiogram. Atrial septal defects, including patent foramen ovales, should be closed during cardiopulmonary bypass. Their absence should be confirmed by a bubble study in all patients, as their presence in the setting of an LVAD would turn a left-to-right shunt into a right-to-left shunt and lead to hypoxia. Because aortic regurgitation is likely to progress on a continuous-flow LVAD, in every patient with more than mild aortic insufficiency, the valve should be repaired or replaced with a bioprosthesis. Presence of a mechanical aortic valve is not a contraindication for an LVAD; however, the valve should be patch-closed or exchanged with a bioprosthesis to prevent left ventricular outflow tract and valve thrombosis. Patients with a bioprosthetic aortic valve or any prosthetic valve in the mitral position do not require any additional procedures. Moderate and severe mitral valve stenosis is extremely rare in LVAD candidates, but if present (Fig. 47.5), it should prompt correction during the surgery. On the other hand, even severe mitral insufficiency does not necessarily require additional mitral valve procedures, as it is prone to improve after LVAD implantation owing to normalization of LV filling pressures and reverse LV remodeling. Tricuspid valve insufficiency is extremely common in this population, but the approach to its management is a subject of controversy. Recent analysis of six studies addressing this issue showed that tricuspid valve repair was associated with longer cardiopulmonary bypass time without any early mortality or morbidity benefits.[28] Other small studies suggest that tricuspid valve repair does not decrease the rate of late right heart failure.[29]

Adverse Events

Table 47.1 lists some of the adverse events post-LVAD placement. Of note, despite frequent hospitalizations for an adverse event, the majority of patients spend greater than 90% of their time out of the hospital.[30]

The two major perioperative complications are surgical bleeding and right ventricular (RV) failure. Early reports noticed an elevated risk of mediastinal bleeding post-LVAD compared to other open-heart procedures.[31] Importantly, bleeding requiring reoperation and the number of units transfused correlated with 1-year mortality in some studies.[32] Significant delayed bleeding requires interruption of anticoagulation and may predispose to pump thrombosis. Conversely, before and during initiation of unfractionated heparin, chest tube output should be meticulously monitored. Cardiac tamponade is suggested by a combination of elevated central venous pressure (CVP) and hypotension and mandates an emergent echocardiogram to look for pericardial effusion or pericardial hematoma in order to differentiate tamponade from RV failure. Although respiratory variation of the pulsatility index has been described to diagnose cardiac

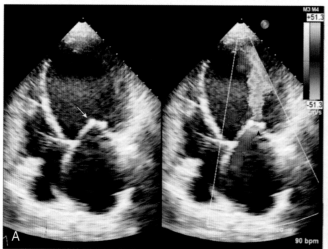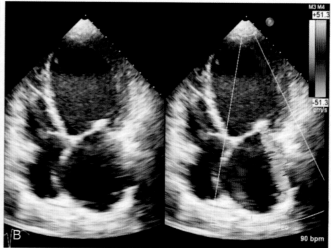

Fig. 47.5 Transthoracic apical four-chamber view of a 47-year-old woman with mitral stenosis, mitral regurgitation, and nonischemic cardiomyopathy. (A) End diastole. The mitral valve leaflets are thickened and have a "hockey-stick" appearance *(arrow)*; the left atrium is enlarged. Color flow mapping shows characteristic aliasing proximal to the stenotic mitral valve *(arrowheads)* and "candle-flame" diastolic left ventricular (LV) inflow. Mitral valve area by pressure half-time was 1.3 cm^2 on transesophageal echocardiography. (B) Systolic frames demonstrate lack of LV contraction and severe mitral regurgitation. The patient underwent left ventricular assist device placement and mitral valve replacement (see Video 47.1).

TABLE 47.1 **Adverse Events Presented per Patient-Year in Individuals With HeartMate II (HM II) LVAD and HVAD**

Adverse Events	Hm II Event Rate	HVAD Event Rate
Bleeding requiring reoperation	0.09–0.23	0.19–0.26
Gastrointestinal bleeding	0.17–0.38	0.23–0.27
Drive-line infection	0.12–0.37	0.08–0.25
Sepsis	0.18–0.35	0.04–0.24
Right hear failure	0.16–0.36	0.04–0.33
Stroke	0.083–0.13	0.12–0.2
Ischemic stroke	0.031–0.06	0.09–0.11
Hemorrhagic stroke	0.052–0.07	0.08–0.09
Pump thrombosis	0.024–0.027	0.07–0.08
De novo aortic insufficiency	0.22–0.32	NR[a]

LVAD, Left ventricular assist device; *NR*, not recorded.

[a]One report[73] suggests low incidence of de novo aortic insufficiency in HVADs equipped with Lavare cycle not available in the United States.

Modified from Slaughter MS, et al. Advanced heart failure treated with continuous-flow left ventricular assist device. *N Engl J Med.* 2009;361(23):2241–2251; Jorde UP, et al. Results of the destination therapy post-Food and Drug Administration approval study with a continuous flow left ventricular assist device: a prospective study using the INTERMACS registry (Interagency Registry for Mechanically Assisted Circulatory Support). *J Am Coll Cardiol.* 2014;63(17):1751–1757; Jorde UP, et al. Prevalence, significance, and management of aortic insufficiency in continuous flow left ventricular assist device recipients. *Circ Heart Fail.* 2014;7(2):310–319; and Soleimani B, et al. Development of aortic insufficiency in patients supported with continuous flow left ventricular assist devices. *ASAIO J.* 2012;58(4):326–329.

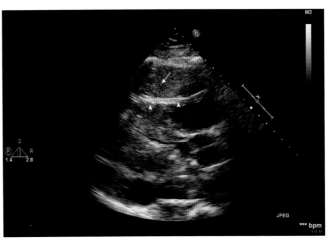

Fig. 47.6 A transthoracic echocardiogram from a patient with refractory hypotension shortly post–left ventricular assist device implantation. Parasternal long-axis view shows a large anterior hematoma *(arrow)* and posterior pericardial effusion causing compression of the right ventricle free wall *(arrowheads)* and small LV cavity (see Video 47.2).

tamponade,[33] it and other physical examinations findings, such as pulsus paradoxus, are not reliable and an echocardiogram is always needed (Fig. 47.6). Emergent drainage or hematoma evacuation is the only definitive treatment of cardiac tamponade.

Approximately 1 out of 5 patients develop some form of RV failure after LVAD surgery. Unfortunately, it is difficult to predict this prior to LVAD implantation.[34] INTERMACS defines early RV failure as a need for a prolonged (>14 days) course of inotropes or placement of a right ventricular assist device (RVAD). With a functioning LVAD in place, cardiac output is dependent on the ability of the RV to provide sufficient preload to the left side of the heart; however, increased RV preload may unmask preexisting RV failure. Changes in RV geometry are also important. Although multiple algorithms were suggested to predict the development of RV failure, they performed poorly when applied to individual patients.[35] The presence of elevated CVP and significant RV dilation raises concerns that additional RV support may be required perioperatively. Patients with low pulmonary artery pressure in the setting of high CVP have, in fact, already developed RV failure. Patients with significant RV failure despite initial treatment, including inhaled nitric oxide, should not leave the operating room without an RVAD. In a study by Takeda et al., the development of RV failure requiring an RVAD identifies patients with a poor prognosis.[36] Those with an unplanned RVAD had only a 49% chance to be weaned from

RVAD support and 6-month survival in the unweaned subgroup was dismal (13%). The availability of the percutaneously placed Impella RP (Abiomed, Inc.) offers a new and enticing temporary mechanical support option for the failing RV. This platform has the ability to be removed at the bedside without requiring a repeat trip to the operating room to reopen the chest.[37]

Pharmacologic treatment of early and late RV failure consists of optimization of preload, augmentation of RV contractility, and reduction of pulmonary vascular resistance. If the patient is hypotensive and vasoplegic, a preferential vasoconstrictor is vasopressin, which does not increase pulmonary vascular resistance as all other vasopressors do.[38] LVAD speed must be optimized to avoid any left heart contribution to elevated pulmonary pressure. Care must be taken to optimize the speed to keep the interventricular septum midline and allow the RV to have a geometric shape conducive to contraction. Nitric oxide followed by sildenafil[39] in combination with milrinone are used as pharmacologic agents to lower pulmonary artery pressures. Macitentan is currently being evaluated for treatment of pulmonary hypertension in post-LVAD patients.[40] Occasionally, late refractory RV failure dictates placement of an RVAD and heart transplantation listing if pulmonary vascular resistance is permissive. The importance of the RV in the management of LVAD patients cannot be overstated.

With intermediate and long-term use, common LVAD complications are infection and gastrointestinal bleeding. The relative immunosuppression of critical illness and the presence of large amounts of foreign material leave LVAD patients particularly susceptible to infectious complications. Infections in LVAD patients can be classified into VAD-specific, VAD-related, and non-VAD infections.[41] LVAD-specific infections can occur in the device pocket or surrounding surgical area, along the percutaneous drive lines, and inside the device itself. Goldstein et al. found that 19% of patients with a continuous-flow device had a percutaneous site infection (PSI) at 1 year.[42] Trauma of the driveline exit site is important in the pathogenesis of PSI.

In the same study, young age was the only risk factor identified in the development of a PSI. This is likely due to a more active lifestyle in younger patients, predisposing to driveline trauma. Mean time to the first PSI was 6.6 months.[42] This highlights the importance of ongoing driveline care in the prevention of infection postdischarge. The majority of the PSIs were bacterial (87.5%), with *Staphylococcus* and *Pseudomonas* emerging as the most common organisms.[34] No pathogen is isolated in 11.5% of patients.[43]

Evaluation of LVAD patients with a suspected infection should include a complete blood count, blood cultures, and chest radiograph. All patients with purulent drainage from a surgical site or driveline should have samples sent for Gram stain, KOH, and routine bacterial and fungal cultures. When physical examination is equivocal for the extent of the infection or a surgical collection is suspected, imaging with a CT or ultrasound scan may be helpful. For patients with positive blood cultures with a pathogen known to cause endocarditis, an echocardiogram should be obtained. A consensus statement recommends diagnosis of VAD-related endocarditis according to several major and minor criteria similar to the modified Duke criteria.[41]

Management of device-related infections is challenging owing to the formation of an antibiotic-resistant biofilm on the surface of the device that is virtually resistant to penetration with antimicrobial agents. A prolonged course of culture-guided antibiotics is usually required. The risk of superinfection and morbidity is high. In one study of 40 superficial PSIs, 13 (32.5%) progressed to deep infections.[43] When the infection spreads deep along the driveline or to the pocket, surgical drainage with removal of infected tissue and obtaining a deep culture is necessary. The use of sustained-release antibiotic beads has been reported by some groups.[44] The most severe form of infection, VAD-related endocarditis, is rare. Urgent listing for transplantation or pump exchange once the blood cultures are sterile is required and suppressive antibiotics are necessary as long as the LVAD is still in place. Because prevention of LVAD-related infections is extremely important, methicillin-resistant *Staphylococcus aureus* (MRSA) decontamination, in addition to meticulous care of the driveline exit site, is strongly emphasized.[45]

Gastrointestinal (GI) bleeding in LVAD patients is common. The observed higher GI bleeding rate in continuous-flow LVADs does not obviate the importance of antithrombotic management in thrombosis prevention (discussed later). The rate of GI bleeding following continuous-flow LVAD implantation ranges from 23 to 63 events per 100 patient-years[46,47] and is disproportionately high compared to patients receiving warfarin for other indications (i.e., anticoagulation for mechanical valves, which carries a major bleeding risk of 1.2–2.6 events per 100 patient-years).[48,49] Formation of GI tract AVMs and acquired von Willebrand deficiency syndrome have been proposed as mechanisms responsible for this discrepancy. The latter condition is caused by destruction of large biologically active multimers of von Willebrand factor by the pump and resolves after cardiac transplantation.[50] In the Study of Reduced Anti-Coagulation/Anti-Platelet Therapy in Patients with the HeartMate II LVAS (US-TRACE) trial, deescalation of double antithrombotic therapy to a single or even no agent still resulted in a subsequent major bleeding event in 43%

of patients within 1 year. This illustrates the intrinsic predisposition of continuous-flow LVAD recipients to bleeding complications even with minimal or no antithrombotic therapy.[51]

Aspirin dose is an important factor that can potentially contribute to bleeding. Saeed et al. retrospectively compared different regimens of aspirin therapy.[52] While the rate of thrombotic events was similar in patients with a HeartMate II LVAD, bleeding episodes were three times more likely for the group taking aspirin 325 mg compared to 81 mg. However, in the Action in Diabetes and Vascular Disease: Preterax and Diamicron MR Controlled Evaluation (ADVANCE) trial, low-dose aspirin was found to be associated with HVAD thrombosis and strokes.[53,54] This is an example of a device-specific thrombotic and bleeding profile requiring a device-specific therapy.

Most LVAD bleeding events are managed therapeutically with blood transfusion and proton pump inhibitors. Initial evaluation of overt bleeding should include endoscopy in an attempt to locate and manage the source of blood loss. The upper GI tract is responsible for 40% to 50% of bleeding events from gastric erosions, ulcers, or AVMs. In one meta-analysis,[55] obscure bleeding was present in 19% of patients; it was speculated that most of these cases originated from angiodysplasias in the duodenum or jejunum. Endoscopic maneuvers to stop bleeding are usually successful in the short term; however, in up to 50% of patients, rebleeding occurs.[56] Capsule endoscopy has limited diagnostic accuracy but should be considered for recurrent and obscure bleeding events. Similarly, octreotide should be considered for all patients with GI bleeding and angiodysplasias, although experience with this agent is primarily reported in case reports and case series.[57,58]

Pump thrombosis is a potentially fatal complication of continuous-flow LVADs. According to the INTERMACS registry, the peak of pump thrombosis occurs within the first 3 months after LVAD insertion. An abrupt increase of pump thrombosis in 2010 to 2012 still remains poorly understood but was possibly related to a loosening of anticoagulation requirements, changing thrombosis definition, changes in thrombosis screening, or device design changes. All potential causes of thrombosis could be classified as related to the patient, pump, or management.[59] Pump-related factors are unique for each device and stem from abnormal flow and interactions between the blood components and LVAD surface. For example, in the HeartMate II pump, globular clots were reported on the inflow bearings and in regions of sharp angulation.[60] In contrast, laminar fibrin deposits develop on the impeller of HVAD pumps when a thrombotic event occurs.[61] Outflow graft kinking or impingement of the inflow cannula by the interventricular septum (Fig. 47.7) or LV free wall can also result in altered flow patterns and thrombosis.[62] Patient-related factors include a preexisting or acquired hypercoagulable state, infection, sepsis, or dehydration.[59] Subtherapeutic INR is the most commonly encountered management-related factor. Similarly, erythropoietin use is associated with LVAD thrombosis and should be avoided.[63] Hypertension with a MAP greater than 90 mm Hg with the potential to decrease pump flow is another risk factor identified in the ADVANCE study.[53]

Pump thrombosis has a diverse spectrum of clinical presentations. Asymptomatic device alarms or hemolysis with darkening

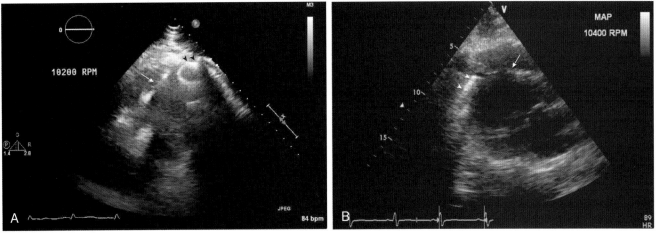

Fig. 47.7 In this patient with HeartMate II left ventricular assist device the inflow cannula *(arrowheads)* was malpositioned and the tip was occasionally impinged by interventricular septum *(arrows)*, causing symptoms (see Video 47.3). (A) Apical four-chamber view showing the circular-appearing left ventricular device inflow cannula abutting the interventricular septum. (B) Parasternal long-axis view showing the inflow cannula abutting the interventricular septum.

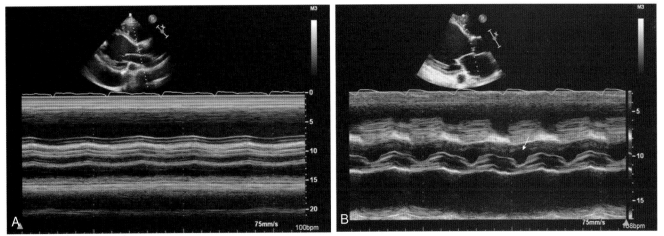

Fig. 47.8 M-mode echocardiograms from the same patient in Fig. 47.7 with a (A) normally functioning HeartMate II left ventricular assist device and (B) pump thrombosis. In A, the aortic valve is closed on each beat. In B, the left ventricle is now distended and the aortic valve opens on every beat *(arrow)*. Pump thrombosis was confirmed during a device exchange (see Video 47.4).

of the urine might be the only sign of pump thrombus.[64] On the other side of this spectrum are patients with thromboembolic events, new HF, and cardiogenic shock. Understanding that elevation of plasma lactate dehydrogenase (LDH) level is related to pump thrombosis allows early diagnosis of this condition by routine measurement of LDH levels.[59] Release of LDH is likely caused by blood cell destruction secondary to deposition of thrombotic material on different pump components.

In addition to LDH level, all patients with a suspected pump thrombus should be admitted to the hospital, started on unfractionated heparin or bivalirudin, and should have a chest radiograph and echocardiogram. Findings suspicious for pump thrombus include poor LV uploading, worsening of mitral regurgitation (MR) and one-to-one opening of a previously closed aortic valve (Fig. 47.8). CT angiogram may be useful to evaluate the position of the inflow cannula and the outflow graft.

An echocardiographic ramp study has proven valuable in HeartMate II patients with an LV end-diastolic dimension slope absolute value of less than 0.16, which is highly suggestive of obstructive thrombus.[59] The same benefit of an echocardiographic ramp study was not demonstrated for HeartWare patients. Instead, the log files should be reviewed for presence of power spikes (Fig. 47.9).[65] If the peak power is elevated less than 200% and growth rate of the power curve is less than 1.25, then thrombolysis might be helpful. On the other hand, outcomes of thrombolysis for HeartMate II thrombosis were unsatisfactory. This highlights the importance of pump- and patient-specific treatment decisions. Emergent pump exchange or cardiac transplantation is the recommended treatment for HeartMate II and HVAD thrombosis with red alarms, pump stoppage, or shock.[65] While controversial, emerging data indicate that it may be useful to exchange a HeartMate II pump even in the absence of pump malfunction or hemodynamic compromise. In a study by Levin et al.,[66]

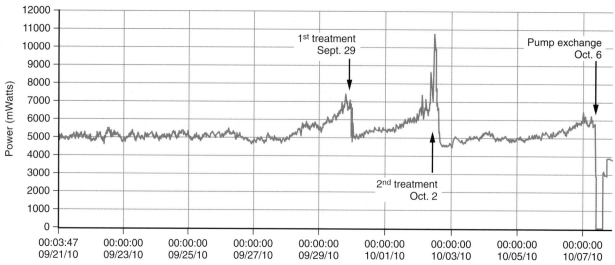

Fig. 47.9 HVAD power consumption during pump thrombus and after multiple treatments. A device thrombus in which the patient received two unsuccessful doses of tissue plasminogen activator (on September 29 and October 2) before eventually requiring a pump exchange on October 6. (Modified from Jorde UP, et al. Identification and management of pump thrombus in the HeartWare left ventricular assist device system: a novel approach using log file analysis. *JACC Heart Fail.* 2015:3[11]:849–856.)

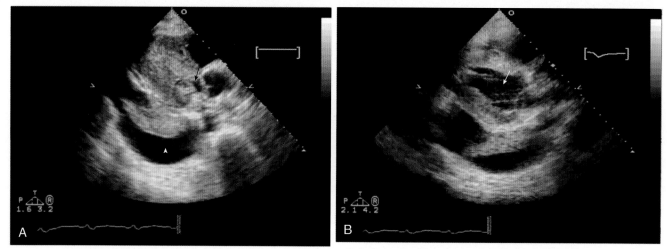

Fig. 47.10 A patient with a left ventricular assist device (LVAD) had recalcitrant ventricular tachycardia. (A) Parasternal long-axis view demonstrates almost complete obliteration of LV cavity *(arrow)*. A large pleural effusion was an incidental finding *(arrowhead)*. (B) The study was repeated after administration of intravenous fluids and LVAD speed decrease. LV cavity size has increased to 4 cm *(arrow)*. The patient was no longer in ventricular tachycardia after improvement in the LV chamber size (see Video 47.5).

HeartMate II patients with an LDH level greater than 700 U/L refractory to medical therapy who underwent device exchange through a subcostal approach had a lower 1-year risk of stroke and death compared to those who were managed with continued medical therapy (87.5 vs. 49.5%).

LVAD patients with sustained ventricular tachycardia (VT) may tolerate the arrhythmia without hemodynamic collapse. However, VT should be managed urgently to avoid deterioration of RV function. The majority of patients will have some symptoms at presentation, although they may not be specific. The correct diagnosis relies entirely on obtaining an electrocardiogram. The majority of VT occurs within the first 30 days of device

implantation[67] and might be caused by electrolyte abnormalities, β-blocker withdrawal, and the proarrhythmic effect of inotropes. A history of preoperative VT[68] and the absence of β-blockade[67] were identified as predisposing factors for VT in the early postoperative setting. Possible mechanisms of monomorphic VT include creation of a reentrant loop around the inflow cannula or preexistent scars. An LVAD-specific cause of VT is a suction event.[69] This occurs when the LV wall comes in contact with the inflow cannula in the setting of volume depletion or too high a pump speed. Rapid identification by echocardiogram is essential so that the speed can be decreased or volume given to correct this mechanical cause of VT (Fig. 47.10).

Management of VT consists of discontinuing proarrhythmic drugs, correction of electrolyte abnormalities, appropriate use of β-blockers and antiarrhythmic drugs, and timely echocardiogram to rule out suction. LVAD speed might need to be adjusted in the presence of suction events. In situations in which VT cannot be controlled, VT ablation can be attempted.

Late aortic insufficiency (AI) has emerged as a complication of long-term therapy with continuous-flow devices. The pathogenesis of AI relates to the loss of aortic valve opening followed by fusion of the leaflets. At least moderate AI is expected to develop in 38% of patients after 3 years if an aortic valve opening strategy is not prospectively used.[70] Persistent recirculation of blood from the LVAD to the LV and back to the LVAD creates a closed loop. Although patients may present with symptoms of HF, the clinical significance of less than severe AI post-LVAD is unknown. An increase in LVAD flow might be the first clue to the development of this condition. Diagnostic evaluation is complicated by the fact that traditional echocardiographic methods of AI assessment underestimate its severity.[71] The best management approach is unknown. However, in severe symptomatic cases, use of transcatheter or surgical aortic valve replacement has been described.[72]

FUTURE DIRECTIONS

The field of MCS has advanced considerably in the previous two decades. An entirely new paradigm related to continuous-flow devices has emerged. Careful patient selection and prompt recognition and management of complications have been shown to improve outcomes.[10,14] Research on smaller, minimally invasive pumps, hemocompatible pumps, and fully implantable pumps without a driveline are ongoing. The ultimate goal of therapy with an LVAD is to provide uncomplicated long-term hemodynamic support appropriate to circulatory demands.

The full reference list for this chapter is available at ExpertConsult.com.

48

Heart Transplantation for Advanced Heart Failure

Daniel E. Westerdahl, Jon A. Kobashigawa

OUTLINE

Heart failure (HF) continues to be a leading cause of morbidity and mortality in the United States. Approximately 5.7 million Americans are currently living with HF; that number is expected to increase to more than 8 million by 2030. For the 915,000 new cases of HF diagnosed each year, 5-year mortality remains at approximately 50%.[1] The gross annual cost for managing HF is approximately $30.7 billion and is expected to reach $70 billion by 2030.[2] Strategies to avert these costs should focus on prevention considering that 75% of new HF cases are preceded by a history of hypertension.[3] Technologic advances continue to improve therapeutic options and outcomes for patients living with advanced HF (AHF). Ultimately, heart transplantation provides the best long-term outcomes for AHF patients.

IDENTIFYING ADVANCED HEART FAILURE

The cardiac intensivist must be adept at identifying, stabilizing, and treating the AHF patient. Depending on the practice environment and patient population, proficiency begins with:

1. Identifying AHF patients (Box 48.1)[4]
2. Determining which patients with AHF are potential heart transplant candidates
3. Managing critically ill heart transplant candidates, which includes:
   - Intensification of intravenous diuretics, vasodilators, and inotropes
   - Interpretation of hemodynamics to guide therapy

BOX 48.1 Diagnostic Criteria and Clinical Events Identifying Patients With Advanced Heart Failure

1. Diagnostic criteria
   a. Advanced NYHA functional class (NYHA class III-IV)
   b. Episodes of HF decompensation, characterized by either volume overload or reduced cardiac output
   c. Objective evidence of severe cardiac dysfunction shown by one of the following:
      i. LVEF <30%
      ii. Pseudo-normal or restrictive mitral inflow pattern
      iii. PCWP >16 mm Hg and/or RAP >12 mm Hg
      iv. Elevated BNP or NT-proBNP plasma levels in the absence of noncardiac causes
   d. Severe impairment of functional capacity shown by one of the following:
      i. Inability to exercise
      ii. Distance walked in 6 minutes ≤300 m
      iii. Peak oxygen consumption (VO$_2$) <12–14 mL•kg•min
   e. History of ≥1 HF hospitalizations in the past 6 months
   f. Presence of all of the previous features despite "attempts to optimize" therapy, unless these are poorly tolerated or contraindicated, and cardiac resynchronization therapy when indicated

2. Clinical events that suggest AHF
   a. Frequent (≥2) HF hospitalizations or ED visits in the past 12 months
   b. Progressive decline in renal function
   c. Cardiac cachexia
   d. Intolerance to ACE inhibitors because of hypotension or worsening renal function
   e. Intolerance to β-blockers because of hypotension or worsening HF
   f. Frequent systolic blood pressure <90 mm Hg
   g. Persistent dyspnea with dressing or bathing requiring rest
   h. Inability to walk 1 block on the level ground because of dyspnea or fatigue
   i. Escalation of diuretics to maintain euvolemia (furosemide dose >160 mg/day or use of metolazone)
   j. Progressive decline in serum sodium levels (<133 mEq/L)
   k. Frequent ICD shocks

ACE, Angiotensin-converting enzyme; *BNP*, B-type natriuretic peptide; *ED*, emergency department; *ICD*, implantable cardioverter-defibrillator; *LVEF*, left ventricular ejection fraction; *NT-proBNP*, N-terminal pro-B-type natriuretic peptide; *NYHA*, New York Heart Association; *PWCP*, pulmonary capillary wedge pressure; *RAP*, right atrial pressure; *VO$_2$*, oxygen consumption.
Modified from Yancy CW, Jessup M, Bozkurt B, et al. 2013 ACCF/AHA Guideline for the Management of heart failure: A Report of the American College of Cardiology Foundation/American Heart Association Task Force on practice guidelines. *Circulation* 2013;128(16):e240-327; and Metra M, Ponikowski P, Dickstein K, et al. Advanced chronic heart failure: a position statement from the Study Group on Advanced Heart Failure of the Heart Failure Association of the European Society of Cardiology. *Eur J Heart Fail.* 2007;9(6-7):684–694.

- Identification of optimal timing for mechanical circulatory support (MCS)
4. Proficiency in the immediate postoperative care following heart transplantation
5. Competency in the management of longer-term posttransplant complications that require cardiac intensive care unit (CICU) support;
   - Primary graft dysfunction
   - Acute and chronic rejection
   - Managing the denervated heart
   - Cardiac allograft vasculopathy
   - Complications of immunosuppression

EPIDEMIOLOGY

Of the almost 6 million Americans living with HF, approximately 200,000 patients have AHF or American College of Cardiology/American Heart Association (ACC/AHA) stage D heart failure.[5] Once an AHF or stage D patient is identified and determined to be high risk for rehospitalization, heart transplant or mechanical circulatory support candidacy should be determined. Critical to optimal patient outcomes is timely selection of the right intervention for the right patient. The limited supply of donor hearts warrants strict selection criteria, ensuring that those who are listed for heart transplantation are most likely to benefit. Box 48.2 outlines common elements used for evaluation of potential cardiac transplant candidates.

HEART TRANSPLANTATION INDICATIONS/CONTRAINDICATION

Box 48.3 outlines common indications for heart transplantation. It is important to have a solid background in these indications to ensure that necessary treatment is not delayed and that unnecessary testing and treatment is not performed. In addition, the intensivist must recognize that severe HF or suboptimally treated HF is an insufficient indication for heart transplantation. Many patients considered for advanced therapies may still have stage C HF and require only medical optimization.

Furthermore, the HF team must understand when heart transplantation is not an option or unlikely to be successful for a patient. Absolute and relative contraindications exist (Box 48.4); practice varies among transplant centers.

Recognizing risk factors and comorbidities helps determine the safety and appropriateness of transplantation for AHF patients and is critical to optimizing posttransplant outcomes. Members of every transplant center must work through their individual policies and determine what is an acceptable amount of risk while maintaining optimal outcomes.

Age

Age greater than 72 years is considered a relative contraindication to heart transplantation, based on work by Mancini and Lietz.[6] There are limited data on septuagenarians, but Goldstein et al.[7] reviewed 332 patients older than 70 years who underwent heart

---

BOX 48.2   Evaluation of Potential Cardiac Transplant Candidates

1. Detailed medical history and thorough physical examination
2. Laboratory evaluation
   - Complete blood count
   - Renal function tests
     - Blood urea nitrogen/creatinine
     - Creatinine clearance
     - Glomerular filtration rate
   - Liver function tests
     - Alkaline phosphatase
     - Bilirubin
     - Albumin
     - Transaminases
   - ABO blood type and antibody screen
   - Serologies for:
     - Hepatitis A, B, C
     - HIV (human immunodeficiency virus)
     - Cytomegalovirus
     - Epstein-Barr virus
     - Herpes simplex viruses I, II
     - *Toxoplasma gondii*
     - Syphilis
   - Skin test for tuberculosis with controls
   - Right heart catheterization
   - Left heart catheterization/coronary angiography, if indicated
   - Echocardiogram or other form of ventriculography, if indicated
   - Electrocardiogram
   - Chest radiograph
   - Carotid ultrasound, if indicated
   - Pulmonary function tests
   - Exercise testing with measured oxygen consumption, VO_2
   - Histocompatibility leukocyte antigen typing/panel reactive antibody
3. Psychosocial/financial consultation

BOX 48.3   Commonly Accepted Indications for Heart Transplantation

Cardiogenic shock with low probability of recovery
- Refractory volume overload and inability to wean ventilator
- Inability to wean temporary mechanical circulatory support
- Intraaortic balloon pump, ventricular assist device, ECMO
- Inability to wean continuous inotropic support

NYHA class IIIb or IV despite maximal medical and surgical therapy
- Including hypertrophic and restrictive cardiomyopathies
- Complex congenital heart disease not amenable to surgical or procedural intervention

Severe functional limitations secondary to underlying cardiac condition
- Peak oxygen consumption $VO_2 \leq 1214$ mL/kg/min, or marked serial decline over time in the context of age appropriate controls
- 6-minute walk test <300 m

Ischemic heart disease with refractory CCS class III or IV angina pectoris despite optimal medical, surgical, and/or interventional therapy

Recurrent life-threatening ventricular arrhythmias despite optimal medical, electrophysiologic, and surgical therapy

Localized cardiac tumors with low likelihood of metastasis

CCS, Canadian Cardiovascular Society; *ECMO,* extracorporeal membrane oxygenation; *NYHA,* New York Heart Association.

---

transplantation and demonstrated median unadjusted survival of 8.5 years compared to 9.8 years in over 5800 sexagenarians. They concluded that select heart transplant candidates over the age of 70 years still derive great benefit from cardiac transplantation. It is generally accepted that heart transplant programs develop specific donor and recipient criteria in the context of their local organ availability and quality to ensure optimal outcomes and a high probability of transplantation for all patients listed.

Weight

There continues to be worse outcomes in patients at the extremes of the body mass index (BMI) spectrum, BMI less than 18.5 kg/m^2 and greater than 35 kg/m^2.[8,9] It is a class IIa recommendation[10] that patients achieve BMI less than 35 kg/m^2 before listing for heart transplantation. Additionally, there is a growing body of literature demonstrating safety and improved long-term outcomes in morbidly obese AHF patients who undergo bariatric surgery, some of whom are able to then go onto heart transplantation.

Diabetes Mellitus

Patients with diabetes mellitus (DM) who have no or minimal end-organ damage have excellent short- and intermediate-term outcomes with heart transplantation. Steroids will cause postprandial hyperglycemia, leading to worsened blood glucose control. Tacrolimus and cyclosporine will likely lead to end-organ damage, most commonly nephrotoxicity and/or neurotoxicity. The guidelines have adopted a class IIa recommendation stating a relative contraindication to heart transplantation in patients with DM and end-organ damage or persistent HbA1c levels greater than 7.5%.

Renal and Hepatic Impairment

AHF often leads to worsening renal and hepatic function. Cardiorenal syndrome and hepatic congestion can rapidly progress to irreversible stages. While no single test is an optimal predictor of recovery following heart transplantation, current guidelines recommend assessing renal function using estimated glomerular filtration rate (eGFR) or creatinine clearance. Evaluation often includes 24-hour proteinuria assessment, renal ultrasonography, and consultation with a nephrologist. The liver is more challenging than the kidney to predict degree of irreversible damage. Screening tools such as assessment of hepatic synthetic function (e.g., international normalized ratio [INR], platelets, albumin) are often misleading. Imaging of the liver, including abdominal ultrasound and abdominal computed tomography (CT), can often yield inconsistent results. The liver biopsy is being debated as a gold standard. Optimal liver biopsy specimens still have up to a 25% rate of discordance for fibrosis staging and an inherent risk of sampling bias.[11] Newer imaging techniques—such as ultrasound elastography/fibroscan, perfusion imaging with CT, and magnetic resonance elastography (MRE) may improve disease assessment. Transplantation candidates with marginal hepatic and renal function are not only at risk during the perioperative period but have higher long-term morbidity and mortality.

BOX 48.4 Commonly Accepted Contraindications for Heart Transplantation

Absolute Contraindications

Systemic illness with a life expectancy of <2 years despite HT, including

- Active or recent solid organ or blood malignancy within 5 years (e.g., leukemia, low-grade neoplasms of prostate with persistently elevated prostate-specific antigen)
- AIDS with frequent opportunistic infections
- Systemic lupus erythematosus, sarcoid, or amyloidosis that has multisystem involvement and is still active and not amenable to treatment
- Irreversible renal or hepatic dysfunction in patients considered for only HT
- Significant obstructive pulmonary disease (FEV_1 <1 L/min)
- Fixed pulmonary hypertension
- Pulmonary artery systolic pressure >60 mm Hg
- Mean transpulmonary gradient >15 mm Hg
- Pulmonary vascular resistance >6 Wood units

Relative Contraindications

- Age >72 years
- Any active infection (with exception of device-related infection in VAD recipients)
- Active peptic ulcer disease

- Severe diabetes mellitus with end-organ damage (neuropathy, nephropathy, or retinopathy)
- Severe peripheral vascular or cerebrovascular disease
  - Peripheral vascular disease not amenable to surgical or percutaneous therapy
  - Symptomatic carotid stenosis
  - Ankle brachial index <0.7
  - Uncorrected abdominal aortic aneurysm >6 cm
- Morbid obesity (body mass index >35 kg/m^2) or cachexia (body mass index <18 kg/m^2)
- Creatinine >2.5 mg/dL or creatinine clearance <25 mL/min[a]
- Bilirubin >2.5 mg/dL, serum transaminases >3×, INR >1.5 off warfarin
- Severe pulmonary dysfunction with FEV_1 <40% normal
- Recent pulmonary infarction within 6–8 weeks
- Difficult-to-control hypertension
- Irreversible neurologic or neuromuscular disorder
- Active mental illness or psychosocial instability
- Drug, tobacco, or alcohol abuse within 6 months
- Heparin-induced thrombocytopenia within 100 days

[a]May be suitable for HT if inotropic support and hemodynamic management produce a creatinine <2 mg/dL and creatinine clearance >50 mL/min. Transplantation may also be advisable as combined heart-kidney transplantation.
FEV₁, Forced expiratory volume in 1 second; *HT,* heart transplantation; *INR,* international normalized ratio; *VAD,* ventricular assist device.
Modified from Mancini D, Lietz K. Selection of cardiac transplantation candidates in 2010. *Circulation.* 2010;122:173–183.

Pulmonary Function

Severe chronic lung disease increases the risk of complications during the perioperative period and, independently, decreases the patient's functional capacity and chance for survival following transplantation. Patients with pulmonary dysfunction on immunosuppressive therapy demonstrate an increased incidence of pulmonary infection. Data are limited, but a single-center review of over 600 heart transplant patients demonstrated patients with FEV_1 (forced expiratory volume in one second)/FVC (forced vital capacity) ratio of 70% or less had significant prolongation of intubation and a significant reduction in 3-year survival compared to patients with FEV_1/FVC ratio greater than 70%. Similar outcomes were seen in patients with a diffusing capacity of the lungs for carbon monoxide (DLCO) less than 60%. Caution should be exercised when evaluating patients with abnormal pulmonary function tests for heart transplantation.

Pulmonary Hypertension

Left ventricular (LV) dysfunction is the most common cause of pulmonary hypertension worldwide. Pulmonary hypertension increases the risk for right ventricular failure during the perioperative period and significantly worsens mortality.[12] Patients under consideration for heart transplantation should undergo right heart catheterization (RHC). Several key parameters are determined at the time of RHC, including pulmonary vascular resistance (PVR), transpulmonary gradient (TPG), and the diastolic pulmonary gradient. Pulmonary artery (PA) systolic pressure greater than 50 mm Hg and a TPG greater than 15 mm Hg or a PVR greater than 3 Wood units is a class I recommendation to perform a vasodilator challenge. If these parameters can be corrected during initial hemodynamic measurement (e.g., with

the administration of intravenous nitroprusside or an inotropic agent), it can safely be assumed that these abnormalities are secondary to the marked degree of cardiac dysfunction. Many AHF centers use indwelling PA catheters to allow for inpatient hemodynamic optimization. Select patients with severe cardiac dysfunction may require temporary MCS (tMCS) to fully unload the LV and allow for optimization of hemodynamics. This strategy may improve patient selection for durable MCS and, ultimately, patient outcomes. Durable MCS has been successful in lowering LV filling pressures over months, leading to negative remodeling. This strategy may provide marginal candidates the opportunity to become acceptable for heart transplantation. RHC should be routinely performed on patients based on risk factors and the clinical severity of disease in those who are being considered for heart transplantation. During episodes of decompensation or if patients are found to have unacceptably high PA pressures, admission to the CICU with PA catheter placement for medical optimization can be very helpful prior to transplantation. Young donor hearts with a naïve right ventricle (RV) have limited exposure to elevated pulmonary pressures and are at high risk for acute RV failure when transplanted into individuals with pulmonary hypertension. Patients with irreversible pulmonary hypertension may be considered for combined heart-lung transplantation.

Peripheral Vascular Disease and Cerebrovascular Disease

Severe symptomatic cerebrovascular or peripheral vascular disease can significantly hinder recovery and cardiac rehabilitation following heart transplantation. Registry data of over 1000 transplant patients with a history of symptomatic cerebrovascular disease document an increased risk of stroke and functional decline following transplantation.[13] As part of the routine pretransplant evaluation, carotid Doppler ultrasound should be performed in patients with coronary artery disease or in patients older than 40 to 50 years. If significant carotid occlusive disease is identified, surgical correction should be strongly considered before transplantation. History and/or clinical signs or symptoms of peripheral vascular disease (PVD) should warrant appropriate screening and assessment, which may include lower extremity arterial Doppler evaluation and assessment of ankle-brachial indexes.

Infection

Transplanting in an individual with active infection is extremely high risk. The critical importance of immunosuppression immediately postoperatively leaves little room for error. It is routine to consult with an infectious disease specialist prior to transplantation if there are any active infectious concerns. Inpatient transplant candidates are particularly at risk for the development of a nosocomial infection. Meticulous attention to ongoing indications for indwelling lines or Foley catheters can help to avoid preventable infections. Practicing consistent sterile precautions while performing line maintenance can help prevent catheter-related infections. Using a very low threshold at the first sign of fever or leukocytosis to initiate a thorough investigation is recommended. At times, it is necessary to defer a patient's candidacy or downgrade a patient's listing status. An extensive infectious workup is performed on all potential transplant candidates. Finally, a thorough dental examination should be conducted before listing to identify patients with poor dentition and subclinical sources of infection. It is also important to recognize that patients who test positive for cytomegalovirus, *Toxoplasma gondii*, Epstein-Barr virus, hepatitis, human immunodeficiency virus (HIV), or prior tuberculosis (TB) infections can still be considered for heart transplantation. A transplant infectious disease physician can be instrumental in guiding therapy for this patient population, especially after the initiation of immunosuppression.

Malignancy

Transplantation significantly increases the incidence of malignancy, largely related to the effects of chronic immunosuppression. The prognosis, rate of progression, type of malignancy, response to treatment, and likelihood of widespread metastases must be thoroughly discussed and considered prior to proceeding with heart transplantation. Ongoing studies are needed to guide this decision process, especially for individuals with chemotherapy-induced cardiomyopathy.

Frailty

With an increasingly older population undergoing heart transplantation, accurate assessment of frailty is a growing area of interest. Frailty is a clinically recognized syndrome of decreased physiologic reserve that is often unmasked with only minor stressors. It is defined as a positive response to three or more of the following five components: weak grip strength, slowed walking speed, poor appetite, physical inactivity, and exhaustion. Frailty

is an independent predictor of increased all-cause mortality in patients with AHF who are referred for heart transplantation.[14] The difficulty with evaluating frailty is a lack of standardization. Flint et al.[15] raise concern that not all frailty can be considered the same. They suggest that some frail patients may be appropriately treated with advanced therapy while others may not; therefore the current definition needs additional refinement and further study.

Psychosocial Issues

A comprehensive team evaluating all aspects of transplant candidacy, including psychosocial factors, is critical to optimizing patient outcomes and appropriate patient selection. A robust social support system is essential to the success of any patient undergoing heart transplantation. The vital nature of medication adherence, consistent follow-up, and early recognition of abnormal signs or symptoms are paramount to quality of life and long-term survival. The International Society for Heart and Lung Transplantation (ISHLT) guidelines provide a class IIa recommendation that "any patient for whom social supports are deemed insufficient to achieve compliant care in the outpatient setting may be regarded as having a relative contraindication to transplant."[16] Every heart transplant candidate should receive a careful and thorough evaluation by qualified professionals. Psychiatric conditions, including active substance abuse or prior substance abuse without clearly documented abstinence, may profoundly increase the risk of posttransplant complications. Tobacco use and alcohol abuse should be categorized with illicit drugs in estimating the scope of substance abuse. Marijuana has gained increasing attention as individual states have passed laws legalizing its use. The psychological stress of heart transplantation and its long-term sequela demand patient investment and commitment. Therefore it is important that psychosocial issues be addressed prior to heart transplantation.

Finances

The financial burden of heart transplantation varies significantly by region and insurance coverage. The estimated average 2014 billed charges associated with heart transplant in the United States[17] are as follows:

    30 days pretransplant: $50,900
    Procurement: $97,200
    Hospital transplant admission: $771,500
    Physician during transplant: $88,600
    180 days posttransplant discharge: $198,400
    Immunosuppressants and other medications: $35,600
    Total: $ 1,242,200

These figures do not include the nonmedical costs associated with food, lodging, transportation to and from a transplant center, need for child care and lost wages for the patient and family member who may be required to leave work to function as a primary caretaker. While most insurers cover the expenses incurred in the transplant procedure itself, coverage varies dramatically for medications and long-term care. A comprehensive transplant team will have dedicated financial specialists who can assess the costs of future care based on an individual's insurance coverage. The goal of the financial team is to ensure that the

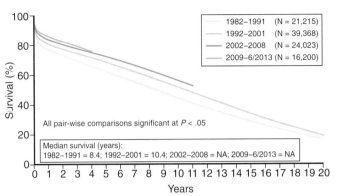

Fig. 48.1 Kaplan-Meier long-term survival for adult heart transplants performed between January 1982 and June 2013. Recipient survival improves with each successive 5 to 10 years; however, the major gains in survival are limited to the first 6 to 12 months, with the long-term attrition rate being unchanged. (Modified from Lund LH, Edwards LB, Kucheryavaya AY, et al. The registry of the International Society for Heart and Lung Transplantation: thirty-second official adult heart transplantation report—2015; focus theme: early graft failure. *J Heart Lung Transplant.* 2015;34: 1244–1254.)

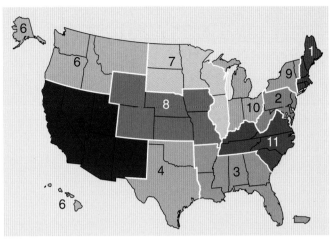

Fig. 48.2 Map of the 11 United Network for Organ Sharing regions in the United States. (Modified from Quader M, Wolfe L, Katlaps G, Kasirajan V. Donor heart utilization following cardiopulmonary arrest and resuscitation: influence of donor characteristics and wait times in transplant regions. *J Transplant.* 2014;2014:519401.)

family is prepared and capable of dealing with the financial burden of heart transplantation. Undergoing heart transplantation is physically, emotionally, and psychologically challenging. The burdensome financial strains add to the complexity and, ultimately, can lead to nonadherence to treatment plans and protocols, resulting in poor outcomes.

OVERVIEW OF HEART TRANSPLANTATION

Heart transplantation remains the most effective treatment for selected patients with AHF. Once transplanted, survival is significantly improved, as shown in Fig. 48.1.

Survival at 1, 10, and 20 years is nearly 90%, 50%, and 20%, respectively.[18] This is a dramatic improvement for AHF patients living with New York Heart Association (NYHA) class IV, stage D heart failure whose 5-year survival approaches zero.[4] Heart transplantation is limited primarily by a worsening supply-demand mismatch. As recently as 2012, nearly 2000 heart transplants were performed nationwide, yet over 3300 patients were on the waiting list with a 1- to 2-year survival of 50%.

Patients with AHF awaiting heart transplantation face not only the challenges of their disease process but the limitations of donor availability, regional differences in wait times (Fig. 48.2 and Table 48.1), and an increasingly complex donor allocation system. Since 2004, the annual number of cardiac transplants performed in the United States has slowly increased to approximately 2600 per year.

The median wait time for a patient listed as status 1A in Region 7 is approximately 90 days. The criteria required for patients to become listed as status 1A are presented in Table 48.2. It has been nearly a decade since the last revision of the heart allocation policy in the United States. Although during that time advances in medical therapy and drastic improvements in MCS options have helped to prolong survival, the status 1A

TABLE 48.1 Median Wait Time by Region for Status 1A Patients Awaiting Heart Transplantation and Mean Heart Transplant Volume Relative to a Region's Population

Region	Total Population	HTx Population	Mean HTx Volume/y	Median 1A Wait Time (d)
1	13,936,692	158,371	88	59.6
2	30,917,426	110,026	281	74.3
3	48,262,570	165,851	291	40.0
4	29,874,023	140,915	212	47.6
5	52,294,441	115,176	337	34.6
6	15,521,147	242,517	64	72.6
7	25,513,744	125,683	203	90.3
8	19,601,598	141,018	139	80.3
9	20,196,272	133,750	151	58.3
10	27,974,919	136,463	205	68.6
11	33,498,321	140,160	239	67.6

Modified from Quader M, Wolfe L, Katlaps G, Kasirajan V. Donor heart utilization following cardiopulmonary arrest and resuscitation: influence of donor characteristics and wait times in transplant regions. *J Transplant.* 2014;2014:519401.
HTx, Heart transplantation.

mortality rate remains unacceptably high.[19] An updated heart allocation policy with a six-tier system has been accepted and implemented in 2018.

The wait for heart transplantation is becoming longer for candidates due to several factors: a surge in the number of candidates, an increase in survival with the use of MCS as a bridge to transplant, and a plateau of acceptable donor hearts. The allocation of such a scarce resource warrants an investment in research and technology to help expand the donor pool.

In an effort to deliver the best outcomes with the highest quality of life to patients, intensivists must recognize the role

TABLE 48.2 United Network for Organ Sharing (UNOS) Heart Allocation Algorithm

Status Level	Category

Status 1A	Transplant candidate must be admitted to listing transplant center hospital and have at least one of the following devices or therapies in place
	I. Mechanical circulatory support for acute hemodynamic decompensation that includes at least one of the following:
	   a. Candidates with implanted left and/or right ventricular assist device may be listed for 30 days under this criterion at any point after being implanted if treating physicians determine they are clinically stable—admittance to hospital not required.
	   b. Total artificial heart
	   c. Intraaortic balloon pump
	   d. Extracorporeal membrane oxygenator (ECMO)
	II. Mechanical circulatory support with objective medical evidence of significant device-related complications
	III. Continuous mechanical ventilation
	IV. Continuous infusion of a single high-dose intravenous inotrope or multiple intravenous inotropes in addition to continuous hemodynamic monitoring of left ventricular filling pressures

Status 1B	Transplant candidate listed must have at least one of the following devices or therapies in place: I. Left and/or right ventricular assist device implanted II. Continuous infusion of intravenous inotropes
Status 2	A transplant candidate who does not meet the criteria for status 1A or 1B
Status 7	A transplant candidate who is considered temporarily unsuitable to receive a heart transplant

Modified from Kilic A, Emani S, Sai-Sudhakar C, Higgins R, Whitson B. Donor selection in heart transplantation. *J Thorac Dis.* 2014;6(8):1097–1104.

BOX 48.5 Indications of Intolerance of Current Medical Management

Worsening Cardiovascular Symptoms
- Easy fatigability
- Increasing frequency and severity of angina
- Exertional dyspnea/shortness of breath at rest
- Orthopnea/paroxysmal nocturnal dyspnea
- Dysrhythmia (tachycardia, palpitations)

Worsening Cardiovascular Physical Signs
- Hypotension/narrow pulse pressure
- Resting tachycardia/frequent ventricular ectopy/atrial fibrillation
- Elevated jugular venous pressure
- Prominent S_3/S_4
- Loud murmur of mitral/tricuspid regurgitation
- Hepatomegaly/ascites/hepatojugular reflux
- Edema/anasarca
- Diminished peripheral perfusion (cyanosis/delayed capillary refill)

Worsening Objective Measures of Cardiac Performance
- Diminished renal perfusion (prerenal azotemia/rising serum creatinine)
- Hepatic congestion (elevated liver function tests)
- Decreased end-organ perfusion (metabolic acidosis/elevated serum lactate)
- Deteriorating left ventricular function by echocardiogram
- Decreased left ventricular ejection fraction by radionuclide ventriculography
- Worsened cardiomegaly/pulmonary edema on chest radiograph
- Diminished maximal oxygen consumption VO_2 on exercise testing
- Abnormal parameters on right heart catheterization
- Elevated central venous pressure
- Worsening pulmonary arterial hypertension/pulmonary vascular resistance
- Declining cardiac output/cardiac index
- Increasing arteriovenous oxygen difference $(A - VO_2)$

of the multidisciplinary cardiovascular care team (Fig. 48.3), which includes cardiothoracic surgeons, mechanical circulatory support teams, interventional/structural cardiologists, critical care teams, AHF cardiologists, and supportive/palliative care physicians. Such a collaborative approach is fundamental for optimal patient care.[20] Several randomized controlled trials have demonstrated that multidisciplinary team-based care for patients with AHF can reduce mortality by 25% to 46%, HF hospitalization by 25%, and all-cause hospitalizations by 20% to 30%.[21] Additional studies have confirmed that the implementation of team-based care for AHF decreases length of stay and improves quality of life.[22,23]

PRETRANSPLANT PATIENT CARE

Pretransplant patient management starts with early recognition of patients with AHF. There are several levels of care that a patient with AHF awaiting heart transplantation may require; the physician must determine which will be sufficient. Many patients can be managed in the outpatient setting and remain

listed as status 2. Frequent outpatient visits and assessment of adequate metabolic, cellular, and nutritional health are critical in preventing irreversible end-organ damage. The common symptoms, physical signs, and objective measures of cardiopulmonary status are listed in Box 48.5.

There is no single parameter that identifies an individual who would benefit from heart transplantation. LV ejection fraction (LVEF) was previously thought to be the primary indicator of worsening prognosis and survival, but we now know that LVEF fails to consistently predict outcomes and, alone, is an inadequate indication for heart transplantation. Nearly 50% of HF patients have HF with preserved ejection fraction (HFpEF). The field of AHF must find better ways of predicting outcomes and obtaining objective data points that can assist in predicting outcomes for this patient population. Two diagnostic tests, RHC and cardiopulmonary exercise testing (CPET), provide reliable, objective data that are helpful in evaluating patients with AHF.

RHC has a class I recommendation for all adult candidates in preparation for listing for heart transplantation. In addition, an RHC should periodically be performed on candidates awaiting heart transplantation at a frequency that is personalized to each individual situation. With the development of ambulatory PA pressure monitoring systems, such as the CardioMEMS[24] (Abbott) device, future guidelines may need to consider alternatives to recurrent invasive procedures.

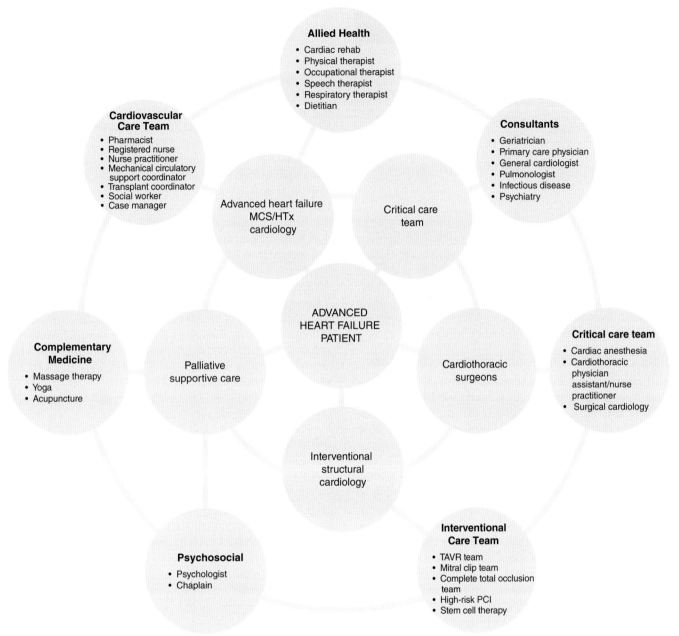

Fig. 48.3 An integrated model of team-based care for advanced heart failure patients incorporating multidisciplines while maintaining the patient at the center of the care plan. *HTx*, Heart transplant; *MCS*, mechanical circulatory support; *PCI*, percutaneous coronary intervention. (Modified from Fendler TJ, Swetz KM, Allen LA. Team-based palliative and end-of-life care for heart failure. *Heart Fail Clin.* 2015;11(3):479–498.)

Recent trials have built upon the foundational work of Mancini and colleagues on the use of CPET as a tool for predicting outcomes in AHF patients.[25] They found that a peak VO_2 of less than 14 mL/kg per minute can be used to predict a 1-year mortality benefit with heart transplantation in patients with AHF. CPET has been integrated into recent scientific statements.[26–28] Multiple studies have demonstrated the utility of measuring exercise capacity and oxygen consumption to assist in determining the degree of cardiac dysfunction and prognosis.[29] As our knowledge and understanding of the pathophysiology of AHF have matured, we have developed a better understanding of why the functional reserve capacity in AHF patients is limited. Exercise capacity in AHF patients is impaired by abnormal O_2 uptake in the lungs, progressive anemia limiting O_2 transport to skeletal muscle, reduced cardiac output in the setting of chronotropic and inotropic incompetence, and impaired vasoreactivity. The careful measurement of both ventilatory and peripheral O_2 uptake patterns can provide both prognostic value and quantification of disease severity.[30]

The use of HF prognosis scores such as the Heart Failure Survival Score (HFSS) or the Seattle Heart Failure Model (SHFM) may be used to predict morbidity and mortality in ambulatory AHF patients and assist in discriminating patients who should be listed for transplantation.[31] Predicted patient survival of less

---

BOX 48.6   Acute Precipitants of Acute Decompensated Heart Failure

Dietary indiscretion: high salt intake
Pulmonary infections
Medication changes or nonadherence
Arrhythmias and antidysrhythmic medications
Anemia
Thyroid dysfunction

Data from Tsuyuki RT, McKelvie RS, Arnold JMO, et al. Acute precipitants of congestive heart failure exacerbations. *Arch Intern Med.* 2001;161.19:2337–2342.

than 80% at 1 year by the SHFM or in the medium- to high-risk range by the HFSS is considered a reasonable threshold for listing for cardiac transplantation. Risk calculators such as the SHFM[32] were developed for predicting events in outpatient cohorts, which limits their applicability to hospitalized AHF patients. While survival scores can be helpful in prognostication, listing patients for heart transplantation based only on survival risk scores is a class III recommendation and should be avoided.

Acute Precipitants of Heart Failure Exacerbations

As HF progresses toward the advanced stages, patients become increasingly more susceptible to decompensation. Events that may have been well tolerated early in the disease process become increasingly difficult for patients to manage without inpatient care. Box 48.6 lists acute precipitants of acute decompensated HF, which is also discussed in greater detail in Chapter 18.[33] Many of the precipitating conditions are easily reversible but should lead the clinician to quickly review optimization of guideline-directed medical therapy (GDMT), indications for implantable cardioverter defibrillators (ICDs), and cardiac resynchronization therapy (CRT), and ensure that there is no reversible structural abnormality contributing to the patient's condition. These strategies should have been used earlier in the course of the disease, but in a recent review[34] of over 1000 consecutive patients listed for heart transplant, only 51% of the patients had an ICD in place at the time of being listed. Patients who suffer decompensation due to arrhythmia may benefit from an electrophysiology evaluation. Options include ablative procedures, optimization of antidysrhythmic regimens, and, in some cases, surgical sympathectomy to treat potentially lethal ventricular arrhythmias. If loss of sinus rhythm is thought to have been a precipitant of the decompensation, a robust attempt should be made to establish and maintain sinus rhythm. Based on the 2013 ACC/AHA guidelines, amiodarone and dofetilide are the preferred antidysrhythmic drugs largely based on their neutral effect on mortality in the HF population.

Guideline-Directed Medical Therapy

It is relatively common for patients presenting to the hospital with decompensated HF to have their β-blocker withheld. Only when there is cardiogenic shock, tissue hypoperfusion, and/or the initiation of inotropic therapy should β-blockers be withheld. Patients taking β-blockers who develop decompensated HF should be maintained on their medication if at all possible. Hemodynamic

goals may necessitate dose adjustment; however, every effort should be made to continue β-blocker therapy.

The deescalation of GDMT is a disservice to HF patients in terms of mortality, but is clinically indicated on occasion. Renal dysfunction, symptomatic hypotension, and electrolyte disturbances are the most frequent reasons for discontinuing angiotensin-converting enzyme (ACE) inhibitors, angiotensin II receptor blockers (ARBs), sacubutril/valsartan (an angiotensin receptor neprilysin inhibitor [ARNI]), and aldosterone antagonists. Patients who can no longer tolerate GDMT should be recognized as individuals in need of advanced therapy. Patients with renal dysfunction warrant special attention with frequent laboratory assessment when initiating or adjusting dosages of the above medications. In general, systolic blood pressure less than 80 mmHg, serum creatinine greater than 2.5 mg/dL in men and greater than 2.0 mg/dL in women, or a serum potassium level greater than 5.0 mmol/L should give pause to clinicians when considering initiation of an ACE inhibitor, ARB, ARNI, or aldosterone antagonist. Although patients with serum sodium less than 132 mM/L are at increased risk for symptomatic hypotension with ACE inhibitors, they derive the greatest benefit. Hydralazine and isosorbide dinitrate have a unique class I recommendation for use in African Americans with NYHA class III to IV HF with reduced ejection fraction (HFrEF) but are still a class IIa recommendation for any symptomatic patient with HFrEF who cannot take ACE inhibitors, ARBs, or ARNIs.

Other Common Heart Failure Drugs

Digoxin remains a controversial drug with a class IIa recommendation for patients with HFrEF to reduce hospitalizations for HF. Guidelines recommend 0.125 to 0.25 mg daily, with even lower doses for patients greater than 70 years old, impaired renal function, or low lean body mass. Serum levels between 0.5 and 0.9 ng/mL are suggested, as higher drug levels are unlikely to provide additional benefit and are more likely to lead to toxicity, especially when the level is greater than 2 ng/mL. Increased risk for digoxin toxicity occurs with concomitant amiodarone use and close monitoring should be done in patients with labile renal function. In addition, calcium channel blockers are not recommended for patients with HFrEF and should be avoided, with the exception of amlodipine for the treatment of hypertension or angina. Last, anticoagulants are not recommended in patients with chronic HFrEF without atrial fibrillation, a prior thromboembolic event, or an embolic event from a presumed cardiac source.

Medical Therapy in Advanced Heart Failure

The natural disease course in AHF leads to progressive functional decline with many of the clinical signs and symptoms listed in Box 48.5. One of the many challenges in treating AHF patients is understanding that a successful strategy to treat one patient does not always translate into a successful strategy for the next patient. As previously mentioned, a low threshold for hospitalization, intensification of therapy, and avoidance of end-organ damage are important in slowing the disease progression.

As AHF progresses, therapy is often escalated from intravenous diuretics to intravenous inotropic agents. Technological advances have made the role of tMCS increasingly important. It is common for patients who are failing intravenous inotropic agents to undergo placement of an intraaortic balloon pump (IABP) or tMCS as a temporizing measure to determine if a patient can be successfully bridged to a more long-term solution (heart transplantation or durable MCS). Again, this advanced stage of HF is frequently characterized by the deescalation of therapy that initially was well tolerated. Several common clinical problems arise during this stage, which is discussed in greater detail here.

Many patients present acutely with decompensated HF and in critical condition, requiring admission to a CICU. Recognizing the level of required care to gain control of and stabilize progression of the disease is a critical skill set that can determine life or death for this patient population. If inappropriately triaged, patients are at risk of suffering compromised end-organ function, which ultimately worsens posttransplant morbidity and mortality. Data from the Evaluation Study of Congestive Heart Failure and Pulmonary Artery Catheterization Effectiveness (ESCAPE) trial[35] played a significant role in the decreased use of invasive hemodynamic monitoring with PA catheters. The guidelines provide a class III recommendation for the *routine use* of invasive hemodynamic monitoring in normotensive patients with acute decompensated HF. However, invasive hemodynamic monitoring to guide therapy in patients who have respiratory distress or clinical evidence of impaired perfusion is still a class I recommendation. The role for invasive hemodynamic monitoring in AHF patients is a critical step in determining the reversibility of elevated pulmonary pressures and increased pulmonary vascular resistance. While PA catheters are not therapeutic, the data they provide can help guide therapy and prognosis and possibly improve outcomes before and after heart transplantation.

Relief of Congestion

Symptomatic relief for patients with AHF can often be achieved using loop diuretics in high doses or in continuous infusions. Both strategies proved comparable in the Diuretic Optimization Strategies Evaluation (DOSE) trial, albeit at low infusion doses.[36] As AHF progresses and diuretic resistance develops, effective diuresis often necessitates the combination of loop diuretics and metolazone or intravenous thiazides. When creatinine rises and diuretic resistance develops, the intensivist must recognize worsening cardiorenal syndrome. Cardiorenal syndrome may require support from inotropic infusions or the use of tMCS to help relieve congestion and improve renal function. In some refractory cases, the administration of nesiritide has been successful at promoting diuresis. Nesiritide gained popularity following the Vasodilation in the Management of Acute CHF (VMAC) trial,[37] but subsequently lost favor when the Acute Study of Clinical Effectiveness of Nesiritide in Decompensated Heart Failure Trial (ASCEND-HF) trial[38] published its findings. Ultrafiltration (UF) has been studied in both the Ultrafiltration versus IV Diuretics for Patients Hospitalized for Acute Decompensated CHF (UNLOAD) trial[39] and the Cardiorenal Rescue Study in Acute Decompensated Heart Failure (CARRESS-HF) trial,[40] with mixed results. Ongoing enrollment in the Aquapheresis Versus Intravenous Diuretics and Hospitalization for Heart Failure

(AVOID-HF) trial may help to determine if early use of UF will reduce heart failure events and has a role in pretransplant patient care.

Pleural effusions and ascites are common signs of congestion. Patients can experience significant relief following thoracentesis or paracentesis. It is imperative to understand that restoration of normal volume status markedly enhances the response to vasodilators. Decongesting a patient may afford the opportunity to reinitiate GDMT, but previously ineffective doses may result in effective or even excessive vasodilation. Although it is common for the initiation of GDMT to lead to a rise in creatinine, diuretics should not be withheld. Many effectively treated patients will experience an increase in creatinine and blood urea nitrogen, often by as much as 50%, which is acceptable. One strategy to deal with worsening renal function is to slow the rate of diuresis if the patient is no longer volume overloaded and to avoid excessive vasodilation. If the patient is in a low-output state, cardiac output must be optimized before effective diuresis can be achieved without compromising end-organ function.

Role for Intravenous Inotropic and Vasodilator Therapy

Most AHF patients awaiting heart transplantation will require inotropic support to be successfully bridged to MCS or heart transplantation. The guiding principal when using inotropes is to apply as low a dose as possible for the shortest necessary duration to achieve the clinical goal. Some patients will require the placement of long-term IV access and the initiation of home inotrope infusion. Most cardiac intensivists are most comfortable using dobutamine and milrinone for inotropic support. In patients with hypotension, dopamine—and occasionally epinephrine—can provide blood pressure and inotropic support. Data from De Backer et al.[41] compared dopamine with levophed in over 1600 patients presenting with shock and noted no significant difference in mortality; however, 24% of patients on dopamine compared to 12% of patients on levophed experienced arrhythmias ($P = .01$). Furthermore, a subgroup analysis found that in 280 cardiogenic shock patients, 28-day mortality was significantly higher in those treated with dopamine compared to those treated with levophed ($P = .03$). There are situations in which isoproterenol may also be considered for very-short-term support.

Understanding the physiology and side-effect profiles of these medications allows precision therapy for AHF patients. In general, the adverse effects of these medications are duration dependent and dose dependent; combining agents at lower doses may help avoid adverse events. Patient dependence upon continuous IV inotropic support is a poor prognostic indicator and signals the very final stages of AHF. The United Network for Organ Sharing (UNOS) status listing acknowledges the increased morbidity and mortality associated with continuous IV inotropes; thus these patients are given higher priority on the waiting list. Caution must be exerted when transitioning off inotropic support. Patients frequently become overly sensitive to afterload reduction in the setting of intravascular depletion or while titrating down inotropic support. Therefore, special attention should be given to assessing the patient's volume status and tolerance of vasodilators. The role for PA catheter-guided management of hemodynamics with special attention to the SVR can help avoid this clinical scenario. Renal vascular vasodilation and renal vascular congestion can both lead to a rise in serum creatinine. Anticipating and differentiating between these events can help prevent patient mismanagement. "Start low and go slow" is an appropriate strategy when it comes to oral vasodilator dosing prior to discontinuation of inotropic therapy. In the clinical scenario in which inotropic weaning is unsuccessful, a plan for palliative care, bridge to MCS, or bridge to transplantation should be put in place. When a patient is discharged on inotropic support that is not palliative, ICD placement should be considered given the increased risk for arrhythmia-related, sudden cardiac death.

Not all AHF patients will require inotropic support. PA catheter placement may provide hemodynamic data that suggest significantly elevated SVR. In this situation, the use of intravenous vasodilators, such as nitroprusside or nitroglycerin, can offer important clinical benefit. Patients with ischemic cardiomyopathy or pulmonary hypertension complicated by severe right heart failure may respond well to intravenous nitroglycerin. Nitroprusside has also been used in this setting but caution must be exercised in patients with renal failure, as they are at higher risk for the development of thiocyanate toxicity.

Mechanical Circulatory Support

MCS continues to play an increasing role in the treatment of AHF. In the past 9 years, over 15,000 patients have been implanted in the United States, and the current rate of implantation exceeds 2000 patients per year.[42] Approximately 30% of those recipients were listed for heart transplantation at the time of implant and an additional 23% were implanted with the plan of bridge-to-transplant (BTT) strategy. Technology is advancing rapidly in this field and, while 1-year survival now approaches 80%, it is still well below the 90% survival at 1 year for heart transplantation. Durable and temporary devices, including extracorporeal membrane oxygenators (ECMOs), will likely play an increasing role in improving survival to heart transplantation. MCS is discussed in much greater detail in Chapters 49 and 50, including both percutaneously and surgically implanted options.

Immediate Pretransplant Considerations

In 1984, the United States created the Organ Procurement and Transplant Network (OPTN) to help develop a system that would guide organ allocation. The UNOS is the only nonprofit organization that has ever run the OPTN and has been managing it since the initial contract was awarded in 1986. The UNOS has helped to develop an organ-sharing system in which donor hearts are allocated based on degree of illness in the recipient, blood type compatibility, size disparity, and length of time that the candidate has been actively waiting for transplantation. The algorithm for listing patients has evolved over the years: in 1988 there were two tiers; in 1989, there were three tiers; and in 2006, the system was modified for broader organ sharing. The current heart allocation system is based on 3 tiers of medical urgency: status 1A, status 1B, and status 2. Status 1A is given the highest priority on the waiting list; status 2 represents the more stable candidate, generally

awaiting transplant at home. The field of heart transplantation has recognized the need to decrease time on the waiting list and related mortality. In 2015, a new system with six tiers was proposed and has undergone public comment and expert refinement.[43] As of 2017, the OPTN and UNOS approved the revised adult allocation system with ongoing modification. As of 2018, the new system better incorporates the advances of MCS and its increasing role in helping to successfully bridge candidates to heart transplantation.

ABO Blood Type

Organ donors and transplant recipients are paired based on ABO blood type matching. There are 3 categories of ABO matching: ABO identical, ABO compatible, and ABO incompatible.[44] ABO blood type plays an important role in expected wait times for status 1A patients. This should be considered when listing critically ill patients who may need MCS to successfully bridge them to transplant.

Body Weight

Current guidelines from the ISHLT provide a class I recommendation that adult heart donors' body weight be within 30% of the recipients. Further, they recommend that a female-to-male donation be within 20%. The guidelines state that a male donor of average weight (70 kg) can be safely used for any recipient regardless of weight.[45]

Heart Transplantation Morbidity and Mortality

The driving forces of morbidity and mortality in heart transplantation are highly related to the time from transplantation. Understanding this temporal relationship may help guide the initial work-up and treatment for heart transplant patients who present with nonspecific symptoms, especially in the CICU (Fig. 48.4).

For cardiac intensivists taking care of heart transplant patients, it is important to recognize that most infections and rejection episodes are treatable. Furthermore, advances in both durable and tMCS are expanding rescue options and the candidate pool.

POSTTRANSPLANT PATIENT CARE

Hemodynamics

The physiology of the transplanted heart is far different than that of most other cardiac patients. In the immediate postoperative period, the transplanted heart usually requires higher-than-normal filling pressures. PA catheters play a critical role in targeting optimal filling pressures for every posttransplant patient. In general, optimal right-sided preload is usually a right atrial pressure between 8 and 15 mm Hg and optimal left-sided preload is a pulmonary capillary wedge of 15 to 20 mm Hg. The elevated filling pressures are thought to be driven by the dramatic decrease in ventricular compliance and diastolic dysfunction after transplantation. Given the degree of diastolic dysfunction and limited stroke volume following heart transplantation, a heart rate of 100 to 120 beats/min is targeted to maintain optimal cardiac output.

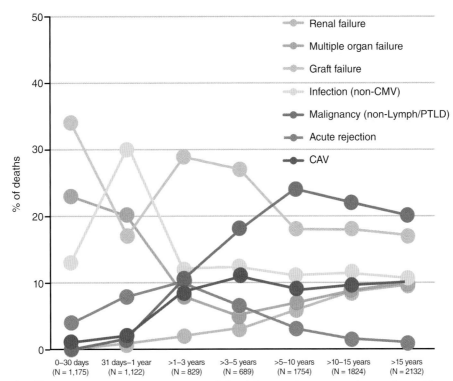

Fig. 48.4 The seven most common causes of death in post–heart transplant patients. Time from transplant on the x-axis demonstrates significant variation in the most common etiology leading to death. *CAV,* Cardiac allograft vasculopathy; *CMV,* cytomegalovirus; *PTLD,* posttransplantation lymphoproliferative disorder. (Modified from Lund LH, Edwards LB, Kucheryavaya AY, et al. The registry of the International Society for Heart and Lung Transplantation: thirty-second official adult heart transplantation report—2015; focus theme: early graft failure. *J Heart Lung Transplant.* 2015;34:1244–1254.)

Inotropic Support

Approaches to postoperative inotropic support in heart transplantation patients vary by center. Unfortunately, there are few data to guide protocols. Isoproterenol use is uncommon in the CICU, but it is used in doses of 0.25 to 5.00 μg/min for the newly admitted postoperative heart transplant patient. Some institutions argue that the potential lusitropic effect of isoproterenol enhances diastolic relaxation. Typically, heart transplant recipients will require some degree of inotropic support: dobutamine (3.0 to 10.0 μg/kg per minute), milrinone (0.37 to 0.75 μg/kg per minute), dopamine (1.0 to 5.0 μg/kg per minute), and/or epinephrine (1.0 to 5.0 μg/min) are commonly used. The β-adrenergic receptors of the denervated heart are extremely sensitive to β-adrenergic agonists. The duration of inotropic support is often affected by the donor/recipient age, ischemic time, and effectiveness of cardioplegia. Many transplant programs have implemented critical care protocols for inotropic weaning that typically occurs over 2 to 5 days.

Ventilation

In uncomplicated heart transplantation, the critical care team is often able to rapidly wean sedation, assess the neurologic status, and provide the patient a spontaneous breathing trial prior to extubation within the first 6 to 12 hours postoperatively. Individuals with severe RV dysfunction, volume overload, marginal

pulmonary function, or high inhaled nitric oxide requirements will typically be weaned more slowly prior to attempted extubation. Prolonged intubations increase the risk for ventilator-associated pneumonia, especially in the posttransplant population who are significantly immunosuppressed.

IMMEDIATE POSTOPERATIVE COMPLICATIONS

The first 72 hours following heart transplantation is critical for both the short- and long-term prognosis of the patient. Major complications are discussed later. Vital to the success of the intensive care team is the ability to anticipate problems before they reach an irreversible point and respond with urgent intervention.

Cardiac Denervation

One major difference in heart transplant recipients is their arrival to the CICU with a denervated heart. The cardiac physiology in a denervated heart is unique and deserves special attention.[46] Normal cardiac physiology involves both sympathetic and parasympathetic innervation by the autonomic nervous system. During heart transplantation, there is complete transection of neural axons to the heart, resulting in loss of cardiac norepinephrine reserves. Afferent denervation impairs the response to changes in cardiac filling pressures. Sympathetic and parasympathetic regulation is diminished by efferent denervation, resulting in an elevated resting heart rate and decreased inotropic and chronotropic responses to exercise. Normal sinoatrial (SA) node activity is often impaired after heart transplantation. Initially, many patients suffer from relative sinus bradycardia. This is often a result of trauma to the SA node following surgery, prolonged ischemic time, or amiodarone use in the recipient prior to heart transplantation. This is often treated with temporary cardiac pacing through surgically placed epicardial pacing wires. Terbutaline has been used with mixed results to temporarily increase resting heart rates following weaning from inotropes. Most patients are able to discontinue terbutaline within the first month after transplant; less than 5% of patients will require pacemaker implantation.

Arrhythmias

Sinus tachycardia is the most commonly encountered arrhythmia and is considered the normal physiologic response to denervation. Postoperative atrial arrhythmias (including atrial tachycardia, atrial flutter, and atrial fibrillation) occurred at rates up to 50% in older series.[47] Surgical technique may have reduced the occurrence rate, as the bicaval approach has increasingly replaced the biatrial anastomosis. Arrhythmias may be triggered by postoperative inflammation originating from suture lines or from high-dose inotropic support in the immediate postoperative period. The denervated heart is especially sensitive to AV nodal blocking agents. Attempts at reducing inotropes should be the initial intervention followed by the cautious consideration of calcium channel blockers and, less preferably, β-blockers. If there is concern for LV dysfunction, amiodarone should be considered.

Digoxin is unlikely to be effective in cardiac transplant patients given that its primary mechanism of action is through its effect on vagal tone. Extreme caution must be applied if considering adenosine, as it can result in prolonged ventricular asystole. If adenosine is considered in a heart transplant patient, we recommend no more than 3 mg via a peripheral IV or 1.5 mg via a central IV. Additionally, it should be kept in mind that rate controlling agents such as verapamil, diltiazem, and amiodarone can significantly increase immunosuppression drug levels.

Vasoplegia Syndrome

Vasoplegia syndrome (VS) is rare but can be lethal following heart transplantation. It consists of severe refractory hypotension, metabolic acidosis, and low systemic vascular resistance.[48] VS is seen following cardiac surgery using cardiopulmonary bypass and is not unique to heart transplantation. Risk factors include preoperative intravenous heparin, ACE inhibitors, and calcium channel blockers. The incidence of VS may also be increased in individuals who are bridged to transplant with MCS. The pathophysiology is thought to be related to the upregulation of several vasodilatory mechanisms, including circulating interleukin-1,[49] endothelial injury,[50] and dysregulation of nitric oxide synthesis. In addition, an association between vasodilatory shock and vasopressin deficiency was described by Argenziano et al.[51] Treatment approaches include hemodynamic support with vasopressors.[52] Norepinephrine, vasopressin, and pure α-adrenergic agonists, such as phenylephrine, have typically been able to restore mean arterial blood pressure. When refractory hypotension is present

despite optimal vasopressor support, methylene blue has been used to treat VS following heart transplantation.[53] Methylene blue can be given as a single infusion over 20 minutes, typically 2 mg/kg as described by Leyh et al.[54] Following infusion of methylene blue, patients may develop greenish discoloration of the urine and, occasionally, the skin. Pulse oximetry is unreliable because of light emission interference by methylene blue. A 25% mortality has been seen when methylene blue is used in individuals with severe renal insufficiency and G6PD deficiency.

Hyperacute Rejection

Assessing compatibility for both ABO blood group and major histocompatibility antigens prior to transplantation has dramatically decreased the incidence of hyperacute rejection. Hyperacute rejection occurs when circulating preformed antibodies to the donor heart are present, resulting in graft failure within minutes to hours of transplantation. Immediate MCS is typically required in the form of ECMO. Plasmapheresis and aggressive immunosuppression focusing on eliminating or removing the preformed antibodies provides the best chance of survival for these individuals. Antithymocyte globulin (ATG), intravenous immunoglobulin (IVIG), and complement inhibitors such as eculizumab have been used to treat this complication. For patients in cardiogenic shock, ECMO support may be indicated while antirejection therapy is being administered.

Right Ventricular Failure

RV failure is another common complication in the immediate postoperative period. Several factors contribute to the likelihood of RV failure. In most younger donor hearts, the RV is naïve to elevated PA pressures and is, therefore, susceptible to acute RV failure at time of implantation into a recipient with pulmonary hypertension. This principal was demonstrated in animal models in the 1950s by Guyton et al.[55] Several early posttransplant deaths in the 1960s were attributed to acute RV failure in patients with known pulmonary hypertension. In the 1970s, the risk of death from acute RV failure following heart transplantation was reported by Griepp et al.[56] See Box 48.7 for goals in the treatment of acute RV failure adapted from Stobierska-Dzierzek et al.[57]

RV failure is characterized by progressive congestive symptoms with impaired RV filling and/or reduced cardiac output. Increased RV afterload or preload leads to ventricular dilatation

---

BOX 48.7 Goals in the Treatment of Acute Right Ventricular Failure

1. Preserving coronary perfusion through maintenance of systemic blood pressure.
2. Optimizing right ventricular preload.
3. Reducing right ventricular afterload by decreasing pulmonary vascular resistance.
4. Limiting pulmonary vasoconstriction through ventilation with high inspired oxygen concentrations (100% FiO_2), increased tidal volume, and optimal positive end-expiratory pressure ventilation.

Modified from Stobierska-Dzierzek B, Awad H, Michler RE. The evolving management of acute right-sided heart failure in cardiac transplant recipients. *J Am Coll Cardiol* 2001;38(4):923–931.

and tricuspid valve insufficiency. Patients who are bridged to heart transplant with MCS are at increased risk for perioperative RV failure because of the technically more challenging surgical approach, increased blood product requirements, and prolonged ischemic time. Focal cardiac tamponade, acute respiratory distress syndrome (ARDS), and the presence of pulmonary hypertension can all cause acute RV failure. The failing RV often results in worsening venous congestion and subsequent renal, hepatic, and intestinal dysfunction. Treatment of RV failure includes volume optimization, inotropic support, afterload reduction, and mechanical circulatory support. Inhaled nitric oxide (iNO) is commonly used postoperatively for heart transplant patients with elevated pulmonary pressures and RV dysfunction. The normal dose of iNO is 20 to 40 ppm and is typically weaned off prior to extubation. iNO can be very effective in the short term but has limitations with longer-term use. Therefore, other modalities to unload the right ventricle (such as milrinone, isoproterenol, nesiritide, and sildenafil) are also utilized.

Primary Graft Dysfunction

Primary graft dysfunction (PGD), compared to secondary graft dysfunction, occurs when there is no discernible cause (such as hyperacute rejection or pulmonary hypertension) leading to RV failure. In 2013, the ISHLT held a consensus conference on PGD to better define the clinical condition and its management.[58] PGD can involve the isolated RV, LV, or manifest as biventricular

dysfunction. It is graded with a 3-tier grading system: mild, moderate, or severe. Risk factors for the development of PGD involve donor, recipient, and surgical factors. Box 48.8 provides a comprehensive list of risk factors. Universal acceptance of the PGD definition has allowed the development of targeted treatment modalities with the goal of reducing mortality (Table 48.3). While the management of PGD is predominantly supportive with escalation of appropriate inotropic and mechanical support, there may be a role for therapies such as plasmapheresis that require future study. Until then, intensivists should focus on preventing PGD from occurring. Box 48.9 describes several preventive measures to decrease the incidence of PGD.

Nephrotoxicity

Kidney function is a major predictor of both mortality on the waiting list and 1-year mortality after transplant. Studies have demonstrated that for every 1 mg/dL increase in creatinine, there is a 58% increase in graft failure at 1 year.[59] Data from the UNOS registry suggest a serum creatinine greater than 2.5 is associated with twice the mortality risk at 1 year. Acute kidney injury (AKI) is commonly encountered in the CICU following heart transplantation. Over 30% of patients develop clinically significant AKI following cardiac surgery.[60] The pathophysiology of AKI following cardiac surgery is multifactorial, including, but not limited to, cellular ischemia leading to tubular and vascular endothelial injury, loss of autoregulation of glomerular filtration rate at

---

BOX 48.8 Risk Factors for Development of Primary Graft Dysfunction

Donor Risk Factors
Age
Cause of death
Trauma
Cardiac dysfunction
Inotropic support
Comorbidities: diabetes, hypertension
Downtime of cardiac arrest
Drug abuse: alcohol, cocaine, amphetamines
Left ventricular hypertrophy
Valvular disease
Hormone treatment
CAD/wall motion abnormalities on TTE
Sepsis
Alternate list/marginal donor allocation—not increased risk
Troponin trend
Hypernatremia

Recipient Risk Factors
Age
Weight

Mechanical support
Congenital heart disease as etiology of heart failure
Multiple reoperations
LVAD explant
Comorbidities: renal dysfunction, liver dysfunction (high MELD), DM
Ventilator dependent
Multiorgan transplant
Elevated PVR
Allosensitization
Infection
Retransplant

Surgical Procedural Risk Factors
Ischemia time
Donor-recipient sex mismatch
Weight mismatch
Noncardiac organ donation
Experience of procurement team and center volume
Cardioplegic solution
Increased blood transfusion requirement
Elective vs. emergency transplant

Donation of all noncardiac organs, with the exception of lung donation, was associated with decreased incidence of PGD using data from the UNOS. Alternative study shows a high degree of correlation between heart and lung PGD in patient undergoing a paired transplant.
Single-center study showed an incidence of 36% of PGD in the group that received an emergency heart transplant, whereas the incidence was 16% in those for which the transplant was done electively.
CAD, Coronary artery disease; *DM*, diabetes mellitus; *LVAD*, left ventricular assist device; *MELD*, Model for End-stage Liver Disease; *PGD*, primary graft dysfunction; *PVR*, peripheral vascular resistance; *TTE*, transthoracic echocardiogram; *UNOS*, United Network for Organ Sharing.
Modified from Kobashigawa J, Zuckermann A, Macdonald P, et al. Report from a consensus conference on primary graft dysfunction after cardiac transplantation. *J Heart Lung Transplant*. 2014;33(4):327.

TABLE 48.3 **Definition of Severity Scale for Primary Graft Dysfunction (PGD)**

1. PGD-left ventricle (PGD-LV):	*Mild PGD-LV: One* of the following criteria must be met:	I. LVEF ≤40% by echocardiography, *or*
		II. Hemodynamics with RAP >15 mm Hg, PCWP >20 mm Hg, CI <2.0 L/min/m² (lasting >1 h) requiring low-dose inotropes
	Moderate PGD-LV: Must meet one criterion from I *and* another criterion from II:	I. *One* criterion from the following:
		i. Left ventricular ejection fraction ≤40%, *or*
		ii. Hemodynamic compromise with RAP >15 mm Hg, PCWP >20 mm Hg, CI <2.0 L/min/m², hypotension with MAP <70 mm Hg (lasting >1 h)
	Severe PGD-LV:	II. *One* criterion from the following:
		i. High-dose inotropes: Inotrope score >10 *or*
		ii. Newly placed IABP (regardless of inotropes)
		Dependence on left or biventricular mechanical support, including ECMO, LVAD, BiVAD, or percutaneous LVAD. Excludes requirement for IABP.
2. PGD-right ventricle (PGD-RV):	Diagnosis requires either both I and ii, or iii alone:	i. Hemodynamics with RAP >15 mm Hg, PCWP <15 mm Hg, CI <2.0 L/min/m²
		ii. TPG <15 mm Hg and/or pulmonary artery systolic pressure <50 mm Hg, *or*
		iii. Need for RVAD

BiVAD, Biventricular assist device; *CI,* cardiac index; *ECMO,* extracorporeal membrane oxygenation; *IABP,* intraaortic balloon pump; LVAD, left ventricular assist device; PCWP, pulmonary capillary wedge pressure; RAP, right atrial pressure; RVAD, right ventricular assist device; TPG, transpulmonary pressure gradient.

Inotrope score = dopamine (×1) + dobutamine (×1) + amrinone (×1) + milrinone (×15) + epinephrine (×100) + norepinephrine (×100) with each drug dosed in μg/kg/min.

Modified from Kobashigawa J, Zuckermann A, Macdonald P, et al. Report from a consensus conference on primary graft dysfunction after cardiac transplantation. *J Heart Lung Transplant.* 2014;33(4):327.

BOX 48.9 **Preventive Measures to Reduce Primary Graft Dysfunction**

- Improved donor management
- Better matching of donor to recipient
- Better preservation
- Gradual wean of inotropes
- Increase use of nitric oxide
- Decrease ischemic time
- Decrease transfusion requirements
- Improved procurement techniques
- Improve recipient selection

Modified from Kobashigawa J, Zuckermann A, Macdonald P, et al. Report from a consensus conference on primary graft dysfunction after cardiac transplantation. *J Heart Lung Transplant.* 2014;33(4):327.

mean arterial blood pressures less than 80 mm Hg, initiation of a systemic inflammatory response, and hemolysis-related kidney injury due to the generation of plasma-free hemoglobin and iron. Furthermore, anemia, red blood cell (RBC) transfusions, and the need for surgical reexploration can potentiate AKI. Preservation of kidney function and maintenance of adequate urine output is one of the most critical jobs of the cardiac intensivist. In the setting of escalating dosages of diuretics, there may be a role for short-term nesiritide to promote diuresis and maintain urine output. Intensivists must avoid nephrotoxic medications, prevent hypotensive episodes, and maintain cuvolemia to help ensure successful recovery of kidney function following heart transplantation. Preservation of kidney function allows for optimization of immunosuppression and enhances graft survival. Despite best efforts, transplant patients may require continuous renal replacement therapy (CRRT) or even intermittent hemodialysis (IHD). Most patients will regain renal function within 6 months. Long-term hemodialysis can significantly decrease quality of life. Individuals with an eGFR less than 30 prior to transplant should be considered for dual organ (heart/kidney) transplantation.

IMMUNOSUPPRESSION: EARLY VERSUS LATE

The adaptive immune system is a highly modifiable, specialized, and effective defense system. When targeted appropriately, the adaptive immune system helps to preserve human life. If inappropriately targeted, it can lead to the demise of an individual and a transplanted organ. The amplification of the immune system begins at the moment of the first surgical incision. Tissue factors trigger the upregulation of cytokines that increase the production of both cellular and humoral components of the immune system. The immune system becomes primed to target and destroy anything foreign. Even the most identical donor/recipient matched organ carries the risk for rejection for the life of the recipient. A recipient's immune system will constantly survey the donor heart for markers (antigens) that would identify it as foreign.

The strategy adopted by most transplant centers is early use of multiple drugs that sequentially and synergistically decrease the chance of rejection while attempting to reduce the overall toxicity and side effects of the medications. Immunosuppression may be divided into "early" and "maintenance" immunosuppression. Early immunosuppression refers to therapeutics used at the time of transplantation. Maintenance immunosuppression is often started within hours of heart transplantation but is continued long term. There is considerable overlap between early immunosuppression regimens and treatment for established rejection episodes. The commonly used drugs are listed in Table 48.4.

TABLE 48.4 Pharmacology of Commonly Used Immunosuppressive Agents

Agent	Mechanism of Action	Administration	Toxicity
Antithymocyte globulin (ATG) Both rabbit- and equine-derived preparations available **Induction Therapy**	Targets multiple epitopes on T-cells, leading to a significant reduction in functional T-cell immunity, plasma cells, and NK cells[67]	IV Infusion rATG can be dosed at 1.5 mg/kg for 5–7 days for a total 7.5 mg/kg Equine antithymocyte globulin (ATGAM) can be dosed 10–15 mg/kg/day	Anaphylaxis Serum sickness Toxic epidermal necrolysis Leukopenia Thrombocytopenia Hemolysis Infection Fevers/rigors
Basiliximab **Induction Therapy**	Chimeric antibody receptor antagonist of interleukin 2 (IL-2). Disrupts lymphocyte proliferation	IV 20 mg on POD 0 and POD 4 Retrospective analysis comparing ATG and basiliximab showed worsened long-term survival at 5 and 10 years in the basiliximab group[68]	Infection Lymphoproliferative disorders Leukopenia Polycythemia Diabetes mellitus Anaphylaxis Capillary leak syndrome
Cyclosporine	Binds to cyclophilin, inhibits calcineurin-dependent transcription and translation of cytokine genes, particularly interleukin (IL)-2	PO or IV Oral to IV dose adjustment is 3:1 Oral dosage 3-6 mg/kg/day Targeted to 12-hour trough level	Renal dysfunction Hypertension Gingival hyperplasia Hirsutism Tremor Headache Paresthesias Flushing
Tacrolimus	Binds to FK-binding protein, inhibits calcineurin-dependent transcription and translation of cytokine genes, particularly IL-2	PO or IV Oral to IV dose adjustment is 5:1 Oral dosage 0.05–0.15 mg/kg/day Targeted to 12-hour trough level	Renal dysfunction Hypertension Tremor Headache Hypomagnesemia Hyperkalemia Flushing Paresthesias Glucose intolerance
Azathioprine	Inhibits purine ring biosynthesis, decreasing synthesis of DNA and RNA	PO or IV No significant oral to IV adjustment Oral dosage 1–2 mg/kg/day White blood cell (WBC) count to remain >4000/mm^3	Macrocytic anemia Leukopenia Pancreatitis Cholestatic jaundice Hepatitis
Mycophenolate mofetil	Inhibits inosine monophosphate dehydrogenase, inhibiting the de novo pathway for guanine nucleotide biosynthesis	PO or IV No significant oral to IV adjustment Oral dosage 2000–3000 mg/day	Gastrointestinal distress Leukopenia
Sirolimus	Binds to FK-binding protein, inhibits IL-2- and IL-6-driven events	PO Oral dosage 0.5–2 mg/day Targeted to 24-hour trough level	Oral ulcers Dyslipidemias Poor wound healing Bone marrow suppression Lower extremity edema Pleural and pericardial effusions Pulmonary toxicities Nephrotoxicity
Everolimus	Binds to FK-binding protein, inhibits IL-2- and IL-6-driven events	PO Oral dosage 1.5 mg/day divided into 2 doses	Similar to sirolimus but less severe wound healing impairment
Corticosteroids	Lymphocytolysis, inhibits release and action of various interleukins, interferes with antigen receptor interactions	PO or IV with methylprednisolone Oral dosage 0.0–0.1 mg/kg/day divided into 2 doses, which is then tapered to daily	Cushingoid habitus Glucose intolerance Hyperlipidemia Hypertension Cataracts Myopathy Osteoporosis Poor wound healing Salt and water retention Peptic ulcer disease

Modified from Yamani MH, Taylor DO. Heart Transplantation. Cleveland Clinic Center for Continuing Education. August 2010. http://www.clevelandclinicmeded.com/medicalpubs/diseasemanagement/cardiology/heart-transplantation/. Accessed October 31, 2017.

Early: Induction Versus Noninduction

Early immunosuppression in highly sensitized patients (with elevated levels of circulating antibodies to class I/class II human leukocyte antigens) may begin prior to heart transplantation; these patients are often referred for desensitization therapy. These individuals are at highest risk for the development of rejection. Certain transplant centers specializing in desensitization have implemented protocols that focus on reducing an individual's level of sensitization. Current desensitization strategies include bortezomib, plasmapheresis, rituximab, and IVIG. New studies are looking at the use of monoclonal antibodies such as eculizumab in highly sensitized individuals. The goal is to decrease the likelihood of rejection and, ultimately, to improve long-term survival.

Heart transplant patients typically receive high-dose steroids at the time of transplantation followed by a relatively slow taper. Approximately 50% of transplant programs utilize induction therapy. The decision to use induction therapy balances the risk of increased infection against the benefit of potentially decreased rejection. Individuals at a higher risk for rejection typically will undergo induction therapy, most commonly with ATG.

Transplant recipients typically receive standard triple therapy immediately following surgery. Standard triple drug therapy consists of a calcineurin inhibitor (CNI; most commonly tacrolimus, with less use of cyclosporine), an antiproliferative (mycophenolate mofetil, mycophenolic acid, or azathioprine), and steroids. Many transplant programs have a renal-sparing protocol for patients with underlying renal dysfunction. Induction therapy with ATG allows the clinician to safely withhold the calcineurin inhibitor for the first 3 to 5 days in an effort to avoid nephrotoxicity.

As immunosuppression regimens transition from early to maintenance therapy, immunosuppressive medications are weaned to target lower therapeutic drug levels and reduce the risk of associated morbidity. Approximately 50% of patients are weaned off of corticosteroids by 1 year.

Maintenance

The first year of maintenance immunosuppression is driven, in part, by biopsy results, echocardiographic findings, and patient tolerance of medications. Typical maintenance therapy will include tacrolimus, mycophenolate, and low-dose prednisone. Some individuals are switched to proliferation signal inhibitors (PSIs), such as sirolimus or everolimus, instead of antiproliferative agents once adequate wound healing has occurred. There are multiple indications to switch to a PSI, which are discussed later. PSI use is discouraged in the first 6 months given their association with poor wound healing and significant nephrotoxicity. Newer laboratory tests, such as a T-cell immune function assay, may hold promise in allowing clinicians to target the lowest effective doses of immunosuppressive medications. This strategy promises to reduce the complications and side effects associated with higher dosages of the medications. Once a patient has stabilized on an outpatient maintenance regimen, the incidence of rejection drops dramatically between years 1 and 3.[61]

LONG-TERM COMPLICATIONS OF HEART TRANSPLANTATION

Cardiac Allograft Vasculopathy

When patients present with LV dysfunction and a negative workup for rejection, the diagnosis of cardiac allograft vasculopathy (CAV) must be considered. CAV is a unique process with a pathophysiology different from traditional atherosclerosis. CAV occurs along a spectrum but continues to be a leading cause of long-term mortality beyond the first postoperative year.[63] The development of CAV within the first 12 months confers a much higher mortality compared to individuals with no evidence of CAV. Early CAV is typically a diffuse process, affecting the distal vessels in the coronary vascular bed with little hope for successful intervention. Late development of CAV is much more likely to involve the proximal vessels and to be focal in nature. The pathophysiology suggests that both acute and chronic rejection play a significant role in the development of CAV. While many programs have various prophylactic regimens for CAV, the guidelines provide class I recommendations only for statin therapy and strict control of cardiovascular risk factors.[62] The treatment of CAV with percutaneous intervention and, in rare situations, coronary bypass surgery is largely dependent on lesion location and length. Treatment beyond revascularization includes optimization of immunosuppression and the use of PSIs. Sirolimus and everolimus decreased progression of CAV; CAV is a clear indication to switch a patient from antimetabolites to PSIs. Patients with progressive CAV may develop such severe graft dysfunction that retransplantation is the only therapeutic option.

Infection

Infections are a common complication following heart transplantation. Recognizing the duration of time from transplant, the degree of posttransplant immunosuppression, and the presence of intravascular devices can assist in generating a differential diagnosis. Although a transplant recipient is at an increased risk of unusual infections, the microbiology is generally dictated by the time from transplant (Fig. 48.5).[63] In general, infections that trigger an acute decompensation causing septic shock are usually bacterial in nature, with the possible exception of influenza. Although bacteremia is common, the mortality in this population is not higher than in the nontransplant population, likely due to the increased vigilance resulting in earlier identification and the blunted host inflammatory response.[64,65]

Recent health care contact and antibiotic exposure influences the likelihood of resistant gram-positive organisms such as methicillin-resistant *Staphylococcus aureus* (MRSA), vancomycin-resistant enterococcus (VRE), and resistant gram negatives such as *Pseudomonas* and *Acinetobacter*. VRE infrequently causes severe illness; broad spectrum antibiotic therapy with vancomycin and a β-lactam agent with antipseudomonal activity should be considered to be first-line treatment. If the local microbiology has a high percentage of extended-spectrum β-lactamase (ESBL) producers, consideration should be given to a carbapenem as the β-lactam. The presence of indwelling central venous catheters or other endovascular devices warrant MRSA coverage with vancomycin. Additionally, the presence of these devices may

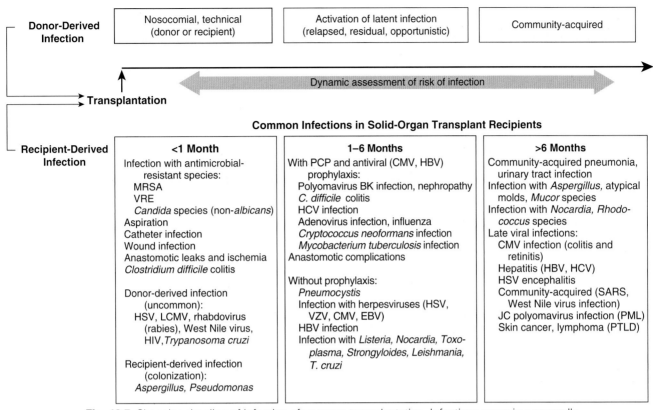

Fig. 48.5 Changing timeline of infection after organ transplantation. Infections occur in a generally predictable pattern after solid-organ transplantation. The development of infection is delayed by prophylaxis and accelerated by intensified immunosuppression, drug toxic effects that may cause leukopenia, or immunomodulatory viral infections, such as infection with cytomegalovirus (CMV), hepatitis C virus (HCV), or Epstein-Barr virus (EBV). At the time of transplantation, a patient's short-term and long-term risk of infection can be stratified according to donor and recipient screening, the technical outcome of surgery, and the intensity of immunosuppression required to prevent graft rejection. Subsequently, an ongoing assessment of the risk of infection is used to adjust both prophylaxis and immunosuppressive therapy. *HBV,* Hepatitis B virus; *HIV,* human immunodeficiency virus; *HSV,* herpes simplex virus; *LCMV,* lymphocytic choriomeningitis virus; *MRSA,* methicillin-resistant *Staphylococcus aureus*; *PCP, Pneumocystis carinii* pneumonia; *PML,* progressive multifocal leukoencephalopathy; *PTLD,* posttransplantation lymphoproliferative disorder; *SARS,* severe acute respiratory syndrome; *VRE,* vancomycin-resistant *Enterococcus faecalis*; *VZV,* varicella-zoster virus. (Modified from Fishman JA. Infection in solid-organ transplant recipients. *N Engl J Med.* 2007;357[25]:2601–2614.)

justify empiric antifungal treatment with an echinocandin. An extensive history of antibiotic exposure, intraabdominal surgery, or total parenteral nutrition use dramatically increases the incidence of candidemia.

The early posttransplant period is the highest risk period for development of opportunistic infections. Immunosuppressive regimens are most intense during the first 6 months after transplant; the use of prophylaxis has significantly reduced the burden of opportunistic infection. Common prophylactic regimens include valganciclovir for cytomegalovirus (CMV), trimethoprim-sulfamethoxazole for *Pneumocystis jiroveci* (PCP), fluconazole for coccidioidomycosis, and nystatin swish and swallow for oral candidiasis. Fungal infections peak in the 2 months after transplant and most commonly occur in individuals who were recently treated with broad spectrum antibiotics. During months 6 through 12, infection is largely related to common

community-acquired pathogens. Patients presenting with shortness of breath, cough, and infiltrates on chest radiographs at 12 months have most likely developed community-acquired pneumonia, whereas at 3 months, opportunistic infections are much more common.

In subacute presentations, the type and degree of immunosuppression used, any recent increase in immunosuppression, and the time from transplant must be used to assess the risk of unusual pathogens. Care must also be taken to consider noninfectious etiologies in these patients with multiple reasons to have sepsis-like syndromes.

Arrhythmias

Late-onset atrial arrhythmias can represent an underlying episode of rejection. Syncope and palpitations should be taken very seriously in this patient population. Severe cases of rejection

TABLE 48.5 International Society for Heart and Lung Transplantation Standardized Cardiac Biopsy Grading: Acute Cellular Rejection

Grade	Description	Prior Classification
0R	No rejection	0
1R, mild	Interstitial and/or perivascular infiltrate with up to one focus of myocyte damage	1A, 1B, 2
2R, moderate	Two or more foci of infiltrate with associated myocyte damage	3A
3R, severe	Diffuse infiltrate with multifocal myocyte damage ± edema ± hemorrhage ± vasculitis	3B, 4

Modified from Stewart S, Winters GL, Fishbein MC, et al. Revision of the 1990 Working Formulation for the Standardization of Nomenclature in the Diagnosis of Heart Rejection. *J Heart Lung Transplant.* 2005;24:1710-1720.

TABLE 48.6 Diagnosis of Antibody-Mediated Rejection

		Immunopathology	
		−	+
Histology	−	pAMR0 *Negative*	pAMR1i *Suspicious*
	+	pAMR1h *Suspicious*	pAMR2 *Positive* pAMR3 *Severe*

The grading scheme stratifies biopsies based on no histologic or immunologic evidence of antibody-mediated rejection (negative, pAMR0); either histologic or immunologic evidence of antibody-mediated rejection (suspicious, pAMR1h or pARMi, respectively); both histologic and immunologic evidence of antibody-mediated rejection (positive, pAMR2); and a final category for severe findings of myocardial destruction (pAMR3).
Modified from Kittleson MM, Kobashigawa JA. Long-term care of the heart transplant recipient. *Curr Opin Organ Transplant.* 2014;19:515–524.

may manifest as bradyarrhythmias with the potential for progression to cardiac arrest and/or asystole. Conduction abnormalities may be present in cases of CAV and/or significant cardiac fibrosis. Ventricular arrhythmias are rarely encountered after heart transplantation, but their development can be ominous. New-onset ventricular arrhythmias may be the first representation of CAV or acute rejection. Every heart transplant patient presenting with a new arrhythmia should undergo thorough evaluation.

Rejection: Acute Cellular Versus Antibody Mediated

The majority of heart transplant recipients demonstrate normal LV and RV function at the time of discharge. Any decrease in cardiac function, whether accompanied by symptoms or not, must be taken seriously and thoroughly evaluated. There are two major causes of decreased cardiac function after transplant: cardiac allograft rejection and cardiac allograft vasculopathy. Patients suffering from acute rejection present with a wide variety of symptoms and clinical findings. If rejection is suspected, aggressive treatment should be initiated as soon as possible, as these patients can quickly decompensate. The gold standard for diagnosing rejection is an endomyocardial biopsy but the sensitivity is limited and results may not be confirmed for up to 72 hours. Waiting for the tissue diagnosis in this patient population before treating is discouraged, as patients may die from a potentially treatable rejection episode.

There are three major types of rejection: hyperacute rejection (discussed earlier), acute cellular rejection (ACR), and antibody-mediated rejection (AMR). Revised grading systems have been adopted by the ISHLT in an effort to standardize definitions. These grading systems are based on histologic grade, including endothelial activation with intravascular macrophages and immunopathology (deposition of complement and human leukocyte antigen) in AMR (Tables 48.5 and 48.6).

Several factors must be considered when there is suspicion of acute rejection:

- Is there ventricular dysfunction?
- Is the patient symptomatic?
- Is there a history of rejection?
- What is the time from transplantation?
- What are the current doses of immunosuppressive agents?
- Are the levels of immunosuppressive agents therapeutic?

Table 48.7 reviews current treatment recommendations for both acute cellular and antibody-mediated rejection.

Side Effects of Immunosuppression: Malignancy, Nephrotoxicity, Drug-Drug Interactions

Major limitations in the field of transplantation are related to the sequelae of chronic immunosuppression. Immunosuppressive drugs decrease the risk of rejection and treat established rejection, but at a price.[66] Starting in years 2 to 3 following transplantation, the incidence of malignancy begins to increase; by year 5, it becomes the leading cause of death. Studies have demonstrated a 2- to 4-fold increase in the incidence of malignancy in heart transplant patients compared to kidney transplant recipients. This likely represents the difference in the degree of immunosuppression required to prevent rejection in the heart and the kidney. The current strategy includes the transition from CNIs and antimetabolites to the use of a PSI, which has been demonstrated to reduce both the incidence and progression of malignancy.

In addition to the side effects of immunosuppression, it is important that the cardiac intensivist is aware of the drug-drug interactions that occur in patients on chronic immunosuppression. Box 48.10 demonstrates how immunosuppression levels are affected by various drugs.

FUTURE DIRECTIONS

Research to address the supply and demand mismatch between donors and potential recipients is generating exciting discoveries in organ preservation techniques, which may result in an increased donor pool. New pharmacotherapeutics hold the promise of

TABLE 48.7 Treatment of Acute Cellular and Antibody-Mediated Rejection

	Asymptomatic	Reduced EF	Heart Failure/Shock
Cellular rejection	Target higher CNI levels Oral steroid bolus + taper MMF → PSI	Oral steroid bolus/taper *or* IV pulse steroids	*Treat based on clinical presentation;* *do not wait for biopsy findings* IV pulse steroids Cytolytic therapy (ATG) Plasmapheresis (before ATG dose) IV immunoglobulin Inotropic therapy IV heparin IABP or ECMO support
Antibody-mediated rejection with no or decreased DSA	Target higher CNI levels MMF → PSI	IV pulse steroids Consider IV immunoglobulin	
Antibody-mediated rejection with increased DSA	Oral steroid bolus + taper MMF → PSI Consider IV immunoglobulin and rituximab	IV pulse steroids IV immunoglobulin Consider ATG, rituximab, or bortezomib	

ATG, Antithymocyte globulin; *CNI,* calcineurin inhibitor; *DSA,* donor-specific anti-human leukocyte antigen antibodies; *ECMO,* extracorporeal membrane oxygenation; *EF,* ejection fraction; *IABP,* intraaortic balloon pump; *IV,* intravenous; *MMF,* mycophenolate mofetil; *PSI,* proliferation signal inhibitor.
Modified from Kittleson MM, Kobashigawa JA. Long-term care of the heart transplant recipient. *Curr Opin Organ Transplant.* 2014;19:515–524.

BOX 48.10 Drugs That Affect the Levels of Tacrolimus, Cyclosporine, Sirolimus, and Everolimus

Decrease Immunosuppression Levels
Antiepileptics
Carbamazepine
Fosphenytoin
Phenobarbital
Phenytoin

Antiretrovirals
Efavirenz
Etravirine
Nevirapine

Other
Antacids containing magnesium, calcium, or aluminum (tacrolimus only)
Deferasirox
Modafinil
St. John's wort
Thalidomide
Ticlopidine
Troglitazone

Increase Immunosuppression Levels
Antimicrobials
Clarithromycin
Erythromycin
Metronidazole and tinidazole
Quinupristin/dalfopristin
Levofloxacin

Antifungals
Clotrimazole
Itraconazole
Ketoconazole
Fluconazole
Posaconazole
Voriconazole

Antiretrovirals
Protease inhibitors (general)
Amprenavir
Atazanavir
Darunavir
Fosamprenavir
Indinavir
Nelfinavir
Ritonavir
Saquinavir
Tipranavir

Modified from Costanzo MR, Dipchand A, Starling R, et al. The International Society of Heart and Lung Transplantation Guidelines for the care of heart transplant recipients, *J Heart Lung Transplant.* 2010;29(8):914–956.

decreasing episodes of rejection without increasing the risk for infection. Identification of biomarkers allowing for earlier detection of rejection are actively being developed. Improved techniques to optimize donor-recipient immunologic matching to help further reduce the risk of rejection are showing significant promise. Technological advances allowing for improved mechanical support options will decrease waiting list mortality for AHF patients. While the field awaits exciting future discoveries, a focus on improved candidate selection and meticulous pre- and post-transplant management will improve outcomes and the quality of life for AHF patients.

Acknowledgments

We thank Dale G. Renlund, Brad Y. Rasmusson, Patrick W. Fisher, and Abdallah G. Kfoury, who contributed to this chapter in previous editions of the book.

The full reference list for this chapter is available at ExpertConsult.com.

49

Emergency Airway Management

Nazish K. Hashmi, Sharon McCartney, Lauren H. Jones, Raquel R. Bartz

OUTLINE

Respiratory distress is a common complication of acute illness. It may result from a primary pulmonary disorder, such as acute respiratory distress syndrome, or be a sequela of another disease, such as volume overload owing to acute renal insufficiency or sepsis. Respiratory distress may necessitate support with control of the airway and positive pressure ventilation. Failure to maintain adequate oxygenation and ventilation can lead to brain injury and death.

REQUIREMENTS FOR SAFE AIRWAY MANAGEMENT

Regardless of the nature of the respiratory distress, a few components to airway management are essential to safe and effective practice. A checklist should be provided at the bedside of critically ill patients so that items are not missed in acute scenarios (Box 49.1). It is also recommended that a time-out be performed prior to securing a patient's airway and essential equipment named and located prior to induction of anesthesia. This will ensure that the operator is prepared and familiar with the surroundings and equipment and will allow safe airway management for the patient.

Supplemental Oxygen

Preoxygenation should be performed on any patient requiring invasive airway management. For any patient who has been rendered apneic, there is a finite period before oxygen desaturation occurs. Preoxygenation is defined as providing supplemental oxygen (inspired fraction of oxygen, FiO_2, approximately 1.0) prior to induction of anesthesia and intubation, allowing for an increased time of apnea before the patient desaturates. It is imperative to perform preoxygenation, allowing safe airway management and preventing hypoxemia; however, preoxygenation of critically ill patients has been found to be less effective than preoxygenation of healthy patients.[1] Preoxygenation can be performed by applying a bag-valve-mask with a one-way inhalation and exhalation port (FiO_2 1.0), face mask at maximal flow rate (FiO_2 0.9), or bilevel positive airway pressure (BiPAP) with FiO_2 set to 1.0.[2] A high-flow nasal cannula has been advocated to preoxygenate healthy patients or patients with mild to moderate hypoxemia but has not been shown to be effective at preoxygenating patients who are critically ill with severe hypoxemia.[3,4] The supine position and obesity both decrease functional residual capacity (FRC), leading to desaturation during apnea. Studies have demonstrated that preoxygenation in the head-up or sitting position improves preoxygenation and lengthens the time before desaturation during intubation in patients.[5–7] If a patient is being supported with BiPAP prior to intubation, it is advised to continue BiPAP as the method of preoxygenation, as derecruitment and alveolar collapse can occur, resulting in shunting and ineffective preoxygenation with its discontinuation. Noninvasive ventilation may also lead to improved preoxygenation with less time to reach an expired fraction of oxygen (FeO_2) greater than 0.9 in patients not previously supported with BiPAP.[8] With adequate preoxygenation, up to 10 minutes of apnea can be maintained prior to desaturation. However, the amount of time before a patient desaturates is also dependent on delivery of oxygen, oxygen demand, oxygen extraction, and functional residual capacity.

Apneic oxygenation was first described by Frumin et al. in 1959 and can allow up to 30 to 55 minutes of adequate oxygenation during apneic periods.[9] Because of the favorable benefits of apneic oxygenation during difficult intubations, a high-flow nasal cannula at 60 L/min has recently been advocated during intubation and in one study has shown to lengthen the time before desaturation during periods of apnea, prior to securing the airway.[10] However, other studies have not shown a difference.[11–13] More clinical trials are needed before this technique becomes standard practice during intubation.

Functioning Intravenous Line

A functioning intravenous (IV) catheter is mandatory during airway control in order to administer induction agents and emergent vasoactive medications. In the event of cardiac arrest with an endotracheal tube in place and loss of a functioning IV, some medications can be administered directly through the endotracheal tube, including naloxone, atropine, vasopressin, epinephrine, and lidocaine (mnemonic: NAVEL).

Monitoring

Airway management should occur in a monitored environment, with continuous blood pressure monitoring (invasive or non-invasive), electrocardiogram (ECG), and pulse oximetry. Ideally, hemodynamic stability should ensue prior to induction of anesthesia and invasive airway management, as induction of anesthesia and institution of positive pressure ventilation can worsen the hemodynamic profile of the patient.

Suction

During airway management, continuous suction should be available and near the patient. After induction of anesthesia, gastric contents can arise from the stomach and suction may be immediately required to withdraw the contents from the oropharynx to prevent aspiration of the gastric contents. Additionally, patients may have secretions obscuring the view of the laryngeal anatomy and preventing instrumentation of the airway. A rigid suction tip (Yankauer) should be used during induction of anesthesia and instrumentation of the airway. If thick secretions are found after endotracheal intubation, a soft endotracheal suction catheter may be used to clear material from the airways.

Vasoactive Medications

Vasopressors and inotropes should be readily available, as hypotension is a common occurrence after induction of anesthesia. Hypotension after airway management is often multifactorial in a patient with respiratory distress and may be related to vasodilatory properties of induction agents, institution of positive pressure ventilation, or reduction in catecholamines after relief from hypoxemia or hypercarbia. Hypotension may be short lived, or may require institution of vasoactive infusions after airway management.

AIRWAY EVALUATION AND PREPARATION

When a patient is going to require invasive mechanical ventilation and airway management, the clinician should assess difficulty of securing the airway. Difficulty can be encountered during any part of the intubation process, including bag-mask ventilation, direct or indirect laryngoscopy, or tracheal intubation. It is important to note that increased difficulty with airway management is encountered in the intensive care unit (ICU) more than in the operating rooms, with three or more attempts at tracheal intubation increasing from 0.9% to 1.9% in the operating room to 6.6% to 9.0% in the ICU.[14]

Definition of a Difficult Airway

Difficult Bag-Mask Ventilation. Unless rapid-sequence intubation is being performed, bag-mask ventilation is often performed prior to intubation in order to maintain adequate oxygenation and ventilation prior to airway instrumentation. Difficulty may be encountered during bag-mask ventilation due to anatomic or operator features and may range along a continuum from no difficulty to impossible. Difficult bag-mask ventilation is signified by manipulations required for effective gas exchange, including adjustments of the head and neck, the use of adjuvants (oral and nasal airways), use of exaggerated jaw lift, and two-handed face-mask application with assistance of a second operator.[14] Impossible bag-mask ventilation may be encountered if no gas exchange exists despite all additional manipulations.

Difficult Laryngoscopy. Laryngoscopic exposure using direct or indirect laryngoscopy is typically graded using the Cormack-Lehane scale (Fig. 49.1). Similar to bag-mask ventilation, difficulty encountered during laryngoscopy proceeds along a continuum from no difficulty to impossible. Generally, a grade 1 view of laryngeal structures indicates no difficulty in laryngoscopy, while a grade 3 or grade 4 view represents difficult or failed laryngoscopy, respectively.[14] It is important to note whether any maneuvers were required to obtain the view (Sellick maneuver, head and neck positioning), as all laryngeal views are vulnerable to non-reproducibility and worsening if the patient's positioning and optimization maneuvers are not reproduced, a circumstance in which the critically ill patient in extremis requiring airway instrumentation may be most at risk. Notably, the incidence of grade 3 and grade 4 laryngeal views increases from 0.8% to 7% in the operating room to 11% in ICUs.[14]

Difficult Tracheal Intubation. Despite a laryngoscopic view that appears favorable to tracheal intubation (i.e., grade 1 or grade

2), difficulty in subsequent tracheal intubation may be encountered. For this reason, difficulty in laryngoscopy and difficulty in tracheal intubation should be assessed independently.[14] Difficulty in tracheal intubation can be defined as one of the following: multiple attempts or more than one operator required; or use of an adjunct, such as a tracheal tube introducer or alternative intubation device required after unsuccessful use of the primary device (i.e., changing from direct to indirect laryngoscopy after unsuccessful attempt).[14]

Failed Airway. A failed tracheal intubation is defined as failure to achieve successful tracheal intubation in a **maximum of three attempts**, regardless of the technique(s) used.[14] In the most extreme circumstances, a failed airway may be encountered where failed oxygenation has occurred (cannot intubate, cannot ventilate) in which the patient cannot be successfully ventilated (by bag-mask ventilation or a supraglottic airway) and cannot be intubated despite multiple techniques.[14]

History

If the patient is able to communicate or there is a family member available to communicate with, it is important to take a history relevant to the airway prior to induction of anesthesia. This focused history will include a history of prior intubations, difficulty with prior intubations, and a history of prior tracheostomies. If the patient has been intubated previously, any available records of that intubation should be reviewed, including equipment used and laryngeal view during intubation. Additional topics pertinent to the airway history include large weight loss or weight gain since prior intubation (large weight gain since last intubation may reflect more difficulty with the current intubation attempt), history of obstructive sleep apnea, radiation therapy to the head and neck (impairing neck mobility and mouth opening), and cervical spine abnormalities (impairing neck mobility).

Physical Examination

A physical examination directed to airway management should always be performed. Three easy-to-perform tests have emerged as highly predictive indicators of intubation difficulty: Mallampati class, thyromental distance, and atlanto-occipital extension. The Mallampati classification evaluates the size of the tongue in relation to the size of the oral cavity (Fig. 49.2). The Mallampati score exists on a continuum; in general, a Mallampati I airway is favorable, whereas a Mallampati IV is less favorable. The thyromental distance—the distance from the anterior larynx (neck) to the mandible (chin)—is a predictor of difficult intubation. Generally, a thyromental distance of greater than or equal to 3 cm or the width of 3 fingerbreaths is acceptable. A thyromental distance that is less than or equal to 3 cm or less than 3 fingerbreaths is a predictor of a difficult intubation. Last, the atlanto-occipital joint extension is an important predictor. Normally, 35 degrees of atlanto-occipital joint extension is possible. If restricted extension is encountered, difficulty with intubation may be predicted. While the presence of one of these factors may indicate some difficulty with intubation, the presence of multiple factors (e.g., Mallampati IV, short thryomental

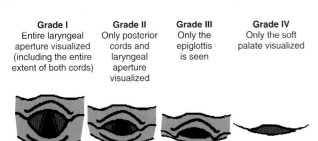

Grade I	**Grade II**	**Grade III**	**Grade IV**
Entire laryngeal aperture visualized (including the entire extent of both cords)	Only posterior cords and laryngeal aperture visualized	Only the epiglottis is seen	Only the soft palate visualized

Fig. 49.1 Four grades of laryngoscopic view. The grading of laryngoscopic view is based on the anatomic features that are visualized during the performance of direct laryngoscopy. (From Cormack RS, Lehane J. Difficult tracheal intubation in obstetrics. *Anesthesia.* 1984;39:1105.)

Class I
Soft palate,
fauces, uvula,
anterior and
posterior pillars

Class II
Soft palate,
fauces, uvula

Class III
Soft palate,
base of uvula

Class IV
Soft palate
not visible
at all

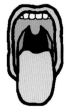 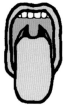 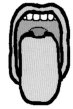 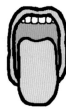

Fig. 49.2 Mallampati classification. Classification of the upper airway relating to the size of the tongue to the pharyngeal space based on the anatomic features seen with the mouth open and the tongue extended. (Modified from Mallampati SR, et al. A clinical sign to predict difficult tracheal intubation: a prospective study. *Can J Anaesth.* 1985;32:429.)

BOX 49.2   Predictors of Difficult Bag-Mask Ventilation

Obesity
Older age
Male gender
Limited mandibular protrusion
Reduced thyromental distance
Mallampati class III or class IV
Presence of a beard
Edentulousness
History of snoring or obstructive sleep apnea
History of neck radiation
Limited head and neck extension

BOX 49.3   Predictors of Difficult Laryngoscopy

Limited mouth opening
Limited mandibular protrusion
Reduced thryomental distance
Mallampati class III or class IV
Limited head and neck extension

---

distance, reduced atlanto-occipital extension) is highly predictive of difficulty with airway management.

The history and physical should be performed together to anticipate the difficulty of bag-mask ventilation, laryngoscopy, or tracheal intubation.[15] Predictors of difficult bag-mask ventilation are described in Box 49.2, and predictors of difficult laryngoscopy are described in Box 49.3.

ANESTHESIA INDUCTION

For most advanced airway management techniques, rendering a patient unconscious with the induction of anesthesia is desired. There are numerous medications to facilitate induction of anesthesia, which will be reviewed here. First and foremost, hemodynamic stability should be achieved prior to induction

of anesthesia, as this process can result in further hypotension and hemodynamic compromise owing to the vasodilatory effects of anesthetic agents and loss of sympathetic drive following withdrawal of endogenous catecholamines.

Induction Agents

Propofol. Propofol is a potent hypnotic agent that is commonly used for the induction and maintenance of anesthesia in the operating room and ICU. Propofol directly activates GABA$_A$ receptors, inhibits the N-methyl-D-aspartate (NMDA) receptor and modulates calcium influx through slow calcium ion channels. Propofol has a rapid onset of action and rapid recovery. The hypnotic effect of propofol is dose related, with small doses causing sedation and increased doses causing unconsciousness and apnea. Propofol decreases cerebral oxygen consumption, reduces intracranial pressure, and has anticonvulsant and bronchodilatory properties. The most common complications of propofol include irritation and discomfort during IV administration and dose-dependent hypotension. Rarely, allergic complications have been reported and are attributed to the metabisulfite found in some formulations, added to retard bacterial and fungal growth.[16] The propofol formulation also includes soybean oil, glycerol, and egg phosphatide.[16] Concern exists for cross-reactivity in patients allergic to egg and/or soybean oil. However, current evidence does not support a direct link and the use of propofol should be used with caution but is not contraindicated in these patients.[17] Propofol is metabolized in the liver by conjugation to glucoronide and sulfate and is eventually excreted via the kidneys. The induction dose of propofol is typically 1 to 2 mg/kg. However, in critically ill patients, this dose may be excessive and 0.1 to 0.4 mg/kg may be effective and safer.

Etomidate. Etomidate is a hypnotic agent first introduced in 1972 after being initially developed as an antifungal agent. Etomidate binds to GABA$_A$ receptors, potentiating the effects of GABA. In addition, etomidate is an agonist at central α_2-receptors, thereby maintaining vascular tone and myocardial contractility following an induction dose.[18] Etomidate maintains cardiovascular stability during induction of anesthesia and may be selected for this profile. Etomidate is metabolized by hepatic esterases and excreted via the kidney. Etomidate has also been found to cause adrenal suppression by 11-β-hydroxylase inhibition even after single-dose administration, but whether this increases mortality in critically ill patients remains unknown.[19] A systematic review and meta-analysis after single-dose administration of etomidate in septic patients suggested that mortality is not increased but was largely based on potentially biased observational data.[20] The standard induction dose of etomidate is 0.2 to 0.3 mg/kg and, while hemodynamic stability is favorable, etomidate can lead to hypotension in any patient maintaining one's cardiac output (CO) with a high level of endogenous catecholamines.

Ketamine. Ketamine is a unique dissociative anesthetic that produces amnesia and analgesia. Ketamine acts by noncompetitive antagonism of the NMDA receptor. Ketamine also acts via a complex interaction with μ- and κ-opioid receptors, is an agonist of dopamine-D$_2$ receptors, interacts with 5-hydroxytryptamine

(5-HT$_2$) receptors, and is an antagonist of muscarinic and nicotinic receptors.[21] Ketamine has sympathomimetic effects and can cause hypertension and tachycardia. In a patient maintaining hemodynamic stability with maximal endogenous sympathetic tone, ketamine can lead to hypotension owing to depletion of catecholamines. The standard induction dose of ketamine is 2 to 5 mg/kg IV or 1 to 5 mg/kg intramuscularly (IM). With small doses of ketamine (0.5–2 mg/kg), respiration and airway reflexes remain intact, which may be advantageous in a difficult airway, as spontaneous ventilation may be maintained. Ketamine is a bronchial smooth muscle relaxant and therefore may be beneficial in asthmatic patients. Ketamine is metabolized in the liver by microsomal enzymes to metabolites that are then altered to the glucoronide form and excreted into the urine. Adverse reactions of ketamine include perceptual abnormalities, disruption of some cognitive and sensorimotor function, mood changes, and delirium/psychosis.

Rapid Sequence Induction

For patients at high risk of aspiration (such as inadequate nothing-by-mouth [NPO] status, esophageal pathology), a rapid-sequence intubation (RSI) should be performed. All other patients should undergo anesthetic induction with bag-mask ventilation attempted, as it is the safest technique and allows maintenance of hemodynamic stability, oxygenation, and ventilation that results in a controlled environment for reliable and safe intubation. RSI differs from other anesthetic induction, as the anesthetic agent and paralytic are given in immediate succession, without attempts at bag-mask ventilation to avoid inflation of the stomach and subsequent aspiration of gastric contents into the trachea. RSI is not well suited for anticipated difficult airways or hemodynamically unstable patients.

Induction Agents. Any of the previously discussed induction agents can be used in RSI. Each will produce a dose-dependent hypnotic state; however, hemodynamic profiles vary. In a multicenter randomized controlled trial, ketamine was found to have a similar hemodynamic profile but less adrenal suppression than etomidate in RSI.[22] Despite the choice of induction agents, a hypnotic state should be obtained after the initial dose of induction agent, as the paralytic will follow in immediate succession and the patient should be rendered unconscious by the time paralysis occurs.

Neuromuscular Blocking Agents. For RSI, a neuromuscular blocking agent with rapid onset is desired. This can be achieved with either a depolarizing neuromuscular blocker, succinylcholine, or a nondepolarizing neuromuscular blocking agent, rocuronium. Succinylcholine is the most commonly used neuromuscular blocker in RSI. It has a rapid onset of action (40–60 seconds) and a short duration, lasting 6 to 10 minutes. Succinylcholine is degraded by pseudocholinesterase. Adverse effects of succinylcholine include hyperkalemia; it is contraindicated in major burns (starting 48 hours after the burn), major crush injuries (starting 48 hours after injury), severe abdominal sepsis, denervation syndromes, muscular dystrophy, and spinal cord injuries.[23] It is also contraindicated in known hyperkalemia and malignant

hyperthermia.[23] The intubating dose (for RSI or otherwise) of succinylcholine is 1 to 2 mg/kg. Alternatively, rocuronium can be used to create similar intubating conditions. A standard intubating dose of rocuronium is 0.6 mg/kg; however, when larger doses are used (1 to 1.2 mg/kg), an onset of action similar to succinylcholine can be achieved (40 to 60 seconds). Unfortunately, the duration of action of rocuronium is longer (37 to 72 minutes) and can be prolonged in myasthenia gravis, hepatic disease, kidney disease, and neuromuscular disease.[23] In a systematic review and meta-analysis, succinylcholine was found to be a superior neuromuscular blocking agent for RSI, leading to superior intubating conditions.[23]

Adjuvant Agents. RSI may be managed with adjuvant medications in order to attenuate the negative physiologic responses that can occur during tracheal intubation. Fentanyl, a centrally acting opioid, may be used to blunt the sympathetic response with pain receptor stimulation that can occur with intubation. With its rapid onset and short duration of action, it is the preferred opioid in this scenario. A dose of 1 to 3 µg/kg can be given a few minutes prior to induction. Fentanyl is metabolized in the liver by oxidation, without active metabolites.[24] Chest wall rigidity, with inability to ventilate the patient, can occur after large doses of fentanyl.

Lidocaine has historically been used to blunt the hemodynamic and sympathetic response to tracheal intubation. The mechanism is not completely understood but may work by suppression of a combination of reflexes. Many have now refuted lidocaine's benefit in tracheal intubation, but it remains commonly used.[24] The typical dose of lidocaine at induction is 1.5 mg/kg. Lidocaine undergoes metabolism by the liver. Excessive lidocaine will lead to local anesthetic toxicity, which can be seen even with nontoxic doses in the setting of liver failure.

TECHNIQUES OF EMERGENCY AIRWAY MANAGEMENT

Emergency airway management in the critically ill patient includes a wide spectrum of techniques, from simple bag-mask ventilation to surgical airway placement.

Bag-Mask Ventilation

Mask ventilation is a basic and, quite possibly, the most important airway management skill. It can be a bridge to definitive airway placement or a temporary rescue maneuver in patients with an unanticipated difficult airway. It is contraindicated in situations in which the risk of aspiration is increased, such as patients with a full stomach. It should also be avoided in patients with unstable cervical spine injuries and severe facial trauma in order to avoid unnecessary head and neck movement.

There are three essential components to effective bag-mask ventilation: choosing an appropriately sized mask, effective positioning of the mask on the patient's face, and coordinated compression of the bag. Bag-mask ventilation will only be effective if the patient has an unobstructed upper airway.[25] The mask is typically held with the left hand and should ideally cover the bridge of the nose, both malar eminences, the mandibular alveolar ridge. The thumb and index finger form a C around the curvature of the mask. The third and fourth digits are on the ramus of the mandible and the fifth digit is placed on the angle of the mandible, with the aim of upward displacement of the mandible.[26] Bag-mask ventilation can be performed by one operator (one-handed technique) or two operators (two-handed technique). With the one-handed technique, the left hand is used to hold the mask, while the right hand remains free to compress the bag (Fig. 49.3). Occasionally, the one-handed technique may be ineffective, such as in obese or edentulous patients. In such instances, the two-handed technique is valuable, in which one operator uses both hands in the same configuration as previously described on both sides of the mandible while the assistant or a ventilator can provide positive pressure ventilation (Fig. 49.4). Effective mask ventilation is confirmed by adequate chest rise and capnography. On most occasions, effective bag-mask

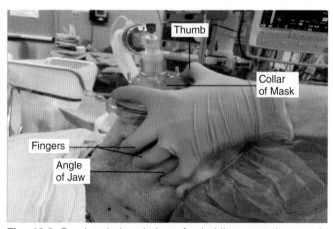

Fig. 49.3 One-handed technique for holding a mask properly on a patient's face. The thumb encircles the upper part of the patient's mask while the second finger is applied to the lower portion of the mask. The third, fourth, and fifth fingers pull the soft tissue under the mandible up toward the mask, providing jaw thrust.

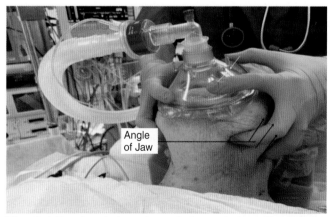

Fig. 49.4 Two-handed mask ventilation technique. The thumbs are hooked over the collar of the mask. The lower fingers are maintaining jaw thrust and the upper fingers are pulling the mandible into the mask while extending the head (arrows indicate direction of force).

ventilation requires placing the patient in the sniffing position with cervical spine and occiput extension. When the sniffing position and adequate jaw thrust are ineffective at relieving airway obstruction, additional devices, such as oropharyngeal and nasopharyngeal airways, may be placed.

Difficult mask ventilation, as defined in 2013 by the American Society of Anesthesiologists (ASA) Task Force on management of the difficult airway, is a situation in which it is not possible to provide adequate mask ventilation owing to either inadequate mask seal, excessive gas leak, or excessive resistance to the ingress or egress of gas.[27] Predictors of difficult mask ventilation include age greater than 55 years, obesity (BMI ≥30 kg/m^2), history of snoring or obstructive sleep apnea, presence of a beard, male gender, lack of teeth, Mallampati class III or class IV, and abnormal mandibular protrusion test (see Box 49.2).[28]

Laryngeal Mask Airway

The laryngeal mask airway (LMA) is the most commonly used supraglottic airway in use. Initially described by Dr. Archie Brain in 1983, the LMA has found its importance in both standard and emergent airway management.[29] It is also a critical component of the ASA difficult airway algorithm. The LMA is typically an oval-shaped silicone mask with an inflatable cuff that is designed to be seated in the hypopharynx. The cuff can be inflated to form a seal around the supraglottic tissues and attached to a bag-valve device or a mechanical ventilator. It comes in various sizes, from 1 (neonate) to 6 (large adult), and is selected according to patient weight. Many variants of the LMA are currently available, including the LMA Fastrach (Teleflex), which is an intubating LMA, and the LMA Proseal (Teleflex), which allows for a better seal with a posterior cuff and has a drainage tube for oral, gastric, and respiratory secretions. The LMA allows for spontaneous and positive pressure ventilation at airway pressures up to 20 cm H_2O (higher with the LMA Proseal).

The insertion of an LMA requires sufficient anesthesia. It is inserted along the hard palate after the posterior aspect of the mask is lubricated and the cuff is deflated. It is advanced until definite resistance is met, at which point the cuff is inflated. Placement is confirmed by chest rise, auscultation, and capnography (Video 49.1). LMA placement is associated with a lower risk of damage to teeth, sore throat, hoarse voice, and.[30,31] It is relatively easy to perform and does not require neuromuscular blockade. While there are many advantages to the use of an LMA, there are a few important disadvantages that may limit its use. It does not protect against laryngospasm and even the newer-generation devices do not eliminate the risk of gastric aspiration. Therefore, it is relatively contraindicated in obese patients or patients with a full stomach at a higher risk of aspiration. It is also relatively contraindicated in patients with supraglottic pathology.[26]

Endotracheal Intubation

Endotracheal intubation is the gold standard of airway management. There are several indications for endotracheal intubation, including critical illness and hemodynamic instability, high risk of aspiration, lung abnormalities, need for lung isolation, need for prolonged mechanical ventilation, and neuromuscular blockade and prone positioning.[26] Endotracheal intubation in the critically ill patient is a high-risk procedure. Unlike the operating room, where intubation is typically an elective procedure with ample time for preoxygenation, ICU intubation is usually urgent or emergent and is required in patients who are desaturating and already hypoxemic, hypercarbic, or both. Preoxygenation may be ineffective in this patient population and intubation may be complicated by hypotension, hypoxemia, and even cardiac arrest.[32] The most common method for standard and emergent intubation is by direct laryngoscopy (DL).

DL involves using a laryngoscope to visualize the glottic opening by aligning the oral, laryngeal, and pharyngeal axes. This is achieved by extension at the atlanto-occipital joint and is referred to as the *sniffing position*. The two most common types of laryngoscope blades used for direct laryngoscopy are the curved Macintosh blade and the straight Miller blade. Techniques of intubation are slightly different with each of these blades. The Macintosh blade is inserted along the right side of the oral cavity, the tongue is swept to the left, and the blade is advanced until the tip is located in the vallecula, hence exposing the glottic opening (Fig. 49.5). The straight Miller blade is inserted lateral to the tongue and advanced along the paraglossal gutter between the tongue and tonsil. The blade is advanced until the epiglottis is visualized, at which point the blade is passed posterior to the epiglottis, revealing the glottic opening (Fig. 49.6). Lifting force is carefully applied during direct laryngoscopy with careful attention to ensure that there is no damage to the teeth and soft tissues. While choice of laryngoscope blades depends on the operator, the Macintosh blade is commonly used in adults while the Miller blade is preferred for pediatric patients.[33] Miller blades are also preferred in patients with short thyromental distance and a large redundant epiglottis.

Video Laryngoscopy

Video laryngoscopy (VL) is an invaluable tool that is now commonly available for standard and difficult airway management both in the ICU and the operating room (Video 49.2). It is also included in the ASA difficult airway algorithm and should be considered in patients with a predicted or previously documented difficult airway. Video laryngoscopes can be classified into three broad groups: those with a design similar to the Macintosh blade, those with highly curved blades, and those with an endotracheal tube guiding channel.

The C-MAC laryngoscope (Karl Storz) is the most commonly available and widely studied video laryngoscope. The laryngoscope is shaped like a Macintosh blade and the process of intubation is identical to that of direct laryngoscopy, including a leftward sweep of the tongue during insertion of the video laryngoscope (Fig. 49.7). A custom-styletted tube is not necessary for intubation with the C-MAC.

In certain situations, such as cervical spine instability or an anteriorly displaced glottic opening, a distally angulated blade is useful in visualizing the glottis. The Glidescope (Verathon) has been the prototype device to use in such patients. The laryngoscope blade has a 60-degree angulation with a camera at the tip; the image is displayed on a stand-alone monitor. Because of such angulation, a custom-styletted tube is necessary with the curve on the stylet matching the angulation of the blade (Fig. 49.8). Other devices with angulated blades include the McGrath MAC laryngoscope (Aircraft Medical) and the D-Blade for the C-MAC device. These devices should be inserted in the midline of the oropharynx (without leftward sweeping of the tongue) under direct vision. The styletted endotracheal tube should be inserted along the right side of the oral cavity in the 3 o'clock

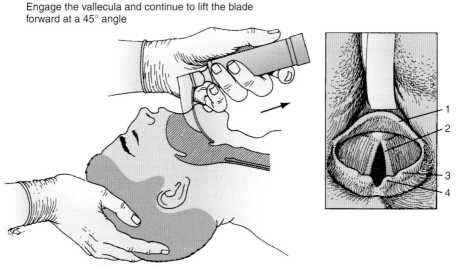

Engage the vallecula and continue to lift the blade forward at a 45° angle

Fig. 49.5 This figure demonstrates the correct position of the curved (Macintosh) laryngoscope blade in the vallecula and the angle of pressure that should be applied (45 degrees from the patient's axial line). The inset demonstrates the laryngeal view obtained when the Macintosh blade is used. *1,* Epiglottis; *2,* vocal cords; *3,* cuneiform part of arytenoid cartilage; *4,* corniculate part of arytenoid cartilage. (From Benumof JL. Conventional [laryngoscopic] orotracheal and nasotracheal intubation [single lumen type]. In: Benumof JL, ed. *Clinical Procedures in Anesthesia and Intensive Care.* Philadelphia: Lippincott-Raven; 1992:127.)

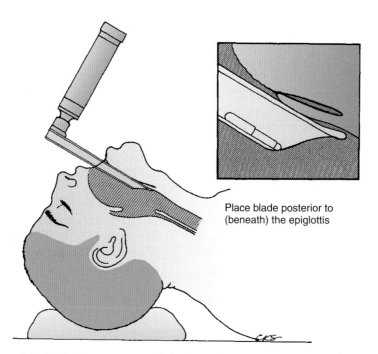

Place blade posterior to (beneath) the epiglottis

Fig. 49.6 A straight (Miller) laryngoscope blade should pass underneath the laryngeal surface of the epiglottis; then the handle of the laryngoscope blade should be elevated at a 45-degree angle similar to that used with a Macintosh blade. By lifting up the epiglottis, the laryngeal aperture should come clearly into view. (From Benumof JL. Conventional [laryngoscopic] orotracheal and nasotracheal intubation [single lumen type]. In: Benumof JL, ed. *Clinical Procedures in Anesthesia and Intensive Care*. Philadelphia: Lippincott-Raven; 1992:128.)

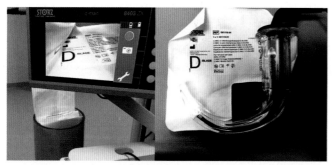

Fig. 49.7 C-MAC video laryngoscope. This video laryngoscope is named based on its similar shape to the Macintosh direct laryngoscopy blade. Advantages of the C-MAC include its ability to be used for direct laryngoscopy (gives adequate exposure for direct visualization of the glottic opening) or as a video laryngoscope in the event that direct visualization is not obtained.

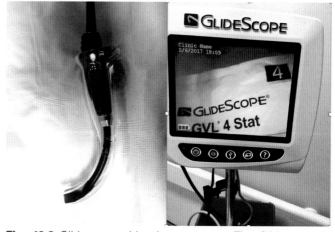

Fig. 49.8 Glidescope video laryngoscope. The Glidescope is similar to the C-MAC video laryngoscope except that it contains a more angulated distal curvature. The traditional Glidescope blade cannot be used for direct laryngoscopy; however, newer blades are available that can be used for both direct laryngoscopy and video laryngoscopy.

position while looking at the patient to avoid oropharyngeal trauma.[34] Once the tip of the endotracheal tube is past the oropharynx, the operator should look at the screen and rotate the endotracheal tube to the 12 o'clock position to prevent the tip of the tube from "hanging up" on the right arytenoid and causing arytenoid trauma.

The last category of video laryngoscope includes those with curved blades and an integrated tube-guiding channel, eliminating the need for a stylet. These include the Airtraq (Prodol Meditec SA) and the King Vision (King Systems). These can be especially useful in patients with limited cervical spine mobility. Other advantages of these laryngoscopes are their small size and ease

of storing and, since they do not need a power source, they are easily transportable (Fig. 49.9).

In a propensity-matched analysis, VL increased the odds for first-attempt intubation compared to direct laryngoscopy by 2.8 times when performed by nonanesthesiologists in a medical ICU. There were also reduced rates of esophageal intubation and arterial desaturation events during the intubation.[35] In a recent systematic review, Lewis et al. evaluated 64 randomized clinical

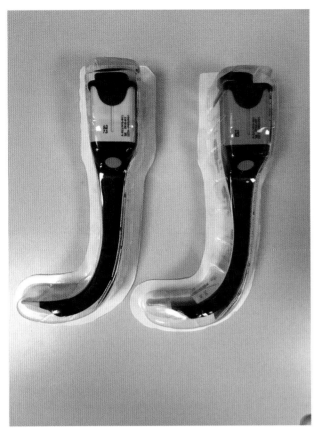

Fig. 49.9 Airtraq video laryngoscope. These laryngoscopes either have an eye piece in which the operator places the eye directly to the top of the laryngoscope for visualization of the glottic opening or a small screen attached for visualization of the glottis.

trials to determine whether VL in adults undergoing general anesthesia reduced the risk of failed intubations and complications when compared with DL. Their analysis revealed that VL aids intubation in patients with known or predicted difficult airway and may reduce the incidence of airway trauma. However, they found no evidence that VL reduces the number of intubation attempts, the development of hypoxia, or the time for intubation compared with DL.[36] Video laryngoscopes can also be used for awake intubations in the morbidly obese[37] or those with upper airway tumors.[38] Indeed, as more intensivists opt for awake intubation of the critically ill patient in the ICU, VL may be more commonly used in lieu of fiberoptic intubation.[39]

DIFFICULT AIRWAY

The difficult airway is one of the most challenging situations that an anesthesiologist and an intensivist can encounter during the management of critically ill patients. According to the ASA, the inability to successfully manage a difficult airway was identified as the cause of 30% of deaths attributed to anesthetic complications.[40] The ASA published its most updated practice guidelines for the management of the difficult airway in 2013.[27] Many other societies, including the Canadian Airway Focus Group,[14,15] have also proposed recommendations for the management of the difficult airway.

The management of a difficult airway begins after an adequate history and physical examination. Previous airway history is elicited, as are existing comorbid conditions. Certain syndromes—such as Down, Treacher-Collins, and Pierre-Robin—and others are associated with a difficult intubation. Other predictors of difficult intubation include obesity, history of obstructive sleep apnea, or other comorbidities, such as the presence of mediastinal masses (see Box 49.3). Coexisting medical conditions, such as respiratory failure and coronary artery disease, may affect the management of a difficult airway. Previous anesthetic and intubation records should also be reviewed. A detailed airway assessment should be performed as described previously in the chapter and supplemented with appropriate additional imaging, such as a computed tomographic (CT) scan of the chest and upper airways in the case of mediastinal or upper airway masses.

The ASA difficult airway algorithm[27] (Fig. 49.10) describes six scenarios that may occur independently or in combination to make airway management difficult. These include:
- Difficulty with patient cooperation or consent
- Difficult mask ventilation
- Difficult supraglottic device placement
- Difficult laryngoscopy
- Difficult intubation
- Difficult surgical access

Difficult mask ventilation, difficult laryngoscopy, and difficult intubation have been described previously in this chapter. When a difficult airway is encountered, four basic management options have been proposed:
- Awake intubation versus intubation after induction of anesthesia
- Noninvasive versus invasive airway management (cricothyrotomy vs. tracheostomy)
- VL as the first choice for airway management
- Spontaneous ventilation versus paralysis during airway management

The decision is tailored to the individual patient's ability to cooperate, the clinical situation (urgent or emergent vs. elective intubation), and the advantages and disadvantages of the particular technique.

Two Limbs of the ASA Difficult Airway Algorithm

The difficult airway algorithm follows two main limbs: awake intubation and intubation in the asleep patient.

In the awake intubation scenario for a difficult airway, appropriate patient selection and preparation is key to success. The patient should be able to cooperate and the airway management should be elective, as in the case of a known difficult airway. One of the key recommendations in the algorithm is to deliver supplemental oxygen throughout the process of managing the difficult airway. Awake fiberoptic intubation is described in detail later in this chapter. If intubation is unsuccessful, other options for airway management include supraglottic devices, transtracheal jet ventilation, or awake tracheostomy. A less desirable option would be to perform the procedure under local infiltration and regional anesthesia or abort the procedure completely. Retrograde intubation is also another option for invasive airway management.

American Society of
Anesthesiologists®
DIFFICULT AIRWAY ALGORITHM

1. Assess the likelihood and clinical impact of basic management problems:
   • Difficulty with patient cooperation or consent
   • Difficult mask ventilation
   • Difficult supraglottic airway placement
   • Difficult laryngoscopy
   • Difficult intubation
   • Difficult surgical airway access
2. Actively pursue opportunities to deliver supplemental oxygen throughout the process of difficult airway management.
3. Consider the relative merits and feasibility of basic management choices:
   • Awake intubation *vs.* intubation after induction of general anesthesia
   • Non-invasive technique *vs.* invasive techniques for the initial approach to intubation
   • Video-assisted laryngoscopy as an initial approach to intubation
   • Preservation *vs.* ablation of spontaneous ventilation
4. Develop primary and alternative strategies:

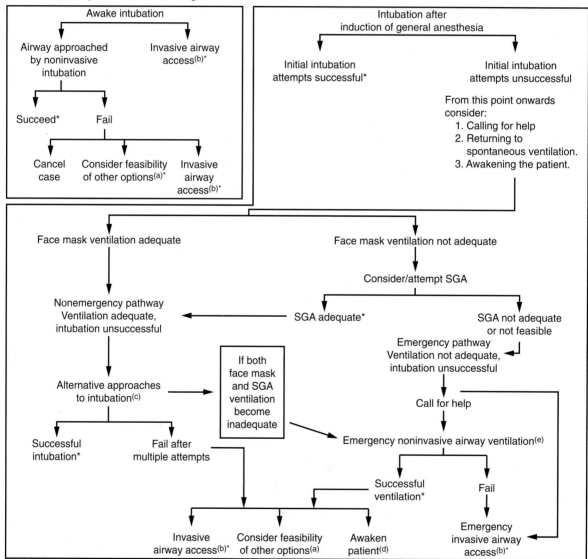

*Confirm ventilation, tracheal intubation, or SGA placement with exhaled CO$_2$.

a. Other options include (but are not limited to): surgery utilizing face mask or supraglottic airway (SGA) anesthesia (e.g., LMA, ILMA, laryngeal tube), local anesthesia infiltration or regional nerve blockade. Pursuit of these options usually implies that mask ventilation will not be problematic. Therefore, these options may be of limited value if this step in the algorithm has been reached via the Emergency Pathway.
b. Invasive airway access includes surgical or percutaneous airway, jet ventilation, and retrograde intubation.
c. Alternative difficult intubation approaches include (but are not limited to): video-assisted laryngoscopy, alternative laryngoscope blades, SGA (e.g., LMA or ILMA) as an intubation conduit (with or without fiberoptic guidance), fiberoptic intubation, intubating stylet or tube changer, light wand, and blind oral or nasal intubation.
d. Consider re-preparation of the patient for awake intubation or canceling surgery.
e. Emergency non-invasive airway ventilation consists of a SGA.

Fig. 49.10 American Society of Anesthesiologists difficult airway algorithm. *ILMA,* Intubating laryngeal mask airway; *LMA,* laryngeal mask airway; *SGA,* supraglottic airway. (From Apfelbaum JL, Hagberg CA, Caplan RA, et al. Practice Guidelines for Management of the Difficult Airway: An updated report by the American Society of Anesthesiologists Task Force on Management of the Difficult Airway. *Anesthesiology.* 2013;118:251–270.)

The asleep limb of the algorithm provides considerations for the unanticipated difficult airway, after general anesthesia has been induced. It may also be appropriate when managing the airway in an uncooperative patient. The algorithm is activated after the initial intubation attempts are unsuccessful, at which point the primary clinician calls for help. At this point, adequacy of mask ventilation is assessed. If mask ventilation is easy, alternative approaches to airway management are sought, including VL, using an alternative blade, supraglottic airway–guided intubation, use of an intubating stylet or tube exchanger, asleep fiberoptic intubation, and blind nasal or oral intubation. If this fails, a surgical airway should be considered. Alternatively, the patient is mask ventilated until paralysis wears off and subsequently awakened. The most challenging situation arises when mask ventilation is inadequate. At this point, supraglottic device placement should be considered and ventilation attempted. If supraglottic airway placement is unsuccessful, a "cannot intubate, cannot ventilate" situation exists. This is considered an airway emergency and the physician should call for additional help at this time. Other possible options for airway management at this time including the rigid bronchoscope, retrograde intubation, or jet ventilation. However, these specialty tools are rarely immediately available outside the operating room. If these options are unavailable or ineffective, an emergency surgical airway should be established.[27]

Techniques for Difficult Airway Management
Awake Flexible Fiberoptic Bronchoscopy.
Indirect laryngoscopy using the flexible fiberoptic bronchoscope is one of the most useful skills in the armamentarium of the anesthesiologist or the intensivist. It can be used in the awake and asleep patient and is considered a gold standard for difficult airway management.

There are several important indications for awake intubations, including[33]:
- Previous history of difficult intubation
- Predicted difficult mask ventilation
- Physical examination findings predictive of difficult intubation, such as small mouth opening, receding mandible, macroglossia, and a short neck
- Limited range of motion of cervical spine (cervical spine fusion, ankylosing spondylitis, rheumatoid arthritis)
- Congenital airway anomalies
- Morbid obesity
- Mediastinal masses
- Upper airway masses and obstruction, including tongue, tonsils, larynx, and thyroid masses
- Airway pathology, such as tracheomalacia
- Facial or airway trauma
- Unstable cervical spine, including presence of a cervical spine stabilizing device, such as a halo
- Severe hemodynamic instability

While many other techniques may be used for awake intubation, flexible fiberoptic bronchoscopy is perhaps the most widely used (Video 49.3). The advantages of an awake technique include the ability of the patient to protect one's own airway, maintain pharyngeal tone, and monitor one's own neurologic symptoms (in patients with cervical spine injury). The caveat is that the

---

> ### BOX 49.4 Checklist for Awake Fiberoptic Intubation
>
> **Equipment**
> ECG, blood pressure, and pulse oximetry measurement
> Oxygen source: nasal cannula or face mask
> Fiberoptic bronchoscope
> Light source and video monitor
> Ovassapian airway and other oral airways
> Atomizer
> Suction
> Endotracheal tubes of multiple sizes
>
> **Pharmacologic Preparation**
> Lidocaine 4% for nebulization and for spraying the vocal cords
> Oxymetazoline spray
> Viscous lidocaine 2% for topicalization of the oropharynx
> Sedatives (based on provider preference)
> - Dexmedetomidine
> - Midazolam
> - Analgesia: fentanyl
> Antisialagogue: glycopyrrolate

---

patient must be cooperative and must be well topicalized (described in detail later in the chapter). While there are no absolute contraindications, it is difficult to perform in pediatric patients or uncooperative adults. It is also relatively contraindicated in patients with true local anesthetic allergy[41] (Box 49.4).

Preprocedure preparation. The success of a flexible fiberoptic intubation hinges heavily on appropriate patient preparation and preparedness for emergencies during the procedure. Every patient undergoing an intubation must have basic monitoring, including at least a three-lead ECG, pulse oximetry, and blood pressure monitoring. In addition, there must be good intravenous access. The patient should receive supplemental oxygen during the procedure.

The intubating physician should ideally be accompanied by an assistant, preferably another expert at airway management. In an urgent or emergent situation, a surgeon trained in performing a cricothyrotomy and tracheostomy should be readily available or even present at the time of the initial attempt.

A variety of airway equipment should be present for the procedure, ideally organized in a difficult airway cart. A nasal cannula and face mask should be used for preoxygenation. An appropriately sized working fiberoptic bronchoscope with a suction port, light source, and video monitor is the primary tool for this procedure. The bronchoscope should be lubricated and an antifogging solution should be applied to the tip of the scope to avoid fogging upon insertion. Some authors recommend placing the endotracheal tube in a warm water bath, which makes the plastic softer and the insertion less traumatic to the vocal cords.[26] Suction should be attached to the bronchoscope and must be in working condition. Multiple sizes and styles of endotracheal tubes should be in the cart and the appropriately sized tube should be loaded on the bronchoscope. Laryngoscope light handles and blades of various sizes and designs, endotracheal tube stylets, exchange catheters, gum-elastic bougie, and Magill forceps should be stored in the cart. In case of an unforeseen emergency, a variety of supraglottic airways in different sizes, esophageal tracheal Combitube, and a video laryngoscope should be readily available. Other equipment that should be in the airway cart include an emergency percutaneous cricothyrotomy kit, a nebulizer, atomization devices, a variety of oral airways (including the Ovassapian airway), and local anesthetic for topicalization.

Topicalization. Adequate topicalization of the airway by local anesthetic, commonly lidocaine, is the cornerstone of a successful intubation. Lidocaine is an amide local anesthetic. It is available in various concentrations, but the 2% and 4% are commonly used for airway topicalization. Cocaine is a potent vasoconstrictor in addition to being a local anesthetic and should be considered in nasal fiberoptic intubation.

There are a variety of devices used to topicalize the airways. We prefer to use a nebulizer to administer the 4% lidocaine to the pharynx, larynx, and tracheobronchial tree. The nebulizer delivers a fine mist of lidocaine at low oxygen flows and can be delivered with a mouthpiece device or a face mask. The patient is instructed to "pant like a dog" to allow the local anesthetic to reach the vocal cords. A standard dose is 4 mL of 4% lidocaine. However, a single method may not be adequate to achieve airway anesthesia. An atomizer can be used to deliver local anesthetic to the pharyngeal pillars, the oropharynx, and the vocal cords.

Another technique involves placing a cotton gauze or Q tip soaked in 4% viscous lidocaine in the oral cavity as deep as the patient can tolerate. The local anesthetic is allowed to drip in the oropharynx and laryngopharynx. An alternative is having 2% lidocaine in a syringe attached to the injection port of the bronchoscope, which allows for the "spray-as-you-go" approach and allows spraying of the vocal cords and other deeper structures during the intubation. In the nasal fiberoptic approach, local anesthetic–soaked pledgets are placed in the nare(s) identified for the intubation. A vasoconstrictor, such as oxymetazoline or phenylephrine, is sprayed in the nare(s) to prevent bleeding. Some physicians prefer to perform nerve blocks to anesthetize the airway. A variety of nerves—which are branches of the trigeminal, glossopharyngeal, and vagus nerves—supply the airway and should be blocked prior to airway instrumentation. The most common sites of blockade are the glossopharyngeal nerve at the palatoglossal arch, the superior laryngeal nerve at the superior cornu of the thyroid, and transtracheal lidocaine (Fig. 49.11).[42] Despite the technique(s) used for topicalization, vigilance must be maintained to avoid local anesthetic toxicity, especially in smaller patients, in whom a moderate amount of 4% lidocaine may result in toxic doses.

Premedication. The goal of premedication is to relieve the patient's anxiety and to reduce secretions, allowing for a clean

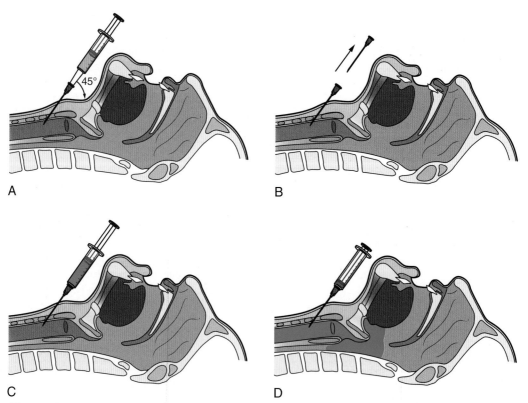

Fig. 49.11 Translaryngeal anesthesia (midsagittal view of the head and neck). (A) The angiocatheter is inserted at the cricothyroid membrane, aimed caudally. An aspiration test is performed to verify the position of the tip of the needle in the tracheal lumen. (B) The needle is removed from the angiocatheter. (C) The syringe containing local anesthetic is attached and the aspiration test is repeated. (D) Local anesthetic is injected, resulting in coughing and nebulization of the local anesthetic (shaded area). (From *The Retrograde Cookbook*. University of California, Irvine Medical Center, Department of Anesthesia.)

and dry airway during the procedure. Most endoscopists prefer to give an antisialogue, such as glycopyrrolate 0.2 mg, barring any contraindications, approximately 30 minutes prior to topicalization. Glycopyrrolate is the preferred anticholinergic drug, since it does not cross the blood-brain barrier, avoiding sedative effects. Some endoscopists also give histamine (H_2) receptor blocker or proton pump inhibitors (PPI) for aspiration prophylaxis. Sedatives are generally avoided in these patients. If needed, low doses of short-acting benzodiazepines, such as midazolam, are preferred for their rapid onset and short duration of action. Low-dose fentanyl or remifentanil are well tolerated during the procedure. However, opiates should be avoided in patients with a high risk of respiratory depression or those in respiratory failure. Low-dose propofol, ketamine, or dexmedetomidine can be safely titrated to the patient's hemodynamics and respiratory rate.[33]

Procedure: orotracheal intubation. The patient should be positioned supine or sitting in a beach chair–like position. The endoscopist should be at the head of the supine patient or in front of the sitting patient.

After appropriate topicalization, premedication, and patient education, the indirect laryngoscopy is performed via the oral or nasal route. Prior to bronchoscopy, an appropriately sized endotracheal tube (ETT) is loaded and secured to the bronchoscope (Fig. 49.12). The scope is inserted in the midline via the oral cavity. Typically, an assistant can gently grasp the patient's tongue and provide gentle traction while the endoscopist maneuvers the scope past the base of the tongue, while staying in the midline. Some physicians prefer the use of oral airways—such as the Ovassapian, Berman, or Williams airways—to guide

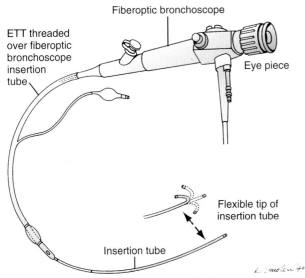

Fig. 49.12 Fiberoptic bronchoscope (FOB) with endotracheal tube (ETT) threaded over the insertion end of the FOB. The ETT is secured to the body of the FOB with a piece of tape. The distal (insertion) end of the FOB is lubricated with a silicone-based fluid; the cuff of the ETT is deflated. The tip of the FOB can be flexed in only one plane. To maneuver the FOB in other planes, the scope itself must be longitudinally twisted. (From Zupan J. Fiberoptic bronchoscopy in anesthesia and critical care. In: Benumof JL, ed. *Clinical Procedures in Anesthesia and Intensive Care*. Philadelphia: Lippincott-Raven; 1992:258.)

the bronchoscope. However, these may induce gagging in awake patients. Once the scope is positioned in the oropharynx, the tip is flexed to visualize the epiglottis and vocal cords. Once the tip passes beyond the epiglottis, it is directed toward the anterior commissure of the vocal cords and then flexed posteriorly to enter the trachea. The trachea is identified by the presence of anterior tracheal rings. The bronchoscope is advanced until the carina is visualized. At this point, the ETT is directed gently over the fiberoptic scope into the trachea. Occasionally, the tube impinges on the right arytenoid and resistance is met during advancement. At this point, it should be withdrawn slightly and rotated counterclockwise so that the Murphy eye is positioned posteriorly. The ETT is positioned above the carina and the depth confirmed while the scope is withdrawn.[26]

Flexible fiberoptic bronchoscopy can be combined with other airway devices in the most challenging airway situations. It can be combined with an Aintree catheter through a regular LMA or by itself with an intubating LMA, such as a Fastrach or the Ambu Aura-i (Ambu A/S). It can also be combined with DL or VL to lift a redundant epiglottis or in cases of upper airway edema.[33]

Laryngeal Mask Airway in the Difficult Airway. The LMA is a critical component of the difficult airway algorithm. It is used as a rescue tool in a "cannot intubate, cannot ventilate" scenario. The LMA is successful in these scenarios because of how it is designed. It seats in the hypopharynx and does not rely on direct laryngeal visualization. Therefore many factors that are associated with a difficult laryngoscopy do not affect placement and ventilation through the LMA.

The use of an LMA as a conduit for intubation was initially described in 1984.[43] It soon gained popularity for airway management after failed intubation attempts. The LMA was incorporated as a rescue tool in the ASA's practice guidelines for difficult intubation in 1993. A review of the use of the LMA in the ASA difficult airway algorithm was published in 1996. It recommended that the LMA be considered in other situations than just as a rescue in the emergency pathway: as a conduit for fiberoptic bronchoscopy during awake intubation (awake limb of the difficult airway algorithm), as an aid to endotracheal intubation in the anesthetized patient (asleep limb of difficult airway algorithm), and for definitive airway placement in nonemergency situations (as a rescue ventilatory device in the emergent pathway, after which it can be used as a conduit for tracheal intubation).[44] Based on these recommendations, the LMA has now found its place in the difficult airway algorithm as more than just a rescue device.

The Fastrach Intubating LMA (LMA North America; Fig. 49.13) was designed to facilitate blind or fiberoptic tracheal intubation through it. It is available only in adult size. It consists of a curved, rigid conduit with a 13-mm internal diameter attached to the end of the LMA. The angle of the metal tube is such that it fits the oropharyngeal space without requiring cervical extension. Proximally, the shaft forms a standard 15-mm connector for the anesthesia circuit and acts as a guiding handle to stabilize the LMA during intubation. The LMA is inserted in a standard fashion. Once it seats appropriately and placement is

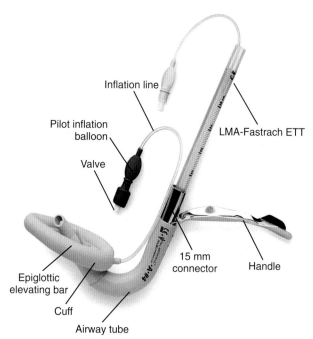

Fig. 49.13 Fastrach laryngeal mask airway. *ETT,* Endotracheal tube.

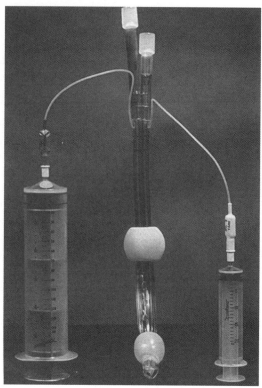

Fig. 49.14 Two longitudinally fused tubes comprise the Combitube; both cuffs are inflated with their corresponding syringes. Lumen No. 1 is the longer tube located on the left and lumen No. 2 is on the right. (From Wissler RN. The esophageal-tracheal Combitube. *Anesthesiol Rev.* 1993;20:147–151.)

confirmed by capnography, the intubating LMA is rotated in the sagittal plane until resistance to ventilation is minimal and then gently lifted using the rigid handle during passage of the ETT. ETT placement is confirmed by auscultation and capnography, after which the rigid intubating LMA is removed to prevent pressure on surrounding tissues.

Many new devices with improved features for endotracheal intubation are now available. These include the Ambu Aura-i (Ambu A/S), i-gel (Intersurgical Ltd.), and the air-Q (Cookgas LLC; Mercury Medical), among others. The air-Q and i-gel are popular for airway management and as a conduit for endotracheal intubation in the pediatric population.[45]

Esophageal-Tracheal Double-Lumen Airways. In the era of VL, esophageal-tracheal double-lumen airways are rarely encountered in the hospital but are still used by emergency medical personnel in the field. Two such devices, the Combitube (Covidien) and the EasyTube (Rüsch EasyTube, Teleflex Medical), are widely described in the literature and can be used in the emergent or elective setting. These devices can be encountered in patients who have required airway management in the prehospital setting, such as in trauma or cardiac arrest.

The Combitube (Fig. 49.14) is a double-cuff, double-lumen tube. The oropharyngeal balloon is in the middle portion of the tube, while the tracheal cuff is at the end. It is inserted blindly until the printed rings lie at the teeth. Both cuffs are then inflated. It is available in two sizes, 37 Fr and 41 Fr. The pharyngeal lumen is closed distally and has eight perforations between the esophageal and tracheal cuffs. These perforations allow ventilation when the tube is positioned in the esophagus (Fig. 49.15). When the device is placed in the trachea, ventilation occurs through the tracheal lumen (Fig. 49.16). The esophageal lumen allows for

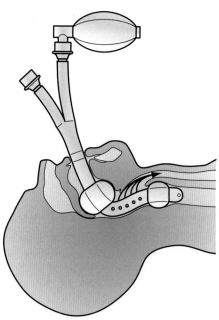

Fig. 49.15 Typical ventilator pattern when the Combitube is blindly placed in the esophagus. (Modified from Wissler RN. The esophageal-tracheal Combitube. *Anesthesiol Rev.* 1993;20: 147–151.)

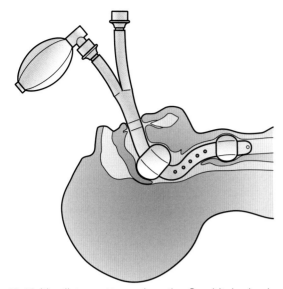

Fig. 49.16 Ventilator pattern when the Combitube is placed in the trachea. Tracheal positioning of the Combitube is rare; more than 97% of the time the Combitube will enter the esophagus when placed blindly. (Modified from Wissler RN. The esophageal-tracheal Combitube. *Anesthesiol Rev.* 1993;20:147–151.)

passage of a suction catheter into the stomach, hence decreasing the risk of aspiration. The blind insertion, standard sizing, and no preparation make this device ideal for use in the prehospital environment where there is limited space and lighting. It can also be placed with ease by untrained personnel and does not require neck extension. The disadvantages include inability to suction the trachea when placed in the esophagus and a higher incidence of oral complications, similar to the LMA.[33]

The EasyTube is similar in construct to the Combitube. The main difference is that it is made of nonlatex material and has a proximal lumen that ends below the oropharyngeal balloon, allowing passage of a tube exchanger or bronchoscope. A study comparing insertion times of these two devices showed shorter insertion times with the EasyTube.[46]

Retrograde Intubation. Retrograde intubation is a well-established technique that involves endotracheal intubation over a flexible guidewire placed percutaneously through the cricothyroid membrane and guided cephalad through the larynx and pharynx out of the mouth. It is indicated when the view of the vocal cords is obstructed by blood or secretions, in patients with an unanticipated difficult airway, and limited airway opening, such as in maxillofacial trauma or trismus. It can also be used in lieu of fiberoptic intubation in developing countries where resources are limited. It has been described as an alternative approach for tracheal intubation in the ASA difficult airway algorithm. It is a minimally invasive technique that can be accomplished rapidly in both the supine and seated positions.

The classic description of the procedure involves puncturing the cricothyroid membrane and using an epidural catheter as a guidewire. Practically, an intravenous catheter can be used along with a standard guidewire, which can pass through it. Ideally, the wire should be twice as long as the ETT. An 18-g catheter

can accommodate a guidewire that is 0.038 inches in diameter and 110 cm long. Commercial kits are also available. Once the patient is positioned, the nondominant hand stabilizes the cricothyroid cartilage while the dominant hand is used to insert an 18-g angiocatheter attached to a saline-filled syringe through the cricothyroid membrane. Once air bubbles are seen in the syringe, the needle is removed and local anesthetic can be instilled through it to achieve a transtracheal block. The guidewire is advanced until it exits out of the nose or mouth. This may be assisted by DL. An ETT or an exchange catheter can be passed over the wire into the trachea. Complications include bleeding; injury to the esophagus, oropharynx, and trachea; subcutaneous emphysema; pneumomediastinum; and pneumothorax.[26]

Invasive Airway Access

Transtracheal jet ventilation. Transtracheal jet ventilation is an invasive technique used for oxygenation and ventilation in the management of a difficult airway. Jet ventilation through a rigid bronchoscope is commonly used in the operating room during interventional pulmonology procedures and laryngeal surgery. It is mentioned in the ASA difficult airway algorithm as a rescue modality during the emergent management of the difficult airway. It is not readily available outside the operating room, thus limiting its usefulness.

A needle cricothyrotomy is performed using a large catheter, ideally 12 Fr or 16 Fr in size. A special 6 Fr catheter (Cook Critical Care) designed to prevent kinking is also available. The technique for catheter insertion is identical to retrograde intubation; in this case, however, the bevel is directed caudad (Fig. 49.17). The jet ventilator is attached to the catheter and the lung is insufflated. Expiration occurs passively as the lung and chest wall recoil when insufflation is released. Expiration occurs through the glottis. Having an unobstructed upper airway is vital to preventing complications. If the upper airway is obstructed, an oropharyngeal or nasopharyngeal airway should be placed to promote egress of oxygen. An urgent surgical airway is mandated once adequate oxygenation and ventilation is established. Oxygen saturation and chest recoil should be monitored to assess adequacy of translaryngeal insufflation.[33]

Adequate time for expiration should be allowed in order to prevent hypercarbia and barotrauma. Barotrauma may result in a pneumothorax from delivering high pressure oxygen. Other complications include subcutaneous and mediastinal emphysema, bleeding, aspiration, and injury to the trachea and esophagus. Transtracheal jet ventilation should not be performed in patients with laryngeal injury and is relatively contraindicated in coagulopathic patients or those with distorted anatomy.[26]

Cricothyrotomy. Cricothyrotomy is an invasive, life-saving procedure. It is included in the ASA difficult airway algorithm for emergency airway management when all other techniques have failed and the patient is at risk of decompensation.[27] Percutaneous cricothyrotomy kits are readily available and should be included in emergency airway supplies.

There are relatively few contraindications to a cricothyrotomy. Patients with preexisting laryngeal diseases have a high incidence of complications with the procedure. There is a high incidence

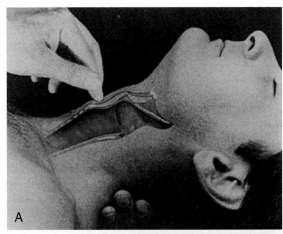

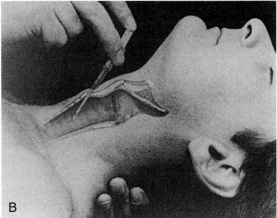

Fig. 49.17 (A) A 14-gauge angiocatheter passing through the cricothyroid membrane at an angle approximately 30 degrees caudad from the skin. (B) After achieving this position, the metal stylet is withdrawn and a syringe is applied to the catheter to confirm intratracheal position; aspiration of air is the expected endpoint if the 14-gauge catheter is truly in the tracheal lumen. (From Benumof JL, et al. Transtracheal ventilation. In: Benumof JL, ed. *Clinical Procedures in Anesthesia and Intensive Care.* Philadelphia: Lippincott-Raven; 1992:199.)

of subglottic stenosis in patients who have been translaryngeally intubated for greater than or equal to 7 days. It may be difficult to perform in patients with distorted neck anatomy. Patients with coagulopathy may experience bleeding.

In children younger than 6 years, the cricothyroid membrane is the narrowest portion of the airway, and the thyroid isthmus nearly approaches the cricothyroid membrane. Therefore cricothyrotomy is contraindicated in this group of patients and a tracheostomy is the preferred approach.

The procedure can be performed percutaneously or open. The percutaneous technique is preferred by anesthesiologists and intensivists. This procedure employs the Seldinger technique and can be easily performed using commercially available kits. The patient's neck is extended and the cricoid cartilage is palpated. The cricothyroid membrane is identified and punctured at a 45-degree angle directed caudad with an 18-g needle and catheter attached to a saline-filled syringe. When free air is aspirated, the needle is in the trachea. Next, the needle and syringe are removed and a guidewire is inserted 2 to 3 cm into the trachea through the catheter. The catheter is removed and a curved dilator with the airway cannula is advanced over the wire, maintaining control of the guidewire. Once the airway cannula is seated, the guidewire and dilator are removed together, the cuff is inflated, and bag-mask ventilation attempted. Placement is confirmed by auscultation.[26]

A surgical cricothyrotomy is performed when equipment for the percutaneous approach is not available (Fig. 49.18). It only requires a No. 20 scalpel and an ETT. The neck is extended and a horizontal stab incision is made through the skin and cricothyroid membrane. If the anatomy is not palpable, a vertical skin incision should be made. Once the cricothyroid membrane is identified, an incision is made in its lower half and a tracheal hook inserted to exert upward and outward light traction on the thyroid cartilage. The ETT is inserted, the cuff inflated, and low-pressure ventilation is initiated to confirm placement.[47]

The procedure is usually performed emergently. Complications include injury to the posterior tracheal wall or esophagus, vocal cord damage, thyroid laceration, bleeding, and subcutaneous or mediastinal emphysema from placement of the airway in subcutaneous tissue. Subglottic stenosis is a known late complication.

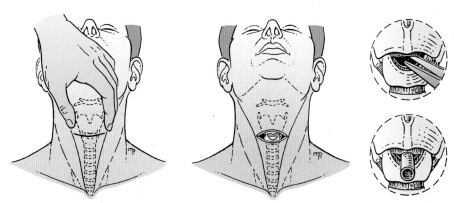

Fig. 49.18 Horizontal skin incision *(left)*, incision of cricothyroid membrane *(middle)*, dilation of the opening *(upper right)*, and introduction of a ventilation tube *(lower right)*. (From Biro P, et al. Transtracheal access and oxygenation techniques. *Acta Anesth Scand.* 1998;42:169.)

Tracheostomy. Emergent tracheostomy is rarely performed because of the high incidence of bleeding associated with it. Tracheostomy differs from cricothyrotomy in the location of entry into the airway. In a tracheostomy, the airway is entered at or below the first tracheal ring. In the emergent situation, a vertical incision is made in the neck along the midline. This minimizes bleeding and avoids the anterior jugular veins. The skin and subcutaneous tissues are incised with the scalpel through the platysma and strap muscles. Once the tracheal rings are exposed, a horizontal incision is made between the first and second tracheal rings. The tracheostomy tube is rapidly introduced into the trachea and ventilation is initiated. An elective tracheostomy is shown in Fig. 49.19.

EMERGENCY AIRWAY MANAGEMENT COMPLICATIONS

Elective airway management has become increasingly safe over the years, with a low incidence of minor complications. Complications are more likely to occur in a difficult airway or the failed intubation. The incidence of failed intubation is approximately 1 in 1000 to 2000 in the elective setting,[48] compared to 1 in 50 to 100 in the emergency department (ED) and ICU.[49] Emergency airway management is a precarious procedure, generally required in the sickest of patients. An analysis of emergency intubation in the ED by Mort showed a 7-fold increase in cardiac arrest and 14-fold increase in hypoxemia when more than two laryngoscopic

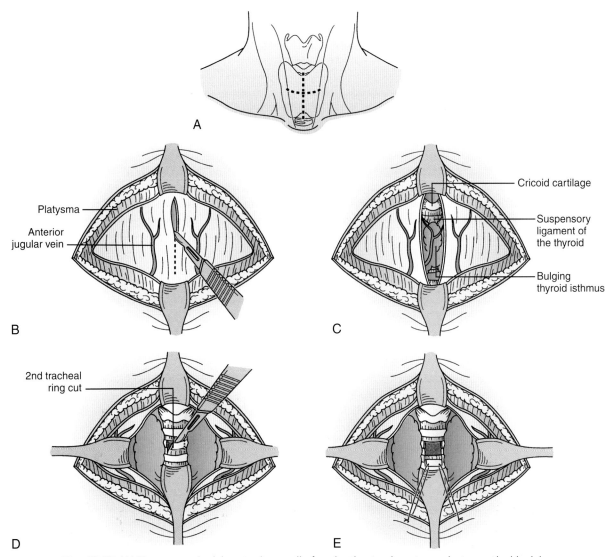

Fig. 49.19 (A) Transverse incision made usually for elective tracheostomy, but a vertical incision allows for less bleeding when an emergent procedure is done. (B) The strap muscles are separated and (C–D) thyroid isthmus retracted caudally. (E) After the second tracheal ring is cleaned off, an inferiorly based flap is developed in the tracheal wall and sutured to the skin to allow easy access to the trachea while the tract matures. (Neifeld JP. Head and neck. In: Greenfield LJ, et al, eds. *Surgery: Scientific Principles and Practices.* Philadelphia: Lippincott-Raven; 1997:644.)

attempts were made.[50] Complications from emergency airway management can be put into two main categories: (1) hemodynamic alterations and associated complications and (2) airway-related complications.

Hemodynamic Complications

Intubation is a significant stressor for the critically ill patient; it can cause major hemodynamic changes that can ultimately result in cardiac arrest and anoxic brain injury from severe hypoxemia.

Hyperdynamic Response to Airway Management. Laryngoscopy and airway manipulation can result in a brisk hyperdynamic response that may manifest as hypertension and tachycardia. The patients at the highest risk include those with neurologic injuries, trauma, sepsis, and patients younger than 50 years.

The hyperdynamic response is indicative of many physiologic variables, including level of consciousness, nature of the airway manipulation, underlying cardiovascular disease, and intravascular volume status. Tachycardia and hypertension may persist beyond the intubation in patients with altered autonomic responses, such as diabetics, patients in renal failure, and those with underlying cardiovascular disease. Postintubation manipulation of the airway, such as with suctioning or ventilator dyssynchrony, may also result in a catecholamine surge.

Patients in the cardiac ICU (CICU) with respiratory failure are typically on the verge of cardiopulmonary arrest. The hyperdynamic response may increase myocardial oxygen consumption, promoting myocardial ischemia and infarction in the diseased heart. Elevated catecholamines sensitize the myocardium to ectopy, predisposing to arrhythmias that may be poorly tolerated. In patients with underlying aortic disease, such as aortic dissections and aneurysms, tachycardia and hypertension may exacerbate the extent of the dissection or cause aortic rupture. In postcardiotomy patients, this response may result in bleeding and potentially cause tamponade. Other morbidities associated with the hyperdynamic response include acute right ventricular (RV) and left ventricular (LV) failure, altered flow dynamics in underlying valvular heart disease, and increased cerebral blood flow and pressure increasing the risk of an intracranial hemorrhage in the susceptible patient. Postintubation, the patient may experience hypotension and subsequent cardiovascular collapse. A combination of induction agents, opiates, local anesthetics, paralytics, and vasoactive medications tailored to the individual patient should be used to prevent the hyperdynamic response.[50,51]

Hypotension. Hypotension in the postintubation setting is due to the combination of a myriad of hemodynamic alterations. The vasodilatory and occasional myocardial depressant effects of induction agents—as well as attenuation of the sympathetic response from hypoxia and hypercarbia—may contribute to hypotension. In patients with hypovolemia, hemorrhage, sepsis, and underlying myocardial depression, especially RV dysfunction, the initiation of positive pressure ventilation and positive end expiratory pressure (PEEP) will also contribute to postintubation hypotension.[52] Positive pressure ventilation will decrease venous return to the right heart, which will lower the preload. It also increases RV afterload, resulting in reduced LV filling pressures

and hence, decreased stroke volume. Postintubation hypotension is associated with poor outcomes and prolonged hospital length of stay, especially in traumatized and neurologically injured patients.[53]

Bradycardia. Bradycardia may result from vagotonic stimulation due to prolonged laryngoscopy and, in severe and prolonged hypoxemia, during failed intubations. Patients with intrinsic atrioventricular (AV) nodal disease and those on AV nodal blocking drugs—such as β-blockers, calcium channel blockers, and amiodarone—are prone to bradycardia. High-dose opiates (such as fentanyl) or sedatives (such as dexmedetomidine) may also predispose to bradycardia by drastically reducing the sympathetic tone. Hypoxemia is the primary cause of bradycardia in the pediatric population, especially infants. Bradycardia results in reduced CO and, therefore, hypotension. Several database analyses have noted that bradycardia preceded cardiac arrest in 90% of cases.[50,54] With the aggressive implementation of the ASA difficult airway algorithm and the availability of rescue devices, such as the LMA and fiberoptic bronchoscopy, the incidence of bradycardia and cardiac arrest following intubation has decreased by up to 50%.[55]

Arrhythmias. Arrhythmias may occur during airway instrumentation or immediately after it. The most common are supraventricular tachycardias, such as atrial fibrillation or atrial flutter with rapid ventricular response. An abnormal rhythm is usually poorly tolerated in the critically ill patient, especially in patients with underlying cardiac disease.

Certain drugs, such as succinylcholine,[50] have been associated with dysrhythmias. In the postcardiotomy patient, epinephrine and dopamine infusions may also predispose to rhythm disturbances.

Cardiac Arrest. Emergent intubation outside the operating room is associated with a high risk of cardiac arrest. It can be precipitated by a multitude of factors, such as multiple attempts, failed intubation, hypoxemia, and aspiration. Most patients in the ICU already have a low cardiovascular reserve and may not be able to tolerate the hemodynamic changes associated with induction and intubation. The Adult Cardiac Life Support (ACLS) algorithm should be followed during a cardiac arrest. The best way to prevent and respond emergently to a cardiac arrest after intubation is to preempt it in the sickest patient and to be prepared with appropriate medications and defibrillator prior to intubation.

Airway-Related Complications

The end result of most airway-related complications is hypoxemia. It can occur as a result of multiple intubations in the case of a difficult airway, esophageal intubation, aspiration, and mainstem bronchus intubation.

Hypoxemia. Hypoxemia is the most common complication of endotracheal intubation in the critically ill patient. Unlike in an elective intubation, the rapidly decompensating patient in the CICU is unlikely to get effective preoxygenation. Noninvasive ventilation should be optimized prior to attempting laryngoscopy.

Modalities such as the standard cannula, high-flow nasal cannula, and the non-rebreather mask should be used in these patients. Mask ventilation may be limited in patients who are obese, have facial trauma, poor dentition, beard, older age, and in patients who require a rapid sequence intubation.[56] A recent study compared pre- and periprocedure oxygenation using a high-flow nasal cannula with a non-rebreather in patients with mild to moderate hypoxemia and found significantly less hypoxemia during intubation on the high-flow device.[3]

The patient's underlying diagnosis may also predispose to hypoxemia. It is more likely during intubation in patients with pulmonary disease such as pneumonia and chronic obstructive pulmonary disease (COPD). Hypoxemia may also occur during the airway management of patients with ischemic and embolic stroke, cardiogenic shock, acute myocardial infarction, congestive heart failure (CHF), and upper gastrointestinal bleeding.[57]

The physiologic consequences of hypoxemia vary with the peripheral capillary oxygen saturation (S_pO_2) and partial pressure of oxygen (PaO_2). A hyperdynamic response with hypertension and tachycardia is seen in mild hypoxemia. However, once the oxygen saturation is below 60% or the PaO_2 is around 30 mm Hg, the heart rate starts to decrease and the patient may progress to profound bradycardia and asystole.

Esophageal Intubation. The lack of recognition of esophageal intubation is a rare but catastrophic complication. It leads to severe hypoxemia, increases the risk of regurgitation and aspiration, and can cause severe anoxic brain injury and death. Failure to recognize an esophageal intubation is not just limited to inexperienced proceduralists or resident physicians. Because of its grave consequences, the use of multiple modalities to confirm ETT placement, such as capnography, should be used. The proceduralist should have a low threshold to verify placement using a fiberoptic bronchoscope if the index of suspicion for esophageal intubation is high.[57] At the author's institution, use of a video laryngoscope during emergency airway management is the preferred approach. This allows a supervising physician to verify ETT placement through the vocal cords as the proceduralist intubates, reducing the chances of a missed esophageal intubation.

Regurgitation and Aspiration of Gastric Contents. Emergency airway management increases the risk of regurgitation and aspiration compared to elective intubation. The incidence of regurgitation is anywhere from 1.6% to 8.5%, while the aspiration risk is from 0.4% to 5%.[54] Patients at risk of aspiration include those with full stomachs, such as trauma or pregnant patients; obese individuals; and patients with gastrointestinal pathology, such as ileus, bowel obstruction, gastroparesis, and gastrointestinal bleeding. In these patients, an RSI is preferred. However, awake intubation or intubation in the lightly sedated patient can also help to maintain airway reflexes and prevent aspiration.

Mainstem Bronchial Intubation. Mainstem bronchial intubation is a common occurrence during elective and emergency intubations. Typically, the ETT is placed into the right mainstem bronchus and can lead to atelectasis, lobar collapse, hypoxemia,

and barotrauma due to overdistension. Placement of an ETT in the CICU should always be verified with a postprocedure chest radiograph[58] in addition to capnography and auscultation. The definitive tool for verification and optimal positioning of the ETT is fiberoptic bronchoscopy. Another quick method is the palpation of the cuff above the sternal notch, but this is subject to operator interpretation.

EXTUBATING THE PATIENT WITH A DIFFICULT AIRWAY

Planned tracheal extubation of the patient with a known difficult airway should be conducted in a controlled manner with providers present who are skilled in airway management. The ASA Task Force on Management of the Difficult Airway states that planned extubation is a logical extension of the intubation process and therefore should be planned with a goal-oriented strategy.[27] The checklist for emergency airway management, outlined in Box 49.1, should be included in the planning process for extubation of patients with known difficult airway and the need for emergent reintubation should be anticipated, as reintubation of critically ill patients is a common event in the ICU setting. Demling and colleagues studied the incidence of emergent reintubation of ICU patients and found that 4% to 12% required emergent reintubation.[59] In this study, risk factors for reintubation included a history of previous difficult intubation, airway edema secondary to surgical manipulation and/or volume resuscitation, morbid obesity, and an immobilized or unstable cervical spine.[59]

Preparation for planned extubation in the critically ill patient requires optimization and, ideally, resolution of the pathophysiologic processes that required ventilatory support. These may include hypoxia, hypercarbia, interstitial lung disease, acute respiratory distress syndrome (ARDS), or many other causes of respiratory failure in the ICU setting. In addition, other physiologic parameters—such as neurologic function, respiratory function, respiratory muscle strength, hemodynamic stability, acid-base status, renal function and fluid balance, and the mechanics of the upper airway—must be considered prior to planned extubation. Sedative and analgesic medication dosing and frequency must be adjusted prior to extubation with the pharmacokinetics of these medications taken into consideration in the time leading up to a planned extubation. Sedative drugs that cause loss of pharyngeal tone include benzodiazepines, opioids, and adjunctive analgesics, such as α_2-agonists. Ideally, time should be allowed for sufficient clearance of these medications prior to extubation to maximize pharyngeal muscle tone.[60]

Anticipation of challenges following extubation should also guide planning and preparation for extubation. For example, patients with preexisting obstructive sleep apnea, obesity, or upper airway pathology may benefit from an upright position at extubation combined with immediate continuous positive airway pressure (CPAP) therapy following extubation. Thus, a CPAP or bilevel positive airway pressure (BiPAP) machine should be readily available at extubation for such patients. In addition, planning for extubation of a patient who required VL for intubation should include a video laryngoscope at the bedside in anticipation of a repeated difficult intubation. Any airway adjuncts used during establishment of the patient's airway at intubation should also be available at the time of extubation.

An airway exchange catheter (AEC) may be used at extubation for patients identified as having difficult airways. This technique involves utilization of a thin, flexible, open lumen AEC such as the Cook AEC (3.7 mm 11 Fr, 4.7 mm 14 Fr, 6.3 mm 19 Fr; Cook Critical Care) inserted into the ETT lumen, then extubation of the ETT over the AEC, followed by an observation period while the AEC remains in place in the airway secured with waterproof tape to the patient's forehead for up to 1 hour. Should the need for reintubation arise, a skilled provider may utilize DL or VL to guide an ETT over the AEC into the appropriate position in the trachea. In an observational analysis of 278 patients requiring reintubation following extubation in the ICU setting, the first-pass success rate of an attending anesthesiologist performing reintubation without an adjunctive device such as an AEC was 14%, whereas the first-pass success rate of reintubation using an AEC was 87%.[61] During usage of an AEC, one must remain cognizant of the depth of insertion of the AEC, which is recommended to be inserted to the depth of the ETT. In an emergency scenario, the open-lumen feature of the AEC allows for oxygenation using an adapter that is commonly supplied within the AEC kit. However, it is recommended that oxygen insufflation through an AEC occur only during an emergency scenario owing to reports of barotrauma following jet insufflation through an AEC.[62]

Following extubation of a critically ill patient, close observation is necessary to detect signs of impending respiratory failure, upper airway obstruction, hypoxia, hypercapnia, and need for reintubation. Although staff in critical care settings have advanced airway management skills, inexperienced staff may not recognize early signs of impending airway obstruction in the postextubation period.[63] Of particular note in the CICU, signs of hypercarbia and hypoxia may manifest as subtle changes in pulmonary arterial pressures, hemodynamic instability, and acid–base status and, thus, may not present as visible respiratory retractions or audible stridor. Therefore, observation by a skilled practitioner is critical to identify patients who may require intervention following extubation.

MANAGEMENT IN VARIOUS CLINICAL SCENARIOS

When managing the airway of a patient with cardiac disease, maintenance of hemodynamic stability is important. The pathophysiology of the patient's cardiac disease and/or clinical scenario may alter the selection of induction agents or ventilation parameters. Various clinical scenarios and implications for airway management will be reviewed here.

Full Cardiopulmonary Arrest

During airway management of a patient in cardiopulmonary arrest, no induction agents are necessary. However, oxygen, suction, proper preparation, and patient positioning remain important. During cardiopulmonary resuscitation (CPR), management should follow the ACLS guidelines.[64] Airway management may begin with bag-mask ventilation and proceed to endotracheal intubation during prolonged CPR.

Respiratory Failure Owing to Airway Compromise

The airway expert should always be prepared to use transtracheal jet ventilation (TTJV) or to perform an emergent cricothyrotomy for the patient who has a compromised airway. Clinical signs of airway compromise are stridor, chest retractions, carbon dioxide retention, and, ultimately, hypoxia. Airway compromise can occur secondary to tumor, foreign body, trauma, epiglottis, laryngeal edema associated with anaphylaxis or drug allergy, and postoperative complications. Common postoperative causes of stridor include bleeding into a fresh surgical wound following neck surgery (carotid endarterectomy, thyroid, or parathyroid surgery) and soft tissue swelling following operations on the neck (i.e., anterior cervical diskectomy) and massive blood transfusion.

For the stridorous patient with impending airway obstruction, the primary directive should be to maintain airway patency and spontaneous ventilation until the airway is secured (i.e., a partial airway obstruction should not be transformed into a complete airway obstruction). Therefore, a controlled awake technique with topical anesthesia and using a fiberoptic bronchoscope or direct vision is the recommended approach. Blind techniques are not recommended because they may cause complete airway obstruction. Furthermore, emergency airway management in a patient with a suspected difficult airway or with stridor should be performed in the presence of another physician (preferably a surgeon) with particular expertise in obtaining a surgical airway.

Congestive Heart Failure

The patient who has respiratory insufficiency attributable to CHF has, by definition, inadequate CO and invariably manifests a high resting catecholamine state. The high sympathetic output serves to maintain cardiac reserve and vascular tone. One can occasionally temporize the patient with pulmonary edema with high-flow oxygen, noninvasive ventilation (BiPAP), and medical therapy. If the patient requires intubation, however, consideration should be given to initiating support with inotropic agents and invasive monitoring before commencing airway management. Furthermore, only very small doses of induction agents should be administered, as the loss of catecholamines may lead to hemodynamic instability.

Congenital Heart Disease

The maneuvers used to intubate the trachea in a patient with congenital heart disease can significantly alter the pathophysiologic expression of that disease. The airway expert must consider not only the effects of the drugs used on heart rate, rhythm, preload, afterload, and contractility but also the relative effects on pulmonary vascular resistance versus systemic vascular resistance and the resultant pulmonary versus systemic blood flow. Some lesions typically cause a predominant left-to-right shunt, whereas others cause a right-to-left shunt. Several lesions (i.e., hypoplastic left heart, transposition of the great vessels) can cause shunting in either direction, depending on the patient's specific anatomy

TABLE 49.1   Anesthesia Induction Considerations for Patients With Congenital Heart Disease

| | PATHOPHYSIOLOGIC EXPRESSION OF DISEASE | | | |
	Right-to-Left Shunt	Left-to-Right Shunt	Right Ventricular Obstruction	Left Ventricular Obstruction
Lesions responsible	ASD (late) TGV Tetralogy of Fallot[a] Tricuspid atresia	ASD (early) AV canal PDA[b] TAPVR, VSD	Pulmonary stenosis	Coarctation of the aorta Aortic stenosis[c]
Hemodynamic Goals				
Heart rate	↔, ↓[a]	↔	↓	↔, ↓,[c]
Rhythm	Sinus	Sinus	Sinus	Sinus
LV preload	↑	↑	↑	↑
SVR	↑↑	↓↓	↔	↓, ↑,[c]
PVR	↓↓	↑↑	↓↓	↔
Contractility	↔	↔↑	↔	↔
Induction drug considerations	These shunts are increased by decreasing SVR (large induction dose of sodium pentothal) or by increasing PVR (excessive positive-pressure ventilation, hypoxia, acidosis, hypercarbia).	Avoid pulmonary vasodilators; maintain on lower FiO₂; and avoid myocardial depressants. (If chest open, hypotension can be aided by surgically applied PA obstruction.)	Fairly fixed RV output. Will be made worse by increasing the PVR, or by decreasing the perfusion pressure to the hypertrophic RV (do not decrease the SVR or contractility).	Strong ventricle and necessarily so (do not decrease the contractility). For coarctation of aorta, may decrease SVR. For AS, keep rate slower and SVR high.

[a]If dynamic RV obstruction is operative, limit tachycardia.
[b]Occasionally, right-to-left shunt (hypoplastic left heart).
[c]Recommendations for coarctation of the aorta and aortic stenosis are the same except where indicated (HR and ↑ SVR recommendations apply to aortic stenosis).
ASD, Atrial septal defect; *AV*, arteriovenous; *LV*, left ventricular; *PA*, pulmonary artery; *PDA*, patent ductus arteriosus; *PVR*, pulmonary vascular resistance; *RV*, right ventricular; *SVR*, systemic vascular resistance; *TAPVR*, totally anomalous pulmonary venous return; *TGV*, transposition of the great vessels; *VSD*, ventricular septal defect; ↑, slightly increased; ↑↑, significantly increased; ↓, slightly decreased; ↓↓, significantly decreased; ↔, maintained stable without need for increase or decrease.

(caliber of the pulmonary vessels, size of an atrial septal defect, relative ventricular outflow obstruction, and so on) and physiologic state. Table 49.1 shows the common congenital lesions and hemodynamic manipulations that should be attempted.

Lesions that increase pulmonary blood flow are said to cause a left-to-right shunt. Emergency airway manipulations for patients with such lesions are designed to limit pulmonary perfusion and to increase systemic perfusion. This goal is achieved through manipulating pulmonary vascular resistance and systemic vascular resistance (PVR and SVR, respectively). If the PVR/SVR ratio is increased, less blood will flow to the lungs. Increasing PVR promotes the shunting of blood away from the lungs. The goal in these patients is not to increase PVR, but rather to avoid manipulations that decrease PVR. Maneuvers that decrease PVR include any that cause high FiO₂, hypocarbia, alkalosis, low mean airway pressure, and abolition of sympathetic simulation.

In patients with diminished pulmonary blood flow, anesthetic manipulations should be designed to improve flow through the pulmonary vasculature. Pulmonary blood flow can be promoted and right-to-left shunting reduced by decreasing the right heart to left heart pressure ratio. This can be done by maintaining a high FiO₂, promoting hypocarbia (through hyperventilation), eliminating acidosis, maintaining a low mean airway pressure, and achieving a normal or slightly elevated SVR. In the case of a fixed pulmonary outflow obstruction (such as tetralogy of

Fallot), changes in systemic vascular resistance may alter pulmonary blood flow more than similar changes in pulmonary vascular resistance. In a patient with a tetralogy of Fallot, infusion of phenylephrine frequently reduces intracardiac shunting and increases blood flow through the pulmonary system, improving oxygenation.

Valvular Heart Disease

Just as in congenital heart disease, anesthetic drug administration and emergency airway management in valvular heart disease can have a significant impact on the patient's physiology. Other chapters in this textbook have more completely addressed the pathophysiology of the various valvular lesions; thus, the subject will not be duplicated here. Nevertheless, a brief overview of the basic physiology and important hemodynamic goals suggested for safe emergency airway management are provided (Table 49.2).

Aortic stenosis (AS) is the most common cardiac valvular abnormality. The pathophysiology results from obstruction of the LV outflow at the valvular level, which leads to concentric hypertrophy of the LV myocardium. The LV end-diastolic pressure (LVEDP) is generally elevated to promote filling of the hypertrophied LV. Similarly, sinus rhythm is critical because left atrial contraction is required to fill the noncompliant LV. Myocardial contractility is typically preserved and is very important for stability in patients with AS. Hemodynamic goals include

TABLE 49.2   Anesthesia Induction Considerations for Patients With Valvular Heart Disease

	Aortic Stenosis	Aortic Insufficiency	Mitral Stenosis	Mitral Regurgitation
Pathophysiology	Concentric hypertrophy	Dilated LV, volume overloaded Stroke volume and ejection fraction maintained with preload reserve.	Dilated LA, ↑PAP, empty and protected LV May manifest as dyspnea, may be secondary to increased cardiac output (pregnancy or sepsis).	Dilated LA and LV, volume overloaded LV failure may be underdiagnosed because of regurgitant flow to LA despite severely decreased forward stroke volume.
Hemodynamic Goals				
Heart rate	↓↓	↑↑	↓↓	↑↑
Rhythm	NSR	—	Frequently in AF But, NSR→AF = ↓ BP	—
LV preload	↑	↑	↑	↑
SVR	↑↑	↓	↔	↓↓
PVR	↔	↔	↓ (these patients may have severe PA HTN)	↓
Contractility	↔↑	↔↑	↔	↔↑
Induction considerations	Avoid myocardial depression, maintain CA perfusion, pressure (↑SVR, ↑BP). Be prepared to perform cardioversion if an arrhythmia occurs (CPR may be unsuccessful). Treat hypotension with phenylephrine.	Minimize myocardial depression and keep the patient fast, full, and vasodilated. Dobutamine is a reasonable support drug at anesthesia induction.	Avoid tachycardia and extreme changes in preload. Do not decrease contractility. Inadequate sedation can precipitate extreme anxiety and tachycardia. Consider esmolol to treat tachycardia.	MVP is most common cause of isolated MR. Keep the patient fast, full, and vasodilated. Have several methods on hand to increase heart rate.

AF, Atrial fibrillation; *BP,* blood pressure; *CA,* coronary artery; *CPR,* cardiopulmonary resuscitation; *HTN,* hypertension; *LA,* left atrium; *LV,* left ventricle; *MR,* mitral regurgitation; *MVP,* mitral valve prolapse; *NSR,* normal sinus rhythm; *PAP,* pulmonary artery pressure; *SVR,* systemic vascular resistance; ↑, slightly increased; ↑↑, significantly increased; ↓, slightly decreased; ↓↓, significantly decreased; ↔, maintained stable without need for increase or decrease.

maintaining a low heart rate to give the ventricle a longer time to fill and to increase the relative diastolic time when the coronary arteries perfuse the hypertrophic LV. Preload should be high and SVR must be maintained on the relatively high side to augment coronary artery blood flow. Also, it must be recognized that the resistance that the LV ejects against in AS is at the valvular level and is not related to the SVR.

Patients with aortic insufficiency (AI) typically have volume overload physiology; stroke volume and ejection fraction are generally maintained through preload reserve and afterload reduction. The hemodynamic goals here are to maintain the heart rate in a relatively higher range to keep LV preload on the higher side and to minimize SVR to help promote forward flow. Contractility should be maintained but not increased.

Mitral stenosis (MS) is another valvular lesion with specific implications for choice of anesthesia induction. Patients with MS have a dilated left atrium and an underfilled but physiologically normal LV in the absence of other valvular lesions or myocardial disease. Patients with baseline normal sinus rhythm can manifest acute decompensated heart failure if they develop atrial arrhythmias. Thus, such patients should not be made anxious during airway manipulations. Hemodynamic goals for MS include reducing the heart rate, allowing time for blood to flow from the dilated volume-overloaded left atrium through the stenotic mitral valve and into the relatively underfilled LV. Normal sinus rhythm should be maintained (if the patient is in

this rhythm). Preload must be maintained, as hypovolemia will lead to decreased filling of the LV, while increased preload will lead to pulmonary edema.

Mitral regurgitation (MR) is the final valvular lesion with significant hemodynamic considerations for induction of anesthesia for emergency airway management. Patients with this lesion have LV volume overload physiology. The heart rate should be maintained in the higher range and LV preload should be elevated during anesthesia induction. The SVR should be kept low, however, to help the LV to eject blood in a forward direction rather than retrograde through the regurgitant mitral valve. Contractility should be maintained. Pharmacologic methods of increasing the heart rate (with atropine, epinephrine, isoproterenol) should be available in case the rate decreases with the manipulations used to control the airway.

Airway Management for Cardioversion

Direct-current cardioversion is commonly employed in the ICU setting. Synchronized cardioversion is used to convert supraventricular and ventricle arrhythmias to sinus rhythm. When the patient is hemodynamically stable and has an arrhythmia of long duration that does not respond to drug therapy, cardioversion can be performed electively.

Cardioversion is painful; thus, a light general anesthesia is required to allow the patient to undergo the procedure without remembering it or experiencing the pain. When cardioversion is performed electively, the patient should have fasted 8 hours before the procedure and should be monitored with pulse oximetry, blood pressure, and electrocardiogram. Anesthesia should not be induced until the cardiologist is ready to administer the countershock. At this time, the patient is preoxygenated and given small, incremental doses of anesthetic drug until no longer responsive.

Often, more than one shock is required for restoration of normal sinus rhythm and additional doses of intravenous medication may be required. Following the restoration of normal sinus rhythm, the patient is allowed to resume spontaneous ventilation; the mask should be held in place until the patient awakens and has control of the airway and gag response. No muscle relaxants should be used and intubation is not required unless the patient is prone to aspiration or has a full stomach.

If the cardioversion is performed on an emergent basis, it must be remembered that the patient has not fasted and intubation of the trachea may be appropriate. Furthermore, in hemodynamically unstable patients, a drug devoid of myocardial depressor or vasodilator effects, such as etomidate or ketamine, may be superior to propofol.

CONCLUSION

The morbidity and mortality of emergency airway management in critically ill patients can be decreased by carefully preparing the patient and clinician for the planned manipulation and by developing alternative plans before the initiation of airway management. Preparation helps the clinician avoid catastrophic complications, such as failed intubation, aspiration of gastric contents, and hemodynamic compromise.

Acknowledgments

We acknowledge the support and technical expertise of John Newman (Simulation Technology and Media Specialist, Department of Anesthesiology, Duke University Hospital) in the production of the airway videos for this chapter, and Rebecca Klinger (Assistant Professor, Department of Anesthesiology, Duke University Hospital) for performing the awake fiberoptic intubation.

We also acknowledge the contributions of Anushirvan Minokadeh and William C. Wilson, who were the authors of this chapter in the previous edition of the book.

The full reference list for this chapter is available at ExpertConsult.com.

50

Mechanical Ventilation and Advanced Respiratory Support in the Cardiac Intensive Care Unit

Mohamad Kenaan, Robert C. Hyzy

Compared to initial coronary care units dedicated to the monitoring of and rapid intervention in life-threatening ventricular arrhythmias in the setting of acute myocardial infarction (MI), cardiac intensive care units (CICUs) have evolved into models providing care for a broader spectrum of acute cardiovascular conditions along with increasing prevalence of noncardiac comorbidities.[1–5] Recent data suggested a further expansion in the role of CICUs to care for patients with secondary cardiovascular comorbidities presenting with acute noncardiac disease.[2,3] The treatment of respiratory failure and use of advanced respiratory support has become a common indication for CICU admission. For example, an acute MI can be complicated by pulmonary edema in up to 40% of patients admitted to intensive care units. Likewise, there has been an increase in the use of mechanical ventilation in CICUs.[2,3] This chapter provides a summary of commonly available modes of respiratory support, their physiologic effects, indications, and clinical issues related to cardiac patients. It focuses on the high-flow nasal cannula, noninvasive ventilation, and invasive mechanical ventilation. When available, data specific to patients with cardiogenic etiology of respiratory failure will be presented, although further studies are necessary to define best practices for these patients.

BASIC RESPIRATORY PHYSIOLOGY

Among the essential functions of the respiratory system, the two most commonly addressed in the critical care setting are ventilation and oxygenation. In normal respiration, the interplay between respiratory muscle action and chest wall compression with the compliance of the lungs, alveolar surface tension, and transpulmonary pressure determines the lung volumes at various stages of the respiratory cycle. Changes in lung volumes create a pressure differential that allows air to move in and out of the lungs. The tidal volume represents the volume of air inspired and expired with each breath. The tidal volume multiplied by the respiratory rate yields the minute ventilation. With each breath, part of the tidal volume occupies a portion of the respiratory system that is not involved in gas exchange, known as dead space ventilation, while the remaining portion that participates in gas exchange is known as alveolar ventilation. Alveolar ventilation allows gas exchange across the alveolar-capillary membrane down a pressure gradient. At the end of passive expiration, the outward recoil of the chest wall is counterbalanced by the elastic tendency of the lungs to collapse, maintaining the lung volume at the functional residual capacity (FRC). FRC not only helps to prevent atelectasis but also acts as an oxygen reservoir, maintaining steady partial pressure of oxygen (PaO_2). FRC can be affected by various physiologic and pathologic states. Pulmonary edema commonly encountered in the CICU is associated with reduced compliance of the lung and, therefore, decreased FRC.

HEART-LUNG INTERACTIONS

The cardiovascular and respiratory systems are intimately coupled given their complex connection and anatomic containment within the closed space of the thorax. Both spontaneous breathing and positive pressure ventilation can affect cardiovascular parameters by altering intrathoracic pressures, lung volumes, and metabolic demands. Analyzing the respirophasic changes in cardiac preload and afterload as well as the effect of hypoxia and hypercapnia on vascular resistance and myocardial contractility can provide a simplified summary of the complex heart-lung interactions during critical illness (Fig. 50.1). Understanding the hemodynamic alterations with positive pressure ventilation is essential for the management of complex patients in the CICU.[6–8]

Spontaneous Breathing

During spontaneous inspiration, the generation of a negative intrapleural pressure has multiple hemodynamic effects. It leads to an increase in the venous return and right ventricular (RV) preload and stroke volume owing to an increase in the pressure gradient between the right atrium (RA) and the mean venous systemic pressure.[9,10] Such a simplified summary of the effect of spontaneous inspiration on right-sided chamber filling and stroke volume ignores the effects of the inspiratory increase in lung volumes on pulmonary vascular resistance (PVR) and RV afterload. Although alveolar distention during inspiration causes compression of adjacent alveolar vessels and, therefore, an increase in PVR, these changes do not become clinically significant until lung volumes start approaching extremes (residual volume or total lung capacity).[11,12] Alternatively, being subjected to intrathoracic pressure changes, transmural aortic pressure, and left ventricular (LV) afterload increase with reduction in intrapleural pressure.[13,14] Owing to ventricular interdependence, reduced LV diastolic filling coupled with the increased LV afterload result in a mild decrease in stroke volume and systemic blood pressure during inspiration.[15–17] In healthy individuals, the change in LV

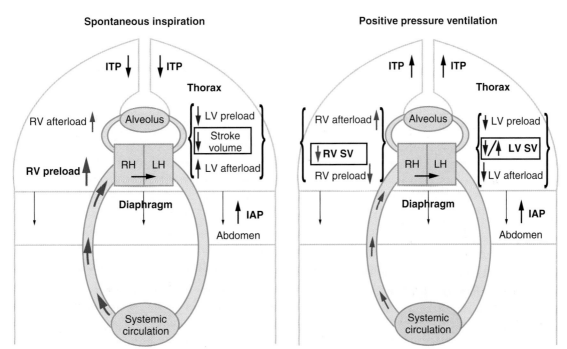

Fig. 50.1 Cardiopulmonary interactions during normal spontaneous inspiration and positive pressure ventilation. *IAP,* Intraabdominal pressure; *ITP,* intrathoracic pressure; *LH,* left heart; *LV,* left ventricle; *RH,* right heart; *RV,* right ventricle; *SV,* stroke volume.

stroke volume is not dramatic and is slightly offset by increased RV stroke volume during the next cycle. However, this effect can be amplified in conditions of exaggerated respiratory work or pathologic states with marked ventricular interdependence.

Positive Pressure Ventilation

To avoid alveolar derecruitment, many contemporary modalities of advanced respiratory support use and maintain positive airway pressure at end expiration. This baseline level of positive airway pressure is partially transmitted to the intrathoracic cavity at varying degrees depending on the compliance of the chest wall and lungs. The increase in intrathoracic pressure, in turn, is reflected as an increase in RA pressure, causing a reduction in the pressure gradient responsible for systemic venous return and ultimately a decrease in RV preload.[18,19] These changes are not as drastic as would be expected owing to a lesser degree of increased mean venous systemic pressure.[18–21] The increased intrapleural pressure and distention of the alveoli also lead to an increase in PVR and RV afterload.[22,23] Both effects translate to a reduction in RV stroke volume in patients treated with positive pressure ventilation.

The effects of positive pressure ventilation on the LV can be more complex and variable. Although the reduction in RV preload could potentially allow the interventricular septum to shift to the right and possibly improve LV compliance, this is usually offset by the increased RV afterload causing RV dilation, which, along with decreased RV stroke volume and increased lung volumes, result in decreasing LV preload.[24,25] Additionally, the increased intrapleural pressure leads to a reduction of LV afterload.[26,27] These changes can improve cardiac output (CO) or affect it adversely depending on the patient's specific loading conditions, underlying cardiac disease, and myocardial performance. For example, in hypovolemic patients or those with preload-dependent cardiac conditions such as cardiac tamponade, RV infarction, or aortic stenosis, positive pressure ventilation is likely to decrease CO. However, by decreasing afterload, improving myocardial oxygen demand and shifting the preload to a more optimal relationship on the Starling curve, patients with LV systolic dysfunction may demonstrate improvement in CO. Last, patients with severe pulmonary hypertension and RV dysfunction can experience deleterious hemodynamic effects and possible circulatory collapse with positive pressure ventilation owing to multiple factors, including increased RV afterload and worsened RV ischemia, in addition to medications needed for induction and sedation of mechanically ventilated patients. Mechanical ventilation is also associated with major humoral and autonomic changes that can have a significant effect on the cardiovascular system.[28–31] These effects can be complex and are beyond the scope of this chapter.

INDICATIONS FOR ADVANCED RESPIRATORY SUPPORT IN THE CARDIAC INTENSIVE CARE UNIT

No studies have specifically evaluated the indications for mechanical ventilation and advanced respiratory support in CICUs. Several multicenter studies including medical and surgical intensive care units have been conducted in the past decade to shed light on

the indications for mechanical ventilation. In the largest study of 412 ICUs, which included 1638 patients receiving mechanical ventilation, acute respiratory failure was the most common indication, accounting for 66% of the total study population (70% in the United States) with cardiogenic pulmonary edema being the third most prevalent cause of acute respiratory failure (13% of patients). Other causes for requiring advanced respiratory support included acute exacerbation of chronic respiratory disease (13%), coma, and neuromuscular disorders.[80] More recent, smaller multicenter prospective studies conducted in single countries have shown similar trends.[81,82] Despite a stable trend in the indications for mechanical ventilation, Esteban et al. showed an increase in the use of noninvasive ventilation (11.1% in 2004 compared to 4.4% in 1996).[83]

The most common need for mechanical ventilation in the CICU continues to be cardiogenic pulmonary edema due to various myocardial, pericardial, arrhythmic, or valvular disorders. The increases in cardiac filling pressures can flood the alveoli with transudative fluids and lead to significant ventilation-perfusion mismatch that causes significant hypoxia, increased work of breathing, and possible ventilatory failure and hypercapnia that can be further exacerbated by bronchial edema. Other indications for mechanical ventilation in the CICU include the following:

- States that result in loss of upper airway reflexes, increased risk of aspiration or hypoventilation/apnea, such as cardiac arrest, cardiogenic shock, or heavy sedation
- Management of respiratory comorbidities with acute or chronic pulmonary disease
- Concomitant neuromuscular disease
- Nosocomial and iatrogenic complications leading to respiratory failure (pulmonary embolism, hospital-acquired pneumonia, critical illness polyneuropathy, pneumothorax)
- Deep sedation required for procedures or in some patients with incessant unstable arrhythmias (ventricular tachycardia/electrical storm)

COMMON MODALITIES OF ADVANCED RESPIRATORY SUPPORT IN THE CARDIAC INTENSIVE CARE UNIT

As patients have presented with more complex cases and in attempts to reduce the need for endotracheal intubation, technological advancements have allowed the development of less invasive methods to treat respiratory failure. This was previously limited to noninvasive ventilation (NIV), but the more recent introduction of high-flow oxygen delivery via nasal cannula (HFNC) has provided a possible alternative in a select patient population.

HIGH-FLOW NASAL CANNULA OXYGEN

The limitations of conventional low-flow oxygen delivery (up to 15 L/min) provided by nasal prongs or face masks have been well recognized. In some patients with acute respiratory failure, the needed inspiratory flow could exceed 30 L/min and up to 120 L/min.[32,33] This mismatch of flow provided by conventional low-flow devices results in an inconsistent fraction of inspired oxygen (FiO_2) and insufficient oxygenation for the demands of critically ill patients. A high-flow nasal cannula system delivers optimally heated and humidified oxygen at up to 60 L/min with an adjustable FiO_2 in the driving gas.

Physiologic Effects of High-Flow Nasal Cannula Oxygen

In addition to improved patient comfort, evidence suggests that adequate heating and humidification of the inspired gas protects from some of the adverse effects of breathing dry and cold air, including mucosal inflammation, impaired mucociliary clearance, and bronchoconstriction.[34-38] Moreover, HFNC oxygen appears to be associated with improved oxygenation compared to conventional oxygen therapy with low-flow nasal cannula or face masks. The ability of HFNC oxygen to maintain flow rates equivalent to the inspiratory rates of patients with acute respiratory failure minimizes the dilution of delivered oxygen by entrainment of room air and allows for sustaining a constant and more reliable FiO_2.[39-42] An additional advantage is the ability of the HFNC systems to generate a small amount of positive airway pressure attributed to the resistance to expiratory flow generated by the continuous high flow of delivered gas. Studies conducted on healthy volunteers, postoperative patients, and critical care patients demonstrated variable degrees of positive airway pressure, ranging from 3 cm H_2O and up to 10 to 12 cm H_2O depending on flow rates, open-mouth breathing, and specific vendors.[41,43-47] Another benefit provided by HFNC therapy is to washout carbon dioxide from anatomic dead space, thus minimizing reinhalation of expired gas and improving alveolar ventilation. These physiologic effects, along with improving thoracoabdominal synchrony, are credited with the decreased work of breathing associated with the use of HFNCs.[34,35,48-50]

Effect of High-Flow Nasal Cannula Oxygen on Clinical Outcomes

Although the evidence regarding the improvement in clinical outcomes with HFNC therapy is not conclusive, several studies have shown promising results. In a randomized, multicenter trial of 310 patients, Frat and colleagues compared the impact of HFNC therapy to conventional oxygen therapy through a low-flow face mask or noninvasive ventilation on the rate of invasive mechanical ventilation for acute hypoxic respiratory failure. Patients randomized to HFNC demonstrated the lowest need for invasive mechanical ventilations (38% for the HFNC vs. 47% and 50% for conventional therapy and NIV, respectively) and the highest rate of ventilator-free days at 28 days in addition to the lowest 90-day mortality rate.[51] Another randomized trial comparing postextubation treatment with HFNC to NIV when used for postsurgical patients who were at high risk for or who developed acute respiratory failure showed that the HFNC was not inferior to NIV in regard to the requirement for reintubation.[52] These findings were not replicated in a meta-analysis of 14 trials that demonstrated no difference in mortality and intubation rates when treating acute hypoxic respiratory failure with HFNC compared to usual care.[53] The paucity of data about the use of the HFNC is more apparent in the CICU patient population. Patients with cardiogenic pulmonary edema were excluded from the randomized study by Frat et al. and were underrepresented in the other trials.[51] However,

given the improvement in oxygen delivery and generation of low levels of positive airway pressure, the HFNC would theoretically be of significant benefit in the treatment of cardiogenic pulmonary edema. In a small series reported by Carratala-Perales et al., five patients demonstrating persistent hypoxemia with conventional therapy were successfully treated for acute decompensated heart failure using HFNC therapy.[54]

HFNC oxygen therapy is highly promising as a treatment for mild to moderate acute hypoxic respiratory failure in CICUs. Further trials are necessary to help define the patient population that would benefit from this therapy, optimal flow-rate titration, predictors of therapy failure to avoid delays in escalation of therapy to mechanical ventilation, best rescue measures, and possible contraindications or adverse effects.

NONINVASIVE VENTILATION

NIV refers to forms of mechanical ventilatory support that do not require endotracheal intubation. These devices commonly use full oronasal masks or nasal masks that use a silicone rim to form a tight seal. NIV can be delivered in the form of continuous positive airway pressure (CPAP) providing a baseline supra-atmospheric pressure throughout the respiratory cycle improving alveolar recruitment, lung compliance, and oxygenation, or bilevel positive airway pressure (BiPAP) that adds noninvasive inspiratory positive airway pressure (IPAP) to the baseline expiratory positive airway pressure (EPAP), which would also improve ventilation.

Noninvasive Ventilation in Cardiogenic Pulmonary Edema

As NIV became more widely available, its role in the treatment of pulmonary edema was readily recognized and early data from small studies were promising. These studies suggested that the use of CPAP in patients with heart failure could be associated with improvement in oxygenation, reduction in work of breathing, and overall improvement in cardiac performance and CO.[55-58] In addition to these physiologic effects, small randomized trials emerged associating the use of NIV for the treatment of acute decompensated heart failure and pulmonary edema with lower rates of invasive ventilation and improved surrogates of treatment failure. However, these trials were too underpowered to show an effect on mortality when compared to standard therapy.[59-63] The conclusions of seven meta-analyses or systematic reviews, albeit with overlapping studies analyzed and different outcomes assessed, yielded similar encouraging results correlating the use of NIV with improved in-hospital mortality and a reduced need for invasive ventilation.[64-70]

In the largest multicenter randomized controlled study, the Three Interventions in Cardiogenic Pulmonary Oedema (3CPO) trial, Gray et al. compared the use of CPAP and noninvasive intermittent positive-pressure ventilation (NIPPV) with standard oxygen therapy in 1069 patients presenting to the emergency department with acute pulmonary edema with the primary endpoint being 7-day mortality and the composite outcome of mortality and need for invasive ventilation.[71] As in smaller trials, NIV (CPAP or NIPPV) was associated with improvement in physiologic and subjective parameters but there was no statistically significant difference in 7-day mortality (9.8% for standard therapy vs. 9.5% for NIV, $P = .87$) compared to standard therapy. There were also no differences in the secondary outcomes of 30-day mortality (16.4% vs. 15.2%, $P = .64$) or in the need for intubation (2.8% vs. 2.9%, $P = .90$). However, the study was performed in patients undergoing treatment in the emergency department and did not enroll patients in other hospital settings. In addition, the overall mortality and intubation rates were lower than demonstrated in other studies, suggesting a less critically ill patient population. Most important, there was considerable crossover of about 15% from the standard therapy group to NIV that could have reduced adverse outcomes in the standard therapy group, particularly when assessing the need for intubation. Although some trials have suggested faster correction of gas-exchange abnormalities and improvement in dyspnea scores, the majority of meta-analyses and small randomized trials have demonstrated no difference in hospitalization outcomes, including mortality, when comparing CPAP to BiPAP.[63–67,72] These results were replicated in the 3CPO trial.

Safety of Noninvasive Ventilation and Risk of Myocardial Infarction

The 3CPO trial reconfirmed the safety of using NIV in patients with cardiogenic pulmonary edema. Initial concerns about the increased risk of acute MI with NIPPV/BiPAP led to the termination of a trial by Mehta et al.[73] Likewise, a weak signal was noted in a meta-analysis that included this study.[65] However, subsequent studies that included the 3CPO trial did not find an association between the use of NIV and risk of acute MI.[70–72,74,75] On the contrary, data have emerged to suggest comparable physiologic and clinical effects of NIV in the treatment of pulmonary edema complicating acute MI. In a retrospective study of 206 patients, including 26% who had an acute MI, NIV-associated improvement in oxygenation and reduction in the need for invasive ventilation was unaffected by the underlying cause of pulmonary edema.[76]

Although the beneficial effect of NIV on mortality in patients with acute cardiogenic pulmonary edema is yet to be proven in a large randomized trial, NIV remains a valuable adjunct therapy with a favorable safety profile. Early introduction of NIV in the appropriate patient population (e.g., adequate level of consciousness, able to tolerate mask, acceptable level of secretions, synchronous breathing with respirator) remains a helpful and widely used rescue treatment for respiratory failure in the CICU. The modality used and the device-patient interface depends on patient-specific characteristics, gas exchange abnormalities, and system availability. Newer studies have evaluated the use of adaptive servoventilation (ASV) in acute cardiogenic pulmonary edema. ASV provides both positive expiratory pressure and pressure support during inspiration with automatic adjustments in the settings based on the analysis of the patient's breathing. Only limited data about the use of ASV in heart failure are available so far. Small trials have suggested a favorable hemodynamic effect, sympathetic modulation, and possible reduction in rate of intubation when compared to standard oxygen therapy in the treatment of acute pulmonary edema.[77–79] These results are not conclusive and no trials comparing ASV to other forms of NIV have been conducted.

INVASIVE MECHANICAL VENTILATION

Invasive mechanical ventilation requiring tracheal intubation remains the most commonly used method of advanced respiratory support in the CICU.[80–82] The correction of gas exchange impairment is the paramount goal of mechanical ventilation as the underlying etiology of respiratory decompensation is addressed. To simplify the approach to mechanical ventilation, management of the impairments in gas exchange can be separated into oxygenation and ventilation.

Oxygenation

Maintaining adequate tissue oxygenation and efficient aerobic metabolism is of utmost importance in preserving tissue viability and improving outcomes of critically ill patients. When considering tissue oxygenation, oxygen delivery is determined as follows:

$$DO_2 = CO \times [(1.3 \times Hb \times SaO_2) + (0.003 \times PaO_2)]$$

Since most of the oxygen content in blood is bound to hemoglobin, the oxygen delivery rate (DO_2) is therefore directly proportional to CO, hemoglobin concentration (Hb), and hemoglobin oxygen saturation (SaO_2). Thus, the optimization of CO and oxygen-carrying capacity of blood are as essential as increasing SaO_2 or PaO_2 in critically ill patients. Likewise, it is crucial to consider the interactions between these factors. In some patients, changes in mechanical ventilation to improve SaO_2 could lead to a decrease in CO that would overall adversely affect tissue oxygenation.

Goal Oxygen Level

In most critically ill patients, the goal is to maintain SaO_2 above 90% to 92%. Considering the sigmoid shape of the oxyhemoglobin dissociation curve, it is usually not necessary to achieve a normal PaO_2 of 100 mm Hg or greater. In the absence of significant abnormalities of pH or temperature, the curve approaches the flat portion at a PaO_2 close to 60 mm Hg. As a result, a goal PaO_2 of 65 to 80 mm Hg is reasonable. In fact, potential harm related to hyperoxia can include direct lung injury from interstitial fibrosis, atelectasis, and tracheobronchitis.[84,85] Hyperoxia can also be associated with unfavorable cardiovascular effects related to systemic vasoconstriction, coronary vasoconstriction, and reduced coronary blood flow.[86,87] With meta-analyses reporting potentially worse outcomes in patients with acute MI when routinely treated with oxygen, the multicenter, randomized Air Versus Oxygen in Myocardial Infarction (AVOID) trial suggested an association between increased early myocardial injury by peak creatine kinase level and infarct size by cardiac magnetic resonance imaging performed at 6 months when patients presenting with ST elevation MI were treated with supplemental oxygen (8 L/min) in the absence of hypoxia.[88–90] To define the goal PaO_2 or peripheral capillary oxygen saturation (SpO_2), other studies not specific to CICU patients have demonstrated that conservative oxygenation strategies are safe, feasible, and could be associated with improved outcomes—including ventilator-free days and, possibly, mortality rate.[91–94] The definition of conservative oxygenation was not identical in these trials, but general targets included PaO_2 as low as 55 to 85 mmHg and SpO_2 as low as 90% to 92% in the studies assessing safety. More liberal targets of PaO_2 of 70 to 100 mm Hg and SpO_2 of 92% to 95% were used in trials demonstrating possible outcome improvements. Future studies addressing optimal oxygenation targets in CICU patients are needed.

Adjusting/Improving Oxygenation

In mechanically ventilated patients, oxygenation is mostly determined by the FiO_2 and mean airway pressure, which, in turn, is dependent on peak inspiratory pressure, positive end expiratory pressure (PEEP), and inspiratory time.[95] Hypoxemia is often corrected by the increased FiO_2 provided by mechanical ventilation. Maintaining PEEP can allow the recruitment of atelectatic or consolidated alveoli, therefore improving ventilation-perfusion matching, lung compliance, and increasing FRC, which acts as an oxygen reservoir. Thus initiating and optimizing PEEP can help reduce FiO_2 requirements, avoid toxic oxygen levels, and improve overall oxygenation but needs to be accompanied by close monitoring of the hemodynamic effects of positive pressure ventilation.

When hypoxemia remains refractory to increased FiO_2 and PEEP, other therapies targeted at improving oxygenation and reducing oxygen consumption can be considered. Heavy sedation and utilization of neuromuscular blocking agents can help maintain oxygen consumption to vital organs and reduce ventilator dyssynchrony. The evidence for the use of neuromuscular blockade is heavily weighted toward patients with acute respiratory distress syndrome (ARDS).[96-99] In the randomized controlled ARDS et Curarisation Systematique (ACURASYS) trial and subsequent meta-analyses, use of neuromuscular blockade in early ARDS was associated with improved mortality.[98,100] However, the risk of critical illness polyneuropathy should be weighed against the potential benefits. Although some of the currently used neuromuscular blockers, such as atracurium and cisatracurium, have minimal cardiovascular effects, these agents have not been well studied in the CICU population.[101]

Another rescue technique used in refractory hypoxemia is inverse ratio ventilation (IRV), which requires reversing the inspiratory/expiratory time ratio (I:E). Usually, the longer expiratory phase provides more comfort and reduces auto-PEEP. By prolonging the inspiratory time, the increase in mean airway pressure allows further alveolar recruitment and possible improvement in oxygenation although without conclusive association with improvement in clinical outcomes and mortality.[102-105] IRV can have unfavorable pulmonary effects, including increased gas trapping, auto-PEEP, and possible aggravation of ventilator-induced lung injury as well as a negative impact on venous return and CO.[106,107] It is also associated with discomfort to patients and requires heavy sedation or neuromuscular blockade. The use of inhaled pulmonary vasodilators (nitric oxide or prostacyclin) can improve oxygenation by selective pulmonary vasodilation in well-ventilated lung regions, thus improving ventilation-perfusion matching. Although the limited adverse effects of inhaled nitric oxide can be readily avoided, it remains a very costly intervention without improvement in ventilator-free days or mortality.[108-110] Last, prone ventilation may improve oxygenation due to mechanisms related to better ventilation-perfusion matching, increased FRC, improved clearance of secretions, and changes in regional diaphragmatic motions. Prone ventilation has regained clinical use after the results of the Proning Severe ARDS Patients (PROSEVA) trial in severe ARDS demonstrating that prone ventilation was associated with an improvement in mortality and ventilator-free days.[111] This study was performed in a select patient population with ARDS and severe hypoxemia at experienced centers that were routinely using prone ventilation and excluded hemodynamically unstable patients.

Ventilation

Carbon dioxide elimination is primarily dependent on alveolar ventilation, which is a function of minute ventilation and dead space. Assuming a stable dead space, carbon dioxide clearance is inversely proportional to minute ventilation. In mechanically ventilated patients, factors affecting carbon dioxide production, such as the metabolic state, are rarely manipulated. Therefore partial pressure of carbon dioxide (PCO_2) can be altered by adjusting the respiratory rate and tidal volume. Controlling PCO_2 is important owing to its regulation of pH as well as its pulmonary vasomodulatory effect. Abnormal pH can have significant cardiovascular effects. Marked acidosis can impair cardiac contractility and responsiveness to vasopressors.[112,113] Marked alkalosis reduces the threshold for ventricular arrhythmias in susceptible patients.[114] However, mild changes in pH can be well tolerated and permissive hypercapnia has emerged as a management strategy in the treatment of ARDS.

Delivery of Invasive Mechanical Ventilation

Mechanical ventilators have evolved significantly to optimize improvement in gas exchange while minimizing ventilator-associated lung injury (VALI). With technological advancements, the terminology has become more complex, contributing to possible confusion for the clinician. Modern mechanical ventilation allows the manipulation of every aspect of inspiration while expiration is not altered except for the magnitude of PEEP applied.

Given the lack of significant evidence regarding the superiority of one mode of mechanical ventilation over another in improving clinical outcomes, including mortality, the selection of the initial mode is usually based on clinical familiarity, institutional preference, and available technology. The commonly used mechanical ventilation methods/modes and some more advanced alternatives are briefly discussed in the next section.

Volume-Controlled Ventilation

In volume-controlled ventilation, for all ventilator-initiated breaths, the patient receives a preset tidal volume determined by the preset flow rate over a set inspiratory time. The clinician selects the tidal volume, respiratory rate, peak inspiratory flow rate (therefore, inspiratory time and I:E ratio) in addition to PEEP and FiO_2. Airway pressures (peak, plateau, and mean) are not directly adjusted and are dependent on patient variables (compliance and airway resistance) as well as ventilator settings. Volume-controlled ventilation can be delivered in one of several modes:

- **Continuous mandatory ventilation (CMV):** Minute ventilation is entirely determined by the ventilator settings since the patient is unable to initiate spontaneous breaths. This mode completely eliminates the work of breathing and is used when there is no incentive to allow possible patient-triggered increases in minute ventilation.

- **Assist control ventilation (AC):** AC allows the clinician to set minimum minute ventilation (set respiratory rate and tidal volume) that can be augmented via patient-triggered, ventilator-assisted breaths beyond the set respiratory rate. In patient-triggered breaths, the ventilator delivers the full preset tidal volume.

- **Intermittent mandatory ventilation (IMV) and synchronized intermittent mandatory ventilation (SIMV):** IMV maintains minimum minute ventilation (set respiratory rate and tidal volume) that can be augmented via unassisted patient-generated breaths. SIMV is more commonly used and synchronizes the ventilator breaths with the patient inspiratory effort. SIMV allows greater patient control over the level of support, improves patient-ventilator synchrony, and preserves respiratory muscle function.[115] In some patients, the reduction in mean airway pressure and intrapleural pressure associated with SIMV can attenuate the negative hemodynamic effects of positive pressure ventilation.[116] These advantages have to be weighed against the increased oxygen consumption associated with spontaneous breathing in critically ill patients.

Pressure-Controlled Ventilation

In pressure-controlled ventilation, the ventilator maintains a set airway pressure for a given inspiratory time. The clinician would set the inspiratory pressure level, PEEP, I:E ratio, respiratory rate, and FiO_2. In this mode, the peak airway pressure is constant (inspiratory pressure + PEEP) while the tidal volume can be variable depending on patient characteristics (compliance, airway/tubing resistance) and driving pressures. Pressure-controlled ventilation can be delivered using the same modes of volume-controlled ventilation explained earlier, including CMV, AC, and SIMV.

In general, pressure-controlled ventilation is associated with lower peak airway pressures compared to volume-controlled ventilation, but the difference is less significant when the option of ramp flow is used in volume-controlled ventilation. Pressure-controlled ventilation can also allow better synchrony with the ventilator and more homogenous gas distribution. However, those advantages do not seem to translate to statistically significant improvement in patient outcomes, including mortality, work of breathing, or oxygenation.[117–120]

Pressure Support Ventilation

Pressure support ventilation (PSV) is a flow-limited mode of spontaneous but supported ventilation when the ventilator transitions from PEEP during expiration to a higher inspiratory pressure target that is maintained until the inspiratory flow decreases to a predetermined percentage of its peak value. In addition to setting the PEEP and FiO_2, the clinician also selects an inspiratory pressure support level. All breaths are patient triggered; therefore, tidal volume, respiratory rate, and minute ventilation are dependent on patient mechanics and ventilator settings. Thus it is not a mode of ventilation that is suited for patients requiring full ventilator support. It can be combined

with SIMV to provide some support for patient-triggered breaths. Alternatively, PSV is used for weaning from mechanical ventilation because it tends to be a comfortable mode with more patient control. However, there is no evidence that PSV improves weaning.

Alternative Modes of Mechanical Ventilation

Pressure-Regulated Volume-Controlled/Adaptive Pressure-Controlled Ventilation. This is a mode of ventilation that delivers pressure-controlled breaths with a target tidal volume. Unlike pressure-controlled ventilation, this mode guarantees a specific average tidal volume by adjusting the inspiratory pressure depending on patient mechanics and effort. The algorithm allows a variation in the flow of gas to maintain a constant airway pressure equal to the set inspiratory pressure. Although this ventilation mode theoretically delivers a stable tidal volume at lower peak airway pressure, there is no evidence that it improves patient outcomes and could be associated with increased work of breathing in some scenarios.[121]

Airway Pressure Release Ventilation. Airway pressure release ventilation (APRV) delivers pressure-controlled, time-triggered, and time-cycled breaths with the ventilator shifting between high levels of continuous airway pressure (P_{high}) delivered for a long duration (T_{high}) alternating with time-cycled "releases" to a lower pressure (P_{low}) and shorter duration (T_{low}). The maintenance of high constant pressure (P_{high}) aids in improving alveolar recruitment and oxygenation with the intermittent releases allowing for ventilation. The tidal volume is usually determined by the difference between P_{high} and P_{low} (driving pressure), the number of releases, and patient mechanics. In ARPV, spontaneous breathing can occur at any phase, which is a distinguishing feature of APRV compared to other modalities with inverse ratio ventilation, such as pressure-controlled ventilation with extreme I:E inverse ratio. Biphasic intermittent positive airway pressure (also referred to as BiLevel or BiPhasic) is a specific type of APRV that is characterized by a longer T_{low} compared to traditional APRV. BiLevel is designed to allow more spontaneous breaths to occur at P_{low} to potentially allow unrestricted spontaneous breathing and promote weaning.

APRV has been studied most in patients with acute lung injury and ARDS. Compared to conventional ventilation modes, ARPV appears to be associated with improved alveolar recruitment, enhanced ventilation-perfusion matching and, therefore, better oxygenation while maintaining lower peak airway pressures.[122–124] The effect of APRV on clinical outcomes of patients with ARDS has been variable, with none of the studies showing improvement in mortality. In a randomized controlled trial comparing APRV with pressure-controlled ventilation, Putensen et al. demonstrated an improvement in oxygenation and a reduction in ventilator and ICU days with APRV.[125] However, these results could not be replicated in a subsequent larger randomized prospective trial or a retrospective international cohort study.[126,127] Despite initial concerns about the hemodynamic effects of sustained high airway pressure, APRV appears to be hemodynamically well tolerated. In one study, switching from pressure-controlled ventilation with IRV to APRV correlated with an increase in cardiac output and decrease in vasopressor use. However, this could have been related, in part, to decreased sedation and neuromuscular blockade.[128]

Adaptive Support Ventilation.   In adaptive support ventilation (ASV), using the patient's demographic data and an estimated expiratory constant from "test breaths," the ventilator calculates the optimal respiratory rate to achieve the desired minute ventilation delivered by pressure-controlled breaths. This technology provides a mode with automatic selection and adjustment of most ventilator settings (except for PEEP and FiO_2) with changing patient condition providing a single mode of support from initial intubation to weaning.

High-Frequency Oscillatory Ventilation.   High-frequency oscillatory ventilation (HFOV) uses an oscillatory pump to deliver very low tidal volumes at high frequency at a relatively constant pressure (P_{aw}). It results in homogenous distribution of ventilation and, therefore, improves alveolar recruitment and oxygenation while reducing atelectrauma. HFOV has been studied in ARDS in two large multicentered trials with no mortality benefit in one and potential harm found in the other.

Mechanical Ventilation in Select Patient Populations

Mechanical Ventilation in Acute Myocardial Infarction and Cardiogenic Shock.
The increased use of mechanical ventilation in the CICU has been well documented.[2,3] Acute pulmonary edema, cardiogenic shock (60%), incessant ventricular arrhythmias, or cardiopulmonary arrest (30% to 60%) are some of the complications of MI that frequently necessitate advanced respiratory support and mechanical ventilation.[129,130]

The hemodynamic effects of positive pressure ventilation have raised concerns regarding possible worsening of clinical outcomes of patients with MI and/or cardiogenic shock managed by mechanical ventilation. Several retrospective studies, including studies with contemporary rates of timely percutaneous coronary intervention, associated the need of mechanical ventilation in patients with acute MI with in-hospital mortality ranging from 29% to as high as 51%.[4,129–132] However, these data cannot be used to infer a causal relationship between mechanical ventilation and increased mortality. Mechanically ventilated patients had other characteristics that are associated with worse outcomes in patients with acute MI, including lower LV ejection fraction, larger infarct size, older age, cardiogenic shock, and evidence of multiorgan dysfunction.

Conversely, established data suggest that positive pressure ventilation could have favorable effects in patients with significant LV dysfunction and myocardial ischemia by reducing LV afterload owing to decreased transmural (or transthoracic) pulmonary pressure; reducing LV preload thereby unloading the congested heart; decreasing work of breathing and overall metabolic demand; reversing hypoxia-related pulmonary vasoconstriction; and improving oxygenation and oxygen supply to the ischemic myocardium.[133] In small studies assessing the effects of PEEP on cardiac performance, CO and stroke index improved with the addition of PEEP to patients with elevated LV filling pressures.[134–136] Likewise, small studies have suggested that

the use of mechanical ventilation in cardiogenic shock patients treated with an intraaortic balloon pump (IABP) is safe and could be associated with improved outcomes. In a nonrandomized, prospective trial of 28 patients treated with IABP for cardiogenic shock complicating MI, 10 patients were placed on mechanical ventilation with PEEP of 10 cm H_2O immediately after placement of an IABP. There was a statistically insignificant improvement in weaning off mechanical circulatory support with an IABP and survival to discharge in the mechanically ventilated group when compared to those treated with supplemental oxygen therapy.[136] In a more recent retrospective analysis of patients greater than 60 years of age with cardiogenic shock complicating acute MI, the use of mechanical ventilation with PEEP was associated with enhanced beneficial effects of IABP on LV function at the expense of increased pulmonary infections and renal insufficiency. There was no difference in mortality between the two groups.

In patients with MI complicated by cardiogenic shock, mechanical ventilation can be safely used in well-selected patients with potential improvement in hemodynamic factors that may influence patient outcomes. Unfortunately, there is no evidence to guide best practices, settings, and modes of mechanical ventilation in this patient population. Recent small studies suggest that noninvasive ventilation can be safe in the management of some patients with cardiogenic shock.[131] Future research is necessary to define the prognostic indicators and settings of mechanical ventilation for cardiac patients that would improve outcomes.

Pulmonary Arterial Hypertension.
Patients with pulmonary arterial hypertension (PAH) and RV dysfunction are among the most susceptible to the adverse hemodynamic effects of positive pressure ventilation. The decreased RV preload and associated increased afterload can drastically reduce RV stroke volume, shift the interventricular septum to the left, and reduce LV stroke volume and CO. The decrease in systemic arterial pressure may also exacerbate RV ischemia. Some of the medications used for sedation can be associated with increased pulmonary vascular resistance and decreased systemic arterial pressure. It is not uncommon for the initiation of mechanical ventilation in patients with PAH to precipitate cardiovascular collapse.[137,138] In a recent retrospective analysis of a heterogeneous group of PAH patients, mechanical ventilation was associated with an in-hospital mortality of 39.1% as compared to 12.6% in patients treated with noninvasive ventilation.[139] Although these data cannot establish causality, they support the European Society of Cardiology (ESC) 2015 guidelines for treatment of PAH recommendation that "intubation should be avoided in patients with RV failure, as it frequently results in hemodynamic collapse."[140] If possible, noninvasive respiratory support should be considered while balancing the detrimental effects of severe hypoxia, hypercarbia, and acidosis of insufficiently treated acute respiratory failure in PAH. If invasive mechanical ventilation is unavoidable, preemptive administration of vasoactive agents and inotropes should be considered prior to induction of anesthesia to avoid hypotension and worsening of RV contractility. Anesthetics that minimize systemic hypotension and pulmonary vasoconstriction should be used. Airway pressure should be maintained at the minimum

required level to support adequate oxygenation and mechanical ventilation modes that achieve lower airway pressures should be selected. Last, the use of pulmonary artery catheterization should be considered on an individualized basis, as it has been associated with better outcomes and reduced mortality in critically ill patients with PAH.[138]

Acute Respiratory Distress Syndrome. Although less commonly encountered in the CICU, ARDS can affect patients with cardiovascular comorbidities or develop as a complication during their admission for a different primary diagnosis. Cardiac intensivists should be well equipped to provide evidence-based management to these patients. A full discussion about management of ARDS is beyond the scope of this chapter. However, ventilation strategies for ARDS recognize the risk of VALI associated with alveolar overdistention and cyclic atelectasis that occurs with conventional ventilation. The initial treatment of patients with ARDS requires full-support ventilator modes with a focus on the concepts of lung protective ventilation and open-lung ventilation.

Lung protective ventilation or low tidal volume ventilation has been associated with lower mortality and a reduction in the duration of mechanical ventilation compared to conventional mechanical ventilation.[141] It is based on providing a low tidal volume (goal 6 mL/kg of predicted or ideal body weight) to avoid alveolar overdistention and decrease VALI. The tidal volume is further adjusted to maintain a plateau airway pressure of less than 30 mm H_2O. While avoiding auto-PEEP, the respiratory rate is changed to maintain adequate minute ventilation while accepting some degree of hypercapnia and respiratory acidosis (permissive hypercapnia). The added strategy of open-lung ventilation uses high PEEP to improve oxygenation and has been associated with improved hospital and ICU mortality.[142–144] Theoretically, this strategy reduced VALI by allowing the recruitment of new alveoli and keeping them open, thereby reducing alveolar overdistention and atelectrauma. Lung protective ventilation utilizing tidal volumes in the vicinity of 6 mL/kg ideal body weight has been increasingly advocated for use in all patients undergoing invasive mechanical ventilation. Future studies will be required to determine the utility of this approach in patients with respiratory failure due to reasons other than ARDS.

COMPLICATIONS OF MECHANICAL VENTILATION

The complications of mechanical ventilation are associated with adverse patient outcomes. Established prophylactic measures should be used to avoid these complications. Equally important, appropriately timed discontinuation of mechanical ventilation is imperative to minimize these complications. Complications of mechanical ventilation can be grouped into six categories.

Pulmonary Complications

- *Barotrauma:* Barotrauma results from alveolar rupture and can cause pneumothorax, subcutaneous emphysema, or pneumomediastinum. Using lung protective ventilation and avoiding hyperventilation can reduce the risk of barotrauma.

- *Volutrauma:* Volutrauma is more descriptively referred to as VALI with pathophysiologic and clinical characteristics similar to ARDS. VALI results from alveolar overdistention and cyclic alveolar atelectasis and expansion (atelectrauma). Preventive measures have been studied best in ARDS patients and include lung-protective ventilation and open-lung ventilation.

- *Auto-PEEP:* Auto-PEEP can occur in the setting of high minute ventilation, increased airway resistance, and prolonged inspiratory time settings.

Ventilator-Associated Infections

Ventilator-associated pneumonia (VAP) develops more than 48 to 72 hours after endotracheal intubation and has been associated with increased mortality and morbidity. Risk factors include prolonged intubation/reintubation, older age, ARDS, prior antibiotic exposure, use of agents that increase gastric pH, aspiration, and malnutrition. There are a number of important interventions to minimize the risk of VAP, including the following:

- Elevating the head of the bed to 30 degrees[145]
- Subglottic secretion suctioning using specially designed endotracheal tubes[146]
- Proper oral care and decontamination of the oropharynx with chlorhexidine[147]

Complications Related to the Endotracheal Tube

Elevated endotracheal tube cuff pressure can cause mucosal injury and possibly lead to tracheal stenosis or tracheomalacia.

Hemodynamic Effects of Positive Pressure Ventilation

Depending on the underlying cardiovascular comorbidities and volume status, positive pressure ventilation can result in worsening cardiac performance.

Sedation and Neurologic Effects

Oversedation is commonly encountered in mechanically ventilated patients. Daily sedation holidays are necessary to minimize sedation.

Muscle Weakness

Early mobilization and physical therapy improves recovery of independent functional status.[148]

WEANING OF INVASIVE MECHANICAL VENTILATION

The best preventive measure against the complications of mechanical ventilation is to discontinue mechanical ventilator support as soon as possible. Clinicians occasionally delay extubation even when mechanical ventilation is no longer needed. Studies have shown that a large proportion of patients tolerate discontinuation of mechanical ventilation on the first attempt. In another study, less than half of the patients who had an unplanned extubation required reintubation and less than one-third needed reintubation if the self-extubation occurred during the weaning phase.[149–151]

Hemodynamic Effects of Weaning

Recognizing the dynamic effects of the weaning process on the cardiovascular system plays a role in the successful discontinuation of mechanical ventilation. Weaning can reverse the beneficial effects of mechanical ventilation in patients with LV dysfunction and has been equated to stress testing.[152] With the withdrawal of positive pressure ventilation, the increased LV filling pressure and afterload can overwhelm a dysfunctional LV. The increased work of breathing increases oxygen demand in the setting of limited cardiopulmonary reserve while the sympathetic surge associated with weaning contributes to increased myocardial oxygen consumption and further elevation in LV afterload. Recent data have emphasized the role of diastolic dysfunction in weaning failure as a less recognized but important factor.[153]

Readiness to Discontinue Mechanical Ventilation

In the multistep process of weaning, patients should be regularly assessed for the readiness to undergo a weaning trial. The mode of the weaning trial should be determined. Finally, cardiac and noncardiac reasons for failure to wean should be identified and addressed.

To assess readiness for weaning, several factors need to be considered:
- Reversal/improvement of underlying reason for mechanical ventilation
- Hemodynamic stability (no or low requirements of hemodynamic support)
- Adequate mental status with intact respiratory drive (spontaneous awakening trial)
- Adequate gas exchange (pH >7.25) and oxygenation on acceptable ventilator support (PaO$_2$ >60 mm Hg on FiO$_2$ <40% to 50%, and PEEP of no more than 5 to 8 mm H$_2$O or PaO$_2$/FiO$_2$ >150)
- A weaning screen or "weaning parameters" can supplement clinical judgment in assessing readiness for liberation from mechanical ventilation but should not be solely depends on deciding whether or not to extubate the patient. Weaning parameters include the following:
  - *Rapid shallow breathing index (RSBI):* RSBI is the ratio of respiratory rate to tidal volume. RSBI is the most studied parameter. RSBI greater than 105 is associated with low likelihood for successful extubation.
  - Minute ventilation: less than 10 L/min
  - Negative inspiratory force (NIF): less than −20 to −30 mm H$_2$O
  - Respiratory rate
  - Tidal volume and vital capacity

Once considered clinically appropriate to undergo a spontaneous breathing trial (SBT), the patient is transitioned to completely unassisted breathing (T-piece or T-tube) or minimally supported modes of ventilation, such as CPAP or PSV for at least 30 minutes while closely monitoring for discomfort, work of breathing, and hemodynamic instability. Evidence suggests that there is no difference between using PSV or T-piece in successful weaning, reintubation, or ICU mortality.[149,150,154–156] If the patient performs well during the SBT and demonstrates adequate mental status and the ability to clear secretions, the decision is made to discontinue mechanical ventilation.

Weaning Mechanical Ventilation in Cardiac Patients

While weaning the cardiac patient from mechanical ventilation, special attention should be given to the reversed hemodynamic effects of withdrawing positive pressure ventilation. Given that these effects can be difficult to predict, several modalities have been studied to aid in predicting the successful withdrawal of mechanical ventilation and to identify cardiac etiologies for failure to wean.
- Significant tachycardia and hypotension can be suggestive of worsening cardiac performance due to change in loading conditions or worsening ischemia.
- *Pulmonary artery catheter (PAC):* Although the placement of pulmonary artery catheters to aid in extubation is rarely indicated, in patients who already have a PAC, a significant increase in pulmonary artery occlusive pressure or a decrease in mixed venous oxygen saturation is likely associated with a cardiac etiology in failure to wean.[157,158]
- *Echocardiography:* Echocardiography can be used as a surrogate to estimate filling pressures, although it can be difficult to perform during an SBT while the patient is in distress.
- *Cardiac biomarkers:* As opposed to the absolute value of B-type natriuretic peptide (BNP) or N-terminal pro B-type natriuretic peptide (NT pro-BNP), a 12% increase in levels correlates with development of weaning-induced pulmonary edema.[159]

When a cardiac etiology for failure to wean is suspected, treatment is targeted to the underlying cause, including the use of diuretics, relieving ischemia, the use of vasodilators, and assessing the need for inotropes or afterload reducers to optimize hemodynamics and volume status prior to the next attempted wean.[160–162] In some cases, it can be helpful to initiate afterload reduction (nitroprusside) or preload reduction (nitrates) during the weaning trial if significant hypertension is noted. Similarly, extubating to elective NIV has been linked to lower rates of postextubation respiratory failure in high-risk patients.[163]

▮ SUMMARY

The CICU has evolved to provide care for patients with significant active respiratory conditions and pulmonary comorbidities. Optimal patient care in the CICU requires adequate knowledge of the various respiratory support modalities, including (but not limited to) mechanical ventilation with good understanding of the indications, limitations, hemodynamic consequences, and adverse effects of these supportive therapies. The paucity of evidence about the best treatment options in the CICU remains obvious and problematic. Further efforts should be targeted toward clinical trials that better address these questions.

The full reference list for this chapter is available at ExpertConsult.com.

51

Cardiopulmonary Resuscitation and Critical Care After Cardiac Arrest

Jacob C. Jentzer, Clifton W. Callaway

This chapter reviews the clinical care of a patient with cardiac arrest. Cardiac arrest consists of complete or nearly complete cessation of blood flow and is fatal unless reversed in seconds or minutes. The cardiac intensivist may manage initial resuscitation of a patient to reverse cardiac arrest. In addition, post–cardiac arrest patients are critically ill; the intensivist must care for the aftermath of this event. Understanding unique aspects of this particular set of patients can improve outcomes and more efficiently deliver appropriate care for each patient.

EPIDEMIOLOGY AND OUTCOMES OF CARDIAC ARREST

Out-of-hospital cardiac arrest (OHCA) affects nearly 1000 adult Americans each day; when including in-hospital cardiac arrest (IHCA), more than 500,000 adults suffer cardiac arrest each year in the United States.[1] The most common cause of OHCA is cardiac disease, particularly coronary artery disease (CAD) and other structural heart diseases, such as cardiomyopathy.[2] Cardiac arrest may be the initial manifestation of cardiac disease in up to half of patients dying from cardiovascular causes.[2] IHCA etiology varies according to the type and location of patient,[3] but progression of respiratory distress to cardiac arrest is most common in many hospitals.[4]

Survival after cardiac arrest has increased steadily over the past 15 years despite the lack of novel therapeutics as a result of multiple improvements in the systems of care.[5,6] Only 25% to 30% of patients with OHCA initially achieve return of spontaneous

circulation (ROSC) and are admitted to the hospital.[6] About 40% to 50% of IHCA patients achieve ROSC initially.[7] The majority (approximately 60% to 70%) of cardiac arrest patients (either OHCA or IHCA) who initially achieve ROSC subsequently die in the hospital, with rates of survival in the United States of approximately 12% for OHCA and 24% for IHCA.[6,7] Marked regional differences in initial ROSC rates and subsequent hospital and overall mortality exist for patients with both OHCA and IHCA, attributable to differences in baseline patient characteristics, cardiac arrest circumstances, and peri-arrest care.[8,9]

Predictors of favorable and unfavorable cardiac arrest outcomes have been identified (Table 51.1).[10,11] These variables are often not available or reliable in clinical practice, limiting their utility for clinical decision making. The most important clinical distinction in cardiac arrest patients is between those with shockable rhythms, such as ventricular fibrillation (VF) or pulseless ventricular tachycardia (VT), and those with nonshockable rhythms, such as asystole or pulseless electrical activity (PEA). Patients with shockable arrest rhythms generally have more favorable outcomes, higher rates of underlying (reversible) cardiac etiology, lower rates of comorbidities, and fewer clinical adverse prognostic signs. Nonshockable rhythms may result from prolonged VF or cardiac failure after defibrillation of VF, but also may result from noncardiac etiologies such as hypoxia, sepsis, pulmonary embolus, hypovolemia, or other toxic-metabolic derangements. These situations are associated with worse outcomes, lower rates of reversible etiology, and higher rates of comorbidities. Over time, rates of shockable rhythms in OHCA have declined and now

TABLE 51.1 Favorable and Unfavorable Prognostic Indicators for Patients With Cardiac Arrest

Favorable Prognostic Indicators	Unfavorable Prognostic Indicators
Shockable rhythm (VT, VF)	Nonshockable rhythm (asystole, PEA)
Witnessed collapse	Unwitnessed collapse
Public location	Private/home location
Immediate initiation of CPR by bystander	Delayed initiation of bystander CPR or lack of bystander CPR
Younger age	Older age
Higher end-tidal CO_2 during CPR	Lower end-tidal CO_2 during CPR
Cardiac etiology (e.g., acute coronary occlusion)	Noncardiac etiology (e.g., respiratory arrest)
Fewer comorbidities	More comorbidities
Shorter interval from collapse to initiation of CPR (shorter no-flow interval)	Longer interval from collapse to initiation of CPR (longer no-flow interval)
Shorter interval from start of CPR to ROSC (shorter low-flow interval)	Longer interval from start of CPR to ROSC (longer low-flow interval)
Received fewer doses of epinephrine	Received more doses of epinephrine
Mild lactic acidosis on presentation or rapidly clearing lactic acidosis	Severe lactic acidosis on presentation or slowly clearing lactic acidosis
No/mild shock on presentation (i.e., normotension not needing vasopressors)	Severe shock on presentation (i.e., hypotension requiring vasopressors)
Mild or no coma on presentation	Deep coma on presentation
Preserved brainstem reflexes	Missing brainstem reflexes
Reactive EEG pattern	Unreactive or malignant EEG pattern
No abnormal movements	Seizures or myoclonus
Normal head CT	Brain edema on head CT
Lack of respiratory failure	Hypoxemic respiratory failure

CO_2, Carbon dioxide; *CPR*, cardiopulmonary resuscitation; *CT*, computed tomography; *EEG*, electroencephalogram; *PEA*, pulseless electrical activity; *ROSC*, return of spontaneous circulation; *VF*, ventricular fibrillation; *VT*, ventricular tachycardia.
Modified from Rab T, Kern KB, Tamis-Holland JE, et al. Cardiac arrest: a treatment algorithm for emergent invasive cardiac procedures in the resuscitated comatose patient. *J Am Coll Cardiol.* 2015;66:62–73; and Maupain C, Bougouin W, Lamhaut L, et al. The CAHP (Cardiac Arrest Hospital Prognosis) score: a tool for risk stratification after out-of-hospital cardiac arrest. *Eur Heart J.* 2016;37:3222–3228.

account for only 25% to 30% of initial rhythms reported.[6] Rates of shockable rhythms are higher in witnessed OHCA and OHCA occurring in public places.

INTENSIVE CARE IMPLICATIONS OF INITIAL CARDIOPULMONARY RESUSCITATION

Evidence-based guidelines have been widely disseminated for cardiopulmonary resuscitation (CPR), electrical therapy, pharmacologic therapy, and mechanical support to reverse cardiac arrest.[12-15] Cardiac intensivists should understand how different parts of the initial resuscitation can influence subsequent organ dysfunction or recovery. During cardiac arrest, the heart is not generating adequate forward flow to maintain brain and organ perfusion, leading to tissue ischemia and progressive metabolic abnormalities. Immediately after restoration of pulses, there is potential for reperfusion injury when oxygenated blood arrives in acidotic, metabolically depleted tissues.

CARDIOPULMONARY RESUSCITATION

Closed-chest cardiac massage (chest compressions) can produce enough forward blood flow to the brain and organs to decrease the extent of ischemic injury and to delay metabolic deterioration.[14] The quality of chest compressions varies between providers; minimizing interruptions of chest compressions is now recognized as an important determinant of patient survival.[16] High-quality chest compressions are defined as a rate between 100 and 120

compressions per minute with a depth of at least 2 inches in adults, including full recoil.[17,18] Minimizing interruptions of compressions required to deliver a defibrillation shock or to place an airway are examples of preventable decrements to organ perfusion during CPR.[19,20]

Recent guidelines recommend a 30:2 ratio of chest compressions to rescue breaths during CPR prior to placement of an advanced airway with continuous chest compressions performed thereafter.[14] One logical step to further reduce interruptions of CPR is to provide continuous chest compressions with no rescue breaths, sometimes called compression-only CPR or cardiocerebral resuscitation. Initial observational studies suggested that OHCA victims treated with continuous chest compressions rather than standard CPR had improved outcomes.[21,22] However, a subsequent randomized clinical trial showed that continuous compressions with no interruptions prior to advanced airway placement is not superior to a 30:2 ratio.[23]

Mechanical chest compression devices have been developed to prevent a decrease in CPR quality over time from rescuer fatigue. While safe and effective, in randomized studies these devices are not superior to manual CPR from highly trained providers.[24] The role for these devices probably includes prolonged resuscitation efforts, CPR in settings in which manual CPR is difficult or dangerous (e.g., under fluoroscopy or in a moving ambulance), or when there are insufficient personnel to perform all procedures.

Another factor to consider during CPR is the adverse hemodynamic consequences of positive-pressure breathing. Increased intrathoracic pressure resulting from positive-pressure ventilation impairs venous return and forward cardiac flow, particularly with high inspiratory pressures or prolonged inflation.[25] For this reason, rescue breaths should be given quickly and should not be excessively large; the rate of rescue breaths should only be 10 to 12 per minute with an advanced airway in place to avoid hyperventilation.[14] At the time of arrest, the lungs are full of oxygenated air and a patient may tolerate longer pauses between rescue breaths. As cardiac arrest progresses, the oxygen reservoir in the lungs is depleted, but pulmonary blood flow is low during CPR; thus relatively minimal ventilation can still provide adequate gas exchange. In many cases, the amount of air entry into the lungs produced by the mechanical effect of chest compressions is adequate for gas exchange if supplemental oxygen is applied with or without positive-pressure breathing using a bag-valve mask.

Physiologic monitoring during resuscitation, which may be available particularly in cardiac intensive care unit (CICU) patients, can help guide the quality of CPR. End-tidal carbon dioxide monitoring is particularly useful once an advanced airway is placed. End-tidal carbon dioxide in the setting of CPR primarily reflects the amount of pulmonary blood flow; low end-tidal carbon dioxide readings imply poor pulmonary blood flow from ineffective CPR.[26,27] Therefore a low end-tidal carbon dioxide reading (<10 to 20 mm Hg) not only suggests the need to improve CPR quality but also portends a poor prognosis for achieving ROSC.[27] Failure to detect any significant end-tidal carbon dioxide suggests esophageal intubation and requires assessment of the endotracheal tube position. An abrupt, sustained increase in end-tidal carbon monoxide (>40 mm Hg) typically reflects ROSC.[26] During prolonged CPR, maintenance of a relatively high end-tidal carbon dioxide suggests acceptable forward flow and a more favorable prognosis. Arterial blood pressure monitoring can directly demonstrate the pressure generated by chest compressions; restoring and maintaining an adequate diastolic blood pressure (perhaps >40 mm Hg, which is a surrogate for aortic relaxation pressure and partly determines coronary perfusion pressure) appears to be a major determinant of ROSC. Bedside cardiac ultrasound can often be performed using a subxiphoid (subcostal) imaging window at the time of pulse/rhythm check during CPR, but providers must be cautious that attempts to gain better images do not compromise or interrupt the ongoing life-saving interventions. For pulseless patients with an organized cardiac rhythm (i.e., PEA), absence of detectable cardiac contraction portends a very low likelihood of gaining ROSC. Specific complications, such as cardiac tamponade from pericardial effusion, can be readily identified. Several diagnostic algorithms using cardiac ultrasound in PEA have been proposed; in practice, however, interpretation of ultrasound images during CPR can be challenging.[28]

DEFIBRILLATION

Timely defibrillation for patients with shockable rhythms is essential for achieving successful ROSC.[14] The success rate of defibrillation decreases over time, accompanied by changes in the VF waveform morphology. VF waveform analysis may predict

defibrillator shock success and prognosis.[29] Immediately after initiation of VF, VF is high amplitude with much power in lower frequencies ("coarse VF"). This early VF is readily defibrillated; this early period is called the *electrical phase* of VF.[30] After several minutes, myocardial ischemia causes VF to become lower amplitude with power distributed among both high and low frequencies ("fine VF"). This situation is less likely to result in successful defibrillation with rescue shocks, but it can be improved with CPR and perfusion. This period is called the *circulatory phase* of VF. With very prolonged VF, the *metabolic phase* of VF develops due to accumulation of metabolic by-products of anaerobic metabolism and successful defibrillation becomes far less likely. Within several minutes of VF onset, modern biphasic defibrillators have an 85% to 90% first-shock success rate for converting VF with little increase in success when shock energies are increased.[14] For this reason, multiple "stacked" shocks are not recommended if the first shock fails. Different manufacturers have differing recommendations about escalating energy levels if the first shock fails. Regardless of cardiac arrest duration, defibrillation should be performed as soon as possible for patients with an initial rhythm of VF.[14] Randomized trials failed to show a benefit of a predefined period of chest compressions with the goal of improving coronary perfusion prior to defibrillation, even for patients with unwitnessed OHCA.[31] Using automated VF waveform analysis to guide a shock-first or CPR-first strategy likewise failed to improve survival in OHCA.[32] On the contrary, continuation of chest compressions during defibrillator charging with immediate resumption of chest compressions after defibrillation may be beneficial.[19]

AIRWAY MANAGEMENT

Optimal airway management during cardiac arrest remains controversial. Various observational studies report either improvement or worsening of outcomes in patients receiving an advanced airway, including either supraglottic airways (such as laryngeal mask airways [LMA] and laryngeal tubes) or endotracheal tube, during CPR when compared to bag-valve mask alone.[33] These studies are difficult to interpret because arrest duration, the need for CPR interruption for airway placement, and whether specific airways were selected because of skill level of the providers or the anatomy of the patient are often not known or not taken into account in the analyses. Given the aforementioned adverse hemodynamic effects of positive-pressure ventilation and the fact that supplemental oxygen alone is adequate during the early phases of cardiac arrest, advanced airways are unlikely to provide a significant benefit during the initial stages of resuscitation.[34] For prolonged resuscitation, placement of an advanced airway is likely appropriate to ensure adequate gas exchange and allow measurement of end-tidal carbon dioxide.[15] Supraglottic airways are employed more often by prehospital providers or during early CPR owing to the ease and rapidity of placement when compared to a standard endotracheal tube. Supraglottic airways can be placed blindly without laryngoscopy, eliminating any need to interrupt chest compressions. After return of pulses, emergency airways may be replaced with an adequate endotracheal tube for anticipated intensive care support.

DRUG THERAPY

Drug therapies for cardiac arrest are largely unproven.[28] Studies comparing prehospital providers who can administer intravenous drugs to providers who cannot administer drugs failed to show a difference in outcome for OHCA.[35,36] Similarly, placement of an intravenous (IV) line for medication administration failed to improve OHCA outcomes in a randomized study.[37] No specific drug has been shown to improve survival compared to placebo when applied to all OHCA patients.[28] It is important to note that drug circulation is markedly reduced during CPR, leading to reduced medication efficacy. Placement of a peripheral or central IV line can be time consuming during CPR; use of a rapidly deployable intraosseous (IO) cannulation kit is preferable.

For patients with persistent VF after one or more defibrillation attempts, use of an antidysrhythmic drug may increase the success of subsequent defibrillation. Amiodarone 300 mg (5 mg/kg) and lidocaine 100 mg (1.5 mg/kg) are the antidysrhythmics most studied. Initial trials suggested a higher VF conversion and ROSC rate with amiodarone compared to placebo and compared to lidocaine.[38,39] These data only indicate that amiodarone can lead to a higher hospital admission rate but not any improvement in long-term survival; amiodarone was more frequently associated with hypotension and/or bradycardia than lidocaine. A recent large randomized controlled trial of amiodarone versus lidocaine versus placebo did not detect any difference in survival among these drugs across the entire study population, though there was higher survival in subgroups of patients treated with antidysrhythmic drugs.[40] Among patients with a witnessed collapse, either amiodarone or lidocaine increased survival compared with placebo, perhaps indicating that these drugs are more effective when administered earlier. Alternative antidysrhythmic agents, such as sotalol and nifekalant, have not shown clear superiority to the standard antidysrhythmic agents.[41] Multiple trials found no effect of magnesium sulfate as an adjunctive antidysrhythmic agent for drug-refractory VF.[41] Atropine is not effective for restoring ROSC in patients with asystole or bradycardic PEA but still remains a first-line therapy for hemodynamically unstable bradyarrhythmias with a pulse.[15]

Vasopressor drugs can increase coronary artery perfusion during CPR. Achieving return of pulses requires adequate coronary perfusion pressure (typically >15 mm Hg), which may be difficult to achieve with chest compressions alone.[42] Vasopressor drugs constrict peripheral vessels, increase central aortic and coronary pressure, and improve rates of ROSC.[43] Vasopressor agents have not been shown to improve survival, however, either compared to each other or to placebo.[28] Epinephrine remains the standard vasopressor recommended based largely on its short-term effects, with bolus doses of 1 mg recommended because of tradition and demonstrated lack of superiority from higher doses.[15,44] The limited placebo-controlled trials of epinephrine during CPR clearly show an increased rate of ROSC and hospital admission but lacked power to detect any difference in long-term survival.[45] In support of epinephrine administration, observational studies in both OHCA and IHCA have shown that a longer time to first epinephrine dose in nonshockable rhythms is associated with worse outcomes.[46]

Epinephrine has potentially deleterious physiologic effects. The potent β-adrenergic agonist effects may facilitate defibrillation of VF in some circumstances but can trigger myocardial ischemia and promote recurrent arrhythmias. Excessive β-adrenergic activation may contribution to cardiac stunning in post-arrest myocardial dysfunction (PAMD).[47] Interestingly, despite the favorable effect of early epinephrine in nonshockable rhythms, more rapid administration of epinephrine is associated with worse outcomes in shockable rhythms.[48] Epinephrine may also have direct injurious effects on other organs: its primary mechanism of action is to constrict blood flow in tissues in order to divert flow to the heart. This may also restrict perfusion of the brain. Observational studies find worse neurologic and overall outcomes in patients who receive epinephrine during CPR.[36] Total cumulative dose of epinephrine is clearly associated with worse neurologic outcomes.[49,50] This effect may be due to a direct harmful effect of epinephrine itself or simply a marker for more severe or prolonged cardiac arrest.

Vasopressin is a nonadrenergic vasopressor that is more effective during acidemia and therefore could be more efficacious during cardiac arrest. Initial studies suggested that use of vasopressin as an alternative or a supplement to epinephrine during cardiac arrest may be associated with better outcomes, but larger subsequent studies failed to show any clinical difference between the drugs.[51] Therefore vasopressin remains an alternative to epinephrine but is equally unproven regarding its benefit.

Other resuscitation drugs have theoretical benefit based on physiologic arguments but lack supporting clinical data (Table 51.2).[28] Intravenous calcium is recommended only as an adjunctive therapy during cardiac arrest owing to hyperkalemia. Metabolic acidosis (and often superimposed respiratory acidosis) typically develops during prolonged cardiac arrest owing to reduced tissue perfusion with anaerobic lactic acidosis that is exacerbated by markedly reduced ventilation during CPR owing to limited pulmonary blood flow. Reversal of acidosis can improve cardiovascular responsiveness to catecholamines and improve cardiac performance and vascular tone, but there is no clinical trial evidence supporting the use of intravenous bicarbonate or other buffers as part of advanced life support.[52] One theoretical concern regarding the use of intravenous bicarbonate is that it triggers overproduction of carbon dioxide, which can exacerbate intracellular and systemic acidosis if it is not cleared by ventilation (which is typically inadequate during CPR). Use of thrombolytic therapy—when there is no availability of primary percutaneous coronary intervention (PCI)—is a logical strategy for suspected pulmonary embolus or acute myocardial infarction (MI), which are among the most common causes of cardiac arrest. Despite this, clinical trials of empiric thrombolytic therapy during cardiac arrest have not shown a clinical benefit.[53]

TEAM MANAGEMENT

Potentially more important than the specific medical therapies during resuscitation is team management. Cardiac arrest is inherently a chaotic circumstance; an organized approach to

TABLE 51.2 Effective and Ineffective Therapies During Resuscitation From Out-of-Hospital Cardiac Arrest

Intervention	Effect on Survival
Compression-only CPR	No benefit
Mechanical chest compression devices	No benefit
Impedance threshold device	No benefit
Active compression/decompression CPR	No benefit
Delayed vs. immediate CPR	No benefit
Single vs. multiple stacked shocks	No benefit
Advanced airway placement	Uncertain
Prehospital intravenous line placement	No benefit
Epinephrine vs. placebo	No benefit, possible harm
High vs. standard epinephrine dose	No benefit
High-dose epinephrine vs. high-dose norepinephrine	No benefit
Epinephrine vs. vasopressin	No benefit
Amiodarone vs. lidocaine	Uncertain
Lidocaine vs. placebo	Possible benefit
Amiodarone vs. placebo	Possible benefit
Atropine vs. placebo	No benefit
Aminophylline vs. placebo	No benefit
Sodium bicarbonate vs. placebo	No benefit
Magnesium sulfate vs. placebo	No benefit
Calcium chloride vs. placebo	No benefit
Extracorporeal CPR vs. conventional CPR	Possible benefit
Prehospital cooling	No benefit

CPR, cardiopulmonary resuscitation.
Modified from Jentzer JC, Clements CM, Wright RS, White RD, Jaffe AS. Improving survival from cardiac arrest: a review of contemporary practice and challenges. *Ann Emerg Med.* 2016;68:678–689.

management provides the best likelihood of successful resuscitation. One of the most crucial aspects is ensuring minimally interrupted, high-quality CPR. Regularly rotating rescuers performing chest compressions maintains CPR quality by avoiding fatigue. For multi-provider resuscitation, having a team leader who provides team members with clearly defined roles to avoid duplication of effort is essential. Clear, efficient, closed-loop communication is essential to prevent errors; team members must be empowered to provide feedback to each other.

OVERVIEW OF POST–CARDIAC ARREST CARE

Immediately after restoration of pulses, patients remain fragile and may have ongoing organ injury. In many cases, the precipitating cause of the cardiac arrest may not have been reversed during resuscitation. In fact, only primary dysrhythmias, hypoxia, or large airway obstructions are likely to have been completely resolved by the time that pulses are restored. Therefore post–cardiac arrest care has two major priorities: (1) damage control and resuscitation of the injured organ systems, particularly the heart and brain; and (2) identification and treatment of the precipitating cause of cardiac arrest. Implementing post–cardiac arrest intensive care is best organized with an understanding of the post–cardiac arrest syndrome.

POST–CARDIAC ARREST SYNDROME

As many as 60% of patients who are admitted to the intensive care unit (ICU) after resuscitation from cardiac arrest still die in the hospital.[54] Initially termed *postresuscitation disease,* the constellation of abnormalities arising after resuscitation from cardiac arrest has more recently been termed post–cardiac arrest syndrome (PCAS).[55] PCAS has four major components: anoxic brain injury, systemic ischemia-reperfusion injury (IRI), post-arrest myocardial dysfunction (PAMD), and persistent precipitating pathology (Table 51.3).[55] Anoxic brain injury is the primary source of in-hospital mortality after cardiac arrest and will be discussed separately. The systemic IRI response is central to the pathophysiology of brain and other organ injury after cardiac arrest. During the no-flow state of cardiac arrest and the low-flow state of CPR, brain and tissue ischemia initiates direct hypoxic organ damage mediated by lack of metabolic energy substrates and accumulation of by-products of anaerobic metabolism. This most severely affects organs with a high resting metabolic rate, such as the brain and heart, and occurs in direct proportion to the duration of the no-flow and low-flow state. PAMD can lead to sustained hypoperfusion during the hours and days after restoration of circulation. Finally, the persistent precipitating pathology can lead to recurrent arrest if not corrected.

Systemic IRI occurs with reperfusion of previously ischemic organs.[55] The abrupt influx of oxygen-rich blood and rapid restoration of tissue metabolic function results in unbalanced metabolism, often with accumulation of damaging molecules (e.g., free calcium or oxygen free radicals) or depletion of other protective molecules (e.g., antioxidants or buffers). IRI is a stereotyped tissue response that also occurs in MI after reperfusion therapy. Effects peak 24 to 48 hours after reperfusion. IRI can trigger programmed cell death pathways in cells that survived the initial anoxic insult.

The principal difference between systemic IRI after cardiac arrest and single-organ IRI, such as myocardial reperfusion, is that multiple organs and tissues are affected simultaneously. This situation triggers a systemic inflammatory response and coagulopathy with increased production of inflammatory cytokines, such as interleukin-6 (IL-6), mimicking the systemic inflammatory response syndrome (SIRS) of severe infection and sepsis.[56,57] One conceptualization of this syndrome is a diffuse activation of the endothelium in many parts of the body, which appears to be associated with PCAS severity and outcomes.[58,59] The degree of elevation of IL-6 and other cytokines and the extent of activation of coagulation factors may be useful as surrogate markers of PCAS severity.[60]

PAMD may be a manifestation of IRI to the heart as well as a consequence of acute cardiac disease (persistent precipitating pathology).[47] PAMD is associated with loss of myocardial microcirculatory function as measured by coronary flow reserve.[61] In addition, treatments administered during resuscitation, such as epinephrine or high-energy defibrillation, may contribute to post-resuscitation dysfunction.[47] PAMD also peaks 24 to 48 hours after reperfusion and may be reversible.[62,63]

Causes of death in patients admitted to the ICU after cardiac arrest follow a typical timing and etiology pattern.[64,65] A minority

TABLE 51.3 Components and Driving Pathophysiologic Processes of the Post–Cardiac Arrest Syndrome[55]

Pathophysiologic Processes	Post–Cardiac Arrest Syndrome Components
Anoxic Cell/Tissue Injury • Anaerobic cellular metabolism	**Systemic Ischemia-Reperfusion Response** • Systemic inflammatory response
Ischemia-Reperfusion Injury • Cellular sodium/calcium overload • Reactive oxygen species • Intracellular acidosis • Initiation of apoptosis	**Post–Cardiac Arrest Myocardial Dysfunction** • Post-defibrillation stunning • Ischemia-reperfusion injury • Cardiac depression from cytokines • β-Adrenergic downregulation
Systemic Inflammatory Response • Vasoplegia • Microvascular/endothelial dysfunction • Cytokine-mediated cell/tissue injury • Dysregulation of coagulation system • Mitochondrial dysfunction • Abnormal energy metabolism • Capillary leak	**Persistent Precipitating Pathology** • Myocardial ischemia/infarction • Cardiomyopathy • Respiratory failure • Sepsis or distributive shock • Toxic/metabolic derangement • Obstructive process (PE/tamponade) • Massive hemorrhage
Neurohormonal Dysregulation • Adrenergic surge with β-adrenergic receptor downregulation • Hypothalamic-pituitary-adrenal axis dysfunction	**Anoxic Brain Injury** • Hypoxic-ischemic encephalopathy • Excitotoxic neuronal injury • Hyperthermia-mediated injury • Secondary neuronal apoptosis

Modified from Neumar RW, Nolan JP, Adrie C, et al. Post-cardiac arrest syndrome: epidemiology, pathophysiology, treatment, and prognostication. A consensus statement from the International Liaison Committee on Resuscitation (American Heart Association, Australian and New Zealand Council on Resuscitation, European Resuscitation Council, Heart and Stroke Foundation of Canada, InterAmerican Heart Foundation, Resuscitation Council of Asia, and the Resuscitation Council of Southern Africa); the American Heart Association Emergency Cardiovascular Care Committee; the Council on Cardiovascular Surgery and Anesthesia; the Council on Cardiopulmonary, Perioperative, and Critical Care; the Council on Clinical Cardiology; and the Stroke Council. *Circulation.* 2008;118:2452-83.

of deaths occur early, within the first day after ROSC. These early deaths occur primarily from cardiovascular causes, such as recurrent cardiac arrest, refractory shock, and multiorgan failure. Early deaths are more common in patients resuscitated from IHCA, who typically have more severe premorbid illness. Cardiovascular and respiratory failure are the most important nonneurologic drivers of outcome after cardiac arrest.[66] Later deaths during the days and weeks after cardiac arrest result from progression of multiple organ dysfunction or from neurologic injury.

Perceived irreversible anoxic brain injury contributes to over 70% of in-hospital deaths after cardiac arrest. A formal diagnosis of brain death occurs in 10% to 15% of cases,[67] whereas withdrawal of life-sustaining therapies (WLST) owing to poor anticipated neurologic prognosis is the major cause of death among patients resuscitated from OHCA.[68] Accurately determining the extent of brain injury is essential to avoid inappropriate or premature WLST in patients who are not irreversibly brain injured. Therefore rigorous neurologic prognostication is a major component of post–cardiac arrest intensive care. This topic will be discussed in the next section.

ORGANIZATION OF POST–CARDIAC ARREST CARE

As in other critically ill patients, care of patients after resuscitation from cardiac arrest can be divided into three distinct phases: early, middle, and late (Fig. 51.1). The next section describes each phase and the organ-specific priorities for patient management during each phase.

The early (salvage) phase of post-arrest care occurs during the first few hours: for OHCA, this is in the ambulance, emergency department (ED), and ICU; for IHCA, this may begin in the ward and transition to the ICU. This phase focuses on damage control to prevent worsening brain injury and other organ injury. Major goals during this early phase include the following:

- Stabilization of hemodynamics and pulmonary function
- Restoration of normal organ homeostasis
- Prevention of acute deterioration and other complications
- Identification/treatment of the triggering etiology
- Initiating targeted temperature management (TTM)

The middle (optimization/stabilization followed by deescalation) phase of post–cardiac arrest care occurs during the subsequent 24 to 72 hours in the ICU and focuses on supporting organ function to allow neurologic recovery. Major goals during this middle phase include the following:

- Optimizing and maintaining organ homeostasis
- Prevention/management of critical illness complications
- Maintenance of TTM, followed by rewarming

The late (recovery/convalescent) phase of post–cardiac arrest care occurs after 72 hours, when TTM has been completed. Major goals during this late phase include the following:

- Accurate neurologic assessment
- Liberation from ICU
- Initiating rehabilitation to restore the prior level of functioning
- Definitive long-term treatment of the precipitating pathology (secondary prevention of cardiac arrest)

ACUTE STABILIZATION

Immediately after ROSC, patients resuscitated from cardiac arrest are critically ill, at risk of rearrest, and frequently electrically and hemodynamically unstable. The initial early phase of postresuscitation care involves damage control and salvage of organ function to prevent further hypoperfusion that can exacerbate organ injury (especially brain injury). As in other diseases causing brain injury, even a single episode of hypoxemia

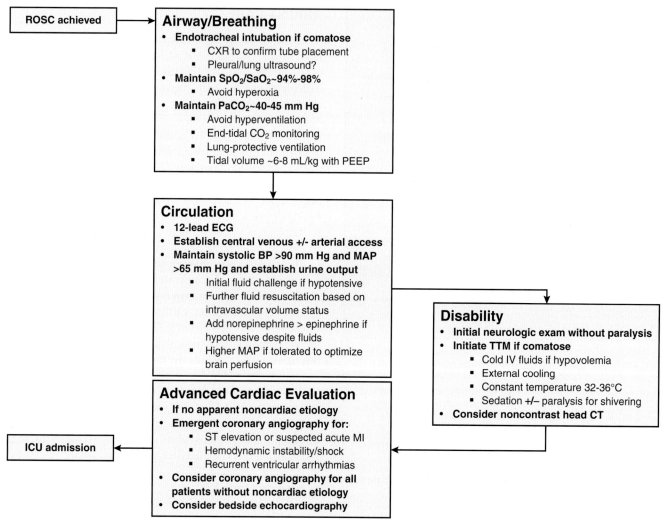

Fig. 51.1 Phases of care after cardiac arrest. *TTM,* Targeted temperature management.

Fig. 51.2 Early management priorities after resuscitation from cardiac arrest. BP, Blood pressure; *CT,* computed tomography; *CXR,* chest radiograph; *ECG,* electrocardiogram; *ICU,* intensive care unit; *MAP,* mean arterial pressure; *MI,* myocardial infarction; *PEEP,* positive end-expiratory pressure; *ROSC,* return of spontaneous circulation; TTM, targeted temperature management.

or hypotension is associated with significantly increased risk of mortality.[69] An additional goal in this early phase of care is to identify and begin treatment of the triggering etiology of cardiac arrest.

Several immediate procedures are appropriate during stabilization for most patients resuscitated from cardiac arrest (Fig.

51.2).[28,70] A safe and definitive airway should be established for patients requiring mechanical ventilation: this may require replacement of emergency supraglottic airways or simply confirmation of placement for endotracheal tubes. Continuous blood pressure monitoring and anticipated frequent blood gas sampling will require arterial catheter placement. Adequate intravenous

---

BOX 51.1 Focused Neurologic Examination for Comatose Patients After Resuscitation From Cardiac Arrest

Breathing
Breathing over set ventilator rate

Brainstem Reflexes
Pupils' response to light (constrict to light)
Corneal reflexes (blink when cornea brushed)
Oculocephalic reflex (eyes move when head is turned)
Gag when throat is stimulated (suction posterior pharynx)
Cough when airway is stimulated (suction endotracheal tube)

Motor Response
Motor response of arms and legs to stimulation (none, extension, flexion, withdrawal, purposeful movement, communicating)

---

access usually requires a central venous catheter. Temperature is a critical variable in brain-injured patients; a core temperature monitor (esophageal, bladder, or central venous) should be placed if the patient is comatose.

NEUROLOGIC CONSIDERATIONS

Most patients resuscitated from cardiac arrest lasting more than a few minutes are comatose (i.e., not following commands on examination). A focused neurologic examination (Box 51.1) performed in the absence of confounding drug effects has prognostic value and should be performed in all patients prior to administration of sedative or paralytic drugs if possible.[71] If uncertain whether a patient has had paralytic drugs (i.e., after prehospital intubation), a nerve stimulator should be used to confirm muscle response. Sedatives, shock, and acidosis may worsen the neurologic examination; clinicians should assume that the patient's examination is confounded when there is concern for these factors.

With optimal care, most OHCA survivors awaken and are able to return to a normal or near-normal level of functioning.[72,73] Brain recovery requires days to be evident, making it perilous to make any prognostic statement during the early phase after cardiac arrest.[74,75] The most conservative approach is to treat patients as if they have a chance to awaken for at least a few days while additional data are accumulated.

Baseline characteristics of the patient, circumstances of the cardiac arrest, and subsequent resuscitation are associated with the probability of good recovery (see Table 51.1).[10,11] Several groups have combined these variables into prognostic scores to estimate probability of recovery after OHCA[11,76] or IHCA.[77] However, these variables, particularly the historical variables gathered during the emergency, are often imprecisely known during the acute phase or are imprecisely defined for OHCA.[78] The IHCA scores may be more reliable yet may lack the ability to predict subsequent survival prior to cardiac arrest.

In order to avoid using unreliable historical factors, other groups examined stratification of patients based on illness severity scores.[66,71,79-82] A combination of initial neurologic examination

(using Full Outline of Unresponsiveness motor and brainstem subscales)[83] and cardiopulmonary failure (using Serial Organ Failure Assessment cardiovascular and respiratory subscales)[84] provides a rapid and parsimonious stratification of post–cardiac arrest patients into different illness severities with different likelihoods of survival (Fig. 51.3).[71,72] This examination and assessment of the patient provides a starting point for prognostication by providing a pretest estimate of odds of survival, which can be revised as more data are gathered. This initial estimate of prognosis can also be used to set realistic expectations about outcomes and to help determine the aggressiveness of care in specific circumstances. For example, patients who remain unresponsive to pain with missing brainstem reflexes on their best neurologic exam in the first 6 hours after ROSC (deep coma) have very poor outcomes and nearly always die from neurologic causes regardless of other treatments for shock or organ failure, including coronary revascularization.[71,85]

Early objective neurologic testing can be useful for further risk stratification in patients with deep coma, but no single modality is completely definitive by itself. Computed tomography (CT) scan of the brain can demonstrate brain edema (defined by a reduced ratio of gray matter to white matter [GWR] <1.2) in over 20% of post-ROSC patients. This finding suggests a severe brain injury and poor outcomes, although the cutoffs that are nonsurvivable remain controversial.[86] A small percentage (<4%) of patients have unsuspected intracranial hemorrhage on CT scan. Where available, an early electroencephalogram (EEG) can supplement the clinical examination in comatose patients; an EEG is particularly important for patients with abnormal movements and suspected myoclonus.[87] An early EEG showing a malignant pattern, such as burst-suppression or status epilepticus combined with deep coma and/or brain edema on head CT, portends a grim prognosis.[88]

TTM is recommended for all patients with coma after cardiac arrest. A large body of preclinical data, several clinical trials of variable quality, and many observational implementation studies suggest that TTM is associated with better brain recovery after cardiac arrest.[54,89-91] One clinical trial found no difference in outcome when patients were maintained at 36°C versus 33°C for 24 hours after cardiac arrest.[92] Current research seeks to determine whether temperatures lower than normal body temperature are actually beneficial or if the TTM treatment is preventing deleterious effects of fever. Fever is well known to be detrimental for other types of acquired brain injuries.

Measurement and control of patient temperature should begin as soon as possible. Benefits of TTM regimens in preclinical studies decline with delays of more than 6 hours after ROSC.[93] However, clinical trials have found no advantage to initiating TTM in the ambulance prior to ED arrival; possible harm was suggested using large boluses of cold IV fluids.[94,95] Therefore TTM is an intervention to initiate in the ED for OHCA or during transition to the ICU from a ward for IHCA. Induction of TTM can occur concurrently with coronary angiography or other procedures. Patients usually present with some degree of mild hypothermia (core temperature 35°C) after ROSC because of equilibration of peripheral and core blood compartments. If the patient temperature is below the selected target temperature,

PCAC Category 1	Category 1 Awake	Early Survival
FOUR Score M + B = 8 *Any SOFA CV + R score*	*Follows commands or makes purposeful movements (e.g., pulling at tubes and lines.*	**~80%**
PCAC Category 2 *FOUR Score M + B = 4-7* *SOFA CV + R score <4*	**Category 2 Coma without severe shock** Does not follow commands or make purposeful movement but brainstem reflexes are present. Modest vasopressor requirements and reasonable oxygenation on standard mechanical ventilation.	**Early Survival** **~60%**
PCAC Category 3 *FOUR Score M+B = 4-7* *SOFA CV + R score ≥ 4*	**Category 3 Coma with cardiopulmonary dysfunction** *Does not follow commands or make purposeful movement but brainstem reflexes are present. High vasopressor requirements or very difficult to oxygenate (e.g., requiring high ventilator settings).*	**Early Survival** **~30%**
PCAC Category 4 *FOUR Score M+B < 4* *Any SOFA CV + R score*	**Category 4 Coma with loss of brainstem reflexes** *Does not follow commands or make purposeful movement and multiple brainstem reflexes are lost (e.g., no pupil response or gag or cough).*	**Early Survival** **<10%**

Fig. 51.3 Pittsburgh Cardiac Arrest Categories (PCAC) and Hospital Survival after Out-of-Hospital Cardiac Arrest. To determine the PCAC, first examine coma and brainstem reflexes (best motor response to voice or pain, pupil reaction to light, corneal response, gag, cough, spontaneous breathing) to determine the Full Outcome of UnResponsiveness (FOUR) score, motor and brainstem subscores (out of 8 possible points), and determine severity of shock (vasopressor requirements to keep systolic blood pressure >100 mm Hg) and pulmonary status (can you oxygenate the patient) to determine the Sequential Organ Failure Assessment (SOFA) score cardiovascular (CV) and respiratory (R) subscores (out of 8 possible points).

the patient should not be rewarmed too fast: gradual passive rewarming at rates less than 0.25°C per hour up to the target temperature is appropriate rather than rapid rewarming. When initial patient temperature is higher than the selected target temperature, cooling as rapidly as possible is reasonable.

Various surface and endovascular methods of controlling temperature are available; no method has demonstrated an advantage. Clinicians should select devices for their institution based on nursing and provider preferences. In the ED, cooling blankets and ice packs are often simpler to use than feedback-controlled TTM devices. However, once a patient reaches target temperature and transitions to the ICU, a feedback-controlled device is necessary for precise control. If a patient also requires fluid resuscitation and has no pulmonary edema, rapid bolus of refrigerated IV fluids will facilitate cooling.[94] Fluids must be administered via a central line or quickly enough via peripheral lines to enter the core blood compartment in order to alter core temperature.

Suppression of shivering is essential to maintain target temperatures below normal, particularly during induction of cooling. Absence of heat generation because of severe brain injury is actually an adverse prognostic indicator.[96] Sedative and paralytic drugs are highly effective at suppressing shivering but can confound neurologic assessment. Institutional shivering protocols are useful to ensure adequate shivering suppression and consistent care.[97] Opioid analgesics (e.g., fentanyl) and sedative medications (e.g., dexmedetomidine or propofol) may effectively suppress shivering. Adjunctive agents, such as high-dose IV magnesium sulfate or high-dose buspirone, are advocated to reduce sedative requirements, with limited supporting evidence.[97] Acetaminophen can be useful as an antipyretic. Skin surface counterwarming can be an effective nonpharmacologic adjunctive method for suppression of shivering. When these measures fail to suppress shivering, neuromuscular blockade is indicated to allow stable TTM; observational studies suggest a possible benefit of neuromuscular blockade during TTM.[98]

CARDIOVASCULAR CONSIDERATIONS

Cardiovascular failure is the most prognostically important nonneurologic organ failure after resuscitation from cardiac arrest.[66] The shock state that develops after resuscitation from cardiac arrest is dynamic and the dominant pathophysiology changes over time.[47] Immediately after ROSC, patients are often normotensive or even hypertensive owing to residual effects of vasopressors given during CPR. This situation is self-limited and may help reperfusion. Thus treatment with antihypertensive drugs during this phase is not recommended. Hypotension and shock often occurs in a delayed fashion after a period of several minutes or even a few hours, creating a "honeymoon period" of transient hemodynamic stability. Many patients develop a low-output state with cardiogenic shock driven by PAMD, peaking at approximately 6 to 8 hours after ROSC.[99] This subsequently transitions to a mixed shock state with pathologic vasodilation resembling the SIRS, on top of residual PAMD.[47,99] The shock state may transition to a purely vasoplegic state after 24 to 48 hours, as PAMD resolves and inflammatory vasodilation peaks. Vasopressor requirements often peak at around 24 hours after ROSC; vasopressor dependence may persist for up to 48 to 72 hours.[99]

Cardiovascular assessment should identify and correct the triggering cause of cardiac arrest.[70] The first step is to obtain a 12-lead electrocardiogram (ECG), looking for evidence of myocardial ischemia or infarction. Up to 25% to 30% of patients resuscitated from OHCA have evidence of ST elevation myocardial infarction (STEMI) on ECG.[100] All patients who are otherwise candidates for aggressive care should be treated with emergent coronary angiography and reperfusion therapy, as with all other STEMI patients.[101,102] Coma and cardiac arrest are not contraindications to reperfusion therapy for STEMI, and coronary angiography is preferred over thrombolytic therapy.[101,102] In addition, acute coronary events remain the most likely cause of arrest for patients with a suspected cardiac etiology of OHCA whose ECG does not show STEMI. Pulmonary embolism (PE) is another common and treatable etiology of OHCA, particularly for patients with witnessed PEA arrest. Clinical predictors of PE in patients resuscitated from OHCA remain uncertain, but a CT angiogram of the chest is appropriate when PE is suspected.[103] Bedside cardiac ultrasound can identify focal wall motion abnormalities or right heart strain that will increase suspicion for acute coronary events or PE, as well as identifying effusions or structural abnormalities. Immediate echocardiography should be considered for all patients with uncertain etiology of arrest and/or significant hemodynamic instability.[28]

Hypotension, shock, and high vasopressor requirements all predict adverse clinical and neurologic outcomes in patients resuscitated from cardiac arrest.[47,66,104] Early hemodynamic stabilization is a critical component of early salvage resuscitation after cardiac arrest. The injured brain has an impaired blood flow autoregulation capacity and may have an increase in the critical closing pressure of the cerebral microvasculature. Therefore early hypotension leads to worsening brain ischemia and extension of brain injury. While the optimal arterial pressure target for patients resuscitated from cardiac arrest remains unclear, patients who are unable to maintain a systolic blood pressure of at least 90 to 100 mm Hg and/or a mean arterial pressure (MAP) of at least 65 to 70 mm Hg have worse outcomes.[70,101] These cutoffs define the minimal acceptable hemodynamic goals for patients after resuscitation from cardiac arrest. Some early hemodynamic optimization protocols have targeted a MAP of 80 to 100 mm Hg, based on observational data suggesting failure of cerebral blood flow autoregulation below 80 mm Hg.[105]

Given the pathophysiologic similarities between SIRS and the shock that develops after resuscitation from cardiac arrest, some early hemodynamic stabilization protocols after cardiac arrest mimic those for septic shock (Fig. 51.4).[28,47,105] Capillary leak may lead to a relative hypovolemia during the initial phase after ROSC. Fluid resuscitation is generally the first-line therapy for hypotensive patients after resuscitation from cardiac arrest.[70,106] Due to underlying PAMD, cardiac arrest patients may be at increased risk of pulmonary edema with aggressive fluid resuscitation, warranting assessment of preload responsiveness. Patients may require several liters of fluid resuscitation over the first 24 hours after ROSC to maintain adequate circulating volume.[99] For patients who have severe hypotension or who remain hypotensive after initial fluid resuscitation, vasopressors should be administered to maintain adequate MAP for organ perfusion. Norepinephrine is a reasonable first-line vasopressor for all patients at a usual dose of 0.05 to 0.5 μg/kg per minute;

epinephrine can be used as an alternative agent at this same dose, particularly for patients with bradycardia or evidence of low cardiac output (CO).[70,101] Dopamine has been associated with increased arrhythmias and mortality in other populations of critically ill patients with shock and is not recommended.[107]

Serum lactate production is a measure of end-organ perfusion: in the immediate phase after ROSC, the severity of lactic acidosis typically reflects the duration and magnitude of low-flow status during cardiac arrest. Higher initial and worst lactate level and lower arterial pH are associated with worse outcomes.[10,108] As in patients with sepsis, the rate of lactate clearance during the post-ROSC period is a measure of resuscitation effectiveness.[109] Persistent lactic acidosis should prompt fluid resuscitation in patients with evidence of fluid responsiveness. If lactic acidosis persists despite adequate fluid and vasopressor therapy, inotrope therapy should be considered if there is objective evidence of reduced CO.[47] Inotropic support in septic shock patients with low central venous oxygen saturation has unclear relationships to outcomes and no relevant studies exist in post–cardiac arrest patients. Due to the frequent development of PAMD, reduced CO is more common in patients resuscitated from cardiac arrest than in septic patients and inotropic support is more likely to be appropriate.[47] Low central venous oxygen saturation (<60%) typically implies a decreased CO, and may be an indication for inotropic support when there is persistent lactic acidosis or evidence of other organ hypoperfusion, such as decreased urine output. Dobutamine is the first-line inotropic agent and is typically effective at reversing PAMD and improving CO at a low dose (≤5 μg/kg per minute).[110] Low-dose epinephrine may be effective as an alternative inotrope but can aggravate lactic acidosis and may be harmful when used at high doses as a vasopressor.[111] Restoration of a normal serum lactate and adequate urine output greater than 0.5 mL/kg/h implies adequate organ perfusion and should be the goal of resuscitation and inotropic support.

Cardiogenic shock frequently occurs after cardiac arrest due to acute MI, leading to a much worse prognosis than when either is present alone. In fact, OHCA appears less prognostically important than shock in post-MI patients.[112,113] Even in the absence of STEMI, patients with cardiogenic shock after OHCA require emergent coronary angiography with PCI when indicated; multivessel intervention may be beneficial.[101,114,115] Outcomes for patients with cardiogenic shock remain poor with supportive care alone and no specific therapy beyond reperfusion therapy has proven benefit for these patients (see Chapter 13). Vasopressor support with norepinephrine and inotropic support with dobutamine are recommended for patients with cardiogenic shock; high-dose dopamine or epinephrine may be harmful.[107,111,115] TTM may provide beneficial hemodynamic effects in appropriately selected patients with cardiogenic shock after OHCA.[116] Mechanical circulatory support is often considered when medical therapy is inadequate to restore hemodynamics and organ perfusion.[117] Unfortunately, no studies demonstrate a clear mortality benefit of mechanical circulatory support devices. The IABP-SHOCK-II trial randomized patients with cardiogenic shock due to pump failure from acute MI despite reperfusion to intraaortic balloon pump (IABP) insertion or medical therapy alone. Nearly half

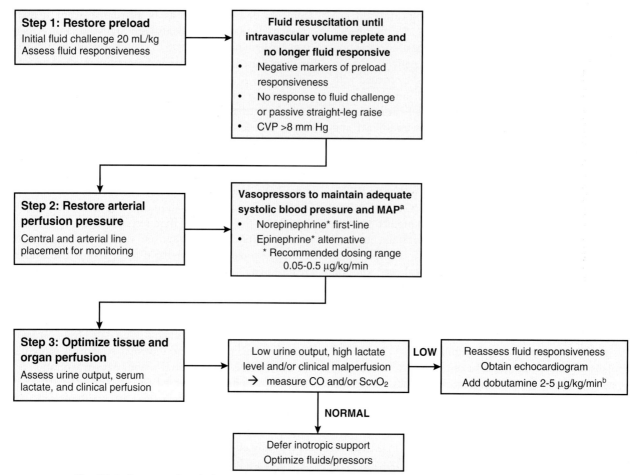

Fig. 51.4 Suggested early hemodynamic optimization strategy for patients with hypotension or hypoperfusion after return of spontaneous circulation after cardiac arrest. *CO,* Cardiac output; *CVP,* central venous pressure; *MAP,* mean arterial pressure; *ScvO₂,* venous oxygen saturation (normal >70%). ªWe suggest a systolic blood pressure goal of > 90–100 mm Hg and a MAP goal of >65–70 mm Hg. ᵇLow-dose epinephrine 0.01–0.05 µg/kg/min is an alternative.

of the patients enrolled in this study had OHCA, but there was no clear clinical benefit of IABP in either the entire population or this subgroup.[118] More advanced mechanical circulatory support devices, such as the Impella (Abiomed) or TandemHeart (Cardiac Assist) have not been systematically explored in patients with OHCA; preliminary studies in patients with cardiogenic shock demonstrate improvements in hemodynamics, but no clear effect on mortality (see Chapter 13).[117]

The mechanical circulatory support device that has been studied the most in OHCA patients is venoarterial extracorporeal life support (ECLS).[119,120] By providing up to 4 to 5 L/min of flow, ECLS can be an effective mechanical circulatory support strategy for patients with severe shock and is easier to deploy rapidly at the bedside than other devices. ECLS can be used in OHCA patients as part of one of two distinct strategies: during CPR (extracorporeal CPR [ECPR]) or for persistent shock after ROSC. Guidelines and approaches for ECLS in refractory shock after ROSC in OHCA patients do not differ substantially from use of ECLS in other shock states except that OHCA patients should demonstrate evidence that they do not have severe anoxic brain injury. This is one instance in which use of early neurologic

prognostication, as discussed earlier, can be applicable for guiding decision making.

ECPR involves cannulation for ECLS during ongoing CPR for patients with refractory cardiac arrest. Patient selection for ECPR is challenging; developing an ECPR program requires complex multidisciplinary cooperation and substantial infrastructure. Candidates for ECPR should be young and free from severe comorbidities, with a witnessed arrest from a shockable rhythm (or nonshockable rhythm from a likely reversible cause, such as PE) and bystander CPR. A shorter no-flow time and less severe lactic acidosis are favorable, as is a body habitus conducive to rapid cannulation.[121] The decision to initiate ECPR should occur rapidly during cardiac arrest. Few patients receiving more than 20 to 30 minutes of conventional CPR survive with good neurologic outcomes; thus the goal should be to initiate ECPR within this time frame if possible.[122] Patients with a high end-tidal carbon dioxide level (persistently >20 mm Hg) during prolonged CPR are generally more favorable candidates for ECLS, as this implies that high-quality effects CPR has occurred. Mechanical CPR devices can facilitate ongoing high-quality CPR during cannulation for ECLS. Patients treated with ECPR should undergo coronary angiography and TTM. With ECPR, TTM, and coronary angiography, up to 1 in 4 highly selected OHCA patients with refractory arrest may survive with good neurologic function.[123] Use of ECPR remains controversial and has not yet been tested in randomized trials. Appropriate patient selection remains challenging.[120]

After initial resuscitation from cardiac arrest, patients remain at risk of recurrent cardiac arrest, which occurs in 5% to 10% of patients.[69] Recurrent cardiac arrest can be due to untreated primary pathology or due to a secondary complication. Patients with OHCA due to a ventricular arrhythmia may have recurrent ventricular arrhythmias as part of electrical storm, as discussed in Chapter 23. Emergent coronary angiography is recommended for these patients, given that ongoing ischemia is the most common etiology even without ECG evidence of STEMI.[101] Patients may require antidysrhythmic drug infusion after ROSC, though receipt of antidysrhythmics during CPR does not mandate continuing infusions. Few data exist to guide appropriate use of antidysrhythmic drugs after resuscitation from cardiac arrest. Antidysrhythmic drug infusion is reasonable for patients with significant ventricular ectopy or nonsustained ventricular arrhythmias after resuscitation from a VT/VF arrest prior to or during coronary angiography. For patients with an acute coronary event who have been revascularized and are not having recurrent ventricular arrhythmias, a benefit of ongoing antidysrhythmic drug therapy is less likely. Patients without recurrent arrhythmias probably do not benefit substantially from ongoing antidysrhythmic drug infusion, which can produce hypotension and bradycardia. Recurrent PEA arrest often occurs due to profound shock and multiorgan dysfunction with metabolic abnormalities and often is a preterminal event. If a reversible etiology is suspected as the cause for recurrent cardiac arrest, then institution of ECLS may be warranted in highly selected patients without definite evidence of severe brain injury.

OTHER ORGAN CONSIDERATIONS

Respiratory failure is common after resuscitation from OHCA, and the majority of patients are intubated during CPR.[66] All patients who remain comatose after ROSC should be endotracheally intubated, even if the initial airway strategy was an LMA or other supraglottic device. Placement of a nasogastric tube is appropriate in the early phase to allow gastric decompression and facilitate administration of enteral medications. A chest radiograph is warranted to confirm tube placement and exclude complications such as pneumothorax. Lung ultrasound can be a useful adjunct, particularly when there is a delay in obtaining a chest radiograph. Appropriate monitoring using pulse oximetry is recommended after obtaining an arterial blood gas to confirm the results.[70] Use of end-tidal carbon dioxide monitoring may facilitate titration of ventilation to optimal carbon dioxide levels, recognizing that reduced CO due to PAMD can increase the gap between end-tidal carbon dioxide and partial pressure of carbon dioxide (P_aCO_2) levels (i.e., dead space ventilation). The injured brain is highly susceptible to perturbations in arterial oxygen and carbon dioxide tensions; stabilization of oxygenation and ventilation is necessary to avoid worsening brain injury. As in other critically ill patients, low tidal volume ventilation with less than or equal to 6 to 8 mL/kg ideal body weight using at least 5 to 10 cm H_2O of applied positive end-expiratory pressure (PEEP) appears beneficial in patients resuscitated from OHCA; this ventilatory approach may reduce the risk of lung injury and pneumonia.[70,124]

Hypoxemia early after ROSC should be avoided to prevent exacerbation of cerebral hypoperfusion and anoxic brain injury. Studies have consistently demonstrated that arterial hypoxemia after ROSC is associated with worse neurologic outcomes; thus an adequate fraction of inspired oxygen is required to maintain partial pressure of oxygen (P_aO_2) greater than 60 mm Hg and oxygen saturation levels (S_pO_2) greater than 90%.[125] Hyperoxia, defined by excessively high P_aO_2 (>300 mm Hg) during the early post-ROSC period, is associated with brain injury and worse clinical outcomes.[125] The proposed mechanism for this association between hyperoxia and brain injury is exacerbation of reactive oxygen species production with worsened IRI. Subsequent studies have not consistently shown this association between hyperoxia and brain injury; thus the clinical focus should be on avoiding hypoxemia using adequate supplemental oxygen. Supplemental oxygen should be titrated to achieve an S_pO_2 of 94% to 99% and a P_aO_2 of 80 to 150 mm Hg in most patients.[70] Increasing the P_aO_2 is an effective method for improving brain tissue oxygenation, but it remains unknown whether titration of P_aO_2 to target a specific level of brain tissue oxygenation is effective in OHCA patients (as has been demonstrated in selected patients with traumatic brain injury).

Arterial carbon dioxide tension is an important determinant of cerebral vascular tone; the injured cerebral vasculature continues to respond to P_aCO_2. Hyperventilation leading to low P_aCO_2 (<35 to 40 mm Hg) can trigger cerebral vasoconstriction and worsen brain hypoperfusion and should be avoided. On the contrary, mild hypoventilation allowing a mildly elevated P_aCO_2 (45 to 50 mm Hg) may facilitate cerebral vasodilation and improve cerebral perfusion, especially when the MAP is relatively low. Clinical studies show a U-shaped relationship between P_aCO_2 and neurologic outcomes after cardiac arrest, suggesting an optimal P_aCO_2 target in the range of 45 to 50 mm Hg.[125,126] Cerebral oximetry measures increase when P_aCO_2 is allowed to rise and decrease when P_aCO_2 is reduced by hyperventilation.[127] As in patients with acute respiratory distress syndrome (ARDS), permissive hypercapnia targeting a P_aCO_2 of 45 to 50 mm Hg during mechanical ventilation may be beneficial in OHCA patients.

Restoration of renal perfusion to allow adequate urine output (>0.5 to 1 mL/kg per hour) is an important goal of hemodynamic stabilization. Electrolyte abnormalities are common as both a cause and consequence of cardiac arrest; they can also be exacerbated by TTM. Hypokalemia is the most common electrolyte disorder triggering cardiac arrhythmias, often caused by diuretic therapy. Potassium supplementation to maintain a serum potassium of at least 3.5 mEq/L is warranted acutely. Hyperkalemia is another cause of cardiac arrest, particularly in patients with renal failure; hyperkalemia can be caused by acidosis in the post-ROSC setting. Acute treatment to lower serum potassium, coupled with IV calcium administration to stabilize cardiac membranes, is warranted in the presence of serum potassium above 6 mEq/L or when hyperkalemic ECG changes are present. Magnesium supplementation is often provided, especially in the presence of hypokalemia or hypomagnesemia. Careful administration of bicarbonate therapy may be needed to maintain an adequate arterial pH for patients with lactic acidosis who are receiving permissive hypercapnia. Hyperglycemia is common as part of the stress response to cardiac arrest and may be harmful to the injured brain; insulin is appropriate to control hyperglycemia while avoiding hypoglycemia.

MIDDLE PHASE OF POST-RESUSCITATION CARE

The second phase of post–cardiac arrest care is the stabilization/ optimization and de-escalation phase. This corresponds clinically to the maintenance and rewarming phases of TTM. The primary goal of this phase is to support organ function and maintain physiologic homeostasis while protecting the brain to allow neurologic recovery. High-quality critical care is essential to prevent complications of critical illness in these vulnerable patients. Care bundles and management protocols can facilitate optimal care delivery, even if few data support each individual bundle component.

TARGETED TEMPERATURE MANAGEMENT

Brain injury after resuscitation from cardiac arrest consists of an initial anoxic insult due to the no-flow and low-flow state, causing cerebral ischemia; this is followed by a more severe secondary wave of injury due to IRI.[55,128] It is important to note that the majority of neuronal injuries and deaths occurs in a delayed fashion, typically 24 to 48 hours after ROSC. This creates a time window for therapeutic intervention to allow neuroprotection. Extensive preclinical and human studies have consistently demonstrated a harmful effect of elevated body temperature on various forms of brain injury, including anoxic brain injury after cardiac arrest.[128] Dysregulation of central thermoregulatory mechanisms and induction of inflammatory cytokines leads to frequent development of pyrexia in patients resuscitated from cardiac arrest. Cooling the body after cardiac arrest may reduce the severity of the secondary wave of injury that occurs from neuronal IRI and prevent the harmful effects of subsequent fevers. The mechanisms by which elevated temperatures produce brain injury and hypothermia causes neuroprotection are complex and incompletely understood.[128] Hypothermia can also reduce infarct size in animal models of MI-induced cardiac arrest.

Cooling to maintain mild hypothermia in the range of 32 to 36°C is one of the only therapies associated with reduced severity of brain injury and improved outcomes after OHCA.[101] Two landmark studies from 2002 demonstrated that cooling to 32 to 34°C for 12 to 24 hours in comatose patients after resuscitation from witnessed VF OHCA improved neurologically intact survival compared to standard supportive care without increasing rates of major complications.[90,91] Therapeutic hypothermia, now called TTM, rapidly became the standard of care and is recommended by guidelines for all comatose patients resuscitated from cardiac arrest.[70,89,101] Limited data exist to support use of TTM in patients

with nonshockable arrest rhythms or IHCA, but the potential benefit and low risk of complications from TTM warrant consideration of this therapy for eligible patients with these conditions. There are few contraindications to TTM, such as uncontrolled bleeding or refractory shock; little is known about the safety of TTM in pregnant patients.

Patients in the standard care arm of the original hypothermia trials almost universally developed fevers, leading to uncertainty about the relative benefit of hypothermia versus active fever suppression after cardiac arrest. A subsequent trial compared TTM to 33°C versus 36°C in a more heterogeneous group of OHCA patients, including patients with nonshockable rhythms.[92] There were no significant differences in any major complications or outcomes between the two target temperature groups; no specific subgroup seemed to show a benefit of 33°C versus 36°C. Patients with shockable versus nonshockable rhythms and shorter versus longer ischemic time had similar outcomes with either target temperature. Patients with significant shock may have worse outcomes at 33°C versus 36°C, which argues for caution in the use of 33°C for hemodynamically unstable patients with shock.[129] Overall, this study does not refute the benefit of TTM as a therapeutic strategy but implies that the goal temperature is not the critical determinant of outcomes in the population studied. Current guidelines advise use of a higher target temperature in patients with bleeding complications and suggest considering a lower target temperature in patients with more severe neurologic injury.[101] Proposed advantages of each target temperature are listed in Table 51.4.[130] Some experts propose that cooling patients to a lower-than-normal body temperature (even 36°C) may not be beneficial beyond strict maintenance of normothermia (37°C) with active fever suppression. Whether a different TTM target temperature or duration or a rigorous fever-prevention strategy might be beneficial remains open to speculation. Until this is demonstrated by randomized controlled trials, we recommend applying TTM for resuscitated cardiac arrest patients. Current guidelines recommend TTM to 32 to

TABLE 51.4 **Advantages and Disadvantages of Common Goal Temperatures During Targeted Temperature Management**	
Goal Temperature 33°C	**Goal Temperature 36°C**
Easier to maintain goal temperature	Easier and more rapid to achieve goal temperature
Potentially greater neurologic protection	Less marked physiologic disturbances may reduce risk of minor complications
Randomized trials demonstrate benefit versus standard care	Improved hemodynamic stability and reduced vasopressor requirements
Preferred for severe brain injury	Preferred for patients at risk of bleeding
Fever unlikely if patient exceeds goal temperature (greater buffer)	Better outcomes for patients with significant shock
Less shivering and need for sedation/paralysis at goal temperature	

TABLE 51.5	Common Complications of Targeted Temperature Management
Organ System	**Common Complications**
Neurologic	Shivering
	Decreased sedative clearance
Cardiovascular	Bradycardia
	Decreased cardiac output
	Peripheral vasoconstriction
	Increased need for vasopressors and inotropes
	Endothelial dysfunction
Pulmonary	Pneumonia
	Decreased CO_2 production
Renal	Autodiuresis with hypovolemia
	Loss of potassium, magnesium, phosphorus
Gastrointestinal	Impaired gut motility/ileus
	Gastrointestinal bleeding
	Decreased hepatic metabolism with slowed lactate and drug clearance
Hematologic	Impaired platelet and clotting factor function
	Hypocoagulable state
Immune	Impaired immune function with immunosuppression
	Increased risk of infection
Endocrine	Insulin resistance and hyperglycemia

CO₂, Carbon dioxide.

36°C for 24 hours after ROSC, followed by up to 48 to 72 hours of active fever suppression to maintain temperature below 38°C.[101] If 36°C is used as the goal temperature for TTM, care should be taken to ensure that the patient does not exceed this temperature during TTM. TTM is considered a safe and low-risk therapy, but a number of predictable complications are known to occur (Table 51.5).[128]

Methods for cooling and maintenance of TTM differ among centers. Simple surface-cooling methods, such as ice packs and cooling blankets, with or without refrigerated IV fluids, are effective for inducing hypothermia but can be unreliable for accurately maintaining a target temperature during TTM. Various computer-controlled temperature management devices circulate temperature-controlled water through surface pads or endovascular balloons based on patient temperature. These devices make induction and maintenance of TTM easier and less complicated. No device has demonstrated a clinical benefit compared to any other method or device. A randomized trial comparing surface cooling devices and intravascular cooling devices found similar induction and maintenance of TTM and similar clinical outcomes after OHCA.[131]

Difficulty cooling a patient to target temperature or difficulty maintaining the target temperature is most often due to shivering. Suppression of shivering during TTM may guide the selection of analgesics and/or sedatives in the ICU, as discussed earlier.[97] Most patients receiving TTM are treated with opioid analgesics and/or sedatives, which also promotes patient comfort on mechanical ventilation. Short-acting sedative agents are typically recommended, such as propofol and dexmedetomidine, though hypotension and bradycardia are common side effects of these drugs, respectively. Fentanyl is a commonly used opioid analgesic, most often administered as a continuous infusion.

Benzodiazepines can be used for sedation, but drug accumulation due to impaired clearance and accumulation in fat can promote delirium and delay neurologic recovery or awakening.[75] Some studies suggest improved outcomes in OHCA patients treated with neuromuscular blockers during TTM, via an uncertain mechanism.[98] Fever worsens many forms of acquired brain injury. Therefore even after patients complete their TTM regimen, fever should be actively suppressed to maintain temperature below 38°C for up to 72 hours.[101]

NEUROLOGIC COMPLICATIONS

Comatose patients resuscitated from cardiac arrest have a wide spectrum of brain injury that can manifest with a number of specific neurologic complications. An EEG and brain imaging can help characterize brain injury.

Seizures occur in approximately 25% of OHCA patients but can often be nonconvulsive or clinically undetectable owing to neuromuscular blockade.[132] Comatose OHCA patients with seizures have a worse prognosis owing to both the greater initial severity of brain injury and extension of brain injury by the hypermetabolic effects of the seizure itself.[132] Status epilepticus is a severe manifestation that has a particularly poor prognosis.[133] Status myoclonus, characterized by frequent single jerks of the whole body, is distinct from status epilepticus both clinically and on EEG. Status myoclonus, in which these jerks are repetitive and sustained over 30 minutes, is often associated with a nonsurvivable neurologic injury (malignant pattern), but other myoclonus patterns distinguished by EEG (benign pattern) may be survivable.[87,134] Various other malignant patterns on EEG are associated with an unfavorable prognosis.[132,133] Because many clinically relevant EEG patterns are not associated with a clinical correlate, continuous EEG monitoring is suggested. Some centers have developed aggressive seizure treatment protocols with the goal of suppressing seizures to avoid worsening brain injury. It remains uncertain whether seizure suppression improves outcomes given the severe brain injury that often triggered the seizures. A step-wise approach to antiepileptic drug therapy for seizure suppression may be considered, starting with deep sedation using benzodiazepines and propofol followed by sequential addition of specific antiepileptic drugs, such as valproic acid, levetiracetam, phenytoin/fosphenytoin, or lacosamide. No clinical studies have clearly demonstrated superiority of a particular antiepileptic drug after cardiac arrest. All antiepileptic drugs can produce or aggravate hypotension, particularly with rapid infusion. When post–cardiac arrest seizures are successfully suppressed with drug therapy, some patients may awaken with good neurologic function.[135]

Cerebral edema is common after the global anoxic injury that occurs during cardiac arrest. A head CT scan may identify a reduced GWR, as discussed earlier. Markedly reduced GWR, below 1.2, suggests brain edema and a very poor prognosis.[86] Brain edema can lead to elevations in intracranial pressure (ICP), although the epidemiology of this complication after cardiac arrest is not well described. Measures to reduce ICP are effective in populations with traumatic brain injury and other neurologic insults but are understudied in cardiac arrest patients with elevated ICP. Head of bed elevation, hyperventilation, and osmotherapy with mannitol or hypertonic saline can lower ICP. Studies in patients with traumatic brain injury have demonstrated that brain tissue oxygen saturation can be critically low despite apparently adequate systemic oxygen delivery. It is likely that this phenomenon also occurs after cardiac arrest. The most effective methods for increasing brain tissue oxygen levels are to increase the arterial oxygen tension (to facilitate diffusion) and to increase MAP using vasopressors; increasing cardiac index with inotropes does not consistently improve brain tissue oxygen levels. When ICP is elevated, osmotherapy can improve brain tissue oxygen levels, but hyperventilation may fail to improve cerebral tissue oxygenation due to triggering of cerebral vasoconstriction. Future studies will be needed to determine whether principles of neurocritical care developed to treat other brain injuries can be successfully applied to patients after cardiac arrest.

CARDIOVASCULAR CONSIDERATIONS

Cardiovascular diseases, including acute MI or cardiomyopathy, trigger the majority of cardiac arrests. OHCA may be the first manifestation of cardiovascular disease.[2] Shock with the need for vasopressors is the most common and prognostically important organ failure after cardiac arrest.[47,66] Most patients resuscitated from cardiac arrest require vasopressors during the post-ROSC phase and lactic acidosis from hypoperfusion is common.[47,108,109] Hypotension and shock and/or higher vasopressor requirements are strong predictors of poor outcomes in patients resuscitated from OHCA.[104,136] Hypotension and shock severity can drive worsening outcomes directly by exacerbating anoxic brain injury and are also a marker for a more severe initial insult.

The pathophysiology of shock after cardiac arrest is dynamic and heterogeneous, with inter- and intrapatient variability over time. Post–cardiac arrest shock is a mixed shock state with both cardiogenic and vasoplegic components.[47,99] Cardiogenic shock develops from the interaction between the precipitating pathology and superimposed PAMD, peaking at 6 to 8 hours after ROSC and typically resolving in survivors over the ensuing 24 hours.[47,99] Vasoplegia with vasodilatory shock driven by IRI and SIRS develops in a more delayed fashion, starting around 12 hours after ROSC and progressing over the subsequent 24 hours. The nadir cardiac output typically occurs during the early phase (6 to 8 hours), but vasopressor requirements often peak later (24 hours) and the need for vasopressors may last up to 48 to 72 hours.[99] Vasopressor requirements and vasoplegia correlate with levels of endotoxemia and inflammatory cytokines, such as IL-6, more than with cardiac systolic function.[60,137–139] Similar to patients with sepsis, patients resuscitated from cardiac arrest may require several liters of fluid resuscitation over the first 24 to 48 hours to maintain adequate filling pressures,[99] though the hemodynamic benefit of these fluids must be balanced with the risks of edema. Metabolic derangements, such as lactic acidosis or relative adrenal insufficiency, can worsen hypotension and shock severity. See Fig. 51.4 for an algorithmic approach to hemodynamic stabilization after ROSC.

Reversible myocardial stunning is frequently identified in patients resuscitated from cardiac arrest.[47,63] Differentiating reversible PAMD from underlying structural heart disease (persistent precipitating pathology) is challenging clinically. Echocardiography can define cardiac function and identify reversible etiologies of arrest. At least two-thirds of patients have some left ventricular (LV) systolic dysfunction after resuscitation from cardiac arrest, with right ventricular (RV) systolic dysfunction and LV diastolic dysfunction less frequently reported.[47,139–141] Patients with PAMD may have global LV dysfunction and/or regional wall motion abnormalities depending on the underlying structural heart disease. PAMD itself typically produces global LV dysfunction. Studies examining LV systolic function after cardiac arrest have shown an average LV ejection fraction (LVEF) of approximately 35% to 40% initially, which may increase by 10% or more prior to hospital discharge.[47,63,139] In IHCA patients with a previously documented LVEF, one study showed a reduction in LVEF by 25% from baseline independent of baseline LVEF. In this study, patients with lower prearrest LVEF had lower hospital survival.[142] Most studies of PAMD have not shown a consistent association between LVEF and mortality, although a few studies have shown independent associations between markers of diastolic dysfunction and mortality.[139,140] For this reason, repeat echocardiography prior to hospital discharge may be appropriate in cardiac arrest survivors with evidence of PAMD to establish a new baseline and to determine potential need for a defibrillator. Little is known about long-term myocardial recovery after PAMD.

The pathophysiology of reversible PAMD (stunning) is complex and likely differs between patients. The major pathophysiologic mechanisms for PAMD are global myocardial ischemia with subsequent IRI and a SIRS-like state.[47,55] IRI causes PAMD in animal models. Myocardial stunning also occurs in humans after cardiopulmonary bypass, a clinical IRI state. Cellular calcium overload and acidosis as well as reactive oxygen species leading to mitochondrial dysfunction appear pathogenic; sodium-hydrogen exchanger inhibitors and cyclosporine reduce PAMD in animal models.[47] Inflammatory cytokines, such as tumor necrosis factor-α (TNF-α), can depress myocardial function and drive vasoplegia, microvascular dysfunction, and capillary leak. In animal models, TNF-α antagonists decrease PAMD.[47] PAMD is greater in VF arrest compared to asphyxial arrest, and VF itself may produce some degree of stunning owing to depletion of myocardial energy substrates. More important, defibrillator shocks produce significant myocardial stunning and likely represent a major cause of PAMD in patients resuscitated from VF. β-Agonist toxicity from high-dose epinephrine is another major contributor to PAMD via mechanisms that overlap with stress cardiomyopathy (apical ballooning or takotsubo syndrome).[47] Excessive activation of β-receptors can trigger direct myocardial toxicity, myocyte apoptosis, and receptor down-regulation to impair systolic function in a regional or global manner, perhaps explaining the association of higher epinephrine doses with adverse OHCA outcomes.

Hypothermia has numerous well-known effects on the cardiovascular system that can exacerbate cardiovascular dysfunction in OHCA survivors treated with TTM. As with other complications of TTM, these are more severe at a lower target temperature, such as 33°C. During hypothermia, CO decreases as the result of a decrease in heart rate and stroke volume.[143,144] This may or may not be associated with a change in serum lactate or venous oxygen saturation depending on the associated reduction in tissue metabolic rate and oxygen demands. Peripheral vasoconstriction also occurs, leading to an increase in systemic vascular resistance and LV afterload. Echocardiographic findings may not be consistently affected by hypothermia or specific target temperature.[143] Vasopressor requirements are higher at a lower target temperature, and outcomes for patients with significant shock may be worse at a lower target temperature.[129,144] One study of patients with cardiogenic shock after OHCA suggested improvements in selected hemodynamic parameters during TTM, emphasizing the complexity of systemic hemodynamic changes after OHCA.[116] Marked bradycardia may occur during hypothermia, yet rarely requires therapy; a lower heart rate during TTM may be associated with a more favorable outcome.[145]

Coronary angiography in patients resuscitated from OHCA reveals obstructive CAD in over 70% of patients.[100] Approximately 25% to 30% of patients with OHCA have ST elevation myocardial infarction (STEMI), most of whom have an occluded coronary artery.[100] Of OHCA patients without ST elevation, about 25% have an occluded coronary artery.[100] Identification of patients with an acutely occluded coronary artery as the cause of OHCA is critically important, as coronary angiography with reperfusion is likely to provide a substantial benefit in these patients. Studies of coronary angiography after OHCA consistently demonstrate that patients who receive a coronary angiogram have better survival and neurologic outcomes. However, these patients also have a lower clinical risk profile, reflecting selection bias in observational studies.[54,85,146–148] Early coronary angiography (within 6 to 24 hours) after OHCA appears particularly beneficial. Reperfusion drives the apparent benefit of coronary angiography; patients receiving early coronary angiography with reperfusion have the best outcomes.[146,147]

The ECG is the first-line test for identification of STEMI in OHCA patients, but ST elevation on ECG has poor sensitivity (as low as 60%) for identifying acute coronary occlusion in this population.[149] Use of additional ECG abnormalities, such as ST depression or QRS prolongation, may identify a greater percentage of patients with acute coronary occlusion, but 15% to 20% of patients with acute coronary occlusion after OHCA have a nearly normal ECG.[149] Clinical predictors of acute coronary occlusion after OHCA include preceding angina, known CAD, major CAD risk factors (such as smoking), clinical evidence of heart failure, a shockable arrest rhythm, and a brief arrest requiring few doses of epinephrine.[150,151] Small serum cardiac troponin elevations are common after OHCA and may reflect supply-demand mismatch injury to the heart, but significantly elevated or rising troponin suggests acute coronary occlusion.[150] Higher initial and peak serum troponin levels are associated with acute coronary occlusion, although precise cutoffs are hard to define.[150] Echocardiographic wall motion abnormalities have not been systematically evaluated as a predictor of CAD or coronary occlusion after OHCA. Composite risk scores have been used to improve identification of coronary occlusion after OHCA; one such risk score incorporates the presence of ST elevation, shockable arrest, preceding angina, clinical heart failure, and shockable arrest rhythm.[151]

Appropriate patient selection for coronary angiography after OHCA is important and most patients with unexplained OHCA of presumed cardiac etiology warrant coronary angiography.[152] Current guidelines strongly recommend emergent coronary angiography (within 2 hours) for patients with STEMI, clinically suspected acute MI, cardiogenic shock, or recurrent ventricular arrhythmias.[101] The decision to perform coronary angiography in these patients should be independent of the presence of coma.[102] Patients with ischemic ECG abnormalities other than ST elevation, markedly elevated serum troponin, shockable arrest rhythm, significant hemodynamic instability, frequent ventricular ectopy, or other risk factors for CAD and coronary occlusion should be considered for coronary angiography (Fig. 51.5). Some authors and guidelines have proposed coronary angiography for all OHCA patients without a contraindication, although the timing remains uncertain.[152] In general, patients with higher severity of illness and/or higher likelihood of coronary occlusion are likely to benefit from coronary angiography sooner (i.e., urgently or emergently).

One important consideration when selecting patients without a strong indication for coronary angiography is the anticipated severity of brain injury.[10] Patients who are likely to have severe brain injury are less likely to benefit from reperfusion. One study showed that patients who were unresponsive to pain with missing brainstem reflexes on examination did not benefit from early coronary angiography and almost always died of brain injury independent of coronary angiography.[85] If the decision is made to forego acute coronary angiography and a clear noncardiac cause of arrest is not determined, patients should undergo coronary angiography and appropriate treatment of CAD prior to hospital discharge.

Cardiac arrhythmias are common in OHCA patients, both as triggers for OHCA and in the post-resuscitation phase. For patients with shockable arrest rhythms, continuation of antidysrhythmic drug infusion after ROSC has not been systematically evaluated. For patients with recurrent ventricular arrhythmias or frequent ectopy despite coronary angiography and reperfusion, antidysrhythmic drug therapy is appropriate. No clinical benefit has been demonstrated for suppression of ventricular ectopy after OHCA. Amiodarone and lidocaine are used most frequently, with lidocaine considered less effective for suppressing arrhythmias but less likely to cause hemodynamic instability. The pharmacokinetic properties of these drugs have not been thoroughly studied in patients undergoing TTM, but hepatic lidocaine clearance is likely to be reduced. Bradycardia is common during TTM and may be exacerbated by amiodarone.

OTHER ORGAN CONSIDERATIONS

Mechanical ventilation will be necessary for most patients during this phase of care. Hypoxemic respiratory failure is the second most common and prognostically relevant manifestation of multiorgan failure.[66] Patients are almost universally intubated during CPR or due to coma from anoxic brain injury, but lung disease is common as a cause or consequence of arrest. Aspiration during emergent intubation is very common and may progress to pneumonia in up to half of OHCA patients.[153] Acute lung

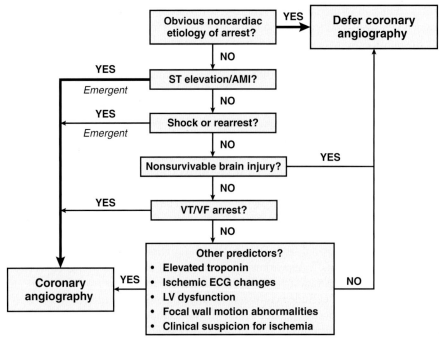

Fig. 51.5 Suggested approach to patient selection for emergent coronary angiography after out-of-hospital cardiac arrest. Emergent coronary angiography is defined as within 2 hours and routine coronary angiography is defined as within 24 hours. See Table 51.1 for clinical predictors of severe neurologic injury. *AMI,* Acute myocardial infarction; *ECG,* electrocardiography; *LV,* left ventricular; *VF,* ventricular fibrillation; *VT,* ventricular tachycardia.

injury and ARDS are common due to aspiration and the SIRS response after ROSC, often aggravated by cardiogenic pulmonary edema due to fluid resuscitation in the setting of underlying structural heart disease and PAMD. Lung contusions from CPR are frequently recognized and can progress to overt acute lung injury or pulmonary hemorrhage with hemoptysis, particularly in anticoagulated patients.

The severity of hypoxemic respiratory failure, defined by the P_aO_2/F_iO_2 (PF) ratio, is an important independent predictor of outcomes.[66] Patients resuscitated from cardiac arrest should be considered a population at high risk of developing ARDS and should be treated with lung-protective ventilation.[70] Ventilator settings appropriate for established ARDS are reasonable for cardiac arrest patients, especially if they have significant hypoxemic respiratory failure. Many patients who are intubated after OHCA will meet oxygenation criteria for ARDS (a PF ratio <200).[66] We recommend low tidal volume ventilation (<8 mL/kg) for all mechanically ventilated cardiac arrest patients, with less than 6 mL/kg recommended for those patients with evidence of lung injury or significant respiratory failure; permissive hypercapnia is appropriate.[124] Adequate PEEP of at least 5 to 10 cm H_2O is beneficial to allow use of a moderate F_iO_2 less than 60% when possible.[124] Deep sedation is often required to allow low tidal volume ventilation due to strong patient respiratory efforts driven by brain injury and metabolic acidosis. As in other patients with severe ARDS, cardiac arrest patients with a PF ratio less than 100 may benefit from early neuromuscular blockade.[98] Prone positioning is another option for patients with persistent hypoxemia.

Ventilator weaning in comatose patients should commence after patients complete TTM, depending on patient mental status and clinical condition. Patients who remain comatose may still undergo spontaneous breathing trials to maintain respiratory muscle function, but extubation is rarely appropriate for patients whose Glasgow Coma Scale score remains below 8. Pulmonary effects of TTM are not well described, although a decrease in systemic oxygen demand and carbon dioxide production may reduce ventilatory requirements. Lung mechanics may be impaired by rib and/or sternal fractures, though these fractures rarely prevent extubation in awake patients. Pain control using acetaminophen, systemic or topical nonsteroidal antiinflammatory drugs, topical anesthetics, and judicious use of opioids is beneficial. Low-dose ketamine infusion or local nerve blocks can be helpful for appropriately selected patients with pain limiting ventilator weaning. After extubation, meticulous pulmonary toilet and incentive spirometry are critical to maintain lung expansion and prevent recurrent respiratory failure.

Acute kidney injury (AKI) occurs in a significant number of patients after cardiac arrest, though the need for renal replacement is uncommon.[66] AKI after cardiac arrest results primarily from initial ischemic time complicated by subsequent shock and SIRS. AKI has generally not been an independent risk factor for mortality when corrected for shock.[66] Initial creatinine on presentation, predominantly reflecting chronic kidney disease, may be a more significant mortality predictor than rises in creatinine from AKI. Major risk factors and preventive strategies for AKI after cardiac arrest have not been well described, but contrast exposure from coronary angiography does not appear to be a major contributor.

Electrolyte abnormalities are common after cardiac arrest and may be significantly exacerbated by TTM. Hypothermia impairs renal tubule function, preventing absorption of fluid and electrolytes by the kidney. This produces a "cold diuresis," leading to excessive urine production with loss of fluid and electrolytes during hypothermia, particularly at lower target temperatures. For this reason, maintaining urine output above 1 mL/kg per hour is appropriate for hemodynamic resuscitation during TTM at low temperatures to ensure adequate renal perfusion. Hypovolemia and deficiencies of potassium, magnesium, phosphorus, and calcium all occur during TTM, requiring frequent electrolyte monitoring and supplementation. Hypokalemia is further exacerbated by intracellular shifts that can reverse during rewarming, triggering hyperkalemia. For this reason, moderate potassium supplementation to a serum potassium level of 3.5 mEq/L is typically recommended during TTM. Metabolic acidosis after cardiac arrest is most often due to lactic acidosis, which should clear with restoration of adequate perfusion. Bicarbonate therapy is unlikely to be beneficial for most patients.

Gastrointestinal system dysfunction is less frequently reported after cardiac arrest. Liver injury may occur from ischemic hepatitis as manifested by elevated serum transaminases and subsequent jaundice; this is typically mild and rarely progresses to liver failure.[66] Studies of multiorgan dysfunction after cardiac arrest have not demonstrated an independent prognostic effect of hepatic dysfunction after cardiac arrest.[66] Intestinal dysfunction is likely common after cardiac arrest, but rarely reported. Ileus is common from ischemia and medication effects, along with the antimotility effects of hypothermia. Mechanically ventilated OHCA patients warrant consideration of pharmacologic stress ulcer prophylaxis. Early initiation of low-volume enteric tube feeding is recommended for most mechanically ventilated patients but has not been evaluated in post–cardiac arrest patients. Delaying initiation of tube feeding until vasopressor requirements decline, lactic acidosis clears, and TTM is completed seems reasonable. Patients with a severe global ischemic insult may develop nonocclusive mesenteric ischemia with intestinal mucosal sloughing and significant lactic acidosis, carrying a poor prognosis. Translocation of gut bacteria and endotoxemia due to loss of intestinal mucosal integrity may be an important contributor to SIRS.[138] Initiation of tube feeding after rewarming and shock resolution may preserve gut mucosal integrity; provision of nutritional support will combat malnutrition and aid in recovery.

Intraabdominal organ injury, such as hepatic or splenic laceration, is a potentially lethal but uncommon complication of CPR (1% to 2% of cases). Depending on severity, solid-organ laceration or injury can present acutely or subacutely and mild cases are likely clinically silent. A dramatic presentation of major solid-organ laceration from CPR is hemorrhagic shock, which may result in post-ROSC hypotension or recurrent cardiac arrest with PEA (particularly in anticoagulated patients). Bedside ultrasound (such as a Focused Abdominal Sonography in Trauma exam) may reveal free fluid in the abdomen, though exclusion of ruptured abdominal aortic aneurysm is also warranted. Shock or recurrent arrest with a dropping hemoglobin and/or fluid-responsive hypotension with abdominal distention is characteristic. Hemorrhagic shock after resuscitation from nontraumatic cardiac arrest in the absence of an obvious cause

of blood loss should be evaluated with an abdominal CT scan. Extreme cases may produce abdominal compartment syndrome with a tense abdomen, fluid-responsive hypotension, oliguria, and increased plateau airway pressures on the ventilator. Delayed hemorrhage from solid-organ injury may occur in patients who are subsequently started on anticoagulation.

Hematologic dysfunction is a less frequent complication after cardiac arrest. Thrombocytopenia may occur but is rarely severe and does not appear to affect prognosis.[66] More commonly, patients are treated with antiplatelet and anticoagulant drugs for treatment of acute MI. Hypothermia impairs platelet and clotting factor function, increasing bleeding risk. TTM should be avoided in patients who are actively bleeding, although patients with mild bleeding may be treated with TTM using a higher goal temperature. Bleeding complications requiring transfusion are infrequent, although a nonspecific decline in hemoglobin with resultant anemia is more common (as in other populations of critically ill patients). The appropriate hemoglobin threshold for transfusion in cardiac arrest patients has not been established but likely depends on the presence of active bleeding or myocardial ischemia. As with other critically ill patients, pharmacologic and mechanical venous thromboembolism prophylaxis is appropriate owing to limited mobility during TTM.

Infection is common after OHCA, occurring in more than half of patients, with nearly one-third of patients having evidence of bacteremia.[154,155] The majority of infections are pulmonary in origin from ventilator-associated or aspiration pneumonia. This fact supports using aggressive prophylactic measures against ventilator-associated pneumonia.[153] Early pneumonia is frequent due to aspiration of oropharyngeal contents during intubation; empiric or prophylactic antibiotics are appropriate and appear beneficial.[153,156,157] Patients frequently have vascular and/or urinary catheters after cardiac arrest, leading to an elevated risk of catheter and line infections. Hypothermia impairs humoral and cellular immune function, potentially increasing the risk of infection while masking fever. Elevation of inflammatory cytokines, particularly IL-6, appears to predict prognosis and associated shock and multiorgan failure severity.[60,137,138] The magnitude of inflammatory cytokine production does not appear to be significantly modified by goal temperature during TTM.[137] Endotoxemia is frequent and associated with degree of vasopressor requirements, presumably due to loss of mucosal barrier integrity.[138] Delayed fevers after completion of TTM are common and may be due to nosocomial infection or noninfectious SIRS. Fever suppression and infectious workup are appropriate, with consideration of empiric antibiotics when applicable.

Endocrinologic abnormalities include hyperglycemia and adrenal suppression. Hyperglycemia is frequent owing to the effects of stress hormones and hypothermia, which produce peripheral insulin resistance.[158] Elevated blood glucose appears to worsen brain injury and clinical outcomes, justifying insulin treatment for patients with blood glucose above 200 mg/dL to maintain moderate blood glucose control in the range of 140 to 180 mg/dL without causing hypoglycemia.[159] No further benefit from lower glucose control has been demonstrated. As in patients with septic shock, cardiac arrest patients sometimes have absolute or relative adrenal corticosteroid insufficiency, which may be associated with increased shock severity and/or adverse prognosis.[160] A small study failed to show a benefit of routine hydrocortisone supplementation in patients with shock after cardiac arrest, though the subset of patients with baseline low levels of cortisol may have benefitted from it.[161] Testing for hypocortisolemia and considering treatment for patients with shock is reasonable.

LATE PHASE OF POST-RESUSCITATION CARE

The final phase of post–cardiac arrest care is the recovery/convalescence phase. This phase begins after patients are rewarmed from TTM and extends through hospital discharge and beyond. The goals of this final phase of post–cardiac arrest care are neurologic assessment, ICU liberation, and rehabilitation to restore the prior level of functioning, along with secondary prevention of cardiac arrest if applicable. Patients may show signs of neurologic recovery and awakening, but many will remain comatose, requiring further neurologic assessment to determine their likelihood of awakening. Patients resuscitated from cardiac arrest have been critically ill, mechanically ventilated in the ICU for days, and will require substantial rehabilitation and optimization to allow liberation from the ICU.

NEUROLOGIC PROGNOSTICATION

Determining the most likely functional outcome for a patient who has survived the initial phases of cardiac arrest is a high priority for the treating team and for the family of the patient. Most long-term survivors of cardiac arrest have favorable functional recovery.[73,162] This is due in part to the fact that many surrogate decision makers elect to withdraw life-sustaining treatment in patients who are expected to have functional impairments.[163] This fact makes accurate prognostication critically important, because any bias toward pessimism could inappropriately increase mortality.

This section reviews the key features of clinical examination and neurologic testing that are believed to have strong relationships to outcome. Selecting and interpreting specific findings should be based on the availability of tests at given institutions and the expertise and experience of the clinical team. In some locations, this requires collaboration between intensivists, neurologists, neuroradiologists, or neurophysiologists.

Guidelines for prognostication of functional recovery after cardiac arrest have synthesized a large and complex literature.[101,133,164] These reviews highlight several limitations in the existing literature. First, a significant amount of data on the association of specific tests or clinical findings with outcome were collected several decades ago when intensive care and overall outcomes were quite different. The relevance of those associations with patients receiving modern intensive care is uncertain. Second, almost all studies of the associations between tests and patient outcomes did not blind the treating team to the results of the test. This situation can lead to a self-fulfilling prophecy in which a poor test result or clinical finding sometimes leads to WLST and thus inflates the apparent negative predictive value (the inverse of the false-positive rate) of the test. Third, all reviews

agree that no single clinical finding or test provides certainty of good or poor outcome. Consequently, guidelines recommend that clinicians should usually employ multiple signs or tests in order to make a prognosis for an individual patient. Finally, very few studies examine the incremental value of combining tests or clinical findings. Thus there is little guidance on the specific order in which a clinician should perform testing or what is the most efficient strategy for patient evaluation. In general, it will take at least 72 hours after ROSC to provide sufficiently accurate neurologic testing to warrant WLST. A few highly selected patients with multiple incontrovertible objective adverse findings may warrant withdrawal of care prior to this time point.

The clinical examination evolves over time after cardiac arrest. While the initial neurologic examination in the first 24 hours after cardiac arrest cannot exclude the possibility of recovery, a rapidly improving examination is a favorable finding associated with higher odds of recovery.[71] Persistent absence of corneal and pupil responses more than 72 hours after cardiac arrest has a strong association with poor outcome.[133] Caution is advised if the patient has had sedatives, which are very potent at reducing corneal reflexes. In contrast, the motor response to stimulation (flexion, extension, or other response) is unreliable for determining outcomes, particularly after TTM.

One of the most ominous clinical signs after cardiac arrest is status myoclonus or myoclonic status epilepticus. This syndrome is a repetitive jerk of the face, trunk, or extremities lasting for more than 30 to 60 minutes. In many cases, this physical sign is related to widespread damage to the cerebral cortex. Myoclonus can appear with or without epileptiform activity on EEG. Persistent status myoclonus with a suppression-burst pattern (or other malignant pattern) on EEG over the first 72 hours after cardiac arrest is associated with very low odds of recovery.[87,88,133] It is important to note that not all myoclonic jerks are malignant status myoclonus and a minority (~10%) that can be recognized on EEG may be survivable.[87,134] Likewise, myoclonic jerks may be confused with epileptiform activity, which might be treatable and survivable.[135] Accurate assessment of clinical myoclonic jerks, including neurophysiologic characterization to distinguish them from epileptiform activity or more benign myoclonus, is crucial. EEG and neurologic consultation is essential.

In some patients, clinical examination will be consistent with brain death: apnea with absence of brainstem reflexes and absent motor response (other than spinal reflexes). This situation may occur in up to 10% to 15% of patients admitted to intensive care.[67] Local law and custom will dictate the specific testing and confirmation required to diagnose irreversible brain death. In general, the dynamic neurologic examination shortly after cardiac arrest and the potential for confounding factors to alter the examination (shock, toxins, acidosis, or other metabolic derangements) make it difficult or impossible to confidently make this diagnosis for 24 to 48 hours after cardiac arrest. Exceptions would include cases in which imaging reveals irreversible structural brain injury, such as massive cerebral edema with herniation or radiographically confirmed absence of cerebral blood flow. Patients who progress to brain death may have declared their wish to become organ donors, which increases the importance of correct recognition of this situation.

Neurophysiologic studies, including EEG and somatosensory evoked potentials (SSEPs), can predict functional recovery. Malignant EEG patterns, such as epileptiform discharges, are associated with reduced likelihood of good recovery but are potentially survivable with treatment.[135] This fact has prompted some groups to recommend routine continuous EEG monitoring as part of the care for post–cardiac arrest patients. The EEG finding that is most strongly associated with favorable odds of recovery is a reactive EEG background.[165] Return of EEG reactivity implies electrically intact regions of cerebral cortex and can be a harbinger of awakening.

SSEPs are typically performed at 48 to 72 hours after ROSC, when rewarming is completed. Absence of an SSEP elicited in the parietal cortex by median nerve stimulation has extensive literature relating it to poor neurologic outcome.[133] This cortical response normally occurs 20 ms after the median nerve is stimulated and is called the N20 response. Absence of the N20 response implies damage to the thalamocortical projections in the parietal region, a situation of cortical damage that typically precludes awakening. A few case reports of patients who awakened after documented absent N20 responses included antecedent sedation with midazolam and fentanyl as well as TTM at lower temperatures (33°C). Repeating an SSEP test may be warranted if these potential confounders are present or other data suggest that the patient may be more viable.

Imaging of the brain can reveal areas of anoxic damage. CT imaging of the brain early after cardiac arrest can reveal cerebral edema that is immediately life threatening.[86] Progression of cerebral edema over the first few days after arrest can reveal structural compromise to the brain, including herniation, but CT scan is not very sensitive or specific as a prognostic test and will not typically demonstrate the subtle findings of anoxic brain injury. Magnetic resonance imaging (MRI) with diffusion-weighted images (DWI) can more clearly reveal damaged areas with restricted diffusion on DWI sequences. These changes increase over the first days after resuscitation and are most prominent 4 to 10 days after cardiac arrest. Thus MRI is typically performed in patients who remain comatose beyond 72 hours.[166] More extensive DWI changes in the cerebral cortex are associated with lower probability of good functional recovery.[167,168] Clinicians can assess the anatomic areas of restricted diffusion with consideration of the functional role of each area: damage to highly fluent areas (e.g., speech and motor cortex) are likely to be more clinically devastating than damage to less fluent areas (e.g., prefrontal cortex or small areas of occipital cortex). Research studies and specialized examinations of the brain have used magnetic resonance spectroscopy to assess brain metabolism, but the current literature on these techniques is limited.

Blood biomarkers used for making prognosis include enzymes released from neurons (neuron-specific enolase [NSE]) or from glia (S-100B).[133,165] This literature is confusing because the analytic standards for these markers are not standardized between laboratories and the optimal cutoff for predicting outcome remains controversial. In addition, there is large regional variation in use: NSE levels are commonly measured in Europe but rarely used in the United States. Levels of NSE that are persistently elevated after 72 hours have the highest association with poor outcome; higher peak values and/or a rising rather than falling pattern are likewise concerning for poor outcomes.[133,165] S-100B levels are highest at hospital admission, with higher levels associated with worse outcome.[133,165] Many other blood and CSF biomarkers have been examined in laboratory studies but none are in widespread use at this time.

Algorithms for prognostication propose sequences for testing and time windows when different clinical, neurophysiologic, imaging, or biomarker tests might be useful.[133,164,165] Each patient will differ and individual patients may require none, some, or all of these evaluations. In some cases, prognosis remains indeterminate despite extensive testing and some patients awaken after extended periods of observation. While the most conservative strategy is always to prolong observation in the absence of clear indicators of poor outcome, prolonged intensive care support increases the risk of devastated patients surviving in a persistent vegetative state. Therefore prognostic evaluation during the first week of recovery is warranted. In general, a combination of early assessments within the first 24 hours (clinical examination, head CT, EEG) is supplemented by further assessments at 48 to 72 hours (repeat clinical examination, SSEP, EEG, MRI, NSE), as dictated by evolution of the patient's clinical condition (Fig. 51.6).

Long-term support for patients who remain on mechanical ventilation or who remain too comatose to protect their own airway after 1 week may require tracheostomy and feeding tube placement. The clinician and surrogate decision makers will need to decide if this is consistent with the wishes of the patient, depending on the anticipated likelihood and extent of neurologic recovery. A few interventions in the ICU may ameliorate complications and improve recovery from coma. Specifically, early mobilization, physical therapy, and occupational therapy can help stimulate comatose patients. In other patients who are not expected to awaken but who are going to receive long-term support, therapists can begin early to minimize complications of long-term dependency. Padding and splints to reduce pressure ulcers and contractures are examples of these interventions. Finally, some studies have reported on the use of stimulant medications, such as amantadine, methylphenidate, or modafinil to promote arousal in patients who remain comatose.[169]

CARDIOVASCULAR CONSIDERATIONS

Evaluation for the etiology of cardiac arrest begins with the initial clinical assessment, supplemented by additional testing—including ECG, echocardiogram, and coronary angiography. All patients resuscitated from cardiac arrest should have an ECG and echocardiogram. The majority of patients warrant coronary angiography prior to hospital discharge, particularly if they had a shockable arrest rhythm and/or have significant or new regional wall motion abnormalities or LV systolic dysfunction. These tests are most appropriate for patients with OHCA, who are more likely to have a cardiac etiology and/or unknown cause than patients with IHCA. For patients whose ECG, echocardiogram, and coronary angiogram do not reveal a cause of cardiac arrest, a cardiac MRI with contrast can help to identify occult structural heart diseases, such as hypertrophic cardiomyopathy,

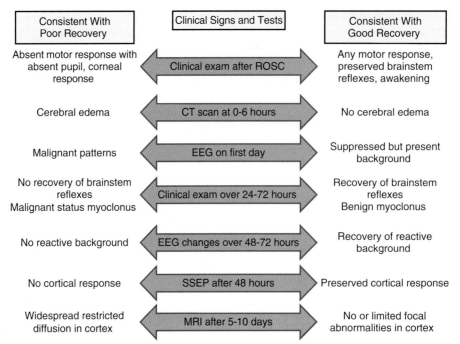

Consistent With Poor Recovery	Clinical Signs and Tests	Consistent With Good Recovery
Absent motor response with absent pupil, corneal response	Clinical exam after ROSC	Any motor response, preserved brainstem reflexes, awakening
Cerebral edema	CT scan at 0-6 hours	No cerebral edema
Malignant patterns	EEG on first day	Suppressed but present background
No recovery of brainstem reflexes Malignant status myoclonus	Clinical exam over 24-72 hours	Recovery of brainstem reflexes Benign myoclonus
No reactive background	EEG changes over 48-72 hours	Recovery of reactive background
No cortical response	SSEP after 48 hours	Preserved cortical response
Widespread restricted diffusion in cortex	MRI after 5-10 days	No or limited focal abnormalities in cortex

Fig. 51.6 Prognostic signs and tests that are useful for patients after cardiac arrest. Some patients who improve quickly or who are clearly devastated may not require each test. No single test or sign is completely accurate for predicting outcome; each institution should develop comfort with execution and interpretation of a particular sequence or combination of testing that is customized for individual patients. *CT,* Computed tomography; *EEG,* electroencephalography; *MRI,* magnetic resonance imaging; *ROSC,* return of spontaneous circulation; *SSEP,* somatosensory evoked potential.

myocarditis, or cardiac sarcoidosis. For patients with a shockable arrest rhythm but no identifiable structural heart disease, further workup is appropriate guided by the clinical history in conjunction with a heart rhythm specialist. Advanced testing—such as provocative testing for coronary vasospasm, cardiac electrophysiology testing (programmed electrical stimulation), drug or exercise provocation studies, and occasionally genetic testing—may be appropriate. This testing should be performed prior to hospital discharge from the index event.

Patients who have suffered a cardiac arrest are at elevated risk of recurrent cardiac arrest, with high rates of recurrent events despite antidysrhythmic drug treatment. Development of the implantable cardioverter-defibrillator (ICD) dramatically reduced mortality rates in survivors of shockable OHCA and remains the standard of care for secondary prevention of cardiac arrest. All patients with an unprovoked cardiac arrest due to a shockable rhythm warrant consideration of secondary prevention ICD implantation prior to hospital discharge unless their life expectancy is less than 6 to 12 months.[170] Cardiac arrest from ventricular arrhythmias developing within the first 48 to 72 hours of acute MI is considered to be provoked and therefore not typically an indication for secondary prevention ICD implantation. When there is uncertainty about whether a shockable cardiac arrest was provoked or whether the provoking event is likely to recur, the bias should be toward ICD placement. In some of these patients, a wearable defibrillator may be considered as a bridging therapy until a final decision regarding ICD implantation can be made; the role for a wearable defibrillator in patients with

cardiac arrest due to acute MI remains uncertain. Patients with cardiomyopathy and significant LV systolic dysfunction (i.e., LVEF <35%) who have suffered a nonshockable cardiac arrest typically should be considered for ICD implantation, although this is technically considered primary prevention.[170] A meta-analysis of secondary prevention ICD clinical trials suggested that the majority of the benefit of an ICD is in patients with LV systolic dysfunction (LVEF <35%), but ICD is typically offered to appropriate candidates regardless of LVEF.[171] There is no evidence that antidysrhythmic drugs reduce long-term mortality after cardiac arrest, although amiodarone may reduce arrhythmic death and reduce the risk of ICD shocks.[172,173] In appropriate candidates, catheter ablation prior to ICD implantation may reduce the risk of ICD shocks.[174]

FOLLOW-UP AND CHRONIC/POST-DISCHARGE ISSUES

Cardiac arrest survivors share with all critically ill patients a variety of post-ICU physical and psychological problems.[175] In addition, there are a number of unique issues for post–cardiac arrest patients. The transitions from ICU to hospital floor and post–acute care hospital care are opportunities to detect and initiate treatment for these problems. It is now clear that functional recovery from the acute event continues for months or years after the initial hospitalization.[176,177] Unfortunately, many patients who return to a relatively normal neurologic baseline are unable to return to work owing to persistent disability.

A number of neurologic and cognitive deficits are observed in survivors of cardiac arrest, although the majority of cardiac arrest survivors have good functional status.[73] Up to one-quarter of patients arriving for outpatient cardiac rehabilitation after surviving a cardiac arrest and one-half of all survivors exhibit cognitive deficits on detailed testing.[178–180] Memory and executive function are commonly impaired; these deficits can reduce the ability to complete complex tasks.[178] Interestingly, visual problems are also reported with high frequency in cardiac arrest survivors, perhaps related to the particular sensitivity of the occipital cortex to hypoperfusion and hypoxia.[181] Detection of these impairments usually requires formal testing with specific instruments. However, many instruments are brief, portable, and within the scope of occupational therapy, psychiatry, neurology, or physiatry. Each institution should explore which testing is available and what providers should routinely evaluate the patient recovering from cardiac arrest.

Anxiety and depression also are common during recovery from cardiac arrest.[182–184] These emotions seem paradoxical given that survivors are celebrating recovery from a high mortality event; as a result, patients may be less likely to complain about or acknowledge their negative emotions. Nevertheless, these factors can interfere with return to normal activity and participation in rehabilitation and can reduce quality of life. Consequently, it is incumbent on clinicians to screen and intervene when appropriate.

Treatments exist for the post-ICU problems experienced by cardiac arrest survivors. Appropriate disposition of patients after acute care hospitalization is complex. In many instances, patients do not receive evaluation and referral to outpatient support or inpatient rehabilitation that can increase the likelihood of successful reintegration into the community.[185] For example, a number of patient support groups and online forums exist that can be useful for patients wishing to discuss their experiences or anxieties. Therapists are now designing specific outpatient or inpatient interventions to help with specific symptoms.[186,187] Family support for patients with cognitive impairment may be a critical factor to help patients remain in the community.[188] Clinical evaluation for deficits should be coupled with a plan for referral and service for the surviving patient.

The full reference list for this chapter is available at ExpertConsult.com.

52

Palliative Care in the Cardiac Intensive Care Unit

Milla J. Kviatkovsky, Briana N. Ketterer, Sarah J. Goodlin

BURDEN OF HEART FAILURE

The burden of heart failure (HF) includes frequent deteriorations often requiring hospitalization, high mortality, and significant symptoms, reducing the quality of life. HF contributes to more than 10% of deaths in the United States.[1] Despite advances in therapy, the number of deaths attributable to HF today is similar to the numbers in 1995.[2] Patients who survive a hospitalization for HF have age-adjusted 28-day and 1-year case fatalities of 10.4% and 29.5%, respectively. After three or four hospitalizations for HF, patients older than 85 years and patients younger than 65 years have a 50% 6-month mortality rate.[3]

Symptoms are prevalent throughout the course of HF; most HF hospitalizations are associated with increased dyspnea, fatigue, or other cardiovascular symptoms. Heart failure patients are predominantly elderly, most of whom have more than four comorbid conditions. Some patients with HF will be hospitalized for unrelated issues and HF management complicates their care. The majority of patients with chronic HF are also frail and may have cognitive impairment, complicating intensive care management. Communication and decision making with the patient and family should acknowledge mortality and address palliation in addition to life extension.

This chapter addresses palliative and end-of-life concerns encountered in the intensive care unit (ICU). Care for the patients with advanced HF who are without further options for advanced therapies is specifically addressed. Fig. 52.1 illustrates the trajectory of HF, incorporating palliative and care supportive throughout the course of the illness. HF results in severe impairment of function that might result in cardiac intensive care unit (CICU) admission, but appropriate medications and treatment often can rescue the patient. This chapter is particularly relevant to patients who do not recover with aggressive treatment (see Fig. 52.1, time point 4), or who may no longer have options for advanced therapies (such as left ventricular assist device [LVAD] or transplant).

Approximately 5% to 10 % of all patients with HF have stage D disease[4]; a larger number of patients have stage C HF with significant comorbidities. Patients with American College of Cardiology/American Heart Association (ACC/AHA) stage D HF have refractory HF. These patients experience rest symptoms despite optimal medical management and are refractory to conventional therapy, which may also include advanced treatment strategies, such as inotropes or LVADs.[2,4] Patients with ACC/AHA stage C HF who have significant comorbidities and complications (frailty, COPD, dementia) are also approaching the end of life. Life expectancy is limited for HF patients even when advanced therapies are used. Patients who receive cardiac transplant have an average 10-year survival and about 70% LVAD device recipients survive 2 years, though newer devices may improve length of life. Patients with HF and reduced left ventricular ejection fraction (HFrEF) receiving continuous inotropic support have an average 6-month survival.[5–7] Options for an approach to patients in these groups are presented in Fig. 52.2. Comprehensive HF management should weave in palliative interventions throughout the course of care for communication and shared decision making, including advanced care planning, and symptom management. When appropriate, end-of-life care should include hospice care.

DEFINING HOSPICE AND PALLIATIVE CARE

Palliative care is a philosophy of care as well as a care delivery system that often employs a multidisciplinary team involving physicians, advanced care practitioners, nurses, social workers, and—most notably—the patient and the patient's family. All clinicians provide palliative care when suffering and the burden of illness are addressed. Palliative care emphasizes alleviation of physical, psychosocial, and spiritual symptom burden to enhance quality of life. Palliative care should be provided throughout the course of all serious illnesses, and does not necessitate end of

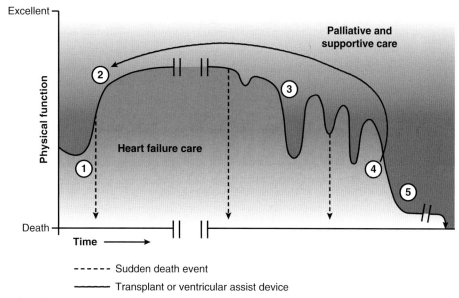

Fig. 52.1 Comprehensive heart failure care. Time point 1 illustrates initial diagnosis of heart failure, in which care emphasizes initiation of evidence-based therapies, education of patient and family about the disease, and how to manage it. Time point 2 is the plateau phase, in which treatment has been initiated and quality of life is improved from initial diagnosis. Patients remain in this stage and benefit from medical management, a variable length of time until time point 3, with oscillating exacerbation and rescue with decline in physical function, increased need for supportive care, and perhaps increasing frequency of hospitalizations. Time point 4 is generally a crossroad phase in which advanced therapies, such as a left ventricular assist device or transplant, may bring patients back to a new plateau. Alternatively, progression of disease to time point 5 occurs, characterized by low function, frailty, and significant need for palliative therapies, with variable length of time until death. (From Goodlin SJ. Palliative care in congestive heart failure. *J Am Coll Cardiol.* 2009;54:386–96.)

life or a set prognosis. Palliative care consultation in the CICU results in increased referrals of patients to hospice.[8] Hospice and palliative care often go hand in hand. Hospice is a model of care targeting those in the last 6 months of life, while palliative care is provided at any time and concurrently with life-prolonging treatment. Thus, in the CICU, palliative care and advanced treatment of HF are *not* mutually exclusive but instead are synergistic and beneficial to all stakeholders (patients, family, providers, and the hospital itself). We recommend early consultation of in-patient palliative care teams for patients with life-shortening illness. Clinicians based in the CICU provide many components of palliative care; however, when hospice referral is appropriate, palliative care consultants can facilitate continuity of care. Incidentally, ICU palliative care consultations benefit the health care system via reduced length of stay and cost saving of an estimated $7700 per hospitalization for HF.[8,9]

Hospice care incorporates palliative care and supportive services 24 hours a day, 7 days a week. The majority of hospice care is delivered as intermittent visits in the home or patient's residence (including long-term care settings). The hospice benefit also includes "general inpatient care" for severe symptoms or crises that cannot be managed in the home, "continuous care" that delivers 8 to 24 hours of skilled care in the home for a few days to manage acute problems or provide training to caregivers, and respite care for the primary caregiver. Physical, social, spiritual, and emotional care are provided via an interdisciplinary team.

Individuals who qualify for hospice have a likely life expectancy of 6 months or less. Patients are eligible for hospice via Medicare (and most other insurers) with two physician certifications of 6 months or less of life if the illness runs its natural course, although patients can be repeatedly certified for the hospice benefit when they live longer than 6 months. The patient must elect the hospice benefit and agree to not be hospitalized for the hospice diagnosis. More information can be obtained at https://www.medicare.gov.

When the hospice diagnosis is HF, the traditional guidelines include HF New York Heart Association (NYHA) class IV with either symptoms at rest or inability to carry out minimal activities due to dyspnea despite optimal medical treatment. These criteria are outdated and serve more as a guideline, as more weight is given to the physician's statement regarding prognosis based on the complexity of HF, including the number of associated hospitalizations; decline in self-care; frailty; and other comorbidities, such as cancer or markers of disease severity, including hyponatremia, elevated N-terminal prohormone brain natriuretic peptide (NT-proBNP), cachexia, and use of inotropes.

PROGNOSTICATION

The American Heart Association/American College of Cardiology (AHA/ACC) 2013 and the European Society of Cardiology (ESC) 2013 HF guidelines recommend ongoing discussion with patients

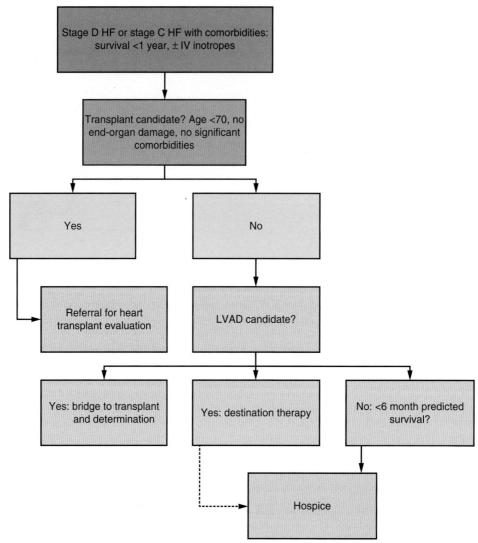

Fig. 52.2 Decision tree for patients with stage D heart failure or stage C with comorbidities and <1 year predicted survival. *HF,* Heart failure; *IV,* intravenous; *LVAD,* left ventricular assist device.

and families about prognosis for functional capacity and survival, palliative and hospice care, and discussions regarding implanted device deactivation.[2] Ideally, these topics should be addressed throughout the course of the patient's HF progression, and should be readdressed with changes in clinical status. Patients and their families may also request to have these discussions. Fig. 52.2 provides a decision tree, with various branch points when hospice might be considered. Several risk models can assist with prognostication. We suggest that clinicians identify which model is most useful for the specific patient and circumstance at hand, bearing in mind that the tools reflect aggregate data and provide only estimates. Table 52.1 lists prognostic models and their characteristics.[3,5,10–14] One out of five patients do not want to know their prognosis; thus it is important to begin communication by asking what the patient wants to know.

COMMUNICATION STRATEGIES

Communication with patients and families about prognosis is an important skill for all clinicians. Communication about goals

and end-of-life planning should occur throughout the continuum of care of a patient with HF. HF patients are at risk for rapid deterioration and sudden cardiac death; thus, conversations should occur early in their care and be readdressed on a regular basis. Despite these previous conversations, many patients hospitalized with HF and their families may be surprised that they are at risk of imminent death. One model to approach these patient-centered conversations is "Ask-Tell-Ask" (Table 52.2). This model begins the conversation with asking the patient for the patient's understanding of the current situation or worries or concerns. Then the clinician shares information. Finally, the clinician asks what the patient or family understood and asks for their questions.[15] Table 52.2 provides example phrases to facilitate these conversations.

Often, this point in the care continuum presents a crossroad for medical providers. When patients in the CICU are nearing the end of their life or may not have options for advanced HF therapies, the medical team guides shared decision making. This starts by identifying the patient's values and priorities, then sets joint clinician and patient goals, and assesses how the available

TABLE 52.1 Outpatient Models for Heart Failure Prognostication

Model	Outcome	Variables, Limitations, Advantages	Example Patient	Survival vs. Mortality
Seattle Heart Failure Model[13]	Continuous risk score expressed as predicted life expectancy and percentage chance of survival (1-, 2-, and 5-year mortality)	Accounts for NYHA functional class, ischemic etiology, diuretic dose, LVEF, SBP, sodium, hemoglobin, percent lymphocytes, uric acid, cholesterol. Not derived from HF population. Most commonly used, validated in HF patients	65 yo male w/ ischemic cardiomyopathy; EF 30%; NYHA class IV; SBP 90; on ACEi, BB, statin; with ICD in place	1-year mortality, 11%; 2-year, 20%; 5-year, 43%
Heart Failure Survival Score[2]	All-cause mortality	Peak VO$_2$, LVEF, serum Na, mean BP, HR, ischemic etiology, QRS duration/morphology Limitation: difficult to acquire VO$_2$ data	LVEF 40%; SBP 90; serum Na 135; known ischemic cardiomyopathy; IVCD of 124 ms; resting HR of 90 beats/min (VO$_2$ max not known)	Score: 7.25 Medium risk: 72% predicted 1-year survival

Inpatient Models for Heart Failure Prognostication

Model	Outcome	Variables, Limitations, Advantages	Example Patient	Survival vs. Mortality
EVEREST Risk Model[29]	Combined endpoint mortality or persistently poor QOL over 6 months postdischarge	Age, DM, h/o stroke, h/o arrhythmia, BB use, BUN, Na, BNP, KCCQ score		
EFFECT[12]	30-day and 1-year mortality	Age, SBP, RR, Na, hemoglobin, BUN, h/o CVA, h/o dementia, h/o COPD, h/o cirrhosis, h/o cancer Limitation: no EF requirement	Predicted 30-day survival for 62 yo male, RR, 20 beats/min; SBP, 100 mm Hg; BUN, 30; hemoglobin, 10; serum Na, 132; + CVD + COPD + dementia	Score: 122 High risk: 26%–32.7% 30-day mortality
ADHERE[11]	In-hospital mortality	BUN, SBP, serum Cr Limitation: no EF requirement	Mean BUN <43 mg/dL; SBP <115 mm Hg; intermediate risk 3%–5.5% in-hospital mortality Compared to mean BUN >43 mg/dL, SBP <115 mm Hg, serum Cr >2.75 mg/dL	High risk Predicted in-hospital mortality: 21.9%
ESCAPE Discharge[14]	6-month mortality	BNP, CPR, or mechanical ventilation during hospitalization, BUN, Na, age >70 y, loop diuretic use, BB use, 6-min walk distance	75 yo male, BUN >40, 6-min walk <300 ft, Na >130 mEq, no h/o CPR/mechanical ventilation, on 40 mg furosemide BID, not tolerating BB, with BNP 650 pg/mmol	Score: 5 Predicted 6-month mortality: 66.4%

Commonly used Heart Failure Prognostication models separated by their clinical utility in the outpatient versus inpatient setting. Example patient and associated risk stratification is provided to illustrate differences and guide decisions regarding which model is most suited for specific patient in question.
ACEi, Angiotensin-converting enzyme inhibitor; *BB*, β-blocker; *BID*, twice daily; *BNP*, brain natriuretic peptide; *BP*, blood pressure; *BUN*, blood urea nitrogen; *COPD*, chronic obstructive pulmonary disease; *CPR*, cardiopulmonary resuscitation; *Cr*, creatinine; *CVA*, cerebrovascular accident; *CVD*, cardiovascular disease; *DM*, diabetes mellitus; *EF*, ejection fraction; *HF*, heart failure; *h/o*, history of; *HR*, heart rate; *ICD*, implantable cardioverter-defibrillator; *IVCD*, intraventricular conduction delay; *KCCQ*, Kansas City Cardiomyopathy Questionnaire; *LVEF*, left ventricular ejection fraction; *Na*, sodium; *NYHA*, New York Heart Association; *QOL*, quality of life; *RR*, respiratory rate; *SBP*, systolic blood pressure; *yo*, year old.

treatment options might approach those goals while supporting the patient's values. It is important to depict what the course might be with each option. Identifying values and aligning treatment options with them limits confusion and avoids care that is not beneficial or may be harmful, while prioritizing the patient and the family.[16] In part, this raises an ongoing ethical debate questioning whether just because we *can* do something we *should* do it.[17] These conversations are challenging for patients and providers. It is important to recognize emotions both on the part of the clinician and the patient and family. Naming

surprise, sadness, anger, and other emotions is essential to being able to conduct a discussion. Voicing "I Wish" statements such as "I wish things were different," is one way for providers to empathetically align with patients and acknowledge that the outcome is not something anyone desired. Designation of surrogate decision makers and early conversations acknowledging and planning for possible death are important. Planning for "the worst," including undesired states and death, is often easiest when done as a dichotomous discussion that includes clinicians' hope for the best outcomes.

SYMPTOM MANAGEMENT IN HEART FAILURE

The most common complaints of end-stage HF patients are dyspnea, depression, pain, edema, and fatigue. Other symptoms also include feelings of uncertainty, anxiety, and worry about what to expect. In assessment and management of symptoms, medications are often added in a stepwise fashion to target specific symptoms (Fig. 52.3). Table 52.3 lists therapies that may be added to assist with symptom management.

In advanced HF, one of the most distressing symptoms is dyspnea. Dyspnea is a complex symptom that takes into account pulmonary congestion and neurohormonal activation and renin-angiotensin-aldosterone system (RAAS) disarray, along with increased proinflammatory cytokines.[18] Therefore, in addition to decongestion strategies via diuresis and vasodilation, treatment strategies focus on blocking or modifying the neurohormonal and cytokine abnormalities. When at all possible, it is beneficial to continue β-blockers and angiotensin-converting enzyme (ACE) inhibitors (or angiotensin receptor blockers [ARBs]). Dose adjustments may be needed in the setting of volume overload, hypotension, and acute kidney injury. The use of "medical air" and fans to stimulate the respiratory centers on the face can aide in alleviating the symptom of air hunger. Use of oxygen is not recommended in patients who are not hypoxemic. Opiates and benzodiazepines can also improve the sensation of dyspnea. Opiates are appropriate at all phases of HF while benzodiazepines have more limited utility, especially in the frail and elderly.

Depression in the HF population is present in 9% to 77.5% of patients.[19] Depression correlates with decreased quality of life and increased pain, as well as worsened prognosis. Selective serotonin reuptake inhibitors (SSRIs) are the mainstay of therapy, although at low doses, sertraline was not better than frequent phone contact. Depression remission was significantly associated with improvements in Kansas City Cardiomyopathy Questionnaire (KCCQ) scores in particular subscales of physical and mental self-assessment.[20] In addition, controlled-release paroxetine in a small population of patients with HF was associated with significant improvement in depression (69% vs. 23%; $P = .018$) and improvement in psychological aspects of quality of life.[21] Overall, this highlights the importance of addressing comorbid depression in HF.

In one study, 84% of advanced HF patients had pain.[22] Opiates are useful for pain in that they also simultaneously treat symptoms of dyspnea. Topical and nonpharmacologic therapies, including physical therapy and exercise, should be used to manage pain in the CICU. Last, intravenous (IV) inotropes should be considered for palliation of symptoms and improved functional capacity in select circumstances with the caveat that there is increased risk of sudden cardiac death.

DISCONTINUATION OF THERAPIES

Implanted Electric Devices

Implantable cardioverter-defibrillators (ICDs) do not improve symptoms and should not be implanted when patients approach end of life, for example, when life expectancy is less than 1 year. It is not uncommon for ICDs to fire at the end of life; some studies suggest 10% to 20% of patients receive shocks during the last weeks to months of life.[23,24] Deactivation of ICDs should be discussed before implantation and as end of life nears, especially

TABLE 52.2	Examples of "Ask-Tell-Ask" Strategies in Advanced Heart Failure
Ask	"Tell me what you understand about your heart failure."
	"Tell me how you think things are going."
	"Under what circumstances would you not want your life to be prolonged?"
	"What are you concerned or worried about?"
	"What is important to you?"
Tell	"Given everything we have talked about, and that you wish to let death occur naturally, I would like to talk about how to achieve that and manage your symptoms."
	"I would like to talk about all of your options so you can make a choice."
	"I would like to talk about the plan for turning off the shock function of your cardiac defibrillator."
	"I would like to talk about what it would look like if we turned your LVAD off."
	or
	"I would like to talk about what it would be like if we kept your LVAD on."
Ask	"Tell me what you understood from our discussion. When you tell your family about what we talked about, what will you tell them?"
	"What questions do you have?"

LVAD, Left ventricular assist device.

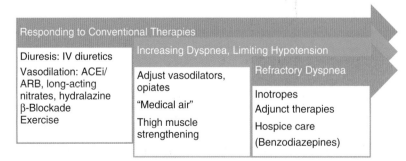

Fig. 52.3 A summative approach to symptom management in heart failure. *ACEi,* Angiotensin-converting enzyme inhibitor; *ARB,* angiotensin receptor blocker; *IV,* intravenous.

TABLE 52.3 Heart Failure Symptom Management

Medication	Advantages	Cautions	Dosing/Titration
Dyspnea/Pain			
Morphine	Reduces preload	Renal excretion, toxic metabolites, delirium	Low doses often sufficient for dyspnea
Hydromorphone	Less toxic metabolites	Accumulation of metabolites	Titrate to pain or dyspnea
Methadone	GI excretion	Prolongs QTc interval at high doses	Accumulates in tissues; reduce dose/frequency after 4–5 days
Fentanyl	Hepatic metabolism; no active metabolites; available in oral formulation as lozenges and lollipops	Transdermal use for moderate to severe pain has long half life	Transdermal patch not for opioid-naive patients; require 8 hours to reach dose IV recommended over morphine in ICU patients
Benzodiazepines	Benefit if opiate refractory	Confusion and falls in elderly	
NSAIDs	Oral not recommended, consider topical use	Sodium and fluid retention, worsening renal function	
Nonpharmacologic: physical therapy, heat/cold therapy, topical analgesics, acupuncture, fan as "medical air"	Physical therapy, thigh muscle strengthening, getting patients up and out of bed	Few to none	
Depression			
SSRIs: sertraline,[21] paroxetine[22]	No evidence of harm compared to TCAs	Potential hyponatremia, orthostatic hypotension, some prolong QTc interval	Therapeutic benefit may be patient and dose specific
TCAs	Should be used by experienced clinician	QTc prolongation, can prolong RR interval, anticholinergic	ECG and serum level monitoring
Functional Decline			
Inotropes		Risk of sudden cardiac death as a result of ventricular arrhythmias	Average life expectancy 6 months
Physical therapy	Maintain function, reduce deconditioning		

ECG, Electrocardiogram; *GI,* gastrointestinal; *ICU,* intensive care unit; *IV,* intravenous; *NSAIDs,* nonsteroidal antiinflammatory drugs; *QTc,* corrected QT; *RR,* respiratory rate; *SSRIs,* serotonin reuptake inhibitors; *TCAs,* tricyclic antidepressants.

if patients choose to die naturally. This discussion should be revisited when patients with HF have a change in clinical status or transition to comfort care.[10,25] Cardiac resynchronization therapy (CRT) provides symptom relief in HF by pacing the ventricles simultaneously and improving left ventricular ejection fraction. Thus, generally, it should be continued until the end of life. Standard pacemaker function for bradycardia and heart block is also generally continued, but it is appropriate to plan for management of all electrical device functions as the end of life approaches. Unfortunately, many people approach death before they have the opportunity to discuss deactivation of their device.[23,24] Hospitals and hospice agencies should have protocols in place for ICD deactivation at the end of life.

Left Ventricular Assist Devices

LVADs are being used more frequently for destination therapy (DT) in addition to bridging therapy. All patients receiving an LVAD should plan for adverse events and undesired outcomes with their family or a designated surrogate in the process of obtaining an LVAD. As more patients undergo DT LVAD implantation, an increasing number will ultimately die. The discussion regarding device-related death should be introduced when first discussing the potential for LVAD placement. We recommend that every institution that implants LVADs also have a discontinuation protocol that can be applied and adapted when the need arises. Notably, hospice enrollment for LVAD patients is location and hospice specific, making knowledge of your local hospice agencies and policies key to a smooth transition. LVAD discontinuation can result in rapid decompensation and death at a time when patients are likely awake and alert. The most common triggers for LVAD discontinuation are infection, stroke, cancer, renal failure, and impending pump failure.[26] Most patients die within 20 minutes of device deactivation.[27] Therefore patients and families should be forewarned and a thoughtful plan for management should be in place.

CONCLUSIONS

Comprehensive HF management involves not only care of symptoms but also planning for the future and disease progression. The variable trajectory has notoriously made HF a challenging arena for advance care planning. Individuals with HF are at risk for sudden changes in their disease trajectory with hospitalizations, ICU stays, advanced therapies, and sudden cardiac death. Meanwhile, there are others who live for years with HF symptoms. A palliative care model addresses the patient, the patient's symptoms, the family, and planning for what is to come. Hospice provides respite for caregivers and grief counseling for family after the death of their loved one; some hospice agencies are able to use advanced therapies at home, such as home inotropes or LVADs. Ultimately, the emphasis is shared decision making and symptom management that focuses on patient-centered values and goals. Enrollment in hospice may be appropriate for increasing numbers of patients living with HF, but all CICUs should anticipate death and have plans to manage devices, HF, and other symptoms and to support HF patients and families who approach the end of life in the CICU. We implore CICU providers to begin the planning process early, engage HF patients and their families often in the decision-making process, and build processes in collaboration with palliative care clinicians and hospice agencies to provide a smooth transition at the end of life.

The full reference list for this chapter is available at ExpertConsult.com.

Page numbers followed by "*f*" indicate figures, "*t*" indicate tables, and "*b*" indicate boxes.